Food and Culture

8E

SeAnne Safaii-Waite, PhD, RDN, LD
Associate Professor Emerita Foods and Nutrition, University of Idaho
Adjunct Professor, University of Missouri

Nina Mukerjee Furstenau
Food and Culture Author, Retd. University of Missouri, Director Food Systems Communication, Science and Agricultural Journalism

Kathryn P. Sucher, ScD, RDN
Department of Nutrition and Food Science San Jose State University

Marcia Nahikian-Nelms, PhD, RDN, LD, CNSC
Medical Dietetics, College of Medicine, The Ohio State University

Pamela Goyan Kittler, MS
Food, Culture, and Nutrition Consultant

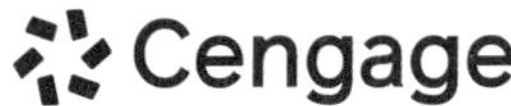

Australia • Brazil • Canada • Mexico • Singapore • United Kingdom • United States

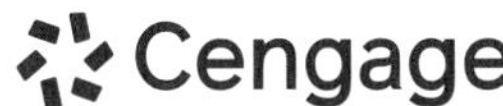

***Food and Culture,* 8e**
SeAnne Safaii-Waite, Nina Mukerjee Furstenau
Kathryn P. Sucher, Marcia Nahikian-Nelms, Pamela Goyan Kittler

SVP, Product: Cheryl Costantini

VP, Product: Thais Alencar

Portfolio Product Director: Maureen McLaughlin

Senior Portfolio Product Manager: Courtney Heilman

Product Assistant: Olivia Pan

Senior Learning Designer: Paula Dohnal

Senior Content Manager: Samantha Rundle

Director, Product Marketing: Danae April

Product Marketing Manager: Taylor Shenberger

Content Acquisition Analyst: Ann Hoffman

Production Service: Lumina Datamatics Ltd.

Designer: Chris Doughman

Cover and Interior Image Source: fcafotodigital/Getty Images

Last three editions, as applicable: ©2017, © 2012, © 2008

Copyright © 2024 Cengage Learning, Inc. ALL RIGHTS RESERVED.

Unless otherwise noted, all content is Copyright © Cengage Learning, Inc.

No part of this work covered by the copyright herein may be reproduced or distributed in any form or by any means, except as permitted by U.S. copyright law, without the prior written permission of the copyright owner.

For product information and technology assistance, contact us at **Cengage Customer & Sales Support, 1-800-354-9706 or support.cengage.com.**

For permission to use material from this text or product, submit all requests online at **www.copyright.com**.

Library of Congress Control Number: 2023901804

Student Edition:
ISBN: 978-0-357-72958-8

Loose-leaf Edition:
ISBN: 978-0-35772959-5

Cengage
200 Pier 4 Boulevard
Boston, MA 02210
USA

Cengage is a leading provider of customized learning solutions. Our employees reside in nearly 40 different countries and serve digital learners in 165 countries around the world. Find your local representative at **www.cengage.com.**

To learn more about Cengage platforms and services, register or access your online learning solution, or purchase materials for your course, visit **www.cengage.com.**

Printed in the United States of America
Print Number: 01 Print Year: 2023

Contents

Preface

The population of the United States is increasingly heterogeneous, moving toward a plurality of ethnic, religious, and regional groups. Each of these groups has traditional food habits that differ—slightly or significantly—from the so-called typical American majority diet. Effective nutrition counseling, education, and food service require that these variations be acknowledged and understood within the context of culture. It is our goal to provide dietitians, nutritionists, health professionals, and food service professionals with the broad overview needed to avoid ethnocentric assumptions and the nutrition specifics helpful in working with each group discussed. We have attempted to combine the conceptual with the technical in a way that is useful to other health professionals as well.

We would like to draw attention specifically to the area of nutrition counseling as diet is key to disease prevention and life long health. The Academy of Nutrition and Dietetics recommends multicultural competency in the area of nutrition, counseling, and medical nutrition therapy due to the sensitivity and influence of culture on individual food intake, attitudes, and behavior. A model (Harris-Davis & Haughton, 2000) recommended for multicultural nutrition competencies specifically lists the following:

1. Understand food selection, preparation, and storage with a cultural context.
2. Have knowledge of cultural eating patterns and family traditions such as core foods, traditional celebrations, and fasting.
3. Familiarize self with relevant research and latest findings regarding food practices and nutrition-related health problems of various ethnic and racial groups.
4. Possess specific knowledge of cultural values, health beliefs, and nutrition practices of particular groups served, including culturally different clients.

This book offers information fundamental to these competencies.

New to this Edition

Content has been revised to acknowledge diversity and inclusivity with efforts to recognize and reduce implicit bias. Throughout this textbook, cultural words have not been italicized when they are explained within the sentence. This was a careful choice to avoid framing closely held terms as "foreign." At times, italics are used for clarity and for scientific terms. Also, authentic menus, recipes, longevity, and comfort food highlights have been included. Outdated counseling approaches have been removed and replaced with information that embraces cultural humility.

- Chapter 1. Food and Culture—Updated population data and added information on culinary research and comfort foods.
- Chapter 2. Traditional Health Beliefs and Practices—Updated data on the use of complementary and alternative medicine (CAM).
- Chapter 3. Intercultural Communications—Updated to introduce the term Cultural Humility and LEARN Guidelines.
- Chapter 4. Food and Religion—Updated demographics data on religious affiliation in the United States and expanded information on specific religions based on new data.
- Chapter 5. Native Americans—Updated U.S. Census data on Native American population and other demographics. Updated information on current diets, nutritional status, and medical disorders related to diet and nutrition. New information on the indigenous foodways and the food sovereignty movement, comfort foods, longevity foods, and new recipes for students to try.
- Chapter 6. Northern and Southern Europeans—Updated U.S. Census population and other demographics on European groups. Updated information on current diets, nutritional status, medical disorders related to diet and nutrition, comfort foods, longevity foods, and new recipes for students to try.
- Chapter 7. Central Europeans, People of the Former Soviet Union, and Scandinavians—Updated U.S. Census population and other demographics on central and eastern European groups. Updated information on current diets, nutritional status, medical disorders related to diet and nutrition, comfort foods, longevity foods, and new recipes for students to try.
- Chapter 8. Africans, African Americans, and Black Americans—Updated U.S. Census population and other demographics on African Americans and more recent

immigrant groups from Africa. Updated information on current diets, nutritional status, medical disorders related to diet and nutrition, comfort foods, longevity foods, and new recipes for students to try.

- Chapter 9. Mexicans and Central Americans—Updated U.S. Census population and other demographics on Mexicans and Central American groups. Updated information on current diets, nutritional status, medical disorders related to diet and nutrition, and new recipes for students to try.
- Chapter 10. Caribbean Islanders and South Americans—Updated U.S. Census population and other demographics on Caribbean and South American groups. Updated information on current diets, nutritional status, medical disorders related to diet and nutrition, comfort foods, longevity foods, and new recipes for students to try.
- Chapter 11. East Asians—Updated U.S. Census population and other demographics on East Asian groups. Updated information on current diets, nutritional status, medical disorders related to diet and nutrition, comfort foods, longevity foods, and new recipes for students to try.
- Chapter 12. Southeast Asians and Residents of Oceania—Updated U.S. Census population and other demographics on East Asian groups. Updated information on current diets, nutritional status, medical disorders related to diet and nutrition, comfort foods, longevity foods, and new recipes for students to try.
- Chapter 13. People of the Balkans and the Middle East—Updated U.S. Census population and other demographics on Balkan and Middle Eastern groups. Updated information on current diets, nutritional status, and medical disorders related to diet and nutrition, comfort foods, longevity foods, and new recipes for students to try.
- Chapter 14. South Asians—Updated U.S. Census population and other demographics on South Asian groups. Updated information on current diets, nutritional status, and medical disorders related to diet and nutrition, comfort foods, longevity foods, and new recipes for students to try.
- Chapter 15. Regional Americans—Updated U.S. Census regional population and other demographics. Updated information on current diets, nutritional status, and medical disorders related to diet and nutrition.

Organization of the Text

The first four chapters form an introduction to the study of food and culture. Chapter 1 discusses methods for understanding food habits within the context of culture, changing demographics, and the ways in which ethnicity may affect nutrition and health status. Chapter 2 focuses on the role of diet in traditional health beliefs. Some intercultural communication strategies are suggested in Chapter 3, and Chapter 4 outlines the major Eastern and Western religions and reviews their dietary practices in detail.

Chapters 5 through 14 profile North American ethnic groups and their cuisines. We have chosen breadth over depth, discussing groups with significant populations in the United States, as well as smaller, more recent immigrant groups who have had an impact on the health care system. Other groups with low numbers of immigrants but notable influences on American cooking are briefly mentioned.

Groups are considered in the approximate order of their arrival in North America. Each chapter begins with a history of the group in the United States and current demographics. Worldview (outlook on life) is then examined, including religion, family structure, and traditional health practices. This background information illuminates the cultural context from which ethnic foods and food habits emerge and evolve. The next section of each chapter outlines the traditional diet, including ingredients, some common dishes, meal patterns, special occasions, the role of food in the society, and therapeutic uses of food. The final section explains the contemporary diet of the group, such as adaptations made by the group after arrival in the United States and influences of the group on the American diet. Reported nutritional status is also reviewed. Special call outs to foods or behaviors that may contribute to health aging and longevity are found at the end of each chapter. Those, along with comfort foods and recipes, provide a more personal connection to each chapter.

One or more cultural food group tables are found in each of the ethnic group chapters. The emphasis is on ingredients common to the populations of the region. Important variations within regions and unique food habits are listed in the "Comments" column of the table. Known adaptations in the United States are also noted. The tables are intended as references for the reader; they do not replace either the chapter content or an in-depth interview with a client.

Chapter 15 considers the regional American fare of the Northeast, the Midwest, the South, and the West. Each section includes an examination of the foods common in the region and general nutritional status. Canadian regional fare is also briefly considered. This chapter brings the study of cultural nutrition full circle, discussing the significant influences of different ethnic and religious groups on North American fare.

Before You Begin

Food is so essential to ethnic, religious, and regional identity that dietary descriptions must be as objective as possible to prevent inadvertent criticism of the underlying culture. Yet as members of different ethnic and religious groups, we recognize that our own cultural assumptions are unavoidable and, in fact, serve as a starting point for our work. One would be lost without such a cultural footing. Any instances of bias are unintentional.

Any definition of a group's food habits implies homogeneity in the described group. In daily life, however, each member of a group has a distinctive diet, combining traditional practices with new influences. We do not want to stereotype the fare of any cultural group. Rather, we strive to generalize common U.S. food and culture trends as a basis for understanding the personal preferences of individual clients.

We have tried to be sensitive to the designations used by each cultural group, though sometimes there is no consensus among members regarding the preferred name for the group. Also, there may be some confusion about dates in the book. Nearly all religious traditions adhere to their own calendar of events based on solar or lunar months. These calendars frequently differ from the Gregorian calendar used throughout most of the world in business and government. Religious ceremonies often move around according to Gregorian dates, yet usually they are calculated to occur in the correct season each year. Historical events in the text are listed according to the Gregorian calendar, using the abbreviations for before common era (BCE) and common era (CE).

We believe this book will do more than introduce the concepts of food and culture. It should also encourage self-examination and individual cultural identification by the reader. We hope that it will help dietitians, nutritionists, other health care providers, and food service professionals work effectively with members of different ethnic, religious, and regional groups. If it sparks a gustatory interest in the foods of the world, we will be personally pleased. *De gustibus non est disputatum!*

Ancillary Package

Additional instructor resources for this product are available online. Instructor assets include an Instructor's Manual, Educator's Guide, PowerPoint® slides, Transition Guide, Guide to Teaching Online, and a test bank powered by Cognero®. Sign up or sign in at https://faculty.cengage.com/ to search for this title. Then, you can save the title for easy access and download the resources that you need.

For this revision, the Instructor's Manual will be updated to reflect content changes from the new edition of the textbook and the order of the content will be rearranged based on the new instructor supplement template.

For this revision, the PowerPoint® slides will be updated to reflect content changes from the new edition of the textbook and reorganized to include the mandatory content and activity slide types based on the new instructor supplement template.

For this revision, the Transition Guide will be updated to reflect content changes from the new edition of the textbook.

For this revision, the test bank powered by Cognero® will be updated to reflect content changes from the new edition of the textbook.

Acknowledgments

We are forever indebted to the many researchers, especially from the fields of anthropology and sociology, who did the seminal work on food habits that provided the groundwork for this book, and to the many nutrition professionals who have shared their expertise with us over the years. We especially want to thank the many colleagues who have graciously given support and advice in the development of the numerous editions: Carmen Boyd, MS, LPC, RD, Missouri State University; Bonny Burns-Whitmore, DrPH, RD, California State Polytechnic University, Pomona; Arlene Grant-Holcomb, RD, MAE, California State Polytechnic University, San Luis Obispo; Carolyn Hollingshead, PhD, RD, University of Utah; Tawni Holmes, PhD, RD, University of Central Oklahoma; Claire G. Kratz, MS, RD, LDN, Montgomery County Community College; Yvonne Moody, EdD, Chadron State College; Sudha Raj, PhD, Syracuse University; Stacey A. Roush, MS, Montgomery County Community College; Dana Wassmer, MS, RD, Cosumnes River College; Judith Dodd MS, RDN, LDN, Sudha Raj, Sheila Barrett, Shelley DePinto, Emily Shupe, Stacey Gomes, Amy Loverin, Donna Winham, Jill Comess, Emily Shupe, Jane Burrell, Pao Ying Hsiao, Michelle Abich, Samantha Coogan, Dawn Matusz, Danielle Kronmuller, Slavko Komarnytsky, and Donna M. Winham, DrPH, Arizona State University. We are grateful for the expertise of Gerald Nelms, PhD, as his development of the discussion starters during the 6th edition revision was an important contribution to the pedagogy for this text.

About the Authors

SeAnne Safaii-Waite is a registered dietitian nutritionist and is an Associate Professor Emeritus of Nutrition and Dietetics at the University of Idaho and adjunct professor at the University Missouri. She received her bachelor's degree in dietetics from North Dakota State University, her master's degree in Community Health from the University of Oregon and a doctorate of philosophy from the University of Idaho in Adult Learning and Organizational Leadership. She has worked extensively in the areas of child nutrition, diabetes education, Alzheimer's Disease and healthy aging around the world. She has served on various state and national leadership committees and has written grants collaboratively to fund various community health nutrition interventions. She is the author of *Medical Nutrition Therapy Simulations* (2019), co-author of *The Alzheimer's Prevention Food Guide* (2017), and a contributing author to *Food Science An Ecological Approach*, 2nd ed (2019). Her leadership in dietetics has been recognized by the Academy of Nutrition and Dietetics with several awards and she is recipient of the prestigious University of Idaho Community Outreach and Engagement award. She and her husband John are active supporters of various food insecurity organizations and enjoy leading a very active lifestyle cycling, running, skiing, and just about anything that gets them outdoors.

For my husband John and our children to encourage them to never stop writing.

Nina Mukerjee Furstenau is an author and journalist with a research focus on food and identity. She was director of food systems communication at the University of Missouri Science and Agricultural Journalism program from 2010–2018, and has served as part of a USAID human nutrition project in Mozambique and Ghana where she conducted field interviews on food story with native populations. She has written the books, *Green Chili & Other Impostors* (2021), *Tasty! Mozambique* (2018), and *Biting Through the Skin: An Indian Kitchen in America's Heartland* (2013); published essays and articles on food in publications such as the *Atlanta Journal Constitution, Feast, and Sauce*; and written a chapter for the *Routledge Handbook on Food and Landscape* (2018). Among other recognitions, Nina won the M.F.K. Fisher Book Award for culinary cultural literature. She received her B.A. from The Missouri School of Journalism, and her M.A. from the University of Missouri. Nina was a Fulbright Global Scholar in Kolkata, India, in 2018–19, researching heritage foods, and long ago in 1980, was a Peace Corps volunteer in Tunisia where her love of heritage foods and human nutrition emerged. She is currently the FoodStory book series editor for the University of Iowa Press.

For my husband Terry, my constant support.

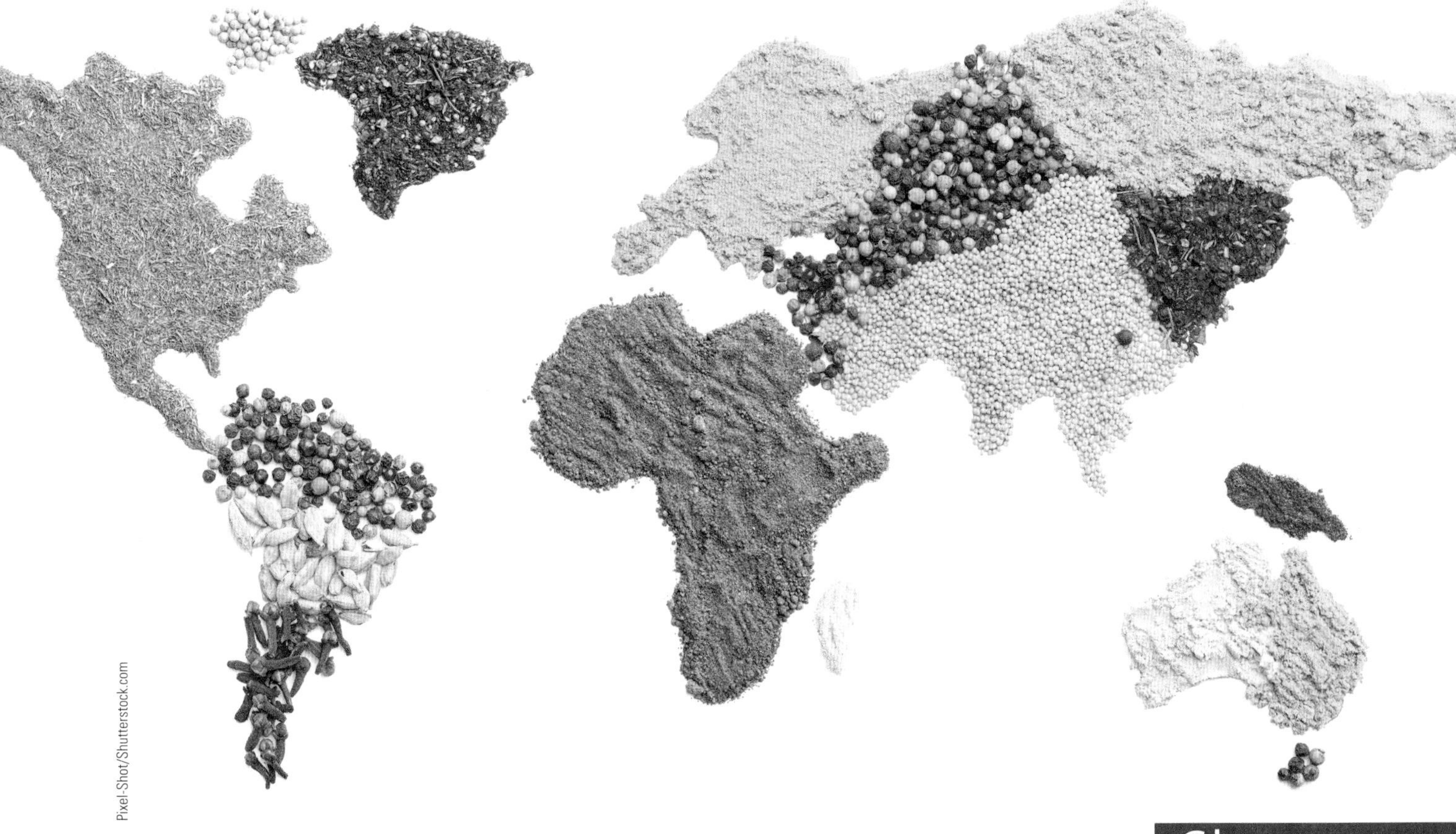

Pixel-Shot/Shutterstock.com

Chapter 1

Food and Culture

Learning Objectives

1.1 List the fastest-growing ethnic groups in the United States.

1.2 Define the "Omnivore's Paradox."

1.3 Explain symbolic meanings that can be assigned to food.

1.4 Describe how food choices can reveal cultural identity and self-identity.

1.5 Explain acculturation, enculturation, biculturation, and assimilation.

1.6 List the components of the core and complementary foods model.

1.7 Define flavor principles.

1.8 Outline the components of the developmental perspective of food culture.

1.9 Identify ways that health care providers can become more skilled in intercultural communication.

What do Americans eat? Meat and potatoes, according to popular myth. There's no denying that per person in the United States, an average of over half a pound of beef, pork, lamb, or veal is eaten daily, and more than one hundred and twenty pounds of potatoes (mostly as chips and fries) are consumed annually. Yet, the American diet is as diverse as its population, and we should no longer describe the U.S. population as White, Anglo-Saxon, and Protestant, or the diet as consisting of mostly meat and potatoes.

The U.S. Census and other demographic data show that just under 40 percent of Americans are not White, and 13.5 percent are foreign-born.[1] Asian Americans recorded the fastest population growth rate among all racial and ethnic groups in the United States between 2000 and 2019, growing 81 percent from about 10.5 million to 18.9 million people. Latinx people grew the second-fastest, followed by Native Hawaiians and Pacific Islanders (henceforth in this text referred to as Southeast Asians/residents of Oceania) at 70 and 61 percent, respectively. The U.S. Black population grew as well by 20 percent. There was virtually no change in the White population.[2]

Each American ethnic, religious, or regional group has its own culturally based food habits. Many of these customs have been modified through contact with American culture and, in turn, changed and shaped American food habits. Today, a fast-food restaurant or street stand is as likely to offer pizza, tacos, egg rolls, or falafel as it is hamburgers. The intricate interplay between past and present food habits, the old and new, and the traditional and innovative is the hallmark of the American diet.

What Is Food?

Food, as defined in the dictionary, is any substance that provides the nutrients necessary to maintain life and growth when ingested. When most animals feed, they repeatedly consume those foods necessary for their well-being, and they do so in a similar manner at each feeding. Humans, however, do not feed. They eat.

It is said that this, and cooking, sets humans apart from other animals. Plus, we bring our minds (memories, associations) with us to every food we eat. Aroma becomes an intimate reminder of a past event and sound (such as the sizzle of roasting meat) can conjure not only saliva but bring people to mind who may have once cooked for us. Taste can make a favorite dish never measure up to the way our mothers (or fathers) once cooked it, even if it is made by a skilled chef. What we bring to the table—our senses—can trigger an entire world: an edible archive of our life. Consider, too, that all humans across any geography and period use the same senses to eat. In this way, food and human culture are connected across geography, culture, and time in a tangible, sensory way.

Eating is also distinguished from feeding by the ways humans use food. Humans not only gather or hunt food, but they also cultivate plants and raise livestock. Agriculture means that some foods are regularly available, alleviating dependence on natural cycles for sustenance. This permits the development of specific customs associated with foods that are the foundation of the diet, such as wheat or rice. Humans also cook, softening tough foods, including raw grains and meats, and combine foods to create new textures and taste sensations. This greatly expands the number and variety of edible substances available. Humans often use utensils to eat meals and institute complex rules, commonly called manners, about how meals are consumed. And, significantly, humans share food. Standards for who may dine with whom, who prepares the food, how diners are seated and where, not to mention who grows the food and many more complexities, in each eating situation are well defined in every culture.

The term *food habits* (also called food culture or foodways) refers to how humans use food, including everything from how it is selected, obtained, and distributed to who prepares it, serves it, and eats it. The significance of this process is unique to humankind. Why don't people simply feed on the diet of our primitive ancestors, surviving on foraged fruits, vegetables, grains, and the occasional insect or small mammal thrown in for protein? Why do people choose to spend their time, energy, money, and creativity on eating? The answers to these questions, according to some researchers, can be found in the basic biological and psychological constitution of humans.

This book touches on the striking diversity of traditional diets around the world, and which of those ranges of food came to the United States with immigrant populations, trade routes, food fads, and more. It also addresses pre-European-contact Indigenous heirloom foods passed down through generations and which foods folded into ever-new, tasty creations. All of them have impacts on health, reveal culture, and connect people.

Food for Thought

As suggested by their names, not even hamburgers and French fries are American in origin. Chopped beef steaks first showed up in print in 1834 in America on the menu at New York's Delmonico Restaurant, where the chopped and formed "Hamburg steak" was a prominent item. The German city of Hamburg was known at the time for exporting high-quality beef.[3] Other foods considered typically American also have foreign origins, for example, hot dogs, apple pie, and ice cream.

Data from the 2016 Canadian census indicate more than 250 different ethnic origins were documented. English, Scottish, French, and Irish origins are still among the most common (20 million), however, their share in the population has decreased. The most common newer groups include individuals from China (1.8 million), India (1.4 million), and the Philippines (837,130). Communities of Edo, Ewe, Malinke, Wolof, and Djiboutian from Africa, and Hazara, Kyrgyz, Turkmen, Bhutanese, and Karen from Asia, are among the newest groups in Canada.[4]

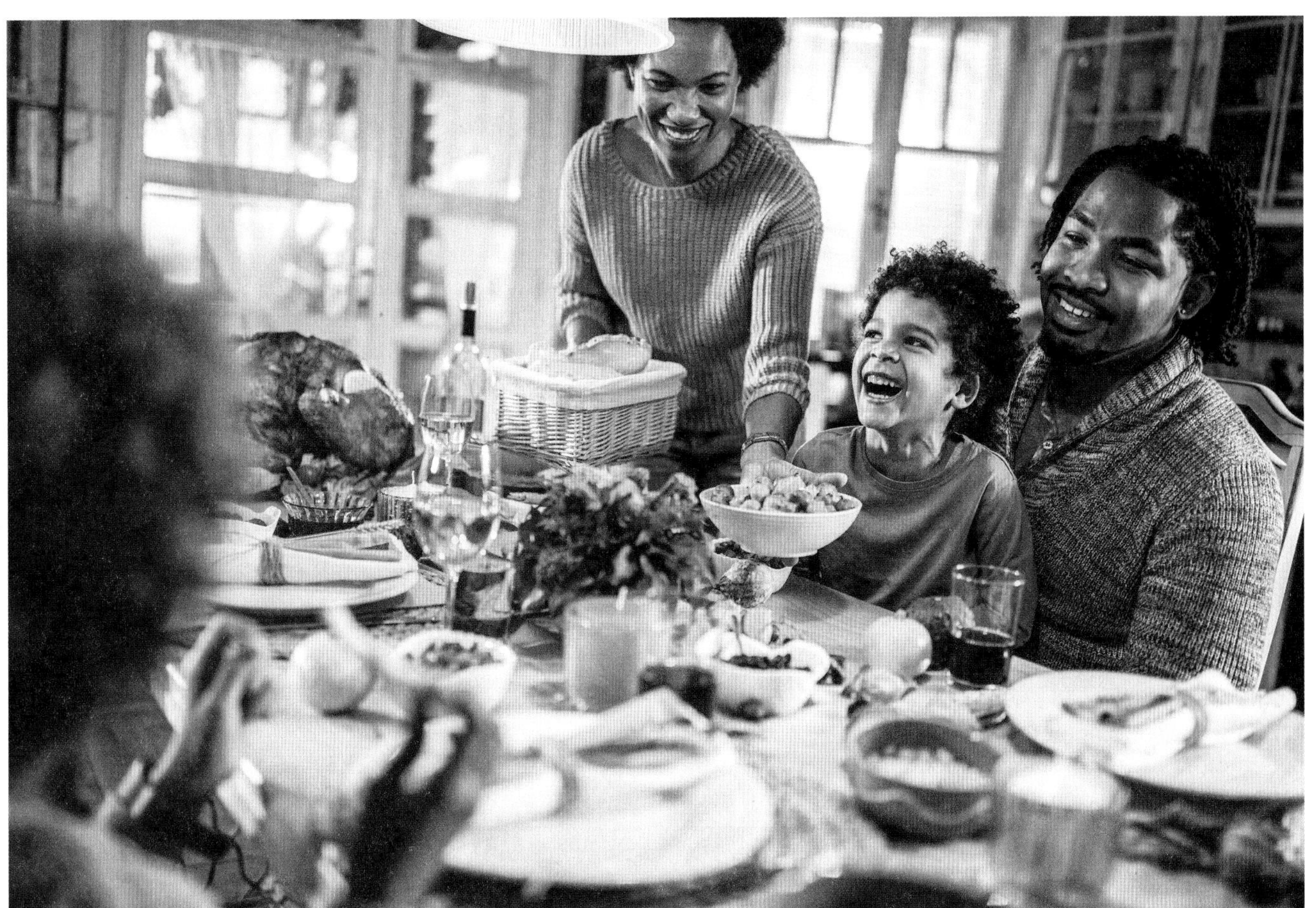
iStock.com/Skynesher

▲ **Humans create complex rules, commonly called manners, about how food is to be eaten.**

Food for Thought

It is thought that children are less likely than adults to try new foods, in part because they have not yet learned cultural rules regarding what is safe and edible. A child who is exposed repeatedly to new items loses the fear of new foods faster than one who experiences a limited diet.[5,6]

The Omnivore's Paradox

Humans are omnivorous, meaning that they can consume and digest a wide selection of plants and animals found in their surroundings. The primary advantage of this is that they can live in various climates and terrains. Because no single food provides the nutrition necessary for survival, humans must be able to eat enough of a variety of items, yet cautious enough not to ingest foods that are harmful and possibly fatal. This dilemma, the need to experiment combined with the need for caution, is known as the omnivore's paradox.[7] It results in two contradictory psychological impulses regarding eating—an attraction to new foods, but a preference for familiar foods. The food habits developed by a community provide the framework that reduces the anxiety produced by these opposing desires. Rules about which foods are edible, how they are procured and cooked, how they should taste, and when they should be consumed provide guidelines for both testing new foods (based on previous experience with similar plants and animals or flavors and textures) and maintaining food traditions through ritual and repetition.

Self-Identity

The choice of which foods to ingest is further complicated by another psychological concept regarding eating—the incorporation of food. This means that consumption is not just the conversion of food into nutrients in the human body, but also includes gaining the food's physical properties as well—hence one interpretation of the phrase "You are what you eat." In most cases, this refers to the physical properties of a food expressed through incorporation. For example, some Asian Indians eat walnuts, which look like miniature brains, to make them smarter, and weight lifters may dine on rare meat to build muscle. In other cases, the character of the food is incorporated. Some Native Americans believe that because milk is a food for infants it will weaken adults. The French say a person who eats too many turnips becomes gutless, and some Vietnamese consume gelatinized tiger bones to improve their strength.

It is a small step from incorporating the traits associated with a specific food to making assumptions about a total diet. The correlation between what people eat, how others perceive them, and how they characterize themselves is striking. In one study, eating was a powerful way to mark symbolic class boundaries. People used food knowledge, adventurousness, and openness to give themselves a certain cache and establish belonging in a social class to which they were not born. Some used ethical eating to establish their distinction from those around them, or employed healthy eating for distinct moral boundary marking. Healthy eating as a topic seems to have become pervasive, across social class groups, perhaps due to the dissemination of healthy eating messages, good news for those involved in the field of nutrition.[8]

Food choice is influenced by self-identity, a process whereby food likes or dislikes are accepted and internalized as personal preferences. Culinary practices can be a force for social order, as well as a point of cultural resistance. Food can shape ideas ranging from nationalism to gender and sexuality norms, suggesting that eating "right" is a gateway to becoming an American, a good citizen, and an ideal person. Eating in America has long been a place for people to distinguish themselves from Europeans. In fact, the first cookbook published on American shores, *American Cookery* by Amelia Simmons, 1796, placed recipes using indigenous corn flour made into Johnny cake and slapjack made "before the fire" or on a hot griddle, just pages away from fancy wheat flour English cakes with 30 ingredients. Though cooking patterns still resembled old English tradition, simple recipes, simply made with available bountiful ingredients, were the order of most lives and a sure break from the motherland of America's first European settlers. The tension between how to balance the sumptuous with the simple in American life had begun.[9] *American Cookery* has been seen as using food as another declaration of independence.[10]

Research suggests that children choose foods eaten by admired adults (e.g., teachers), fictional characters, peers, and especially older siblings. Group approval or disapproval of food can also condition a person's acceptance or rejection. This may explain why certain relatively unpalatable items, such as chili peppers or unsweetened coffee, are enjoyed if introduced through socially mediated events, such as family meals or workplace snack breaks. Although the mechanism for the internalization of food preference and self-identity is not well understood, it is considered a significant factor in the development of food habits.[11] The consumption of organic vegetables, for example by those who identify themselves as green (people who are concerned with ecology and make consumer decisions based on this concern), can mean an intention to eat organic items independent of other attitudes, such as perceived flavor and health benefits.[12,13]

Food as self-identity is especially evident in the experience of dining out. Researchers suggest that restaurants often serve more than food, satisfying both emotional and physical needs. A diner may consider the menu, atmosphere, service, and cost or value when selecting a restaurant, and most establishments cater to a specific clientele. Some offer quick, inexpensive meals and children's play equipment to attract families. Business clubs feature a conservative setting suitable for financial transactions, and the candlelit ambiance of a bistro might be considered conducive to romance. The same diner may choose the first in her role as a mother, the second while at work, and the last when meeting a date. In Japan, restaurants serve as surrogate homes where company is entertained, preserving the privacy of family life. The host chooses and pays for the meal ahead of time, all guests are provided the same dishes, and the servers are expected to partake in the conversation. Ethnic restaurants appeal to those individuals seeking familiarity and authenticity in the foods of their homeland or those interested in novelty and culinary adventure. Conversely, exposure to different foods in restaurants is sometimes the first step in adopting new food items at home.[14]

Symbolic Use of Food

The development of food habits clearly indicates that for humans, food is more than just nutrients. Humans use foods symbolically, due to relationship, association, or convention. Bread is an excellent example—it is called the staff of life in several cultures; one breaks bread with friends, bread represents the body of Christ in the Christian sacrament of communion, and a person with money has "a lot of bread." White bread was traditionally eaten by the upper classes, dark bread by the less wealthy, but whole wheat bread is consumed today by people concerned more with health than status. In many cultures, bread is shared by couples as part of the wedding ceremony or left for the soul of the dead. Superstitions about bread also demonstrate its importance beyond sustenance. Greek soldiers took a piece from home to ensure their safe, victorious return; English midwives placed a loaf at the foot of the mother's bed to prevent the woman and her baby from being stolen by evil spirits; and sailors traditionally brought a bun to sea to prevent shipwreck. The base grain in other cultures, such as rice in Asia and corn (maize) in Mesoamerica, also have a symbolic value that carries throughout the culture. "Have you had rice?" means have you eaten in India, and rice is symbolically the first solid food eaten at a baby's annaprashan ceremony (meaning "first feeding" or "grain initiation" in Sanskrit), and more. Corn to many Native Americans plays a mythological role as a diety, or as a special gift to people from the Creator. Its sacred pollen can be a spiritual offering. It can be the symbolic use of food that is valued most by people, not its nutritional composition.

Food for Thought

The inability to express self-identity through food habits can be devastating. A study of persons with permanent feeding tubes living at home or in nursing facilities found they frequently avoided meals with families and friends. They missed their favorite foods, but more importantly, they mourned the loss of their self-identities reinforced by these daily social interactions.[15]

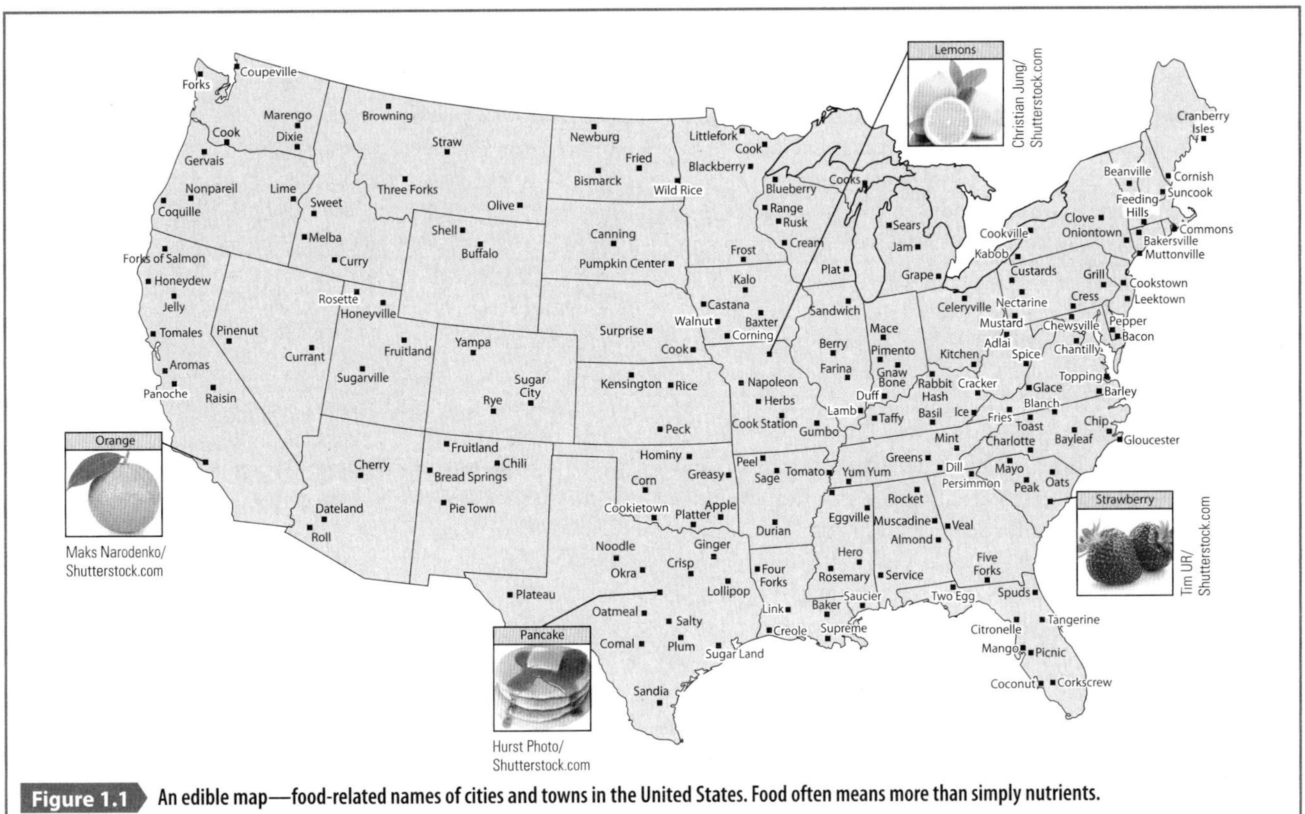

Figure 1.1 **An edible map—food-related names of cities and towns in the United States. Food often means more than simply nutrients.**

Source: From *All Over the Map: An Extraordinary Atlas of the United States: Featuring Towns That Actually Exist!* by David Jouris, copyright © 1994 by David Jouris. Used by permission of Ten Speed Press, an imprint of Crown Publishing Group, a division of Random House, Inc.

Cultural Identity

An essential symbolic function of food is cultural identity. What one eats defines who one is, culturally speaking, and, conversely, who one is not. In the Middle East, for example, a person who eats pork is probably Roman Catholic or Orthodox Christian, not Jewish or Muslim (pork is prohibited in Judaism and Islam). Ravioli served with roast turkey may suggest an Italian American family celebrating Thanksgiving, not a Mexican American family, who would be more likely to dine on tamales, pozole, flan, and turkey. The food habits of each cultural group are often linked to religious beliefs or ethnic behaviors. Eating is a daily reaffirmation of cultural identity (Figure 1.1).

Foods that demonstrate affiliation with a culture are usually introduced during childhood and are associated with security or good memories. Such foods hold special worth to a person, even if other diets have been adopted due to changes in residence, religious membership, health status, or daily personal preference. They tend to be the favorite foods of childhood, or linked to a specific person, place, or time. They may be eaten during cultural holidays and for personal events, such as birthdays or weddings, or during times of stress. These items are sometimes called comfort foods because they satisfy the basic psychological need for food familiarity. A survey of more than 1,000 North Americans noted that the top comfort foods were potato chips (24 percent), ice cream (14 percent), cookies (12 percent), pizza and pasta (11 percent), beef/steak burgers (9 percent), fruits/vegetables (7 percent), soup (4 percent), and other (9 percent). There were gender differences in this finding: women preferred ice cream, chocolate, and cookies. Men chose ice cream, soup, and pizza/pasta, more hot "main" foods than sweet. Loneliness, depression, and guilt were all found to be key drivers of comfort eating for women. Men in the survey, however, typically reported that they ate comfort food when feeling jubilant. In addition to eating comforting foods when low, many times comfort food is eaten as a reward for success.[16] Occasionally, a person embraces a certain diet as an adult to establish an association with a group. A convert to Judaism, for instance, may adhere to the kosher dietary laws. African Americans may choose to eat soul food, which is rooted in the cultures of the African diaspora.

The reverse is also true. One way to establish that a person is not a member of a certain cultural group is through diet. Researchers suggest that when one first eats the food of another cultural group, a chain of reasoning occurs, beginning with the recognition that one is experiencing a new flavor and ending with the assumption that this new flavor is an authentic marker of other group members.[17] Ethnic groups may be denigrated by using food stereotyping, and such slurs are found in nearly all cultures.

Foods that come from other cultures may also be distinguished as foreign to maintain group separation. Kafir, a derogatory Arabic term for "infidel," was used to label some items found in areas they colonized, including the knobby kaffir lime (termed more appropriately the makrut lime) of Malaysia, and kaffir corn (millet) in Africa. Similarly, when some non-Asian foods were introduced to China, they were labeled barbarian or Western and named after items already familiar in the diet. Thus, sweet potatoes were called barbarian yams, and tomatoes became barbarian eggplants.[18] Less provocative place names are used, too, though the origins of the food are often incorrect, such as Turkey wheat (the Dutch term for native American corn, which was thought to come from Turkey) and Irish potatoes (which are indigenous to Peru but were brought to the United States by immigrants from Ireland). The powerful symbolic significance of food terms leads occasionally to renaming foreign items in an attempt to assert a new cultural identity. Turkish coffee (it was the Ottomans of Turkey who popularized this thick, dark brew from Africa and spread it through their empire) became Greek coffee in Greece after tensions between the two nations escalated in the 1920s. Examples in the United States include renaming sauerkraut "liberty cabbage" during World War I, and more recently, calling French fries "freedom fries" when France opposed the United States in the invasion of Iraq.

Food for Thought

A child's rejection of foods, or fussy/picky eating behavior, peaks at around 2–3 years of age. This happens just when there are rapid improvements in a child's ability to categorize food from non-food items. The perception of the food, a child's emotional feeling toward that food or toward eating in general, the environment around eating, and other factors all contribute to pickiness.[19] Usually it takes a child 10–15 tries of a new food before they will accept it.[20,21]

The appropriate use of food and the behaviors associated with eating, also known as etiquette, is another expression of group membership. In the United States, entirely different manners are required during a business lunch at an expensive restaurant, when eating in the school cafeteria or at a barbeque, or when dining with a date. Discomfort can occur if a person is unfamiliar with the rules, and if a person deliberately breaks the rules, he or she may be ostracized or shunned.

Another function of food symbolism is to define status—a person's position or ranking within a particular cultural group. Food can be used to signify economic social standing: champagne, Kobe beef, and truffles suggest wealth; trendy, hip restaurants suggest upward mobility; and beans, potatoes, and minestrone soup are considered more accessible, easy to prepare, and commonly eaten regardless of social status. Status foods are characteristically used for social interaction. In the United States, a spouse may appreciate a box of chocolates from their partner—but not a bundle of broccoli. Wine is considered an appropriate gift to a hostess—a gallon of milk is not.

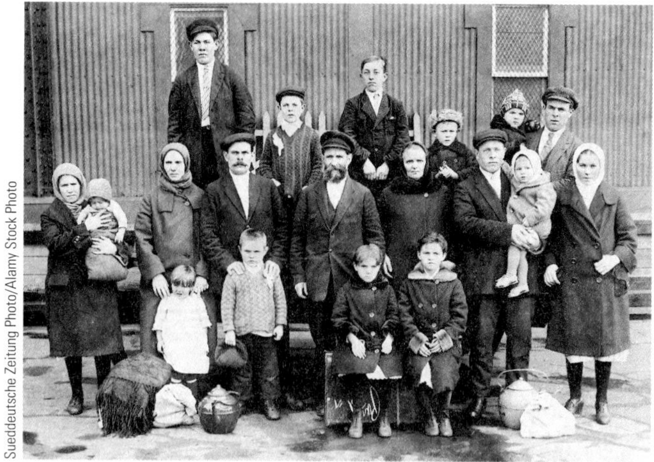

Sueddeutsche Zeitung Photo/Alamy Stock Photo

▲ **Typically, first-generation immigrants remain emotionally connected to their ethnicity, surrounding themselves with a reference group of family and friends who share their cultural background.**

In general, eating with someone connotes social equality with that person. Many societies regulate commensalism (who can dine together) as a means of establishing class relationships. Men may eat separately from women and children, or servants may eat in the kitchen, away from their employers. In India, the separate social castes did not traditionally dine together, nor were people of higher castes permitted to eat food prepared by someone of a lower caste. This class segregation was also seen in some U.S. restaurants that excluded Black and Latinx Americans before civil rights legislation of the 1960s.

What Is Culture?

When referring to humans, culture can be broadly defined as the values, beliefs, attitudes, and practices accepted and socially learned by members of a group or community. It is present in all or most members of the community, and absent or rare in other social groups of the same species. There is evidence of this definition of culture in other mammals (such as dolphins, meerkats, whales), fish, and birds.[22] Culture is not inherited; it is learned and then passed from generation to generation through language and socialization in a process called enculturation. Yet culture is not rigid and does change over time in response to group dynamics.[23]

Ethnicity is the identification of a group based on perceived cultural distinctiveness that makes the group into a "people."[24] Unlike national origin (which may include numerous ethnic groups), ethnicity is a social identity associated with shared behavior patterns, including food habits, dress, language, family structure, and often religious affiliation.[23,25] Members of the same ethnic group usually have a common heritage through locality or history and participate together with other cultural groups in a larger social system. As part of this greater community, each ethnic group may have different statuses or positions of power. Diversity within each cultural group is also common due to racial, regional, or economic divisions as well as different rates of acculturation to the majority culture.[25]

Food for Thought

Ethnocentric is the term applied to a person who uses his or her values to evaluate the behaviors of others. It may be done unconsciously or in the conscious belief that their habits are superior to those of another culture. *Ethnorelativism* occurs when a person assumes that all cultural values have equal validity, resulting in moral paralysis and an inability to advocate for a belief. *Prejudice* is hostility directed toward persons of different cultural groups because they are members of such groups; it does not account for individual differences.[26–28]

The Acculturation Process

When people from one ethnicity move to an area with different cultural norms, adaptation to the new majority society begins. This process is known as acculturation, and it takes place along a continuum of behavior patterns that can be very fluid, moving back and forth between traditional practices and adopted customs. It occurs at the micro level, reflecting an individual's change in attitudes, beliefs, and behaviors, and at the macro level, resulting in group changes that may be physical, economic, social, or political in nature.[29,30] Typically, first-generation immigrants remain emotionally connected to their culture of origin. They integrate into their new society by adopting some majority culture values and practices but generally surround themselves with a reference group of family and friends from their ethnic background. For example, Asian Indians living in the United States who consider themselves to be mostly or very Asian Indian may encourage their children to speak English and allow them to celebrate American holidays, but may not permit them to date non-Asian Indian peers.

Other immigrants become bicultural, which happens when the new majority culture is seen as complementing, rather than competing with, an individual's ethnicity. The positive aspects of both societies are embraced, and the individual develops the skills needed to operate within either culture. Asian Indians who may call themselves Indo-Americans or Asian Indian Americans fall into this category, eating equal amounts of Indian and American foods, and thinking and reading equally in an Indian language and English.

Assimilation occurs when people from one cultural group shed their ethnic identity and fully merge into the majority culture. Although some first-generation immigrants strive toward assimilation, due perhaps to personal determination to survive in a foreign country or to take advantage of opportunities, most often assimilation takes place in subsequent generations. Asian Indians who identify themselves as being "mostly American" do not consider Asian Indian culture superior to American culture, and they are willing to let their children date non-Indians. It is believed that ethnic pride is reawakened in some immigrants if they become disillusioned with life in America, particularly if the disappointment is attributed to prejudice from the majority society. A few immigrants exist at the edges of the acculturation process, either maintaining total ethnic identity or rejecting both their culture of origin and that of the majority culture.[31]

Acculturation of Food Habits

Culturally based food habits are often the last practices people change through acculturation. Unlike speaking a foreign language or wearing traditional clothing, eating is usually done in the privacy of the home, hidden from observation by others. Adoption of new food items does not generally develop as a steady progression from the traditional diet to the diet of the majority culture. Instead, research indicates that the consumption of new items is often independent of traditional food habits.[29,30] The lack of available native ingredients may force immediate acculturation, or convenience or cost factors may speed change. Samoans and people from southern India may be unable to find the fresh coconut cream needed to prepare favorite dishes, for instance, or an Iranian may find the cost of saffron prohibitive. Additionally, many traditional African dishes are plant-based and incorporate gluten-free grains, nuts and seeds, and spices such as fonio, egusi, berbere, and sorghum, which may not be readily sourced in the United States. Some immigrants, however, adapt the foods of the new culture to the preparation of traditional dishes.[29] Tasty foods are easily accepted—fast food, pastries, candies, and soft drinks; conversely, unpopular traditional foods may be the first to go. For example, Mexican children living in the United States may quickly reject certain cuts of meat, such as tripe, that their parents still enjoy. It is the foods most associated with ethnic identity that are often the slowest to be acculturated. Other groups will probably never eat pork, regardless of where they live. People from several Asian countries may insist on eating rice with every meal, even if it is the only Asian food on the table.[32–34]

Cultural Food Habits

Food functions vary culturally, and each group creates categories reflective of their priorities. In the United States, food has been typically classified by food group (protein, dairy, cereal and grain, vegetables and fruits), by the percentage of important nutrients (as identified in Dietary Reference Intake [DRI] for energy, protein, fat, carbohydrates, vitamins, and minerals), or according to recommendations for health. American models, especially the Dietary Guidelines for Americans 2010 and the newer model, MyPlate, outline current dietary recommendations to support health guidelines. These categories also suggest that Americans value food more for its nutritional content and impact on health than for any symbolic use. But only limited information is provided about U.S. food habits; although these schemes list what foods people eat, they reveal nothing about how, when, or why foods are consumed.

Culturally based categories are commonly used by members of each culture. Examples found in both developing and industrialized societies include cultural superfoods, usually staples that have a dominant role in the diet; prestige foods, often protein items or expensive or rare foods; body image foods, believed to influence health, beauty, and well-being; sympathetic magic foods, whose traits, through the association of color or form, are incorporated; and physiologic group foods, reserved for, or forbidden to, groups with certain physiologic status, such as gender, age, or health condition.

Researchers have proposed numerous models to understand the food habits of different cultures. Some of these models are helpful in understanding the role of food within a culture, including:

1. Core and complementary foods model: frequency of food consumption;
2. Food-flavor principles: ways a culture traditionally prepares and seasons its foods;
3. Meal patterns and meal cycles: daily, weekly, and yearly use of food; and
4. Developmental perspective of food culture: changes in food functions that emerge during structural growth in a culture.

Core and Complementary Foods Model

Foods selected by a culture can be grouped according to how often they're consumed. Core foods are staples regularly included in a person's diet, usually daily.[35] These typically include complex carbohydrates, such as rice, wheat, corn, yams, cassava, taro, or plantains. Foods widely but less frequently eaten are termed secondary foods. These items, such as chicken, lettuce, or apples, are consumed once a week or more, but not daily. Foods eaten only sporadically are called peripheral foods. These foods are characteristic of individual food preference, not cultural group habits.

A slightly different version of this model suggests that in many cultures the core food is always served with fringe, or complementary, items to improve palatability (Figure 1.2).[36] Because most starchy staples are bland and uniform in texture, these flavorful foods, eaten in small quantities, encourage consumption of the core food as the bulk of the diet. Legumes, for example, are sometimes a complementary food and sometimes a secondary food. It has been hypothesized that these core and complementary food pairings often combine to provide nutritionally adequate meals, especially when legumes are included. Another example is in cultures where grain is a core food and additional sources of vitamins A and C are required. Rice, breads and pastas, and corn are frequently prepared with leafy green vegetables, abundant herbs, or tomatoes, which are high in these needed nutrients. Chinese rice with pickled vegetables, Italian noodles with tomato sauce, Mexican corn tortillas with salsa, and Middle Eastern pilaf with parsley and dried fruit are examples. When the core diet is almost adequate nutritionally, the addition of secondary foods—including legumes (soybean products in China; beans or lentils in Italy; red or pinto beans in Mexico; chickpeas, fava beans, and lentils in the Middle East; and lentils in India), small amounts of meats, poultry, fish, and cheeses or yogurt—can provide the necessary balance.

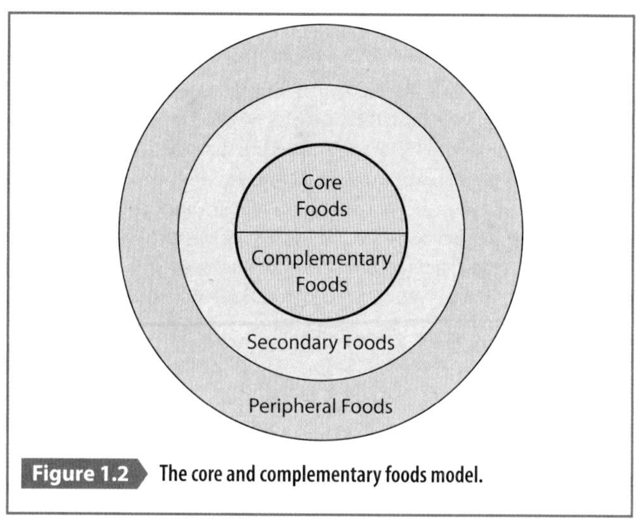

Figure 1.2 The core and complementary foods model.

Changes in food behaviors are believed to happen most often with peripheral foods and then core foods. A person who is willing to omit foods that she or he rarely eats is typically much more reluctant to change those eaten daily and associated with her or his cultural identity. Although little has been reported on the significance of complementary foods in diet modification, presumably, if complementary items were altered or omitted, the core would no longer be palatable. The complementary foods provide the flavor familiarity associated with the core.

Flavor Principles

The significance of food flavor cannot be overestimated. The ways foods are prepared and seasoned are only second in importance to the initial selection of ingredients. It is no less than the transformation of feeding into eating.

Foods demonstrate variability according to location. Much is made, for example, of wine terroir—the soil texture, natural minerals, drainage, source of water, sun exposure, average temperature, and other environmental factors in which grapes are grown for wine production. Each region and vineyard are distinctive, often producing appreciable differences in the resulting product. Yet this variation is insignificant when compared to how foods in general are processed for consumption. Every technique, from preparation for cooking (e.g., washing, hulling or peeling, chopping, pounding, squeezing, soaking, leaching, and marinating) to cooking (e.g., baking, roasting, grilling, stewing, toasting, steaming, boiling, and frying) and preserving (e.g., drying, curing, canning, pickling, fermenting, and freezing), alters the original flavor of the ingredient. Nevertheless, location and manipulation practices alone do not equal cuisine. How it is seasoned is also a factor.

Historians and scientists speculate there are several reasons why herbs and spices have assumed such an essential role in food habits. Foremost is palatability. Salt, one of the most widely used seasonings, prompts an innate human taste response. It is enjoyed by most people and physiologically craved by some. Researchers also suggest that the burn of chili peppers (and perhaps other spices) may trigger the release of pleasurable endorphins (not to mention adding critical vitamin C to diets). Another debunked theory on the popularity of seasoning is that it was used to disguise the taste of spoiled meats, though this is far-fetched (it is next to impossible to disguise the taste and aroma of rancid meat and, in addition, people would be sickened if it were eaten). There is ample evidence, however, as well as ancient medical systems such as Ayurveda in India, that assert various health benefits from spices and herbs. Not only do spices enhance the flavor, aroma, and color of food and beverages, they appear to possess antioxidant, anti-inflammatory, glucose- and cholesterol-lowering properties, and some effects that affect cognition and mood, among other traits. While a recent study shows little evidence that spice use reduces infection with antimicrobial effects,[37] other properties of individual spices are beginning to be documented by Western scientists. Other researchers in older studies speculate that eating chili peppers (and, by extension, other hot seasonings such as mustard, horseradish, and wasabi) is a benign form of risk-taking that provides a safe thrill,[38] while a recent study in China shows spicy food cravings stimulate certain brain regions when compared to non-cravers.[39]

Unique seasoning combinations, termed *flavor principles*, typify the foods of cultural groups worldwide. They are so distinctive that few people mistake their use. For example, a dish flavored with soy sauce is Asian and not European. These seasoning combinations are often found in the complementary foods of the core and complementary foods model, providing the flavors associated with the starchy carbohydrates that are the staples of a culture. They usually include herbs, spices, vegetables, and a fat or oil, although many variations exist. A principal flavor combination in West Africa is tomatoes, onion, and chili peppers that have been sautéed in palm oil. In the Pacific Islands, a flavor principle is coconut milk or cream with a little lime juice and salt. Yams taste like West African food when topped with the tomato mixture and like Southeast Asia/Oceania food when served with the coconut sauce. Some widely recognizable flavor principles include:

- Asian Indian: garam masala (a spice blend, often coriander, cumin, fenugreek, turmeric, black pepper, cayenne, cloves, cardamom, and chili peppers)
- Brazilian (Bahia): chili peppers, dried shrimp, ginger root, and palm oil
- Chinese: soy sauce, rice wine, and ginger root
- French: butter, cream, wine, bouquet garni (selected herbs, such as tarragon, thyme, and bay leaf)
- German: sour cream, vinegar, dill, mustard, and black pepper
- Greek: lemon, onions, garlic, oregano, and olive oil
- Italian: tomato, garlic, basil, oregano, and olive oil
- Japanese: soy sauce, sugar, and rice wine vinegar
- Korean: soy sauce, garlic, ginger root, black pepper, scallions, chili peppers, and sesame seeds or oil
- Mexican: tomatoes, onions, chili peppers, and cumin
- Puerto Rican: sofrito (seasoning sauce of tomatoes, onions, garlic, bell peppers, cilantro, capers, pimento, annatto seeds, and lard)
- Russian: sour cream, onion, dill, and parsley
- Scandinavian: sour cream, onion, mustard, dill, and caraway
- Thai: fermented fish sauce, coconut milk, chili peppers, garlic, ginger root, lemongrass, and tamarind

It would be incorrect to assume that every dish from each culture is flavored with its characteristic seasoning combinations, or that principal flavor seasoning is limited to just those listed. It is common to find regional variations as well. In China, northern cuisine often includes seasonings enhanced with soybean paste, garlic, and sesame oil. In the south, fermented black beans are frequently added, although in the Szechwan region hot bean paste, chili peppers, or Szechwan (fagara) pepper is more common. In the specialty cuisine of the Hakka, the addition of red rice wine is distinctive. Further, in any culture where the traditional seasoning combinations are prepared at home, not purchased, modifications to suit each family are customary.[40] For example, in India, garam masala is often unique to each family's preferred mix of spices. Flavor principles are therefore more of a marker for each culture's cuisine rather than a rigid rule.

Food for Thought

A few cuisines have extremely limited seasonings, including the fare of the Inuits. Broadly speaking, cuisines offering large portions of meat and other protein foods tend to be less seasoned than those with a higher proportion of grains, fruits and vegetables, and legumes.

The sprig of parsley added to a plate of food may have originated to sweeten the breath, but also because of folklore incorporating the length of time it took to germinate the plant—parsley, it was said, had to travel to the Underworld and back before it could grow. This idea then led to depictions of Persephone (Queen of the Underworld in Greek mythology) carrying a parsley sprig to Hades and back to get it to germinate, which led to ideas of death and protection. The idea of protection landed parsley on your plate of food today to safeguard the meal from evil.

In many homes, few meals are eaten as a family. The term *grazing* refers to grabbing small amounts of food throughout the day to consume. There are an estimated 7 million vending machines in the United States, with over 100 million customers daily.

Meal Patterns and Meal Cycles

People in every culture dine on at least one meal each day, and meal patterns and meal cycles reveal clues about complex social relations and the significance of certain events in a society.[41] The first step in decoding these patterns and cycles is to determine what types of food constitute a meal within a culture.

In the United States, for instance, cocktails and appetizers or coffee and dessert are not considered meals. A meal should consist of a main course and side dishes; typically, a meat, vegetable, and starch. In the western African nation of Cameroon, a meal is a snack unless cassava paste is served. In many Asian cultures, a meal is not considered a meal unless rice is included, no matter how much other food is consumed. A one-pot dish is considered a meal if it contains all the elements of a full meal. For example, American casserole dishes often feature protein, vegetables, and a starch, such as tuna casserole (tuna, peas, and noodles). In England, it could be shepherd's pie (ground beef, green beans, and tomato sauce topped with mashed potatoes).

The elements that define a meal must also be served in their proper order. In the United States, appetizers come before soup or salad, followed by the entrée and then by dessert. In France, the salad is served after the entrée. All foods are served simultaneously in Vietnam so that each person may combine flavors and textures according to taste. In addition to considering the proper serving order, foods must also be appropriate for the meal or situation. Some cultures do not distinguish which foods can be served at different meals, but in the United States, eggs and bacon are considered breakfast foods, while cheese and olives are popular in the Middle East for the morning meal. Soup is commonly served at breakfast in Southeast Asia, but in the United States soup is a lunch or dinner food, and in parts of Europe fruit soup is sometimes served as dessert. Cake and ice cream are appropriate for a child's birthday party in the United States, wine and cheese are not.

Other aspects of the meal message include who prepares the meal and what culturally specific preparation rules are used. In the United States, ketchup goes with French fries; in Great Britain, vinegar is sprinkled on chips (fried potatoes). Observant Jewish people consume meat only if it has been slaughtered by an approved butcher in an approved manner and has been prepared in a particular way. (See Chapter 4, "Food and Religion," for more information on Judaism.)

Who eats the meal is also important. A meal is frequently used to define personal relationships. Americans are comfortable inviting friends for dinner, but they usually invite acquaintances for just drinks and appetizers. For a family dinner, people may include only some of the elements that constitute a meal, but serving a meal to guests requires that all elements be included in their proper order.

The final element of what constitutes a meal is portion size. In many cultures, one meal a day is designated the main meal and usually contains the largest portions. The amount of food considered appropriate varies, however. A traditional serving of beef in China may be limited to one ounce added to a dish of rice. In France, a three- or four-ounce filet is more typical. In the United States, a six- or even eight-ounce steak is not unusual, and some restaurants specialize in twelve-ounce or larger cuts of prime rib. American tradition is to clean one's plate regardless of how much is served, while in other cultures, such as those in the Middle East, it is considered polite to leave some food to demonstrate that enough was provided by the host.

Just as individual meals have cultural differences, the number of meals and when they are eaten also varies. In much of Europe, a large main meal is customarily consumed at noontime, for example, while in most of the United States today the main meal is eaten in the evening. In less wealthy societies, only one meal per day may be eaten, whereas in wealthy cultures three or four meals are standard.

The meal cycle in most cultures also includes feasting or fasting, and often both. Feasting celebrates special events, occurring in nearly every society where a surplus of food can be accumulated. Religious holidays such as Christmas and Passover; secular holidays such as Thanksgiving and the Vietnamese New Year's Day, known as Tet; and even personal events such as births, marriages, and deaths are observed with appropriate foods. In many cultures, feasting means simply more of the foods consumed daily and is considered a time of plenty when everyone has enough to eat. Special dishes that include costly ingredients or are time-consuming to prepare also are characteristic of feasting. The elements of a feast rarely differ from those of an everyday meal. There may be more everyday foods or several main courses with additional side dishes and a selection of desserts, but the meal structure does not change. For example, Thanksgiving typically includes turkey and often another entrée such as ham or a casserole (meat); several vegetables; bread or rolls, potatoes, sweet potatoes, and stuffing (starch); as well as pumpkin, mincemeat, and pecan pies or other dessert selections. Appetizers, soups, and salads may also be included.

Fasting may be partial or total. Often it is just the elimination of some items from the diet, such as the Roman Catholic omission of meat on Fridays during Lent or a Hindu personal fast day when only foods cooked in milk are eaten. Complete fasts are less common. During the holy month of Ramadan, Muslims are prohibited from taking food or drink from dawn to sunset, but they may eat in the evening. Yom Kippur, the day of atonement observed by many Jews, is a total fast from sunset to sunset. (See Chapter 4 for more details on fasting.)

Developmental Perspective of Food Culture

Trends in food, eating, and nutrition also reflect structural changes in society. The developmental perspective of food culture (Table 1.1) suggests how changes may alter how consumers obtain food, as well as types of food and variety. Globalization is defined as the integration of local, regional,

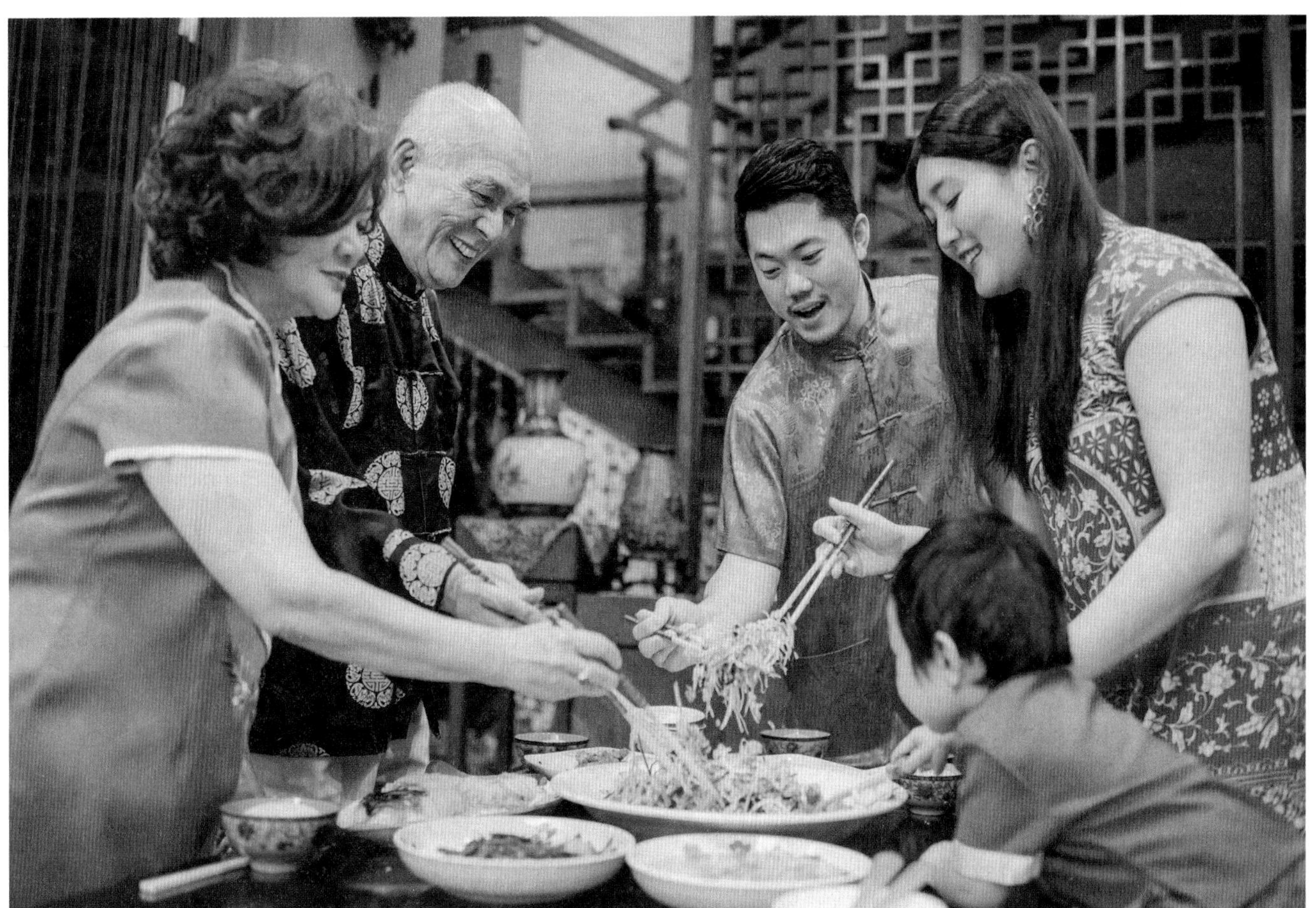
Edwin Tan/E+/Getty Images

▲ **Special dishes that include costly ingredients or are time-consuming to prepare are characteristic of feasting in many cultures.**

and national phenomena into an unrestricted worldwide organization. The parallel change in cultural food habits is consumerization, the transition of a society from producers of indigenous foods to consumers of mass-produced foods. Traditionally seasonal ingredients, such as strawberries, become available any time of year from a worldwide network of growers and suppliers. Specialty products, such as ham and other deli meats, which were at one time prepared annually or only for festive occasions, can now be purchased presliced, precooked, and prepackaged for immediate consumption.

The social dynamic of modernization with new technologies results in socioeconomic shifts, such as during the Industrial Revolution when muscle power was replaced by fuel-generated engine power or during the 1990s with

Food for Thought

Feasting functions to redistribute food from wealthy to less wealthy, to demonstrate status, to motivate people toward a common goal (e.g., a political fundraising dinner), to mark the seasons and life-cycle events, and to symbolize devotion and faith (e.g., Passover, Eid al-Fitr, Holi, and communion).

From 2001–2018 added sugar intake in the United States among children 2–8 years old and adolescents and teens 9–18 years old declined 3 to 4 percent across sociodemographic factors, but remain above recommended levels. The decline was due mainly to decreases in added sugars from sweetened beverages. The decline also roughly coincides with the reforms in the national school lunch and breakfast programs aimed at improving the nutritional quality of foods in schools.[42]

Table 1.1 Developmental Perspective of Food Culture

Structural Change	Food Culture Change
Globalization: Local to worldwide organizations	Consumerization: Indigenous to mass-produced foods
Modernization: Muscle to fueled power	Commoditization: Homemade to manufactured foods
Urbanization: Rural to urban residence	Delocalization: Producers to consumers only
Migration: Original to new settings	Acculturation: Traditional to adopted foods

Source: Adapted from Sobal, J. 1999. Social change and foodways. In *Proceedings of the Cultural and Historical Aspects of Food Symposium.* Corvallis: Oregon State University.

the rise of the information age. Cultural beliefs, values, and behaviors are modified in response to the structural changes that take place. Food habits changed, with foods becoming more processed and meals pre-prepared instead of cooked at home. The fresh milk from the cow in the barn becomes the plastic gallon container of pasteurized milk sold online over the Internet to a consumer who has limited time to shop.

Urbanization occurs when a large percentage of the population abandons the low density of rural residences in favor of higher-density suburban and urban residences. Often, income levels do not change in the move, but families who previously survived on subsistence farming become dependent on others for food. Delocalization occurs when the connections among growing, harvesting, cooking, and eating food are lost, as meals prepared by anonymous workers are purchased from convenience markets and fast-food restaurants.

Finally, the migration of populations from their original homes to new regions or nations creates a significant shift from a home-bound, culture-bound society to one in which global travel is prevalent and immigration common. Traditional food habits are in flux during acculturation to the diet of a new culture and as novel foods are introduced, they become accepted into the majority cuisine. Often, new traditions emerge from the contact between diverse cultural food habits.

The developmental perspective of food culture assumes that cultures progress from underdeveloped to developed through the structural changes listed. Deliberate efforts to reverse that trend can be seen in the renewed popularity of farmers' markets in the United States and attacks on fast-food franchises in Europe. Other evidence of resistance includes the work of the Slow Food movement—mobilizing against the negative effects of industrialization—and the seed banks that have opened throughout the world to promote genetic diversity and save indigenous plant populations.[43–45]

Individual Food Habits

Each person lives within his or her culture, mostly unaware of the influences exerted by that culture on food habits. Eating choices are typically made according to what is obtainable, what is acceptable, and what is preferred: the diet is determined by availability and by what each person considers edible or inedible. Beyond that, factors that influence an individual's food selection are taste, cost, convenience, self-expression, well-being, and variety, which are explained in the consumer food choice model, discussed later in the chapter.

Food Availability

A person can select a diet only from available foods. Local ecological considerations such as weather, soil, and water conditions; geographic features; indigenous vegetation; the native animal population; and human manipulation of these resources through the cultivation of plants and domestication of livestock determine the food supply at a fundamental level. A society living in the cool climate of northern Europe is not going to establish rice as a core food, just as a society in the hot wet regions of southern India is not going to rely on oats or rye. Seasonal variations are a factor, as are climactic events, such as droughts, that disrupt the food supply.

The political, economic, and social management of food at the local level is typically directed toward providing a reliable and affordable source of nourishment. Advances in food production, storage, and distribution are examples. However, the development of national and international food networks has often been motivated by other needs, including profit and power. The complexity of the food supply system has been examined by many disciplinary approaches. Historians trace the introduction and replacement of foods as they spread regionally and globally. Economists describe the role of supply and demand, the commodity market, price controls, trade deficits, and farm subsidies (as well as other entitlements) on access to food. Psychologists investigate how individual experience impacts diet; political scientists detail how fear of biotechnology, bioterrorism, and disease (such as the mad-cow or bovine spongiform encephalopathy scare in Europe) can alter acceptability. Sociologists document how social structures and relations affect the obtainment of food; legal experts debate the ethics of food policies for people who are not able to afford food, are incarcerated, and are terminally ill. This is only a small sampling of the factors influencing food availability. However, except in regions where serious food shortages are anticipated for various reasons including conflict, availability issues are usually not at the forefront of individual food choice for much of the world.

Edible or Inedible?

The consideration of edible or inedible was one of the earliest food habit models, describing the individual process that establishes the available, appropriate, and personal food habits. Each person's choice of what to eat is generally limited to the foods found in this model.[46]

1. ***Inedible foods:*** These foods are poisonous or are not eaten because of strong beliefs or taboos (or taboo foods, from the Tongan word *tabu*, meaning "marked as holy"). Foods defined as inedible vary culturally. Examples of frequently prohibited foods include animals useful to the cultural group, such as cattle in India; animals dangerous to catch; animals that have died of unknown reasons or disease; animals that consume garbage or excrement; and plants or animals that resemble a human ailment (e.g., strawberries or beef during pregnancy to protect the infant, as described later).
2. ***Edible by animals, but not by me:*** These foods are items such as rodents in the United States or sometimes corn in France (where it is used primarily as an animal feed grain). Again, the foods in this category vary widely by culture.

3. ***Edible by humans, but not by my kind:*** These foods are recognized as acceptable in some societies, but not in your own culture. Some rural South Africans who consider termites a delicacy are repulsed by the idea of eating scorpions, a specialty enjoyed by some Chinese.[47,48]
4. ***Edible by humans, but not by me:*** These foods include all those accepted by a person's cultural group but not by the individual, due to factors such as preference (e.g., tripe, liver, raw oysters), expense, or health reasons (a low-sodium or low-cholesterol diet may eliminate many traditional American foods). Other factors, such as religious restrictions (as in kosher law or halal practices) or ethical considerations (vegetarianism), may also influence food choices.
5. ***Edible by me:*** These are all foods accepted as part of an individual's dietary domain.

There are always exceptions to how foods are categorized. It is generally assumed, for instance, that poisonous plants and animals will always be avoided. In Japan, however, fugu (blowfish or globefish) is considered a delicacy despite the deadly toxin contained in its liver, intestines, testes, and ovaries. These organs must be deftly removed by a certified chef as the last step of cleaning (if they are accidentally damaged, the poison spreads rapidly through the flesh). Eating the fish supposedly provides a tingle in the mouth prized by the Japanese. Several people die each year from fugu poisoning.

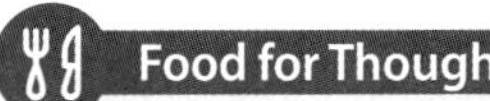

Food for Thought

Among the most universal of food taboos is cannibalism, although anthropologists have discovered numerous examples of prehistoric human consumption in European and New World excavations.

There are approximately 2,000 edible insect species, including beetles, caterpillars, bees, ants, crickets, grasshoppers, and locusts. For hundreds of years, native cultures in Asia, South America, Africa, and Europe included the consumption of various insects. In Western societies today, due to cultural biases, edible insects currently have greater potential as animal feed.[49]

Determinants of Food Choice and Dietary Change Model

An individual's dietary likes and dislikes are established before he or she sets foot in a restaurant, deli, or supermarket. The food choice model (Figure 1.3) explains the factors that influence individual decisions.[50]

Food selection is primarily motivated by taste. Taste is defined broadly by the sensory properties detectable in foods: color, aroma, flavor, and texture. Humans anticipate a specific food will have certain sensory characteristics; deviations can signal that the item is poisonous or spoiled. Many of these expectations are developed through early exposure to culturally acceptable and unacceptable foods. For example, most core foods are pale white, cream, or brown in color; however, some West Africans prefer the bright orange of

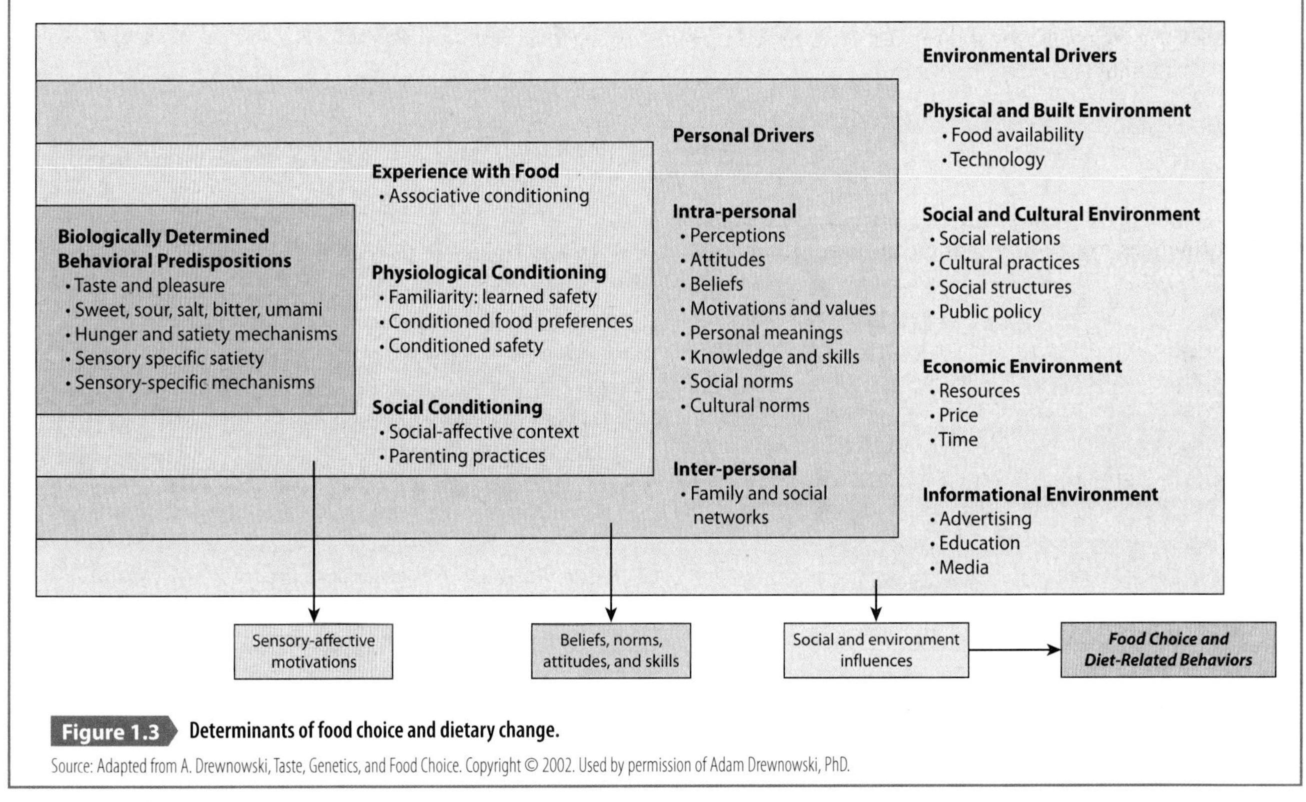

Figure 1.3 Determinants of food choice and dietary change.

Source: Adapted from A. Drewnowski, Taste, Genetics, and Food Choice. Copyright © 2002. Used by permission of Adam Drewnowski, PhD.

sweet potatoes, and Southeast Asians/residents of Oceania consider lavender appropriate for the taro root preparation called poi. Should the core item be an unanticipated color, such as green or blue, it may be rejected. Similarly, each food has a predictable smell. Pleasurable aromas may trigger salivation, while those considered disgusting, such as the odor of rotting meat, can trigger an immediate gag reflex in some people. Again, which odors are agreeable and which are disagreeable are due, in part, to which foods are culturally accepted: Strong-smelling fermented meat products (muktuk) are esteemed by some Inuit and some rural Filipinos. Strong-smelling cheese (controlled rotting of milk) appeals to many Europeans, but even mild cheddar may evoke distaste by many Asians and Latinx, though cultural tastes are changing. Appropriate texture is likewise predictable. Ranging from soft and smooth to tough and coarse, each food has its expected consistency. New textures may be disliked: Some Americans object to gelatinous bits in liquid, as found in tapioca pudding or bubble tea, yet these foods are popular in China. Conversely, some Asians find the thick, sticky consistency of mashed potatoes unappetizing. Okra, which has a mucilaginous texture, is well-liked in the U.S. South but can be considered too slimy by those living elsewhere.

Food for Thought

Humans can detect approximately 10,000 different odors, though genetics may determine which odors can be detected. For example, nearly 50 percent of people cannot smell androstenone (also called boar pheromone), which is found in bacon, truffles, celery, parsnips, boar saliva, and many human secretions; however, researchers have found people can be taught to perceive it through daily sniffing.[51] Some people, 22 to 50 percent of the population, also can smell the sulfuric odor in their urine in as little time as 15 minutes after eating asparagus.[52]

The human tongue has receptors for the perception of sweet, sour, salty, bitter, and umami (a sensation produced by several amino acids and nucleotides and often described as a meaty flavor found in aged cheese, wine, mushrooms, and more). It is hypothesized that food choice in all societies is driven, in part, by an inborn preference for the taste of sugars and fats. These nutrients are indicative of foods that are energy dense; a predisposition for sweets and foods high in fat ensures adequate calorie intake, an evolutionary necessity for omnivores with a wide selection of available foods. Sugars and fats are especially pleasurable flavor elements, associated with palatability and satiety (including the texture factor provided by fats, called mouthfeel).

Preferences for sweets (especially when combined with fats) are found during infancy and childhood and peak in early adolescence. The opposite is true for bitterness, which is associated with toxic compounds found in some foods and is strongly disliked by most children. The ability to detect bitterness decreases with age, however, and many adults consume foods with otherwise unpleasant sulfides and tannins, including broccoli and coffee. Some remain especially sensitive to certain bitter compounds, affecting their other preferences as well; they tend to dislike sweet foods and opt for bland over spicy items. Sourness alone is rarely well-liked but is enjoyed when combined with other flavors, especially sweet. It has been suggested that a preference for the sweet-sour taste prompted human ancestors to seek fruit, an excellent source of vitamins and minerals.[53,54]

Unlike the tastes of sweet, bitter, and sour, babies generally are indifferent to salt until about four months of age. Similar to sugar, children prefer higher concentrations of salt than adults. Their preference for salt is shaped by the frequency of exposure to it after birth, and perhaps perinatally. Excess consumption of salt during pregnancy has been shown to impair cardiovascular function and enhance salt preference in adulthood.[55]

Finally, taste is influenced by flavor principles, the characteristic combinations of core and complementary foods, as well as traditional grouping of meal elements. These traditions are important in providing an expected taste experience and satisfying a need for familiarity with food habits.

Cost is often the second most important influence on food choice, and income level is the most significant sociodemographic factor in predicting selection. In cultures with a limited food supply due to environmental conditions or in societies where a large segment of the population is disadvantaged, food price may be more of a driver than taste, nutritional sufficiency, and well-being. The wealthier the society, the less disposable income is spent on food, and, as income increases, food choices change. Typically, the people of less wealthy cultures survive on a diet dependent on grains or tubers and limited amounts of protein, including meat, poultry, fish, or dairy foods. Only a small variety of fresh fruits or vegetables may be available. People with ample income consistently include more meats, sweets, and fats in their diet (a trend seen in the global popularity of American fast foods), plus a wider assortment of fruits and vegetables.[56,57] When nutritious food is available and affordable, the prestige of certain food items, such as lobster or prime rib, is often linked to cost. Protein foods are most associated with status, although difficult-to-obtain items, such as truffles, can also be pricey.

In the United States, affordability has been found to limit the purchasing of healthy foods, and in some cases, even families with government subsidies find it difficult to meet nutritional needs.[58,59] It is estimated that in 2020 10.5 percent (13.8 million) of households were considered to be food insecure.[60]

A subsistence farmer may have greater access to fresh foods than a person with the same limited income living in a city. In urban areas, supermarkets with a less expensive selection of foods often choose to locate outside low-income neighborhoods, creating a situation where residents may have access only to higher-priced convenience stores or small, independently run groceries with a limited selection.[59,61–63] Further, access to healthful restaurant dining varies. Studies suggest that predominantly Black American and low-income neighborhoods have more fast-food restaurants per square mile than White neighborhoods, with fewer healthy options.[64–67]

Convenience is a major concern in food purchases, particularly by members of urbanized societies. In some cultures, everyone's jobs are near home, and the whole family joins in a leisurely midday lunch. In urbanized societies, people often work far from home; therefore, lunch is eaten with fellow employees. Instead of a large, home-cooked meal, employees may eat a quick fast-food meal. Furthermore, family structure can necessitate convenience. In the United States, the decreasing number of extended families (with help available from elder members) and increasing number of households with single parents, along with couples whom both work outside the home and unassociated adults living together, all reduce the possibility that any adult in the household has the time or energy to prepare meals. However, studies show that home cooking in the United States is increasing, especially among men, though women still cook much more. The percentage of college-educated men in the United States who cook increased from about 38 percent in 2003 to 52 percent in 2016. College-educated women who cook also increased from about 65 percent in 2003 to 69 percent in 2016. Men with less than a high school education who cook did not change (33 percent), and women with less than a high school education who do the family cooking stayed the same (72 percent).[68] Research indicates that a higher amount of family meals is correlated with more positive health indicators.[69] Furthermore, the quality of dietary intake improves when there is a reduction in spending on food away from home.[70] Convenience generally spurs the increasing number of takeout foods and meals purchased at restaurants. In 2020, the restaurant industry's share of the U.S. food dollar was 51 percent.

Self-expression, how we indicate who we are by behavior or activities, is important for some individuals in food selection, particularly as a marker of cultural identity. Although the foods associated with ethnicity, religious affiliation, or regional association are predetermined through the dietary domain, it is worth noting that every time a person makes a food choice he or she may choose to follow or ignore convention. Ethnic identity may be immediate, as in persons who have recently arrived in the United States, or it may be remote, a distant heritage modified or lost over the generations through acculturation. An individual who has just immigrated to the United States from Japan, for instance, may be more likely to prefer traditional Japanese cuisine than a third- or fourth-generation Japanese American.

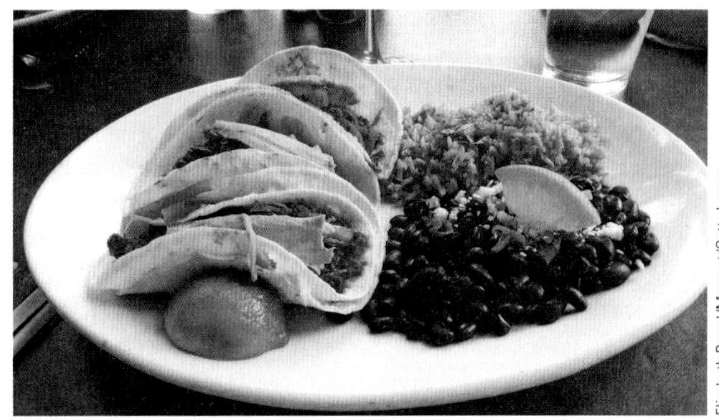

Elizabeth Beard/Moment/Getty Images

▲ **Regional fare differs throughout the United States and can be consumed for self-expression. The southwestern foods shown here represent one of many distinct regional cuisines.**

Food for Thought

Though the physiological response to disgust, nose wrinkling, retraction of the lips, gaping, gagging, and even nausea seems instinctual, it is a cognitively sophisticated feeling that develops in children between the ages of four and seven years old. Which items are disgusting in a culture is learned from parents and peers.[71]

A fifth type of tongue receptor has been found for *umami* (from the Japanese for "savory"). It is the taste associated with such foods as meats, mushrooms, and cheeses.[72] In addition to salt, other flavor preferences may be passed on perinatally.[73]

In 1901, the average American family spent nearly half (45 percent) of their income on food. Today, that figure has decreased to 27 percent of total income on average, and in the highest income brackets it is just 7 percent of income.[74]

Food for Thought

The status of food can change over time. In early years, lobster was so plentiful it piled up on beaches after storms, and colonists considered it fit only for Native Americans, prisoners, or starving settlers.

Religious beliefs are similar to ethnic identity in that they may have a great impact on individual food habits or an insignificant influence depending on religious affiliation and degree of adherence. Many Christian denominations have no food restrictions, but some, such as the Seventh-day Adventists, have strict guidelines about what church members may eat. Judaism requires that only certain foods be consumed in certain combinations, yet most Jewish people in the United States do not follow these rules strictly (see Chapter 4).

A person may also choose foods associated with a specific region. In the United States, the food habits of New England differ from those of the Midwest, the South, and the West, and local specialties such as Pennsylvania Dutch, Cajun, and Tex-Mex may influence the cooking of all residents in those areas.

Self-identity can be another factor in food selection, as discussed previously. An environmentalist may be a vegetarian who prefers organic, locally grown produce, while a gourmet or foodie may patronize small markets in ethnic neighborhoods throughout a city searching for unusual ingredients. Advertising has been directly related to self-expression, especially self-identity. Research indicates that in blind taste tests people often have difficulty discriminating between different brands of the same food item. Consumer loyalty to a particular brand is believed more related to the sensual and emotional appeal of the name and packaging.[75,76] For example, similar-tasting flake cereals such as Wheaties® (which touts itself as the "breakfast of champions"), Special K®, and Total® target sports enthusiasts, dieters, and health-conscious individuals, respectively.

Advertising also promises food-provided pleasure, appealing to the desire of consumers to be seen as popular, fun-loving, and trendy. The exploitation of sex to sell hamburgers and beer is common, as are suggestions that eating a chocolate or drinking a soft drink will add zest to living. A study of television food ads targeting children found that 75 percent were associated with "good times," 43 percent with being "cool and hip," and 43 percent with feelings of happiness.[77-79] Such advertising is a reflection of a larger trend: food as entertainment, the vicarious enjoyment of eating through reading about it or watching food-related programs on television, also called food porn.[80] In the United States, nearly 150 food and wine magazines are published monthly, and magazines that do not have food as the primary focus often have a food section. Food coverage is one segment of print media that continues to grow. In addition, almost 500 million food and wine books are sold annually, digital food blogs are very popular, and numerous network cooking and dining shows air daily with millions of viewers. The impact of this media on food choice is not yet fully known. Food entertainment may popularize certain ingredients, such as kale or mangoes, or cuisines, such as Spanish fare, or updated traditional American dishes like spicy meatloaf and macaroni and cheese. They may also set such a high standard of preparation and presentation that some home cooks feel inadequate, choosing to dine out or select prepackaged items instead of making meals from scratch.

Physical and spiritual well-being is another food choice consideration for some individuals. Physiological characteristics, including age, gender, body image, and state of health, often impact food habits. Preferences and the ability to eat and digest foods vary throughout the life cycle. Pregnant and lactating women commonly eat differently than other adults. In the United States, women are urged to consume more food when they are pregnant, especially dairy products. They are also believed to crave unusual food combinations, such as pickles and ice cream. They may avoid certain foods, such as strawberries, because they are believed to cause red birthmarks.

In some societies with subsistence economies, pregnant women may be allowed to eat more meat than other family members; in others, pregnant women avoid beef because it is feared that the cow's cloven hoof may cause a cleft palate in the infant. Most cultures also have rules regarding which foods are appropriate for infants; milk is generally considered wholesome, and sometimes any liquid resembling milk, such as nut milk, is also believed to be nourishing.

Puberty is a time for special food rites in many cultures. In the United States, adolescents are particularly susceptible to advertising and peer pressure. They tend to eat quite differently from children and adults, rejecting those foods typically served at home and consuming more fast foods and soft drinks. A rapid rate of growth at this time also affects the amount of food that teenagers consume.[81]

The opposite is true of older adults. As metabolism slows, caloric needs decrease. In addition, they may develop a reduced tolerance for fatty foods or highly spiced items. Eating problems tend to increase as we age, such as the inability to chew certain foods or disinterest in cooking and in dining alone. It is predicted that the shift toward an older population in the next two decades will result in a change in the types of foods purchased (an increase in fruits, vegetables, fish, and pork because older adults consume these items more often than younger adults do) and reductions in the total amount of food consumed per capita (because older adults eat smaller amounts of food).[82,83]

Gender has also been found to influence eating habits. In some cultures, women are prohibited from eating specific foods or are expected to serve the largest portions and best pieces of food to men. In other societies, food preference is related to gender. Some people in the United States consider steak to be a masculine food and salad to be a feminine one, or that men drink beer and women drink white wine. Research has shown that gender differences affect how the brain processes satiation responses to chocolate, suggesting that men and women may vary in the physiological regulation of food intake—perhaps accounting for some food preferences.[84,85]

A person's state of health also has an impact on what is eaten. A chronic condition such as lactose intolerance or a disease such as diabetes or celiac disease requires an individual to restrict or omit certain foods. An individual who is sick may not be hungry or may find it difficult to eat. Even minor illnesses may result in dietary changes, such as drinking ginger ale for an upset stomach or hot tea for a cold. Those who are on weight-loss diets may restrict foods to only a few items, such as grapefruit or cabbage soup, or a certain category of foods, such as those low in fat or carbohydrates. Those who are exceptionally fit may practice other food habits, including carbohydrate loading or consumption of high-protein bars. In many cultures, specific foods are often credited with health-promoting qualities, such as ginseng in Asia or chicken soup in eastern Europe. Corn in Native American culture may be selected to improve strength or stamina. Well-being is not limited to physiological conditions; spiritual health is equally dependent on diet in some cultures where the body and mind are considered one entity. A balance of hot and cold or yin and yang foods may be consumed to avoid physical or mental illness. (Refer to Chapter 2, "Traditional Health Beliefs and Practices.")

Food for Thought

Meals and snacks prepared at home are lower in calories per eating occasion and lower in total fat, saturated fat, cholesterol, and salt per calorie than foods prepared away from home. Because of larger portion sizes and preparation methods compared to home-cooked meals, IHOP's Breakfast Country Chicken Fried Steak & Eggs with Sausage Gravy contains 1,441 kcalories, close to one full day's requirement.[86]

One aspect of food as entertainment is competitive eating as a televised sport. Elite eaters can make more than $50,000 a year in winnings, with records such as 46 dozen oysters in 10 minutes; 8.4 lb of baked beans in 2 minutes, 47 seconds; and 11 lb of cheesecake in 9 minutes. Stories about hot-dog king, Joey Chestnut, put his net worth for eating like a champion at $1.5 million.[87,88]

Old age is a cultural concept; among some Native Americans and Southeast Asians, individuals become elders in their forties.[89]

Lactose intolerance, the inability to digest the milk sugar lactose, develops as a person matures. It is believed that only 15 percent of the adult population in the world (those of northern European heritage and African tribes such as the Maasai) can drink milk after weaning age without some digestive discomfort.

The final factor in consumer food choice is variety. The omnivore's paradox states that humans are motivated psychologically to try new foods. Further, the desire for new flavors may also have a physiological basis. Sensory-specific satiety (unrelated to actually ingesting and digesting food) results when the pleasure from a certain food flavor decreases after a minute or two of consumption. The introduction of new food, or even the same food with newly added seasoning, arouses the enjoyment of eating again, encouraging the search for new flavor stimuli.[90,91] In addition, hunger increases the probability that a new food will be liked.[92] Marketers take advantage of the innate human drive for diet diversity by continually reformulating and repackaging processed food products to attract consumers.

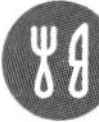

Food for Thought

Research on sensory-specific satiety suggests people eat less food when consuming a monotonous meal, and may overeat and gain weight when abundant variety is available.[93]

Many of the eldest Japanese people practice *hara hachi bu* or eating until they are 80% full.[94]

Interest in the foods of other regions or cultures is associated with the desire for new taste experiences, and also with increased income and educational attainment. Wealth permits experimentation and education can increase wealth. Nutritional knowledge, also affected by educational attainment, encourages the health-promoting benefits of dietary diversity. Some researchers have found that attitudes about the healthfulness of certain foods are important in food selection, and parents may purchase foods they consider healthy for their children even if they would not select those items for themselves.[95]

The nutrition knowledge of the person who plans meals in the home impacts food selection for all household members.[96] Whether accurate or not, nutritional knowledge does not always translate into knowledge-based food choice; a poll found that a majority always read labels (59 percent highly agree) on packaged foods before buying them for the first time. The Nutrition Facts panel (69 percent) and the ingredient list (67 percent) are the two places where most consumers look for information about food healthfulness. Still, taste is the primary consideration when making a food purchase, followed by price. The healthiness factor ranks third following these two primary factors.[97,98]

The consumer food choice model's influence on individual food habits is interrelated. The inborn preference for foods high in sugar, fat, and salt can encourage the consumption of items specifically formulated to enhance those taste experiences. These foods are often convenient, and items such as soft drinks and sandwich meats may cost less than fruit juice or fresh pork or beef (though certainly, some processed items are more expensive than homemade equivalents). Advertisers exploit the need for convenience and the desire to try new foods. A person may be aware of nutrition messages encouraging a reduction in the number of sugars and fats in the diet, as seen in the Dietary Guidelines for Americans, but this nutrition knowledge is often overridden by the primary factor in consumer food choice: taste.

Furthermore, influences on choice may change for each person as she or he matures. Food selection in infants (within the dietary domain of available foods provided by parents) is based almost exclusively on taste factors, with a strong resistance to new items. Children become more interested in self-expression as they grow and become sensitive to family and peer pressure. Young adults continue to be concerned with taste and self-expression, to which cost and convenience are typically added, especially in families with children. For middle-aged adults, increased income may lessen cost issues; and in older adults, health problems may become a more significant factor in food choice than even taste.

Nutrition and Food Habits

The Need for Cultural Competency

In recent years, the significance of culturally based food habits on health and diet has been recognized, and the need for intercultural competencies in the areas of nutrition research, assessment, counseling, and education has been cited.[99,100] The Campinha-Bacote model of competence outlines a process for cultural competency in health care, involving steps of cultural awareness, cultural knowledge, cultural skill, cultural encounter, and cultural desire.[101] Accurate data collection required for assessment and education is dependent on respect for different values and a trusting relationship between respondent and researcher; effective intercultural communication is a function of understanding and accepting a client's perspective and life experience.[102] New standards of nutrition care issued by professional accreditation organizations reflect similar guidelines.[103] Looking toward the future, it has been proposed that health care professionals should move beyond the theoretical concepts to cultural sensitivity and relevance to the practicalities of cultural competency. Language skills, managerial expertise, and leadership are needed to guide diverse communities in healthy lifestyle changes, serve hard-to-reach populations, and effect change in the health care system.

Diversity in the U.S. Population

The growing need for cultural competency is being driven by current demographic trends. Since the 1970s, the United States has moved increasingly toward a cultural plurality, where no single ethnic group is a majority. In 1980, only Hawaii and the District of Columbia had plurality populations. Since that time, California, New Mexico, and Texas have joined the list. Pluralities also exist in several metropolitan area populations, including Chicago, Houston, Los Angeles, Miami, New York City, and Philadelphia. Nationwide, demographers estimate that non-Hispanic Whites will become less than 50 percent of the total population by the year 2060.

This change can be seen in the difference in projected ethnic group growth from 2016 to 2060 (see Figure 1.4). Gains for the Asian population are expected at more than four times the national average and more than three times the national average for the Latinx population.

In actual numbers, Latinx surpassed Black Americans as the largest U.S. minority population in 2008, and now represent 17.8 percent of the total population, whereas Black Americans make up approximately 13.3 percent. Asian Americans are the third largest minority at nearly 6 percent of the total U.S. population. Smaller numbers of Southeast Asians/residents of Oceania and American Indian/Alaska Native (AI/AN on Figure 1.4) are less than 2 percent, and mixed races are 2.6 percent. Notably, many U.S. ethnic populations have an average age significantly lower than that of the total population. Predicted demographic changes are often seen first among children and young adults.[104]

This profile of the general U.S. population is notably different from that of health care professionals, who are mostly White. Among registered dietitians in 2020, 80 percent reported being White, and the next largest was Latinx at 6 percent. Three percent reported as Black American, 5 percent Asian, 2 percent other, and 3 percent did not answer.[105] Researchers note that clients from minority populations prefer to receive health care in settings with minority health care providers; that minority health care providers are more likely to work in underserved areas; and that people from minority groups are more likely to participate in research studies when the investigator is from the same cultural background.[106,107]

Food for Thought

"Respect for diverse viewpoints and individual differences" is an Academy of Nutrition and Dietetics value.

Diversity in the Canadian Population

The Canadian census reported more than 250 different ethnicities in 2016. British Isles and French ancestry remain the most common, with nearly 20 million reporting European origins, though this share in the total population is declining. Canadians of Aboriginal ancestry were 6.2 percent or just over 2 million

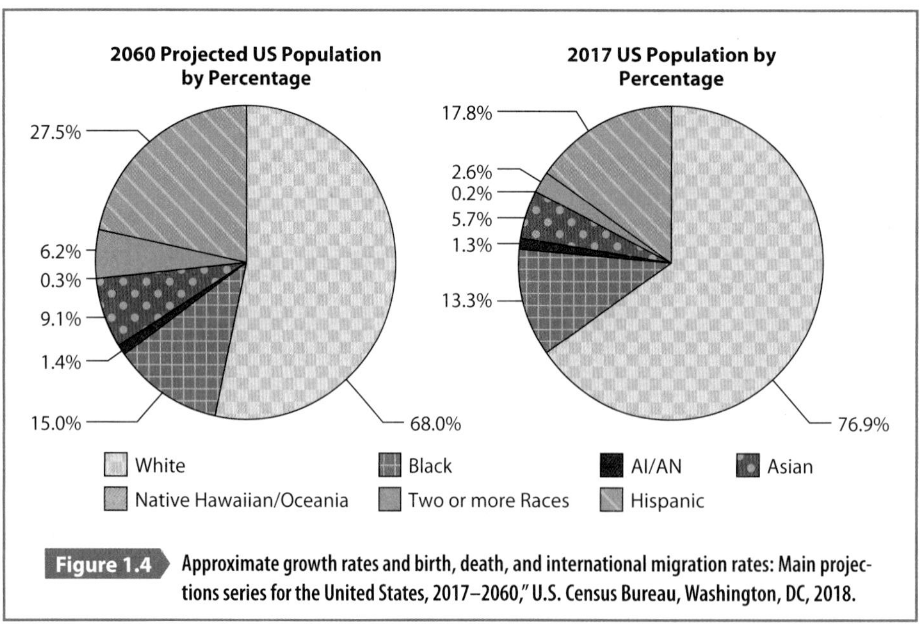

Figure 1.4 Approximate growth rates and birth, death, and international migration rates: Main projections series for the United States, 2017–2060," U.S. Census Bureau, Washington, DC, 2018.

people. Of the three main Aboriginal groups, First Nations (Native North Americans) was the largest with 1.5 million people. Within this group, Cree (356,660), Mi'kmaq (168,480), and Ojibway (125,725) were the most common ancestries. Métis ancestry was reported by 600,000 people, and Inuit ancestry was reported by 79,125 people. Among the 20 most common non-Indigenous and non-European ancestries: Chinese ancestry was reported by 1.8 million people, ancestry from India was reported by about 1.4 million people, and Filipino origins were reported by 837,130 people. Four in 10 reported more than one origin. Immigration growth in Canada has risen dramatically in recent years. For example, close to 70 percent of individuals who reported Asian origins are foreign-born. Nearly all recent immigrants to Canada have settled in urban areas, particularly Toronto, Vancouver, and Montreal.[108]

Ethnicity and Health

Health is not enjoyed equally by all in the United States. Disparities in mortality rates, chronic disease incidence, and access to care are prevalent among many U.S. cultural groups. Poor health status in the United States is also associated with poverty (see Cultural Controversy—Does Hunger Cause Obesity? later in this chapter), low educational attainment, and immigrant status: Immigrant health has been found initially better than similar U.S.-born populations in some research, and is shown to decline with length of stay.[56,109,110]

Food for Thought

Acculturation is so complex that it has been difficult to develop accurate assessments for use in health care and research. Neither U.S. nativity nor the number of years in residence has proved completely indicative, and it has been suggested that acculturation is sometimes based more on ethnic stereotyping than on cultural differences.[111,112]

Acculturation to the majority culture is believed to be a significant factor in health independent of socioeconomic status. First noted in heart disease rates, a modernized Western lifestyle has also been linked to increased blood cholesterol levels, increased blood pressure levels, obesity, type 2 diabetes, and some cancers.[110] The stress of adaptation to the pressures of a fast-paced society is believed to be significant.[91] Hereditary predisposition to developing certain health conditions most probably plays a significant role. It is important to note, however, that acculturation is difficult to define accurately and is not an inherent risk factor in itself.[113] Some changes in diet such as increased availability of fruits and vegetables can be beneficial. Better educational opportunities and health care services can also promote health.

The effects of ethnicity and race on health status are not well delineated, and researchers caution that the research results can be misleading.[114] The Human Genome Project determined that there is no genetic basis for use of the term *race* and that 99.9 percent of all humans have the same genes. Race is simply a category used to describe groups of individuals.[115,116] Many studies do not explain how participants are categorized. Individuals may self-select differently than investigators, and self-identity may change over time. Even official classifications may vary and change. In the United States, the Office of Management and Budget is responsible for defining the categories used in all government work, including the Census. In 1997, the standards were revised to include five classifications for race: American Indian or Native American, Asian, Black or African American, Native Hawaiian or other Southeast Asians/residents of Oceania, and White. Before the revision, there were only four groupings because Asians were combined with Southeast Asians/residents of Oceania, or as "other" in earlier census days. Additionally, the two categories for ethnicity were expanded in 1997 (ethnic members may be of any race): Hispanic and Non Hispanic. These changes from earlier definitions can lead to difficulties in interpreting data trends. Further, the factor of ethnicity is not sufficiently separated from socioeconomic status in many studies, calling into question whether a stated finding is due to ethnicity or whether it is due to income, occupation, or educational status. For example, an evaluation of the incidence of type 2 diabetes in the Black Women's Health Study indicates a strong relationship between individual and neighborhood socioeconomic status and type 2 diabetes even when controlling for factors such as education and income.[117]

Nevertheless, ethnicity data suggesting risks and disparities can be useful to health care providers as long as the caveats above are considered and care is taken to avoid stereotyping a patient by group membership. For example, Table 1.2 illustrates that not all Asians or Hispanics have the same prevalence of type 2 diabetes.

Table 1.2 Percentage of Population Diagnosed with Diabetes

Adult Diabetes by Race/Ethnic Background 2019	
Non-Hispanic Whites	7.4
Asian Americans	9.5
Hispanics	11.8
Non-Hispanic Blacks	12.1
American Indians/Alaska Natives	14.5
Among Asian Americans	
Chinese	5.6
Filipinos	10.4
South Asians	12.6
Other Asian Americans	9.9
Among Hispanic Adults	
Central and South Americans	8.3
Cubans	6.5
Mexican Americans	14.4
Puerto Ricans	12.4

Source: Centers for Disease Control and Prevention. 2019. National diabetes statistics report: Estimates of diabetes and its burden in the United States, 2019. Retrieved from https://www.diabetes.org/about-us/statistics/about-diabetes#:~:text=The%20rates%20of%20diagnosed%20diabetes%20in%20adults%20by,of%20American%20Indians%2FAlaskan%20Natives%2012.1%25%20of%20non-Hispanic%20blacks (accessed May 16, 2022).

Ethnicity can be a significant factor in the development of certain disease conditions, the way they are experienced, and how they are ultimately resolved. (See Chapter 2 for further information.) The growth of ethnic groups in the U.S. population since the mid-1980s, the rapid movement toward cultural pluralism, and the undeniable connection between heritage and health require the need for cultural competency among American health care providers.

Intercultural Nutrition Care

The study of food habits has specific applications in determining nutritional status and implementing dietary change. Even the act of obtaining a twenty-four-hour dietary intake record has cultural implications. (See Chapter 3, "Intercultural Communication.") Questions such as what was eaten at breakfast, lunch, and dinner not only ignore other daily meal patterns but also make assumptions about what constitutes a meal. Snacks and the consumption of food not considered a meal may be overlooked. Common difficulties in data collection, such as underreporting or overreporting food intake, may also be culturally related to the perceived status of an item, for example, or portion size estimates may be an unknown concept, complicated by the practice of sharing food from other family members' plates. Terminology can be particularly troublesome. Words in one culture may have different meanings in another culture or even among ethnic groups within a culture.

Stereotyping is another pitfall in culturally sensitive nutrition applications, resulting from the overestimation of the association between group membership and individual behavior. Stereotyping occurs when a person ascribes the collective traits associated with a specific group to every member of that group, discounting individual characteristics. A health professional knowledgeable about cultural food habits may inadvertently make stereotypical assumptions about dietary behavior if the individual preferences of the client are neglected. Cultural competency in nutrition implies not only familiarity with the food habits of a particular culture, but recognition of intraethnic variation within a culture as well.

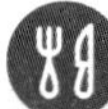

Food for Thought

Sometimes culturally based food habits have vital nutritional benefits. One example is the use of corn tortillas with beans in Mexico. Neither corn nor beans alone supplies the essential amino acids (chemical building blocks of protein) needed to maintain optimum health. Combined, they provide complete protein.

Researchers suggest that health care providers working in intercultural nutrition become skilled in careful observation of client groups, visiting homes, neighborhoods, and markets to learn where food is purchased, what food is available, and how it is stored, prepared, served, and consumed. Participation in community activities, such as reading local newspapers and attending neighborhood meetings or events, is another way to gather relevant information. Informant interviewing reveals the most data about a group; individual members of the group, group leaders, and other health care professionals serving the group are

Cultural Controversy

Does Hunger Cause Obesity?

One of the most perplexing problems in nutrition education and policy is why socioeconomic status is associated with overweight and obesity rates in the United States. Rates of individuals with a body mass index (BMI) over twenty-five but below thirty (considered overweight), and those with a BMI over thirty (considered obese), have doubled in Americans since the late 1970s. Low income and lower levels of education are associated with increased overweight/obesity incidence, regardless of ethnic heritage. The risk declines parallel to socioeconomic improvement in most studies. Additionally, overweight and obesity rates are higher in all other ethnic groups (except for Asians) than in Whites. Because poverty rates are also higher for all other ethnic groups (in some cases more than three times the rate for White people), it may be that socioeconomic status contributes to some of the disparity in the risk of overweight and obesity between ethnic groups.[118,119]

Researchers suggest that those with food insecurity who often do not have enough preferred foods to eat may be at risk for being overweight or obese through the overconsumption of inexpensive, less nutritious foods high in fats or sugar. First postulated by a physician in 1995, it was observed that in the cycle of food assistance, where monthly allocations run out and food shortages occur episodically, a person may compensate by eating larger portions of higher-calorie foods when available.[120,121] Further research has strengthened the hypothesis, finding that high-energy density diets (those that include more fast foods, snacks, and desserts than fruits, vegetables, and lean protein) are cheaper, more palatable, and more filling than healthier choices.[121–123] As with obesity in adults, obesity in children is associated with lower household incomes, lower education levels of parents, and consumption of high-energy-density foods; family meals, which improve the quality of dietary intake in adolescents (including reductions in snacking), are significantly more frequent in higher-income families.[124–126] Biological factors, such as the taste preference for sweets and fats; psychological factors, including the comfort provided in such items; and an obesogenic environment that promotes consumption of energy-dense items in super-sized quantities may be other variables. Studies show that food insecurity and being overweight go hand in hand, and that the prevalence of being overweight remains higher in food-insecure children.[127]

potential sources.[128,129] Combining qualitative approaches such as in-depth, open-ended interviews with clients and quantitative measures through questionnaires is one of the most culturally sensitive methods of obtaining data about a group. Qualitative information obtained through the interviews should alert the researcher to nutrition issues within the group and guide the development of assessment tools; the quantitative results should confirm the data provided through the interview in a larger sample. (See Chapter 3 for more information.)

Cultural perspective is particularly important when evaluating the nutritional impact of a person's food habits. Ethnocentric assumptions about dietary practices should be avoided. A food behavior that on first observation is judged detrimental may have a limited impact on a person's physical health. Sometimes other moderating food habits are unrecognized. For instance, a dietitian may be concerned that an Asian patient is getting insufficient calcium because she eats few dairy products. Undetected sources of calcium in this case might be the daily use of fermented fish sauces or broths rich in minerals made from vinegar-soaked bones.

Likewise, a food habit that the investigator finds repugnant may have some redeeming nutritional benefits. Examples include the consumption of raw meat and organs by the Inuits, which provides a source of vitamin C that would have otherwise been lost during cooking, and the use of mineral-rich ashes or clay in certain breads and stews in Africa and Latin America. In addition, physiological differences among populations can affect nutritional needs.

Thus, diet should be carefully evaluated within the context of culture.[130] When diet modification is necessary, it should be attempted in partnership with the client and respectful of culturally based food habits. Adoption of dietary recommendations is associated with an approach that is compatible with the client's traditional health beliefs and practices. (See Chapter 2 for more information.) A study evaluating women's beliefs about weight gain during pregnancy found that Black women indicated that a lower amount should be gained than the recommendations and that prepregnancy weight had no effect on how much should be gained.[131] Having this information could certainly impact the content and approach for nutrition counseling given during pregnancy. In an older example, educators developed a food guide for Caribbean Islanders living in the United States that grouped cultural foods into three categories: growth, protection, and energy, reflecting client-group perceptions of how food affects health.[132]

The American Paradox

Food habits are so intrinsic to culture that food-related images are often used to describe them. Melting pot suggests a blending of different ethnic, religious, and regional groups to produce a smooth, uniform identity; stew implies a cooking of various populations to achieve a bland sameness with

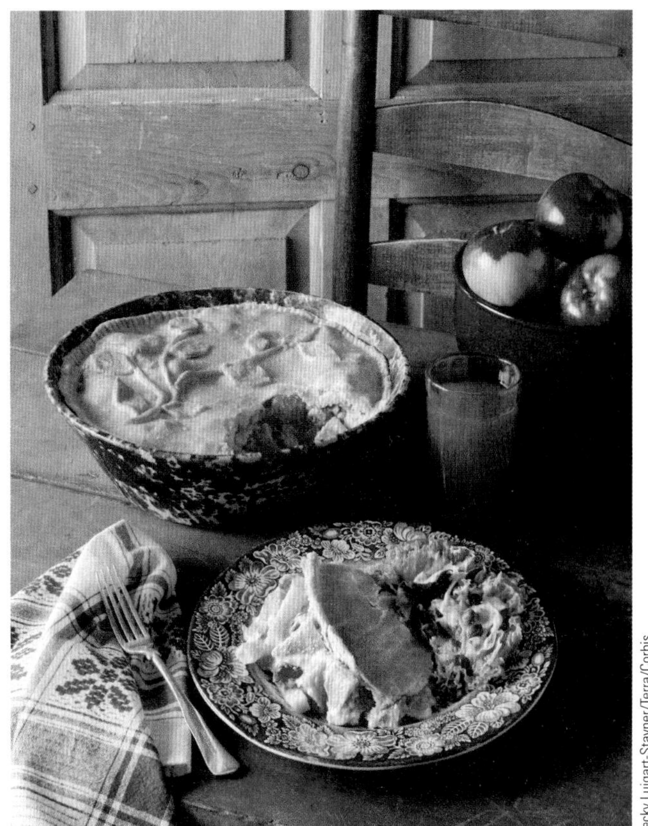

Becky Luigart-Stayner/Terra/Corbis

▲ **Asian tofu is the main ingredient in this vegetarian adaptation of shepherd's pie, a traditional British entrée popular in the United States.**

only just a touch of cultural integrity; and tossed salad allows for maintenance of cultural identity, randomly mixed and coated with a glistening unity. A more accurate metaphor for the American population is the omnivore's paradox. The nation was founded by immigrants, and most citizens today are proud of a heritage that, to paraphrase the inscription on the Statue of Liberty, accepts the tired, the poor, and the huddled masses yearning to be free. Yet many Americans are also suspicious of cultural differences and comfortable with what is familiar. The same can be said for food habits in the United States.

The American paradox, in culinary terms, is that although foods from throughout the world are available, and often affordable, consistency and conservatism are also needed. At one end of the spectrum, people who are exposed to new foods through travel and those who crave new taste experiences have driven the rapidly expanding market for imported fruits, vegetables, and meat products, cheeses, and condiments. Increasing interest in global flavors has driven growth in new regional food restaurants in the United States, far surpassing the growth of restaurants highlighting European traditions. A survey found the top five regions influencing menus in 2022 to be Southeast Asian (Vietnamese, Singaporean, Filipino), South American (Argentinian, Brazilian, Chilean), Caribbean (Puerto Rican, Cuban, Dominican), North African (Moroccan, Algerian, Libyan),

Cultural Foods in the United States: A Timeline*

Pre-17th century

- Regional Native American cuisines develop.

1500s

- Columbian Exchange: New World foods from the Caribbean and Central/South America (corn, potatoes, tomatoes, chili peppers, peanuts, vanilla, chocolate, etc.) are brought to Europe, Africa, Asia; Old World foods (wheat, rice, sugar, beef, pork, apples, etc.) introduced to the Caribbean and Central/South America.
- Ponce de Leon discovers Florida and most likely brings tomatoes, among other foods, to North America.

1620s

- British traditional midday meal introduced, with meat, fowl, or fish as its centerpiece served with cornbread or biscuit. Steamed or boiled pudding is the first course; dessert of fruit pie or cake follows. It is eaten with a knife, spoon, and fingers.
- First Thanksgiving occurs in 1621 at Plymouth colony, a three-day meal combining European and Native American hunting and harvest feast traditions featuring fowl and venison.
- Dutch colonists at New Amsterdam (present-day Manhattan) introduce coleslaw, doughnuts, cookies, and waffles.

1660s

- Yams, watermelon, okra, black-eyed peas, eggplant, and sesame seeds brought with enslaved Africans who also introduce the New World foods peanuts and chili peppers to North America.

1680s

- German Mennonites settle in Pennsylvania, creating Pennsylvania Dutch fare and popularizing dishes such as scrapple, apple butter, and funnel cakes.
- William Penn founds first brewhouse in Philadelphia, featuring English-style ales.

1760s

- England takes control of Canada from France: French Canadians migrate to New England (Franco-Americans) and Louisiana (Cajuns), bringing fish stews, pork pates, boudin sausages, French toast, and other specialties.
- An English plantation owner in New Smyrna, Florida imports 1,500 indentured servants from Italy, Greece, and Minorca to work his indigo fields, who in turn bring eggplant, lemons, and olives to the region.

1770s

- Boston Tea Party occurs; coffee emerges as a protest beverage.
- Thomas Jefferson experiments with crops found in Europe, such as broccoli, cauliflower, eggplant, savoy cabbage, and olives.

1790s

- Pineapples introduced to what is now Hawaii by the Spanish.
- *American Cookery* by Amelia Simmons in 1796 is the first American cookbook; includes recipes for stuffed turkey, a "tasty Indian pudding," "pomkin" pudding (pie), "American citron" (watermelon) preserves, and cornmeal johnnycakes or hoecakes.

1800s

- First shipment of bananas arrives in the United States.
- First recipe for tomato-based ketchup published in 1812, called "love-apple or tomato catchup."

1820s

- First regional American cookbook published in 1824, *The Virginia Housewife, or Methodical Cook*, by Mary Randolph, with recipes for southern specialties; also, foreign dishes, such as ropa vieja and "gazpacho" (Spain), polenta and vermicelli (Italy), curry "after the East Indian manner," and "gumbo—a West Indian dish" (Caribbean).

*References for Timeline

Davidson, A. 1999. *The Oxford companion to food*. New York: Oxford University Press.

Hess, K. 1992. *The Carolina rice kitchen*. Columbia: University of South Carolina Press.

Katz, S. H. (Ed.). 2003. *Encyclopedia of food and culture*. New York: Scribner's.

Trager, J. 1995. *The food chronology*. New York: Henry Holt.

Randolph, M. 1993. *The Virginia housewife, or, methodical cook. A facsimile of an authentic early American cookbook*. New York: Dover.

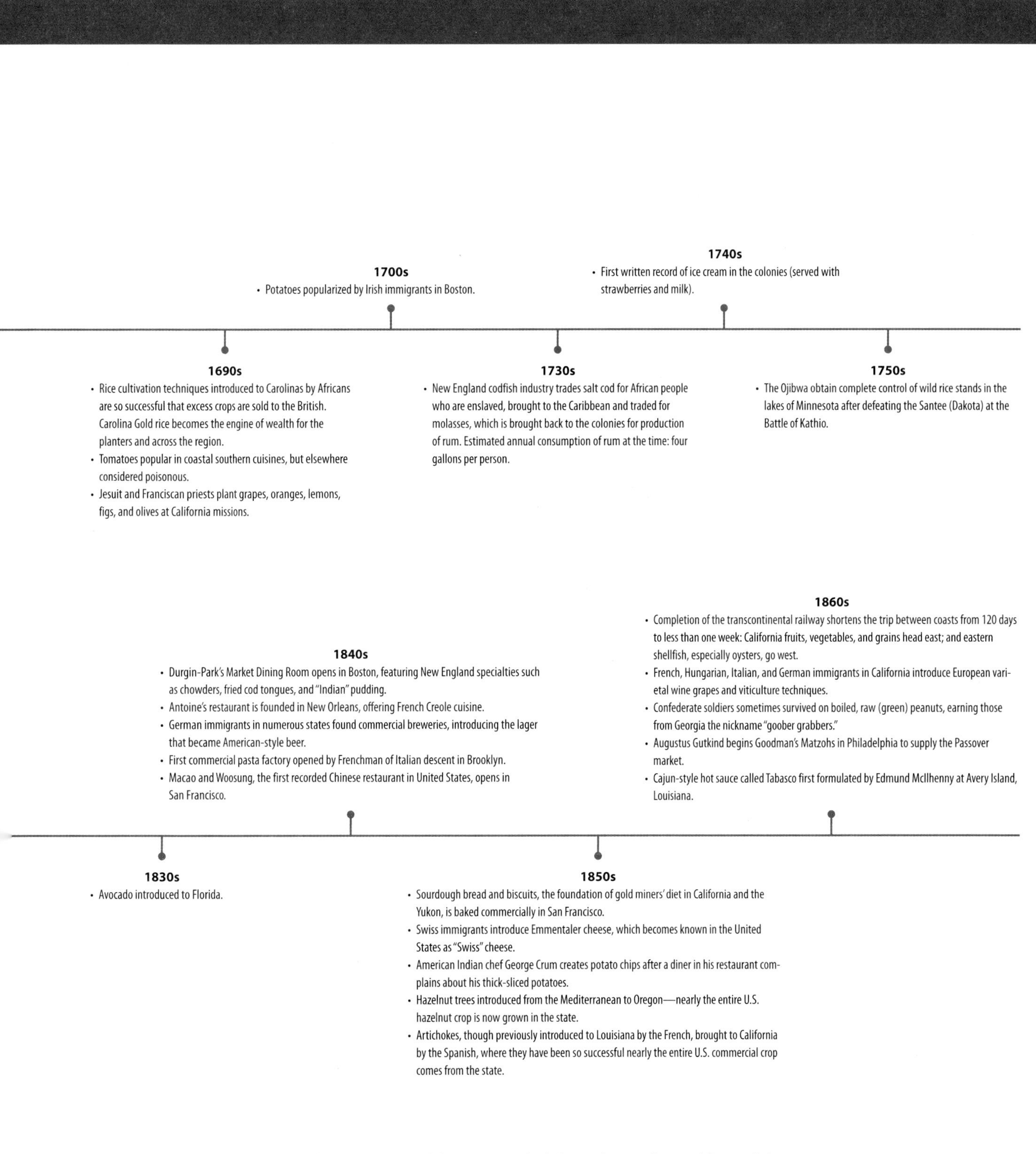

Simmons, A. 1996. *American cookery, or the art of dressing viands, fish, poultry, and vegetables, and the best modes of making puff-pastes, pies, tarts, puddings, custards and preserves, and all kinds of cakes from the imperial plumb to plain cake. A facsimile of the second edition*. Bedford, MA: Applewood Books.

Smith, A. F. 1994. *The tomato in America*. Columbia: University of South Carolina Press.

Cultural Foods in the United States: A Timeline* *(Continued)*

1870s

- *Jewish Cookery*, first cookbook on the subject in the United States, by Esther Levy published in Philadelphia.
- Chinese Pekin ("Peking") ducks imported by New York farms.
- Acceptance of four-tined fork makes using a knife to eat outmoded; American-style use (transferring the fork from right hand to left when cutting foods) is established.
- Buffalo (a Plains Indian staple), which numbered 30 to 70 million, are reduced to approximately 1,500 animals, in part due to prestige of smoked buffalo tongue in urban areas and desire by leaders and politicians to subdue the Native population.
- Navel oranges introduced to California from Brazil, by way of the U.S. Department of Agriculture (USDA) in Washington, DC.

1880s

- Luchow's restaurant opens in New York City, popularizing dishes found in German American homes and local beer gardens, such as smoked eel, bratwurst, weinerschnitzel, spatzle, and German-style beers.
- Oscar F. Mayer, a German American butcher, opens sausage shop in Chicago, later selling wieners to grocery stores throughout the region.
- B. Manischewitz Co. begins production of kosher products in Cincinnati.
- Italian immigrants from Naples introduce spaghetti made with olive oil and tomato paste.

1890s

- Asian immigrants move into San Joaquin valley of California, planting large tracts of land. By the 1940s, Japanese farmers are growing two-thirds of all vegetables in the state, creating shortages when they are interned during World War II.
- Chili powder, combining ground dried chili pepper bits with other seasonings, such as cumin and oregano, is invented in Texas—though attribution is uncertain. Chili stews of beef or goat popular in the region.

1900s

- Chop suey, a Chinese American vegetable and meat dish that may have come originally from southern China (*tsap seui*), is popular in "chow-chows" (Chinese restaurants) in California and New York.
- Foods prepared in the "French fashion" are popular, particularly among the upper classes who can afford to employ cooks knowledgeable in their preparation and dine at expensive restaurants.
- Pistachio tree from the Middle East introduced in California and Texas.
- Coca-Cola, combining extracts from African kola nuts, South American coca leaves, and fruit syrups, goes on sale in Atlanta as a fountain drink.
- The Kellogg brothers at a Seventh-day Adventist spa create cereal flakes as a substitute for meat—a year later they add malt sweetener to increase appeal.
- Loma Linda Foods begins production of health breads and cookies for patients at the Seventh-day Adventist Loma Linda Hospital.
- Broccoli introduced to California by Italian immigrants.
- World's Fair in St. Louis popularizes German hamburger sandwiches and frankfurters (later dubbed hot dogs).
- First American pizzeria opened by Italian immigrant in New York City.

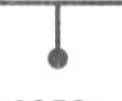

1950s

- Trader Vic's restaurants in California popularize Polynesian food, such as luau dishes and pupu platters, as well as the mai tai cocktail, claimed to have been invented by the owner.
- USDA publishes Basic 4 Food Guide.

1960s

- Beef consumption reaches 99 lb per person in the United States, surpassing pork consumption for the first time.
- Frieda's Finest founded to market specialty produce using samples and recipes in supermarkets; popularizes items such as Chinese gooseberries (renamed kiwifruit), Jerusalem artichokes (as sunchokes), radicchio, spaghetti squash, blood oranges, cactus pears, and other items.
- Julia Child debuts her cooking show, *The French Chef*, on public television, demystifying gourmet cooking and promoting French cuisine.
- The first Taco Bell fast-food restaurant opens in Downey, California.
- Benihana of Tokyo opens teppanyaki-style restaurant in New York.
- Term *soul food* coined for traditional African American cuisine.
- In Atlanta, Lester G. Maddox is ordered by the federal government to serve African Americans at his Pickrick Restaurant—he closes the business instead.
- Catfish farming introduced in Arkansas, dramatically increasing production and popularizing the fish nationwide.
- *Foods of the World* cookbooks from Time-Life Books begin with publication of *The Cooking of Provincial France* by M. F. K. Fisher—the series introduces international cuisine through twenty specialized volumes (African cooking to wines and spirits) followed in the 1970s with seven volumes on regional American fare.

1970s

- Falafel stands and restaurants proliferate with increased immigration of Middle Easterners.
- Chez Panisse restaurant opens in Berkeley, California, emphasizing fresh, locally grown ingredients, leading to development of a new California cuisine and promoting regional fare nationally.
- Nissin Foods USA founded in California to market instant noodle products popular in Japan, such as Top Ramen.
- Vietnamese refugees open small restaurants in California, Texas, and other locations, featuring traditional pho, sandwiches, and other items.
- Small numbers of immigrants arrive from Thailand, and many open restaurants, introducing fish sauces such as nuoc mam and noodle dishes, including pad thai.
- Paul Prudhomme opens K-Paul Louisiana Kitchen in New Orleans, popularizing Cajun cooking nationwide, one of the first regional food trends.

1910s

- George Washington Carver extols the virtues of peanuts, soybeans, and sweet potatoes; he popularizes peanut butter, formerly considered a food for people who were sick and aging adults.
- U.S. pasta production increases when imported supplies from Italy are cut off during World War I.
- American cheese first processed in Chicago by J.L. Kraft & Bros. (Canadian Mennonite immigrants) by melting bits of cheddar with an emulsifier to produce a smooth, mild cheeselike food.
- The fortune cookie created in California.

1920s

- La Choy Food Products founded to sell canned and jarred bean sprouts.
- Polish baker Harry Lender opens first bagel plant outside New York, and popularity begins to spread beyond eastern European enclaves.
- Aplets candy, based on the recipe for Turkish delight, invented by two Armenian immigrants in Washington State.
- Marriott Corp. gets its start as a root beer, tamale, and chili con carne stand in Washington, DC.
- The Russian Tea Room opens in New York, popularizing blinis, caviar, tea in samovars, and other Russian specialties.
- Colombo Yogurt is founded by Armenian immigrants in Massachusetts.

1930s

- Fritos corn chips first marketed in Texas based on a tortillas fritas (fried tortilla strips) recipe purchased from a Mexican restaurant owner.
- Spam is created, becoming a status food in Hawaii and the best-selling canned meat worldwide.
- Goya Foods is founded in New York by Spanish immigrants to import olives and olive oil, later tapping into the growing Latinx food market.

1940s

- Influx of Greek immigrants seeking asylum in areas such as New York, Detroit, and Chicago popularize items such as souvlaki and gyros in family-run restaurants and street stands.
- Ed Obrycki's Olde Crab House in Baltimore converts from tavern to restaurant serving Maryland specialties such as soft-shell crab and crab cakes.
- Domestic servants and some housewives take jobs to support the U.S. war effort during World War II, leading to an increased consumption of convenience foods.
- *The Gentleman's Companion, Being an Exotic Cookery Book or, Around the World with Knife, Fork and Spoon* by Charles Baker, a two-volume set, published in 1946, describing dishes and drinks from throughout Europe and Asia—a second two-volume set on the foods and beverages of South America published in 1951.
- Balducci's specialty food shop (founded as a vegetable stand in 1916 by an Italian immigrant) opens in New York, offering an international assortment of foods from Europe, Asia, and Latin America as well as regional specialties, such as rattlesnake and Cajun andouille.
- The McDonald brothers offer franchises of their hamburger stand, founded in 1940 in Pasadena, California.

1980s

- Ethiopian restaurants become popular in some cities where immigrants have settled, introducing items such as injera and berbere.
- Yaohan supermarkets of Japan open in California catering to Asian population and offering ingredients such as bean sprouts, daikon, seaweed, pickled plums, fresh fish, and prepared items, including sushi.
- Korean immigrants, especially in Los Angeles, introduce Korean barbecue, kimchi, and other specialties through restaurants and markets.
- Fresh fugu fish (which can be highly toxic) is imported for first time for use in American Japanese restaurants under FDA supervision.

1990s

- Salsa becomes the favorite U.S. condiment when sales exceed those of ketchup.
- The term *fusion food* is used for combining the ingredients and preparation techniques of two or more cultural cuisines, such as Thai chicken pizza.
- Chicken consumption per capita first tops beef consumption.
- USDA and Department of Health and Human Services (DHHS) release first version of the Food Pyramid.
- The Food Network begins television broadcasting.
- Spanish tapas restaurants become trendy.

2000s

- Americans consume an average of one tortilla per person each day—representing 30 percent of all bread sales, nearly equal to white bread.
- There are more Chinese restaurants in the United States than McDonald's, Wendy's, and Burger King restaurants combined.
- $1 out of every $7 in grocery purchases is spent on ethnic items in 2005.
- Wine is neck-and-neck with beer as favorite U.S. alcoholic beverage.

and West African (Nigerian, Ghanan, Western Saharan).[133] One development is the success of fast-casual ethnic restaurant chains, such as Chipotle, Qdoba Mexican Grill, and Baja Fresh. One survey reveals that Korean fast-casual dining is rising in popularity and is well established in Hawaii, Nevada, and California. According to a survey using data from Google, interest in Japanese foods is highest in Hawaii, as well as in the Carolinas, followed by California, Washington, and New York. Foods from India are most popular in New Jersey, but also in great demand in Washington, Maryland, and Massachusetts. Fremont, California ranks Indian food as in the most demand. Thai food has the most interest in Fairbanks, Alaska, but is also hugely popular in Washington and Oregon. Chinese and Mexican food are uniformly loved across the United States.[134] On average, both men and women make five food away-from-home purchases per week, many times purchasing from global restaurants.[135] At the other end of the American continuum of cuisine, some people find considerable satisfaction in the uniformity of a meat-and-potatoes diet. A national trends survey found "plain" American food well-liked by respondents, and nearly one-third of consumers said fusion foods such as Korean tacos were a good way to try out new international flavors.[136,137]

Food for Thought

One example of a multicultural culinary creation is the California roll with its addition of avocado to traditional Japanese crab sushi. It is called "American sushi" in Japan.

Discussion Starters

Who Are You? And What Do You Eat?

- Write a short description of your cultural identity. What is your race? What is your ethnicity? What about your parents and your grandparents? Where is your family originally from? Think about your high school friends and classmates. What was their race? Their ethnicity?
- Next, write a description of what you eat. What are your favorite foods? When living at home, what foods did your family typically eat? If your parents cooked meals, what would they typically cook?

Now, form groups of three to four and share your descriptions. Imagine that your instructor asks you to a "potluck," a social gathering where everyone invited is supposed to bring something for everyone else to eat. What do you want the other members of your group to bring? What foods might they bring that you would like to try?

In response to the ambivalence produced by the American paradox, the rising interest in new foods, and the continued desire for familiar flavors, multicultural foods fare is often adapted to American tastes and standardized for national consumption. Spicing is reduced, protein elements (particularly meats and cheeses) are increased, more desserts and sweets are offered, and items considered distasteful to the American majority are eliminated. In considering the three most popular international cuisines in the United States, it is unlikely a consumer will find roasted kid at an Italian restaurant, 1,000-year-old eggs at a Chinese takeout counter, or tripe soup at a Mexican drive-up window. Many Americans are convinced that spaghetti with meatballs, fortune cookies, chop suey, and nachos are authentic dishes, yet they are all items created in the United States for American preferences.[138] Even cultural foods prepared at home from cookbooks are often modified for preparation in American kitchens with American ingredients, losing much of their original content and context. Only in ethnic, religious, and regional enclaves largely isolated from outside influences are traditional food habits maintained. Otherwise, over time, even significant symbolic practices can lose their meaning under the pressure of acculturation.

In many ways, U.S. cooking adapts to current and emerging food trends. Whole foods, plant-based diets, and online delivery of meal ingredients or full meal subscription services, all reflect cultural changes on the dinner table. Trends for 2022 include more fusion cuisine, especially foods that combine savory spices and heat with sweetness (such as Korean-based fried chicken), deep dives into regional Indian food (such as dishes from Gujarat, Kerala, Kashmir, Tamil Nadu, and Awadh), robusta coffee (more resistant to climate pressure and less expensive than arabica beans) made into Vietnamese coffee made with sweetened condensed milk, nostalgic candies from China and South Korea such as ppopgi, seaweeds made into pasta and salsa dishes, meat grown in laboratories from animal cells, and every kind of mushroom.[139] Alternative meats and poultry are on the rise, as are fish burgers, plant-based dairy, and drinks that claim to manage and treat conditions such as hypertension, weight, and diabetes.[137]

Hamburgers, hot dogs, and fried chicken are clearly derived from other cultural fare, yet they are changed through the lens of the American paradox. Cheese melted over burgers on a sesame seed bun, chili con carne poured over frankfurters, and cornmeal-crusted chicken served with cream gravy and buttermilk biscuits are nearly unrecognizable compared to their European and African origins. And while the tamale pie in Texas, ahi burger in Hawaii, tofu lasagna in a vegetarian home, and avocado turkey croissant sandwich in the university cafeteria are not authentic ethnic fare, they are authentic American foods. It is the unexpected and exciting ways in which the familiar and the new are combined that make the study of food habits in the United States such a pleasurable and appetizing challenge.

Review Questions

1. Define the terms *food* and *food habits*. How does the omnivore's paradox influence a person's food choices and food habits?
2. List four factors that may influence an individual's choice of foods. Pick one and explain how this factor influences food choices.
3. Define the terms culture and acculturation. Describe an example of a change in food habits that may reflect acculturation.
4. Describe the flavor principles, core foods, and meal patterns of your family's diet.
5. Which of the factors described by the consumer food choice model currently influence your food choices? Which factors do you think will stay the same and which do you think will change as you age?

Reflection

Looking at your behaviors and taste preferences, values, and community, which of the emerging food trends in the United States resonate with you? Which might you participate in?

References

1. U.S. Census. 2020. American community survey. Retrieved from https://data.census.gov/cedsci/table?q=%20first%20generation%20foreign%20born&tid=ACSDP5Y2020.DP02
2. Budiman, A., & Ruiz, N.G. 2021. *Asian Americans are the fastest-growing racial or ethnic group in the U.S.* Pew Research Center. Retrieved from https://www.pewresearch.org/fact-tank/2021/04/09/asian-americans-are-the-fastest-growing-racial-or-ethnic-group-in-the-u-s/
3. Filippone, P.T. 2020. The history of hamburger meat. The Spruce Eats. Retrieved from https://www.thespruceeats.com/history-of-ground-beef-1807605
4. Statistics Canada. 2017. *Ethnic and cultural origins of Canadians: Portrait of a rich heritage.* Retrieved from https://www12.statcan.gc.ca/census-recensement/2016/as-sa/98-200-x/2016016/98-200-x2016016-eng.cfm
5. Moding, K.J., Bellows, L.L., Grimm, K.J., & Johnson, S.L. 2020. A longitudinal examination of the role of sensory exploratory behaviors in young children's acceptance of new foods. *Physiology & Behavior*, 218, 112821.
6. Amsel, P., Trude, A., Castelo, R., Ezeonyebuchi, C., & Black, M. 2019. Preschoolers are more likely to eat foods they know: A cross-sectional analysis of willingness to try new foods and children's food knowledge (P11-047-19). *Current Developments in Nutrition*, 3(Suppl. 1), nzz048-P11.
7. Fischler, C. 1988. Food, self, and identity. *Social Science Information*, 27, 275–292.
8. Beagan, B.L., Power, E.M., & Chapman, G.E. 2015. "Eating isn't just swallowing food": Food practices in the context of social class trajectory. *Canadian Food Studies/La Revue canadienne des études sur l'alimentation*, 2(1), 75–98.
9. Stavely, K., Fitzgerald, K., & Zocalo Public Square. 2018. What America's first cookbook says about our country and its cuisine. *Smithsonian Magazine.*
10. Simmons, A. 1958. *American Cookery: A Facsimile of the First Edition, 1796.* Oxford University Press.
11. Larson, N., & Story, M. 2009. A review of environmental influences on food choices. 38(Suppl. 1), S56–S73.
12. Vabø, M., & Hansen, H. 2014. The relationship between food preferences and food choice: A theoretical discussion. *International Journal of Business and Social Science*, 5(7).
13. Franchi, M. 2012. Food choice: Beyond the chemical content. *International Journal of Food Sciences and Nutrition*, 63(Suppl. 1), 17–28.
14. Almerico, G.M. 2014. Food and identity: Food studies, cultural, and personal identity. *Journal of International Business and Cultural Studies*, 8, 1.
15. Walker, A. 2005. In the absence of food: A case of rhythmic loss and spoiled identity for patients with percutaneous endoscopic gastrostomy feeding tubes. *Food, Culture & Society*, 8, 161–180.
16. Spence, C. 2017. Comfort food: A review. *International Journal of Gastronomy and Food Science*, 9, 105–109.
17. Strohl, M. 2019. On culinary authenticity: Strohl on culinary authenticity. *The Journal of Aesthetics and Art Criticism*, 77(2), 157–167.
18. Anderson, E.N. 2014. Everyone eats. In *Everyone Eats*. New York University Press.
19. Lafraire, J., Rioux, C., Giboreau, A., & Picard, D. 2016. Food rejections in children: Cognitive and social/environmental factors involved in food neophobia and picky/fussy eating behavior. *Appetite*, 96, 347–357.
20. Swindle, T., Sigman-Grant, M., Branen, L.J., Fletcher, J., & Johnson, S.L. 2018. About feeding children: Factor structure and internal reliability of a survey to assess mealtime strategies and beliefs of early childhood education teachers. *International Journal of Behavioral Nutrition and Physical Activity*, 15(1), 1–15.
21. Satter, E. *Family Meals Focus*. Retrieved from https://www.ellynsatterinstitute.org/family-meals-focus-no-110-giving-children-autonomy-with-eating/ (accessed May 16, 2022).
22. Heyes, C. 2020. Culture. *Current Biology: CB, 30*(20), R1246-R1250.
23. Andrews, M., Backstrand, J., Boyle, J., Campinha-Bacote, J., Davidhizar, R.E., Doutrich, D., Echevarria, M., et al. 2010. Theoretical basis for transcultural care. *Journal of Transcultural Nursing*, 21(Suppl.), 53S–136S.
24. Britannica. Retrieved from https://www.britannica.com/topic/ethnicity
25. Bunce, J.A., & McElreath, R. 2022. Ethnicity and cultural dynamics.
26. Sutherland, L.L. 2002. Ethnocentrism in a pluralistic society. *Journal of Transcultural Nursing*, 13, 274–281.
27. Purnell, L.D. 2016. The Purnell model for cultural competence. In *Intervention in Mental Health-Substance Use*. CRC Press, pp. 57–78.
28. Samovar, L.A., Porter, R.E., McDaniel, E.R., & Roy, C.S. 2016. *Communication between cultures*. Cengage Learning.
29. Franzen, L., & Smith, C. 2009. Acculturation and environmental change impacts dietary habits among adult Hmong. *Appetite*, 52, 173–183.
30. Mezzich, J.E., Caracci, G., Fabrega, H., & Kirmayer, L.J. 2009. Cultural formulation guidelines. *Transcultural Psychiatry*, 46, 383–405.
31. Guo, T., & Uhm, S.Y. 2014. Society and acculturation in Asian American communities. *Neuropsychology of Asians and Asian-Americans*. Springer, New York, pp. 55–76.
32. Serafica, R.C. 2014. Dietary acculturation in Asian Americans. *Journal of Cultural Diversity*, 21(4), 145.
33. Aljaroudi, R., Horton, S., & Hanning, R.M. 2019. Acculturation and dietary acculturation among Arab Muslim immigrants in Canada. *Canadian Journal of Dietetic Practice and Research*, 80(4), 172–178.
34. Cuy Castellanos, D. 2015. Dietary acculturation in latinos/hispanics in the United States. *American Journal of Lifestyle Medicine*, 9(1), 31–36.
35. Popovic-Lipovac, A., & Strasser, B. 2015. A review on changes in food habits among immigrant women and implications for health. *Journal of Immigrant and Minority Health*, 17(2), 582–590.
36. Mintz, S., & Schlettwein-Gsell, D. 2001. Food patterns in agrarian societies: The "core-fringe-legume hypothesis." A dialogue. *Gastronomica*, 1, 41–59.

37. Bromham, L., Skeels, A., Schneemann, H., Dinnage, R., & Hua, X. 2021. There is little evidence that spicy food in hot countries is an adaptation to reducing infection risk. *Nature Human Behaviour*, 5(7), 878–891.
38. Rozin, P., & Schiller, P. 1980. The nature and acquisition of a preference for chile peppers by humans. *Motivation and Emotion*, 4, 77–101.
39. Zhou, Y., Gao, X., Small, D.M., & Chen, H. 2019. Extreme spicy food cravers displayed increased brain activity in response to pictures of foods containing chili peppers: An fMRI study. *Appetite*, 142, 104379.
40. Almerico, G.M. 2014. Food and identity: Food studies, cultural, and personal identity. *Journal of International Business and Cultural Studies*, 8, 1.
41. Niva, M., & Mäkelä, J. 2020. Meals in western eating and drinking. *Handbook of Eating and Drinking: Interdisciplinary Perspectives*, 495–508.
42. Ricciuto, L., Fulgoni, V.L., Gaine, P.C., Scott, M.O., & DiFrancesco, L. 2022. Trends in added sugars intake and sources among US children, adolescents, and teens using NHANES 2001-2018. *The Journal of Nutrition*, 152(2), 568–578. https://doi.org/10.1093/jn/nxab395
43. Waters, A. 2010. *In the green kitchen: Techniques to learn by heart*. New York: Clarkson-Potter.
44. Cachelin, A., Ivkovich, L., Jensen, P., & Neild, M. 2019. Leveraging foodways for health and justice. *Local Environment*, 24(5), 417–427.
45. Petrini, C. 2015. *Food & freedom: How the slow food movement is changing the world through gastronomy*. Rizzoli Publications.
46. Armelagos, G.J. 2014. Brain evolution, the determinates of food choice, and the omnivore's dilemma. *Critical Reviews in Food Science and Nutrition*, 54(10), 1330–1341.
47. Martin, D. 2014. *Edible: An adventure into the world of eating insects and the last great hope to save the planet*. Houghton Mifflin Harcourt.
48. Kim, T.K., Yong, H.I., Kim, Y.B., Kim, H.W., & Choi, Y.S. 2019. Edible insects as a protein source: A review of public perception, processing technology, and research trends. *Food Science of Animal Resources*, 39(4), 521.
49. Kim, T.K., Yong, H.I., Kim, Y.B., Kim, H.W., & Choi, Y.S. 2019. Edible insects as a protein source: A review of public perception, processing technology, and research trends. *Food Science of Animal Resources*, 39(4), 521–540. https://doi.org/10.5851/kosfa.2019.e53
50. Drewnowski, A. 2002. Taste, genetics and food choices. In H. Anderson, J. Blundell, & M. Chiva (Eds.), *Food selection from genes to culture*. Levallois-Perret, France: Danone Institute.
51. Garrido, M.D., Egea, M., Linares, M.B., Martínez, B., Viera, C., Rubio, B., & Borrisser-Pairó, F. 2016. A procedure for sensory detection of androstenone in meat and meat products from entire male pigs: Development of a panel training. *Meat Science*, 122, 60–67.
52. O'Neal, C. 2010. Why your pee smells funny after eating asparagus. WebMD.com
53. Mccrory, M.A., Saltzman, E., Rolls, B.J., & Roberts, S.B. 2006. A twin study of the effects of energy density and palatability on energy intake of individual foods. *Physiology & Behavior*, 87, 451–459.
54. Anderson, E.N. 2005. *Everyone eats: Understanding food and culture*. New York: New York University Press.
55. Dingess, P.M., Thakar, A., Zhang, Z., Flynn, F.W., & Brown, T.E. (2018). High-salt exposure during perinatal development enhances stress sensitivity. *Developmental Neurobiology*, 78(11), 1131–1145.
56. Delisle, H. 2010. Findings on dietary patterns in different groups of African origin undergoing nutrition transition. *Applied Physiology, Nutrition, and Metabolism*, 35, 224–228.
57. Klautzer, L., Becker, J., & Mattke, S. 2014. The curse of wealth–Middle Eastern countries need to address the rapidly rising burden of diabetes. *International Journal of Health Policy and Management*, 2(3), 109.
58. Liu, A., Berhane, Z., & Tseng, M. 2010. Improved dietary variety and adequacy but lower dietary moderation with acculturation in Chinese women in the United States. *Journal of the American Dietetic Association*, 110, 457–62.
59. Mukoya, M.N., McKay, F.H., & Dunn, M. 2017. Can giving clients a choice in food selection help to meet their nutritional needs?: Investigating a novel food bank approach for asylum seekers. *Journal of International Migration and Integration*, 18(4), 981–991.
60. Coleman-Jensen, A., Rabbitt, M., Gregory, C., & Singh, A. 2021. Household food security in the United States in 2020. Economic Research Report No. ERR-298.
61. Karpyn, A.E., Riser, D., Tracy, T., Wang, R., & Shen, Y.E. 2019. The changing landscape of food deserts. *UNSCN Nutrition*, 44, 46.
62. Jetter, K.M., & Cassady, D.L. 2005, March. The availability and cost of healthier food items. University of California Agricultural Issues Center AIC Issues Brief 29.
63. Wilson, T.A., Adolph, A.L., & Butte, N.F. 2009. Nutrient adequacy and diet quality in non-overweight and overweight Hispanic children of low socioeconomic status: The Viva la Familia Study. *Journal of the American Dietetic Association*, 109, 1012–1022.
64. Costa, B.V.L., Menezes, M.C., Oliveira, C.D.L., Mingoti, S.A., Jaime, P.C., Caiaffa, W.T., & Lopes, A.C.S. 2019. Does access to healthy food vary according to socioeconomic status and to food store type? An ecologic study. *BMC Public Health*, 19(1), 1–7.
65. Reitzel, L.R., Regan, S.D., Nguyen, N., Cromley, E.K., Strong, L.L., Wetter, D.W., & McNeill, L.Hd. 2014. Density and proximity of fast food restaurants and body mass index among African Americans. *American Journal of Public Health*, 104(1), 110–116.
66. Wedick, N.M., Ma, Y., Olendzki, B.C., Procter-Gray, E., Cheng, J., Kane, K.J., . . . & Li, W. 2015. Access to healthy food stores modifies effect of a dietary intervention. *American Journal of Preventive Medicine*, 48(3), 309–317.
67. Dubowitz, T., Zenk, S.N., Ghosh-Dastidar, B., Cohen, D.A., Beckman, R., Hunter, G., . . . & Collins, R.L. 2015. Healthy food access for urban food desert residents: Examination of the food environment, food purchasing practices, diet and BMI. *Public Health Nutrition*, 18(12), 2220–2230.
68. Taillie, L.S. (2018). Who's cooking? Trends in US home food preparation by gender, education, and race/ethnicity from 2003 to 2016. *Nutrition Journal*, 17(1), 1–9.
69. Rollins, B.Y., Belue, R.Z., & Francis, L.A. 2010. The beneficial effect of family meals on obesity differs by race, sex, and household education: The national survey of children's health, 2003–2004. *Journal of the American Dietetic Association*, 110, 1335–1339.
70. Beydoun, M.A., Powell, L.M., & Wang, Y. 2009. Reduced away-from-home food expenditure and better nutrition knowledge and belief can improve quality of dietary intake among US adults. *Public Health Nutrition*, 12, 369–381.
71. Tybur, J.M., Çınar, Ç., Karinen, A.K., & Perone, P. 2018. Why do people vary in disgust? *Philosophical Transactions of the Royal Society B: Biological Sciences*, 373(1751), 20170204.
72. Zhang, J., Sun-Waterhouse, D., Su, G., & Zhao, M. 2019. New insight into umami receptor, umami/umami-enhancing peptides and their derivatives: A review. *Trends in Food Science & Technology*, 88, 429–438.
73. Nicklaus, S., & Schwartz, C. 2019. Early influencing factors on the development of sensory and food preferences. *Current Opinion in Clinical Nutrition & Metabolic Care*, 22(3), 230–235.
74. USDA. 2020. Food spending and share of income spent on food across U.S. households, 2020. U.S. Bureau of Labor Statistics, Consumer Expenditure Survey. Retrieved from https://www.ers.usda.gov/data-products/ag-and-food-statistics-charting-the-essentials/food-prices-and-spending/
75. Bailey, R.L. 2017. Influencing eating choices: Biological food cues in advertising and packaging alter trajectories of decision making and behavior. *Health Communication*, 32(10), 1183–1191.

76. National Restaurant Association. Facts at a glance. n.d. Retrieved from http://www.restaurant.org/News-Research/Research/Facts-at-a-Glance (accessed January 25, 2015).
77. Folta, S.C., Goldberg, J.P., Economos, C., Bell, R., & Meltzer, R. 2006. Food advertising targeted at school-age children: A content analysis. *Journal of Nutrition Education and Behavior*, 38, 244–248.
78. Henry, A.E., & Story, M. 2009. Food and beverage brands that market to children and adolescents on the Internet: A content analysis of branded web sites. *Journal of Nutrition Education and Behavior*, 41, 353–359.
79. Smith, R., Kelly, B., Yeatman, H., & Boyland, E. (2019). Food marketing influences children's attitudes, preferences and consumption: A systematic critical review. *Nutrients*, 11(4), 875.
80. Duquesne, D. December 1, 2010. Food porn: Love it or hate it? Huffington Post. Retrieved from http://www.huffingtonpost.com/daphne-duquesne/food-porn_b_790549.html#s196042 (accessed January 6, 2015).
81. McKeown, A., & Nelson, R. 2018. Independent decision making of adolescents regarding food choice. *International Journal of Consumer Studies*, 42(5), 469–477.
82. Blisard, N., Lin, B.H., Cromartie, J., & Ballenger, N. 2002. America's changing appetite: Food consumption and spending to 2020. *Food Review*, 25, 1–9.
83. Schwartz, C., Vandenberghe-Descamps, M., Sulmont-Rossé, C., Tournier, C., & Feron, G. 2018. Behavioral and physiological determinants of food choice and consumption at sensitive periods of the life span, a focus on infants and elderly. *Innovative Food Science & Emerging Technologies*, 46, 91–106.
84. Smeets, P.A., De Graaf, C., Stafleu, A., van Osch, M.J., Nievelstein, R.A., & van Der Grond, J. 2006. Effect of satiety on brain activation during chocolate tasting in men and women. *American Journal of Clinical Nutrition*, 83, 1297–1305.
85. Møller, P. 2015. Satisfaction, satiation and food behaviour. *Current Opinion in Food Science*, 3, 59–64.
86. Fast Food Nutrition. 2022. Retrieved from https://fastfoodnutrition.org/ihop/country-fried-steak-eggs-combo/with-sausage-gravy
87. Schlarp, T. 2020. Joey Chestnut net worth: Updated career earnings in 2020, records for hot dog-eating king. The Sporting News. Retrieved from https://www.sportingnews.com/us/other-sports/news/joey-chestnut-net-worth-career-earnings-records-hot-dog-eating/12o0u9vgy93oa1goosu1y1e86x
88. Wilkins, J. 2005, August. This black widow has quite a bite. *San Diego Union-Tribune*, p. D3.
89. Yang, F.M., & Levkoff, S.E. 2005. Ageism and minority populations: Strengths in the face of challenge. *Generations*, 29(3), 42–48.
90. Gutjar, S., Dalenberg, J.R., de Graaf, C., de Wijk, R.A., Palascha, A., Renken, R.J., & Jager, G. 2015. What reported food-evoked emotions may add: A model to predict consumer food choice. *Food Quality and Preference*, 45, 140–148.
91. Vabø, M., & Hansen, H. 2014. The relationship between food preferences and food choice: A theoretical discussion. *International Journal of Business and Social Science*, 5(7).
92. Prescott, J. 2020. Development of food preferences. *Handbook of Eating and Drinking: Interdisciplinary Perspectives*, 199–217.
93. Larson, N., & Story, M. 2009. A review of environmental influences on food choices. *Annals of Behavioral Medicine*, 38(Suppl. 1), S56–S73.
94. Whiting, K. 2021. "Want to live a long, healthy life? six secrets from Japans oldest people". *World Economic Forum*. Retrieved from weforum.org/agenda/2021/09/japan-okanawa-secret-2-longivity-good-health/
95. Sealy, Y.M. 2010. Parents' perceptions of food availability: Implications for childhood obesity. *Social Work in Health Care*, 49, 565–580.
96. Beagan, B.L., Chapman, G.E., Johnston, J., McPhail, D., Power, E.M., & Vallianatos, H. 2014. *Acquired tastes: Why families eat the way they do*. UBC Press.
97. Food Labeling Survey. 2019. International Food Information Council Foundation and the American Heart Association. Retrieved from https://foodinsight.org/wp-content/uploads/2019/01/IFIC-FDN-AHA-Report.pdf
98. Goody, C.M., & Drago, L. 2010. Introduction: Cultural competence and nutrition counseling. In *Cultural food practices*. Chicago: American Dietetic Association.
99. Henderson, S., Horne, M., Hills, R., & Kendall, E. 2018. Cultural competence in healthcare in the community: A concept analysis. *Health & Social Care in the Community*, 26(4), 590–603.
100. Fleckman, J.M., Dal Corso, M., Ramirez, S., Begalieva, M., & Johnson, C.C. 2015. Intercultural competency in public health: A call for action to incorporate training into public health education. *Frontiers in Public Health*, 3, 210.
101. Andrews, M.M., & Boyle, J.S. (Eds.). 2008. *Transcultural concepts in nursing care* (5th ed.). Philadelphia, PA: Lippincott, Williams & Wilkins.
102. McCabe, C.F., O'Brien-Combs, A., & Anderson, O.S. 2020. Cultural competency training and evaluation methods across dietetics education: A narrative review. *Journal of the Academy of Nutrition and Dietetics*, 120(7), 1198–1209.
103. Zamora, A.N., & Anderson, O.S. 2022. A call for competence in the social determinants of health within dietetics education and training. *Journal of the Academy of Nutrition and Dietetics*, 122(2), 279–283.
104. Census.gov. 2021. National population estimates. Retrieved from https://www.census.gov/quickfacts/fact/table/US/PST045221
105. Academy/Commission on Dietetic Registration Demographics. 2020. Academy of Nutrition and Dietetics. Retrieved from https://www.cdrnet.org/academy-commission-on-dietetic-registration-demographics
106. Pamies, R.J., Hill, G.C., Watkins, L., Mcnamee, M.J., & Colburn, L. 2006. Diversity and the health-care workforce. In D. Satcher & R.J. Pamies (Eds.), *Multicultural medicine and health disparities*. New York: McGraw-Hill.
107. Valentine, P., Wynn, J., & McLean, D. 2016. Improving diversity in the health professions. *North Carolina Medical Journal*, 77(2), 137–140.
108. Statistics Canada. 2017. Census in brief: Ethnic and cultural origins of Canadians, portrait of a rich heritage. Retrieved from https://www12.statcan.gc.ca/census-recensement/2016/as-sa/98-200-x/2016016/98-200-x2016016-eng.cfm
109. Goel, M.S., Mccarthy, E.P., Phillips, R.S., & Wee, C.C. 2004. Obesity among US immigrant subgroups by duration of residence. *Journal of the American Medical Association*, 292, 2860–2867.
110. Popkin, B.M. 2015. Nutrition transition and the global diabetes epidemic. *Current Diabetes Reports*, *15*(9), 1–8.
111. Fox, M., Thayer, Z., & Wadhwa, P.D. 2017. Assessment of acculturation in minority health research. *Social Science & Medicine*, 176, 123–132.
112. Doucerain, M.M., Segalowitz, N., & Ryder, A.G. 2017. Acculturation measurement: From simple proxies to sophisticated toolkit.
113. Nelson-Peterman, J.L., Toof, R., Liang, S.L., & Grigg-Saito, D.C. 2015. Long-term refugee health: Health behaviors and outcomes of Cambodian refugee and immigrant women. *Health Education & Behavior*, 42(6), 814–823.
114. Bonham, V.L., Green, E.D., & Perez-Stable, E.J. 2018. Examining how race, ethnicity, and ancestry data are used in biomedical research. *JAMA*, 320(15), 1533–1534.
115. Hamilton, J.A. 2008, Fall. Revitalizing difference in the Hap Map: Race and contemporary human genetic variation research. *Journal of Law and Medical Ethics*, 471–477.
116. Frank, R. 2014. The molecular reinscription of race: A comment on "Genetic bio-ancestry and social construction of racial classification in social surveys in the contemporary United States". *Demography*, 51(6), 2333–2336.
117. Krishnan, S., Cozier, Y.C., Rosenberg, L., & Palmer, J.R. 2010. Socioeconomic status and incidence of type 2 diabetes: Results from the Black Women's Health Study. *American Journal of Epidemiology*, 171, 564–570.

118. Davis, G.C., & Carlson, A. 2015. The inverse relationship between food price and energy density: Is it spurious? *Public Health Nutrition*, 18(6), 1091–1097.
119. Drewnowski, A. 2018. Nutrient density: Addressing the challenge of obesity. *British Journal of Nutrition*, 120(s1), S8–S14.
120. Ribeiro, G., Camacho, M., Santos, O., Pontes, C., Torres, S., & Oliveira-Maia, A.J. 2018. Association between hedonic hunger and body-mass index versus obesity status. *Scientific Reports*, 8(1), 1–9.
121. Tester, J.M., Rosas, L.G., & Leung, C.W. 2020. Food insecurity and pediatric obesity: A double whammy in the era of COVID-19. *Current Obesity Reports*, 9(4), 442–450.
122. Barosh, L., Friel, S., Engelhardt, K., & Chan, L. 2014. The cost of a healthy and sustainable diet—who can afford it? *Australian and New Zealand Journal of Public Health*, 38(1), 7–12.
123. Jones, N.R., Conklin, A.I., Suhrcke, M., & Monsivais, P. 2014. The growing price gap between more and less healthy foods: Analysis of a novel longitudinal UK dataset. *PloS One*, 9(10), e109343.
124. Ferreira, V.A., & Magalhães, R. 2019. Social Inequalities, poverty and obesity. In *Psychology of health-biopsychosocial approach*. IntechOpen.
125. Purnell, T.S., Calhoun, E.A., Golden, S.H., Halladay, J.R., Krok-Schoen, J.L., Appelhans, B.M., & Cooper, L.A. 2016. Achieving health equity: Closing the gaps in health care disparities, interventions, and research. *Health Affairs*, 35(8), 1410–1415.
126. Drewnowski, A. Obesity, diets, and social inequalities. 2009, May. *Nutrition Reviews*, 67(Suppl. 1), S36–S39.
127. Eisenmann, J.C., Gundersen, C., Lohman, B.J., Garasky, S., & Stewart, S.D. 2011. Is food insecurity related to overweight and obesity in children and adolescents? A summary of studies, 1995–2009. *Obesity Reviews*, 12(5), e73–e83.
128. Stang, J., & Bayerl, C.T. 2010. Position of the American Dietetic Association: Child and adolescent nutrition assistance programs. *Journal of the American Dietetic Association*, 110, 791–799.
129. Nelms, M., & Sucher, K.P. 2015. Nutrition therapy and pathophysiology. Cengage.
130. Thompson, F.E., & Subar, A.F. 2017. Dietary assessment methodology. *Nutrition in the Prevention and Treatment of Disease*, 5–48.
131. Groth, S.W., & Kearney, M.H. 2009. Diverse women's beliefs about weight gain in pregnancy. *Journal of Midwifery and Women's Health*, 54, 452–457.
132. Stowers, S.L. 1992. Development of a culturally appropriate food guide for pregnant Caribbean immigrants in the United States. *Journal of the American Dietetic Association*, 92, 331–336.
133. National Restaurant Association. 2021. Global foods, flavors continue to thrive into 2022: U.S. consumers are on the hunt for exotic items at home and in restaurants. Retrieved from https://restaurant.org/education-and-resources/resource-library/global-foods-flavors-continue-to-thrive-into-2022/
134. Williams, C. 2020. Most popular ethnic cuisines in America according to Google. *Chefs Pencil*. Retrieved from https://www.chefspencil.com/most-popular-ethnic-cuisines-in-america/
135. Saksena, M.J., Okrent, A.M., Anekwe, T.D., Cho, C., Dicken, C., Effland, A., . . . & Tuttle, C. 2018. *America's eating habits: Food away from home* (No. 281119). United States Department of Agriculture, Economic Research Service.
136. Pillsbury, R. 2018. *No foreign food: The American diet in time and place*. Routledge.
137. Sloan, E.A. 2021. The top 10 food trends of 2021. *Food Technology*, 75, 23–35.
138. Brown, M. 2021. The hidden, magnificent history of chop suey: Discrimination and mistranslation have long obscured the dish's true origin. *Gastro Obscura*. Retrieved from https://www.atlasobscura.com/articles/chop-suey-history
139. Severson, K. 2021. How will Americans eat in 2022? The food forecasters speak. *The New York Times*. Retrieved from https://www.nytimes.com/2021/12/28/dining/food-trends-predictions-2022.html

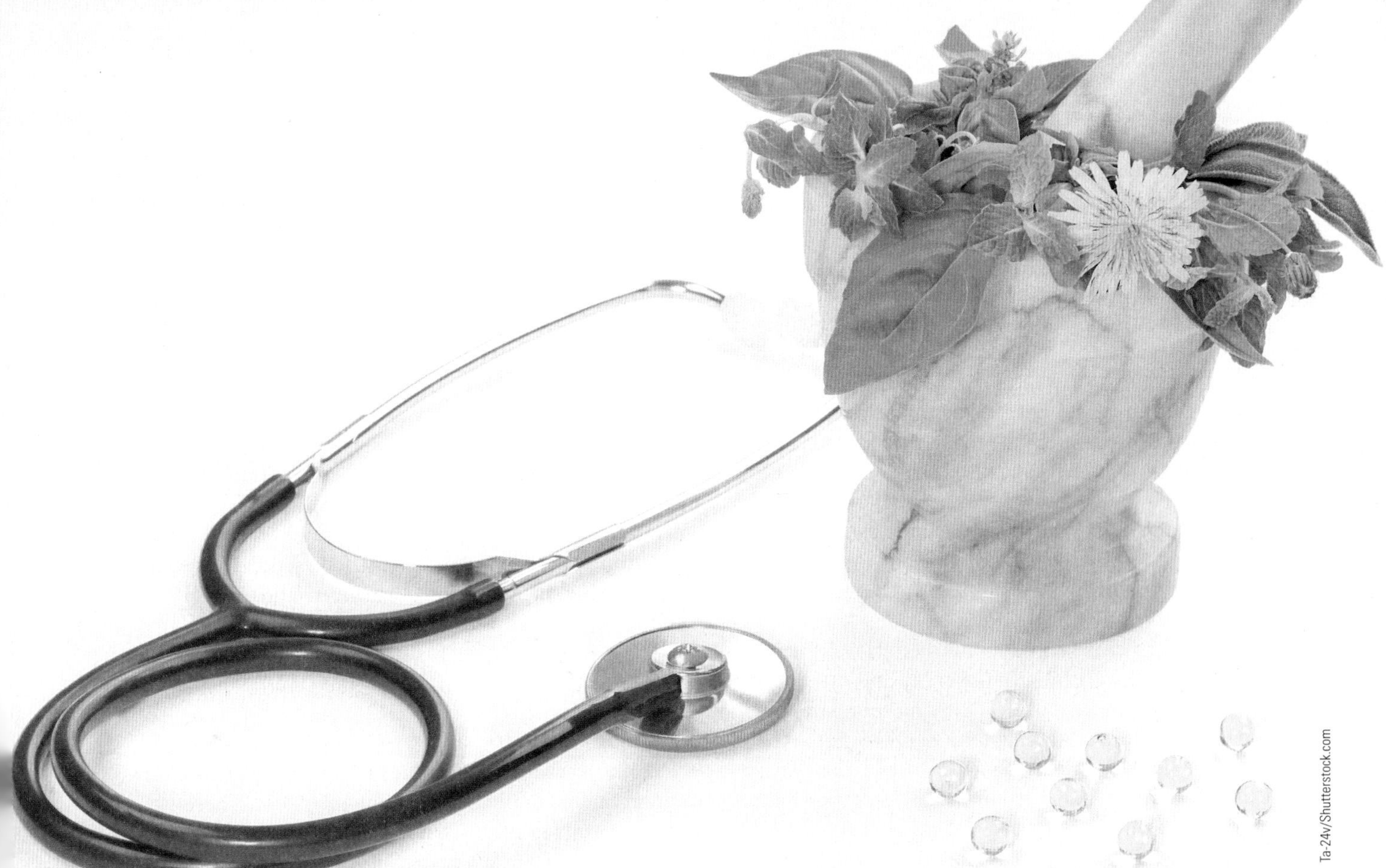
Ta-24v/Shutterstock.com

Chapter 2
Traditional Health Beliefs and Practices

Learning Objectives

2.1 Identify how definitions of health, sickness, and disease vary across cultures.

2.2 Define the biomedical model and complementary therapies.

2.3 Compare the common values of the majority American culture with those of other cultural groups.

2.4 Compare the impact of multiple cultures in the United States on the health care system.

2.5 Differentiate health maintenance habits in various cultural groups.

2.6 Explain how hot and cold or yin and yang worldviews affect what is eaten.

2.7 List the alternative and folk medical healing therapies in the cultures reviewed.

2.8 List botanicals and how they are used in healing therapies.

2.9 Define pluralistic health care systems.

Health and illness in America are usually considered the specialty of mainstream biomedicine. *Biomedicine* is the term used to describe the conventional system of health care in the United States and other Western nations based on the principles of the natural sciences, including biology, physiology, and biochemistry. Furthermore, health promotion is based on scientific findings of researchers regarding diet, exercise, and lifestyle issues such as smoking cessation and stress management; disease is treated according to the latest technologies. In reality, health care is pluralistic in the United States, as well as in most other countries. Many people in the United States never consult a physician or allied health care provider when physical or emotional symptoms occur, relying on home remedies and popular therapies found readily on the Internet rather than seeking professional help. Complementary and alternative medicine (CAM) is popular with many Americans. The National Center for Complementary and Alternative Medicine recently published data gathered from the National Health Interview Survey and estimates that approximately 33 percent of all adults and approximately 11 percent of all children used some form of CAM during the year 2012. However, there may have been changes to this statistic since the 2012 survey, influenced by the 2020–22 pandemic and other factors. There is a lower use of complementary therapies in Hispanic (22%) and non-Hispanic Black adults (19%) compared non-Hispanic White adults (38%). The most popular CAM therapies included natural products, deep breathing, yoga, tai chi, meditation, chiropractic and osteopathic interventions, special diet, guided imagery, and massage.[1] Consumer spending on such practices and products has more than tripled in the past decade, from $11 billion annually to nearly $40 billion,[2] but the costs of complementary therapies are often challenging to determine because they are not used alone but in combination with other therapies. When biomedical care is sought, it is often in conjunction with these other systems. The term *integrative medicine* is used when there is a combination of conventional biomedicine and CAM treatments that have demonstrated scientific evidence of safety and effectiveness.

Culture determines how a person defines health, recognizes illness, and seeks treatment. Traditional health beliefs and practices can be categorized in various ways: through the etiology of illness (due to personal, natural, social, or supernatural causes) or by the cures that are employed (the use of therapeutic substances, physical forces, or magico-religious interventions). There is no consensus, however, on these classifications. In this chapter, home remedies, popular approaches such as folk and alternative traditions, and professional systems (including U.S. biomedicine, traditional Chinese medicine, and Asian Indian Ayurvedic medicine) are reviewed within the cultural context of health and illness. Specific beliefs and practices are detailed in the following chapters on each American ethnic group.

Worldview

Cultural Outlook

Each cultural group has a unique outlook on life, based on a common understanding and ranking of values. These standards typically represent what is considered worthy in a life well lived. They are a collective expression of preferences and priorities—not absolutes—and individuals within a society may hold a spectrum of beliefs. However, expectations about personal and public conduct, assumptions regarding social interaction, and assessments of individual behavior are determined by this cultural outlook or worldview. This perspective influences perceptions about health and illness as well as the role of each within the structure of a society.[3–5] Traditional White American values, which are shared to some degree by many other ethnic groups in the United States, emphasize individuality and control over fate (refer to Table 2.1).

Table 2.1 Comparison of Common Values

Majority American Culture	Other Cultural Groups
Mastery over nature	Harmony with nature
Personal control over the environment	Fate
Doing—activity	Being/becoming
Time dominates	Personal interaction dominates
Human equality	Hierarchy/rank/status
Individualism/privacy	Group welfare
Youth	Elders
Self-help	Birthright inheritance
Competition	Cooperation
Future orientation	Past or present orientation
Informality	Formality
Directness/openness/honesty	Indirectness/ritual/"face"
Practicality/efficiency	Idealism
Materialism	Spiritualism/detachment

Source: Adapted from E. Randall-David, *Strategies for Working with Culturally Diverse Communities*. Association for the Care of Children's Health, 19 Mantua Rd., Mt. Royal, NY 08061. Copyright 1989.

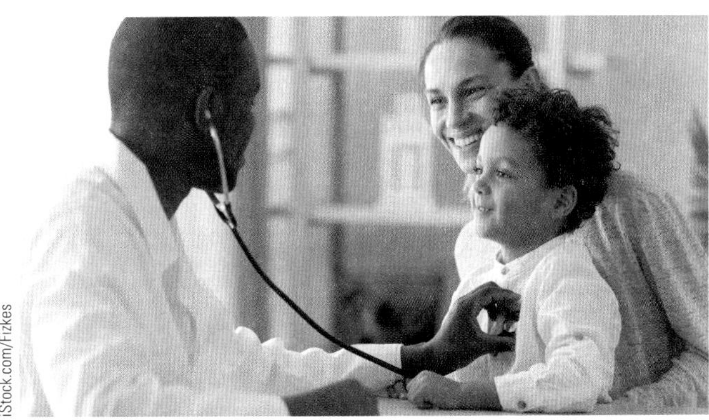

iStock.com/Fizkes

▲ **The concept of preventive health care, such as annual checkups provided by a biomedical professional, is unknown in some cultures where fate is believed to determine health.**

Personal accountability and self-help are considered cultural cornerstones. One older study found that 82 percent of American consumers believe they are directly responsible for their own health.[6] Most other cultures worldwide believe that fate—including the will of God, the actions of supernatural agents, or birthright (i.e., astrological alignment or cosmic karma)—is a primary influence on health and illness. Although most cultures have complex practices regarding the maintenance of health, the concept of preventative health care, such as annual checkups, is unknown in some cultures where fate dominates.

The significance of fate often coincides with differences in perceptions of time. Many Americans place great value on promptness and schedules; they are also future-oriented, meaning they are willing to work toward long-term goals or make sacrifices so that they or their children will reap rewards in the future. One cultural preference in the United States is concentrating on one issue or task at a time in a sequential manner (monochronistic). Planning ahead for things such as appointments is expected. Many other cultural groups live in the present and are often polychronistic, or comfortable doing many things at once. A polychronistic person who is talking with his grandmother while fixing an appliance and watching a baseball game on television may be unlikely to cut the visit short just because he has a medical appointment. Immediate interests and responsibilities, including interpersonal relationships, are more important than being on time.

Most Americans are very task-oriented and desire direct participation in their health care; they feel best when they can do something. Other cultures place a greater value on *being* and feel comfortable with inactivity. In Buddhism, for example, self-worth is based more on personal relationships than on accomplishments. Some of the causes of suffering are attachment, desire, and craving. The whole idea of the provider–client partnership may be alien to Asians, who often expect to be fully directed in their care. While many Americans value patient autonomy and confidentiality, other cultural groups, such as Middle Easterners, believe that the family should be involved in all health care decisions—the welfare of the group outweighs that of the individual.

Many cultures prefer indirect communication, which seems vague and noncommittal to many Americans, who consider honest, open dialogue essential to effective communication (refer to Table 2.2). In addition, Americans often prefer informality, compared to many cultures that expect a formal relationship with everyone but intimate family members. In cultures where identity with a group is more significant than individuality, social status and hierarchy are respected, which can have an impact on the practitioner–client relationship (refer to Chapter 3, "Intercultural Communication," for more information).

Worldview is especially evident in serious, life-and-death health care decisions. Southeast Asians may have little interest in prolonging the life of a terminally ill family member because of a faith in reincarnation. Some African Americans distrust White American health care recommendations regarding do-not-resuscitate orders in part because they contradict the critical role of faith in African American healing. An Orthodox Jewish patient may believe that physicians are mandated to preserve life and that any person who assists death through denial of sustaining care is a murderer; a non-Orthodox Jew may believe that no one should endure uncontrollable pain and thus dying should not be prolonged. Middle Easterners traditionally demand that everything be done to keep a person alive because death is in God's hands, and one must never give up hope. Mexican American family members might view death as part of God's plan for a relative; they might be against anything that would quicken death, or they may expect the practitioner to make the decision. It is beneficial in clinical practice to have a good contextual understanding of culture and traditions related to spirituality during end-of-life treatment options for families.[3,7,8]

Most health care situations are not cases of life or death, and worldview affects many other, less catastrophic aspects of health and illness as well. It is useful to examine the biomedical worldview and understand the perspective of most U.S. health care providers before learning about other traditional health beliefs and practices. Comparisons between biomedicine and other medical systems can reveal areas of potential disagreement or conflict regarding how and why illness occurs and the expectations for treatment before working with a client. Compliance increases with clinical approaches that concur with the client's worldview.[9,10] Recent studies suggest a move toward cultural humility rather than cultural competency (discussed further in Chapter 3). It requires health practitioners to self-reflect on their own culture and clinical interactions and to question their own biases, attitudes, assumptions, and stereotypes that may contribute to a lower quality of care for some patients.[11]

Food for Thought

Some Americans find eating a meal a disruption of daily tasks; others adhere to strict meal schedules. In polychronistic (people-oriented versus task-oriented) societies, meals are usually leisurely events, a chance to enjoy the blessings of food in the company of family and friends.

Table 2.2 Direct and Indirect Communication

Direct Communication	Indirect Communication
1 Openly confront issues or difficulties	1 Focus is not just on what is said but how it is said
2 Communicate concerns straight-forwardly	2 Avoid difficult or contentious issues
3 Engage in conflict when necessary	3 Avoid conflict if possible
4 Express views or opinions in a frank manner	4 Express opinions and concerns diplomatically
Example: Get right to the point during a conversation.	5 Count on the listener to interpret the meaning
	Example: Avoid saying no; say maybe or possibly, even if you mean no.

Source: Peterson, Brooks. 2004. *Cultural intelligence: A guide to working with people from other cultures*. Boston: Intercultural Press.

Biomedical Worldview

Biomedicine is a cultural subdivision of the American worldview. It shares many beliefs with the majority outlook but differs in a few notable areas.[12] There are certainly exceptions to the biomedical worldview within certain specialties, and by some practitioners, yet many of the underlying assumptions are culture-specific. The tendency is for health care providers to enforce their beliefs, practices, and values upon clients, sometimes unknowingly because they are unaware of cultural differences, but more often because they believe their ideas are superior. This process is called *cultural imposition*, and it impacts nearly all client care.[13,14]

Relationship to Nature

Biomedicine adheres to the concept of mastery over nature. Practitioners are soldiers in the war on cancer (or other conditions). They fight infection, conquer disease, and kill pain. Technology is considered omnipotent; its tools are the arsenal used to battle pain and illness.

One factor in this approach is the attitude that health can be measured numerically and that there are standardized definitions of disease. Blood and urine analyses, X-rays, scans, and other diagnostic tests are used to define whether a patient's levels, such as blood sugar, cholesterol, or measures of inflammation, are within normal physical or biochemical range. Results falling within designated parameters mean the patient is functioning normally; if the data are too high or too low, the patient is in an abnormal state that may indicate disease. Diagnosis occurs independently of the idiosyncratic characteristics of the individual, usually without consideration of cultural factors such as ethnic background or religious faith. Symptoms that cannot be linked to a known medical problem are frequently determined to be of psychosomatic origins.[12]

Personal Control or Fate?

The U.S. medical system leaves little room for chance or divine intervention. Scientific rationality dictates that there is a biomedical cause for every condition, even if it is as yet undiscovered. Each individual inherits a certain physiological constitution and has a personal responsibility to make the choices that prevent illness. Receiving immunizations and vaccines, and getting regular checkups are biomedical ways by which individuals can preserve their health. Being obese, smoking cigarettes, consuming immoderate amounts of alcohol, substance abuse, and failing to manage stress are biomedical examples of how individuals may endanger their health.

Food for Thought

Some researchers have noted that although the biomedical community often calls clients whose cultural background differs from the majority "hard to reach," this term is equally applicable to health professionals who refuse to provide culturally appropriate care.

The number of adults over sixty-five years in the United States is expected to double and the number of centenarians (those over 100 years old) is expected to increase 10-fold by the year 2050. Figures among some ethnic groups, such as older African Americans, Asian Americans, Native Americans, and Latinx, show even greater growth potential.

When a person is ill, the biomedical assumption is that they will reliably comply with therapy and that treatment, if undertaken correctly by the patient, will alleviate the condition. The onus of cure is dependent on personal behavior. From the patient's perspective, there is the presumption that health care professionals will provide mistake-free care. Malpractice suits filed when care was less than perfect have led to extensive charting and record-keeping in the U.S. biomedical system.

State of Being

Consistent with the value placed on personal control, biomedical patients are expected to be active partners in their cure. Noncompliance is disliked by biomedical practitioners. Lifestyle changes can help preserve health; taking medications and completing therapeutic regimens can relieve symptomatic pain or cure disease. The biomedical emphasis is on doing, not being. Other worldviews may expect client nonparticipation and acceptance of adverse conditions. Clients are the recipients of healing, not participants in healing.

Role of the Individual

Similar to the American majority worldview, individuality is honored in U.S. biomedicine, and client confidentiality is mandatory. Individuals are seen as a single, biological unit, not as members of a family or a particular cultural group. It is assumed that a person desires privacy, and clients are sometimes encouraged by providers to keep medical matters quiet, even if it means withholding information from relatives. In fact, there can be serious HIPAA (Health Insurance Portability and Accountability Act) violations in releasing patient information to family members without written approval from the patient. Typically, treatment is focused solely on the client, in keeping with the beliefs of personal responsibility and the provider–patient partnership.

Human Equality

A fundamental premise in American biomedicine is that all patients deserve equal access to care, although, practically speaking, cost, location, and convenience prevent many patients from receiving adequate health services. This is a relatively unique perspective; most other societies deliberately ration health care by assessing physical status (e.g., a young person may receive services denied to a terminally ill older person) or through socioeconomic status (e.g., the wealthy can purchase care and those with lower income levels are left to whatever society offers).

The biomedical worldview on human equality differs substantially from the mainstream American outlook in one way, however. A hierarchy of biomedical professionals is strictly observed in the United States, with physicians having the highest status and allied health professionals substantially less. Health care workers outside the professional system, such as clerical and custodial workers, and those beyond the reach of biomedicine, such as folk healers, are accorded even lower standing. Deference to those of superior rank is expected. The client is typically inferior to biomedical professionals within this hierarchy. However, as patients have access to online health information and more engagement in health decision-making and communication, traditional models of the patient–provider relationship are being challenged.[15]

Aging

Biomedicine supports the majority American worldview in its value of youthfulness. Many aspects of health care practice are dedicated to postponing the aging process, from plastic surgery to the technological prolongation of life. The fear of aging is so pervasive in U.S. culture that it influences health care outside the conventional biomedical system as well. Numerous alternative traditions promise everlasting youth through the use of certain products. The emphasis on youthfulness is in direct conflict with other cultural worldviews that honor the wisdom that comes with aging and that hold high esteem for elders. In 2020, the global anti-aging market was estimated to be worth about 58.5 billion U.S. dollars. That market is expected to grow at a rate of 7% between 2021 and 2026.[16]

Perceptions of Time

Biomedicine is future-oriented—that is, what can be done today so that the client will be better tomorrow? Often, treatments are unpleasant, invasive, and even painful at the moment of their application, yet the hope is that they will benefit the client in the future. Long-term management of disease and illness-prevention strategies such as diet is even more oriented toward future benefits.

Although being on time for appointments and taking medications when scheduled are traits valued by clients, biomedical practitioners are often notorious for their disrespect of clients' time. Clients are frequently asked to arrange non-emergency consultations weeks or even months in advance and may be kept waiting on the days of their appointments.

Degree of Formality/Degree of Directness

The established biomedical hierarchy, as well as the emphasis on timeliness, is often reflected in the degree of informality observed in the dialogue between provider and patient. The provider often addresses the client by his or her first name yet expects the patient to use formal titles in return. The provider usually spends limited time on small talk and attempts to get quickly to the problem; the expectation is the patient will also use a direct approach. Extensive medical jargon without explanation is often employed.

Biomedical practitioners value honest, open communication with patients because it enhances their ability to diagnose and treat disease, and it assists in issues such as informed consent. Other cultural worldviews, however, value indirect or intuitive communication with health care practitioners (refer to Chapter 3 for more information). Some cultures also believe that the family, not the patient, should be told about serious conditions.[17]

Materialism or Spirituality?

Each disease, from the biomedical viewpoint, has its own physiological characteristics: a certain cause, specific symptoms, expected test results, and a predictable response to treatment. For many biomedical health care providers, an illness isn't real unless it is clinically significant; emotional or social issues are the domain of other specialists. Biomedicine differs from most traditional health care approaches in its recognition of mind–body duality. Nearly all other cultures consider the mind and body as a unified whole. Somatization refers to the expression of emotions through bodily complaints.[18,19] In biomedical culture, somatic symptoms are often interpreted as a maladaptive emotional response, yet they are the most common presentation of psychological distress in patients worldwide.[20–22] In folk medicine and some alternative traditions, the emotional needs of the patient are addressed through physical therapies. Spiritual intervention is frequently sought concurrently.

What Is Health?

Cultural Definitions of Health

Meaning of Health

The World Health Organization (WHO) describes health as "a state of complete physical, mental, and social well-being, not merely an absence of disease or infirmity." Although comprehensive from a biomedical perspective, this definition does not fit the worldview of many cultural groups because it ignores the natural, spiritual, and supernatural dimensions of health.[23]

Most Native Americans believe that health is achieved through harmony with nature, which includes the family, the community, and the environment. Africans also emphasize a balance with nature and believe that malevolent environmental forces such as those of nature, God, the living, or the dead may disrupt a person's energy and bring illness. Many African Americans, Latinx, Middle Easterners, and some southern Europeans attribute health to living according to God's will. Most Asians believe that health is dependent on their relationship to the universe and that a balance between polar elements, such as yin and yang, must be maintained. Some Southeast Asians are concerned with pleasing their ancestor spirits, who may cause accidents or sickness when angry. Often, residents of Oceania believe that fulfilling social obligations is essential to health and that disharmony with family or village members can result in illness. Many Asian Indians consider mind, body, and soul to be interconnected and believe that spirituality is as important to health as a good diet, getting proper rest, and being in balance with the environment (refer to individual chapters on each ethnic group for more details).

Health in other cultures is less dependent on symptoms than on the ability to accomplish daily responsibilities. Among Koreans, there is a strong desire to avoid burdening their children with their health problems. Mexican men may ignore physical complaints because it is considered weak and unmanly to acknowledge pain. Even within a single culture, socioeconomic differences may contribute to the definition of health; daily aches are tolerated when a weekly paycheck is essential.[12]

Food for Thought

The separation between physical and emotional or psychological health is so embedded in American culture that no English word exists to even express the concept of mind–body unity.

The word *health* comes from the Anglo-Saxon term *hal*, meaning "wholeness."

Health Attributes

As health is defined culturally, so are the characteristics associated with health. Physical attributes are commonly linked with well-being, including skin color, weight maintenance, and hair sheen. Normal functioning of the body, such as regular bowel movements, routine menstruation, and a steady pulse, is expected, as is the use of arms, legs, hands, and the senses. Undisturbed sleep and not being tired also suggests good health.

Harmony within the context of marriage, family, and community is sometimes considered a sign of well-being. The specifics of health characteristics vary culturally. Healthy hair in the United States is advertised as clean, shiny, and flake-free, but in many cultures, oily hair is the norm, and dandruff is not a significant concern. Americans count on a single, strong pulse of about 72 beats per minute when resting, while in other medical systems there is more than one pulse of importance to health, and these pulses are a primary diagnostic tool in illness. Pregnancy is a medical condition in the United States warranting regular exams by biomedical professionals, whereas in many societies' pregnancy is a normal aspect of a healthy woman's cycle, and prenatal care is uncommon. Generally, Americans expect to be content in their lives; many other cultures have no such assumptions and do not link happiness with well-being.

Food for Thought

In traditional Chinese medicine, 15 separate body pulses are identified, each associated with an internal organ and each with its own characteristics.

Body Image

One area of significant cultural variation regarding health is body image. Perceptions of weight, health, and beauty differ worldwide. In the United States, there is significant societal pressure to be thin. Although there is no scientific agreement on the definition of ideal or even healthy weight for individuals, being overweight is usually believed to be a character flaw in the majority of American culture. Even health care professionals reportedly make moral judgments about obesity, depicting overweight persons as weak-willed, ugly, self-indulgent, and fair game for ridicule.[24,25] This stigmatization can be extremely harmful to children and adolescents. The health risks associated with being overweight cause some providers to presume ill health in these clients.[19,26,27] Thinness corresponds to the biomedical worldview regarding mastery of nature, the idea that the mind can control the appetite. However, to many cultures, especially those that may not value thinness as a sign of health, a thin practitioner may be perceived as not understanding weight management as they have not lived with weight issues.[28]

Food for Thought

In Ayurvedic medicine, health is a balance between the body, mind, spirit, and environment.

Historically, thinness has been associated with poor diet and disease. In many cultures today, including those of some Africans, Caribbean Islanders, Filipinos, Mexicans, Middle Easterners, Native Americans, and residents of Oceania, being overweight is traditionally a protective factor that is indicative of health as well as an attribute of beauty. Some Black Caribbean Islander and Puerto Rican women also report a larger body size as attractive to family and peers. Some Hispanic women value a heavier profile for themselves, and even if they opt for a slimmer body personally, they may prefer plump children.[29,30] Researchers have found that some young African American and Latinx women purposefully contest the dominant culture's emphasis on thinness, focusing more on self-acceptance and being caring and attentive. However, ethnic identification may serve as a protective factor. Several studies have suggested that acculturative stress has been linked to body dissatisfaction.

Researchers have found that attitudes about weight sometimes change when an immigrant enters a culture with different attitudes regarding health and beauty. More acculturated Hispanic women and children were more likely to choose a thinner figure as ideal than those who were less acculturated, ideal body image for Samoan women in Hawaii varied with whether they identified with Western or non-Western culture, and Puerto Ricans living on the mainland United States expressed a desire for thinness that is between that of their country of origin and that of the majority culture in their new homeland. Likewise, higher heritage acculturation and lower mainstream acculturation may also be associated with pressure from the media to be thin. The religiosity of various cultures may act as a buffer against appearance dissatisfaction and media pressure to be thin.[31] Among some Native Americans, the ideal body size has changed over time. Elders are more likely than younger adults to prefer a heavier profile, and children demonstrate a desire for even thinner bodies.[32] Some studies also suggest the pressure to be thin may be impacting young people more than adults: the percentage of teens engaging in unhealthy weight control behaviors did not vary by ethnicity in a national examination of high school students. Another study found Asian, Hispanic, and Native American adolescent girls reported similar numbers of weight-related concerns as White girls, though African American girls had fewer weight issues. Immigrant adolescents at all levels of acculturation demonstrate internalizing the thin body ideal prominent in the United States, which can impact their sense of body image.[33-35] Some Native American schoolchildren express a high level of body dissatisfaction, and concerns about being overweight were high in a cohort of third-grade children, with Latinx and African American girls reporting the same or greater level of body dissatisfaction than White and Asian girls.[36,37]

Health Maintenance

Health Habits

Just as with health attributes, there are some broad areas of intercultural agreement on health habits. Nearly all people identify a good diet, sufficient rest, and cleanliness as necessary for preserving health. It is in the definitions of these terms that cultural variations occur. For example, the majority of Americans typically identify three meals each day as a good diet. Asians may indicate that a balance of yin and yang foods is a requirement. Middle Easterners may be concerned with sufficient quantity, and Asian Indians may be concerned with the religious purity of the food. To most Americans, keeping clean means showering daily, while some Filipinos bathe several times each day to maintain a proper hot–cold balance.

In the United States, the National Center for Health Statistics describes the trends for dietary intake. The Dietary Guidelines for Americans (2020–2025) recommend an average energy intake of 2240 kilocalories (kcal) for women and 2700 kilocalories for men, depending on age. Some cultural groups would find these data irrelevant to health status. Macronutrient intake may not be associated with disease prevention, and dietary supplement use may not be familiar. Physical labor is often a factor in preserving health, but recreational exercise is rare throughout much of the world. Alcohol consumption is prohibited by several religions. Preventive care is unusual in many cultures.

Culturally specific health practices differ particularly in those beliefs passed on within families. A small survey of U.S. college students from many backgrounds revealed notable variations in health habits beyond general concepts regarding diet, sleep, physical activity, and cleanliness.[40] Dressing warmly (Eastern European, French, French Canadian, Iranian, Irish, Italian, Swedish) and avoiding going outdoors with wet hair (eastern European, Italian) were listed by some. Daily doses of cod liver oil (British, French, French Canadian, German, Norwegian, Polish, Swedish) or molasses (African American, French, French Canadian, German, Irish, Swedish) as a laxative were frequently reported maintenance measures. Natural amulets were traditionally worn in some families to prevent illness, such as camphor bags (Austrian, Canadian, Irish) or garlic cloves (Italian). Faith was important to many of the students, expressed as blessing of the throat (Irish, Swedish) and wearing holy medals (Irish), as well as daily prayer (Canadian, Ethiopian).

Health-Promoting Food Habits

Food habits are often identified as the most important way in which a person can maintain health. Nearly all cultures classify certain foods as necessary for strength, energy, and mental acuity. Some also include items that maintain the equilibrium between body and soul.

General dietary guidelines for health usually include the concepts of balance and moderation. In the United States, current recommendations include a foundation of complex carbohydrates in the form of whole grains, vegetables, and fruits; supplemented by smaller amounts of protein foods such as meats, legumes, and dairy products; and limited intakes of fats, sugar, salt, and alcohol. The Chinese system of yin–yang encourages a balance of those foods classified as yin (items that are typically raw, soothing, cooked at low temperatures, white or light green in color) with those classified as yang (mostly high-calorie foods, cooked in high heat, spicy, red-orange-yellow in color), avoiding extremes in both. Some staple foods, such as boiled rice, are believed to be perfectly balanced and are therefore neutral. Although which foods are considered yin or yang vary regionally in China, the concept of keeping the body in harmony through diet remains the same, usually adjusted seasonally to compensate for external temperature changes and for physiological conditions such as age and gender (refer to Chapter 11, "East Asia").

Aspects of the yin–yang diet theory are found in many other Asian nations, and a similar system of balance focused on the hot–cold classification of foods is practiced in the Middle East, parts of Latin America, the Philippines, and India. Hot-cold concepts also developed out of ancient Greek humoral medicine that identified four characteristics in the natural world (air-cold, earth-dry, fire-hot, water-moist) associated with four body humors: hot and moist (blood), cold and moist (phlegm), hot and dry (yellow/green bile), and cold and dry (black bile). Applied to daily food habits, this system usually focuses on only the hot and cold aspects of food (defined by characteristics such as taste, preparation method, or proximity to the sun) balanced to account for personal constitution and the weather. In Lebanon, it is believed that the body must have time to adjust to a hot food before a cold item can be eaten. In Mexico, the categorization of hot and cold foods is related to a congruous relationship with the natural world. Asian Indians associate a hot–cold balanced diet with spiritual harmony.

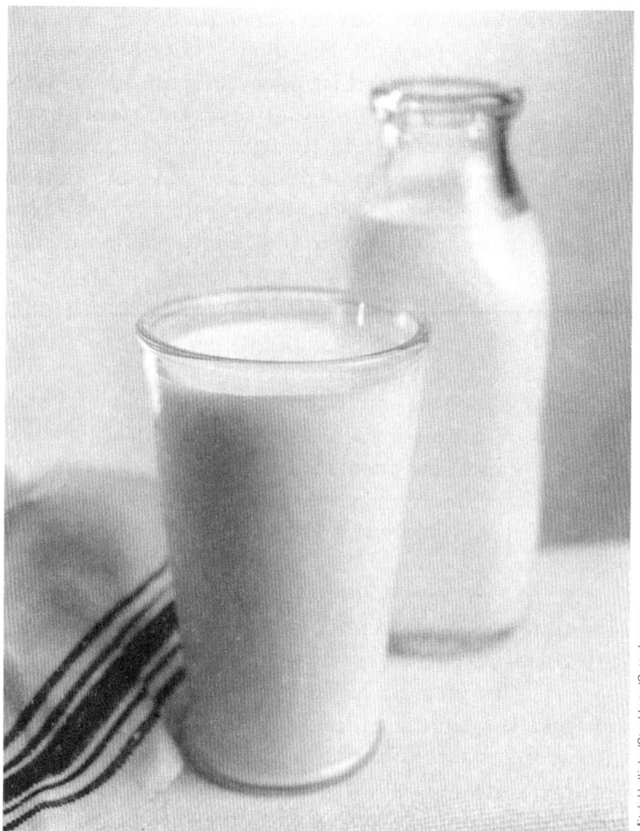

Mitch Hrdlicka/Stockbyte/Getty Images

▲ The health value of specific foods varies culturally. In the United States, it is said that milk builds strong bones. But in certain Native American cultures, milk is considered a weak food. Some Latinos believe milk is only good for children.

Food for Thought

In ancient China, nutritionists were ranked highest among health professionals.

Those Asians who prefer biomedicine and believe that traditional health systems are unsophisticated, usually expand additional foods into the neutral category of humoral medicine.[41–43]

Quantity of food is often associated with health as well. Some African Americans, for example, traditionally eat heavy meals, reserving light foods for ill and recuperating family members. In the Middle East, a poor appetite is sometimes regarded as an illness in itself. As discussed previously, being overweight is frequently associated with well-being in some cultures.

Food for Thought

Historically, ritualistic cannibalism, especially when the heart or liver of a brave and worthy enemy was consumed, is an extreme example of the sympathetic qualities of food.

Food that can provide consolation or a feeling of well-being and is often associated with childhood or home cooking is called comfort food.

In addition to balance and moderation, specific foods are sometimes identified with improved strength or vitality. In the United States, milk is considered to build strong bones, carrots are considered to improve eyesight, and candy is considered to provide quick energy. Chicken soup, a traditional tonic among Eastern European Jews, has become a well-accepted cure-all. Navajos consider milk to be a weak food, but meat and blue cornmeal are strong foods. Asians call strengthening items *pu* or *bo* foods, including protein-rich soups with pork liver or oxtail in China, and bone marrow soup in Korea. Puerto Ricans drink eggnog or malt-type beverages to improve vitality.

The sympathetic quality of a food, meaning a characteristic that looks like a human body part or organ, accounts for many health food beliefs. The properties of a food entering the mouth are incorporated into physical traits. Some Italians drink red wine to improve their blood, and American women sometimes eat gelatin (which is made from animal skin, bones, and other connective tissues) to grow longer, stronger fingernails. Throughout Asia and parts of the United States, ginseng, which is a root that resembles a human figure, is believed to increase strength and stamina. Other foods are believed to prevent specific illnesses. Americans, for instance, are urged to eat cabbage-family (cruciferous) vegetables to reduce their risk of certain cancers. Oatmeal (high in soluble fiber) and fish (high in omega-3 fatty acids) have both been promoted as preventing heart disease.

Some cultures believe that fresh foods prepared at home are the healthiest and, in the United States, the popularity of locally grown items and organic foods (those produced without the use of chemical additives or pesticides) has increased in recent years. Vegetarianism, macrobiotics, customized diets that account for an individual's food sensitivities or allergies, and very low-fat or low-carbohydrate diets are a few of the other ways in which health is promoted by some people through food habits.

Disease, Illness, and Sickness

Cultural Definitions of Disease, Illness, and Sickness

When health is diminished, a person experiences difficulties in daily living. Weakness, pain and discomfort, emotional distress, or physical debilitation may prevent an individual from fulfilling responsibilities or obligations to the family or society. Researchers call this experience illness, referring to a person's perceptions of and reactions to a physical or psychological condition, understood within the context of worldview. In biomedical culture, illness is caused by disease, defined as abnormalities or malfunctioning of body organs and systems. The term *sickness* is used for the entire disease–illness process. When an individual becomes sick, questions such as how the illness occurred, how the symptoms are experienced, and how the illness is cured arise—answered primarily through cultural consensus on the meaning of sickness.

Becoming Sick

During the onset of sickness, physical or behavioral complaints make a person aware that a problem exists. The development may be slow, and the symptoms may take time to manifest into a disease condition. Or, symptoms may occur suddenly, and it is quickly obvious that illness is present.

Except in emergencies, an individual usually seeks confirmation of illness first from family or friends. Symptoms are described and a diagnosis is sought. A knowledgeable relative is often the most trusted person in determining whether a condition is a cause for concern and whether further care should be pursued; in many cultures, a mother or grandmother is the medical expert within a family. This is a major step in the social legitimization of the sickness. If others agree that the person is ill, then the individual can adopt a new role—sick person—within the family or community. In this capacity, the sick person is excused from many daily obligations regarding work and family, as well as social and religious duties. A reprieve from personal responsibility for well-being is also given, with care provided by relatives, healers, or health professionals. The role of a sick person provides a socially accepted, temporary respite from the physical and psychological burdens of everyday life, with the understanding that sickness is not a permanent condition and that recovery should occur.[12]

Explanatory Models

When unexpected events happen, there is a human need to explain the origins and causes of seemingly random occurrences. Explanatory models consistent with a culture's worldview are used to account for why good or evil happens to a person or a community and to calm individual fears of being victimized. In sickness, the explanatory model details the cause of disease, how symptoms are perceived and expressed, how the illness can be healed and prevented from reoccurring, and why one person develops a sickness whereas another remains healthy.[12,44]

Food for Thought

The macrobiotic diet started as a concept by Hippocrates in Greece. It focuses on eating seasonal, local plant foods, exercising, sleeping, and balancing one's life. The macrobiotic diet became popular to promote health in the 19th century by a Japanese physician Dr. Sagen Ishizuka and is based on brown rice, miso soup, and vegetables. It was popularized in Europe as promoting health in the 1920s and has become a diet fad and lifestyle. Serious nutritional deficiencies, including low levels of Vitamin B-12 and iron have been identified in infants and toddlers on this restricted diet.[45]

The etiology of sickness is of central concern because the reason an illness occurs often determines the patient's outlook regarding the progression and cure of the sickness. In biomedical culture, three causes of disease are identified: (1) immediate causes, such as bacterial or viral infection, toxins, tumors, or physical injury; (2) underlying causes, including smoking, high cholesterol levels, glucose intolerance, or nutritional deficiencies; and (3) ultimate causes, such as hereditary predisposition, environmental stresses, obesity, or other factors.[46] The causes of illness are generally more complex. Four theories on the etiology of sickness prevalent in most societies have been described (Figure 2.1): those originating in the patient; those from the natural world; those from the social world; and those due to supernatural causes.[12] It is important to note that in no society do all persons subscribe to any single cause, and there is considerable variation in the degree of belief, intra-culturally as well as interculturally. Additionally, believing in a cause does not necessarily result in a practice associated with that cause.

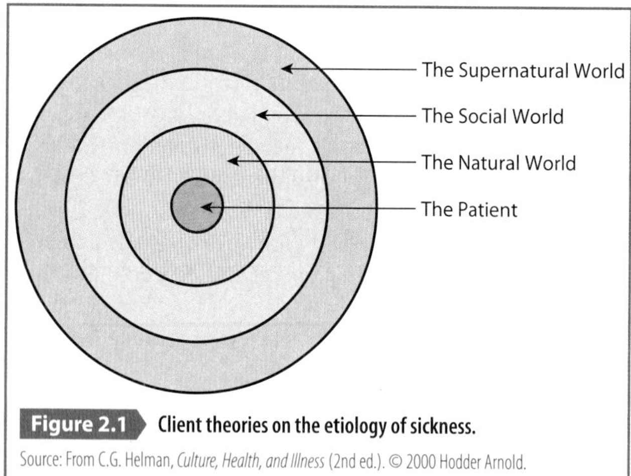

Figure 2.1 Client theories on the etiology of sickness.

Source: From C.G. Helman, *Culture, Health, and Illness* (2nd ed.). © 2000 Hodder Arnold.

Sickness Due to the Patient In the etiology of sickness, the first symptoms that develop within the individual patient are usually attributed to a person's constitution. It is thought that each individual has a genetic (physical or psychological) vulnerability to illness or disease. A person in the United States may be blamed for a heart attack if he is overweight, eats fatty foods, smokes tobacco, and does not exercise. A person who fails to wear a seat belt and then is injured in an auto accident may also be found at fault. Responsibility for sickness falls primarily on the patient, although in many other cultures when a person's actions are unfavorable to health, it is outside forces that are thought to cause an illness or accident in retaliation for the offense.

Sickness Due to the Natural World Etiology in the natural world includes environmental elements such as the weather, allergens, smoke, pollution, and toxins. Viruses, bacteria, and parasites are natural biological agents of sickness. Wind or bad air is of particular concern in many cultural groups, including some Arabs, Chinese, Italians, Filipinos, and Mexicans, because it can enter the body through pores, orifices, or wounds in the body, causing illness. Humoral systems, which associate various body humors with natural elements (as described previously), connect illness and disease with disharmony in the environment. Astrology, which determines an individual's fate (including health status) through planetary alignment at the time of birth, is another natural world phenomenon. Injuries due to natural forces, such as lightning or falling rocks, are sometimes categorized with this group; however, many cultures believe such accidents are the result of the supernatural injunction.

Food for Thought

Regarding the 1918 influenza epidemic, the *New York Post* reported misinformation that epidemics are the punishment nature inflicts for the violation of her laws and ordinances. This outdated belief can still carry over to the current culture.[47]

Fear of the evil eye is mentioned in Talmudic writings, the Bible, and the Qur'an. The concept of protecting yourself and loved from the evil eye is found all over the world.

Sickness Due to the Social World Sickness attributed to social causes occurs around interpersonal conflict within a community. It is common to blame an enemy for pain and suffering. Inadvertent or purposeful malice is the source of illness and disease in many cultures. Among the most common causes is the evil eye.

The evil eye is when an individual stares at a person with envy, resulting in harm to that person even if the gaze is unintentional. Belief in the evil eye is widely held in parts of Africa, Asia, Europe, Greece and the Middle East, India, Latin America, and some areas of the United States. Children are believed to be vulnerable to the evil eye, resulting in colic, crying, hiccups, cramps, convulsions, and seizures. Among adults, the evil eye can cause headaches, malaise, complications in pregnancy and birth, impotence and sterility in men, and insanity. Protections against the evil eye include such practices as placing a red bag filled with herbs on an infant's crib in Guatemala; knotting black or red string around children's wrists in India; leaving children unwashed (making them less admirable) in Iran; wearing a charm in the form of a black hand (mano negro) in Puerto Rico; and painting a house white and blue to blend with the sky, thus avoiding notice, in Greece. Eastern European Jews wear a red string; Sephardic Jews wear a blue string. In Scotland, a fragment of the Bible is kept on the body, and in Muslim areas of Southeast Asia, a piece of the Koran is worn.[12]

Conjury, invoking supernatural forces, is considered to be another frequent social cause of sickness. A person with these powers can direct illness or injury toward an individual, or sell the magic charms or substances necessary for a normal person to inflict harm. Conjury is practiced by witches (called brujos or brujas in Spanish), sorcerers, root doctors, herb doctors, voodoo or hoodoo doctors (refer to Chapter 8, "Africans"), underworld men, and conjure men, most of whom obtain their powers from the devil or other evil spirit. For example, a conjurer might sprinkle graveyard dust under a person's feet, causing him to waste away, known as fading in rural African American tradition. A bundle of sticks placed in the kitchen will cause illness in people who consume food prepared there. A brujo can cause illness in Latinx people through contagious magic, using bits of a person's hair or fingernails when casting a spell. Native American conjury often uses animals or natural phenomena (such as lightning) to attack a person or causes natural objects to be inserted into the body, resulting in pain. The bewitched Native American may behave in inexplicable, disruptive ways and may be abandoned by the community if considered incurable and unable to change undesirable conduct.[12] There is often an overlap between sickness attributed to the social world and that caused by supernatural forces.

Sickness Due to the Supernatural World In the supernatural realm, sickness is caused by the actions of gods, spirits, or the ghosts of ancestors. The will of God is thought to be a prominent factor in illness and disease suffered by many Jews, Christians, and Muslims. Sickness is sometimes considered a punishment for the violation of religious covenants, and at other times, it is viewed as simply a part of God's unknowable plan for humanity. Even those persons who do not follow a specific faith may ascribe illness to fate, luck, or an act of God. Some Africans, Asians, Latinos, Middle Easterners, Native Americans, and residents of Oceania believe that malevolent spirits can attack a person, causing illness. For example, among Cambodians, death can occur when the nightmare spirit immobilizes a person by sitting on his or her chest and causing extreme fright.[48] In other situations, spirit possession takes place. An evil spirit inhabits the body of a person who then exhibits aberrant behavior, such as incoherent speech or extreme withdrawal. Many Southeast Asians associate caretaker spirits with body organs and life forces that may desert a person when angered or frightened, leaving that individual vulnerable to sickness. In addition, the ghosts of ancestors usually protect their living relatives from harm but may inflict pain and illness when ignored or insulted.

A common idea about the cause of sickness in several cultures is soul loss, when the soul detaches from a person's body, usually due to emotional distress or spirit possession. The symptoms typically include general malaise, listlessness, depression, a feeling of suffocation, or weight loss. If left untreated, soul loss can lead to more serious illness.

Folk Illnesses

Since sickness is culturally sanctioned and explained through culture-specific models, it follows that each culture recognizes different disorders. Certain symptoms, complaints, and behavioral changes are associated with specific conditions and are termed folk illnesses or culture-bound syndromes. Examples of such sicknesses are not uncommon, such as cases of soul loss experienced by some Asians, Latinx (who call it susto or espanto), Native Americans, residents of Oceania, and Southeast Asians. Muso, experienced by young Samoan women as a mental illness, and sudden unexpected nocturnal death syndrome (SUNDS) suffered by Cambodians (refer to the previous section, "Sickness Due to the Supernatural World") are examples of folk illness ascribed to evil spirits. Strong emotions, particularly fright or anger, cause many folk conditions, such as stroke precipitated in bilis or colera in some Guatemalans, the cooling of the blood and organs in ceeb, or when frightened, among the Hmong, or the stomach and chest pain of hwabyung in some Koreans. Psychological distress is often expressed through somatic complaints in some cultures; for instance, an Asian Indian may present symptoms of extreme stress as burning on the soles of the feet, or a depressed Asian Indian man may experience that as a loss of semen.

Diet-related folk illnesses are common. High and low blood pressure among some African Americans are examples. Depending on the cultural group, imbalance in the digestive system results in numbness of the extremities (si zhi ma mu) in some Chinese; nausea and the feeling of a wad of food stuck in the stomach (empacho) among Mexicans; and paralysis in some Puerto Ricans (pasmo). Disordered eating such as, anorexia nervosa (a fear of being fat and failure to maintain body weight resulting in a weight 15 percent or more below that recommended) and bulimia nervosa (binge eating followed by the use of self-induced vomiting, laxatives, enemas, or medications to reduce calorie intake, or the use of excessive exercise or fasting) are sometimes described as a culture-bound syndrome in the United States and other Westernized nations. These illnesses are associated with issues such as the drive to thinness, body image, maturity, and control. However, eating disorders are on the rise in Arab and Asian countries in conjunction with industrialization, urbanization, and globalization.[49] In the case of anorexia, it is usually the biomedical culture that identifies the symptoms as a disease state. Many anorectics do not consider themselves ill or in need of medical intervention. Such differences in the definition of sickness account for why some conditions, such as anorexia or other folk illnesses, are difficult to cure with biomedical approaches. Effective treatment of many sicknesses depends on the agreement between the patient, the therapist, and the practitioner regarding how the illness has occurred, the meaning of the symptoms, and how the sickness is healed.[49]

Healing Practices

Biomedical health professionals attempt to diagnose and cure the structural and functional abnormalities found in patients' organs or systems. In contrast, healing addresses the experience of illness, alleviating the infirmities of the sick patient even when disease is not evident. Healing responds to the personal, familial, and social issues surrounding sickness.

Seeking Care

When sickness occurs, a person must make choices regarding healing. Professional biomedical care, if available, is usually initiated when the onset of symptoms is acute or an injury is serious. Nearly all cultural groups recognize the value of biomedicine in emergencies.

Choice of care often depends on the patient's view of the illness in cases when the sickness is not life-threatening. In these situations, home remedies are generally the first treatment applied.[50] Therapies may be determined by the patient alone or in consultation with family members, friends, or acquaintances. If the remedies are ineffective, if other people encourage further care, or if the individual experiences continued disruption of work, social obligations, or personal relationships, professional advice may be sought. The type of healer chosen depends on factors such as availability, cost, previous care experiences, referrals by relatives or friends, and how the patient perceives the problem. If the patient suffers from a folk illness, a folk healer may be sought immediately because biomedical professionals are considered ignorant about such conditions. Otherwise, biomedical care may be undertaken, independently or simultaneously with other approaches. In chronic or recurrent sickness, biomedical, traditional Chinese medicine, and spiritual approaches would be attempted concurrently. The use of multiple approaches is particularly common when there are concerns that a condition is culture-specific.[51,52]

Research suggests that large numbers of Americans obtain health care outside the biomedical system for minor and major illnesses.[53-55] As many as one-third to one-half of patients with intractable conditions (e.g., back pain, chronic renal failure, arthritis, insomnia, headache, depression, gastrointestinal problems), terminal illnesses such as cancer or acquired immune deficiency syndrome (AIDS), and disordered eating seek unconventional treatment. Nearly all do so without the recommendation of their biomedical doctor, integrating multiple therapies on their own. This is partly due to access to biomedical systems for the uninsured or minimally insured. Economic inequality and increasing health disparities in health outcomes help drive the demand for alternative health care. Researchers report these and other inequalities lead the life expectancy of the wealthiest Americans to be 10–15 years longer than the financially disadvantaged population.[56]

Biomedicine is rejected by some people because their experience with care has been impersonal, costly, inconvenient, or inaccessible. Further, conventional treatments may have been painful or harmful. Some clients believe that biomedical professionals are hostile or uninterested in ethnic health issues.[55] Health care professionals may disregard the patients' explanations as to the cause of the health problem or dismiss their complaints as clinically insignificant. Folk healers and other alternative practitioners can provide an understanding of an illness within the context of the patient's worldview and can offer care beyond the cure of disease, including sincere sympathy and renewed hope.

Healing Therapies

There is no consensus concerning the classification of what is called unconventional, alternative, or folk medical care. Home remedies (e.g., herbal teas, megavitamins, relaxation techniques), popular therapies (e.g., chiropractic, homeopathy,

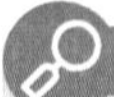

Cultural Controversy

Botanical Remedies

More than 80 percent of the world's population uses herbal remedies to treat illness and optimize health. Technically, a herbal medicine contains only leafy plants that do not have a woody stem. A more comprehensive term is *botanical*, including all therapeutic parts of all plants, from the root (e.g., ginseng), bark (e.g., willow), sap (e.g., from aloe), gum (e.g., frankincense), oil (e.g., from nutmeg), flowers (e.g., echinacea), seeds (e.g., gingko biloba), to the fruit (e.g., bilberries). Botanical remedies often use the whole plant, which practitioners claim is superior to using a single active extract because other components in the plant may work together synergistically in the preparation to enhance the therapeutic value and to buffer any side effects. For this same reason, plants are often combined in formulary mixtures, particularly in traditional Chinese medicine.

Consumers selecting botanical remedies often do so instead of biomedicine because they believe they are safer and more effective than prescription drugs or they are treating chronic conditions for which biomedicine has little to offer in the way of relief. Some proponents note that botanicals have been used for centuries and that reported deaths each year number in only the hundreds, while it is well-known and reported in the United States that prescription medications can cause adverse problems, especially among older adults[57,58] who often use multiple medications (polypharmacy). Polypharmacy has been linked to a broad range of dangerous health outcomes, including falls, frailty, and mortality. The key word regarding botanicals, however, is *reported*. The Dietary Supplement Health and Education Act (DSHEA) passed by Congress in 1994 defines dietary supplements as separate from food and drugs and thus outside the scope of federal monitoring. Manufacturers are exempt from regulations requiring that complaints, injuries, or deaths due to the consumption of their product be documented at the Food and Drug Administration (FDA). Though the FDA retains the right to protect the public from harmful products, the burden of proof is on the government to prove that a particular botanical remedy is unsafe. Many manufacturers have voluntarily adopted good manufacturing processes, and the American Herbal Products Association has created a botanical safety rating system that classifies herbs as (1) safe when consumed appropriately; (2) restricted for certain uses; (3) use only under the supervision of an expert; and (4) insufficient data to make a safety classification.

Unfortunately, the explosive, unregulated growth of the industry has resulted in numerous problems. Of particular concern is the interaction of botanicals when used with biomedical therapies. For example, ginkgo biloba reduces the effectiveness of some prescription drugs, such as certain antacids and antianxiety medications, while potentiating others, including anticoagulants, antidepressants, and antipsychotics.[59] Some botanicals can react adversely with anesthesia, and others can interact with radiation therapy.[60] Further, natural products can be adulterated with pesticides, heavy metals (such as mercury), or prescription drugs (such as warfarin or alprazolam).[61]

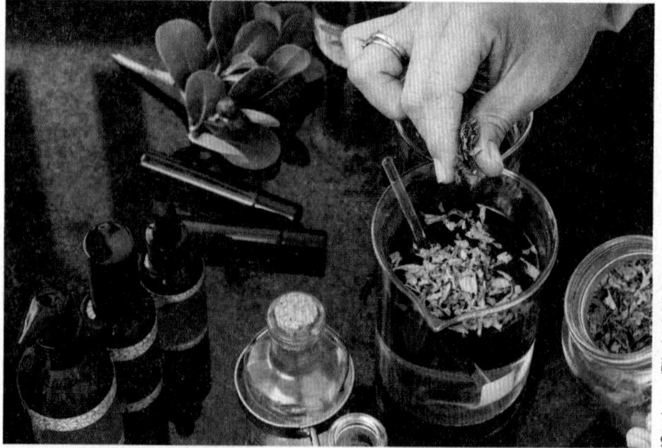

iStock.com/ElizabethAllnutt

▲ Common botanical tinctures.

hypnosis, massage), and professional practices (i.e., those that require extensive academic training in conventionally recognized medical systems, such as biomedicine, traditional Chinese medicine, and Ayurvedic medicine) include a variety of treatments that fall into three broad categories: (1) administration of therapeutic substances; (2) application of physical forces or devices; and (3) magico-religious interventions.[62] Most patients use unconventional therapies without the supervision of a biomedical doctor or any other kind of health care provider. Popular and professional practitioners, when consulted, may use one or several of these treatments in healing a patient.

Administration of Therapeutic Substances Biomedical medication and diet prescriptions are two of the most common types of therapeutics in this category, which also includes over-the-counter medications, health food preparations, prepackaged diet meals, as well as vitamins and mineral supplements. In a 2019 Harris Poll, 86% of Americans take vitamins or supplements. Of this group, only 24% indicated that they had received test results indicating that they had a deficiency.[63] Home remedies and health practitioners other than biomedical professionals often emphasize the use of botanical medicine, which includes whole plants or pieces (particularly herbs), and occasionally animal parts, such as antlers or organs, or certain powdered mineral elements. In many cultures, healers specialize in the use of herbal preparations; often they are elder men or women with intimate knowledge of the natural environment. Root doctors in the American South and the proprietors of botánicas (herbal pharmacies) found in some Latinx neighborhoods are a few examples. In addition to folk healing, both traditional Chinese medicine and Ayurvedic medicine make extensive use of botanical medicine (refer to the chapters on each American ethnic group for more details).

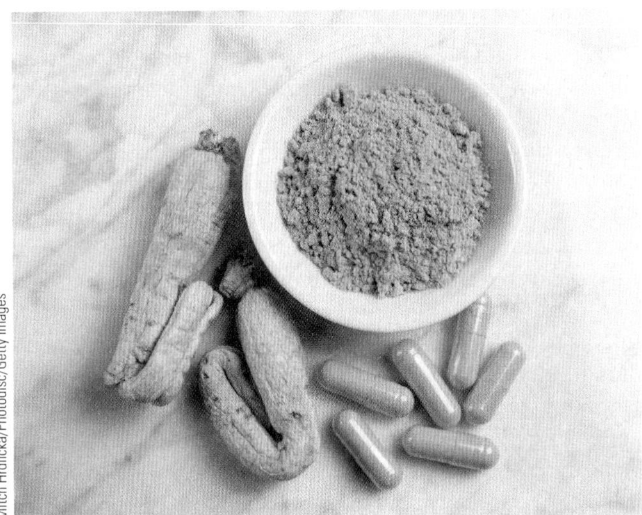
Mitch Hrdlicka/Photodisc/Getty Images

▲ Ginseng, a root found in both North America and Asia, is one of the top ten common herbal remedies used in the United States. It reputedly promotes health through increased strength and vitality, and may be taken specifically to treat digestive upset, anxiety, or sexual impotence.

Homeopathy also prescribes therapeutic substances, such as botanical medicine, diluted venom, bacterial solutions, and biomedical drugs. Originating in Germany, homeopathy is based on the concept that symptoms in illness are evidence that the body is curing itself, and acceleration or exaggeration of the symptoms speeds healing. Naturopathic medicine also focuses on helping the body heal itself, usually through noninvasive natural treatments (including some physical manipulations, as the following section describes), although biomedical drugs and surgery are used in certain cases. Nutritional therapy, based on whole foods and dietary supplements, is the foundation of naturopathic health maintenance and healing.

 **Food for Thought**

Forty percent of pharmacy drugs in Western nations are derived from plants that people have used for centuries, including the top 20 prescription drugs today.[64]

Medications using digitalis, opiates, and salicylates, common today as biomedical therapeutics, were first used by folk healers.

Application of Physical Forces or Devices Manipulations of the body is based on the premise that internal body function improves with adjustments to its physical structure. Chiropractic theory states that misalignments of the spine interfere with the nervous system, interrupting the natural intelligence that regulates the body, resulting in disease and disorder. Osteopathic medicine proposes that blood and lymph flow, as well as nerve function, improves through manipulation of the musculoskeletal system, particularly the correction of posture problems, mobilization of bone joints, and spine alignment. Health problems are treated through the restoration of mobility and improved flexibility.

Several Asian healing therapies can be classified as the application of physical forces or devices. Massage therapy, acupressure, and pinching or scratching techniques are used to release the vital energy flow through the twelve meridians of the body identified in traditional Chinese medicine and in Ayurvedic energy points, which work primarily by relieving primarily by relieving muscle tension so that oxygen and nutrients can be delivered to organs and wastes removed. Coining is a related practice in which a coin or spoon is rubbed across the skin instead of pressing or pinching specific points. Acupuncture is similar to acupressure in that it attempts to restore the balance of vital energy in the body along the meridians, but it differs in that it stimulates specific junctures through the insertion of nine types of very fine needles. The needles do not cause bleeding or pain. Acupuncture is considered useful in correcting conditions where too much heat (yang) is present in the body. In conditions of too much cold (yin), another technique is preferred, called moxibustion, in which a small burning bundle of herbs (e.g., wormwood) or a smoldering cigarette is touched to specific locations on the meridians to restore the balance of energy. A similar method is cupping—the placement of a heated cup or a cup with a scrap of burning paper in it over the meridian points.[65]

The application of electricity is used in various electrotherapies, primarily to stimulate muscle or bone healing, especially in sports medicine. Biofeedback also uses small electric pulses to teach a person how to consciously monitor and control normally involuntary body functions, such as skin temperature and blood pressure, to alleviate health problems, which include insomnia, gastrointestinal conditions, and chronic pain. Hydrotherapy involves the application of baths, showers, whirlpools, saunas, steam rooms, and poultices to relieve the discomforts of back pain, muscle tension, arthritis, hypertension, cirrhosis of the liver, asthma, bronchitis, and head colds. In addition to the hydrotherapeutic qualities, the mineral content of the water is considered stimulating.

Magico-Religious Interventions Spiritual healing practices are associated with nearly all religions. They typically fall into two divisions: those actions taken by the individual and those taken on behalf of the individual by a sacred healer.

In Western religious traditions, God has power over life and death. Sickness represents a breach between humans and God. Healing is interrelated with salvation because both mend broken ties. Living according to God's will is necessary to prevent illness, and prayer is the most common method of seeking God's help in healing. Roman Catholics, for example, make appeals to the saints identified with certain afflictions—St. Teresa of Avila for headaches, St. Peregrine for cancer, St. John of God for heart disease, St. Joseph for terminal illness, and St. Bruno for cases of possession are just a few examples. Pilgrimages to the shrines of these saints are made for special petitions. In Eastern religions, health is determined mostly by correct conduct in this and past lives, as well as in the virtuous behavior of ancestors. Religious offerings are made regularly; for instance, Hindus choose a personal deity to worship daily at a home shrine. Improper actions leading to disharmony within a person, family, community, or the supernatural realm can cause sickness. Healing occurs through the restoration of balance, often including offerings to the deities or spirits of the living and dead who have been offended.[66,67]

Food for Thought

Naturopathic doctors trained in the United States attend a four-year program including the study of many biomedical disciplines. Doctors of chiropractic (DC) are the third largest category of health care practitioners in the United States, following physicians and dentists. Osteopaths are licensed to prescribe medications and perform surgery as doctors of osteopathy (DO) in all 50 states.

Spa therapy is popular throughout Europe, particularly in Germany.

Individual healing practices developed out of religious ritual include meditation, a contemplative process of focus; yoga, the control of breathing and use of systematic body poses to restrain the functions of the mind and promote mind–body unity; and visualization or guided imagery, induced relaxation and targeted willing away of health problems. Each concentrates the power of the mind on reducing health risks, such as stress, high blood pressure, and decreased immune response, or on alleviating specific medical conditions. Hypnotherapy works similarly; although it is generally done with the aid of a hypnotherapist, self-hypnosis can be learned for personal use.

In many cases, the spiritual skills of the individual are inadequate for the problem, and the help of a sacred healer is sought. These health practitioners generally work through interventions with the supernatural world, which may include prayers, blessings, chanting or singing, charms, and conjuring, as well as the use of therapeutic substances (e.g., herbal remedies) and application of physical cures (e.g., the laying on of hands). Faith healers, most of whom get their healing gifts from God, are common among many Christian groups. Some are affiliated with certain denominations and rites, such as the Cajun *traiteurs* of Louisiana, who specialize in treating one or two ailments through prayers and charms associated with Catholicism.[68,69] Others, such as the sympathy healers of the Pennsylvania Dutch who practice powwowing (also known by the German name *Brauche* or *Braucherei*), are considered the direct instruments of God.[70]

Food for Thought

Eighty percent of respondents in a study on faith and healing in the southeastern United States said they believe God acts through physicians to cure illness.[71,72]

Persons with a spiritual calling are often employed to treat illness. *Neng* among the Hmong, Mexican *curanderos* (or *curanderas*), practitioners of Voodoo in the American South, and *espiritos* or *santeros* (or *santeras*) in the Caribbean may communicate with the spirits or saints to heal their patients. Ceremonial invocation is the primary therapy, although charms and spells to counteract witchcraft and botanical preparations to ease physical complaints are used as well.

Shamans, called medicine men or women, or other-gendered "two spirit" people among many Native American groups, are sacred healers with exceptional powers. It is thought that shamanism originated perhaps 20,000 years ago among the hunting and gathering cultures in northern Asia and the Ural-Altaic and spread throughout the world. Typically, shamanism describes the combined role of healer, religious leader, and counselor in indigenous cultures of the Americas, Southeast Asia, Indonesia, Polynesia, and Australia. Remote tribal groups found in Africa, India, and Korea have similar healers. The shaman position is passed on from

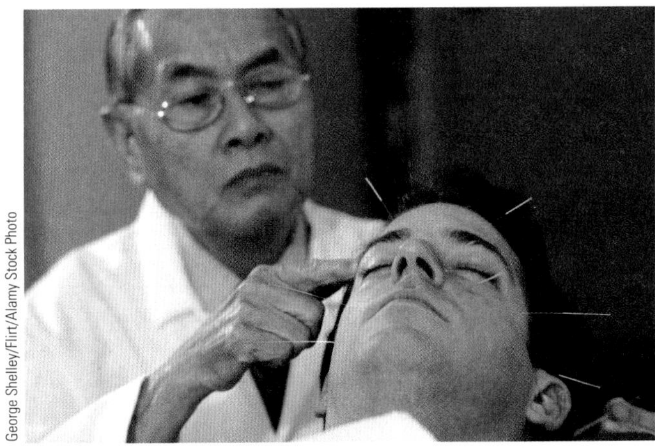

George Shelley/Flirt/Alamy Stock Photo

▲ **Acupuncture attempts to restore the balance of vital energy in the body through inserting and manipulating very thin needles at strategic points.**

generation to generation, or through a calling that could include fainting spells or convulsive fits due to attacks by spirits. Shamans typically complete lengthy apprenticeships and are initiated through a series of trials simulating death and rebirth. In shamanic systems, sickness is due to a spiritual crisis, and healing emphasizes the strengthening of the soul through redirection of the life forces or, in cases of serious illness, retrieval of the soul, which may have been stolen by evil spirits. Shamanic practices include visualization techniques to create harmony between the patient and the universe, singing, chanting, predictions, dream analysis, and séances. Shamans are often expert herbalists.[73]

Pluralistic Health Care Systems

The enduring popularity of traditional health beliefs and practices is consistent with cultural beliefs. Healing sickness, with or without the services of an expert provider, takes place according to a patient's worldview. Humans value what validates their beliefs and discount anything that differs, regardless of statistical data or scientific claims; they give disproportionate authority to persons they like and respect.

Food for Thought

A study of physician beliefs about health and religion found that although 91 percent of respondents said knowledge of a client's faith practices is important in care, only 32 percent ask about religious affiliation.[74]

When Navajos dream frequently of death, it is usually considered a sign of serious illness.

Consultation with a Native American medicine man or woman may take hours to complete; some healing ceremonies take a week to perform and may cost thousands of dollars.[75]

Medical Pluralism

Medical pluralism is the term for the consecutive or concurrent use of multiple health care systems Although it is often assumed that specific ethnic groups, those with lower incomes, the less educated, or recent immigrants are most likely to rely on traditional folk medicine, studies report that the use of healers in some groups increases with education and income level. Further, acculturation is not associated with a rise in the use of biomedical services.[76,77] Medical pluralism is widespread in the United States.

Biomedical Healing

Clients using traditional health practices are generally seeking to alleviate the difficulties experienced in illness through understandable, flexible, and convenient treatment from a warm and caring provider. The personal relationship with the healer is as important as the actual therapy (refer to Chapter 3).

Studies suggest that some unconventional therapies are effective, benefiting the patient physiologically or psychologically, and should be accepted as complementary to biomedical approaches.[78-80] Cooperative monitoring by a biomedical professional can also detect those instances when a home remedy or popular practice is harmful to the patient. Furthermore, biomedical health care providers can adopt certain healing strategies. Understanding the patient's perspective on illness and attending to differences in the patient–provider relationship is one approach.[10] Recommending alternate, experimental biomedical programs in cases of advanced chronic disease is another. A more comprehensive methodology is offered through transcultural nursing theory, developed to provide culturally compatible care that is beneficial, satisfying, and meaningful to clients. This approach identifies three modes of effective care: (1) cultural care preservation and/or maintenance; (2) cultural care accommodation and/or negotiation; and (3) cultural care repatterning or restructuring.[81]

Cultural care preservation and/or maintenance is used when a traditional health belief or practice is known to be beneficial in its effect and is encouraged by the provider. Cultural care accommodation and/or negotiation is accomplished between the provider and the patient (or the patient's family) when there is an expectation for care that is outside the biomedical convention. Cultural care repatterning or restructuring occurs when both provider and patient agree that a habit is harmful to health, and a cooperative plan is developed to introduce a new and different lifestyle. Applied to food habits, the culture care theory acknowledges that some traditional beliefs and practices regarding diet have beneficial or neutral consequences, some have unknown consequences, and some may be deleterious to the health of a client (refer to Chapter 1).

In addition to specific provider approaches, the health care setting can also help promote biomedical healing through services desired by clients in a comfortable, welcoming atmosphere. Some health care organizations are forming therapeutic alliances with community folk healers or combining non-Western practices with biomedicine in an integrative approach. At a minimum, research on traditional practices used by clients and information about alternative community health resources should be available to providers; staff should be encouraged to keep up on current trends through continuing education, diversity training, and refresher workshops. Other useful steps include increasing care accessibility by taking education and services into client communities when possible and providing flexible, nontraditional hours for appointments. Clients also feel more at ease with a staff representative of the community, so to some degree, this preference should be accommodated.[82,83] Successful biomedical healing is dependent on the intercultural knowledge and sensitivity of the health provider and setting. Care must be undertaken in cooperation with the patient, as well as the patient's family and any concurrent traditional providers in use by the patient. Healing should not be the sole domain of home remedies, popular health care approaches, or alternative medical systems. Medical pluralism offers the opportunity for biomedicine to heal sickness through coordinated client care, with an understanding and appreciation for the therapeutic value of traditional health beliefs and practices.

Discussion Starters

What is Your "Worldview" of Health Care?

Culture determines how each of us defines health, recognizes illness, and considers the medical treatment of illness. Reflecting on how we view health and health care can tell us a lot about our cultures. Answer each of the following questions. Don't worry about justifying your beliefs. All you want to do here is reflect on and write down your beliefs. There are no right or wrong answers, as long as the answers honestly express your beliefs.

- **Which most determines a person's health:** The decisions and actions of the person herself or himself? The decisions and actions of one's family and others with whom one has been brought up? The decisions and actions of the government (whether national or local or both)? The will of God? The actions of some other supernatural agency (please identify)? Astrological alignment of the stars and planets? Karma? Fate? Something else?
- **Who is most responsible for a person's health care:** The health care practitioner? The person herself or himself (or, if a child, the parents or adult caregivers)? Someone else?
- **If you became seriously ill or injured and needed dramatic treatment, such as surgery or radiation treatment, who would most influence your decision(s) regarding that treatment:** You alone? Your family? Your church, synagogue, tabernacle, temple, mosque, or other religious congregation? Others?
- **If a loved one is terminally ill—that is, dying from a disease or injury—which of the following would be most important to you:** Trying everything possible to cure your loved one or at least, prolonging that loved one's life? Doing everything possible to relieve any pain that a loved one might be enduring? Praying with that loved one and sustaining her or his faith? Helping your loved one die in a way that she or he wants, which could involve *not* employing life-sustaining measures?
- **Which of the following is the most important way you tell whether you are healthy or not:** By whether or not you have any symptoms of disease? By whether or not you can accomplish daily tasks and meet daily responsibilities? By how you look in the mirror and/or how others perceive how you look?

In small groups of three or four, compare answers for about 10 minutes. Restrain any impulse to criticize. Your task is to gather as much information as possible about each person's worldview relating to health care in the short time that you have. Remember, there are no right or wrong answers. Different cultures exhibit different worldviews.

When members of your group have completed sharing answers, individually write a reflection on what you've learned and how you feel about it (maximum one page).

Review Questions

1. If you become ill, how might your worldview influence your expectations about your illness and its treatment?
2. How does biomedicine in the United States reflect the majority culture?
3. How does the U.S. biomedicine definition of *health* differ from that of the World Health Organization: "a state of complete physical, mental, and social well-being"?
4. Describe three ways that diet may be used to promote or maintain health, using specific examples of foods and practices.
5. What is meant by *folk illnesses* or *culture-bound syndromes*? Using one example, explain how effective treatment for the condition would differ from the conventional biomedical approach.

Reflection

Reflect on your own philosophy of medical care. Do you subscribe to traditional biomedical viewpoints or do you prefer use of complimentary and alternative medicine (CAM) for your own care. Are there certain ailments or symptoms that you choose biomedical care exclusively for treatment? When is CAM most appropriate for you or a family member?

References

1. Lindquist, R., Tracy, M.F., & Snyder, M. (Eds.) 2018. *Complementary and alternative therapies in nursing*. Springer Publishing Company.

2. Nahin, R.L., Barnes, P.M., Stussman, B.J., & Bloom, B. 2009. *Costs of complementary and alternative medicine (CAM) and frequency of visits to CAM practitioners: United States, 2007*. CDC National Health Statistics Report #18.
3. Inbadas, H. 2016. History, culture and traditions: The silent spaces in the study of spirituality at the end of life. *Religions*, 7(5), 53.
4. Suprina, J.S., Matthews, C.H., Kakkar, S., Harrell, D., Brace, A., Sadler-Gerhardt, C., Kocet, M.M., & Association for Lesbian, Gay, Bisexual, and Transgender Issues in Counseling (ALGBTIC). 2019. Best practices in cross-cultural counseling: The intersection of spiritual/religious identity and affectional/sexual identity. *Journal of LGBT Issues in Counseling*, 13(4), 293–325.
5. Pedersen, P.B., Lonner, W.J., Draguns, J.G., Trimble, J.E., & Scharron-del Rio, M.R. (Eds.). 2015. *Counseling across cultures*. Sage Publications.
6. Yankelovich, Inc. 2006. Food for life study. In *The Yankelovich MONITOR*. Chapel Hill, NC.
7. Gysels, M., Evans, N., Meñaca, A.E.A., Toscani, F., Finetti, S., Pasman, H. R., Higginson, I., Harding, R., & Pool, R. 2020. Culture and end of life care: A scoping exercise in seven European countries. *The Ethical Challenges of Emerging Medical Technologies*, 335–350.
8. Boucher, N.A. 2016. Direct engagement with communities and interprofessional learning to factor culture into end-of-life health care delivery. *American Journal of Public Health*, *106*(6), 996–1001.
9. McCalman, J., Jongen, C., & Bainbridge, R. 2017. Organisational systems' approaches to improving cultural competence in healthcare: A systematic scoping review of the literature. *International Journal for Equity in Health*, 16(1), 1–19.
10. Jeffreys, M.R. 2015. *Teaching cultural competence in nursing and health care: Inquiry, action, and innovation*. Springer Publishing Company.
11. Curtis, E., Jones, R., Tipene-Leach, D., Walker, C., Loring, B., Paine, S.J., & Reid, P. 2019. Why cultural safety rather than cultural competency is required to achieve health equity: A literature review and recommended definition. *International Journal for Equity in Health*, 18(1), 174. https://doi.org/10.1186/s12939-019-1082-3
12. Spector, R.E. 2017. *Cultural diversity in health and illness* (9th ed.). Upper Saddle River, NJ: Pearson.
13. Leininger, M.M. 1991. Becoming aware of types of health practitioners and cultural imposition. *Journal of Transcultural Nursing*, 2, 36.
14. Purnell, L.D. 2016. The Purnell model for cultural competence. In *Intervention in Mental Health-Substance Use* (pp. 57–78). CRC Press.
15. Tan, S.S.L., & Goonawardene, N. 2017. Internet health information seeking and the patient-physician relationship: A systematic review. *Journal of Medical Internet Research*, 19(1), e5729.
16. Statista. 2020. Size of the anti-aging market worldwide from 2020 to 2026. Retrieved from https://www.statista.com/statistics/509679/value-of-the-global-anti-aging-market/ (accessed May 10, 2022).
17. Braun, U.K., Beyth, R.J., Ford, M.E., & McCullough, L.B. 2008. Voices of African American, Caucasian and Hispanic surrogates on the burdens of end-of-life decision making. *Journal of General Internal Medicine*, 23, 267–274.
18. Choi, E., Chentsova-Dutton, Y., & Parrott, W.G. 2016. The effectiveness of somatization in communicating distress in Korean and American cultural contexts. *Frontiers in Psychology*, 7, 383.
19. Zhou, X., Min, S., Sun, J., Kim, S.J., Ahn, J.S., Peng, Y., Noh, S., & Ryder, A.G. 2015. Extending a structural model of somatization to South Koreans: Cultural values, somatization tendency, and the presentation of depressive symptoms. *Journal of Affective Disorders*, 176, 151–154.
20. Ots, T. 1990. The angry liver, the anxious heart and the melancholy spleen: The phenomenology of perceptions in Chinese culture. *Culture, Medicine, and Psychiatry*, 14, 21–58.
21. Karkhanis, D.G., & Winsler, A. 2016. Somatization in children and adolescents: Practical implications. *Journal of Indian Association for Child and Adolescent Mental Health*, 12(1), 79–115.
22. Van der Leeuw, G., Gerrits, M.J., Terluin, B., Numans, M.E., van der Feltz-Cornelis, C. M., van der Horst, H.E., Penninx, B.W.J.H., & van Marwijk, H.W.J. 2015. The association between somatization and disability in primary care patients. *Journal of Psychosomatic Research*, 79(2), 117–122.
23. World Health Organization (WHO). Definition of Health n.d. Retrieved from https://www.publichealth.com.ng/world-omihealth-organizationwho-definition-of-health/ (accessed May 10, 2022).
24. Ceballos, N., & Czyzewska, M. 2010. Body image in Hispanic/Latino vs. European American adolescents: Implications for treatment and prevention of obesity in underserved populations. *Journal of Health Care for the Poor and Underserved*, 21, 823–838.
25. Gracia-Arnaiz, M. 2010. Fat bodies and thin bodies: Cultural, biomedical and market discourses on obesity. *Appetite*, 55, 219–225.
26. Tomiyama, A.J., Carr, D., Granberg, E.M., Major, B., Robinson, E., Sutin, A.R., & Brewis, A. 2018. How and why weight stigma drives the obesity 'epidemic' and harms health. *BMC Medicine*, 16(1), 1–6.
27. Dietz, W.H., Baur, L.A., Hall, K., Puhl, R.M., Taveras, E.M., Uauy, R., & Kopelman, P. 2015. Management of obesity: Improvement of health-care training and systems for prevention and care. *The Lancet*, 385(9986), 2521–2533.
28. Lambert, L.J., Raidl, M., & Safaii, S. Perceptions of barriers to weight loss in overweight WIC women. *Topics in Clinical Nutrition Journal*, January–March 2005 20(1).
29. Contento, I.R., Basch, C., & Zybert, P. 2003. Body image, weight and food choices of Latina women and their young children. *Journal of Nutrition Education and Behavior*, 35, 236–248.
30. Crawford, P.B., Gosliner, W., Anderson, C., Strode, P., Becerra-Jones, Y., Samuels, S., Carroll, A.M., & Ritchie, L.D. 2004. Counseling Latina mothers of preschool children about weight issues: Suggestions for a new framework. *Journal of the American Dietetic Association*, 104, 387.
31. Chaker, Z., Chang, F.M., & Hakim-Larson, J. 2015. Body satisfaction, thin-ideal internalization, and perceived pressure to be thin among Canadian women: The role of acculturation and religiosity. *Body Image*, 14, 85–93.
32. Xanthopoulos, M.S., Borradaile, K.E., Hayes, S., Sherman, S., Vander-Veur, S., Grundy, K.M., Nachmani, J., & Foster, G.D. 2011. The impact of weight, sex, and race/ethnicity on body dissatisfaction among urban children. *Body Image*, 8(4), 385–389.
33. McCullough, M.B., Pieloch, K.A., & Marks, A.K. 2020. Body image, assimilation, and weight of immigrant adolescents in the United States: A person-centered analysis. *Journal of Immigrant and Minority Health*, 22(2), 249–254.
34. Eisenberg, M.E., Puhl, R., Areba, E.M., & Neumark-Sztainer, D. 2019. Family weight teasing, ethnicity and acculturation: Associations with well-being among Latinx, Hmong, and Somali Adolescents. *Journal of Psychosomatic Research*, 122, 88–93.
35. Dotse, J.E., & Asumeng, M. 2015. Relationship between body image satisfaction and psychological well-being: The impact of Africentric values. *Journal of Social Science Studies*, 2(1), 320–342.
36. Smith, J.M., Smith, J.E., McLaughlin, E.A., Belon, K.E., Serier, K.N., Simmons, J.D., Kelton, K., Arroyo, C., & Delaney, H.D. 2020. Body dissatisfaction and disordered eating in Native American, Hispanic, and White college women. *Eating and Weight Disorders-Studies on Anorexia, Bulimia and Obesity*, 25(2), 347–355.
37. Bucchianeri, M.M., Fernandes, N., Loth, K., Hannan, P.J., Eisenberg, M.E., & Neumark-Sztainer, D. 2016. Body dissatisfaction: Do associations with disordered eating and psychological well-being differ across race/ethnicity in adolescent girls and boys? *Cultural Diversity and Ethnic Minority Psychology*, *22*(1), 137.
38. Ford, E.S., & Dietz, W.H. 2013. Trends in energy intake among adults in the United States: Findings from NHANES. *The American Journal of Clinical Nutrition*, 97(4), 848–853. https://doi.org/10.3945/ajcn.112.052662
39. Ahluwalia, N., Dwyer, J., Terry, A., Moshfegh, A., & Johnson, C. 2016. Update on NHANES dietary data: Focus on collection, release, analytical considerations, and uses to inform public policy. *Advances in Nutrition*, 7(1), 121–134.

40. Seo, D.C., Torabi, M.R., Jiang, N., Fernandez-Rojas, X., & Park, B.H. 2009. Cross-cultural comparison of lack of regular physical activity among college students: Universal versus transversal. *International Journal of Behavioral Medicine*, 16, 355–359.
41. Anderson Jr., E.N. 1987. Why is humoral medicine so popular? *Social Science & Medicine*, 25(4), 331–337.
42. Logan, M. 1973. Humoral medicine in Guatemala and peasant acceptance of modern medicine. *Human Organization*, 32(4), 385–396.
43. Foster, G.M. 1987. On the origin of humoral medicine in Latin America. *Medical Anthropology Quarterly*, 1(4), 355–393.
44. Kleinman, A., Eisenberg, L., & Good, B. 2006. Culture, illness and care: Clinical lessons from anthropologic and cross-cultural research. *FOCUS*, 4(1), 140–149.
45. Harmon, B.E., Carter, M., Hurley, T.G., Shivappa, N., Teas, J., & Hébert, J.R. 2015. Nutrient composition and anti-inflammatory potential of a prescribed macrobiotic diet. *Nutrition and Cancer*, 67(6), 933–940.
46. Douglas, M.K., & Pacquiao, D.F. (Eds.). 2010. Core curriculum in transcultural nursing and health care. *Journal of Transcultural Nursing*, 21(Suppl. 1).
47. Garrett, L. 1994. *The coming plague: Newly emerging diseases in a world out of balance*. New York: Farrar, Strauss & Giroux.
48. Adler, S.R. 1995. Refuge stress and folk belief: Hmong sudden deaths. *Social Science and Medicine*, 40, 1623–1629.
49. Hoek, H.W. 2016. Review of the worldwide epidemiology of eating disorders. *Current Opinion in Psychiatry*, 29(6), 336–339.
50. Hand, W.D. 1980. *Magical medicine*. Berkeley: University of California Press.
51. Moorehead, V.D., Gone, J.P., & December, D. 2015. A gathering of Native American healers: Exploring the interface of Indigenous tradition and professional practice. *American Journal of Community Psychology*, 56(3), 383–394.
52. Adekson, M.O. 2016. Similarities and differences between Yoruba traditional healers (YTH) and Native American and Canadian Healers (NACH). *Journal of Religion and Health*, *55*(5), 1717–1728.
53. Asuzu, C.C., Akin-Odanye, E.O., Asuzu, M.C., & Holland, J. 2019. A socio-cultural study of traditional healers role in African health care. *Infectious Agents and Cancer*, 14(1), 1–5.
54. Adorisio, S., Fierabracci, A., Rossetto, A., Muscari, I., Nardicchi, V., Liberati, A.M., Riccardi, C., Sung, T.V., Thuy, T.T., & Delfino, D.V. 2016. Integration of traditional and western medicine in Vietnamese populations: A review of health perceptions and therapies. *Natural Product Communications*, 11(9), 1934578X1601100949.
55. Zhang, J.H., Wu, M.S., Wang, Y.F., Jia, Y.M., & Li, E. 2019. Medicine in future and advantages of integrated Chinese and Western medicine. *Chinese Journal of Integrative Medicine*, 25(2), 87–90.
56. Dickman, S.L., Himmelstein, D.U., & Woolhandler, S. 2017. Inequality and the health-care system in the USA. *The Lancet*, 389(10077), 1431–1441.
57. Wastesson, J.W., Morin, L., Tan, E.C., & Johnell, K. 2018. An update on the clinical consequences of polypharmacy in older adults: A narrative review. *Expert Opinion on Drug Safety*, 17(12), 1185–1196.
58. Pazan, F., & Wehling, M. 2021. Polypharmacy in older adults: A narrative review of definitions, epidemiology and consequences. *European Geriatric Medicine*, 12(3), 443–452.
59. Bressler, R. 2005. Interactions between Gingko biloba and prescription medications. *Geriatrics*, *60*, 30–33.
60. King, A.R., Russett, F.S., Generali, J.A., & Grauer, D.W. 2009. Evaluation and implications of natural product use in preoperative patients: A retrospective review. *BMC Complementary and Alternative Medicine*, 9, 38.
61. Colson, C.R., & De Broe, M.E. 2005. Kidney injury from alternative medicines. *Advances in Chronic Kidney Diseases*, 12, 261–275.
62. Murray, R.H., & Rubel, A.J. 1992. Physicians and healers—Unwitting partners in health care. *New England Journal of Medicine*, 326, 61–64.
63. American Osteopathic Association. 2019. Retrieved from https://osteopathic.org/2019/01/16/poll-finds-86-of-americans-take-vitamins-or-supplements-yet-only-21-have-a-confirmed-nutritional-deficiency/ (accessed May 17, 2022).
64. Editors. "Medicinal botany." United States Department of Agriculture, U.S. Forest Service. Retrieved from https://www.fs.usda.gov/wildflowers/ethnobotany/medicinal/index.shtm
65. Mei, M.F. 2011 A systematic analysis of the theory and practice of syndrome differentiation. *Chinese Journal of Integrative Medicine*, 17, 803–810.
66. Sapkota, N., Shakya, D.R., Adhikari, B.R., Pandey, A.K., & Shyangwa, P.M. 2016. Magico-religious beliefs in schizophrenia: A study from Eastern part of Nepal. *Journal of College of Medical Sciences-Nepal*, 12(4), 150–159.
67. Lang, A., LeMay-Boucher, P., & Tomavo, C.C. 2019. Expenditures on malevolent magico-religious powers: Empirical evidence from Benin. *African Studies Review*, 62(4), 154–180.
68. Sonnier, A. 2020. *Cajun TRAITEURS: Faith HEALING on the Bayou the Cajun Traiteur and transmission of Cajun folk healing knowledge* (Doctoral dissertation, California State University, Northridge).
69. Lanoux, G.M. 2015. *The Traiteur: Giving voice to traditional Cajun healing in Louisiana*. University of Louisiana at Monroe.
70. Donmoyer, P. J. 2018. *Powwowing in Pennsylvania: Braucherei and the ritual of everyday life*. Masthof Press & Pennsylvania German Cultural Heritage Center, Kutztown University.
71. Chibnall, J.T., & Brooks, C.A. 2001. Religion in the clinic: The role of physician beliefs. *Southern Medical Journal*, 94, 374–379.
72. Soto-Espinosa, J., & Koss-Chioino, J.D. 2017. Doctors who integrate spirituality and CAM in the clinic: The Puerto Rican case. *Journal of Religion and Health*, 56(1), 149–157.
73. Drury, N. 2019. *The shaman and the magician: Journeys between the worlds* (Vol. 1). Routledge.
74. Gurley, D., Novins, D.K., Jones, M.C., Beals, J., Shore, J.H., & Manson, S.M. 2001. Comparative use of biomedical services and traditional healing options by American Indian veterans. *Psychiatric Services*, 52, 68–74.
75. Mansfield, C.J. 2002. The doctor as God's mechanic? Beliefs in the southeastern United States. *Social Science & Medicine*, 54, 399–409.
76. Marion, L., Douglas, M., Lavin, M.A., Barr, N., Gazaway, S., Thomas, E., & Bickford, C. 2016. Implementing the new ANA standard 8: Culturally congruent practice. *Online Journal of Issues in Nursing*, 22(1).
77. Darnell, L.K., & Hickson, S.V. 2015. Cultural competent patient-centered nursing care. *Nursing Clinics*, 50(1), 99–108.
78. Oh, B., Butow, P., Mullan, B., Beale, P., Pavlakis, N., Rosenthal, D., & Clarke S. 2010. The use and perceived benefits resulting from the use of complementary and alternative medicine by cancer patients in Australia. *Asia-Pacific Journal of Clinical Oncology*, 6, 342–349.
79. Lunny, C.A., & Fraser, S.N. 2010, July. The use of complementary and alternative medicines among a sample of Canadian menopausal-aged women. *Journal of Midwifery and Women's Health*, 55(4), 335–343.
80. Murthy, V., Sibbritt, D.W., & Adams, J. 2015. An integrative review of complementary and alternative medicine use for back pain: A focus on prevalence, reasons for use, influential factors, self-perceived effectiveness, and communication. *The Spine Journal*, 15(8), 1870–1883.
81. McFarland, M.R., & Wehbe-Alamah, H.B. 2018. *Leininger's Transcultural Nursing: Concepts, Theories, Research and Practice*. McGraw Hill Education.
82. Kaptchuk, T.J., & Millar, F.G. 2005. Viewpoint: What is the best and most ethical model for the relationship between mainstream and alternative medicine: Opposition, integration, or pluralism? *Academic Medicine*, 80, 286–290.
83. Yehieli, M., & Grey, M.A. 2005. *Health matters: A pocket guide for working with diverse cultures and underserved populations*. Yarmouth, ME: Intercultural Press.

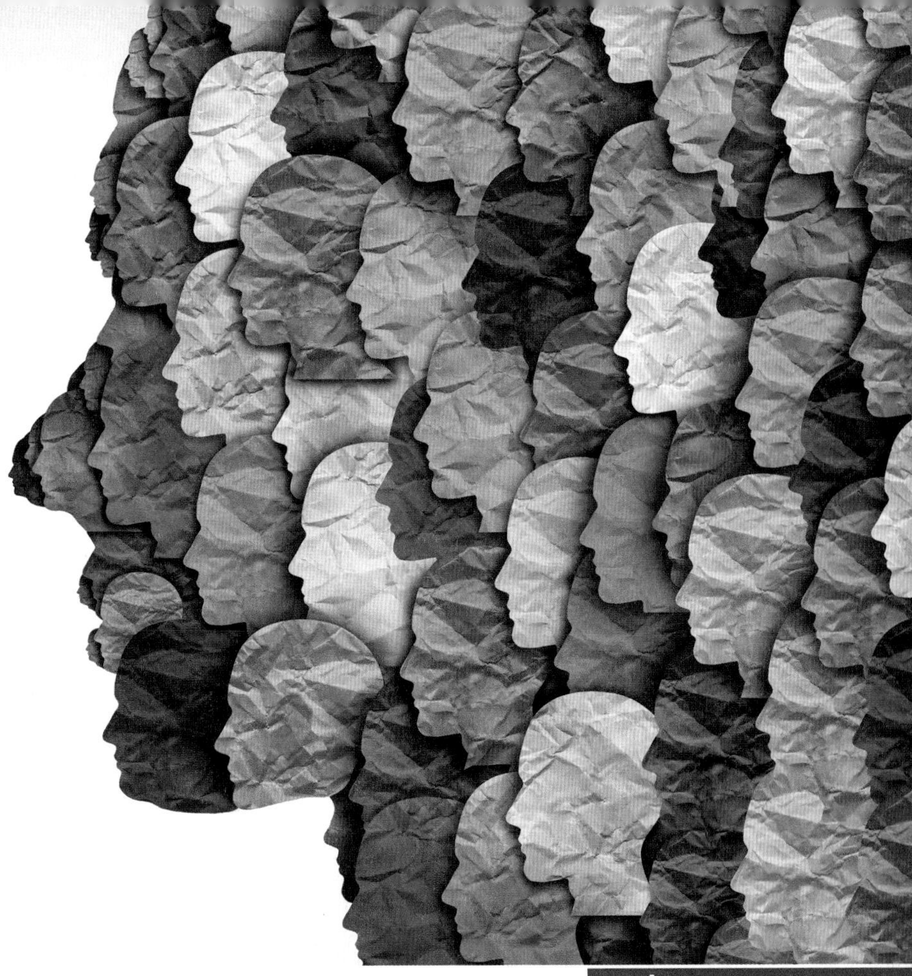

Lightspring/Shutterstock.com

Intercultural Communication

Chapter 3

Learning Objectives

3.1 Identify the different aspects of communication that might vary by culture.

3.2 Define the key elements of the intercultural communication concepts involving the content and relationship between speaker and receiver.

3.3 Explain high-context and low-context elements of communication.

3.4 Describe the effect of power, authority, and status relationships in the healthcare setting.

3.5 Compare time perception and communication in health care across cultural groups.

3.6 Identify the necessary elements of successful intercultural communication.

3.7 Define cultural humility and the assumptions that correspond with this theory.

3.8 Identify successful approaches to use in intercultural counseling.

3.9 List the key influences that reinforce or contradict intercultural nutrition education messages.

The world has always been a global community through social exchanges, travel, wars, and migrations. Communication between people from different cultures is as old as history. Though this is nothing new, it seems even more salient today with international employment, study exchange programs, interdependent economies, and more on the rise.[1]

Whether a person is interacting with people from diverse cultural groups at work and in social settings or traveling to another country for business or pleasure, they need intercultural communication skills to successfully negotiate daily life. Intercultural communication is a specialty in itself. The field encompasses language and the context in which words are interpreted, including gestures, posture, spatial relationships, concepts of time, the status and hierarchy of persons, the role of the individual within a group, and the setting. This chapter presents a broad and limited overview of intercultural communication concepts, as well as information useful in nutrition counseling with individuals or with groups in educational programs. Readers will be introduced to the term *cultural humility* as a form of lifelong active engagement with patients, communities, and colleagues, learning to be careful not to interject personal values into communication. It is a process founded in humility, self-reflection, and self-critique in the life-long communication process.[2]

Food for Thought

"Observe the nature of each country; diet; customs; the age of the patient; speech; manners; fashion; even his silence. . . . One has to study all these signs and analyze what they portend." Hippocratic writings, 5th century BCE

The Intercultural Challenge

Researchers have used an iceberg analogy (refer to Figure 3.1) to describe how a person's cultural heritage can impact communication. Ethnicity, age, and gender are the most visible personal characteristics affecting dialogue—the so-called tip of the iceberg. Beneath the surface, but equally influential, may be the degree of acculturation or assimilation, socioeconomic status, health condition, religion, educational background, group membership, sexual orientation, or political affiliation.

Most people are comfortable conversing with those who are culturally similar to themselves. Communication is sometimes described as one phrase or action leading to the next: in the United States, a person who extends her hand in greeting expects the other person to take her hand and shake it, or when a person says "thank you," a "you're welcome" should follow. Communication comprises a whole series of unwritten expectations regarding how a person should respond, and such expectations are largely cultural in origin. If a person understands the communication action chain and responds as expected, a successful relationship can develop. When a person does not respond as expected, communication can break down, and the relationship can deteriorate.[1]

When meeting a person for the first time, the only data that speakers usually have to work with come from their own cultural norms. They use these norms to predict how that person will respond to their words and what conversational approaches are appropriate. They may also use social roles to determine their communication behavior. Furthermore, speakers modify their words and actions as they get to know a person individually, observing personal cues about communication characteristics that vary from cultural or social customs.[3] An employee, for example, may make certain assumptions about a supervisor based on ethnicity, gender, age, and especially occupational status, and then make adaptations. An employee may start out calling his boss "Mrs. Smith" as a sign of respect for her position but use the more informal "Sue" when she requests that he call her by her first name.

Interpersonal relationships between two individuals are based mostly on personal communication preferences; group interactions commonly depend on cultural or social norms. Misinterpretations at the cultural or social levels of communication are more likely to occur because they are more generalized. As mentioned in Chapter 1, stereotyping occurs if a person misjudges another individual's degree of association with any particular cultural or social group. Assumptions about how a person of a different cultural heritage should communicate can prompt certain types of reactions based on norms in that person's culture: stereotyping can become a self-fulfilling prophecy. The challenge is to increase familiarity with cultural communication behaviors while remaining aware of personal cues and moving toward an interpersonal relationship as quickly as possible.

Intercultural Communication Concepts

Communication uses codes to represent objects, ideas, or behaviors. Thoughts, emotions, and attitudes are decoded into language and nonverbal actions (e.g., gestures, posture, eye contact) to send messages from one person to another.

The two components of the message are the content and the relationship between the speaker and the receiver. Depending on the situation, the content or the relationship may assume greater prominence in the interpretation of meaning. Messages that violate cultural expectations may be accurate in content but hurt the relationship. If the message consistently offends the receiver, the relationship will deteriorate and the message will be disregarded. For example, if a health professional advises a Chinese client to increase calcium intake through increased milk consumption, this is an example worldview of a content message that does little to acknowledge the role of milk in the Chinese diet. Is the client lactose intolerant? Does the client like milk? Does the client classify milk as health-promoting or as a cause of illness?

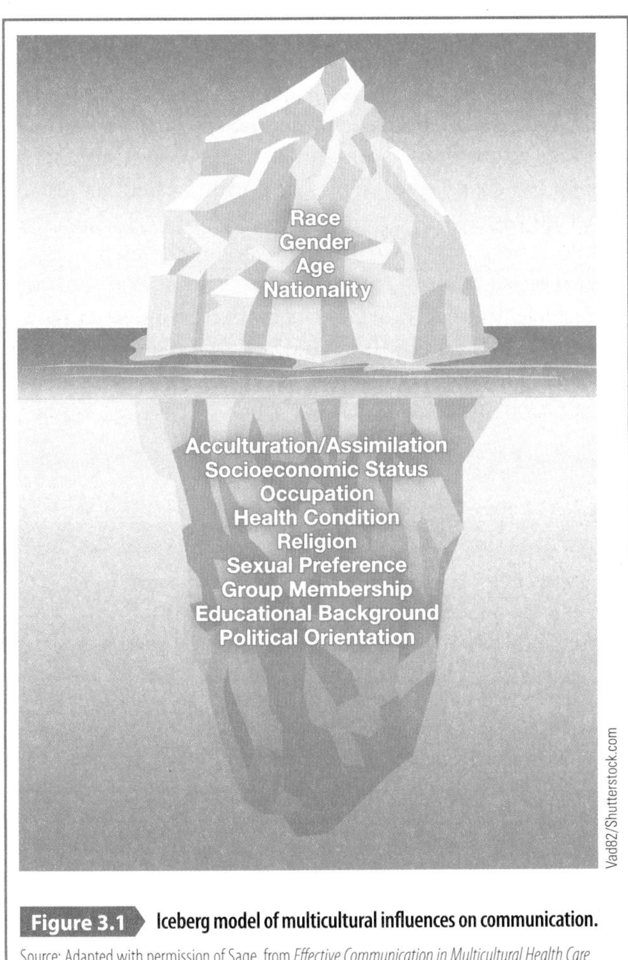

Figure 3.1 Iceberg model of multicultural influences on communication.

Source: Adapted with permission of Sage, from *Effective Communication in Multicultural Health Care Settings*, G.L. Kreps & E.N. Kunimoto, 6. Copyright © 1994. Permission conveyed through Copyright Clearance Center, Inc.

How does milk fit into the balance of the diet according to the client? Unless the provider gains an understanding of how the client conceptualizes the situation, the content of the message may be ignored because the client assumes disinterest or even disrespect for personal beliefs and expectations. Thus, the provider–client relationship is weakened. Messages that demonstrate respect for the individuality of the receiver are called *personal messages* and these improve relationships; those that are disrespectful are termed *object messages* and these often degrade relationships. Communication occurs in a continuum between personal and object messages.[3]

Verbal messages are most useful for communicating content, whereas nonverbal messages usually convey information about relationships. If the nonverbal message is consistent with the verbal message, it can build the relationship and help the receiver correctly interpret the meaning intended by the speaker. When the nonverbal message is inconsistent with the verbal message, both the relationship and the content are undermined. Successful communication is dependent on both verbal and nonverbal skills, each significantly impacted by cultural considerations.

Verbal Communication

The abstract nature of language means it can be correctly interpreted only within context. The cultural aspects of context are so embedded that a speaker often believes they are inherent—that is, that other people must communicate according to the same expectations. Context includes issues common to cultural worldviews, such as the role of the individual in a group and perceptions of power, authority, status, and time. In addition, the context in communication also encompasses the significance of affective and physical expression (termed low or high context) and the level of tolerance for uncertainty and ambiguity (called uncertainty avoidance). Verbal communication occurs within these cultural premises, often operating at an unconscious level in the speaker.

Low- and High-Context Cultures

Conversational context can be defined as the affective and physical cues a speaker uses to indicate meaning, such as tone of voice, facial expression, posture, and gestures.

In most Western cultures, messages usually concern ideas presented in a logical, linear sequence. The speaker tries to say what is meant through precise wording, and the content of the language is more objective than personal along the continuum of personal and object messages. This communication style is termed low context because the actual words are more important than who is receiving the message, how the words are said, or the nonverbal actions that accompany them. Nearly every American has experienced a form of this in the obtuse professional language of attorneys or scientists who fail to convey their message in common, everyday English. Even everyday communication in a low-context culture, is so dependent on words that the underlying meaning is undecipherable if the wording is chosen poorly or deliberately to mislead the recipient. Swiss, German, and Scandinavia are examples of low-context cultures.[4]

In cultures with a high-context communication style, most of the meaning of a message is found in the context, not in the words. In fact, the wording used may be vague,

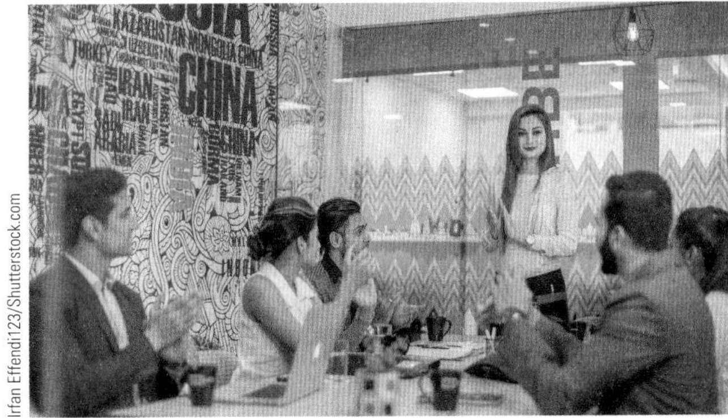

▲ Cultural context is so embedded in the individual that many people believe it is innate and assume all other people share the same background.

circuitous, or incomplete. The content of the language is more personal than objective, dependent on the relationship between speaker and listener. Attitudes and feelings are more prominent in the conversation than thoughts. Communication in high-context cultures is analogous to the expression "reading between the lines." Misunderstandings easily occur if either participant is unfamiliar with the meaning of the nonverbal signifiers being used, such as small eye movements or sounds that are made when in agreement, disagreement, or when upset. When a conversation is uncomfortable some people may squirm, others gasp or grow quiet, and often these reactions depend on the person's culture of origin. High-context cultures are most prevalent among homogeneous populations with a common understanding of the affective and physical expression used in sending the message (refer to the following "Nonverbal Communication" section). Asian, Middle Eastern, and Native American cultures are very high context. Latinx societies are moderately high context. American culture is thought to be toward the low end, but more middle context than many European societies.

In low-context cultures, communication is usually explicit, straightforward, and unambiguous. The focus is on the speaker, who uses words to send messages that are often intended to persuade or convince the receiver. In high-context cultures, indirect communication is preferred. Implicit language is used, and many qualifiers are added; nonverbal cues are significant to interpreting the message. The locus of conversation is the receiver; the speaker adjusts to the listener's feelings.[4] Low-context listeners are often impatient with high-context speakers, wondering when the speaker will get to the point of the conversation. Low-context listeners also frequently miss the affective and physical expression in the message.

Health care situations are often extremely low context. The conversation is focused on the provider who delivers a verbal message to the client with little consideration for the nonverbal message. The communication is high on content and low on relationship. Clients from high-context cultures are likely to be dissatisfied, even offended, by such impersonal, objective interactions. Communication problems may not be evident to a low-context clinician until the client leaves and never returns.

Interactions may range from low- to high-context depending on the situation, regardless of the overall cultural preference. In uncomfortable or embarrassing situations, a low-context communicator may be very sensitive and indirect. In high-context cultures, direct language is frequently used in intimate relationships.

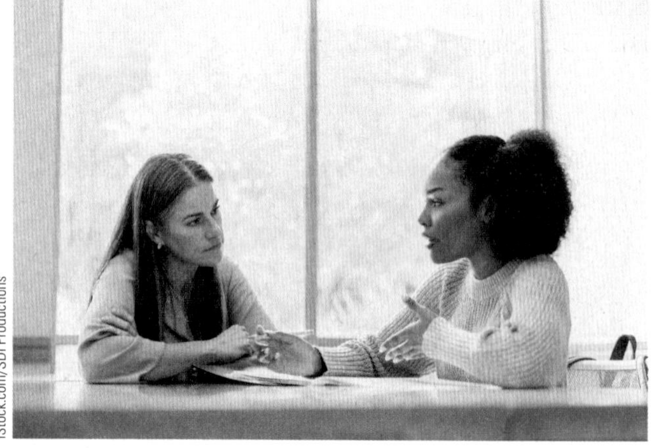

iStock.com/SDI Productions

▲ **Only the person sending the message knows the meaning of the message: the person receiving the message must use what she knows about cultural and social norms, as well as what she knows about the speaker personally, to interpret the message.**

Food for Thought

One area of conflict is due to differences in high- and low-context communication. For example, Black Americans tend to be more high-context than White Americans, using cognitive, affective, and physical responses that may appear disruptive or overly emotional to White individuals. In the United States, the language and symbols of White America has often been the expected mode of communication. This drives other cultures to communicate within that mode.

As an example of low- versus high-context communication in different situations, consider a researcher presenting current nutritional data on spinach to a group of other professionals. She will probably speak in a relatively monotone voice and use scientific jargon. She will sequentially present her points, support her thesis with examples, and then restate her ideas in the conclusion. She will probably stand erect and limit the expressive use of her hands and face. The message is almost entirely in the content of the words she says. In contrast, this same woman might behave very differently when feeding her reluctant toddler spinach for dinner. She might smile and make yummy sounds as she offers him a spoonful or pretends the spinach is a plane coming in for a landing in his mouth. She might give him a spoonful of meat or potato, then try the spinach again. She might even dance around his high chair a little or hum a few bars of the old cartoon theme song about a sailor who liked spinach. She doesn't try to get him to eat spinach by explaining its nutrient content, as she did at her meeting. The message is nonlinear and not dependent on the content of the words she uses. This is not to say that a health care provider should burst out in song when working with a client from a high-context culture. But it does suggest that indirect, expressive approaches may be more effective in some intercultural clinical, educational, or counseling settings. Identification of a culture as either low- or high-context provides a general framework for communication but may be affected by other situational factors.

 **Food for Thought**

Even within low-context cultures, intimate conversations are usually highly contextual; words and phrases may be significantly shortened or abbreviated—just a look may be enough for understanding.

Individuals and Groups

The relationship of the individual to the group is determined in part by whether a culture is low- or high-context. In low-context cultures, the individual is typically separate from the group, and self-realization is an important goal. Self-esteem is dynamic, based on successful mastery or control of a situation. In high-context cultures, the individual is usually defined by group association, and a person desires oneness with the group, not individuation. A mutual dependency exists and self-esteem is based on how well a person can adjust to a situation.[4] Individualism is a prominent characteristic in Australia, Canada, Great Britain, New Zealand, the Netherlands, and the United States. Collectivism is especially valued in the nations of Denmark, Ghana, Guatemala, Indonesia, Nigeria, Panama, Peru, El Salvador, Sierra Leone, Taiwan, Thailand, and Venezuela.

In societies emphasizing individuality, a person must communicate to gain acceptance by the group, whether it is the family, the workplace, or the community. Communication is used to establish the self within an individual or group relationship. When meeting someone new, the action chain in the conversation is flexible, with few expectations. The two people may focus on one or the other speaker and often delve into personal preferences, such as favorite restaurants or sports teams. When group identity is the focus of a society, there is no need for a person to seek acceptance from the group or to communicate individuality. Silence is highly valued. Interactions between strangers tend to be ritualized, and if the action chain is broken, communication cannot continue. The expectation is that each speaker will indicate group affiliation and that such identity conveys all the information needed to know that person.

The role of the individual within the group can have an impact on health care delivery. Within more group-oriented cultures, greater participation is required of their members in matters of health and illness, and it may be expected that relatives will participate in giving patient histories, overseeing physical exams, or making decisions regarding treatment.[5] Middle Easterners expect to go to the hospital with an ill family member to provide care. Next of kin is determined along bloodlines among Latinx, and care decisions are often the responsibility of a grandmother or mother instead of the spouse. Koreans prefer the whole family to make decisions regarding treatment for a terminally ill patient. Some Native Americans are so strongly associated with the group it is difficult for them to communicate individual needs.

Uncertainty Avoidance

Related to the role of the individual in a group is tolerance for uncertainty and ambiguity. Some groups exhibit great discomfort with what is unknown and different; these are defined as high uncertainty avoidance cultures. Members of these cultures may become anxious about behavior that deviates from the norm; high uncertainty avoidance cultures desire consensus. Argentina, Belgium, Chile, Colombia, Costa Rica, Croatia, Egypt, France, Greece, Guatemala, Israel, Japan, Korea, Mexico, Panama, Peru, Portugal, Turkey, Serbia, and Spain are stronger in uncertainty avoidance than the United States, as are most African and other Asian nations. They typically have a history of the central rule and complex laws that regulate individual action on behalf of the group.[4,6]

Cultures with low or weaker uncertainty avoidance include Canada, Denmark, Great Britain, Hong Kong, India, Indonesia, Jamaica, the Netherlands, the Philippines, Sweden, and the United States. People from these nations are usually curious about the unknown and different. They are more informal, willing to accept dissent within a group, and open to change.

It is important to distinguish the differences between risk avoidance and uncertainty avoidance. A person from a high uncertainty avoidance culture may be quite willing to take familiar risks or even new risks to minimize the ambiguity of a situation. But in general, risks that involve change and difference are difficult for people with strong uncertainty avoidance; this is especially a concern when changes threaten acceptance by the group. For example, researchers suggest Black American women may resist certain preparations or seasonings if family members object or if the foods might undermine ethnic identity. Furthermore, weight loss may be avoided if being thin means the potential loss of a peer group that values a larger figure.[4,6,7]

Working with family or peers in a group setting to effect dietary change may be more successful for persons with a low tolerance for uncertainty, especially when the positive value of change is accepted and group consumption patterns are modified.

Power, Authority, and Status

The perception of power, or power distance, can strongly influence communication patterns. In low-context cultures, where individuality is respected, power or status is usually attributed to the role or job that a person fulfills. Power distance is small. People are seen as equals, differentiated by their accomplishments. It is common for an individual to question directions or instructions; the belief is that a person must understand why before a task can be completed. A client may desire a full explanation of a condition and expected outcomes before undertaking a specific therapy. In many high-context cultures, where group identification is esteemed, superiors are seen as fundamentally different from subordinates. Authority is rarely questioned. For example, a health care provider counseling an Ethiopian patient with type 2 diabetes may believe that a culturally sensitive approach is to ask him about his perceptions of the disease. What does he call it? How does he think it can be cured? Unknown to the provider, the Ethiopian man has a large power distance, and he assumes that the provider is the expert. Why would she ask such questions of him? Doesn't she know what she is doing? He expects her to provide all the answers with little participation from him. He may even become uncooperative or fail to return for a follow-up visit because he questions her expertise.

Although there is usually some combination of both small and large power distance tendencies in a culture, one tendency will predominate. Some countries with small power distances include Austria, Canada, Denmark, Germany, Great Britain, Ireland, Israel, the Netherlands, New Zealand, Sweden, and the United States. Those with larger power distance include most African, Asian, Latinx, and Middle Eastern cultures, including (but not exclusively) Egypt, Ethiopia, Ghana, Guatemala, India, Malaysia, Nigeria, Panama, Saudi Arabia, and Venezuela. Client empowerment, particularly in setting goals and objectives, may be resisted by people from groups who come from cultures with a larger power distance; maximum personal responsibility may be preferred by people from groups with a smaller power distance.

Food for Thought

The Inuit conception of time is governed by the tides—one set of tasks is done when the tide is out, another when the tide comes in.

The Arabs say, "Bukra inshallah," which means, "Tomorrow, if God wills."

To many Chinese, the gift of a clock means the same as saying, "I wish you were dead." Each tick is perceived as a reminder of mortality.

Time Perception

Being on time, sticking to a schedule, and not taking too much of a person's time are valued concepts in the United States, but these values are unimportant in societies where the idea of time is less structured. Low-context cultures tend to be monochronistic, meaning that they are interested in completing one thing before progressing to the next. Monochronistic societies are well suited to industrialized accomplishments. Polychronistic societies are often found in high-context cultures. Many tasks may be pursued simultaneously, but not to the exclusion of personal relationships. Courtesy and kindness are more important than deadlines in polychronistic groups.[4] Exceptions occur, however. The French have a relatively low-context culture but are polychronistic; the Japanese can become monochronistic when conducting business transactions with Americans.

Monochronistic persons may see polychronistic behaviors, such as interrupting a face-to-face conversation for a phone call or being late for an appointment, as rude or contemptuous. Yet no disrespect is intended, nor is it believed that polychronistic persons are less productive than monochronistic people.

Nonverbal Communication

High-context cultures place great emphasis on nonverbal communication in the belief that body language reveals more about what a person is thinking and feeling than words do. Yet customs about touching, gestures, eye contact, and spatial relationships vary tremendously among cultures, independent of low- or high-context communication style. As discussed previously, such nonverbal behavior can reinforce the content of the verbal message being sent, or it can contradict the words and confuse the receiver. Successful intercultural communication depends on consistent verbal and nonverbal messages. During personal and group interactions, persons move together in a synchronized manner. Barely detectable motions, such as the tilt of the head or the blink of an eye, are imitated when people are in sync and communicating effectively. How a person moves, however, are usually cultural and often unconscious. Although body language is closely linked to ethnicity, most people believe that the way they move through the world is universal.

Misinterpretations of nonverbal communication subtleties are common and often inadvertent. An earlier review identified more than 7,000 different gestures, and meaning is easily misunderstood when awareness of differences is limited.[8,9]

Touching

Touching includes handshakes, hugging, kissing, placing a hand on the arm or shoulder, and even unintentional bumping. In China, for example, touching between strangers, even handshaking if one person is male and the other female, is uncommon in public. Orthodox Jewish men and women are prohibited from touching unless they are relatives or are married. To Latinx people, touching is an expected and necessary element of every relationship. The *abrazo*, a hug with mutual back-patting, is a common greeting. Touching norms frequently vary according to attributes such as gender, age, or even physical condition. In the United States, it is acceptable for an adult to pat the head of a child, but questionable with another adult. It is admirable to take the arm of an older person crossing the street but rude to do so for a healthy young adult.[10]

Cultures in which touching is mostly avoided include those of the United States, Canada, Great Britain, Scandinavia, Germany, the Balkans, Japan, and Korea. Those in which touching is expected include the Middle East and Greece, Latin America, Italy, Spain, Portugal, and Russia. Cultures that fall in between are those of China, France, Ireland, and India, as well as those in Africa, Southeast Asia, and the Pacific Islands. Health care professionals should take careful note of cultural touching behaviors. Vigorous handshaking is often considered aggressive behavior, and a reassuring hand on the shoulder may be insulting.[10] Of special mention are attitudes about the head. Many cultures consider the head sacred, and an absent-minded pat or playful cuff to the chin may be exceptionally offensive. Conversely, persons from cultures in which frequent touching is the norm may be insulted if someone is reluctant to hug or kiss, or they may be unaware of legal issues regarding inappropriate touching in the United States.

Gesture, Facial Expression, and Posture

Gestures include obvious movements such as waving hello or goodbye or standing to indicate respect when a person enters the room, as well as more indirect motions such as handing an item to a person or nodding the head in acknowledgment. Facial expression includes deliberate looks of attention or questioning and unintentional wincing or grimacing. Even smiling has specific cultural connotations.

Confusion occurs when movements have significantly different meanings to different people. Crossed arms are often interpreted as a sign of hostility in the United States, yet do not have similar negative associations in the Middle East, where it is a common stance while talking. The thumbs-up gesture shows approval in most countries, but in several countries in West Africa and the Middle East, including Iran, Iraq, and Afghanistan, it has the connotation of "up yours!" and is used much like the middle finger is in the United States. The crooked-finger motion used in the United States to beckon someone is considered lewd in Japan; is used to call animals in Croatia, Malaysia, Serbia, and Vietnam; and is used to summon prostitutes in Australia and Indonesia. To many Southeast Asians, it is an insolent or threatening gesture.[11,12]

Some Asians find it difficult to directly disagree with a speaker and may tilt their chins quickly upward to indicate "no" in what appears to Americans to be an affirmative nod. Some Asian Indians, Greeks, Turks, and Iranians shake their heads back and forth to show agreement and nod up and down to express disagreement. Puerto Ricans may smile in conjunction with other facial expressions to mean "please," "thank you," "excuse me," or other phrases. The Vietnamese may smile when displeased.

Good posture is an important sign of respect in nearly all cultures. Slouching or putting one's feet up on the desk is generally recognized as impolite. In many societies, the feet are considered the lowest and dirtiest part of the body, so it is rude to point the toe at a person when one's legs are crossed or to show the soles of one's shoes.

 **Food for Thought**

Studies of human gestures speculate that the handshake, an egalitarian gesture at the point of touching, the hug, and the bow with hands pressed together, offer honor equally between greeters. These differ from the bow in which the lowly give honor to those "on high" in some contexts.[13,14] Though contactless greetings rose in popularity during the 2020 pandemic of Covid-19, the long history of the handshake (3,000-plus years) indicates its resilience as a social convention.[15]

In Japan, the small bow used in greetings and departures is a sign of respect and humility. The inferior person in the relationship always bows lower and longer than the person in the superior position.

Many Asians completely avoid touching strangers, even in transitory interactions, such as returning change after a purchase. This can be offensive to persons who consider physical contact a sign of acceptance, such as African Americans and Latinx people.

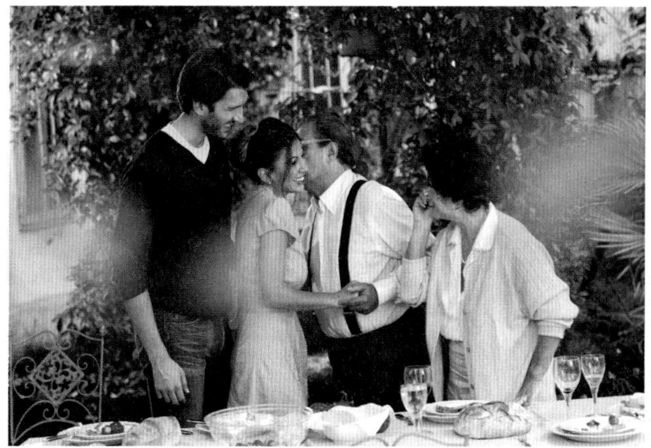

iStock.com/Thomas_EyeDesign

▲ **Touching norms frequently vary according to attributes such as ethnicity, gender, age, or physical condition.**

Eye Contact

The subtlest nonverbal movements involve the eyes. Rules regarding eye contact are usually complex, varying according to issues such as social status, gender, and distance apart. Most Americans consider eye contact indicative of honesty and openness, yet staring is thought to be rude. To Germans, direct eye contact is an indication of attentiveness. To Filipinos, direct eye contact can be an expression of sexual interest or aggression. Among Native Americans, direct eye contact is considered rude, and averted eyes do not necessarily reflect disinterest. When Asians and Latinos avoid eye contact, it is a sign of respect. Middle Easterners believe that the minute motions of the eyes and pupils are the most reliable indicator of how a person is reacting in any situation.[4,16]

 **Food for Thought**

The one-finger salute is considered an insult in many cultures. This gesture dates back to Roman times when it was called *digitus impudicus* (the "impudent finger").

In Japanese culture, closing the eyes and nodding can demonstrate attentiveness.

Spatial Relationships

Each person defines his or her own space—the surrounding area reserved for the individual. Acute discomfort can occur when another person stands or sits within the space identified as inviolate. Middle Easterners prefer to be no more than two feet from whomever they are communicating with so that they can observe their eyes. Latinx people enjoy personal closeness with friends and acquaintances. Intercultural communication is most successful when spatial preferences are flexible.[17]

In addition to distance, the way a person is positioned affects communication in some cultures. It is considered rude in Samoan and Tongan societies, for instance, to speak to a person unless the parties are positioned at equal levels, for example, both sitting or both standing.

Role of Communication in Health Care

Health care providers in the United States take pride in their technical expertise and mastery of knowledge. They spend years understanding biochemical and physiological processes, laboratory assessments, diagnostic data, and therapeutic strategies; yet little of that time is devoted to how valuable information is effectively communicated to the client or members of the health care team. Skills are needed for successful communication with these and other participants, such as extended family members or traditional health practitioners, despite possible differences in language, ethnicity, religious affiliation, gender, age, educational background, occupation, health beliefs, or other cultural factors.

Words are the primary tool of the clinician following diagnosis. Whereas the surgeon depends on the scalpel, most other providers rely on language to inform and guide patients in the treatment and lifestyle changes necessary to maintain or improve health. The surgeon has significant control within the surgical setting; in most cases, the patient is not even conscious. In contrast, the clinician interacts directly with a patient who has independent, sometimes contradictory, ideas about health, illness, and treatment. The provider can control only her or his side of the conversation; if the words are ineffective, the client may reject recommended medications or therapies. Although the actions of the surgeon are generally limited to the patient, the advice of the health care provider often impacts not only the patient but also the patient's family. Dietary modifications, may have long-term implications; if cultural food habits are changed, the new ways of eating may be passed on for generations.

Interaction between Provider and Client

In the time-pressured and cost-constrained setting of health care delivery, object messages are more common than personal messages, and content is considered more relevant than the relationship. Typically, the health care professional relies on the client to provide accurate, detailed information about his or her medical history and current symptoms so that the appropriate diagnosis and treatment can be determined. The client depends on the practitioner to explain any medical condition in terms that are understandable and to describe treatment strategies and expectations clearly. This basic conversation is repeated between providers and their clients daily; it is the essence of clinical health care. In practice, however, this common interaction between provider and client greatly underestimates the complexity of intercultural communication. A recent study looked at the average consultation time with primary care physicians and found that the length of time was 5 minutes or less. Confidence and caring that are established between health care providers and patients in this short amount of time can also contribute to the results of the overall health outcome.[18]

Numerous barriers to the sharing and understanding of knowledge can prevent successful communication in the health care setting. For example, a client may be fearful or in pain when seeking help, more focused on immediate discomfort than on conversing clearly with the provider. During times of stress, a client is also more likely to use her or his mother tongue than English if it is a second language.[19] The provider often assumes the role of the expert, leaving little room for the participation of the client as the authority on what he or she is experiencing physically or emotionally. The provider may rely on medical jargon because it is difficult to interpret many terms without extensive explanations or oversimplification. A provider may be most concerned with the technical aspects of a health problem and inadvertently ignore the interpersonal aspects of the relationship with the patient or may be too rushed to express care and compassion. Furthermore, cultural communication customs may interfere directly with the trust and respect necessary for effective health care. When a primary care provider and patient do not share a language or culture there may be differing views on well-being, health, illness, life, and death. An interpreter can be most useful in these situations because communication can become quite complex.[19,20] The results of ineffective communication in health care can be serious. Noncompliance issues are among the most important for the clinician.

Inadequate communication has been linked to patient dissatisfaction with care, incomprehension with the treatment plan, lower quality of care, and medical errors. Patients may reject recommendations or fail to return for follow-up appointments because they are dissatisfied with their relationship with their health care provider. Patients with diabetes who perceived discriminatory behavior from their health provider due to race, age, socioeconomic status, or gender suffered more symptoms and had higher levels of hemoglobin A1C (a blood test for three-month average sugar levels) than other patients. Conversely, patients who received respectful treatment from health professionals reported significantly better dietary management of their diabetes in

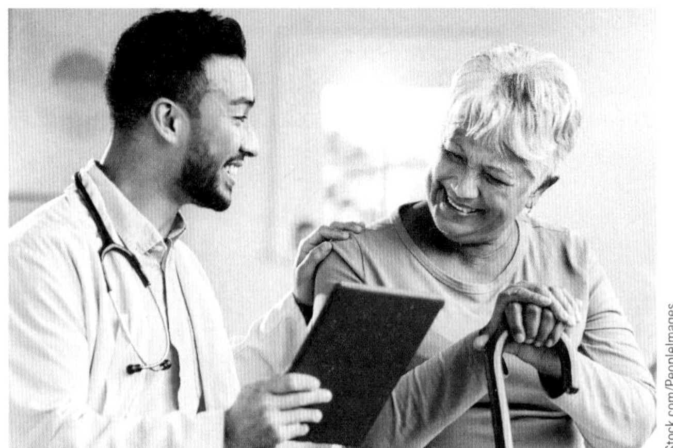

iStock.com/PeopleImages

▲ **The client depends on the practitioner to explain any medical condition in terms that are understandable and to describe treatment strategies and expectations clearly.**

another study. Patients often report better outcomes with traditional healers than with biomedical practitioners because there is more time spent on explanation and understanding of the condition. Development of the interpersonal relationship with the practitioner is crucial to a patient's understanding and accepting treatment strategies, particularly if recommendations conflict with cultural perceptions regarding health and illness.[21]

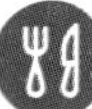

Food for Thought

A framework of cultural competence in health care includes (1) including minority recruitment into the health professions; (2) developing interpreter services and language-appropriate health educational materials; and (3) providing a provider with continuing education on cross-cultural issues.[22]

Participatory research on a Lakota Indian reservation reported that intercultural connections were directly related to the investment of time and commitment to establishing and pursuing meaningful dialogue.[23]

Food for Thought

In one survey, being involved with decision-making was significant for adherence to medical advice for Whites. For racial/ethnic minorities, the most significant factor for medical adherence was being treated with dignity.[24]

Responsibilities of the Health Care Provider

Although communication requires the active participation of at least two persons, the health care provider has certain responsibilities in interactions with clients. All medical encounters can be assumed to be intercultural, since being a physician involves having been socialized into the micro-culture of biomedicine. The provider often assumes the superordinate position in the relationship because they are accorded that status by the client or because the client is distracted by pain or discomfort. In that role, the practitioner must understand what is said by the client and to provide the client with the information needed to participate in treatment. This may require that the clinician be familiar with cultural norms, listen carefully and seriously to the client (observing personal cues), and take action based on what is said by the client. Caring and considered communication can empower the client within the relationship and improve treatment efficacy.[25] One recent study found that a patient's positive experience related to being treated with respect and allowed to maintain a sense of integrity. A negative experience revolved around a patient's feelings of vulnerability. This vulnerability is a direct result of interdependent experiences of disrespect, time constraints, dominance of biomedical culture, and helplessness.[21]

Cultural humility[26] is a theory used in medicine, nursing, and education that takes into account the fluidity of a culture. It offers an alternative framework as opposed to cultural competency, which challenges both individuals and institutions to address inequalities. Cultural humility in health care emphasizes attentive listening, an openness to other cultures, and a large component of self-reflection and self-critique in interacting with others. The following assumptions correspond with the theory:[27,28]

1. All humans are diverse from each other in some way yet part of a global community.
2. Humans are inherently altruistic.
3. All humans have equal value.
4. Cultural conflict is a normal and expected part of life.
5. All humans are lifelong learners.

Cultural humility is viewed as more of an attitude, value, or way of being. Cultural competency focuses on the development of skills or ways of doing.[29]

Successful Intercultural Communication

Effective intercultural communication begins when the speaker is mindful of his or her own communication behaviors and is sensitive to misinterpretations that may result from them. Practitioner knowledge about a culture does not necessarily facilitate effective care without awareness of cultural differences and personal biases. A willingness to listen carefully to a client without assumptions or bias and to recognize that the client is the expert when it comes to information about his or her experience is requisite to successful health care interactions.[29]

The mnemonic CRASH has been suggested as a useful way to remember the components of cultural competency that underlie effective care: C—consider Culture in all patient–practitioner interactions; R—show Respect and avoid gratuitous familiarity and affection; A—Assess/Affirm intracultural differences due to language skills, acculturation, and other factors, recognizing each individual as an expert on his or her health beliefs and practices; S—be Sensitive to issues that may be offensive or interfere with trust in the relationship and show self-awareness regarding personal biases that may cause miscommunication; and H—demonstrate Humility, apologizing quickly and accepting responsibility for communication missteps. With CRASH in mind, the health professional can begin mastery of the communication skills needed to promote understanding and acceptance from clients of many cultural backgrounds.[30]

Intercultural Communication Skills

Reading about culturally based communication differences is an intellectual undertaking. Applying intercultural communication concepts is much more challenging. Successful face-to-face interactions require understanding cultural communication expectations and being familiar with the distinctive style of the other person. Often, there is contradictory information to assimilate. Numerous books, articles, and courses on health care communication are available to supplement this brief overview.

Name Traditions

Determine how clients prefer to be addressed. Americans are among the most informal worldwide, frequently calling strangers and acquaintances by their given names. Nearly all other cultures expect a more respectful approach. This can include the use of titles or prefixes (Mr., Mrs., Miss, Ms., Dr., Sir, Madam, etc.), use of surname, and proper pronunciation. Never use "Dear," "Honey," "Sweetie," "Fella," "Son," or other endearments in place of proper names.

Name order is often different from the United States' pattern of title, given name, middle name, and surname. In many Latin American countries, a married woman uses her given name and her maiden surname, followed by *de* ("of") and her husband's family surname. For instance, a married woman named Ana would use her maiden name of Lopez followed by *de* plus her husband's family surname of Perez. She would then use the name Ana Lopez de Perez. Children typically use their given name, their father's surname, and then their mother's family surname. This causes confusion because while most Latino men prefer to be addressed by their father's family surname, it is often the name that sequentially is placed on the "middle name" line of forms. Persons reading the form often assume the mother's family surname is a Latino's last name.[31]

Middle Easterners use their title, given name, and surname. They may also use bin (for men) or bint (for women), meaning "of" a place or "son/daughter of." This is not to be confused with the given name Ben (although it is pronounced similarly). For example, Abdel Al-Fakeeh bin Saud means Abdel son of Saud. If the grandparent of a Middle Easterner is well known, his or her last name may be added to the name order, following the surname, with another bin. The Vietnamese, Hmong, and Cambodians place the surname first, followed by the given name (although many make the switch to the American name order with acculturation). The Chinese and Koreans use a similar system, including a generation name following the family name and before the given name (the generation name is sometimes hyphenated with the given name, or the two names are run together). For example, a man whose name is Yung and has a generation name of Tsing and a surname of Wai would be referred to as Yung Tsingwai. Married women in China and Korea do not take their husband's surname. In Japan, the surname is followed by san, meaning "Mr." or "Ms." Given names are only used among close friends and intimates. In some Hindu families, a man goes by his given name, preceded by the initial of his father's given name. Muslims in India use the Middle Eastern order, and Christian Indians use the U.S. pattern.[32] There are numerous other name traditions and preferences of address. When in doubt, it is best to ask.

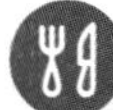

Food for Thought

The use of cultural food potlucks among staff members, students, and other groups can help facilitate cultural understanding among people of diverse backgrounds.[33]

Appropriate Language

Use unambiguous language when working with clients who are limited in English. Choose common terms (not necessarily simple words), avoiding those with multiple meanings, such as "to address," which may mean to talk to someone, to give a speech, to send an item, or to consider an issue. Vague verbs, such as *get*, *make*, and *do*, may confuse. Use specific verbs, such as *purchase*, *complete*, or *prepare*, when directing clients.

Slang and idioms may have no meaning in another culture. Many new English speakers interpret words literally. *How's it going?* makes no sense if one does not understand the meaning of *it* in this context.[38,39] Sports analogies, including *score* and *strike out*, are indecipherable if the game is unfamiliar. Phrases that suggest a mental picture, such as *run that by me* or *easy as pie* or *dodge a bullet*, are barriers to comprehension. The use of slang can make the user sound novel, witty, hip, and "one of the gang," but just as with medical jargon, it is also likely to interfere with communication.[34] Some persons with limited English skills are embarrassed to admit that they do not understand what is being said or to ask that something be repeated. When comprehension is critical, respectfully request clients to repeat instructions in their own words, or ask that they demonstrate a skill so that misunderstandings can be corrected.

Avoid asking questions that can be answered with a simple yes or no. For example, "Do you understand?" will often prompt a positive response in practitioner–client conversations, regardless of comprehension level. It is better to ask leading questions—for example, "What confuses you?" or "Tell me what you don't understand." In some Asian cultures, it is impossible to say no to a request. The Japanese, for instance, have developed many ways to avoid a negative response, such as answering maybe, countering or criticizing the question, issuing an apology, remaining silent, or leaving the room.[35,36]

The direct communication style of the majority of Americans also assumes that each person is saying what he or she means. This can cause difficulties when conversing with persons for whom negotiation is standard practice. For example, a practitioner offers coffee or tea to an Iranian client. She refuses, so he sits down and begins the discussion. The client is upset because she was being polite and had expected the health care professional to ask again, and then insist that she have something to drink.

Typically, Americans not only believe what is said initially; they also consider answers absolute. In some cultures, it is acceptable to make a commitment, then decide later to change the terms of the agreement or decline altogether. People from these groups assume that one cannot predict intervening events or future needs. Further, there can be differences in what is accepted as "truth." In the United States, truth is considered objective and is supported by facts. In many other cultures, truth is subjective, often based on emotions. A Filipino American client may report to the practitioner that she has not lost any weight on her low-calorie diet this week. But when she gets on the scale, she weighs three pounds less. Asked about it, the client explains she is frustrated because she gained one-half a pound yesterday and does not feel she is progressing. Understanding that the definitions of truth vary culturally can help explain some miscommunications.[37,38]

Food for Thought

A professional interpreter reports that unintended results due to limited language skills can be confusing, insulting, or even comic. A friendly physician meant to ask one of his clients, "Cuantos años tiene usted?" ("How old are you?") He mispronounced the word as anos, however, saying, "How many anuses do you have?"[39]

Use of an Interpreter

Language can be the most difficult of all intercultural communication barriers to overcome. Many people are recent immigrants, and others view their stay in the United States as temporary and therefore see no need to learn English.[40]

According to Title VI of the Civil Rights Act of 1964, all persons in the United States are guaranteed equal access to health care services regardless of national origin, which has been interpreted to mean that there can be no discrimination based on language. Most medical institutions have professional interpreters, and in areas where interpreters are unavailable, telephone interpretation services may be an alternative. Through the use of technology, Certified Medical Interpreters are often available at any time and offer a variety of languages.

Unfortunately, it is common for health care providers to resort to nonprofessional interpreters, such as the client's family or friends, to facilitate communication. The inadequacies of such interpretations are numerous. Patients may be reluctant or embarrassed to discuss certain conditions in front of their relatives, or family members may decide that the information provided by the practitioner isn't needed by the patient, so they do not interpret it accurately. Untrained interpreters are often unfamiliar with medical terminology. One study indicated that 23 to 52 percent of phrases were misinterpreted by nonprofessionals; for example, laxative was the term used for "diarrhea" and swelling was confused with "getting fat." The interpreter tended to ignore questions about bodily functions altogether.[29] Even bilingual individuals may not be familiar with all dialects; the terms used in one part of a country may be very different from those used in another region. Ethical issues arise when children are used as interpreters. Children may be frightened of medical procedures, and dependence on a child for communication can invert family dynamics, causing unnecessary intergenerational stress.

Issues regarding informed consent, patient safety, and noncompliance occur when interpretations are inadequate. Some health care providers attempt to use their skills in a foreign language, believing it is better to try to communicate directly than to lose some control through interpreters. Although conversing in the language of the client is often greatly appreciated, it is important for the provider not to overestimate fluency.

When using an interpreter, the practitioner should speak directly to the client, and then watch the client rather than the interpreter during interpretation. If the nonverbal response doesn't fit the comment, confirmation with the interpreter can ensure that the meaning is clear. Sometimes an interpreter may appear to answer for the patient; the interpreter may be very familiar with the patient's history based on previous interpretations for other health providers. Conversely, it may take an interpreter considerably longer to interpret a comment than it takes to say it in English, in part because certain cultural interpretations and explanations may be necessary. The technique of back interpretation, meaning that instructions are repeated back to the clinician, can prevent miscommunication and open the conversation to any further questions by the client. Providers can increase effective communication through an interpreter by using a positive tone of voice and avoiding a judgmental or condescending attitude. Short, direct phrases—avoiding metaphors or colloquialisms—and repeating important information more than once can improve client understanding.[34]

Intercultural Counseling

Practitioner attitude toward outcomes is perhaps the most important element of successful intercultural counseling. A health care provider cannot be open-minded if objectives are completely preplanned. Participation in a relaxed, give-and-take exchange can reveal issues of primary concern to the client. An invitation to share stories, for example, may address concerns that cannot be expressed directly. Mutual commitment to shared goals can be developed by attentive listening to client needs and learning about client expectations. This collaboration in defining and achieving outcomes is the difference between advocacy and manipulation and employs cultural humility. Effective intercultural counseling is an ongoing process of practice and refinement, requiring an open attitude, cultural knowledge, and intercultural communication skills.[29]

Pre-Counseling Preparation

Researchers have made many recommendations regarding effective intercultural communication. The LEARN guideline was developed for health care providers to use in interviews to elicit cultural, social, and personal information related to the patient's illness or disease. There are five steps to reduce communication barriers (Table 3.1).

Table 3.1 The LEARN Guideline

Sequence and Description of Interactions	Example
Listen Active listening is an extremely important skill for a counselor to develop. Some factors related to listening merit emphasis for successful counseling across cultures. You should listen carefully to a client without assumptions or bias and recognize the client as the expert when it comes to information about his or her experience. Not only are you learning, but you are demonstrating to your client that what he or she has to say is important to you. Make sure you come to a common understanding of the issues and problems. All of this information will be important when designing intervention strategies.	Request clarification when necessary by saying, "I didn't quite understand that." Listen carefully to how food decisions are made. Probe to find out who does the food preparation and shopping and determine whether an additional person should be included in the next counseling session.
Explain To clarify that your understanding of the issues is accurate, you should explain back to the client your perception of what has been related. The explanation creates an opportunity to clarify any misunderstandings.	"You feel that diarrhea is a hot ailment, and your baby should not be given a hot food like infant formula but should drink barley water, a cool food. Did I understand you correctly?" Balancing the intake of hot and cold foods is believed to help with healing among several Caribbean and Asian cultures.
Acknowledge The nutrition counselor should acknowledge the similarities and differences between cultures regarding the causes, symptoms, and treatment of the problem.	Both you and your doctor feel that what your baby drinks will help her feel better. You feel your baby needs a cool food like barley water, and the health care providers at this clinic feel that your baby needs a drink with minerals like Pedialyte to get better.
Recommend The client should be given several culturally sensitive options.	An Indian woman who is a vegetarian who wishes to lose weight might be given the following options: "You could start a walking program, reduce the amount of oil or butter used to make lentil dishes, use skim milk for making yogurt, or eat fruits instead of fried snacks."
Negotiate After reviewing the options, the counselor and client should develop a culturally sensitive plan of action. By understanding the powerful influence of the client's culture as well as the equally powerful culture of biomedicine, the need for compromise and mediation become apparent. When the condition is life-threatening or the cultural differences are enormous, Kleinman***** recommends a cultural anthropologist or a respected member of the client's community aid in the negotiation. The health practitioner should decide what is critical and be.	Look to your client to select a starting point: "Which of these options do you think would be a good place to start?" After selecting an option, discuss how it will be implemented.

*Table information is taken from Bauer, K.D., & Liou, D. (2020). *Nutrition counseling and education skill development.* Cengage Learning.[42]

Practically speaking, a health care provider cannot be expected to become an expert in intercultural communication or to fully understand the communication modes best suited to each of the many clients from different cultural heritages. Most patients living in the United States do not expect to be treated as they would in their homeland. But familiarity with intercultural communication attitudes, knowledge, and skills can greatly enhance health care efficacy. The LEARN guideline for health care providers helps elicit cultural, social, and personal information relevant to a given illness.[41,42]

The In-Depth Interview

The in-depth interview is essential in intercultural counseling to determine many of the iceberg issues that may affect communication and cooperation in health care, including ethnicity, age, degree of acculturation or bicultural adaptation, socioeconomic status, health condition, religious affiliation, educational background, group membership, sexual orientation, or political affiliation. However, a client may believe that personal questions about his background are invasive or unnecessary, especially if he comes from a high-context culture. Direct inquiry may even suggest to the client that the practitioner is incompetent because she cannot determine the problem through indirect methods.

One culturally sensitive approach is the respondent-driven interview, in which simple, open-ended questions by the provider initiate conversation. The client can express her understanding and experience in her own words. The practitioner exerts little control over the flow of the response, yet elicits data through careful prompting. Useful questions to ask during the conversation include these:[41]

- What do you call your problem? What name do you give it?
- What do you think caused it?
- Why did it start when it did?
- What does your sickness do to your body? How does it work?
- Will you get better soon, or will it take a long time?

- What do you fear about your sickness?
- What problems has your sickness caused you personally? Your family? At work?
- What kind of treatment will work for your sickness? What results do you expect from treatment?
- What home remedies are common for this sickness? Have you used these home remedies?

Furthermore, information should be requested about traditional healers:

- How would a healer treat your sickness? Are you using that treatment?

For nutritional assessment within the context of the client's condition, questions about food habits are appropriate:

- Can what you eat help cure your sickness or make it worse?
- Do you eat certain foods to keep healthy? To make you strong?
- Do you avoid certain foods to prevent sickness?
- Do you balance eating some foods with other foods?
- Are there foods you will not eat? Why?

Learning about how a client understands his illness, including expectations about how the illness will progress, what the provider should do, and what he has established as therapeutic goals, allows the provider to compare her view of the illness and to resolve any discrepancies that might interfere with care. Demonstrating sincere interest in cultural health beliefs through an open-ended conversation can elicit the information needed to begin assessment and determine the most effective approaches for each individual.

Food for Thought

Successful communication in the interpreter–client relationship is also dependent on intercultural skills. It has been suggested that translators who build rapport and trust are more effective than those who are emotionally detached.[43]

A study on patient participation in decision-making found that 96 percent of clients want care choices offered to them and want their opinions sought. However, 52 percent preferred to leave the final decision to the physician. Well-educated White women were most likely to want shared decision-making; Black Americans and Latinx people were least likely. It is important to remember that individual differences within a culture are important in predicting whether or not to involve the patient's family in decision-making. Avoiding culture-based assumptions about desired family involvement during medical decision-making is central to providing more effective patient-centered care.[44,45]

Health care providers note that age affects intercultural communication because older minority members are often socially isolated and may be unwilling to communicate with health care providers from a different culture.[45]

Demographic data on practitioners show a disproportionate number of Whites (among dietitians, 80 percent are non-Hispanic Whites, 6 percent are Latinx, 5 percent are Asian, 3 percent are Black), suggesting that intercultural counseling will become increasingly prevalent until greater diversity in the health care professions is achieved.[46]

Intercultural Nutrition Assessment

Several difficulties in the collection and analysis of cultural health data have emerged in recent years. Researchers have discovered that standardized assessment tools can introduce systematic bias into results or provide misleading information when used with different cultural populations. Food records and 24-hour recalls are commonly used in counseling environments but are unsuitable for large-scale studies.

Generalized approaches to the use of the 24-hour food recall, food frequency forms, and nutrient databases can produce large errors in assessment.[47,48] Cultural unfamiliarity with concepts, such as fiber; terminology differences, such as using one word for several foods or not having a name for a certain category of food (e.g., there is no Native American word for "vegetables"), or grouping foods by different categories (e.g., by medicinal properties or status); lack of differentiation between meals and snacks; checking "phantom foods" (those not consumed) when not enough traditional items are available for selection; and translation mistakes (e.g., literal translations of food names, use of a brand name for a generic item, or use of the name for a traditional food for a similar American item) are a few ways collected data can be invalidated. Frequent consumption of mixed dishes can result in the omission of some nutrient sources (as when rice is prepared with dried peas or beans, yet reported as rice by some Caribbean Islanders) and overestimation or underestimation of intake due to complications in portion-size estimates. Tremendous variability in the amounts of food eaten has been reported between individuals and cultural groups.[49]

Other assessment tools may be questionable in intercultural settings as well. Health attitudes among White communities are unlikely to be reliable when applied to Mexican Americans, Asian Americans, or other groups. Contradictions between self-administered and interviewer-directed questionnaire responses occur depending on the culture; participants can be more likely to express disagreement about an item when completed individually than when asked about it by the interviewer. Cultural attitudes regarding pleasing authorities can influence answers, calling into question the use of the interview as a valid tool for gathering data in some ethnic groups. In low-literacy populations the opposite was found; self-reported data on food frequency questionnaires were found unreliable when compared to comments made by respondents during follow-up interviews.[51]

A review of acculturation scales and indexes found that many were unsuited for use in dietary interventions or nutrition education programs. Single-item measures of acculturation, including broad questions such as "How long have you lived in the United States?" and "What language do you speak at home?" provide only introductory information about a

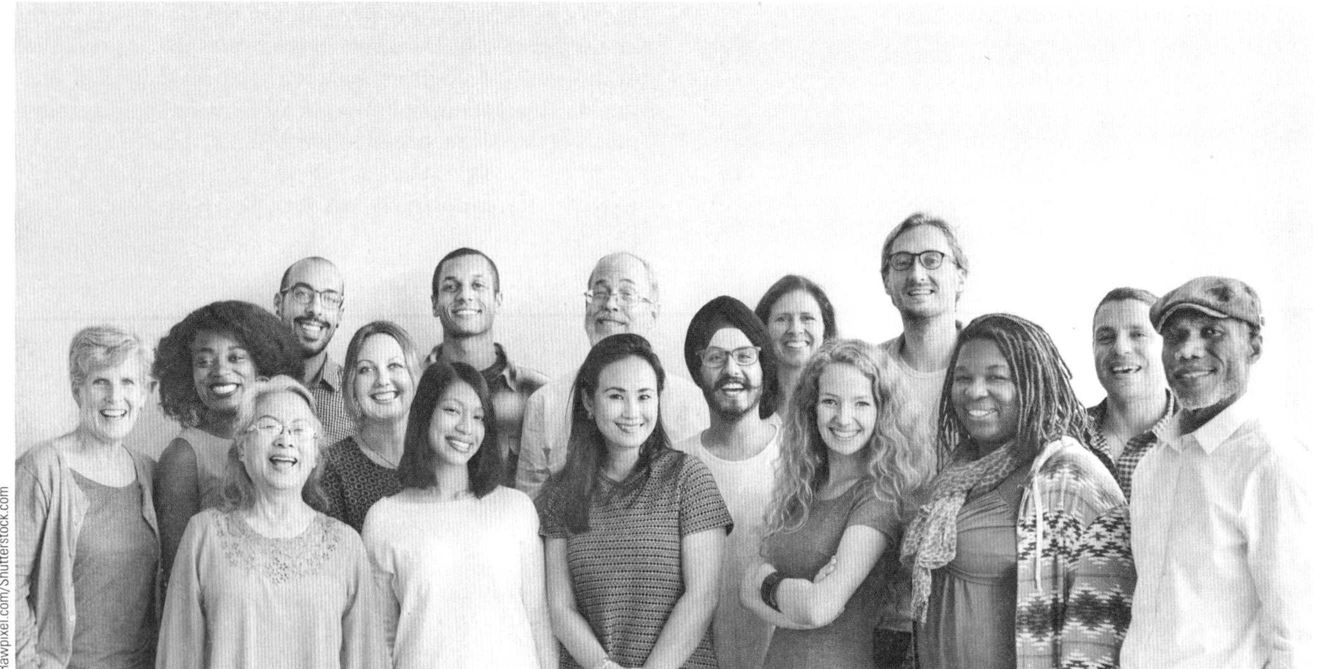

Rawpixel.com/Shutterstock.com

▲ **Standardized height and weight growth curves have not been validated for all ethnic groups and should be applied cautiously with cultural variation in mind.**

client and resulted in outcome discrepancies in data collected on dietary fat intake and acculturation in one study.[52] Acculturation scales are more comprehensive but also do not address questions regarding food habit changes. In addition, acculturation scales are typically validated on homogeneous population samples, such as college students or hospital patients, and may not be fully applicable to a more diverse clientele. Food-based assessments are more promising, but they do not provide data on the psychological or social aspects of acculturation and are usually limited to use with a single cultural group.

Food for Thought

Younger generations are more likely to try new foods today than generations of the past. This is partly due to social media and pop culture. The global ethnic food market was over 45 billion in 2020 and is projected to grow to 98 billion by 2028.[50]

Furthermore, anthropometric measurement tools are sometimes inappropriate for certain populations. Height and weight growth curves are particularly vulnerable to misinterpretation due to cultural variation, especially among Asian groups. Stature prediction equations for Whites were inaccurate for Latinx people and Black Americans.[53,54] The predictive value of waist-to-hip ratios and body mass index (BMI) may vary in some populations.[55-58] Questions about the standard BMI cutoff for overweight and obesity in Asians have been raised due to a high risk for health problems at lower numbers.[59] When the percentage of body fat data was used instead of BMI for calculating obesity in Black Americans and Whites, the difference in rates between women was cut in half (with Blacks still more at risk than Whites), and the gap for men was widened, with far more White men identified as obese. Even physiologic calculations, such as basal metabolic rate equations, may differ culturally.[53,60]

The development of culturally specific techniques and tools is a critical need in nutritional assessment. For an individual client, switching from a quantitative to a more qualitative approach can establish trust and cooperation in initial interviews. The twenty-four-hour recall, for instance, can be conducted in an open-ended manner, requesting simply that all foods consumed the previous day be remembered. This eliminates difficulties with obtaining portion sizes or differentiating meals. The dietitian does not need to predetermine food items or categories. In subsequent meetings, more information, such as frequency and number of given items, can be requested after an explanation of why the information is needed.

When working with many clients of a single cultural heritage, it may be useful to prepare quantitative tools based on qualitative research. This approach is most successful when done by an investigator already familiar with the specific group's food culture. A well-intentioned but culturally biased open-ended question (for example, asking a participant to list "any other foods eaten weekly") may not prompt the recall of foods eaten seasonally, thus underestimating a particular nutrient. The burden of negotiating two different cultural food systems should be on the researcher, not the study participant.[61,62] Detailed interviews with individuals can provide information on appropriate language, categories, concepts, and formatting of the instruments helpful in culturally specific nutritional assessment.

Monthly 24-hour recalls of small, representative samples are useful in determining overall consumption patterns, especially where seasonal variation occurs.[62] Focus groups have been found effective in selecting food items to include and quantification measures in the preparation of multicultural food frequency questionnaires.[49] Guidance from the targeted population is essential.

Access to cultural food composition data and culturally specific anthropometric and physiological measurements is more problematic. Requests for recipes can be used to expand current databases, although this technique may be too time-consuming to complete with every client. Being mindful that data analysis is often approximate and that standardized measurements may be questionable, dietary modifications should be made carefully and cautiously with all clients from cultural backgrounds other than the American majority.

Intercultural Nutrition Education

The biomedical paradigm emphasizes behavioral change accomplished through one-on-one work with an individual. However, many cultural groups prefer learning about nutrition in settings with family members or peers. For example, researchers have found that while White adolescent girls demonstrate poor outcomes when counseled with their mothers, Black adolescent girls show significantly improved outcomes when their mothers participate in weight-loss sessions.[63,64]

Successful nutrition education strategies for groups are as dependent on intercultural communication skills as is nutrition counseling with individuals. For example, researchers have described how culture can affect program outcomes in a group weight-loss setting.[65] Negative results are possible at any phase of the process, from motivation and attendance to skill acquisition and behavior change (see Figure 3.2). At each point, cultural influences may reinforce or contradict the content and context of the educational messages conveyed by the health care practitioner. When communication conflict develops, an inexact period exists when the client is willing to negotiate toward the resolution of the message. If dissatisfaction continues, a poor weight-loss outcome results because the person (1) is never motivated to sign up, (2) drops out of the program before completion, (3) attends but never learns skills, or (4) learns skills but does not apply them in practice. Program designers must do more than superficially modify the program materials and the setting to communicate effectively with a different cultural group. Understanding the cultural health beliefs, attitudes, and values of a target audience; developing education programs within the context of those perceptions; and using culturally appropriate, consistent verbal and nonverbal messages in an accepted medium increase communication efficacy.

Food for Thought

Edible insects are a rich source of protein and other nutrients for many cultures. Insect nutrition profiles are absent from nutrient composition tables and databases, making it challenging to speculate on the contribution of this food to help combat malnutrition.[66]

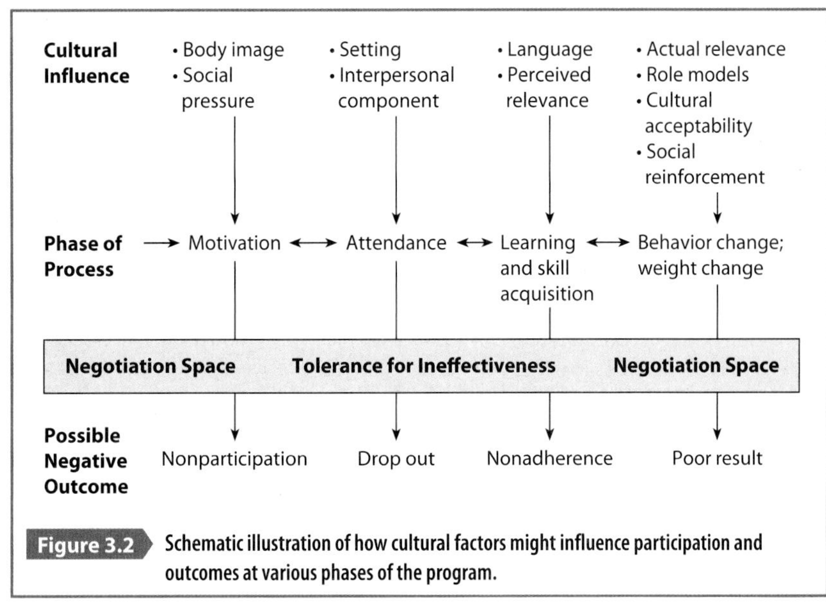

Figure 3.2 Schematic illustration of how cultural factors might influence participation and outcomes at various phases of the program.

Culturally Relevant Program Preparation

Although health education program models typically advise a step-by-step process of planning and execution, the reality is that some aspects of preparation and implementation occur concurrently. A health educator may begin planning with a general idea of goals for a population group, but will probably modify and refine objectives as more information about the target audience is gathered. Ongoing evaluation may suggest better message formats or more suitable influence channels as the effort proceeds. Effective programs are often nonlinear, with each element in planning and implementation connected through feedback and assessment into a continuous improvement loop.

Targeting the Audience

Identification of the target audience in nutrition education efforts is among the most important steps in program planning. Learning about the cultural orientation of the group is key; campaigns to change behaviors without research are usually misdirected.[67] What appear to be significant needs to the health educator may be considered unimportant or too difficult to remedy by members of the target population.

Food for Thought

Content of the message can be critical. For example, some public health advertisements targeting obesity risk, encourage unhealthy weight control and can inadvertently cause subsequent disordered eating behaviors.[68] One older study on the effects of public education efforts to reduce bulimic eating behaviors revealed that some women learned about vomiting as a weight-control method from the campaign.[69]

Definitions of health differ widely among cultures (see Chapter 2, "Traditional Health Beliefs and Practices"). Sometimes, the belief is that illness is a matter of heredity, fate, punishment by God, or is due to supernatural causes. In an older study of health perceptions held by hard-to-reach populations in the United States, it was found that though individuals believed that lifestyle might impact acute infection, there was almost no association between diet or exercise and chronic disease; respondents had limited motivation to improve health behaviors because they felt they had little personal control over their health.[70] Other factors that influence hard-to-reach groups in receiving information on healthy diets and participating in research on healthy lifestyles included mistrust in research or researchers, particularly among Black and Native Americans with a history of being mistreated in medical research, fear of authority, and perceptions that health research presented no personal benefit to them or their community and may cause potential harm, stigma, mistreatment, or exploitation. Other findings were that community gatekeepers such as some health professionals who have the opportunity to encourage health research participation failed to do so due to beliefs that people in lower socioeconomic groups don't have the time, interest, or ability to participate, or have poor communication skills.[71] The role of the individual within the group can also affect responsibility for health maintenance; in some cultures, the extended family is held accountable for the health of each member.

Demographic information about the target audience can guide program development. Primary language should be identified, as well as gender, average age, socioeconomic status, educational attainment, religious affiliation, and other iceberg factors in communication. Assessment of acculturation or bicultural adaptation is equally important. Targeted messages can be more effective when developed for culturally homogeneous populations.[72,73] In many cases, the larger, heterogeneous audience may be stratified into smaller, segmented target groups that share similar cultural beliefs and attitudes.

Involving members of the targeted audience in program planning is one of the best ways to determine cultural orientation.[71] Of special note is the role of community leaders or spokespersons in the process. Seeking the respect, trust, and endorsement of influential persons within the target audience for a particular nutrition education program can open intercultural communication channels otherwise limited to the formal interactions reserved for strangers.[71,74,75] The educator establishes a relationship with the group by asking for permission to present the health message to its members.

Setting Goals and Objectives

The next step in intercultural program planning is to define clear and realistic goals and objectives within the cultural context of the target audience. Even culturally sensitive education messages do not necessarily translate into the sustained modification of food habits without follow-up support, and overly ambitious expectations are a common reason for failure.[76] Nevertheless, strategies emphasizing the continuation of positive cultural dietary patterns or portion control rather than the elimination of certain foods appear to be effective. A barrier to eating healthfully can be when participants believe they have to give up their cultural heritage and conform to the majority culture.[73,77,78] Programs coordinating objectives with cultural beliefs about the role of food in health, such as balancing yin and yang foods in Chinese meals, can reinforce dietary change.[79,80] Consulting health care practitioners in the targeted community can provide information on local needs and concerns useful in defining achievable goals and objectives.

Developing the Message

It is believed that the more fundamental the health message is in relation to a group's survival, safety, or social needs, the more effective it will be interculturally. The message must satisfy the individual's need to gain knowledge or offer a solution to a perceived problem before it is worth the person's time to process the information. Messages should be as direct and explicit as allowed within cultural norms.[81,82] Language relevant to the group should be used in the development of the message, and translation of existing materials should be avoided to prevent inappropriate phrasing and terminology. Common words used by the target audience are effective, although it is important that they not be used in an insincere or condescending way. Written materials should be brief and prepared at the reading level of the target population.

Marketing experts recognize many cultural groups are high-context communicators and have greater abilities than the White American majority culture to send and receive messages through nonverbal modes. Body language must be culturally congruent with the verbal message for successful communication to occur. The use of pictures, cartoons, and photographic images can symbolically enhance the content meaning of a message in a high-context culture, as well as aid target populations with mixed English language skills or reading abilities.

Food for Thought

In one recent study, the barriers to healthy eating and fruit and vegetable consumption include lack of cooking skills, not liking the taste of healthy foods (too boring), preparation time, and willpower.[83]

Educational messages are most effective when they are more personal than objective; the emotional dimension is as important as the content. Many researchers recommend the universally accepted format of storytelling to deliver the message.[84] Actors and other celebrities are especially suited to recounting personal experiences about health issues. Stories can transcend many cultural boundaries; if a message is targeted toward one cultural group yet applicable to many audiences, a spokesperson identified with the intended target group also may have broader appeal when using a narrative approach.

A pilot test of the message with targeted audience members can improve success. Focus groups can be especially useful in assessing the cultural appropriateness of education materials and in identifying any resistance triggers inadvertently included in the message.[85]

Implementation Strategies

Dissemination of a nutrition education message should include analysis of cultural influence channels and media preferences, development of an effective marketing mix, and evaluation of the program. Whether a person hears, sees, and understands a message is dependent on frequency, timing, and accessibility. Exciting, informative, and culturally appropriate messages fail if they never reach the target audience.[86-88]

Food for Thought

Cultural icons incorporated into educational messages should be selected with care. For example, the owl represents wisdom in some Native American cultures; in others, the owl is a symbol of death.[89]

Mass media campaigns are believed to influence a change in health behavior in about 10 percent of the targeted audience, which can be a significant number in a large campaign.

Influence Channels

Influence channels are how message materials are transmitted to the target audience. They include television, video, computers, the Internet, radio, magazines, newspapers, newsletters, direct mail, and telephones. Each cultural group demonstrates distinct media-use patterns and is best approached through those influence channels. Oral traditions are strong among some populations, while written messages are favored by others. Computer-based, interactive nutrition education programs are now an established educational tool, particularly suitable for audiences with low literacy or limited English language skills. The Internet has become a useful technology, offering 24-hour access to health education materials and easy access to group support through bulletin boards and chat rooms, and individualized therapy through e-mail and video conferencing.[90]

Marketing Mix

The four Ps of the marketing mix are product, price, placement, and promotion. They refer to a well-developed message (product) that advances program goals and objectives at a minimal economic or psychological cost to target audience members (price) and presents this message in a method congruent with target audience media preferences (placement) in such a way that the target audience members are encouraged to become more involved in the program, either through phone numbers for further information or through attendance at group meetings (promotion). Attention to all four areas of the marketing mix ensures that the health care message is fully accessible to the target audience.

Evaluation

Process evaluation keeps track of progress throughout the program, especially the identification of larger community conditions that may be presenting barriers to the dissemination of the message. Summative evaluation is used to assess program results after the completion of the effort. Evaluation data are useful in refining intercultural nutrition education strategies both during implementation and in future programs. Publication of culturally sensitive nutrition education program results greatly benefits other health professionals and their clients through shared knowledge about intercultural communication techniques and tools.

Discussion Starters

How Does Dr. Petrocelli Improve His Patient Relations?

Consider this situation: Dr. Petrocelli is a neighborhood doctor in a large U.S. city. His office has been in this urban neighborhood for 40 years. Originally, the neighborhood was ethnically fairly homogeneous: primarily European American and African American. Over the last decade, however, more people of various ethnicities (Asian, Hispanic, and Middle Eastern), mostly immigrants to the United States, have moved into the neighborhood and are seeking health care. Dr. Petrocelli recognizes that sometimes communications with his newer patients are strained, and he worries that he is not fully understanding them and they are not fully understanding him. He's considering several different options along with their drawbacks:

- *Hire an interpreter*. Drawback: To pay this person's salary, he will need to increase the fees for his patients.
- *Continue to rely on the patients' relatives or friends to translate for him*. Drawback: He will continue to worry if the translations are accurate.
- *Start holding an in-depth interview with each of his new patients to get to know them better*. Drawback: These interviews will take a lot of time and could mean that either he will have to extend his hours—and pay his staff overtime—or set a moratorium on taking any new patients until he has completed the interviews. He worries that such a moratorium could mean that some people living in the neighborhood might not receive adequate healthcare.
- *Subscribe to a certified medical interpretation service available online*. Drawback: There is a fee for this service and equipment must be purchased for his clinic. He worries that if he is at a remote clinic or a location without Internet service or it is down, the interpreter service may not be available.

First individually and then in small groups, brainstorm which of these options might be the best—or perhaps better yet, brainstorm a solution to Dr. Petrocelli's problem that combines options or offers a completely different option.

Review Questions

1. Why is communication with another person or group described as an action chain? Give an example of an action chain that might occur when you meet (1) a friend, (2) your new boss, and (3) a young child.
2. Why is it important to become familiar with other cultures' communication behaviors? Give three examples of nonverbal communication behaviors.
3. What is meant by low- or high-context and uncertainty avoidance in describing verbal communications? Name one low-context culture and one high-context culture. How may an individual's relationship to the group differ between high- and low-context cultures? How does uncertainty avoidance differ from risk avoidance? Give an example.
4. What would be the culturally appropriate verbal address for when you meet the following individuals: an African American, a Latin American, a Vietnamese, and an Asian?

Reflection

You are seeing a family from Indonesia who speaks very little English. Your goal is to determine what the family's current eating habits are like using a 24-hour recall. How will you use the LEARN model to ascertain accurate information from this family?

References

1. Ilie, O.A. 2019, June. The intercultural competence. Developing effective intercultural communication skills. In *International Conference Knowledge-based Organization* 25(2), 264–268.
2. Tervalon, M., & Murray-Garcia, J. 1998. Cultural humility versus cultural competence: A critical distinction in defining physician training outcomes in multicultural education. *Journal of Health Care for the Poor and Underserved*, 9(2), 117–125.
3. Hargie, O. 2021. *Skilled interpersonal communication: Research, theory and practice*. Routledge.
4. Broeder, P. 2021. Informed communication in high context and low context cultures. *Journal of Education, Innovation, and Communication*, 3(1), 13–24.
5. Grady, C. 2015. Enduring and emerging challenges of informed consent. *New England Journal of Medicine*, 372(9), 855–862.
6. Merkin, R., Taras, V., & Steel, P. 2014. State of the art themes in cross-cultural communication research: A systematic and meta-analytic review. *International Journal of Intercultural Relations*, 38, 1–23.
7. De Meulenaer, S., De Pelsmacker, P., & Dens, N. 2018. Power distance, uncertainty avoidance, and the effects of source credibility on health risk message compliance. *Health Communication*, 33(3), 291–298.
8. Taylor, K., & Williams, V.R. (Eds.). 2017. *Etiquette and taboos around the world: A geographic encyclopedia of social and cultural customs*. ABC-CLIO.
9. Axtell, R.E. 1991. *Gestures: The do's and taboos of body language around the world*. New York: Wiley.
10. Suvilehto, J.T., Nummenmaa, L., Harada, T., Dunbar, R.I., Hari, R., Turner, R., & Kitada, R. 2019. Cross-cultural similarity in relationship-specific social touching. *Proceedings of the Royal Society B*, 286(1901), 20190467.
11. Mukherjee, S., & Ramos-Salazar, L. 2014. "Excuse us, your manners are missing!" The role of business etiquette in today's era of cross-cultural communication. *TSM Business Review*, 2(1), 18.
12. Anderson, D., Stuart, M., Abadi, M., & Gal, S. 2019. Five everyday hand gestures that can get you in serious trouble outside the U.S. *Business Insider*. Retrieved from https://www.businessinsider.com/hand-gestures-offensive-different-countries-2018-6

13. Corfield, P.J. 2018. Social history as revealed by gesture: Changing eighteenth-century styles of meeting and greeting. *История*, 26(3), 231–238.
14. Al-Shamahi, E. 2021. *The handshake: A gripping history*. Profile Books.
15. Oxlund, B. 2020. An anthropology of the handshake. *Anthropology Now*, 12(1), 39–44.
16. Chen, C., Crivelli, C., Garrod, O.G., Schyns, P.G., Fernández-Dols, J.M., & Jack, R.E. 2018. Distinct facial expressions represent pain and pleasure across cultures. *Proceedings of the National Academy of Sciences*, 115(43), E10013–E10021.
17. Ting-Toomey, S., & Dorjee, T. 2018. *Communicating across cultures*. Guilford Publications.
18. Irving, G., Neves, A.L., Dambha-Miller, H., Oishi, A., Tagashira, H., Verho, A., & Holden, J. 2017. International variations in primary care physician consultation time: A systematic review of 67 countries. *BMJ Open*, 7(10), e017902.
19. Angelelli, C.V. 2019. *Healthcare interpreting explained*. Routledge.
20. Silva, M.D., Genoff, M., Zaballa, A., Jewell, S., Stabler, S., Gany, F.M., & Diamond, L.C. 2016. Interpreting at the end of life: A systematic review of the impact of interpreters on the delivery of palliative care services to cancer patients with limited English proficiency. *Journal of Pain and Symptom Management*, 51(3), 569–580.
21. Rocque, R., & Leanza, Y. 2015. A systematic review of patients' experiences in communicating with primary care physicians: Intercultural encounters and a balance between vulnerability and integrity. *PloS One*, 10(10), e0139577.
22. Betancourt, J.R., Green, A.R., Carrillo, J.E., & Owusu Ananeh-Firempong, I.I. 2016. Defining cultural competence: A practical framework for addressing racial/ethnic disparities in health and health care. *Public Health Reports*.
23. Kavanagh, K., Absalom, K., Beil, W., & Schliessmann, L. 1999. Connecting and becoming culturally competent: A Lakota example. *Advances in Nursing Science*, 21, 9–31.
24. Beach, M.V., Sugarman, J., Johnson, R.L., Arbelaez, J.J., Duggan, P.S., & Cooper, L.A. 2005. Do patients treated with dignity report higher satisfaction, adherence, and receipt of preventative care? *Annals of Family Medicine*, 3, 331–338.
25. Purnell, L.D., & Fenkl, E.A. 2019. Transcultural diversity and health care. In *Handbook for culturally competent care* (pp. 1–6). Springer, Cham.
26. Hook, J.N., Davis, D., Owen, J., & DeBlaere, C. 2017. *Cultural humility: Engaging diverse identities in therapy*. American Psychological Association.
27. Fisher-Borne, M., Cain, J.M., & Martin, S.L. 2015. From mastery to accountability: Cultural humility as an alternative to cultural competence. *Social Work Education*, 34(2), 165–181.
28. Foronda, C. 2020. A theory of cultural humility. *Journal of Transcultural Nursing*, 31(1), 7–12.
29. Mosher, D.K., Hook, J.N., Farrell, J.E., Watkins Jr., C.E., & Davis, D.E. 2016. Cultural humility. In *Handbook of humility* (pp. 107–120). Routledge.
30. McGregor, B., Belton, A., Henry, T.L., Wrenn, G., & Holden, K.B. 2019. Improving behavioral health equity through cultural competence training of health care providers. *Ethnicity & Disease*, 29(Suppl. 2), 359.
31. Dresser, N. 2011. *Multicultural manners: Essential rules of etiquette for the 21st century*. New York: Wiley.
32. Morrison, T., & Conaway, W.A. 2007. *Kiss, bow, or shake hands: Asia: how to do business in 12 Asian countries*. Avon, MA: Adams Media.
33. Burner, O.Y., Cunningham, P., & Hattar, H.S. 1990. Managing a multicultural nurse staff in a multicultural environment. *Journal of Nursing Administration*, 20, 30–34.
34. Samovar, L.A., Porter, R.E., McDaniel, E.R., & Roy, C.S. 2017. *Communication between cultures*. Cengage Learning.
35. Paraskevi-Lukeriya, I. 2017. Refusal strategies in English and Russian. *Вестник Российского университета дружбы народов. Серия: Теория языка. Семиотика. Семантика*, 8(3), 531–542.
36. Beckers, A.M. 1999. *How to say "no" without saying "no": A study of the refusal strategies of Americans and Germans*. The University of Mississippi.
37. Al Shamsi, H., Almutairi, A.G., Al Mashrafi, S., & Al Kalbani, T. 2020. Implications of language barriers for healthcare: A systematic review. *Oman Medical Journal*, 35(2), e122.
38. Meuter, R.F., Gallois, C., Segalowitz, N.S., Ryder, A.G., & Hocking, J. 2015. Overcoming language barriers in healthcare: A protocol for investigating safe and effective communication when patients or clinicians use a second language. *BMC Health Services Research*, 15(1), 1–5.
39. Woloshin, S., Bickell, N.A., Schwartz, L.M., Gany, F., & Welch, H.G. 1995. Language barriers in medicine in the United States. *Journal of the American Medical Association*, 273, 724–728.
40. Johnson, H., Perez., C.A., & Mejia, M.C. 2020 Fact sheet-immigrants in California. Public Policy Institute of California. Retrieved from https://www.ppic.org/publication/immigrants-in-california/ (accessed May 23, 2022).
41. Bauer, K.D., & Liou, D. 2020. *Nutrition counseling and education skill development*. Cengage Learning.
42. Kersey-Matusiak, G. 2018. Cultural competency models and guidelines. *Delivering culturally competent nursing care: Working with diverse and vulnerable populations*, 25.
43. Susam-Saraeva, Ş., & Spišiaková, E. (Eds.). 2021. *The Routledge handbook of translation and health*. Routledge.
44. Alden, D.L., Friend, J., Lee, P.Y., Lee, Y.K., Trevena, L., Ng, C.J., & Limpongsanurak, S. 2018. Who decides: Me or we? Family involvement in medical decision making in eastern and western countries. *Medical Decision Making*, 38(1), 14–25.
45. Levinson, W., Kao, A., Kuby, A., & Thisted, R.A. 2005. Not all patients want to participate in decision making. A national study of public preferences. *Journal of General Internal Medicine*, 20, 531–535.
46. Rogers, D. 2021. 2020 needs satisfaction survey. *JAND 121*(1) 134–138. Retrieved from https://www.jandonline.org/article/S2212-2672(20)31389-7/fulltext (accessed May 23, 2022).
47. Malekshah, A., et al., 2006. Validity and reliability of a new food frequency questionnaire compared to 24h recalls and biochemical measurements: Pilot phase of Golestan cohort study of esophageal cancer. *European Journal of Clinical Nutrition*, 60, 971–977.
48. Cade, J., et al., 2002. Development, validation and utilization of food-frequency questionnaires – a review. *Public Health Nutrition* 5(4), 567–587.
49. Barbieri, P., Crivellenti, L.C., Nishimura, R.Y., & Sartorelli, D.S. 2015. Validation of a food frequency questionnaire to assess food group intake by pregnant women. *Journal of Human Nutrition and Dietetics*, 28, 38–44.
50. Fortune Business Insights. ND. The global ethnic food market is projected to grow from $49.27 billion in 2021 to $98.06 billion in 2028 at a CAGR of 10.33% in forecast period, 2021–2028 Retrieved from: https://www.fortunebusinessinsights.com/ethnic-foods-market-102264 (accessed May 23, 2023).
51. Shim, J.S., Oh, K., & Kim, H.C. 2014. Dietary assessment methods in epidemiologic studies. *Epidemiology and Health*, *36*.
52. Norman, S., Castro, C., Albright, C., & King, A. 2004. Comparing acculturation models in evaluating dietary habits among low-income Hispanic women. *Ethnicity & Disease*, 14, 399–404.
53. Heymsfield, S.B., Peterson, C.M., Thomas, D.M., Heo, M., & Schuna Jr., J.M. 2016. Why are there race/ethnic differences in adult body mass index–adiposity relationships? A quantitative critical review. *Obesity Reviews*, 17(3), 262–275.
54. Misra, A. 2015. Ethnic-specific criteria for classification of body mass index: A perspective for Asian Indians and American Diabetes Association position statement. *Diabetes Technology & Therapeutics*, 17(9), 667–671.

55. Slattery, M.L., Ferucci, E.D., Murtaugh, M.A., Edwards, S., Ma, K.N., Etzel, R.A., & Lanier, A.P. 2010. Associations among body mass index, waist circumference, and health indicators in American Indian and Alaska Native adults. *American Journal of Health Promotion*, 24, 246–254.
56. Yatsuya, H., Folsom, A.R., Yamagishi, K., North, K.E., Brancati, F.L., & Stevens, J. 2010. Atherosclerosis Risk in Communities Study Investigators. Race- and sex-specific associations of obesity measures with ischemic stroke incidence in the Atherosclerosis Risk in Communities (ARIC) study. *Stroke*, 41, 417–425.
57. Huxley, R., Mendis, S., Zheleznyakov, E., Reddy, S., & Chan, J. 2010. Body mass index, waist circumference and waist:hip ratio as predictors of cardiovascular risk—A review of the literature. *European Journal of Clinical Nutrition*, 64, 16–22.
58. Lusky, A., Lubin, F., Barell, V., Kaplan, G., Layani, V., & Wiener, M. 2000. Body mass index in 17-year-old Israeli males of different ethnic backgrounds: National or ethnic-specific references? *International Journal of Obesity and Related Metabolic Disorders*, 24, 88–92.
59. McNeely, M.J., & Boyko, E.J. 2004. Type 2 diabetes prevalence in Asian Americans: Results of a national health study. *Diabetes Care*, 27, 66–69.
60. Adab, P., Pallan, M., & Whincup, P.H. 2018. Is BMI the best measure of obesity? *BMJ*, 360.
61. Block, G., Mandel, R., & Gold, E. 2004. On food frequency questionnaires: The contribution of open-ended questions and questions about ethnic foods. *Epidemiology*, 15, 216–221.
62. Teufel, N.I. 1997. Development of culturally competent food-frequency questionnaires. *American Journal of Clinical Nutrition*, *65*(Suppl.), 1173S–1178S.
63. Lambert, L.J., Raidl, M., & Safaii, S. 2005. Perceptions of barriers to weight loss in overweight WIC women. T*opics in Clinical Nutrition Journal*, 20(1).
64. Quintiliani, L.M., & Whiteley, J.A. 2016. Results of a nutrition and physical activity peer counseling intervention among non-traditional college students. *Journal of Cancer Education*, 31(2), 366–374.
65. Magnus, M., & Gay, M. 2016. Barriers facing multicultural participants in a university weight loss program: A preliminary study. *Mathews Journal of Nutrition & Dietetics*, 1(1), 1–9.
66. Nowak, V., Persijn, D., Rittenschober, D., & Charrondiere, U.R. 2016. Review of food composition data for edible insects. *Food Chemistry*, 193, 39–46.
67. Davis, K.C., & Duke, J.C. 2018. Evidence of the real-world effectiveness of public health media campaigns reinforces the value of perceived message effectiveness in campaign planning. *Journal of Communication*, 68(5), 998–1000.
68. Bristow, C., Allen, K.A., Simmonds, J., Snell, T., & McLean, L. 2022. Anti-obesity public health advertisements increase risk factors for the development of eating disorders. *Health Promotion International*, 37(2), daab107.
69. Swartz, L. 1987. Illness negotiation: The case of eating disorders. *Social Science and Medicine*, 24, 613–618.
70. White, S.L., & Maloney, S.K. 1990. Promoting healthy diets and active lives to hard-to-reach groups: Market research study. *Public Health Reports*, 105, 224–231.
71. Bonevski, B., Randell, M., Paul, C., Chapman, K., Twyman, L., Bryant, J., & Hughes, C. 2014. Reaching the hard-to-reach: A systematic review of strategies for improving health and medical research with socially disadvantaged groups. *BMC Medical Research Methodology*, 14(1), 1–29.
72. Meyer, E. 2016. *The culture map (INTL ED): Decoding how people think, lead, and get things done across cultures*. PublicAffairs.
73. Winham, D.M., Knoblauch, S.T., Heer, M.M., Thompson, S.V., & Der Ananian, C. 2020. African-American views of food choices and use of traditional foods. *American Journal of Health Behavior*, 44(6), 848–863.
74. McCurley, J.L., Gutierrez, A.P., & Gallo, L.C. 2017. Diabetes prevention in US Hispanic adults: A systematic review of culturally tailored interventions. *American Journal of Preventive Medicine*, 52(4), 519–529.
75. Lagisetty, P.A., Priyadarshini, S., Terrell, S., Hamati, M., Landgraf, J., Chopra, V., & Heisler, M. 2017. Culturally targeted strategies for diabetes prevention in minority population: A systematic review and framework. *The Diabetes Educator*, 43(1), 54–77.
76. Rossmann, C. 2017. Content effects: Health campaign communication. *The International Encyclopedia of Media Effects*, 1–11.
77. Kamphuis, C.B., de Bekker-Grob, E.W., & van Lenthe, F.J. 2015. Factors affecting food choices of older adults from high and low socioeconomic groups: A discrete choice experiment. *The American Journal of Clinical Nutrition*, 101(4), 768–774.
78. Vabø, M., & Hansen, H. 2014. The relationship between food preferences and food choice: A theoretical discussion. *International Journal of Business and Social Science*, 5(7).
79. Britannica. n.d. Central Asia and China. Retrieved from: https://www.britannica.com/topic/Buddhism/Central-Asia-and-China
80. Foy, G. 2014. Buddhism in China. *Asia Society*. Retrieved from https://asiasociety.org/buddhism-china
81. Sue, D.W., Sue, D., Neville, H.A., & Smith, L. 2019. *Counseling the culturally diverse: Theory and practice*. John Wiley & Sons.
82. Diller, J.V. 2018. *Cultural diversity: A primer for the human services*. Cengage Learning.
83. McMorrow, L., Ludbrook, A., Macdiarmid, J.I., & Olajide, D. 2017. Perceived barriers towards healthy eating and their association with fruit and vegetable consumption. *Journal of Public Health*, 39(2), 330–338.
84. Simmons, A. (2019). *The story factor: Inspiration, influence, and persuasion through the art of storytelling*. Basic Books.
85. Epstein, J., Santo, R.M., & Guillemin, F. 2015. A review of guidelines for cross-cultural adaptation of questionnaires could not bring out a consensus. *Journal of Clinical Epidemiology*, 68(4), 435–441.
86. Tombleson, B., & Wolf, K. 2017. Rethinking the circuit of culture: How participatory culture has transformed cross-cultural communication. *Public Relations Review*, 43(1), 14–25.
87. Lin, H.C., Swarna, H., & Bruning, P.F. 2017. Taking a global view on brand post popularity: Six social media brand post practices for global markets. *Business Horizons*, *60*(5), 621–633.
88. Li, C., & Tsai, W.H.S. 2015. Social media usage and acculturation: A test with Hispanics the US. *Computers in Human Behavior*, 45, 204–212.
89. Hodge, F.S., Paqua, A., Marquez, C.A., & Geishirt-Cantrell, B. 2002. Utilizing traditional storytelling to promote wellness, in American Indian communities. *Journal of Transcultural Nursing*, 13, 6–11.
90. Zhao, Y., Wang, N., Li, Y., Zhou, R., & Li, S. 2021. Do cultural differences affect users' e-learning adoption? A meta-analysis. *British Journal of Educational Technology*, 52(1), 20–41.

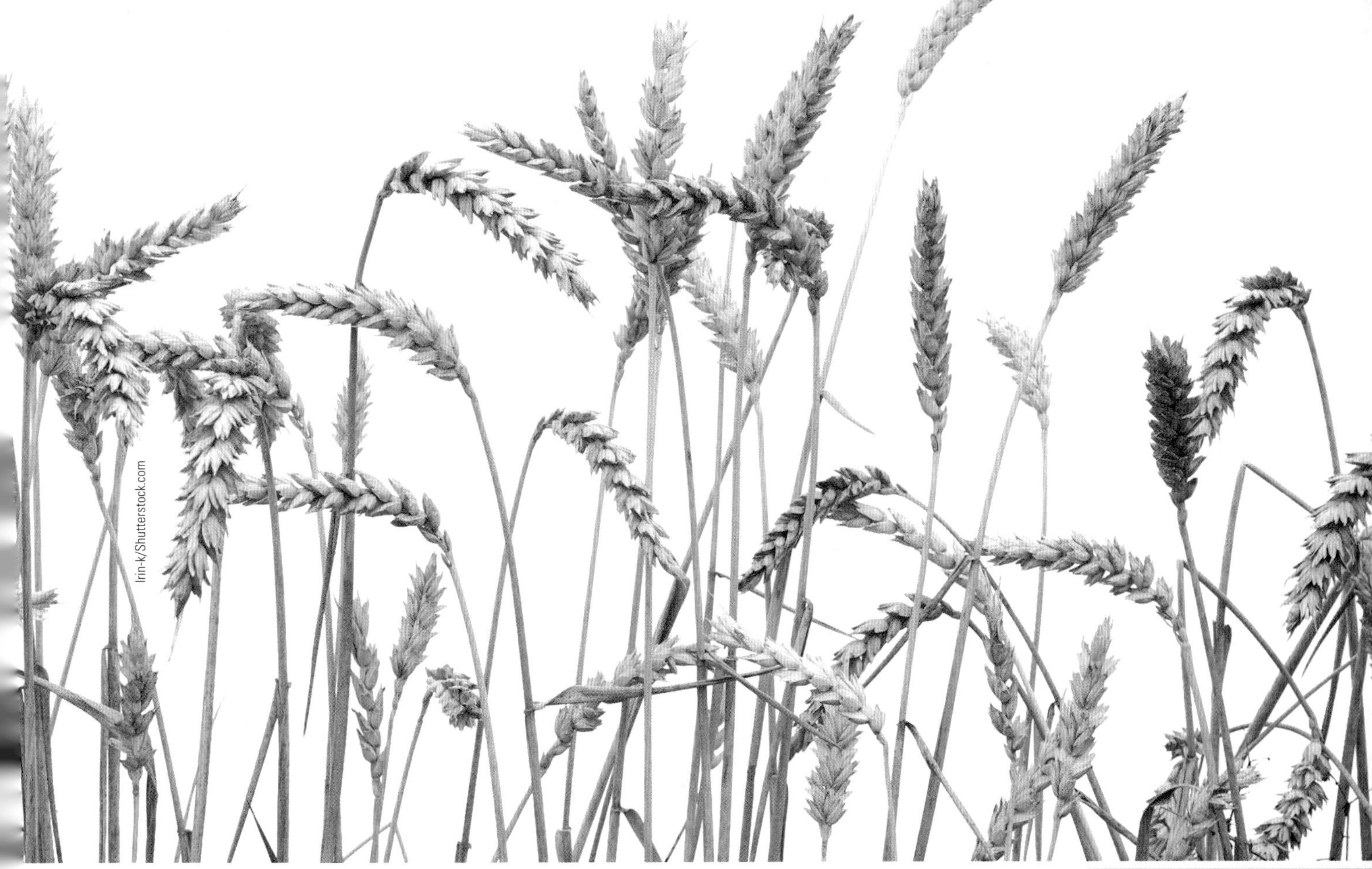
Irin-k/Shutterstock.com

Chapter 4

Food and Religion

Learning Objectives

4.1 Identify the major Western and Eastern religions.

4.2 List the two major subcultures of Judaism and where adherents mainly settled in the United States.

4.3 Define the Jewish dietary laws of kashrut.

4.4 Describe the religious requirements of halal foods according to Islam.

4.5 Identify the Christian religions that have specific laws regarding foods and eating.

4.6 Describe how the concepts of purity and pollution regarding food are related to the Hindu religion.

4.7 Discuss the reasons researchers have offered regarding the meat prohibitions found throughout different cultures.

4.8 Demonstrate how the Buddhist and Hindu principles of reincarnation, karma, and non-violence may relate to maintaining a vegetarian diet.

Religion is an organized set of beliefs and practices of a group of people and can involve cultural perspectives, worldviews, prophecies, and morals. Some religions are centered on a belief in a god, gods, or supernatural forces. Food, because it sustains life, is an important part of religious symbols, rites, and customs—those acts of daily life intended to bring about an orderly relationship with the spiritual or supernatural realm.

In the Western world, Judaism, Christianity, and Islam are the most prevalent religions, whereas Hinduism and Buddhism are common in the East. Western religions, originating in the Middle East, are equated with the belief that God is omnipotent and omniscient. They believe that a person's life is a time of testing and preparation for everlasting life when humans will be held accountable to God for their actions on earth.

The Eastern religions of Hinduism and Buddhism, developed in India, do not teach that God is the lord and maker of the universe who demands that humankind be righteous. Rather, the principal goal of Indian religions is deliverance, or liberation, of the immortal human soul from the bondage of the body. Moreover, nearly all Indian religions teach that liberation, given training, can be experienced in the present life.

This chapter discusses the beliefs and food practices of the world's major religions. Other religions of importance to specific cultures are introduced in the following chapters on each ethnic group. As with any description of food habits, it is important to remember that religious dietary practices vary enormously, even among members of the same faith. Many religious food practices were codified hundreds or thousands of years ago for a specific locale and, consequently, have been reinterpreted over time to meet the needs of expanding populations.

As a result, most religions have areas of curiosity when considered alongside guidelines for modern dietary intake. For example, fish without scales are banned under kosher food laws. Is sturgeon, born with scales they loose with maturity, considered fit to eat for observant Jews? Orthodox Jews say no, whereas many Conservative and Reform Jews say yes: smoked sturgeon can be found at almost any Jewish deli. Hindus might avoid consuming fish with "ugly forms," and fish that are undesirable are identified according to local tradition. In addition, religious food practices are often adapted to personal needs. Catholics, encouraged to make a sacrifice during Lent, traditionally gave up meat but today may choose to give up pastries or candy instead. Buddhists may adopt a vegetarian diet only during the period when as an elder they become a monk or nun. Because religious food prescriptions are usually written in some form, it is tempting to see them as being black-and-white. However, they are among the most variable of culturally based food habits (refer to Table 4.1).[3]

Food for Thought

U.S. law now prohibits the census from including mandatory questions regarding religion. Independent national survey data often differ from religious group records regarding membership.

Christians remain the largest religious group in the United States and Muslims have experienced the greatest increase among religious groups (refer to Figure 4.1).[1] The United States' religious makeup differs from the world as a whole (refer to Figure 4.2).[2]

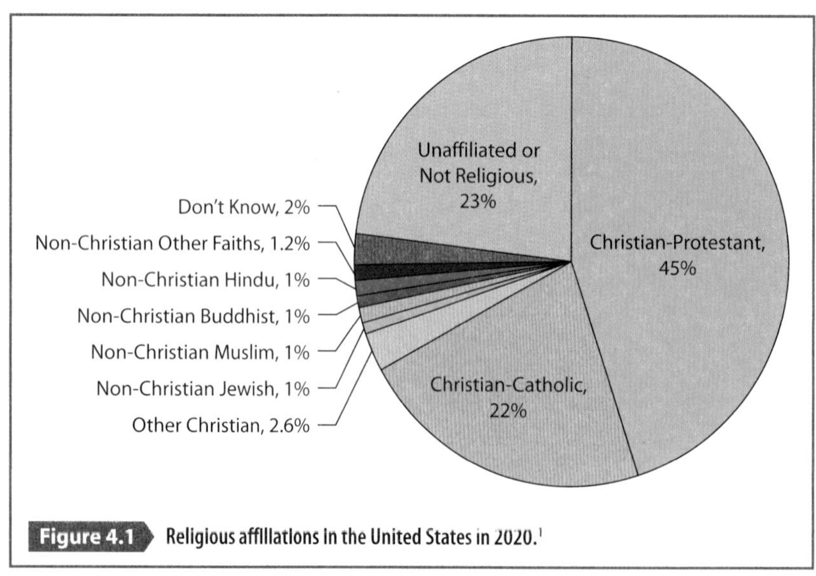

Figure 4.1 Religious affiliations in the United States in 2020.[1]

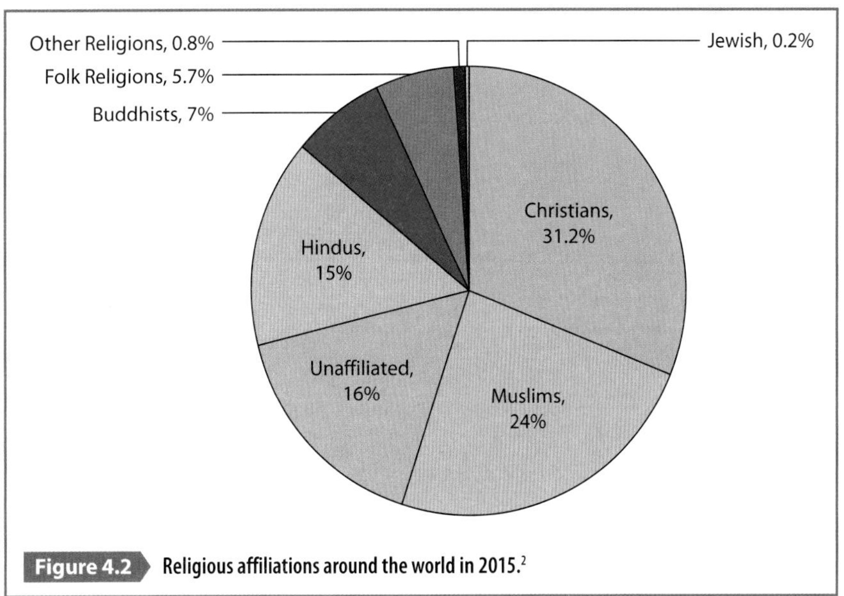

Figure 4.2 Religious affiliations around the world in 2015.[2]

Table 4.1 Common Religious Food Practices

	ADV	BUD	EOX	HIN	JEW	MOR	MUS	RCA
Beef		A		X				
Pork	X	A		A	X		X	
All meat	A	A	R	A	R		R	R
Eggs/dairy	O	O	R	O	R			
Fish	A	A	R	R	R		R	
Shellfish	X	A	O	R	X			
Alcohol	X			A		X	X	
Coffee/tea	X					X	A	
Meat and dairy at the same meal					X			
Leavened foods					R			
Ritual slaughter of meats					+		+	
Moderation	+	+				+	+	

Note: ADV, Seventh-Day Adventist; BUD, Buddhist; EOX, Eastern Orthodox; HIN, Hindu; JEW, Jewish; MOR, Mormon; MUS, Muslim; RCA, Roman Catholic. X, prohibited or strongly discouraged; A, avoided by most devout; R, some restrictions regarding types of foods or when foods are eaten observed by some adherents; O, permitted, but may be avoided at some observances; +, practiced.

Western Religions

Judaism

The Jewish religion, estimated to be about 4,000 years old, started when Abraham received God's earliest covenant for the Jews. Judaism was originally a nation (Judea or Judaea), as well as a religion. However, after the destruction of the capital, Jerusalem, and main sanctuary, the Temple of Solomon, by the Romans in 70 CE, it had no homeland until the birth of Israel in 1948.

During the Diaspora (the dispersion of Jews outside of their homeland), Jews scattered and settled all over the ancient world. Two subcultures of Judaism eventually developed: Ashkenazi, those Jews who prospered in Germany, northern France, and the eastern European countries; and the Sephardim (called Misrahi in Israel), Jews originally from Spain, who now inhabit most southern European and Middle Eastern countries. Hasidic Jews are observant Ashkenazi Jews who believe salvation is to be found in joyous communion with God as well as in the Bible. Hasidic men are evident in larger U.S. cities by their dress, which includes long black coats and black or fur-trimmed hats (worn on Saturdays and holidays only), and by their long beards with side curls.

Food for Thought

In the 2014 Canadian Social Survey, 69.8 percent of the population was identified as Christian, 20 percent had no religious affiliation, and 7.2 percent were identified as non-Christian (refer to Figure 4.3). It is estimated that there are 1,053,945 Muslims (3.2 percent of the population), 550,700 Eastern Orthodox Christians, 329,500 Jews, 498,000 Hindus, 455,000 Sikhs, and 366,800 Buddhists in Canada. Sixteen percent of the population adheres to no religion.[4]

The cornerstone of the Jewish religion is the Hebrew Bible, particularly the first five books of the Bible, the Pentateuch, also known as the books of Moses, or the Torah. It consists of the books of Genesis, Exodus, Leviticus, Numbers, and Deuteronomy. The Torah chronicles the beginnings of Judaism and contains the basic laws that express the will of God to the Jews. The Torah not only sets down the Ten Commandments, but also describes the right way to prepare food, give to charity, and conduct one's life in all ways. The interpretation of the Torah and commentary on it are found in the Talmud. The basic tenet of Judaism is that there is only one God, and His will must be obeyed. Jews do not believe in original sin (that humans are born sinful) but rather that all people can choose to act in a right or wrong way. Sin is attributed to human weakness. Humans can achieve, unaided, their own redemption by asking for God's absolution (if they have sinned against God) or by asking for forgiveness of the person they sinned against. The existence of the hereafter is recognized, but the main concern in Judaism is with this life and adherence to the laws of the Torah. Many Jews belong to or attend a synagogue (temple), which is led by a rabbi, who is a scholar, teacher, and spiritual leader. In the United States, congregations are usually classified as Orthodox, Conservative, or Reform, although American Jews represent a spectrum of beliefs and practices. The main division among the three groups is their position on Jewish laws. Orthodox Jews believe that all Jewish laws, as the direct commandments of God, must be observed in all detail. Reform Jews do not believe that the ritual laws are permanently binding but that the moral law is valid. They believe that the laws are still being interpreted and that some laws may be irrelevant or out of date, and therefore they observe only certain religious practices. Conservative Jews hold the middle ground between Orthodox and Reform beliefs.[5,6]

Food for Thought

The kosher food market was valued at $19.1 billion in 2018 and is projected to reach $25.6 billion by 2026. In the United States, as much as 41 percent of the packaged food in the country is kosher certified. More than 50 percent of kosher food is purchased by non-Jewish people, including Muslims, Seventh-Day Adventists, vegetarians, and those with food allergies, in part due to its reputation for safety and purity.[8,9]

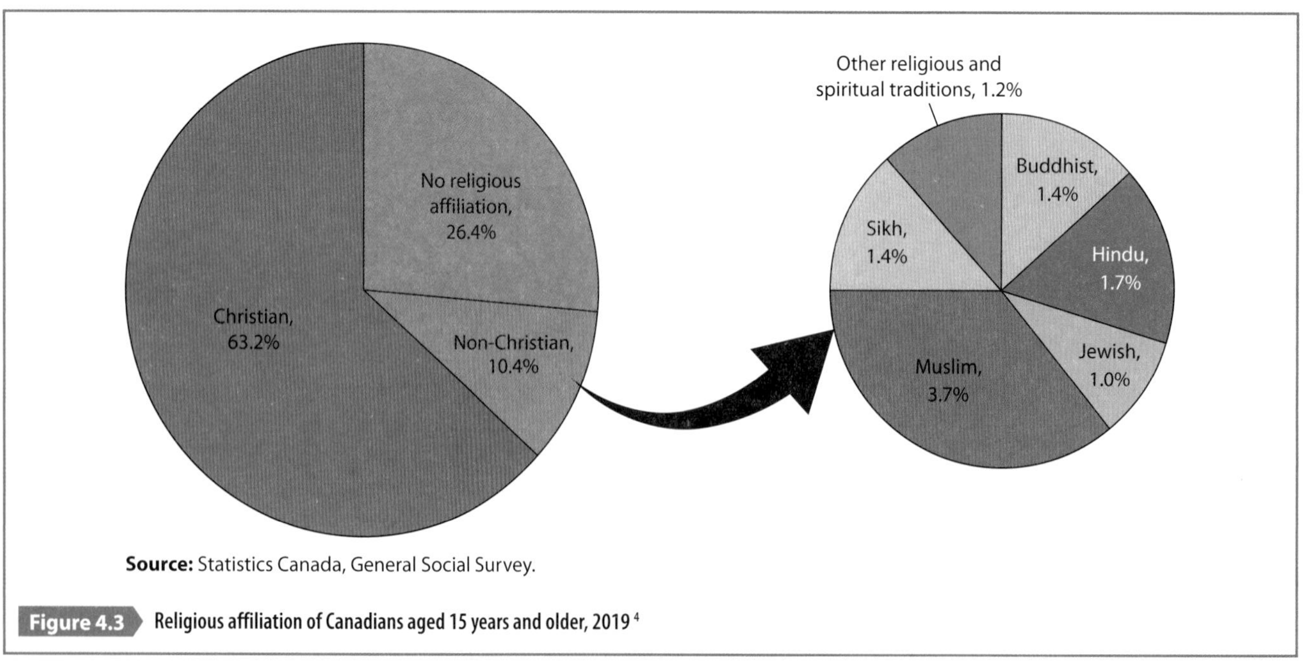

Source: Statistics Canada, General Social Survey.

Figure 4.3 Religious affiliation of Canadians aged 15 years and older, 2019[4]

Immigration to the United States

In the early 19th century, Jewish people, primarily from Germany, sought economic opportunities in the New World. By 1860, approximately 280,000 Jewish people were living in the United States. Peak Jewish immigration occurred around the turn of the century (1880–1920) when vast numbers of Jewish people moved from eastern Europe because of poverty and pogroms (organized massacres practiced by Russia against Jewish people before World War II).

During the Great Depression, Jewish people continued to immigrate to the United States, primarily to escape Nazi Germany. Their numbers were few, however, because of restrictions in the immigration quota system. Today, Jewish people continue to come to the United States, especially from Russia. Some come from Israel as well. The Jewish population in the United States was 5.7 million adults and children in 2020, according to data compiled from local federations; close to half of the Jewish people in the United States live in the northeastern region of the nation.[5,6,7] Large populations are found in New York, California, and Florida. Most Jewish people in the United States are Ashkenazi: 10 percent identify themselves as Orthodox, 34 percent as Conservative, 29 percent as Reform, and the rest are not affiliated with a specific congregation.

Kashrut: Jewish Dietary Laws

Some people in the United States believe that Jewish food consists of dill pickles, bagels and lox (smoked salmon), and chicken soup. In actuality, the foods Jewish people eat reflect the regions where their families originated. Because most Jewish people in the United States are Ashkenazi, their diet includes the foods of Germany and eastern Europe. Sephardic Jewish people tend to eat foods similar to those of southern Europe and Middle Eastern countries, whereas those from India might prefer foods from South Asia. All Orthodox and many Conservative Jewish people follow the dietary laws, kashrut, that were set down in the Torah and further explained in the Talmud.

Kosher or kasher means "fit" and is a popular term for Jewish dietary laws and permitted food items. *Glatt* kosher means that the strictest kosher standards are used in obtaining and preparing food. The laws that provide the foundation for a kosher dietary pattern are collectively referred to as kashrut and are found within the Torah, the Jewish book of sacred texts. Kashrut is one of the pillars of Jewish religious life and is concerned with the fitness of food. Many health-related explanations have been postulated about the origins of Jewish dietary restrictions; however, it is spiritual health, not physical health or any other factor, that is the primary reason for their observance. Jewish people who keep kosher are expressing their sense of obligation to God, to their community, and to themselves, making the seemingly mundane act of eating holy. For food to be considered kosher, it must follow these basic rules (refer Figure 4.4):

- Certain species of animals (and their eggs and milk) are permitted for consumption, while others are forbidden—most notably pork, rabbits, reptiles, and shellfish. Mammals that have split hooves and chew their cud (cows, sheep, goats, bison, and deer) and fish with fins and scales are kosher. The species of kosher birds are listed in the Torah.
- Meat and milk are never combined. Separate utensils are used for each.
- Meat must come from animals that are slaughtered in a specific (and painless) manner known as *shechitah*.
- Fruits, vegetables, and grains are always kosher but must be insect free.
- Wine or grape juice should be certified kosher.

Food for Thought

Most gelatin is obtained from processed pig tissues. Kosher, gelatin-like products are available.

In 2002, the first kosher food in outer space was served to astronaut Ilan Ramon on the space shuttle Columbia.

Tevilah is the Jewish ritual purification of metal or glass pots, dishes, and utensils through immersion in the running water of a river or ocean. Chinese porcelain and ceramic items are exempt.

The prohibition of eating an animal with a sciatic nerve is based on the biblical story of Jacob's nighttime fight with a mysterious being who touched him on the thigh, causing him to limp.

Religious Holidays

The Sabbath The Jewish Sabbath, the day of rest, is observed from shortly before sundown on Friday until after nightfall on Saturday. Traditionally, the Sabbath is a day devoted to prayer and rest, and no work is allowed. All cooked meals must be prepared before sundown on Friday because no fires can be kindled on the Sabbath. Challah, a braided bread, is commonly served with the Friday night meal. In most Ashkenazi homes the meal would traditionally contain fish, chicken, or cholent, a bean and potato dish that can be prepared Friday afternoon and left simmering until the evening meal on Saturday. Kugel, a pudding often made with noodles, is a typical side dish.

Rosh Hashanah The Jewish religious year begins with the New Year, or Rosh Hashanah, which means "head of the year." Rosh Hashanah is also the beginning of a ten-day period of penitence that ends with the Day of Atonement, Yom Kippur. Rosh Hashanah occurs in September or October; as with all Jewish holidays, the actual date varies from year to year because the Jewish calendar is based on lunar months counted according to biblical custom and does not coincide with the secular calendar. For this holiday, the challah is baked in a round shape that symbolizes life without end and a year of uninterrupted health and happiness. In some communities, the challah is

The Union of Orthodox Jewish Congregations
New York, New York

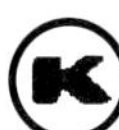
O.K. (Organized Kashrut) Laboratories
Brooklyn, New York

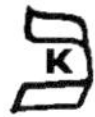
Kosher Supervision Service
Teaneck, New Jersey

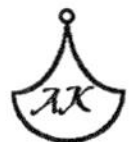
Asian-American Kashrus Services
San Rafael, California

The Heart "K" Kehilla Kosher
Los Angeles, California

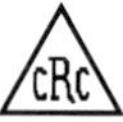

Chicago Rabbinical Council
Chicago, Illinois

Orthodox Vaad of Philadelphia
Philadelphia, Pennsylvania

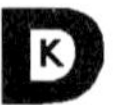
Vaad Hakashrus of Dallas, Inc.
Dallas, Texas

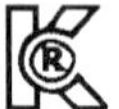
Vaad Harabonim of Greater Detroit and Merkaz
Southfield, Michigan

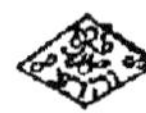
Orthodox Rabbinical Council of S. Florida
(Vaad Harabonim De Darom Florida)
Miami Beach, Florida

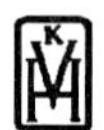
Vaad Harabonim of Massachusetts
Boston, Massachusetts

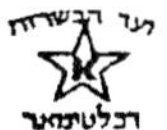
Vaad Hakashrus of the Orthodox Jewish
Council of Baltimore
Baltimore, Maryland

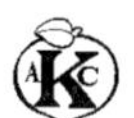
Atlanta Kashruth Commission
Atlanta, Georgia

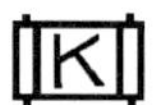
Vaad Hakashrus of Denver
Denver, Colorado

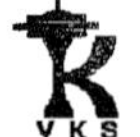

Vaad Harabonim of Greater Seattle
Seattle, Washington

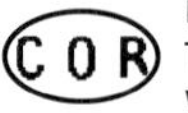

Kashruth Council Orthodox Division
Toronto Jewish Congress
Willowdale, Ontario, Canada

Montreal Vaad Hair
Montreal, Canada

Vancouver Kashruth
British Columbia, Canada

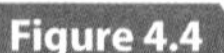
Figure 4.4 **Examples of kosher food symbols.**

formed like a bird representing God's protection. Apples are dipped in honey, and a special prayer is said for a sweet and pleasant year. Some families traditionally consume the head of a fish or a sheep, with the wish that God's will for them is to be at the head, not the tail, of any undertakings in the upcoming year. On the second night, a new fruit, one that hasn't been consumed for a long period, is enjoyed with a prayer for a year of plenty. Often, the fruit is a pomegranate, which reputedly contains 613 seeds, the same as the number of commandments listed in the Torah. No sour or bitter foods are served on this holiday, and special sweets and delicacies, such as honey cakes, are usually prepared.

Yom Kippur, the Day of Atonement Yom Kippur falls ten days after Rosh Hashanah and is the holiest day of the year. On this day, every Jew atones for sins committed against God and those committed against other people and resolves to improve and once again follow all the Jewish laws. Yom Kippur is a complete fast day (no food or water; medications are allowed) from sunset to sunset. Everyone fasts, except boys under 13 years old, girls under 12 years old, persons who are very ill, and women in childbirth. The meal before Yom Kippur is usually bland to prevent thirst during the fast. The meal that breaks the fast is typically light, including dairy foods or fish, fruits, and vegetables.

Sukkot, Feast of Tabernacles Sukkot is a festival of thanksgiving. It occurs in September or October and lasts one week. On the last day, Simchat Torah, the reading of the Torah (a portion is read every week of the year) is completed for the year and started again. This festival is very joyous, with much singing and dancing. Some Jewish families build a sukkah (hut) in their yards and hang fruit and flowers from the rafters, which are spaced far enough apart so that the sky and stars are visible. Meals are eaten in the sukkah during Sukkot.

Hanukkah, the Festival of Lights Hanukkah is celebrated for eight days, usually during the month of December, to commemorate the recapture of the Temple in Jerusalem in 169 CE. Families celebrate Hanukkah by lighting one candle on the menorah (candelabra) each night so that on the last night all eight candles are lit. Traditionally, potato pancakes, called latkes, are eaten during Hanukkah. Other foods cooked in oil, such as doughnuts, are often eaten as well.

Purim Purim, a joyous celebration that takes place in February or March, commemorates Queen Esther's rescue of the Persian Jews from the villainous Haman. It is a mitzvah (good deed) to eat an abundant meal in honor of the deliverance. The feast should include ample amounts of meat and alcoholic beverages. Customarily, people dress in disguise for the day to hide from Haman, to add surprise to gift giving, or to hide from God while overindulging. A food associated with Purim is *hamantaschen* (literally, "Haman's pockets"). A hamantasch is a triangular-shaped pastry often filled with sweetened poppy seeds or fruit jams made from prunes or apricots. Another pastry associated with Purim is kreplach (a triangular or heart-shaped savory pastry stuffed with seasoned meat or cheese and then boiled like ravioli).

Purim challah (a sweet bread with raisins), and fish cooked for the holiday in vinegar, raisins, and spices are often served. Seeds, beans, and cereals are offered in remembrance of the restricted diet eaten by the pious Queen Esther.

Food for Thought

Two breads, or one bread with a smaller loaf braided on top, are usually served on Fridays, the beginning of the Sabbath, symbolic of the double portion of manna (nourishment) provided by God to help sustain the Israelites when they wandered in the desert for 40 years after their exodus from Egypt.

In some less affluent Ashkenazi homes, gefilte (filled) fish became popular on the Sabbath. Similar to the concept of meatloaf, it is made by extending the fish by pulverizing it with eggs, bread, onion, sugar, salt, and pepper, then stewing the balls or patties with more onions.

In some Sephardic homes, matzah is layered with vegetables and cheese or meat for the Passover meal.

Passover Passover, called Pesach in Hebrew, is the eight-day festival of spring and freedom. It occurs in March or April and celebrates the anniversary of the Jewish exodus from Egypt. The Passover seder, a ceremony carried out at home, includes readings from the seder book, the Haggadah, recounting the story of the exodus, the redemption from slavery, and the God-given right of all humankind to life and liberty. A festive meal is a part of the seder; in the United States and Canada, the menu usually includes chicken soup, matzo balls, and meat or chicken. When Moses led the Jewish people out of Egypt, they left in such haste that there was no time for their bread to rise. Today, matzah, a white-flour cracker, is the descendant of the unleavened bread or bread of affliction. During the eight days of Passover, no food that is subject to a leavening process or that has come in contact with leavened foods can be eaten. The forbidden foods are wheat, barley, rye, and oats. Wheat flour can be eaten only in the form of matzah or matzah meal, which is used to make matzo balls. In addition, beans, peas, lentils, maize, millet, and mustard are also avoided. No leavening agents, malt liquors, or beers can be used.

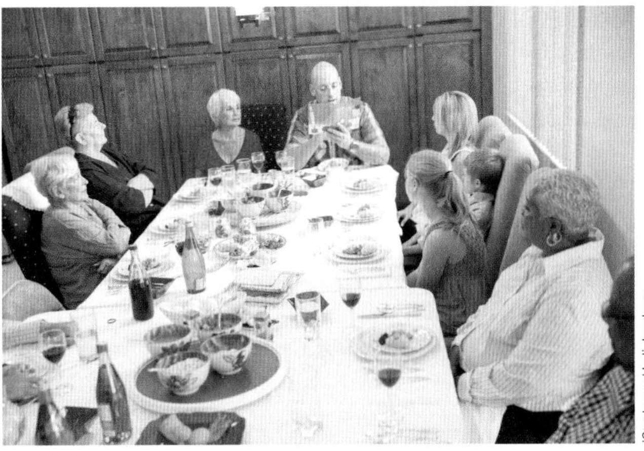

iStock.com/Jodi Jacobson

▲ Typical seder meal.

Because milk and meat cannot be mixed at any time, observant Jewish families have two sets of special dishes, utensils, and pots used only for Passover. The entire house, especially the kitchen, must be cleaned and any foods subject to leavening removed before Passover. It is customary for Orthodox Jewish people to sell their leavened products and flours outside the community before Passover. It is very important that all processed foods, including wine, be prepared for Passover use and be marked "Kosher for Passover."

The seder table is set with the best silverware and china and includes candles, kosher wine, the Haggadah, three pieces of *matzot* (the plural of matzah) covered separately in the folds of a napkin or special Passover cover, and a seder plate.

Shavuot, Season of the Giving of the Torah The two-day festival of Shavuot occurs seven weeks after the second day of Passover and commemorates the revelation of the Torah to Moses on Mount Sinai. Traditional Ashkenazi foods associated with the holiday include blintzes (extremely thin pancakes rolled with a meat or cheese filling, then topped with sour cream), kreplach, and knishes (dough filled with a potato, meat, cheese, or fruit mixture, then baked).

Fast Days

There are several Jewish fast days in addition to Yom Kippur (see Table 4.2). On Yom Kippur and Tisha B'Av, the fast lasts from sunset to sunset and no food or water can be consumed.

Table 4.2 Jewish Fast Days

Tzom	Day after Rosh Hashanah	In memory of Gedaliah, who ruled after the First Temple was destroyed
Yom Kippur	10 days after Rosh Hashanah	Day of Atonement
Tenth of Tevet Seventeenth of Tamuz	December July	Commemorate an assortment of national calamities listed in the Talmud
Ta'anit Ester	Eve of Purim	In grateful memory of Queen Esther, who fasted when seeking divine guidance
Ta'anit Bechorim	Eve of Passover	Gratitude to God for having spared only the firstborn of Israel; usually only firstborn son fasts
Tisha B'Av	August	Commemorates the destruction of the First and Second Temples in Jerusalem

All other fast days are observed from sunrise to sunset. Many Jewish people fast on Yom Kippur, but other fast days are usually observed only by the very observant. Extremely pious Jewish people may add personal fast days on Mondays and Thursdays. All fasts can be broken if it is dangerous to a person's health; those who are pregnant or nursing are exempt from fasting.[5,6]

Additional information about Jewish dietary laws and customs associated with Jewish holidays can usually be obtained from the rabbi at a local synagogue. The Union of Orthodox Jewish Congregations of America also publishes a directory of kosher products.[7–9]

Nutrition Status

Although Judaism is a religion, in many ways the Jewish people are also considered an ethnic group. Few studies have been conducted to determine the nutritional status of Jewish people but certain physiological conditions and medical disorders have been reported to have a higher incidence. Several studies suggest that 60 to 80 percent of Ashkenazi Jewish people are lactase-deficient (lacking the enzyme that allows for easy digestion of the lactose sugar in milk products). Sephardic and Mediterranean Jewish people are also at risk for this condition.[10,11] Research has identified a genetic predisposition to inflammatory bowel disease in Ashkenazi Jews (two to eight times more common).[11]

Food for Thought

The Torah prohibits the drinking of wine made by non-community members because it might have been produced for the worship of idols. Some Orthodox Jewish people extend the prohibition to any grape product, such as grape juice or grape jelly.

Ashkenazi Jewish people traditionally avoided pepper during Passover because it was sometimes mixed with bread crumbs or flour by spice traders.

Christianity

Throughout the world, more people follow Christianity than any other single religion. The three dominant Christian branches are Roman Catholicism, Eastern Orthodox Christianity, and Protestantism. Christianity is founded on recorded events surrounding the life of Jesus—believed to be the Son of God and the Messiah—chronicled in the New Testament of the Bible. The central convictions of the Christian faith are found in the Apostles' Creed and the Nicene Creed. These creeds explain that people are saved through God's grace, through the life and death of Jesus, and through his resurrection as Christ.

For most Christians, the sacraments mark the key stages of worship and sustain the individual worshiper. A sacrament is an outward act derived from something Jesus did or said, through which an individual receives God's grace. The sacraments observed, and the way they are observed, vary among Christian groups. The seven sacraments of Roman Catholicism, for example, are baptism (entering Christ's church), confirmation (the soul receiving the Holy Ghost), Eucharist (partaking of the sacred presence by sharing bread and wine), marriage (union of a man and woman through the bond of love), unction (healing of the mind, spirit, and body), reconciliation (penance and confession), and ordination of the clergy.

Food for Thought

The commemoration of the Last Supper is called Corpus Christi, when Jesus instructed his disciples that bread was his body and wine was his blood. In Spain and many Latin American countries, Corpus Christi is celebrated by parading the bread (called the "Host") through streets covered with flowers.

St. Valentine's Day as we know it contains remnants of both Christian and ancient Roman customs. It is thought the tradition may date back to the spring celebration of Lupercalia, a Roman festival held in mid-February, at which a young man would draw the name of a young woman out of a box to be his sweetheart for a day.

Catholicism

The largest number of persons adhering to one Christian faith in the United States are Catholics. There are over 17,000 parishes in the United States and roughly 51 million Catholic adults in the United States, which accounts for about one-fifth of the total U.S. adult population.[11] The head of the worldwide church is the Pope, considered infallible when defining faith and morals.

Catholics in the United States are racially and ethnically diverse (refer to Table 4.3).[12] The fastest-growing segment of Catholics are Latinx people. Although some Catholics immigrated to the United States during the colonial period, substantial numbers came from Germany, Poland, Italy, and Ireland in the 1800s and from Mexico and the Caribbean in the 20th and 21st centuries. There are small groups of French Catholics

Table 4.3 Hispanics growing as share of adult Catholic population in U.S.

Ethnic background of Catholics in the U.S.	2007	2014
	%	%
White, non-Hispanic	65	59
Hispanic	29	34
Black, non-Hispanic	2	3
Asian, non-Hispanic	2	3
Other, non-Hispanic	2	2
	100	100

Source: Pew Research Center, 2014 U.S. Religious Landscape Study, conducted June 4–Sept. 30, 2014. Figures may not sum to 100% due to rounding. Results exclude non responses.

in New England (primarily in Maine) and in Louisiana. In addition, most Filipinos and some Vietnamese people living in the United States are Catholics. The Catholic religious group is fairly evenly dispersed throughout the United States, with 27 percent living in the South, 26 percent living in the Northeast, 26 percent living in the West, and 21 percent living in the Midwest. Politically, Catholic voters are evenly split between the Democratic and Republican parties.[12]

Feast Days Most Americans are familiar with Christmas (the birth of Christ) and Easter (the resurrection of Christ after the crucifixion). Other Christian feast days celebrated in the United States are New Year's Day, the Annunciation (March 25), Palm Sunday (the Sunday before Easter), the Ascension (40 days after Easter), Pentecost Sunday (50 days after Easter), the Assumption (August 15), All Saints' Day (November 1), and the Immaculate Conception (December 8).

Holiday fare depends on the family's country of origin. For example, the French traditionally serve *bûche de Noël* (a rich cake in the shape of a Yule log) on Christmas for dessert, while the Italians may serve panettone, a fruited sweet bread (refer to individual chapters on each ethnic group for specific foods associated with holidays).

Fast Days Fasting permits only one full meal per day at midday. While taking small amounts of food in the morning or evening is not prohibited, local custom varies as to the quantity and quality of this supplementary nourishment. Abstinence forbids the use of meat, but not of eggs, dairy products, or condiments made of animal fat, and is practiced on certain days and in conjunction with fasting. Only Catholics older than the age of 14 and younger than the age of 60 are required to observe the dietary laws.[12,13]

The fast days in the United States are all the days of Lent, the Fridays of Advent, and the Ember Days (the days that begin each season), but only the most devout fast and abstain on all of these dates. More common is fasting and abstaining only on Ash Wednesday and Good Friday. Before 1966, when the U.S. Catholic Conference abolished most dietary restrictions, abstinence from meat was observed every Friday that did not fall on a feast day. Abstinence is now encouraged on the Fridays of Lent in remembrance of Christ's sacrificial death.

Some older Catholics and those from other nations may observe the pre-1966 dietary laws. In addition, Catholics are required to avoid all food and liquids, except water, for one hour before receiving communion.

Eastern Orthodox Christianity

The Eastern Orthodox Church is as old as the Roman Catholic branch of Christianity, although not as prevalent in the United States. In the year 300 CE, there were two centers of Christianity, one in Rome and the other in Constantinople (now Istanbul, Turkey). Differences arose over theological interpretations of the Bible and the governing of the church, and in 1054 the fellowship between the Latin and Byzantine churches was finally broken. Some of the differences between the two churches concerned the interpretation of the Trinity (the Father, the Son, and the Holy Ghost), the use of unleavened bread for the communion, the celibacy of the clergy, and the position of the pope. In the Eastern Orthodox Church, leavened bread, called phosphoron, is used for Communion, the clergy are allowed to marry before entering the priesthood, and the authority of the pope of Rome is not recognized.

The Orthodox Church consists of 14 self-governing churches, five of which—Constantinople, Alexandria (the Egyptian Coptic Church), Antioch, Jerusalem, and Cyprus—date back to the time of the Byzantine Empire. Six other churches represent the nations where many people are Orthodox (Russia, Romania, Serbia, Bulgaria, Greece, and the former Soviet state of Georgia). Three other churches exist independently in countries where only a small number practice the religion (Poland, Albania, and the Sinai Monastery). Additionally, there are four churches considered autonomous, but not yet self-governing: Czech Republic/Slovakia, Finland, China, and Japan. The Orthodox Church in America was constituted in 1970. The beliefs of the Orthodox churches are similar; only the language of the service differs.[14,15]

The first Orthodox Church in America was started by Russians on the West Coast in the late 1700s. Nearly seven million persons in the United States are estimated to be members of the Orthodox religion today. The major groups associated with this religion adhere to different branches including Greek Orthodox, Russian Orthodox, Ukrainian Orthodox, and Albanian Orthodox. Most states have 1 percent or less of their population identifying as Orthodox Christians except for Alaska which is 5 percent.[16]

Feast Days All the feast days are listed in Table 4.4. Easter is the most important holiday in the Orthodox religion and is celebrated on the first Sunday after the full moon after March 21, but not before the Jewish Passover. Lent is preceded by a

Table 4.4 Eastern Orthodox Feast Days

Feast Day	Date
Christmas	Dec. 25 or Jan. 7
Theophany	Jan. 6 or Jan. 19
Presentation of Our Lord into the Temple	Feb. 2 or Feb. 15
Annunciation	Mar. 25 or Apr. 7
Easter	First Sunday after the full moon after Mar. 21
Ascension	40 days after Easter
Pentecost (Trinity) Sunday	50 days after Easter
Transfiguration	Aug. 6 or Aug. 19
Dormition of the Holy Theotokos	Aug. 15 or Aug. 28
Nativity of the Holy Theotokos	Sept. 8 or Sept. 21
Presentation of the Holy Theotokos	Nov. 21 or Dec. 4

Note: Dates depend on whether the Julian or Gregorian calendar is followed.

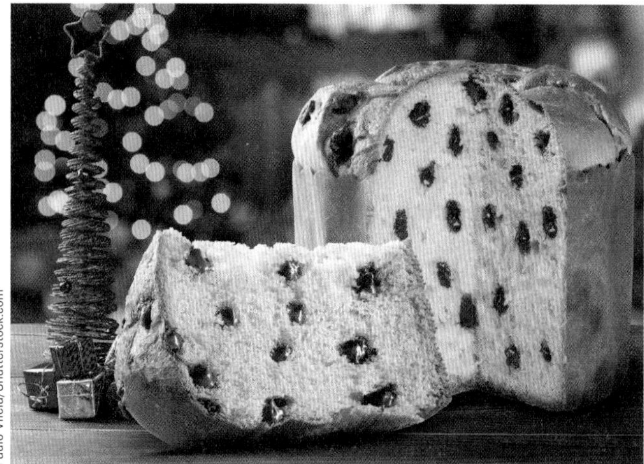

Paulo Vilela/Shutterstock.com

▲ **Italian American Catholics often serve panettone, a sweet bread with dried fruits, on feast days, especially Christmas.**

pre-Lenten period lasting ten weeks before Easter or three weeks before Lent. On the third Sunday before Lent (Meat Fare Sunday), all the meat in the house is eaten. On the Sunday before Lent (Cheese Fare Sunday), all the cheese, eggs, and butter in the house are eaten. On the next day, Clean Monday, the Lenten fast begins. Fish is allowed on Palm Sunday and the Annunciation Day of the Virgin Mary. The Lenten fast is traditionally broken after the midnight services on Easter Sunday. Easter eggs in the Eastern Orthodox religion range from the highly ornate (eastern Europe and Russia) to the solid reddish brown used by the Armenians and red by the Greeks.

Fast Days In the Eastern Orthodox religion there are numerous fast days (refer to Table 4.5). Further, those receiving Holy Communion on Sunday abstain from food and drink before the service. Fasting is considered an opportunity to prove that the soul can rule the body. On fast days, no meat or animal products (milk, eggs, butter, and cheese) are consumed. Fish is also avoided, but shellfish is generally allowed.

Table 4.5 Eastern Orthodox Fast Days and Periods

Fast Days
Every Wednesday and Friday except during fast-free weeks:
Week following Christmas until Eve of Theophany (12 days after Christmas)
Bright Week, week following Easter
Trinity Week, week following Trinity Sunday
Eve of Theophany (Jan. 6 or 18)
Beheading of John the Baptist (Aug. 29 or Sept. 27)
The Elevation of the Holy Cross (Sept. 14 or 27)
Fast Periods
Nativity Fast (Advent): Nov. 15 or 28 to Dec. 24 or Jan. 6
Great Lent and Holy Week: 7 weeks before Easter
Fast of the Apostles: May 23 or June 5 to June 16 or 29
Fast of the Dormition of the Holy Theotokos: Aug. 1 or 14 to Aug. 15 or 28

Note: Dates depend on whether the Julian or Gregorian calendar is followed.

Older or more devout Greek Orthodox followers may not use olive oil on fast days but may eat olives. One recent study looked at the health benefits and consequences of the Eastern Orthodox fasting in monks and found health benefits in terms of body mass index and lipid and glucose profiles for those who followed the strict fasting protocols.[17]

Food for Thought

Lent is the 40 days before Easter; the word originally meant "spring." The last day before Lent is a traditional festival of exuberant feasting and drinking in many regions where Lenten fasting is observed. In France and Louisiana, it is known as Mardi Gras; in Britain, Shrove Tuesday; in Germany, Fastnacht; throughout the Caribbean and in Brazil, Carnival.

The Ethiopian Church is an Orthodox denomination similar to the Egyptian Coptic Church. Timkat (Feast of the Epiphany) in the Ethiopian Church is the most significant Christian holiday of the year, celebrating the baptism of Jesus. Beer brewing, bread baking, and eating roast lamb are traditional.

Protestantism

The 16th-century religious movement known as the Reformation established the Protestant churches by questioning the practices of the Roman Catholic Church and eventually breaking away from its teachings. The man primarily responsible for the Reformation was Martin Luther, a German Augustinian monk who taught theology.[18] He started the movement when, in 1517, he nailed a document containing 95 protests against certain Catholic practices on the door of the castle church in Wittenberg, Germany. A decade later, several countries and German principalities organized the Protestant Lutheran Church based on Martin Luther's teachings.

Food for Thought

Koljivo, boiled whole-wheat kernels mixed with nuts, dried fruit, and sugar, must be offered before the church altar three, nine, and 40 days after the death of a family member in the Eastern Orthodox faith. After the koljivo is blessed by the priest, it is distributed to the friends of the deceased. The boiled wheat represents everlasting life, and the fruit represents sweetness and plenty.

For some, the red Easter egg symbolizes the tomb of Christ (the egg) and is a sign of mourning (the red color). The breaking of the eggs on Easter represents the opening of the tomb and belief in the resurrection.

Luther placed great emphasis on the individual's direct responsibility to God. He believed that every person can reach God through direct prayer without the intercession of a priest or saint; thus, every believer is, in effect, a minister. Although everyone is prone to sin and inherently wicked, a person can be saved by faith in Christ, who by his death on the cross atoned for the sins of all people. Consequently, to Luther, faith was all-important and good works alone could not negate evil deeds. Luther's theology removed the priest's mystical function, encouraging everyone to read the Bible and interpret the scriptures. The beliefs taught by Martin Luther established the foundation of most Protestant faiths.

Other reformers who followed Luther are associated with specific denominations. In the mid-6th century, John Calvin developed the ideas that led to the formation of the Presbyterian, Congregationalist, and Baptist churches; John Wesley founded the Methodist movement in the 18th century. Other denominations in the United States include Episcopalians (related to the English Anglican Church started under King Henry VIII); Seventh-day Adventists; Jehovah's Witnesses; Disciples of Christ; Church of Jesus Christ of Latter-Day Saints (Mormons); Church of Christ, Scientist (Christian Scientists); and Friends (Quakers).

The most significant food ordinance in Protestant churches is the Eucharist, also called Communion or the Lord's Supper. However, other than a liquid and a consecrated bread-like morsel being offered, there is little consistency in the celebration of this ordinance. It can signify an encounter with the living presence of God, a remembrance of the Passover seder attended by Jesus, a continuity of tradition through community, or an individual spiritual experience. Though wine is traditional, many churches switched to grape juice during Prohibition and continue this temperance practice. Some churches offer the wine or juice in a single cup that is shared, while others provide small, individually filled cups. Many liturgical churches, such as the Lutheran Church, offer wafers similar to Catholic practice. Others, such as Methodists, often use a bread pellet. Some organize their members to bake bread (of any type), and many denominations simply cut up white bread of some sort.[19] The primary holidays of the Protestant calendar are Christmas and Easter. The role of food is important in these celebrations; however, the choice of items served is even more varied than Communion practices, determined by family ethnicity and preference rather than a religious rite. Fasting is also uncommon in most Protestant denominations. Some churches or individuals may use occasional fasting, however, to facilitate prayer and worship. Only a few of the Protestant denominations, such as the Mormons and the Seventh-Day Adventists, have dietary practices integral to their faith.

Mormons The Church of Jesus Christ of Latter-Day Saints is a religion that emerged in the United States during the early 1800s. Its founder, Joseph Smith Jr., had a vision of the Angel Moroni, who told him of golden plates hidden in a hill and how to decipher them. The resulting Book of Mormon was published in 1829, and in 1830 a new religious faith was born.

The Book of Mormon details the story of two bands of Israelites who settled in America and from whom certain Native Americans and Pacific Islanders are descended.[20] Christ visited them after his resurrection, and they thus preserved Christianity in its pure form. The two factions did not survive, but the last member, Moroni, hid the nation's sacred writings, compiled by his father, Mormon.

The Mormons believe that God reveals himself and his will through his apostles and prophets. The Mormon Church is organized along biblical lines. Members of the priesthood are graded upward in six degrees (deacons, teachers, priests, elders, seventies, and high priests). From the priesthood are chosen, by the church at large, a council of twelve apostles, which constitutes a group of ruling elders; from these, by seniority, a church president rules with life tenure. There is no paid clergy. Sunday services are held by groups of Mormons, and selected church members give the sermon.[20,21]

To escape local persecution, Brigham Young led the people of the Mormon Church to Utah in 1847. Today, Utah is more than 60 percent Mormon, and many western states have significant numbers of church members. In North America, the estimated total number of adherents was 6.5 million in 2018.[22] The main branch of the church is headquartered in Salt Lake City, but a smaller branch, the Reorganized Church of Jesus Christ of Latter-Day Saints, is centered in Independence, Missouri. All Mormons believe that Independence will be the capital of the world when Christ returns.

Joseph Smith, through a revelation, prescribed the Mormon laws of health, dealing particularly with dietary matters.[20] These laws prohibit the use of tobacco, strong drink, and hot drinks. Strong drink is defined as alcoholic beverages; hot drinks mean tea and coffee. Many Mormons do not use any product that contains caffeine. Followers are advised to eat meat sparingly and to base their diets on grains, especially wheat. In addition, all Mormons are required to store a year's supply of food and clothing for each person in the family.

Many also fast one day per month (donating to those in need the money that would have been spent on food).[23-25] There is some evidence that Millennials who practice Mormonism are less exacting than their parents about some of its religious practices, especially church attendance and dietary restrictions.

Food for Thought

Loma Linda Foods, a brand of plant-based foods, began as a bakery in 1906 providing whole-wheat bread and cookies to the Adventist patients and staff of Loma Linda University Medical Center in Southern California. In 1933, Loma Linda Food Company was producing some of the first meat analogue products prepared from soy and wheat that were available in the United States on a commercial basis.

The American breakfast cereal industry is the result of the dietary and health practices of the Seventh-Day Adventists. In 1886, Dr. John Kellogg became director of the Adventists' sanitarium in Battle Creek, Michigan, and in his efforts to find a tasty substitute for meat, he invented Corn Flakes.

Seventh-Day Adventists In the early 1800s, many people believed that the Second Coming of Christ was imminent. In the United States, William Miller predicted that Christ would return in 1843 or 1844. When both years passed and the prediction did not materialize, many of his followers became disillusioned. However, one group continued to believe that the prediction was not wrong but that the date was actually the beginning of the world's end preceding the coming of Christ. They became known as the Seventh-Day Adventists and were officially organized in 1863.[26]

The spiritual guide for the new church was Ellen G. Harmon, who later became Mrs. James White. Her inspirations were the result of more than 2,000 prophetic visions and dreams she reportedly had during her life. Mrs. White claimed to be not a prophet but a conduit that relayed God's desires and admonitions to humankind.

The Seventh-day Adventist church is one of the fastest-growing churches worldwide, with over 25 million adherents. As of 2020, there were over 1.5 million Seventh-Day Adventists in the United States and 18 million worldwide. Besides the main belief in Christ's advent, or Second Coming, the Seventh-Day Adventists practice the principles of Protestantism. They believe that the advent will be preceded by a monstrous war, pestilence, and plague, resulting in the destruction of Satan and all wicked people; the earth will be purified by holocaust. Although the hour of Christ's return is not known, they believe that dedication to his work will hasten it.[27]

The church adheres strictly to the teachings of the Bible. The Sabbath is observed from sundown on Friday to sundown on Saturday and is wholly dedicated to the Lord. Food must be prepared on Friday and dishes washed on Sunday. Church members dress simply, avoid ostentation, and wear only functional jewelry. The church's headquarters are in Tacoma Park, Maryland, near Washington, DC, where they were moved after a series of fires ravaged the previous center in Battle Creek, Michigan. The church operates over 7,500 schools and over 100 post-secondary institutions and hospitals. Loma Linda University Medical Center in California is world-renowned for its heart and specialty surgeries.

Each congregation is led by a pastor (more a teacher than a minister), and all the churches are under the leadership of the president of the general conference of Seventh-Day Adventists. Adventists follow the apostle Paul's teaching that the human body is the temple of the Holy Spirit. Ellen White believed that her congregation would regain and keep their health if they followed these simple rules along with getting fresh air and exercise:

1. Eat a plant-based, or vegetarian, diet
2. Refrain from alcohol, tobacco, and caffeine
3. Plain, or clean, eating
4. Just two meals a day (breakfast at 7 am and dinner at 1 pm). The time between dinner and the next day's breakfast was intended as a fast.[28–30]

Adventists believe that sickness is a result of the violation of the laws of health. One can preserve health by eating the right kinds of foods in moderation and by getting enough rest and exercise. Overeating is discouraged. Vegetarianism is widely practiced because the Bible states that the diet in Eden did not include flesh foods. Most Adventists are lacto-ovo vegetarians (eating milk products and eggs, but not meat). Some do consume meat, although they avoid pork and shellfish. Ellen White advocated the use of nuts and beans instead of meat, substituting vegetable oil for animal fat, and using whole grains in breads. Like the Mormons, the Adventists do not consume tea, coffee, or alcohol and do not use tobacco products. Water is considered the best liquid and should be consumed only before and after the meal, not during the meal. Meals are not highly seasoned, and hot spices such as mustard, chili powder, and black pepper are avoided. Eating between meals is discouraged so that food can be properly digested. The Adventists' unique lifestyle and dietary practices have been linked with their longevity.[31] In one recent survey of over 63,000 Adventists, abstinence from alcohol occurred in 91 percent of respondents, with 97 percent abstaining from tobacco. Only about 19 percent reported being vegetarian, as most respondents believed that they could pick and choose elements of the global health messages to follow.

According to the book *The Blue Zones*, Loma Linda, California is a community with the highest concentration of Seventh-day Adventists in the United States. Some of its residents live more than 10 years beyond the average American. More than 250 members of the Seventh-day Adventists Church in Loma Linda are 90 or older and another 425 are 80–89. They contribute to their longevity to abstaining from alcohol and tobacco, are frequently vegetarian, favor vegetables, nuts, and fruits, and are often energetic, upbeat, and social.[31,32]

Islam

Islam is the second-largest religious group in the world. Although not widely practiced in the United States, Islam is the dominant religion in the Middle East, northern Africa, Pakistan, Indonesia, and Malaysia. Large numbers of people also follow the religion in parts of sub-Saharan Africa, India, Russia, the former Soviet Union, and Southeast Asia.

Islam, which means surrender to the will of God in the Arabic language, is not only a religion but also a way of life.[33–35] One who adheres to Islam is called a Muslim, "he who submits." Islam's founder, Mohammed, was neither a savior nor a messiah but rather a prophet through whom God delivered his messages. He was born in 570 CE in Mecca, Saudi Arabia, a city located along the spice trade route. Early in his life, Mohammed acquired respect for Jewish and Christian monotheism. Later, the archangel Gabriel appeared to him in many visions. These revelations continued for a decade or more, and the archangel told Mohammed that he was a prophet of Allah, the one true God. Mohammed teachings met with hostility in Mecca, and in 622 he fled to Yathrib. The year of the flight (hegira) is the first year in the Muslim calendar. At Yathrib, later named Medina, Mohammed became a religious and political leader. Eight years after fleeing Mecca, he returned triumphantly and declared Mecca a holy place to Allah.

The most sacred writings of Islam are found in the Qur'an (sometimes spelled Koran or Quran), believed to contain the words spoken by Allah through Mohammed. It includes many legends and traditions that parallel those of the Old and New Testaments, as well as Arabian folk tales. The Qur'an also contains the basic laws of Islam, and its analysis and interpretation by religious scholars have provided the guidelines by which Muslims lead their daily lives.

Muslims believe that the one true God, Allah, is basically the God of Judaism and Christianity but that his word was incompletely expressed in the Old and New Testaments and was only fulfilled in the Qur'an. Similarly, they believe that

Mohammed was the last prophet, superseding Christ, who is considered by Muslims to be a prophet and not the Son of God. The primary doctrines of Islam are monotheism and the concept of the last judgment—the day of final resurrection when all will be deemed worthy of either the delights of heaven or the terrors of hell.

Mohammed did not institute an organized priesthood or sacraments but instead advocated the following ritualistic observances, known as the Five Pillars of Islam:

1. Faith, shown by the proclamation of the unity of God, and belief in that unity, as expressed in the creed, "There is no God but Allah; Mohammed is the Messenger of Allah."
2. Prayer, *salat*, performed five times daily (at dawn, noon, mid-afternoon, sunset, and nightfall), facing Mecca, wherever one may be; and on Fridays, the day of public prayer, in the mosque (a building used for public worship). On Fridays, sermons are delivered in the mosque after the noon prayer.
3. Almsgiving, *zakat*, as an offering to the less fortunate and an act of piety. In some Islamic countries, Muslims are expected to give 2.5 percent of their net savings or assets in money or goods. The money is used to help those in need or to support the religious organization in countries where Islam is not the dominant religion. In addition, zakat is given to those in need on certain feast and fast days (refer to the next section on dietary practices for more details).
4. Fasting, to fulfill a religious obligation, to earn the pleasure of Allah, to wipe out previous sins, and to appreciate the hunger of those in need.
5. Pilgrimage to Mecca, *hajj*, once in a lifetime if means are available. No non-Muslim can enter Mecca. Pilgrims must wear seamless white garments; go without head covering or shoes; practice sexual continence; abstain from shaving or having their hair cut; and avoid harming any living thing.

Food for Thought

For Muslims, prayers are said five times daily (at dawn, noon, mid-afternoon, sunset, and nightfall), facing Mecca, wherever one may be.

There are no priests in Islam; every Muslim can communicate directly with God, so a mediator is not needed. The successors of the prophet Mohammed and the leaders of the Islamic community were the caliphs. No caliphs exist today, though the term is sometimes invoked by a leader of a group or community as a symbol of Islamic unity. A mufti gives legal advice based on the sacred laws of the Qur'an. An imam is the person appointed to lead prayer in the mosque and deliver the Friday sermon.

The following prominent sects in Islam have their origin in conflicting theories on the office of caliph (caliphate): (1) Sunni form the largest number of Muslims and hold that the caliphate is an elected office that must be occupied by a member of the faction of Koreish, the faction of Mohammed. (2) Shi'ia, the second-largest group, believe that the caliphate was a God-given office held rightfully by Ali, Mohammed's son-in-law, and his descendants. The Shiites (followers of Shi'ia Islam) are found primarily in Iran, Iraq, Yemen, and India. This community has a religious hierarchy achieved by scholars in the Islamic tradition. (3) The Khawarij, another sect, believe that the office of caliph is open to any believer whom the faithful consider fit for it. Followers of this sect are found primarily in eastern Arabia and North Africa. (4) The Sufis, ascetic mystics who seek a close union with God now, rather than in the hereafter. Only 3 percent of present-day Muslims are Sufis, and many remain outside mainstream Islam.[33–35,38]

Food for Thought

The Kaaba (in Mecca) is the holiest shrine of Islam and contains the Black Stone given to Abraham and Ishmael by the archangel Gabriel. During the hajj, each pilgrim touches the stone and circles the shrine.

No one claiming title to the office of caliphate has been recognized by all Muslim sects since its abolition by the Turkish government in 1924 following the fall of the Ottoman Empire. The role of the caliphate in modern Islam is uncertain.

The status of fish varies by sect. Most Muslims consider anything from the sea halal; however, some, such as Shiites, eat only fish with scales.[36]

It is estimated that nearly 3.5 million Muslims live in the United States. This number has grown from 2.5 million in 2007, with many coming from the Middle East.[37] Most are Sunnis, with only a small percentage of Shiites, although there is some

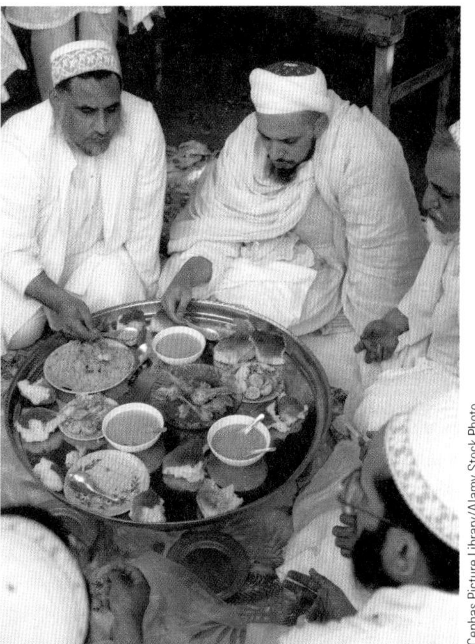

Cephas Picture Library/Alamy Stock Photo

▲ **Islamic laws consider eating to be a matter of worship, and Muslims are encouraged to share meals.**

crossover in worship and religious celebrations. In addition, some Black Americans believe Allah is the one true God; they follow the Qur'an and traditional Muslim rituals in their temple services. The movement was originally known as the Nation of Islam and its adherents identified as Black Muslims. A split in the Nation of Islam resulted in one faction of Black Muslims becoming an orthodox Islamic religion called the World Community of Al-Islam in the West. It is accepted as a branch of Islam. The other Black Muslim faction has continued as the Nation of Islam under the leadership of Louis Farrakhan.[38]

Halal: Islamic Dietary Laws

In Islam, eating is considered to be a matter of worship. Muslims are expected to eat for survival and good health; self-indulgence is not permitted. Muslims are advised against eating more than two-thirds of their capacity, and sharing food is recommended. Food is never to be thrown away, wasted, or treated with contempt. The hands and mouth are washed before and after meals. If eating utensils are not used, only the right hand is used for eating, as the left hand is considered unclean.

Permitted or lawful foods are called halal. Allah alone has the right to determine what may be eaten, and what is permitted is sufficient—what is not permitted is unnecessary.[39] Unless specifically prohibited, all food is edible. Unlawful or prohibited (haram) foods listed in the Qur'an include:

1. All swine, four-footed animals that catch their prey with their mouths, birds of prey that seize their prey with their talons, and any by-products of these animals, such as pork gelatin or enzymes used in cheese making. If the source of any by-product is in question, it is avoided.
2. Improperly slaughtered animals (including carrion). An animal must be killed in a manner similar to that described in the Jewish laws, by slitting the front of the throat; cutting the jugular vein, carotid artery, and windpipe; and allowing the blood to drain completely. In addition, the person who kills the animal must repeat at the instant of slaughter, "In the name of God, God is great." Fish and seafood are exempt from this requirement.
3. Blood and blood products.
4. Alcoholic beverages and intoxicating drugs, unless medically necessary. Even foods that have fermented accidentally are avoided. The drinking of stimulants, such as coffee and tea, is discouraged, as is smoking; however, these prohibitions are practiced only by the most devout Muslims.

A Muslim can eat or drink prohibited food under certain conditions, such as when the food is taken by mistake, when it is forced by others, or there is fear of dying by hunger or disease. The term for a food that is questionably halal or haram is *mashbooh*, and when in doubt, a Muslim is encouraged to avoid the item. Foods that combine halal items with haram items, such as baked goods made with lard or pizza with bacon, ham, or pork sausage topping, are also prohibited. Muslims vary in their observance of the halal diet, with the strictest adherence found among the most orthodox believers. Foods in compliance with Islamic dietary laws are sometimes marked with symbols registered with the Islamic Food and Nutrition Council of America (IFNCA) (Figure 4.5), signifying the food is fit for consumption by Muslims anywhere in the world.[40]

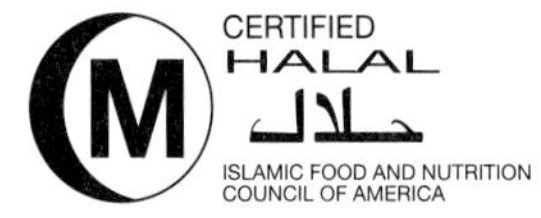

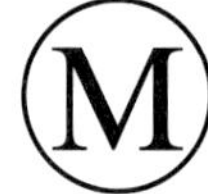

Figure 4.5 Examples of halal food symbols.

New American Perspectives

Islam

My name is Hafsabibi Mojy and I was a student at San Jose State University. I work as a dietitian in a local medical center. Although I immigrated from India to the United States in 1994, I am an observant Muslim, especially when it comes to Islamic food laws. I will shop at specialty stores to buy halal meats, which for me include beef, goat, chicken, veal, and turkey and are more expensive than meat from the supermarket. Most Americans I have met do not know what halal means and they often think I am a vegetarian, probably because I come from India. It is common for me to call myself a "meat-eating vegetarian" as I only eat meat at home or in places where halal is available, but otherwise, I call myself vegetarian when I am at places where halal food is not available.

I fast from sunrise to sunset during Ramadan. It is not hard, but it takes a few days in the beginning to get back to the rhythm of fasting. To me, personally, I get thirsty more than hungry. My favorite Islamic holiday is Eid al-Adha or Feast of Sacrifice. It is the most important feast of the Muslim calendar and lasts for three days. It concludes the Pilgrimage to Mecca. The feast reenacts prophet Ibrahim's obedience to God by sacrificing a cow or ram. The family eats about a third of the meal and donates the rest to the poor. My favorite foods include all Indian meat curry dishes, biryani (spicy rice pilaf with meat or chicken), and kabobs.

Health care that includes dietary modifications may interfere with Islamic food laws. Say, for example, a patient is on a clear liquid diet at a hospital . . . there will be very few choices left to give to a Muslim patient as Jell-O will be excluded (Jell-O, considered a clear liquid because it is liquid at body temperature, contains gelatin which is usually derived from animals and hence will be a non-halal item). Some "vegetarian" dishes contain a chicken-broth base and hence will be considered non-halal. Even a vegetarian burger can have wine in it and will be considered non-halal as all alcoholic products are also prohibited under Islamic food laws.

Feast Days

The following are the feast days in the Islamic religion:

1. Eid al-Fitr, the Feast of Fast Breaking—the end of Ramadan is celebrated with a feast and the giving of alms.
2. Eid al-Adha, the Festival of Sacrifice—the commemoration of Abraham's willingness to sacrifice his son, Ishmael, for God. It is customary to sacrifice a sheep and distribute its meat to friends, relatives, and those in need.
3. Shab-i-Barat, the night in the middle of Shaban—originally a fast day, this is now a feast day celebrated mostly in non-Arab nations, often marked with fireworks. It is believed that God determines the actions of every person for the next year on this night.
4. Nau-Roz, New Year's Day—primarily celebrated by the Iranians, it is the first day after the sun crosses the vernal equinox.
5. Mawlid al-Nabī the birthday of Mohammed.

Feasting also occurs at birth, after the consummation of marriage, at Bismillah (when a child first starts reading the Qur'anic alphabet), after the circumcision of boys, at the harvest, and at death.

Food for Thought

The month of Ramadan can fall during any part of the year as the Muslim calendar is lunar but does not have a leap month.

Fasting hours during Ramadan for Muslims range from 12 to 20 hours. Average calorie consumption during that time reduces to 1220 kcal per day and most see a significant weight loss of about 4-5 pounds providing a healthy means for improving overall health. However, for those with chronic illnesses, fasting should not be undertaken without physician approval.[41]

Fast Days

On fast days, Muslims abstain from food, drink, smoking, and coitus from dawn to sunset. Food can be eaten before the sun comes up and again after it sets. Fasting is required of Muslims during Ramadan, the ninth month of the Islamic calendar. It is believed that during Ramadan, "the gates of Heaven are open, the gates of Hell closed, and the devil is put in chains." At sunset, the fast is usually broken by taking a liquid, typically water, along with an odd number of dates.

All Muslims past the age of puberty (15 years old) fast during Ramadan. Several groups are exempt from fasting, but most must make up the days before the next Ramadan. They include sick individuals with a recoverable illness; people who are traveling; women during pregnancy, lactation, or menstruation; elders who are physically unable to fast; people who are mentally disabled; and those engaged in hard labor. During Ramadan, it is customary to invite guests to break the fast and dine in the evening; special foods are eaten, especially sweets. Food is often given to neighbors, relatives, and needy individuals or families.

Muslims are also encouraged to fast six days during Shawwal, the month following Ramadan; the tenth day of the month of Muharram; and the ninth day of Dhu al-Hijjah, but not during the pilgrimage to Mecca. A Muslim may fast voluntarily, preferably on Mondays and Thursdays. Muslims are not allowed to fast on two festival days: Eid al-Fitr and Eid al-Adha; or on the days of sacrificial slaughter: Tashriq—the twelfth, thirteenth, and fourteenth days of Dhu al-Hijjah. It is also undesirable for Muslims to fast excessively (because Allah provides food and drink to consume) or to fast on Fridays.

Eastern Religions

A reverence for all life, called ahimsa, is fundamental to Asian Indian ideology. It is reflected in the religions native to India, as well as in the vegetarian diet that many Indians follow. For many, the heat of sunrise, the taste of water, and the smell of the earth after rains are all reminders of God. Everything is scared. Each person is imbued with grace. For the Hindu faith and others in Asia, the world is not made of inanimate matter to be wasted for selfish ends.

Hinduism

Hinduism is considered the world's oldest religion, and, like Judaism, it is the basis of other religions such as Buddhism. Most Hindus live in India, its birthplace, though through history Hinduism spread into other regions of Southeast Asia. Hinduism is unique in that it is not a single religion, but a compilation of many traditions and philosophies. The original language of early Hindu sacred books is Sanskrit and they are most appreciated through sound (speech) rather than the written word. In fact, in the Hindu worldview, the universe has sonic origins, and began with the sacred sound vibration OM.

There are two categories of Hindu scriptures: the revealed texts and the remembered texts. The revealed texts were thought to be the divine word heard by a primordial sage and include the Vedas, divided into four sections: the Rig Veda, the Yajur Veda, the Sama Veda, and the Atharva Veda. The Vedas are hymns that are also accompanied by Brahmanas (ritual texts), Aranyakas ("wilderness" texts), and Upanishads (philosophical texts). The remembered texts were created later by humans. They include the epics, the Mahabharata and the Ramayana, the Bhagavad Gita, and the Dharmashastra.[42]

The goal of Hinduism is not to make humans perfect beings or life a heaven on earth but rather to make humans one with the Universal Spirit or Supreme Being. When this state is achieved, there is no cause and effect, no time and space, no good and evil; all dualities are merged into oneness. This goal can be obtained by transforming human consciousness through liberation (moksha) into a new realm of divine consciousness that sees individual parts of the universe as deriving their true significance from the central unity of spirit. To Hindus, all beings are part of God, who is everywhere and in everything. The transformation of human consciousness into divine consciousness can be but is not often achieved in one lifetime. Hindus believe that the soul passes through a cycle of successive lives and each incarnation is dependent on how the previous life was lived (refer Figure 4.6). This is also called the

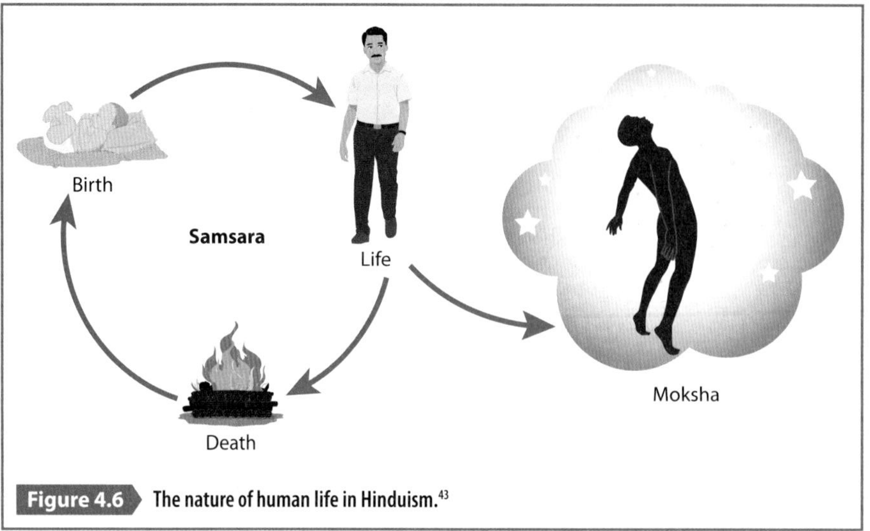

Figure 4.6 The nature of human life in Hinduism.[43]

Cultural Controversy

Meat Prohibitions

Scientists have calculated that animal protein comprised over 50 percent of the total daily calories consumed by prehistoric peoples, a far higher amount than what most Americans eat today.[44,45] In recent studies, however, there is increasing evidence that root foods and nuts were key resources for hunter-gatherers in Europe. Remains identified from at least 28 hunter-gatherer sites across Europe suggest that root foods, including tubers, rhizomes, and bulbs of various plants would have contributed significantly to the Mesolithic diet. Even so, it is believed that only 1 percent of the world population refuses to eat all types of meat, poultry, and fish, and total vegans, who avoid all animal products, equal only one-tenth of 1 percent. Humans favor protein foods, though research shows as the tastiness of protein alternatives rises, preferences for plant-based foods rise. A Gallup poll in 2018 showed that 3 percent of the U.S. population identifies as vegan, up from 2 percent in previous years.[46] In 2022, market research revealed that sales for vegan foods that are direct replacements for milk and meat grew 54 percent in the United States.[47]

Many cultures impose some restrictions on what meats may be consumed, mostly in accordance with prevailing religious dietary laws. The devout of each faith see little reason to ask why a particular food is prohibited. It is considered presumptuous or sacrilegious for humans to question the directives of God or church. This has not deterred researchers from speculating on the rationale of meat taboos. Some have investigated the whole field of taxonomy and how animals are classified as different or unnatural, thus abominable due to their physical characteristics. The Jewish prohibition against pork, for example, has been attributed to the fact that pigs do not chew their cud, marking them as dissimilar from other animals with cloven hooves.[48] This theory is supported by the omnivore's paradox and the psychological need for food familiarity. Others have focused on the use of the term *unclean* in relation to biblical and Qur'anic pork prohibitions, claiming that pork consumption is unhealthful. Many researchers discard this theory because it is thought that ancient populations could not have made the association between eating pork and the slow development of diseases, such as trichinosis, not to mention that other animals that carry fatal illnesses (e.g., spongiform encephalitis or mad-cow disease) are not avoided.

The socioecological theory for why certain meats are avoided suggests that if an animal is more valuable alive than dead or, conversely, if it does not fit well into the local ecology or economy, consumption will be prohibited.[49] Religious dietary codes often reinforce preexisting food practices and prejudices. When reviewing the history of pork in the Middle East, for example, archeological records show it was part of the ancient diet. But by 1900 BCE, pork had become unpopular in Babylonia, Egypt, and Phoenicia, coinciding with an expanding population and deforestation of the region. Pigs compete with humans for food sources. Additionally, they do not thrive in hot, dry climates. Cows, goats, and sheep, on the other hand, can graze over large areas and survive on the cellulose in plants unavailable to human metabolism, and they need no protection from the sun. The nomadic Hebrews were unlikely to have herded pigs in their early history, and by the time they settled there was a broad aversion to pigs by many Middle Easterners. The first followers of Mohammed were also pastoral people, which may explain why the only explicitly prohibited animal flesh in Islam is pork.

The socioeconomic theory is useful in examining other meat prohibitions. In India, where beef is banned for Hindus, cattle are the primary power source in rural farming communities due to the expense of tractors. Further, cattle provide dung that is dried to produce a clean, slow-burning cooking fuel, and cows provide milk for the dairy products important in some vegetarian fare. Even dead cows serve a purpose for their leather. The value of cattle in India is reinforced by religious custom. Horsemeat in Europe is another example. Though horse consumption was frequent in early Europe, other cultures who used the animals for travel and cavalry often banned it. Asian nomads who roamed on horseback consumed horse milk and blood but ate the flesh only in emergencies. It was avoided by the Romans and most Middle Easterners (prohibited for Jews and by custom among Muslims). During the 8th century, when European Christian strongholds came under attack from Muslim cavalry in the south and mounted nomads from the west, Pope Gregory III recognized the need for horses in the defense of the church. He prohibited horsemeat as "unclean and detestable." However, horse consumption was never entirely eliminated, especially during times of hardship, and gradually religious restrictions were eased. By the 19th century, horsemeat had regained favor, especially in France and Belgium, where it is a specialty item today. Despite the initial need for horsepower, the religious prohibition was unsustainable over time because it contradicted prevailing food traditions.

transmigration of souls. This idea is most developed in India and Greece, but has been widespread in the world: occurring in Asia, Africa, Australia, Oceania, among North and South American Indians, and in parts of Europe.

Hindus believe the law of karma, in which a person's past, present, and future actions are interconnected, plays a part in the form of rebirth. In this belief system, each person has the opportunity to get closer to moksha, or release from rebirth, with each cycle. The goal for all souls is liberation.

In the Vedic scriptures, there is one Supreme Being, Brahman, and all the various gods worshiped by humans are partial manifestations of him, or avatars (from the Sanskrit avatāra, meaning "descent," the incarnation or human appearance of a deity). Hindus choose the form of the Supreme Being that satisfies their spirit and make it symbolically an object of love and adoration. This aspect of worship makes Hinduism very tolerant of other gods and their followers; many different religions have been absorbed into Hinduism.

The three most important functions of the Supreme Being (Brahman) are the creation, protection, and destruction of the world, and these functions have become personified in the Hindu trinity: Brahma, Vishnu, and Siva. The Supreme Being as Vishnu is the protector of the world.

Food for Thought

The Seven Social Sins according to Gandhi are politics without principle; wealth without work; pleasure without conscience; knowledge without character; commerce without morality; science without humanity; and worship without sacrifice.[50]

Ganesh got his elephant head when he angered his father, Siva, who cut off his human head. When his mother Parvati, pleaded with Siva to replace his head, Siva used the head of a nearby elephant. Hindus honor Ganesh, the remover of obstacles, through offerings of the foods he favored.

Yoga means "yoke," as in yoking together or union of the mind and body. Yoga has been used for centuries to prepare the body for meditation, or as meditative practice itself.

Karma in Hinduism is the law of action and reaction that governs life. The soul carries with it the impressions it received during its earthly life. These characteristics are collectively called the karma of the soul. Karma literally means "deed or act," and more broadly describes the principle of cause and effect.

Hindus, much like Native Americans, see life as cyclical. Everything from the rotation of the earth and the seasons to the body's digestive process and circulatory system is a cycle. All life goes through birth, life, death, and rebirth, and the world itself passes through repeating cycles. A common version of the creation story is connected to the life of Vishnu. It is described this way: from Vishnu's navel grows a lotus, and from its unfolding petals is born the god Brahma, who creates the world. Vishnu governs the world until he sleeps; then Siva destroys it, and the world is absorbed into Vishnu's body to be created once again. Where the Christian conception of time is strongly linear, having a point of beginning with its creation by God, Hinduism sees time as cyclical. Each cycle begins and passes, but leaves behind the seed from which the next cycle of creation arises. As time passes, the dharma, or righteousness of the first half of the cycle, is used up so that, by the last half, injury, greed, hatred, delusion, and disease arise due to the deterioration of the dharma.[51] This is when Vishnu wakes and the cycle of millennia (or the blink of Vishnu's eye, according to some tales) begins again.

The principles of Hinduism are purity of mind and spirit, self-control, non-attachment, truth, and nonviolence. Purity is both a ceremonial goal and a moral ideal, and all rituals for purification and the elaborate rules regarding food and drink are meant to lead to it. Self-control governs both the flesh and the mind.

Hinduism does not teach its followers to suppress the flesh completely but rather to regulate its appetites and cravings. The highest aspect of self-control is being in the moment with no attachment to the past or future. Complete liberation from this world and union with the divine are not possible if one clings to the good or evil of this existence. The pursuit of truth is indispensable to the progress of humans, and truth is always associated with nonviolence, ahimsa. These principles are considered the highest virtues. India's greatest exponent of this ideal was Mahatma Gandhi, who taught that nonviolence must be practiced not only by individuals, but also by communities and nations.

One common belief of Hinduism is that the world evolved in successive stages, beginning with matter and going on through life, consciousness, and intelligence to spiritual bliss or perfection. Spirit first appears as life in plants, then as consciousness in animals, intelligence in humans, and finally bliss in the supreme spirit. Truth, beauty, love, and righteousness are of higher importance than intellectual values (e.g., clarity, cogency, subtlety, skill) or biological values (e.g., health, strength, vitality). Material values (e.g., riches, possessions, pleasure) are valued least.

The organization of society grows from the principle of spiritual progression. The early Hindu lawgivers tried to construct an ideal society in which people are ranked by their spiritual progress and culture, not according to their wealth or power. The social system reflects this ideal, which is represented by four estates, or castes, associated originally with certain occupations. The four castes are the Brahmins (teachers and priests), the Kshatriyas (soldiers), the Vaisyas (merchants and farmers), and the Śūdras (laborers). Existing outside social recognition are the Scheduled Castes, or Dalits, historically and pejoratively called untouchables (often working as butchers, leather workers, and other occupations thought to be "unclean"), a group of persons who do not fall into the other four categories. The practice of "untouchability" was unlikely part of Hindu scripture, but a corruption of categories of human acts or behaviors. Some scholars translate the texts as seeking to improve (the purity of) the content of individual character (ethical intent, actions, innocence or ignorance, ritualistic behaviors) that became rigid groups through time never intended to be hereditary lineages.[52] Although laws discriminating against Scheduled Castes were repealed in 1949,[53] after centuries of inequity, these groups often remain at the lowest stratum of Indian society. Today, Schedule Caste people have reserved political seats in Parliament and are more integrated into society, but perceptions and prejudices in private matters such as marriage and households are slower to change (refer to Chapter 14).

The practice of untouchability is often associated only with Hinduism but under different names, it appears in other cultures: in Japan (the Buraku), Korea (the Paekchong), Tibet (the Ragyappa), and Burma (pagoda slaves), and some make parallels to how Africans were treated in the United States as well as other nations when they were enslaved and forcibly imported.[54,55]

The castes mark qualities of spiritual progression, in that the most spiritual occupy the top and the least occupy the bottom. A person's good action in this life earns them a promotion to a higher caste in the next life. In each new incarnation, the individual soul moves up or down the spiritual ladder, with moksha or freedom from this cycle, as the goal.

There are thousands of subdivisions of the four main castes in India. The subcastes often reflect a trade or profession, but some scholars contend that the latter was imposed on the former. In daily life, a person's subcaste is very important, whereas what major caste one belongs to makes little difference to non-Brahmins (refer to Chapter 14, "South Asians"). The ideal life of a Hindu is divided into four successive stages, called asramas. The first stage is that of the student and is devoted entirely to study and discipline. The guru becomes an individual's spiritual parent. After this period of preparation, the student should settle down and serve his or her marriage, community, and country. When this active period of citizenship is over, they should retire to a quiet place and meditate on the higher aspects of the spirit. The person can then become a sannyasi, one who has renounced all earthly possessions and ties. This stage is the crown of human life. Though the ultimate aim of life is liberation, on their way to this final goal people must satisfy the animal wants of their bodies, as well as the economic and other demands of their families and communities. However, all should be done within the moral law of dharma (righteousness). Adherence to dharma reflects a unique aspect of Hinduism, namely, that practice is perhaps more important than belief. There are no creeds in Hinduism; it is the performance of duties associated with one's caste or social position that make a person a Hindu. In other words, what you believe is less important than what you do.[56,57] Common practices in Hinduism include rituals and forms of mental discipline. All Hindus are advised to choose a deity on whose form, features, and qualities they can concentrate their mind and whose image they can worship every day with flowers and incense. The deity is only a means of realizing the Supreme Being by means of ritualistic worship. Externally, the deity is worshiped as a king or honored guest. Internal worship consists of prayer and meditation.[56,57]

Food for Thought

Some Hindus break coconuts on temple grounds to symbolize the spiritual experience. The hard shell is a metaphor for the human ego, and once it is cracked open, the soft, sweet meat representing the inner self is open to becoming one with the Supreme Being. Offering coconut symbolizes offering your own self to God.

Hindus can be divided into three broad groups according to their view of the Supreme Being. They are the Vaishnava, the Saiva, and the Sakta, who maintain the supremacy of Vishnu, Siva, and the Sakti (the female and active aspects of Siva), respectively. Different groups are popular in different regions of India. Many Hindus do not worship one avatar exclusively. Vishnu may be worshiped in one of his full embodiments (Krishna or Rama) or partial embodiments. In addition, there are hundreds of lesser deities, much like saints. One is Siva's son, the elephant-headed Ganesh, who is believed to bring good luck and remove obstacles.

There are approximately 2.5 million Hindus in the United States. Partly because Hinduism is relatively recently common in the United States, its beliefs are often misunderstood by other Americans. American Hindus are often deeply concerned by disrespect in the majority culture by businesses and the entertainment industry. The ancient beliefs are often commercialized or misused in public discourse.[58]

Hindu Dietary Practices

In general, Hindus avoid foods believed to hamper the development of the body or mental abilities. Bad food habits will prevent one from reaching mental purity and communion with God. Dietary restrictions and attitudes vary among the castes.

The Laws of Manu (dating from the 4th century CE) state that "no sin is attached to eating flesh or drinking wine, or gratifying the sexual urge, for these are the natural propensities of men; but abstinence from these bears greater fruits." Many Hindus are vegetarians.[59–61] They adhere to the concept of ahimsa, avoiding inflicting pain on an animal by not eating meat. Although the consumption of meat is allowed, the cow is considered sacred and is not to be killed or eaten. If meat is eaten, pork as well as beef is usually avoided. As with most religious food precepts, foods prescribed in Hinduism are not detrimental to health, as suggested by the fact that they have more or less been followed for millennia. Since Hindus believe all living beings are equal, many avoid eating fish and eggs as well as meat. A national study on 641,642 non-pregnant women showed the prevalence of undernutrition and iron deficiency anemia (hemoglobin level less than 12 g/dL) was higher in Hindus than in Muslims, Christians, or others who typically eat meat. Communities with the most restrictive vegetarian diet were more likely to develop iron deficiency anemia. Vitamin B12 deficiency or impairment was found in 51 percent of pregnant Hindu women, and present in 44 percent of their infants at 6 weeks of age.[62]

In the ancient Laws of Manu, there are lengthy considerations. Crabs, snails, crocodiles, numerous birds (e.g., crows, doves, domesticated fowl, ducks, flamingos, parrots, vultures, and woodpeckers), antelopes, camels, boars, bats, porpoises, and fish with ugly forms (undefined) should also be rejected. In addition, the laws make many other recommendations regarding foods that should be avoided, including foods prepared by certain groups of people (e.g., actors, artists, carpenters, cobblers, doctors, eunuchs, innkeepers, musicians, prostitutes, liars, spies, and thieves); foods that have been contaminated by a person sneezing or through contact with a human foot, clothing, animals, or birds; milk from an animal that has recently given birth; and water from the bottom of a boat. No fish or meat should be eaten until it has been sanctified by the repetition of mantras offering it to the gods. Pious Hindus may also abstain from alcoholic beverages. Garlic, turnips, onions, leeks, mushrooms, and red-hued foods, such as tomatoes and red lentils, may be avoided. Despite such lengthy prohibitions, Hindus have always exerted considerable personal discretion regarding taboo foods.[63]

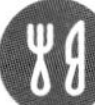

Food for Thought

According to legend, Vishnu rested on a 1,000-headed cobra between the creation and destruction of the world.

Hindus are encouraged to practice moderation—they are advised not to eat too early, not to eat too late, and not to eat too much.

Students studying the Vedas and other celibates are usually vegetarians and may restrict irritating or exciting foods such as honey, chilies, pepper, onions, and garlic.

Intertwined in Hindu food customs is the concept of purity and pollution. Complex rules regarding food and drink are meant to lead to purity of mind and aid spirituality. Pollution is the opposite of purity and should be avoided or ameliorated. Certain substances are considered both pure in themselves and purifying in their application. These include the products of the living cow—milk products, dung, and urine—and water from sources of special sanctity, such as the Ganges River. Pure and purifying substances also include materials commonly employed in rituals, such as turmeric and sandalwood paste. All body products (e.g., feces, urine, saliva, menstrual flow, and afterbirth) are polluting. The use of water is the most common method of purification because water easily absorbs pollution and carries it away.

Feast Days

The Hindu calendar marks eighteen major festivals every year. Additional important feast days are those of marriages, births, and deaths. Each region of India observes its own special festivals; it has been said that there is a celebration going on somewhere in India every day of the year. All members of the community eat generously on festive occasions, and these may be the only days that extremely economically disadvantaged people eat adequately. Feasting is a way of sharing food among the population because the wealthy are responsible for helping everyone celebrate the holidays.

One of the most joyful and colorful of the Hindu festivals is Holi, the festival of color that dates back several centuries before Christ. Though its purpose may have shifted over time, Holi occurs on the spring equinox and celebrates the triumph of good over evil.[64] There are various stories on the origins of Holi—one version has it that an evil king forced his subjects to worship him as their god. But the king's son, Prahlada, continued to worship Lord Vishnu. The angry king plotted with his sister, Holika, to kill his son. Since Holika wore a cloak immune to fire, she lured Prahlada to sit in a pyre with her. But the boy's devotion to Lord Vishnu helped him walk away unscathed while Holika died. Today, large pyres are lit to signify the victory of good over evil. Another story is that Holi commemorates the love of Krishna, a Hindu deity considered a manifestation of Vishnu, and the milkmaid Radha. Mischievous antics ensue: colored powder is thrown (red symbolizes love and fertility, green is for new beginnings, and more), balloons with colored water are

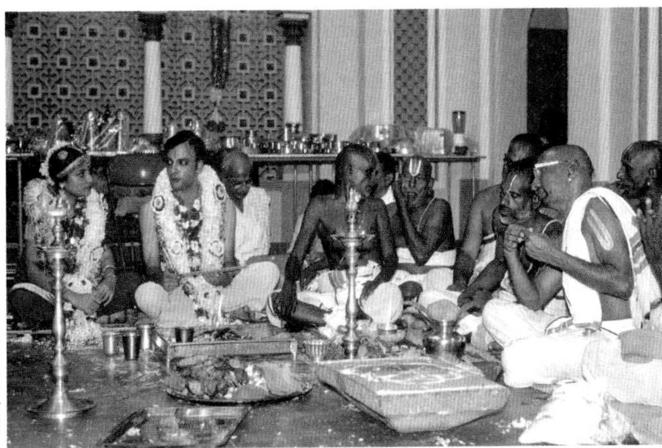

J. Isaac/United Nations

▲ An Indian wedding includes feasting. The numerous religious and secular events celebrated in India serve to distribute food throughout the community.

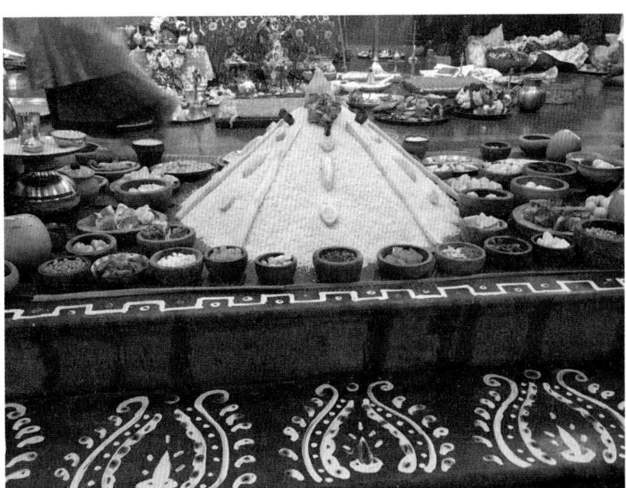

iStock.com/Reddees

▲ After being offered to God, temple food in India is then called prasada, or "favor" or "grace," and served to the community.

pitched off rooftops, and people squirt water guns at passersby. Later on the day of Holi, families gather for festive meals and distribute sweets among neighbors and friends.[65,66]

The ten-day celebration of Dusshera in late September or early October commemorates the victory of Prince Rama (an avatar of Vishnu) over the ten-headed demon Ravana, who abducted Rama's wife, Sita in the epic *Ramayana*. The festival's name, Dusshera, is derived from the Sanskrit words *dasha* (ten) and *hara* (defeat).[67] It is also a grateful tribute to the goddess Durga, who aided Rama. The first nine days are spent in worshiping the deity, and the tenth day is spent celebrating Rama's victory of good over evil.

Diwali or Divali, one of the major festivals in Hinduism, Jainism, and Sikhism, lasts for five days usually falling in late October and November in the Gregorian calendar, varying according to lunar cycles. The name is derived from the Sanskrit term dipavali (row of lights) and commemorates the triumph of light over darkness and knowledge over ignorance. One custom is the lighting of diyas—small earthenware lamps filled with oil—on the night of the new moon to invite the presence of Lakshmi, the goddess of wealth and good fortune.[68] For many, Divali is also the beginning of the new year, when everyone should buy new clothes, settle old debts and quarrels, and wish all people good fortune.

Fast Days

In India, fasting practices vary according to one's caste, family, age, sex, and degree of orthodoxy. A devoutly religious person may fast more often and more strictly than one who is less religious. Fasting may mean eating no food at all or abstaining from only specific foods or meals. The fast days in the Hindu calendar include the first day of the new and full moon of each lunar month; the tenth and eleventh days of each month; the fast (then feast) of Maha Shivaratri; the ninth day of the lunar month Chaitra; the eighth day of Sravana; days of eclipses, equinoxes, solstices, and conjunctions of planets; the anniversary of the death of one's father or mother; and Sundays.

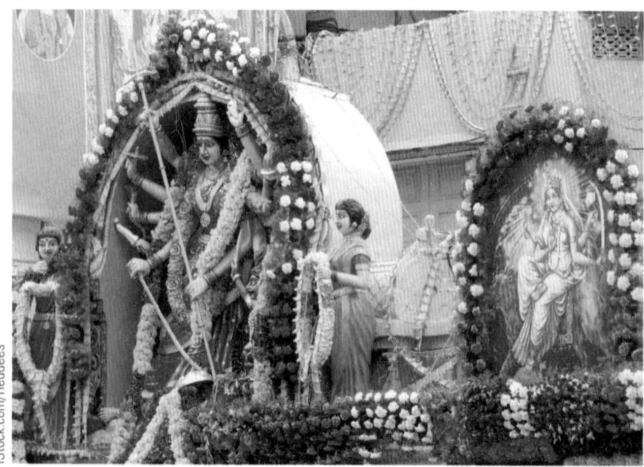

iStock.com/Reddees

▲ **Durga Puja, held annually in the goddess Durga's honor, is one of the great festivals of northeastern India.**

Buddhism

Siddhartha Gautama, who later became known as Buddha (the Enlightened One), founded the Eastern religion of Buddhism in India in the 6th century BCE. Buddhism flourished in India until 500 CE, when it declined and gradually became absorbed into Hinduism, though it is still practiced. Meanwhile, it had spread throughout southeastern and central Asia where it remains a vital religion and has been adapted to local needs and traditions.

Buddhism was a protestant revolt against orthodox Hinduism, but it accepted certain Hindu concepts, such as the idea that all living beings go through countless cycles of death and rebirth, the doctrine of karma, spiritual liberation from the flesh, and that the path to wisdom includes taming the appetites and passions of the body. Buddha disagreed with the Hindus about the methods by which these objectives were to be achieved. He advocated the Middle Way between asceticism and self-indulgence, stating that both extremes in life should be avoided. He also disagreed with the Hindus on caste distinctions, believing that all persons were equal in spiritual potential in *this* life.

The basic teachings of Buddha are found in the Four Noble Truths and the Noble Eightfold Path.[69] The Four Noble Truths are as follows:

1. *Dukkha*—The Noble Truth of Suffering: Suffering is part of living. Persons suffer when they experience birth, old age, sickness, and death. They also suffer when they fail to obtain what they want. At a deeper level, dukkha embodies other concepts, such as dissatisfaction, change, and conditionality.
2. *Samudaya*—The Noble Truth of the Cause of Suffering: This Noble Truth explains that suffering is caused by a person's attachments to their ideas, beliefs, and relationships. For example, when a person clings to their views they may not be open to other information. Buddhism works with a person's views, beliefs, fears, and desires to promote healthy relationships and minimize suffering.
3. *Nirodha*—The Noble Truth of the Cessation of Suffering is the cessation of dukkha. When a person lets go or releases attachment, even for a moment, suffering abates. Buddhism is a practice of letting go until all attachments are relinquished and the person lives in the present moment.
4. *Magga*—The Noble Truth to the Path Leading to the Cessation of Suffering (the Eightfold Path). It is a middle way between the search for happiness through the pursuit of pleasure and the search for happiness through self-mortification and asceticism. By following this path (right view, right thought, right speech, right action, right livelihood, right effort, right mindfulness, and right concentration), a person learns to directly face suffering and disappointment, learn its nature, and thus find freedom.

Food for Thought

For most Hindus, water is often the beverage of choice at meals.

In southern India the rice harvest is celebrated in the festival called Pongal—new rice is cooked in milk, and when it begins to bubble, the family shouts, "Pongal!" ("It boils!").

The Hindu calendar is lunar; thus, its religious holidays do not always fall on the same day each year on the Western calendar. Every three to five years the Hindu calendar adds a thirteenth leap month (a very auspicious period) to reconcile the months with the seasons.

The Noble Eightfold Path (Figure 4.7) can be broken down into three components: wisdom, ethics, and tranquility. The wisdom components include Right View, which leads to clarity about what life offers and doesn't offer. One learns to live in harmony with life just as it is. With Right View, followers develop core values that lead to the practice of Right Intention. Right Intention means to mindfully respond to circumstances with kindness and compassion for oneself and others. From Right Intention follows the components of ethics: Right Speech, Right Action, and Right Livelihood. A Buddhist practitioner may follow a code of conduct known as the Five Precepts. These are (1) abstain from the taking of life, (2) abstain from the taking of what is not given, (3) abstain from sensuous misconduct, (4) abstain from false speech, and (5) abstain from intoxicants because they tend to cloud the mind. To support this practice, followers practice Right Effort, which is releasing negative or compulsive thinking, Right Mindfulness, which is a non-judgmental, clear understanding, and acceptance of moment-to-moment experience and Right Concentration which allows the mind to be collected without distraction. Followers practice meditation to develop these skills so that they can accomplish the Noble Eightfold Path in everyday life. The person who perfects Buddha's teachings achieves nirvana and is called an arahant or bodhisattva, depending on the branch of Buddhism. The mind of an arahant or bodhisattva has no basis for greed, hatred, and delusion, and is characterized by peace, deep spiritual joy, compassion, and a refined awareness. Negative mental states and emotions such as doubt, worry, anxiety, and fear are absent from the enlightened mind. Saints in many religious traditions exhibit some or all of these qualities, and ordinary people also possess them to some degree, although imperfectly developed. An enlightened person can become so in their lifetime, and possess them all completely.[70] In addition, the person is no longer subject to rebirth into the sorrows of existence. Traditionally, the ideal practice of Buddhism—following a life of simplicity and spending a considerable amount of time in meditation—encouraged a monastic lifestyle. Monks own no personal property and are usually vegetarian. To eat, they ask for alms in the form of food. Merit, or good karma, is conferred upon those who give food to monks. In much of the world, this lifestyle is hard to maintain and many Western Buddhists encourage daily meditation practice while also practicing the precepts in everyday activities.

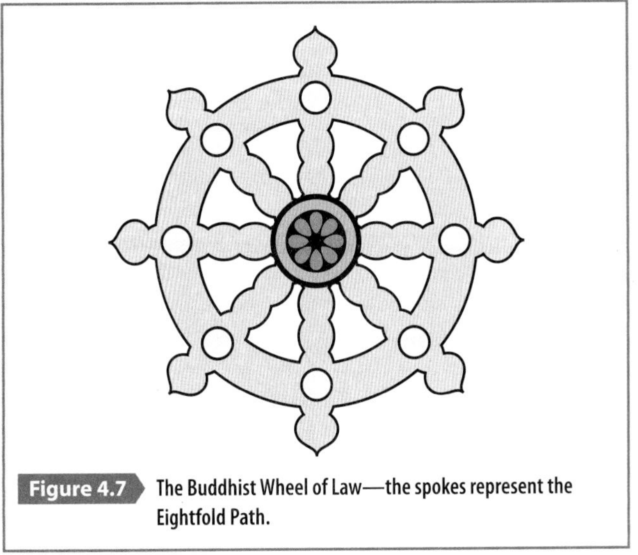

Figure 4.7 The Buddhist Wheel of Law—the spokes represent the Eightfold Path.

Food for Thought

In both Theravada and Mahayana Buddhist temples, worshipers may offer food at the altar, such as apples, bananas, grapes, oranges, pineapples, candy, rice, dried mushrooms, and oil.

A Zen Buddhist monastery, Tassajara, located in central California is famous for its vegetarian restaurant and popular cookbook.

Buddhist monks in Tibet carve sculptures in butter (a few inches in size up to as high as fifteen feet) and parade them during an evening in March, lit by lanterns, for Chogna Choeba, the Butter Lamp Festival. The lamps are made from yak butter and are used in temples to create a warm glowing light.

There are numerous sects in Buddhism and two primary schools of doctrine: Theravada (also known as Hinayana) Buddhism, which is followed in India and Southeast Asia; and Mahayana Buddhism, which is followed in China, Japan, Korea, Tibet, and Mongolia.[71,72] Theravada Buddhism is primarily based on the original doctrines practiced by the Buddha and follows the Pali canon of ancient Indian Buddhism. Theravada places little or no emphasis on deities, teaching that the goal of the faithful is to achieve nirvana. The ideal is the arhat (in Pali: arahant), or perfected saint, who attains enlightenment as a result of their own efforts. In Mahayana, a later form of Buddhism, Buddha is eternal and cosmic, appearing variously in many worlds to make known his truth, called dharma. This has resulted in a pantheon of Buddhas who are sometimes deified and, for some communities, a hierarchy of mystical demons. Central to Mahayana ideology is the idea that anyone can aspire to achieve awakening and become a bodhisattva, one who seeks to be a buddha.[72]

The number of Buddhists in the United States was over 2.2 million in 2014,[73] with the majority being immigrants from Japan, China, and Southeast Asia and their descendants, although non-Asian Westerners are taking up the practice.

Buddhism first came to North America with Chinese immigrants in the 19th century. Many were fleeing the Opium Wars ravaging China, and the discovery of gold in California meant workers were needed to support a booming economy. In the 1880s, Japanese people began to migrate West as well. By the 1930s, most Buddhist schools had built at least one temple in North America. At the same time, European scholars living in British colonies in Asia were producing the first English translations of Asian sacred texts, including the Buddhist sutras. These influenced Europeans, as well as American philosophers such as Ralph Waldo Emerson (1803–1882) and Henry David Thoreau (1817–1862). Books and translations by Daisetsu Teitaro Suzuki (1870–1966), especially on Japanese Zen and Pure Land, introduced many people in the United States to Buddhism for the first time in the 1950s and 1960s, including Beat Generation authors Allen Ginsberg and Jack Kerouac.[74] In 2020, Buddhist Americans made up 1 percent of the population, according to the U.S. Census.

Dietary Practices

Buddhist dietary restrictions vary considerably depending on the sect and country. Buddhist doctrine forbids the taking of life; therefore, many followers are lacto-ovo vegetarians (eating dairy products and eggs, but no meat). Some eat fish, and others abstain only from beef. Others believe that if they were not personally responsible for killing the animal, it is permissible to eat its flesh.

Feasts and Fasts

Buddhist festivals vary according to region. Traditionally, from July to October, Buddhist monks are directed to remain in retreat and meditate, coinciding with the rainy season and the sprouting of rice in the fields. The first day of retreat is a time for worshipers to bring gifts of food and articles of clothing to the monks; the retreat ends with *pravarana*, the end of the rainy season, when worshipers once again offer gifts to the monks, invite them to a meal, and organize processions. On three separate days (which vary according to the regional calendar), Mahayana Buddhists commemorate the birth of Buddha, his enlightenment, and his death; Theravada Buddhists celebrate Magha Puja, the Four Miracles Assembly, in February or March when 1,250 monks gathered, unplanned, to see the Buddha on the night of the full moon of the third lunar month. In April or May, they honor the Buddha on a single holiday called Vesak. Buddhist monks may fast twice a month, on the days of the new and full moon. They also do not eat any solid food after noon.

Discussion Starters

Does Your Religion Affect Your Eating Habits?

Explore your own religious and cultural dietary restrictions. Even if you are not religious, you can probably identify the major religions of your culture, a religion, or multiple religions of your parents, grandparents, or great-grandparents. It's probable that, unless you have made a conscious decision to change your dietary habits from your childhood, you still adhere to at least some of the dietary practices of your family's religion. Answer the following:

- What foods and/or drinks are prohibited by your religion—or were prohibited by your family when growing up?
- Are there certain times during the year when your religion directs you—or your family directed you as a child—to avoid certain foods and drinks or maybe even to fast (not eat at all)?
- Are there certain times during the year when your religion directs you—or when, as a child, your family directed you—to consume particular kinds of foods or drinks?
- Do you observe certain feast days during the year, days when you are supposed to eat a lot?

After answering the questions, seek out others and compare your answers. Don't ask only friends. Contact someone at a local mosque, synagogue, temple, church, or another religious meeting place, and ask to interview someone about her or his religion. Be sure to explain that you are a student studying food and religion. Another way of finding someone of a different culture and religion to interview is to look for local restaurants serving foods of particular ethnic groups: Thai, Chinese, Vietnamese, Korean, Japanese, Mexican, Middle Eastern, Indian, Ethiopian, Cuban, Caribbean, Greek, Italian, French, Cajun, Black American, or another culture. Contact the owner or manager to request an interview, again making sure to explain who you are and your reason for wanting to interview her or him. Because this person may be busy with work, she or he may not be able to talk with you right away. When meeting with the person for the interview, bring them these questions and your answers. Compare your answers with those from your interviewee.

Review Questions

1. What are the basic tenets of Western and Eastern religions?
2. Pick two of the following religions and describe the dietary laws for food preparation and consumption, and any additional laws for holy days: Judaism, Hinduism, and Islam.
3. List the Five Pillars of Faith in Islam and the Four Noble Truths and Noble Eightfold Path in Buddhism.
4. Describe and compare the roles of fasting in Islam and Hinduism, using examples of fasting practices in each faith.

Reflection

After reading this chapter, reflect on how your own religious beliefs or non-beliefs were influenced by your surrounding culture, and how this impacts how you view others with differing belief systems.

References

1. PRRI 2020 American Values Atlas. n.d. The American Religious Landscape in 2020. Retrieved from https://www.prri.org/research/2020-census-of-american-religion (accessed May 25, 2022).
2. Hackett, D., & McClendon, D. April 5, 2017. Pew Research Center (accessed May 26, 2022).
3. Self-described religious affiliation in the United States by percentage—2022. Source: Religious Landscape Study.
4. Religion in Canada (October 28, 2021) Statistics Canada. Retrieved from www150.statcan.gc.ca/n1/pub/11-627-m2021079-eng.htm
5. Baeck, L. 2019. *The essence of Judaism*. Plunkett Lake Press.
6. Goodman, M. 2018. *A history of Judaism*. Princeton, NJ: Princeton University Press.
7. Pew Research Center. (May 11, 2011) "Jewish Americans in 2020." Accessed 12-29-2022 from https://www.pewresearch.org/religion/2021/05
8. Barrow, K. April 13, 2010. More people choosing Kosher for health. *The New York Times*.
9. Kadam, A., & Deshmukh, R. 2020. Kosher food market. Allied Market Research. Retrieved from https://www.alliedmarketresearch.com/kosher-food-market-A06022 (accessed May 26, 2020).
10. Rivas, M.A., Avila, B.E., Koskela, J., Huang, H., Stevens, C., Pirinen, M., . . . & Daly, M. J. 2018. Insights into the genetic epidemiology of Crohn's and rare diseases in the Ashkenazi Jewish population. *PLoS Genetics*, 14(5), e1007329.
11. Schiff, E.R., Frampton, M., Semplici, F., Bloom, S.L., McCartney, S.A., Vega, R., . . . & Levine, A.P. 2018. A new look at familial risk of inflammatory bowel disease in the Ashkenazi Jewish population. *Digestive Diseases and Sciences*, 63(11), 3049-3057.
12. Masci, D., & Smith, G.A. October 10, 2018. Pew Research Center. Retrieved from https://www.pewresearch.org/fact-tank/2018/10/10/7-facts-about-american-catholics/ (accessed May 29, 2022)
13. Clancy, P.M.J. 1967. Fasting and abstinence. In *The New Catholic Encyclopedia*. New York: McGraw-Hill.
14. Fairnbairn, D. 2002. *Eastern orthodoxy through Western eyes*. Louisville, KY: Westminster John Knox Press.
15. Smart, N. 1998. *The world's religions* (2nd ed.). New York: Cambridge University Press.
16. US States by Orthodox Christian Population. n.d. Retrieved from https://www.worldatlas.com/articles/us-states-by-orthodox-christian-population.html (accessed May 29, 2022)
17. Karras, S.N., Persynaki, A., Petroczi, A., Barkans, E., Mulrooney, H., Kypraiou, M., . . . & Naughton, D.P. 2017. Health benefits and consequences of the Eastern Orthodox fasting in monks of Mount Athos: a cross-sectional study. *European Journal of Clinical Nutrition*, 71(6), 743–749.
18. Kolb, R. 2004. Martin Luther. In H.J. Hillerbrand (Ed.), *The encyclopedia of Protestantism*. New York: Rutledge.
19. Sack, D. 2000. *Whitebread Protestants: Food and religion in American culture*. New York: St. Martin's Press.
20. Newell, C. 2000. *Latter days: A guided tour through six billion years of Mormonism*. New York: St. Martin's Press.
21. Douglas, D. 2004. Mormonism. In H.J. Hillerbrand (Ed.), *The encyclopedia of Protestantism*. New York: Rutledge.
22. Mormon Population By State. n.d. World Atlas. Retrieved from https://www.worldatlas.com/articles/mormon-population-by-state.html (accessed May 29, 2022).
23. Milgrom, J. Book of Mormon Central.
24. Riess, J. 2019. *The next Mormons: How millennials are changing the LDS church*. Oxford: Oxford University Press.
25. Knoll, B.R., & Riess, J. 2020. Changing religious and social attitudes of Mormon millennials in contemporary American Society. In *The Palgrave handbook of global mormonism* (pp. 293–320). Palgrave Macmillan, Cham.
26. Greenleaf, F. 2004. Seventh-day Adventists. In H.J. Hillerbrand (Ed.), *The encyclopedia of Protestantism*. New York: Rutledge.
27. Feichtinger, C. 2016. Seventh-day Adventists: An apocalyptic Christian movement in search for identity. In Hunt, Stephen J. (ed.). *Handbook of global contemporary Christianity: Movements, institutions, and allegiance*. Vol. 12. Brill Handbooks on Contemporary Religion.
28. White, E.G.H. 1905. *The ministry of healing*. Hagerstown, MD: Review and Herald Publishing.
29. White, E.G.H. 1923. *Counsels on health*. Hagerstown, MD: Review and Herald Publishing.
30. White, E.G.H. 1938. *Counsels on diet and foods*. Hagerstown, MD: Review and Herald Publishing.
31. Buettner, D., & Skemp, S. 2016. Blue zones: lessons from the world's longest lived. *American Journal of Lifestyle Medicine*, 10(5), 318-321.
32. Eisenbert, R. April 16, 2019. How the oldest people in America's Blue Zone make their money last. *Money & Policy*. Retrieved from https://www.nextavenue.org/oldest-people-americas-blue-zone-make-their-money-last/ (accessed May 31, 2022).
33. Frager, R. 2002. *The wisdom of Islam: An introduction to the living experience of Islamic belief and practice*. Hauppauge, NY: Godsfield Press.
34. Denny, F. 2015. *An introduction to Islam*. Routledge.
35. Ahmed, S. 2015. *What is Islam?* Princeton, NJ: Princeton University Press.
36. Armanios, F., & Ergene, B. A. 2018. *Halal food: A history*. Oxford: Oxford University Press.
37. Mohamed, B. September 1, 2021. Muslims are a growing presence in U.S., but still face negative views from the public. Pew Research Center. Retrieved from https://www.pewresearch.org/fact-tank/2021/09/01/muslims-are-a-growing-presence-in-u-s-but-still-face-negative-views-from-the-public/ (accessed May 31, 2022).
38. Lapidus, I.M. 2014. *A history of Islamic societies*. Cambridge: Cambridge University Press.
39. Saadia, S., & Aziz, F. 2020. The Islamic concept of food and its effects on human beings. *Jihat ul Islam*, 14(1), 35–54.
40. Hussaini, M.M. 1993. *Islamic dietary concepts and practices*. Bedford Park, IL: Islamic Food and Nutrition Council of America.
41. Meo, S. A., & Hassan, A. 2015. Physiological changes during fasting in Ramadan. *Journal of Pakistan Medical Association*, 65(5 Suppl 1), S6–14.

42. Kinnard, J.N. 2015. *The Norton anthology of world religions*, Vol. 1. General Editor, J. Miles; Hinduism Editor, W. Doniger; Buddhism Editor, DS. Lopez, Jr.; Daoism Editor, J. Robson. *Journal of the American Academy of Religion*, 83(2), 591–596.
43. The nature of human life in Hinduism. BBC. Retrieved from https://www.bbc.co.uk/bitesize/guides/zmgny4j/revision/3#:~:text=Reincarnation%20is%20a%20key%20belief,or%20a%20spirit%20or%20soul
44. Cordain, L., Miller, J.B., Eaton, S.B., Mann, N., Holt, S.H.A., & Speth, J.D. 2000. Plant-animal subsistence ratios and macronutrient energy estimations in worldwide hunter-gatherer diets. *Journal of Clinical Nutrition*, 71, 682–692.
45. Derungs, C., Köhl, M., Weibel, R., & Bickel, B. 2018. Environmental factors drive language density more in food-producing than in hunter–gatherer populations. Proceedings of the Royal Society B, 285(1885), 20172851.
46. Reinhart, R.J. 2018. Snapshot: few Americans Vegetarian or Vegan. Gallup. Retrieved from https://news.gallup.com/poll/238328/snapshot-few-americans-vegetarian-vegan.aspx?g_source=link_NEWSV9&g_medium=NEWSFEED&g_campaign=item_&g_content=Snapshot%3a%2520Few%2520Americans%2520Vegetarian%2520or%2520Vegan
47. Good Food Institute. 2022. Plant based foods: 2021 market insights. Retrieved from https://gfi.org/wp-content/uploads/2022/03/2021-U.S.-retail-market-insights_Plant-based-foods-GFI.pdf
48. Douglas, M. 1966. *Purity and danger: An analysis of concepts of pollution and taboo*. New York: Praeger.
49. Harris, M. 1998. *Good to eat: Riddles of food and culture*. Long Grove, IL: Waveland Press.
50. Pandit, B. 2005. *The Hindu mind: Fundamentals of Hindu religion and philosophy for all ages*. Glen Ellyn, IL: Dharma Publishing.
51. Coward, H. Time in Hinduism. *Journal of Hindu-Christian Studies*. Retrieved from https://digitalcommons.butler.edu/jhcs/vol12/iss1/8/
52. Mittal, A. 2016. A brief history of the caste system and untouchability in India." *The Logical Indian*. Retrieved from https://thelogicalindian.com/story-feed/awareness/caste-system-and-untouchability-in-india/
53. Citizens for Justice and Peace (CJP) Editors. 2018. Caste discrimination and related laws in India. Citizens for Justice and Peace (CJP). Retrieved from https://cjp.org.in/caste-discrimination-and-related-laws-in-india/
54. Wilkerson, I. 2020. *Caste (Oprah's Book Club): The origins of our discontents*. Random House.
55. Wagatsuma, H., & DeVos, G. 2021. *Japan's invisible race: Caste in culture and personality*. University of California Press.
56. Flood, G. (Ed.). 2020. *The Oxford history of Hinduism: Hindu practice*. Oxford: Oxford University Press.
57. Flood, G.D. 2020. *Hindu monotheism*. Cambridge: Cambridge University Press.
58. Harvard Divinity School. 2018. Hinduism case study—minority in America. Retrieved from https://rpl.hds.harvard.edu/religion-context/case-studies/minority-america/hindus-american-textbooks#:~:text=There%20are%20around%202.5%20million,Hindu%20immigration%2C%20largely%20from%20India
59. Nikhilananda, S. 2021. *Hinduism: Its meaning for the liberation of the spirit*. Routledge.
60. Cohen, A. B. 2021. You can learn a lot about religion from food. *Current Opinion in Psychology*, 40, 1–5.
61. Sathyamala, C. 2019. Meat-eating in India: Whose food, whose politics, and whose rights? *Policy Futures in Education*, 17(7), 878–891.
62. Chouraqui, J.P., Turck, D., Briend, A., Darmaun, D., Bocquet, A., Feillet, F., . . . & Committee on Nutrition of the French Society of Pediatrics. 2021. Religious dietary rules and their potential nutritional and health consequences. *International Journal of Epidemiology*, 50(1), 12–26.
63. Kilara, A., & Iva, K.K. 1992. Food and dietary practices of the Hindu. *Food Technology*, 46, 94-1-2, 102.
64. Society for the Confluence of Festivals in India. "History of Holi." Retrieved from https://www.holifestival.org/history-of-holi.html
65. Kidangoor, A. 2020. Here's everything you need to know about Holi, the Hindu Festival of Colors." *Time*. Retrieved from https://time.com/5799354/what-is-holi/
66. Zeidan, A. February 14, 2022. Vishu. *Encyclopedia Britannica*. https://www.britannica.com/topic/Vishu
67. Editors of Encyclopedia Britannica. October 26, 2020. Dussehra. *Encyclopedia Britannica*. https://www.britannica.com/topic/Dussehra
68. Editors of Encyclopedia Britannica. May 6, 2022. Diwali. *Encyclopedia Britannica*. https://www.britannica.com/topic/Diwali-Hindu-festival
69. Crosby, K. 2004. Theraveda. In R.E. Buswell (Ed.), *Encyclopedia of Buddhism*. New York: Macmillan Reference.
70. Keown, D. The meaning of nirvana in Buddhism explained: Reaching the end of greed, hatred, and delusion. *The Buddhist Review*: Tricycle. Retrieved from https://tricycle.org/magazine/nirvana/
71. Editors of Encyclopedia Britannica. February 5, 2014. Theravada. *Encyclopedia Britannica*. https://www.britannica.com/topic/Theravada
72. Silk, J.A. August 1, 2017. Mahayana. *Encyclopedia Britannica*. https://www.britannica.com/topic/Mahayana
73. Pew Research Center. 2015. America's Changing Religious Landscape." Pew Research Center: Religion and Public Life. Retrieved from http://www.pewforum.org/2015/05/12/americas-changing-religious-landscape/
74. Tricycle: Buddhism for Beginners. Buddhism comes to America. Retrieved from https://tricycle.org/beginners/buddhism/buddhism-comes-to-america/

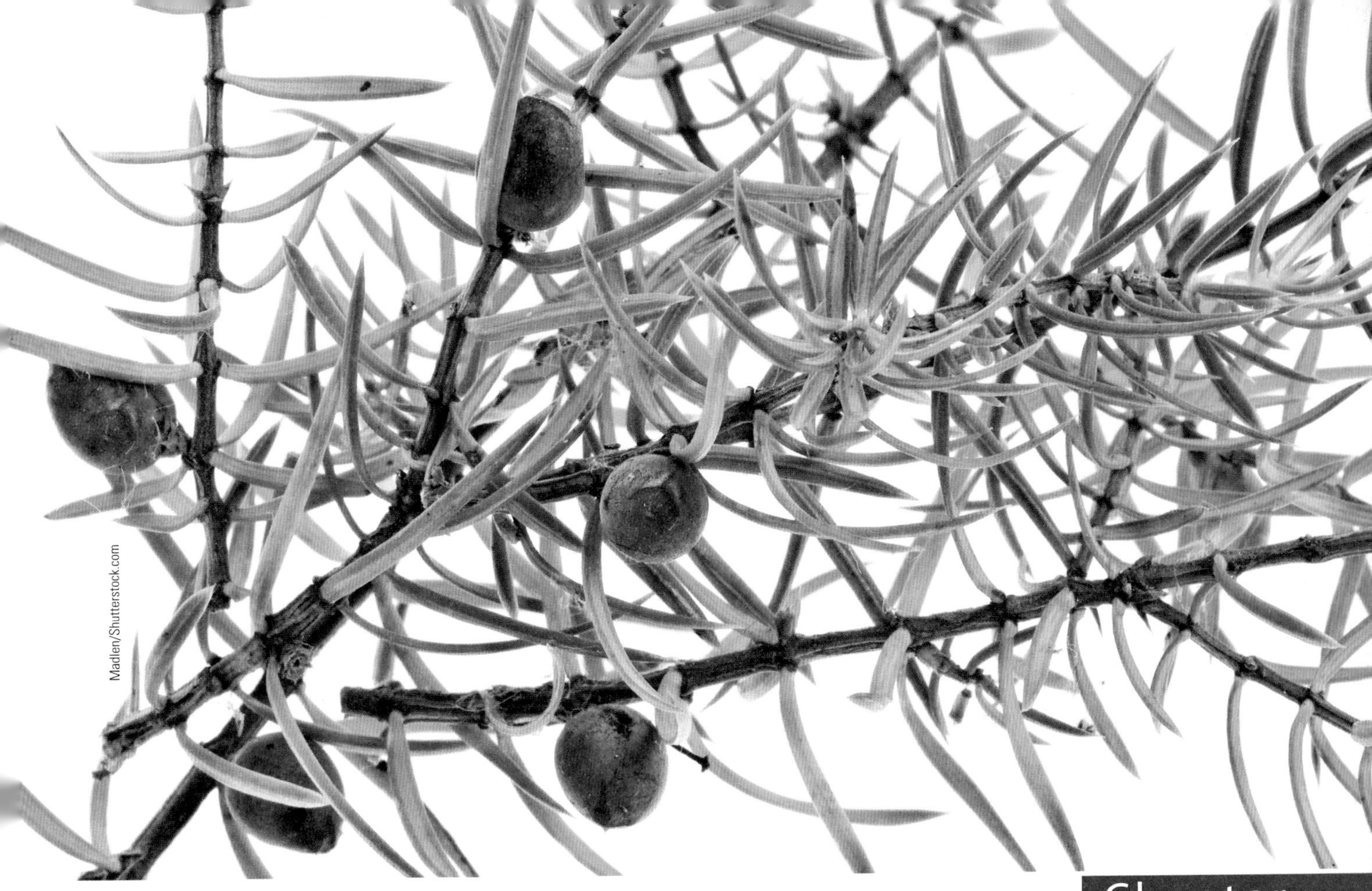

Chapter

5

Native Americans

Learning Objectives

5.1 Explain the designation "Native American."

5.2 Discuss the impact of the interactions between the arriving Europeans and the Native American nations on traditional food resources.

5.3 Analyze how urban versus rural locations of jobs of Native Americans affect socioeconomic status.

5.4 Interpret how the Native American worldview relating to health affects the use of biomedical health services.

5.5 Identify the key components of traditional health beliefs and practices of various Native American groups.

5.6 List indigenous foods commonly used in the different regional Native American cultural groups.

5.7 Identify foods indigenous to the Americas and those introduced from other regions of the world.

5.8 State the core protein food traditionally used in the five Native American regions.

5.9 Compare the meal cycle similarities and differences across regional groups of Native Americans.

5.10 Identify the traditional plants and foods used medicinally by Native Americans.

5.11 Demonstrate the effects of adaptations made to traditional foods in the modern diet of Native Americans.

The designation *Native American*, which includes the greatest number of ethnic groups of any population in the United States, is a term for the indigenous people of the Americas. It is used for Native Americans and Alaska Natives, comprised of Native American, Inuit, and Aleut people. Native Americans comprise 2.2% of the total U.S. population, or currently 7.2 million.[1] Each of the more than 500 Native American and Alaska Native nations have a distinct cultural heritage, which is often determined through "blood," called blood quantum, along with documentation listing tribal ancestor history. Tribal membership may require anywhere from 1/16th to 1/4th native heritage. Many argue that blood represents racial origins, not culture, and that blood quantum is no longer relevant. Culture is defined by kinship, geography, language, religion, lifestyle, and habits, and not by blood. This chapter will focus on Native American culture.[2]

Traditional Native American foods have significantly contributed to today's diet in the United States and beyond. Corn, squash, beans, cranberries, and maple syrup are just a few of the items Native Americans introduced to European settlers. Historians question whether the original colonists would have survived their first years in America without the supplies they obtained and the cooking and agricultural methods they learned from Native Americans. The food traditions of Native Americans have been passed down through generations using both historical story and myth. New Native American cuisine combines both contemporary culinary techniques and flavor combinations with elements of ancestral food tradition. By weaving together the past and present, new Native American cuisine helps restore and disseminate pre-colonial food.[3]

The diet of Native Americans has changed dramatically from its origins, yet recent renewed interest in Native American and Alaska Native culture has prevented the complete disappearance of many traditional foods and food habits. This is noted in the My Plate graphic in Figure 5.1, which focuses on native foods. This chapter reviews both the past and present diet of Native American ethnic groups.

 **Food for Thought**

It has been suggested that native Hawaiians be included as Native Americans; however, the history and culture of these peoples are substantially different from those of Native Americans of the U.S. mainland, Alaska, and Canada, so they are discussed in Chapter 12, "Southeast Asians and Pacific Islanders." Native American cultures of Mexico, Central America, and South America are considered in Chapter 9, "Mexicans and Central Americans," and Chapter 10, "Caribbean Islanders and South Americans."

History of Native Americans

Cultural Perspective

Settlement Patterns

It is hypothesized that the Native Americans came to North America approximately 20,000 to 50,000 years ago across the Bering Strait, which links Asia to Alaska, although some

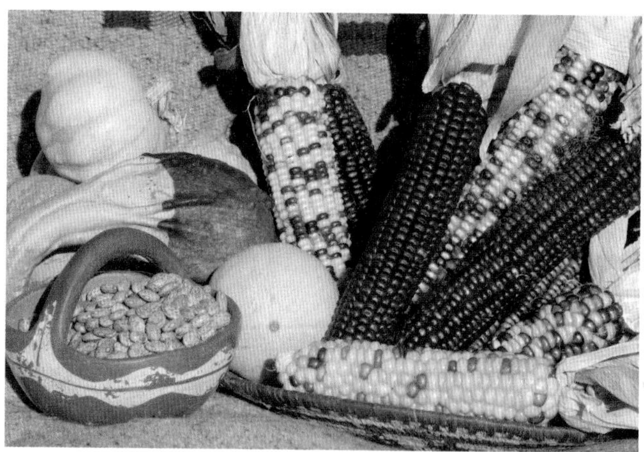

North Wind Picture Archives/Alamy Stock Photo

▲ **Traditional Native American foods (corn and squash shown here) include beans, berries, nuts, fish, jerky, maple syrup, and much more.**

evidence suggests earlier migrations may have occurred. Archaeological research provides little insight into the settlement patterns and diversification of Native American culture in the years before European contact in the 1600s. Furthermore, the Native American languages were entirely verbal, so written historical records are nonexistent. There are, consequently, enormous gaps in what is known of early Native American societies.

The introduction of Spanish horses, firearms, and metal knives changed the lifestyles of many Native nations, especially those that used the new tools to exploit the resources of the Great Plains. This initial interaction between White settlers and plains nations resulted in the development of the stereotype of the buffalo-hunting horseman with a feathered headdress who came to represent all Native American ethnic groups in popular culture. European diseases and the massacre of whole nations reduced the numbers of both Native American individuals and ethnic groups. In addition, many Native Americans were forced to migrate west to accommodate White expansion. The hardships of involuntary relocation and the deaths caused by illness and assault may have caused the extinction of nearly one-quarter of all Native American ethnic groups.

Native American lands dwindled as White settlers moved westward. By the late nineteenth century, the majority of Native Americans lived on lands held in trust for them by the U.S. government, called federal reservations. Still others resided in state reservation communities. Although they were not required by law to live on reservations, there were few other viable Native American communities.

The Bureau of Indian Affairs (BIA) took over the administration of the reservations near the turn of the twentieth century. It established a program of cultural assimilation designed to bring the Native American residents into mainstream U.S. society. Before the 1930s, Native American children were sent to off-reservation boarding schools. Though experiences varied, the children were not allowed to speak their languages, were given Anglo-American names,

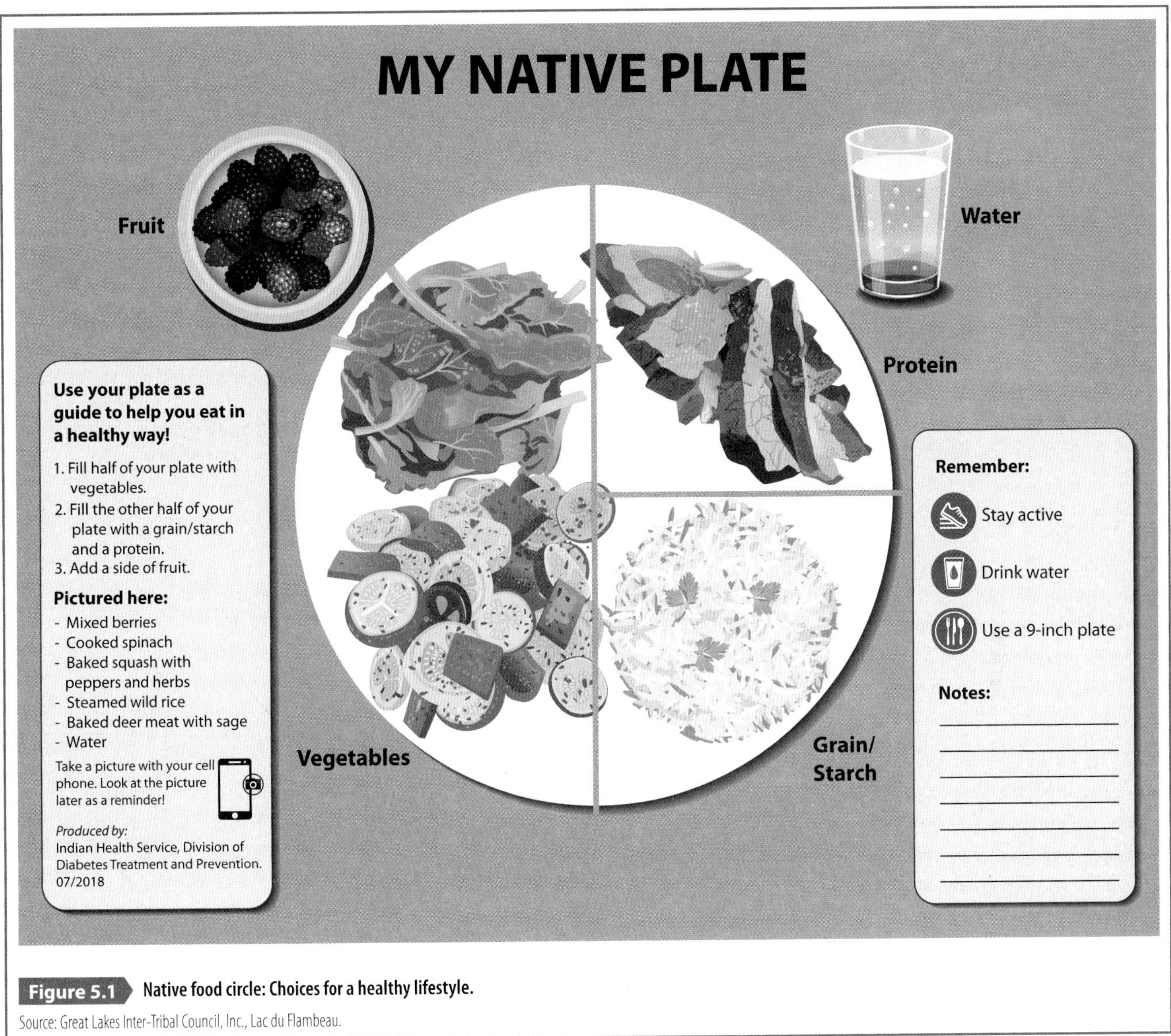

Figure 5.1 Native food circle: Choices for a healthy lifestyle.

Source: Great Lakes Inter-Tribal Council, Inc., Lac du Flambeau.

were taught the importance of private property and materialized wealth, and were forced to convert to Christianity. The first off-reservation boarding school was established in 1879 in Carlisle, Pennsylvania, and founded by Richard Henry Pratt who famously said in a speech in 1892, ".... Kill the Indian in him, and save the man."[4,5] Later, public reservation schools attempted similar indoctrination. However, the BIA program was usually unable to force Native Americans to accept the values of the majority culture. The Native Americans changed their dress, occupation, and social structure but did not fully assimilate. In many cases, their religious beliefs were strengthened, and their involvement in crafts, music, and dance was deepened to support their ethnic identity.

Native American communities would not necessarily identify themselves by the regions outlined in this chapter, but for purposes of categorization, and to showcase the extraordinarily diverse cultures of the various nations, Figure 5.2 depicts seven distinct regions on the map. Currently, there are over 500 federally recognized nations, and more than 100 state-recognized nations.[6]

Current Demographics Many Native Americans left the reservations for employment opportunities available during World War II. According to the Comanche National Museum and Cultural Center, 17 Comanche code talkers (those who spoke native languages that were used as code for sensitive information) enlisted in the army. Thirteen of them landed on the beach on D-Day and survived the war. Many became fluent in English and the ways of the dominant society when they joined the armed services. Others took war-related industry professional jobs. In the 1950s and 1960s, the BIA Employment Assistance Program was a major factor in the continuing out-migration of Native Americans from the reservations to the cities.

The Native American and Alaska Native populations increased from 5.2 million in 2010 to 7.2 million in 2020.

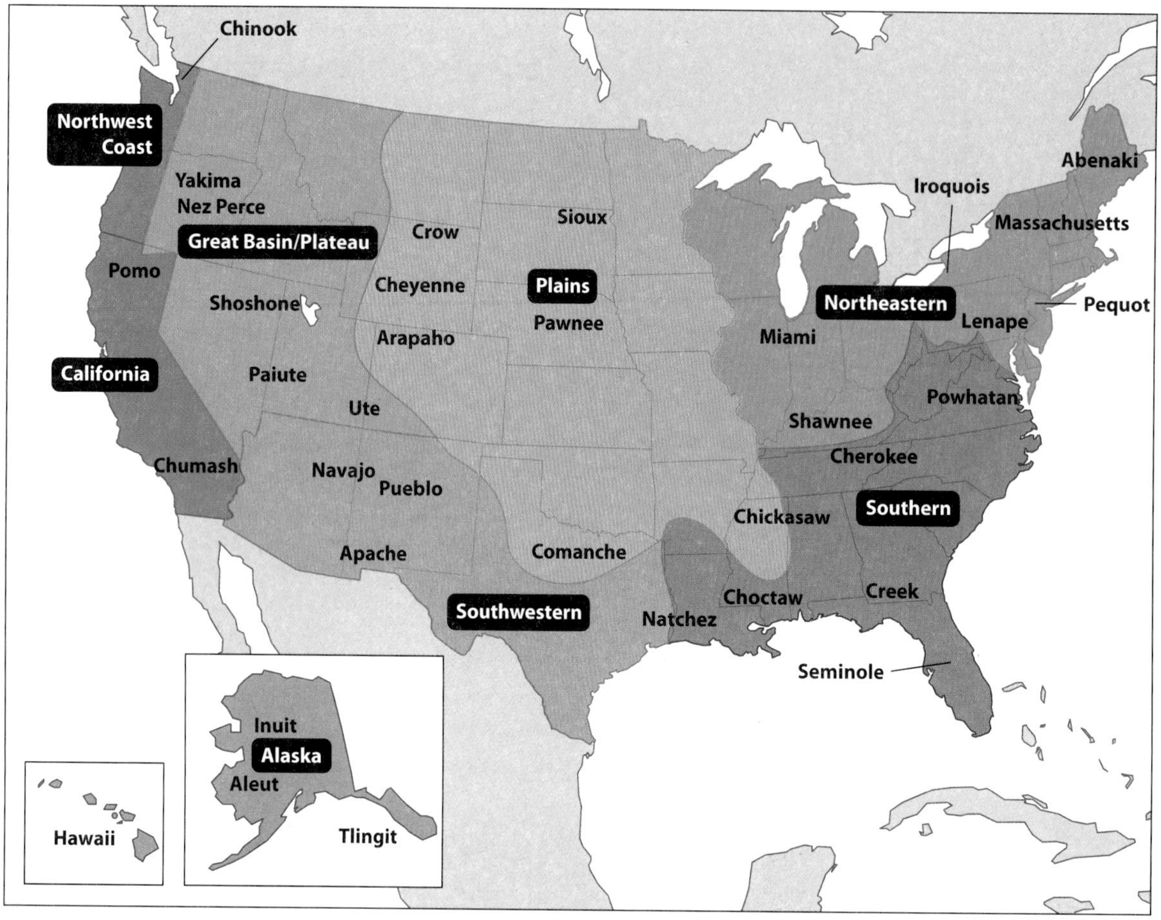

Figure 5.2 Location of some of the Native American nations in the continental United States.

Source: Adapted and reprinted by permission of the publisher from *Harvard Encyclopedia of American Ethnic Groups* edited by Stephan Thernstrom, Ann Orlov, and Oscar Handlin, p. 61, Cambridge, Mass.: The Belknap Press of Harvard University Press, Copyright © 1980 by the President and Fellows of Harvard College.[8]

The Native American and Alaska Native people represent 2.2 percent of the U.S. population, with Alaska and Oklahoma as the states with the highest percentage (20.5 and 14.4 percent, respectively). The vast majority of Native Americans and Alaska Natives today live west of the Mississippi River. Roughly 22 percent live on reservations or other trust lands and 60 percent live in metropolitan areas, which is the lowest metropolitan percentage of any minority population. Native American ethnic identity varies tremendously, from tenacious maintenance of heritage for future generations and reclaiming and celebrating that heritage, to the adoption of many aspects of the majority culture. In 2019, ten states with the largest Native American/Alaska Native populations were: Arizona, California, Oklahoma, New Mexico, Texas, North Carolina, Alaska, Washington, South Dakota, and New York.[7]

Large, urban Native American populations are found in Los Angeles, New York City, Phoenix, Tulsa, Anchorage, Oklahoma City, Albuquerque, and Tucson. Many first-generation urban Native Americans maintain close ties with the reservation of their ethnic group and travel often between the city and tribal land. Members of the second generation living in urban regions are more likely to think of the city as their permanent home.

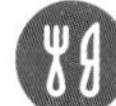

Food for Thought

During the early nineteenth century, the Cherokee had a written language, a bilingual newspaper, *The Cherokee Phoenix*,[9] a school system, a court system, and a Cherokee Nation constitution.[10] They were a prosperous Native nation, and many owned enslaved people.

Socioeconomic Status The socioeconomic status of Native Americans declined drastically with the forced migrations of the nineteenth century. Even those Native American nations that were agriculturally self-sufficient suffered when relocated to regions with poor growing conditions. Further, few Native occupations were valued in the job market outside the reservations. BIA education efforts were generally unsuccessful, and most Native Americans did not find employment until World War II and the development of the BIA Employment Assistance Program. The Indian

Self-Determination and Education Act of 1975 was enacted to promote Native American participation in government and education, but economic improvement continues to be slow. Approximately 32 percent of Native Americans and Alaska Natives work in management and professional occupations.[6] The Apache and Dakota have been active in ranching and rodeo circuits. Today, some of the top-ranked riders in the Professional Bull Riders Circuit are Native. In 2021, the Annual Global Cup included a Native American Team, the USA Wolves. The 2018 rookie of the year came from Utah and is Dine (Navajo).[11] In the Southwest, small-scale agriculture and livestock grazing are still important among some Hopi, Pueblo, and Navajo peoples, and traditional crafts such as weaving, pottery, and silversmithing are significant.[12–14] Some Alaska Natives combine part-time paid employment with subsistence living and often find jobs in the fishing and forestry industries.[15–17]

The overall poverty rate for Native Americans (nearly 21 percent) in 2019 was more than double that of the general population; however, significant tribal differences are seen. In 2019, 84.4 percent of Native Americans and Alaska Natives over 25 years of age had at least a high school diploma, 20 percent of Native Americans and Alaska Natives had attained a bachelor's degree, and 7.6 percent had an advanced graduate degree.[6]

Native American Organizations Even as many tribes in the United States were regaining land or receiving compensation, the U.S. Bureau of Indian Affairs instituted the Urban Indian Relocation Program. Initiated within the bureau in 1948 and supported by Congress from the 1950s on, the relocation program was designed to transform the predominantly rural native population into an assimilated urban workforce. From 1948 to 1980, when the program ended, some 750,000 Native Americans were estimated to have relocated to cities, although not all did so under the official program and not all remained in urban areas permanently. Today, 78% of Native Americans live off-reservation, and 72% live in urban or suburban environments.[18,19] Activists for Native American rights often come from the cities and are not always supported by Native Americans who live on tribal lands. Native American organizations have done much to maintain Native American identity. Most areas with large Native American populations have their own clubs and service associations. Organizations to promote ethnic identity have been founded by the Navajo, Pueblo, Tlingit, Haida, and Pomo. Other groups such as athletic clubs and dance groups serve the social needs of the pan-Native American community.

Food for Thought

Efforts to increase reservation prosperity include utilizing natural resources and establishing gambling operations, which are legal on tribal lands.

Worldview

While indigenous people have a variety of worldviews, researchers have found that most, or perhaps all, Native Americans see the world as a beautiful creation that evokes extremely powerful feelings of gratitude and obliges us to behave as if we are related to one another. Native Americans came to understand the cyclical patterns of life—think of the digestive process, the seasons and rotation of the earth, seasonal migrations of animals, and much more—as opposed to the linear (a person is born, moves through life with a specific goal or end), as fundamental to the way the world functions. More importantly, Native Americans allowed their observations on this reality (much like Buddhist and Hindu belief systems do), to direct the way they live, and inform their beliefs.[20] Harmony with this overarching cycle of nature best describes the Native American approach to life. Each individual strives to maintain a balance among spiritual, social, and physical needs in a holistic approach. Only what is necessary for life is taken from the natural environment; the belief is that the Earth should be cared for and treated with respect. Generosity is esteemed, competitiveness is discouraged, and individual rights are highly regarded. Personal autonomy is protected through the principle of non-interference. Among the Navajo, for example, an individual would never presume to speak for another, even a close family member. For most Native Americans, time is conceptualized as being without beginning or end, and the culture is present-oriented, meaning that the needs of the moment are emphasized over the possible rewards of the future.

Religion Traditional Native American religions vary from an uncomplicated belief in the power of a self-declared evangelist to elaborate theological systems with organized hierarchies of priests. Yet they all share one characteristic: religion permeates all aspects of life. Rather than a separate set of beliefs practiced at certain times in specific settings, religion is an integral part of the Native American holistic worldview. Religious concepts influence both the physical and emotional well-being of the individual.

Many Native American nations have rejected all attempts at Christian conversion, especially in the Southwest. The Navajo, Arizona Hopi, Rio Grande Pueblo, Potawatomi, Lakota, and Dakota have retained most of their historical religious values and rituals, such as sweat lodge purification rites. Other religions unique to Native Americans emerged after European contact, such as the Drum Dance followers and the Medicine Bundle religions, which combine spiritual elements from several different ethnic groups. A Paiute visionary, Wovoka, founded the Ghost Dance religion in the late 1880s, which prophesized an end to White domination through prayer, abstinence from alcohol, and ritual dancing.[21,22] It also encouraged followers to work for wages, farm the land, and educate their children to help Native Americans retain their identity and survive under conquest.[22] Other religions, such as the Native American Church, mix Christianity with traditional beliefs and have been popular since the late nineteenth century. In urban areas where churches have been established to serve all Native American congregations, Roman Catholicism and some forms of Protestantism have risen in popularity. In Alaska, some Native people have become adherents of Russian Eastern Orthodoxy.

Food for Thought

Wounded Knee became a symbol of Native American suffering, brutality, and the loss of the indigenous way of life. The conflict occurred December 29, 1890, when the U.S. Army, worried about the Ghost Dance spiritual movement (which promised peace to Native people and a world returned to them), killed 146 Sioux (some estimates are twice that), half of them women and children. Many see the massacre, which happened on the Pine Ridge reservation in South Dakota, as marking a painful low point, from which much of modern Native American and American life has emerged.[23,24]

Food for Thought

Many Native people prefer to describe themselves in their Native languages: Piikuni for Blackfeet, Ojibwe for Chippewa, and so on. Terms for Native people of the United States, such as "Indian," "Native," "Indigenous," and "American Indian," have come in and out of favor over the years, and different nations and individuals within them have different preferences. In this book, Native American and Indigenous are used, choices governed by a desire for clarity and verisimilitude. The best practice for outsiders is to ask the Native people you are talking with what they prefer.[23,26,27]

The U.S. Census uses the phrase "American Indians and Alaska Natives" (abbreviated AI/AN)[28] and now allows people to self-identify their nation as a write-in under the race section.

Family The primary social unit of Native Americans is the extended family, much like it is in Asian, African, and Middle Eastern cultures. Children are valued highly, and there is great respect for elders. All blood kin of all generations are considered equal; there is no differentiation between close and distant relatives. Aunts and uncles are often considered like grandparents, and cousins are viewed as brothers or sisters, much as they are in India and other cultures. Even other tribal members are sometimes accepted as close kin. In many Native American societies, an individual without relatives is considered poor.

Many Native American nations, such as the Lenape, Hopi, and Iroquois, are matrilineal, meaning that lineage is inherited from the mother. Traditionally, property was often passed down through women in these nations, and decision-making often rested with an elder woman in the family.[27,29] Today, even in matrilineal systems, the men are the family providers and heads of the household; women are typically in charge of domestic matters. Due to the respect for the individual within most Native American groups, men and women hold equal standing. Native

▼ The primary social unit of Native Americans is the extended family, which includes all close and distant kin.

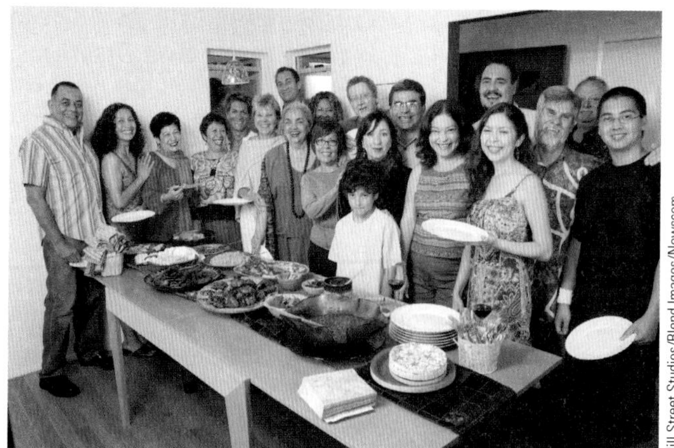

Hill Street Studios/Blend Images/Newscom

American children are expected to assist their parents in running the home.

Traditional Health Beliefs and Practices In Native American culture, health reflects a person's relationship to nature, broadly defined as the family, the community, and the environment. Every illness is due to an imbalance with supernatural, spiritual, or social implications. Treatment focuses on the cause of the imbalance, not the symptoms, and is holistic in approach. Traditional Eastern medical practices embrace similar philosophies. The sick individual is at odds with the universe, and community and family support is focused on restoring harmony, not curing the disease.[27] As explained by the Cherokee medicine man, Sequoyah, "Indian medicine is a guide to health, rather than a treatment. The choice of being well instead of being ill is not taken away from an Indian."[30] Traditional Native American medicine is concerned with physical, mental, and spiritual renewal.

In many Native American belief systems, health is not only a physical state but a spiritual one. Native American groups venerated practices of traditional healers, dubbed medicine men/women or shamans by European settlers, who bridged the natural and spiritual world in a centuries-old health care system using herbs, physical manipulations, and psychotherapy. Ideas on supernatural phenomena manifested a world of wonder for Native Americans. Although witchcraft beliefs were as common among European newcomers to North America as they were to Native Americans, there were completely different societal reactions for a variety of cultural reasons. For example, Native cultures held healers in high regard, whereas witch trials began to take hold in places like Salem, Massachusetts.[30]

Some Navajo believe transgressions committed at ceremonial occasions, evil spirits (especially ghosts), or agents in the form of animals, lightning, and whirlwinds, may cause fainting, hysteria, or other conditions. Witchcraft may also take the form of insidious objects, causing pain where the object is inserted, as well as emaciation. Possession by a spirit may dislodge the soul, resulting in a feeling of suffocation (or possession may be a sign of a gift for healing). Soul loss may also cause mental disorders. Violation of a taboo, whether an actual breach by an individual or contact with evil objects that have committed mythical breaches, results in general seizures.[27,30,34-36] Traditionally, these beliefs are shared by many other Native Americans as well. For example, some Iroquois believe in a similar list of reasons for illness, adding that unfulfilled dreams or desires may also be a contributing factor[34] and some Inuit believe sleep paralysis occurs when the soul is attacked by malevolent spirits or through witchcraft.[35]

Some Native Americans reject the concept that poor nutrition, bodily malfunctions, or an infection by a virus or bacteria can cause sickness. These ailments are attributed to an evil external source instead. Some Dakota, for instance, blame type 2 diabetes on disease-transmitting foods provided by colonizers and other early settlers to eliminate all Native Americans.[34-36] Social conditions created by European and U.S. colonialism can be seen to support this view. For example, in the late seventeenth century during the early days of European contact, warfare and enslavement by Europeans led to outbreaks of pathogens such as dysentery. These outbreaks left Native Americans, depleted by malnutrition, exposure, and lack of palliative care, vulnerable to disease, which spread rapidly. Then, as Native communities were moved off their lands and forced to adapt to new environments, they often became dependent on food programs that did not provide traditional nutrition, and created populations susceptible to diseases such as diabetes. In keeping with this history, an outbreak of serious respiratory infections due to the Hantavirus was explained by Navajo healers as being due to the rejection of traditional ways and the adoption of convenience foods.[34] Some Native Americans attribute alcoholism to soul loss and the cultural changes due to White society.[36]

Small bags of herbs (called "medicine bundles" by certain Plains nations), fetishes, feathers, or symbols may be worn to protect against malevolent forces and as symbolic and ritual aids in healing. Fetishes are representations of animal spirit guides that walk with people through life, teaching, guiding, and, in some cases, protecting them.

Traditional healers often specialize in their practice. Navajo medicine men and women usually exert a positive influence in preventing disharmony through rituals such as the sweat bath to promote peace. They also have negative powers, which can be used to counteract witchcraft or evil acts by a person's enemies. Diagnosticians may be called on to identify the cause of an illness through stargazing or listening (if crying is heard, the patient will die). Hand motions or trembling also may be involved, sometimes including painting with white, blue, yellow, and black colored sand to produce a picture of magical healing power. Other traditional Navajo practitioners are singers, who cure with sacred chanting ceremonies, and healers, who have specific responsibility for the care of the soul. Among the Oneida, dreamers can see the future and diagnose illness.[37] In many Native American groups, herbalists, often women, assist in the treatment of illness through the ceremonial collection and application of wild plant remedies.[38] Refer to "Therapeutic Uses of Food" later in this chapter for examples.

Among California Native Americans, illness was treated first with home remedies. If that proved ineffective, non-sacred healers such as herbalists or masseuses were contacted. If the patient still did not improve, a diviner would be consulted for a diagnosis. If spiritual or supernatural intervention was needed, a shaman (medicine man or woman) was employed. Consultation with native healers is often concurrent with seeking Westernized health care.[26]

Traditional Food Habits

The traditional food habits of Native Americans were influenced primarily by geography and climate. Each Native American nation adopted a way of life that allowed it to maximize indigenous resources. Many were agriculturally based societies, others were predominantly hunters and gatherers, and some survived mainly on fish. Most of each day was spent procuring and preparing food.

Ingredients and Common Foods

Indigenous Foods Archaeological records and descriptions of America by European settlers indicate that Native Americans on the East Coast enjoyed an abundance of food. Fruits, including blueberries, cranberries, currants, grapes, persimmons, plums, and strawberries, as well as vegetables, such as beans, corn, and pumpkins, are mentioned by the New England colonists. They describe rivers so full of life that fish could be caught with frying pans, sturgeon so large they were called "Albany beef," and lobster so plentiful that they would pile up along the shoreline after a storm. Game included deer, moose, partridge, pigeon, rabbit, raccoon, squirrel, and turkey. Maple syrup was used to sweeten foods. Farther south, Native Americans cultivated groundnuts (*Apios americana*, or Indian potatoes) and tomatoes, and collected wild Jerusalem artichokes (a starchy tuber related to the sunflower). Native Americans of the Pacific Northwest collected enough food, such as salmon and fruit, during the summer to support them for the rest of the year. Peoples of the plains hunted buffalo, and those of the northeastern woodlands gathered wild rice; nations of the Southwest cultivated chili peppers and squash amid their corn as noted in Table 5.1.

In many ways, Native Americans have been written out of the early American food story and certainly marginalized. However, Native Americans not only introduced colonizers and other early settlers to indigenous foods but also shared their methods of cultivation and food preparation starting in 1621. For instance, the Wampanoags, who had traded and fought with European explorers since 1524, observed the Pilgrims who arrived in their territory in 1620 for months before their great sachem (chief), Ousamequin, made contact. The contact, including the meeting that is the basis for U.S. Thanksgiving imagery, eventually led to a long history of often brutal colonization for the Native Americans. But it also led to the passing of knowledge of North America's defining indigenous agriculture—the "Three Sisters" of corn, beans, and squash planted in a

Table 5.1 Indigenous Foods of the Americas

Fruits	Berries (blackberries, blueberries, cranberries, gooseberries, huckleberries, loganberries, raspberries, strawberries), cactus fruit (tuna), cherimoya, cherries (acerola cherries, chokecherries, ground-cherries), grapes (e.g., Concord), guava, mamey, papaya, passion fruit (granadilla), pawpaw, persimmon (American), pineapple, plums (American, beach), soursop (guanabana), zapote (sapodilla)
Vegetables	Avocado, bell peppers (sweet peppers, pimento), cactus (nopales, nopalitos), chayote (christophine, chocho, huisquil, mirliton, vegetable pear), pumpkins, squash, tomatillo, tomatoes
Tubers/roots	Arrowroot, cassava (yuca, manioc, tapioca), groundnut, Indian breadroot, Jerusalem artichoke, jicama, malanga (yautia), potatoes, sweet potatoes
Grains/cereals	Amaranth, corn (maize), quinoa, wild rice
Nuts/seeds	Brazil nuts, cashews, hickory nuts, pecans, pumpkin seeds (pepitas), sunflower seeds, walnuts (black)
Legumes	Beans (green beans, most dried beans), peanuts
Poultry	Turkey
Seasonings/flavorings	Allspice, chile peppers (e.g., hot and sweet), chocolate (cocoa), maple syrup, sassafras (filé powder), spicebush, vanilla

NOTE: Foods native to North, Central, or South America. Some items not indigenous to the United States (e.g., pineapple, potatoes) were popularized only after acceptance in Europe and introduction by European settlers. Other foods (e.g., avocado, jicama, tomatillo) have become more common in the United States with the growing Latino population.

mound using fish remains as fertilizer (much like what is now called regenerative agriculture)—and survival for the Pilgrims.[40] The Three Sisters ensured soil health as well as increased soil drainage and provided each plant with appropriate nutrients. Corn, which depletes the soil of nitrogen was planted alongside beans which replenished it, and squash benefited by growing up the available corn stalk without staking.[40,41]

Food for Thought

Thanksgiving is often seen as a heart-warming American origin story. However, its imagery (eastern Native people dressed in the garb of the Plains nations people eating together with kindly Pilgrims in 1621) was embellished. Early settlers often participated in the English Puritan practice of declaring two fast days of prayer each spring and fall to mark a special mercy from God that concluded in a community feast. Native Americans often held food celebrations around harvest. The meal at Plymouth wasn't a particularly special event at the time. It wasn't until 1863 that President Abraham Lincoln declared the last Thursday of November a national day of Thanksgiving, apparently in response to intense lobbying by a magazine editor, Sarah Josepha Hale of *Godey's Lady's Book*. Hale, who rallied readers to foster unity amid the horrors of the Civil War, helped others to propagate the imagery of the grateful Native offering food and land and then exiting American history. Native Americans, many of whom mark the day as the "National Day of Mourning," see this history of colonization differently. Even though the early settlers raided precious seed corn stored for winter use from Wampanoag underground storage barns, the tribe extended a peaceful hand to the newcomers. The Wampanoags had two reasons to do this, researchers say: pity for the newcomers, and their need for allies against their Narragansett rivals after a devasting epidemic (introduced by earlier European slave traders) decimated the Wampanoag population. While about 90 Wampanoags did come to the Pilgrim camp it was because they heard gunshots and came to help. When finding the colonists getting ready for a spring feast, they returned with venison and other foodstuffs to share.[41]

Foods Introduced from Europe Foods introduced by the Europeans, especially the French Jesuits in the North and the Spanish in the South, were well accepted by Native Americans. Apples, apricots, carrots, lentils, peaches, purslane, and turnips were some of the more successful new foods. Settler William Penn noted that he found peaches in every large Native American farm he encountered barely one hundred years after they had been introduced to the Iroquois. The Europeans also brought rye and wheat. However, few Native American nations replaced corn with these new grains.

Livestock made a much greater impact on Native American life than did the new fruits and vegetables. Cattle, hogs, and sheep reduced the Native Americans' dependence on game meats. The Creek and Cherokee of the Southeast fed their cattle on corn and fattened their suckling pigs and young lambs on apples and nuts. The Powhatan of Virginia fed their hogs peanuts, then cured the meat over hickory smoke. Lamb and mutton became staples in the Navajo diet after the introduction of sheep by the Spanish. In addition, the Europeans brought Spanish horses and firearms, which made hunting easier, and metal knives and iron pots, which simplified food preparation. They also introduced the Native Americans to distilled spirits.

Foods Introduced from Africa For millennia, West Africans and Native Americans nourished their communities by growing, gathering, and hunting food. Native Americans had thrived growing corn, beans, and squash as well as fishing, foraging, and hunting. African and Native Americans developed common foodways, including one-pot stews, and both used fermentation for food preservation. Black-eyed peas were not common to Native American diets but were introduced by people from West Africa. They then became so common to Native Americans that some mistakenly thought they originated in North America.

Likewise, Native American corn became a staple among enslaved people from West Africa as can be seen in the common southern food cornbread.[42]

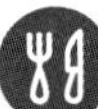

Food for Thought

"I want Indigenous food to be a part of the conversation in the culinary world. There are no other people on the earth that respect [food] more than Indigenous people. How can you have a sense of respect for food and not have a sense of respect for the people that care for the earth the way that Indigenous people do?" ~*Pyet DeSpain, winner of the first season of Fox's Next Level Chef, and operator of a Los Angeles pop-up called Shkodé.*[43,44]

Staples The great diversity of Native American cultures has resulted in a broad variety of cuisines. The cooking of one region is as different from that of another as French food is from German food today. Native American cooking features local ingredients and often reflects the need to preserve foods for future shortages. The only staple foods common to many, though not all, Native American nations are beans, corn, and squash. The cultural food groups are listed in Table 5.2. Corn, a dietary staple for most Native Americans, carries cultural and spiritual significance. Corn stories vary by Native traditions: it was a gift of the creator, it was distributed by crows or blackbirds to the people of the Eastern Woodlands, it was sent from the Great Spirit as a gift of thanks, and more. Corn is celebrated as a symbol of sustenance in ceremonies surrounding planting and harvesting, such as Green Corn feasts. Wheat, the staple grain of Europeans at the time of first contact, carries no such historical significance for Native Americans.[45]

Regional Variations Native American fare has been divided by regions into seven major types: northeastern, southern, plains, southwestern, great basin/plateau, California, and northwest/Alaska Native. Although each area encompasses many different Native American nations, they share similarities in foods and food habits.

Northeastern The northeastern region of the United States was heavily wooded, with numerous freshwater lakes and a long Atlantic coastline. It provided the local Native Americans, including the Iroquois and Powhatan, with abundant indigenous fruits, vegetables, fish, and game. Many of the foods associated with the cooking of New England have their origins in northeastern Native American recipes.

Table 5.2 Cultural Food Groups

Group	Comments	Common Foods	Adaptations in the United States
Protein Foods			
Milk/milk products	High incidence of lactose intolerance among Native Americans with a high percentage of Native American heritage.	No common milk products in traditional diets.	Powdered milk and evaporated milk are typical commodity products, usually added to coffee, cereal, and traditional baked goods; ice cream is popular with some groups. Some reports have been made of frequent milk consumption.
Meat/poultry/fish/eggs/legumes	Meat is highly valued, considered healthful. Meats are mostly grilled or stewed, preserved through drying and smoking. Beans are an important protein source.	*Meat:* bear, buffalo (including jerky, *pemmican*), deer, elk, moose, opossum, otter, porcupine, rabbit, raccoon, squirrel. *Poultry and small birds:* duck, goose, lark, pheasant, quail, seagull, wild turkey. *Fish, seafood, and marine mammals:* abalone, bass, catfish, clams, cod, crab, eel, flounder, frogs, halibut, herring, lobster, mussels, olechan, oysters, perch, red snapper, salmon, seal, shad, shrimp, smelts, sole, sturgeon, trout, turtle, walrus, whale. *Eggs:* bird, fish. *Legumes:* many varieties of the common bean (kidney, navy, pinto, etc.), *tepary* beans.	Beef is well accepted; lamb and pork are also popular. Canned and cured meats (bacon, luncheon meat) may be common if income is limited. Game is rarely eaten. Meats remain a favorite food. Chicken eggs are commonly eaten.
Cereals/Grains	Corn is primary grain; wild rice is available in some areas.	Cornmeal breads (baked, steamed), hominy, gruels, corn tortillas, *piki*, toasted corn; wild rice.	Wheat has widely replaced corn; store-bought or commodity breads and sugared cereals are common.

(Continued)

Table 5.2 Cultural Food Groups (*Continued*)

Group	Comments	Common Foods	Adaptations in the United States
Fruits/Vegetables	Indigenous plants are major source of calories in diet of some Native American nations. Fruits and vegetables are either gathered or cultivated; fruit is a popular snack food.	*Fruit:* blackberries, blueberries, buffalo berries, cactus fruit (tuna), chokeberries, cherries, crab apples, cranberries, currants, elderberries, grapes, groundcherries, huckleberries, persimmons, plums, raspberries, salal, salmonberries, strawberries (beach and wild), thimbleberries, wild rhubarb. *Vegetables:* camass root, cacti (nopales), chile peppers, fiddleheads, groundnuts, Indian breadroot, Jerusalem artichokes, lichen, moss, mushrooms, nettles, onions, potatoes, pumpkin, squash, squash blossoms, sweet potatoes, tomatoes, wild greens (cattail, clover, cow parsnip, creases, dandelion, ferns, milkweed, pigweed, pokeweed, saxifrage, sunflower leaves, watercress, winter cress), wild turnips, yuca (cassava).	Cakes, cookies, pastries are popular. Apples became common after European introduction. Apples, bananas, oranges, peaches, pineapple have been well accepted; canned fruits are popular. Wild berries are still gathered in rural areas. Some traditional vegetables are eaten when available. Green peas, string beans, instant potatoes are common commodity items. Intake of vegetables is low; variety is limited. Potato chips and corn chips often are popular as snacks.
Additional Foods			
Seasonings		Chiles, garlic, hickory nut cream, onions, peppermint, sage, salt, sassafras, seaweed, spearmint, and other indigenous herbs and spices.	
Nuts/seeds	Nuts and seeds are often an important food source; acorns are sometimes a staple.	Acorn meal, black walnuts, buckeyes, chestnuts, hazelnuts, hickory nuts, mesquite tree beans, pecans, peanuts, *piñon* nuts (pine nuts), pumpkin seeds, squash seeds, sunflower seeds, seeds of wild grasses.	
Beverages	Herbal teas are often consumed for enjoyment, therapeutic, or spiritual value.	Teas of buffalo berries, mint, peyote, rose hip, sassafras, spicebush, sumac berries, *yerba buena*; honey and water.	Coffee, tea, soft drinks are common beverages. Alcoholism is prevalent.
Fats/oils	Traditional diets vary in fat content, from extremely low in the mostly vegetarian cooking of California and Nevada Indians to very high in the primarily animal-based fare of Native Alaskans.	Fats rendered from buffalo, caribou, moose, and other land mammals; seal and whale fat.	Butter, lard, margarine, vegetable oils have replaced rendered fats in most regions; seal and whale fat are still consumed by the Inuit and Aleut.
Sweeteners	Consumption of sweets is low in traditional diets.	Maple syrup, other tree saps, honey.	Sugar is primary sweetener; candy, cookies, jams, and jellies are popular.

The clambake was created when the Narragansett and the Penobscot steamed their clams in beach pits lined with hot rocks and seaweed. Dried beans were simmered for days with maple syrup (the precursor of Boston baked beans). The dish that today is called succotash comes from a stew common in the diet of most Native Americans; it combined corn, beans, and fish or game. In the Northeast, it was usually flavored with maple syrup. Clam chowder, codfish balls, brown bread, corn pudding, pumpkin pie, and the dessert known as Indian pudding are all variations of northeastern Native American recipes. In addition to clams, the Native Americans of the region ate lobster, oysters, mussels, eels, and many kinds of saltwater and freshwater fish.[47,48]

Food for Thought

The invention of potato chips in 1853 is attributed to a Native American hotel chef, George Crum. Today, Americans consume an average of seventeen pounds of potato chips per person each year.

Game, such as deer and rabbit, was eaten when available. Wild ducks, geese, and turkeys were roasted with stuffing featuring crab apples, grapes, cranberries, or local mushrooms. Corn, as the staple food, was prepared in many ways, such as roasting the young ears; cooking the kernels or meal in soups, gruels, and breads; steaming it in puddings; or

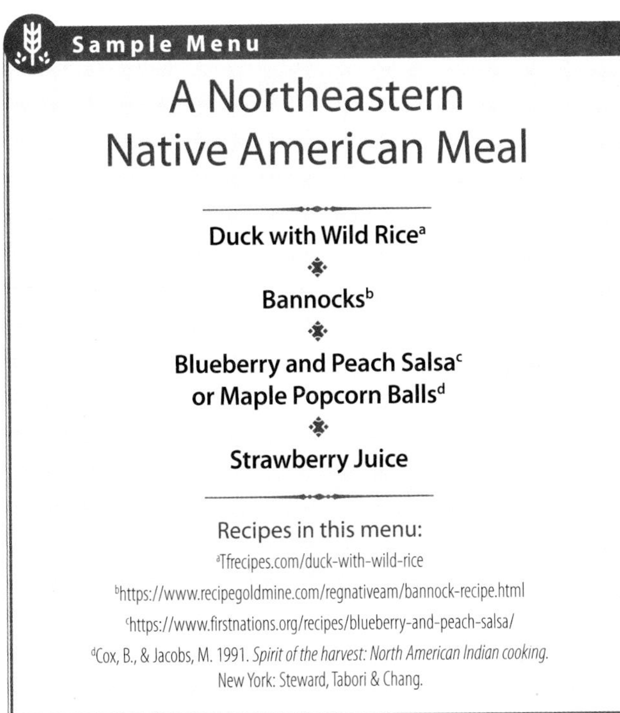

Sample Menu

A Northeastern Native American Meal

Duck with Wild Rice[a]

Bannocks[b]

Blueberry and Peach Salsa[c] **or Maple Popcorn Balls**[d]

Strawberry Juice

Recipes in this menu:

[a]Tfrecipes.com/duck-with-wild-rice

[b]https://www.recipegoldmine.com/regnativeam/bannock-recipe.html

[c]https://www.firstnations.org/recipes/blueberry-and-peach-salsa/

[d]Cox, B., & Jacobs, M. 1991. *Spirit of the harvest: North American Indian cooking.* New York: Steward, Tabori & Chang.

preparing it as popcorn. Breads were often made in a skillet (bannocks). Pumpkins and squash were baked almost daily, and beans were added to soups and stews. Local green leafy vegetables were served fresh. Sweets included cherries stewed with maple syrup, popcorn balls with maple syrup, cranberry pudding, crab apple sauce, and hazelnut cakes.[48–50]

Southern The great variety of foods found in the northeastern region of the United States was matched by the plentiful fauna and lush flora of the South. Oysters, shrimp, and blue crabs washed up on the warm Atlantic beaches during tropical storms. The woodlands and swamplands teemed with fish, fowl, and game, including bear, deer, raccoon, and turtle, as well as ample fresh fruit, vegetables, and nuts. The Native Americans of this region, such as the Cherokee, Creek, and Seminole, were accomplished farmers, growing crops of beans, corn, and squash.

When African people were enslaved and brought to America, they were often housed at the periphery of farms. Initially, a great deal of interaction took place between African arrivals and local Native Americans, who taught them how to hunt the native game without guns and to use the indigenous plants. In addition to African foods and cooking techniques, some of these Native American cooking techniques were later introduced into White southern cuisine by Black cooks as they began to work in kitchens throughout the pre-emancipation South. Many of the flavors typical in modern southern cooking come from traditional Native American foods such as hominy (dried corn kernels with the hulls removed) and grits (made of coarsely ground hominy). The chicken dish known as Brunswick stew is an adaptation of a southern Native American recipe for squirrel. Native Americans also made sophisticated use of native plants for seasoning, and they thickened their soups and stews with sassafras. New recipes from Africa were incorporated into early American cookbooks such as *The Carolina Housewife*, 1847, by "A Lady of Charleston." This cookbook features more than 100 recipes using rice, an ingredient grown by African people that were bought to America for their rice-growing knowledge. Cooking techniques garnered from Africa on how to prepare rice dishes, among other foods and combinations from Native Americans, were learned from enslaved Black people but credited to the White planters in most Southern cookbooks of the era.[47]

Native American staple foods of corn, beans, and squash were supplemented with indigenous woodland fruits and vegetables. Blackberries, gooseberries, raspberries, strawberries, crab apples, grapes, groundcherries, Jerusalem artichokes, leafy green vegetables, persimmons (pounded into a paste for puddings and cakes), and plums were some of the numerous edible native plants. Tomatoes and watermelons were added after introduction by the Spanish into Florida. The Native Americans of the South also used beechnuts, hazelnuts, hickory nuts, pecans, and black walnuts in their cooking. The thick, cream-like oil extracted from hickory nuts was used to flavor corn puddings and gruels, and a traditional Cherokee specialty was kanuche, a soup made from the pureed nuts (often with the addition of corn, hominy, or rice), which is still popular today. Honey was the sweetener used most frequently, and it was mixed with water for a cooling drink. Teas were made from mint, sassafras, or spicebush (Lindera benzoin), and during the summer a tart lemonade-like drink was made from citrus-flavored sumac berries.[51,52]

Food for Thought

The first commercial meat (bison) and fruit bar, the Tanka bar, was started in 2006 on the Pine Ridge Reservation in South Dakota to create a product sourced from and produced by Native people, and to restore the buffalo's place in the lives of the Oglala Lakota. The recipe, based on wasna, a traditional meat and berry food eaten in the Great Plains for hundreds of years, was a way to create a regenerative Native economy based on protein bars.[46]

Plains The Native Americans who lived in the area that is now the American Midwest were mostly nomadic hunters, following the great herds of bison across the flat plains for sustenance. The land was rugged and generally unsuitable for agriculture. Those nations that settled along the fertile Mississippi and Missouri River valleys, however, developed farm-based societies supported by crops of beans, corn, and squash.

Bison meat was the staple food for most plains nations such as the Arapaho, Cheyenne, Crow, Dakota, and Pawnee. The more tender cuts were roasted or broiled, while the tougher ribs, joints, and other bones with marrow were prepared in stews and soups. Pieces of meat, water, and sometimes vegetables would be placed in a hole in the ground lined with cleaned buffalo skin. The stew would then be stone boiled: rocks that had been heated in the fire would be

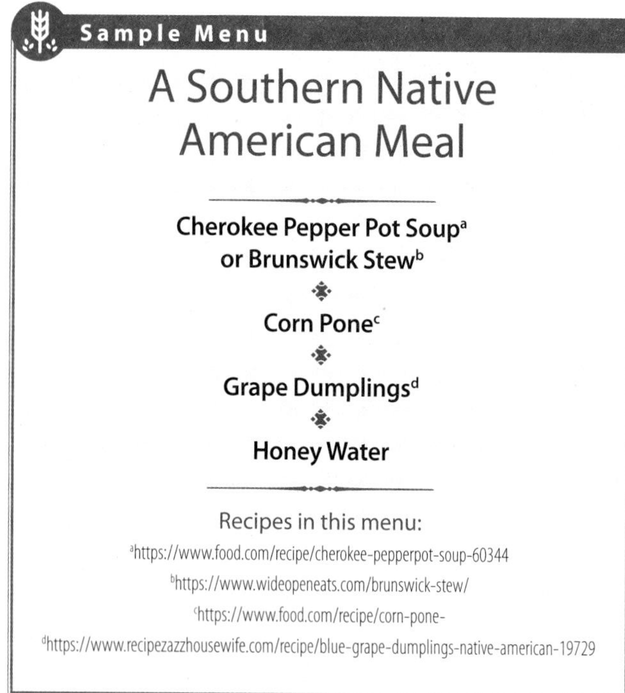

Sample Menu

A Southern Native American Meal

Cherokee Pepper Pot Soup[a]
or Brunswick Stew[b]

Corn Pone[c]

Grape Dumplings[d]

Honey Water

Recipes in this menu:

[a]https://www.food.com/recipe/cherokee-pepperpot-soup-60344
[b]https://www.wideopeneats.com/brunswick-stew/
[c]https://www.food.com/recipe/corn-pone-
[d]https://www.recipezazzhousewife.com/recipe/blue-grape-dumplings-native-american-19729

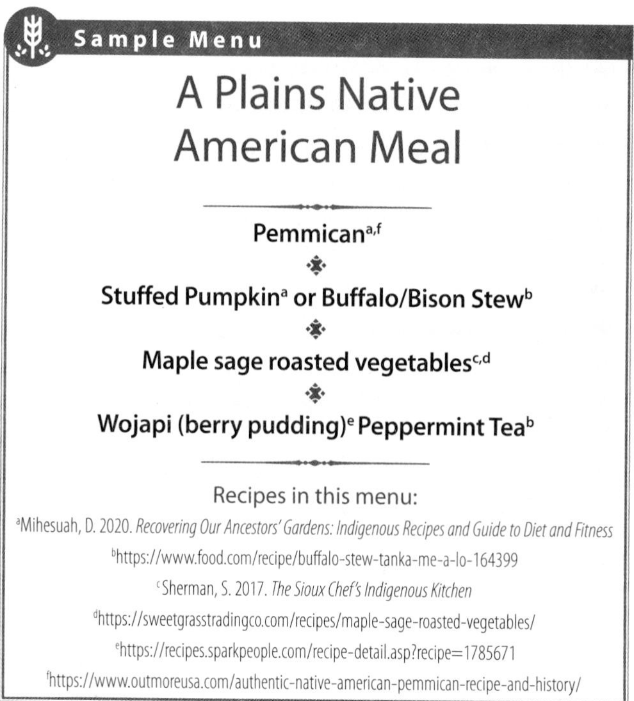

Sample Menu

A Plains Native American Meal

Pemmican[a,f]

Stuffed Pumpkin[a] or Buffalo/Bison Stew[b]

Maple sage roasted vegetables[c,d]

Wojapi (berry pudding)[e] Peppermint Tea[b]

Recipes in this menu:

[a]Mihesuah, D. 2020. *Recovering Our Ancestors' Gardens: Indigenous Recipes and Guide to Diet and Fitness*
[b]https://www.food.com/recipe/buffalo-stew-tanka-me-a-lo-164399
[c]Sherman, S. 2017. *The Sioux Chef's Indigenous Kitchen*
[d]https://sweetgrasstradingco.com/recipes/maple-sage-roasted-vegetables/
[e]https://recipes.sparkpeople.com/recipe-detail.asp?recipe=1785671
[f]https://www.outmoreusa.com/authentic-native-american-pemmican-recipe-and-history/

added to the broth until the mixture was thoroughly cooked. All parts of the bison were eaten, including the liver and kidneys (which were consumed raw immediately after the animal was slaughtered), udder, tongue, and hump. Extra meat was preserved by cutting it into very thin strips and then dehydrating it in the sun or over the fire. This tough, dried meat would keep for several years and was known as jerked buffalo or jerky. The jerky would be pulverized and mixed with water or corn gruel, or, in emergencies, eaten dry. Most often it was shredded and mixed with bison fat and berries, then formed into cakes called pemmican.[53,54,67]

When bison were unavailable, the plains nations would hunt deer, rabbit, and game birds. Fresh leafy green vegetables were consumed in season, and root vegetables, such as wild onions, prairie turnips (*Psoralea esculenta*, also called breadroot, tipsin, and timpsila), and sunchokes (an edible tuber root of a variety of sunflower), also known as Jerusalem artichokes, were eaten throughout the year. Wild rice, a native aquatic grass with an earthy, nutty flavor, was collected in the northern parts of the Midwest. It was served with bison, venison, or duck and used as a stuffing for grouse, partridge, and duck. Wild rice is believed to have traditionally provided as much as 25 percent of the total Ojibwa diet. When made into a sweet dish, wild rice was often prepared with maple syrup.[25,26] Blackberries, shadberries (also called Juneberries or saskatoon berries), cherries, chokecherries, crab apples, grapes, persimmons, and plums were available in some areas, but the most popular fruit was the scarlet buffalo berry (*Shepherdia canadensis*), so called because it was often served in sauces for bison meat or dried for pemmican. In addition, berries were traditionally boiled with bison suet and/or blood to make a thick pudding called wojapi.[47]

Southwestern Some of the oldest Native American settlements in North America were located along the river valleys of the arid Southwest. Despite the semidesert conditions, many Native Americans such as the Hopi, Pima, Pueblo, and Zuni lived in pueblo (Spanish for "town" or "village") communities and were mostly farmers, cultivating beans, chili peppers, corn, and squash. Others, including the Apache and Navajo, were originally roving hunters and gatherers. After the Spanish introduced livestock, some of these nomadic groups began to raise sheep. Mutton has since become associated as a traditional staple food of the region.

Until the arrival of livestock, the diet of the region was predominantly plant-based, providing a nourishing diet when supplemented with small game such as rabbit and turkey. Corn was the primary food, and at least five different colors of corn were cultivated. Each color symbolized one of the cardinal points for the Zuni, and each had its own use in cooking. White corn (east) was ground into a fine meal and used in gruels and breads. Yellow corn (north) was roasted and eaten in kernel form or off the ear. The rarer red (south), blue (west), and black (the nadir, the lowest point beneath the observer) corn was used mostly for special dishes, such as the lacy flat Hopi bread made from blue cornmeal, known as piki. Multicolored corn represented the zenith. The Hopi also attached importance to the color of corn and cultivated twenty different varieties. In many areas, corn was prepared in ways similar to those of the northern Mexican Native Americans—corn tortillas pozole (hominy) and the tamale-like chukuviki (stuffed cornmeal dough packets). Juniper ash (considered a good source of calcium and iron) was often added to cornmeal dishes for flavoring.[45]

Beans were the second most important crop in the southwestern region. Many varieties were grown, including the domesticated indigenous tepary beans and pinto beans from

Mexico. Both squash and pumpkins were commonly consumed, and squash blossoms were fried or added to soups and salads. Squash and pumpkin seeds were also used to flavor dishes, and chile peppers were used as vegetables and to season stews. Cantaloupes (or muskmelons) were also grown after they were introduced by the Spanish, who originally sourced the sweet melon from their homeland in Central and South Asia.

When crops were insufficient, the southwestern Native Americans relied on wild plants, and to add variety, tender amaranth greens were eaten in summer. Piñon seeds (also called pine nuts) flavored stews and soups. Both the fruit (tunas) and the pads (nopales) of the prickly pear cactus were eaten, as were the pulp and fruit of other succulents, such as yucca (the starchy fruit known today as "Navajo bananas") and peaches. A unique food popular with some Apache was the root of the mescal plant, another desert succulent. It would be baked for hours in a covered, stone-heated pit until it developed a soft, sticky texture and a flavor similar to molasses. The beans of the mesquite tree were a staple in some desert regions; they were ground into flour and used in gruels, breads, and sun-baked cakes.

Great Basin/Plateau Unlike the majority of the Native land in the Southwest, the Great Basin/Plateau region includes dense forests, high mountain desserts, and sagebrush-covered hills. The nations of this region were known to be accomplished in hunting, fishing, and gathering. Great Basin/Plateau Native people resided in Washington, Idaho, Utah, and Oregon and include the Yakama, Shoshone-Bannock, Ute, and Warm Springs people.[49,50,61]

Native people in this region ate salmon, trout, whitefish, mollusks, camas bulbs, and wild waterlily seeds (used for flour). Deer, elk, bison, antelope, and moose were prevalent both for food and clothes (hides). Wild root vegetables, seeds, berries, and nuts also supplied the necessary nutrients for survival. The Yakama and Warm Springs peoples have two major food feasts each year to celebrate the bounty of their land. The Salmon Feast is hosted in the spring during the salmon runs and the Huckleberry Feast in the summer when huckleberries are in season. Much of their food was dried to preserve it for the entire year.[56,57]

The Coeur d' Alene people traveled with the seasons to gather and hunt food. Their permanent villages were set up close to Lake Coeur d'Alene as well as near important waterways such as the St. Joe and Coeur d' Alene Rivers. Travel by water was important and the tribe developed an estimated 30 types of canoes. These canoes helped transport the harvest of traditional foods such as balsamroot, s-qawts water potato, blue camas, and many others. When Lewis and Clark came to the Great Basin/Plateau area, they wrote in their journals about the blue fields they encountered—and they got to taste the bounty, too, as the Nez Perce tribe fed the expedition blue camas when they arrived undernourished. Over time, many of these traditional foods ceased to be available. The majority of the blue camas fields are currently being used for other commodity crop production and salmon are less common due to the damming of rivers.[54,55,58,59]

California Before the arrival of colonists, approximately a million Indigenous people lived in what is now California. The vast geography supports more than 100 federally recognized nations and six language groups. A variety of food was available year-round from both land and sea.

For those who lived south of the Bernardino Mountains, antelope, deer, fish, and rabbits were a primary source of meat that was boiled, roasted, or sun-dried. Acorns, cacti pinon nuts, screw beans, and fish were also consumed by nations such as the Cahuillas. Native people along the Pacific coast, such as the Chumash, also ate fish, shellfish, and marine animals.

Hoopa Valley is home to the Hupa tribe many of whom are artists known for their fine baskets and carved arts. The Hupa traditionally consumed a variety of freshwater eels, sturgeon, and trout. They would grind acorns into meal to make bread as well as collect berries (California is known for its manzanita berries), nuts, and other plants.[59,60,62]

The Costanoans/Ohlone (meaning "coast-dwellers") of the San Francisco area relied more on the ocean rather than freshwater fish. They consumed shellfish, speared fish, muscles, abalone, and beached whales. In addition, their diet included seaweed, acorns, and squash. The Costanoans/Ohlone practiced controlled burning early on which helped to expand the grazing area for animals and generated more effective growth for plants.[59,60,63–65]

Northwest Coast/Alaska Natives This culinary region incorporates a diverse geographic area. The climate of the Northwest coast is temperate. The luxuriantly forested hills and

Sample Menu

A Southwestern Native American Meal

Green Chili Stew[a,b]

Blue Cornmeal[a,c] or Frybread[d]

Pueblo Piñon/Feast Day Cookies[e] and Navajo Peach Crisp[f]

Recipes in this menu:

[a]Bitsoie, F. and Fraioli, J. 2021. *New Native Kitchen: Celebrating Modern Recipes of the American Indian.*

[b]https://www.recipegoldmine.com/regnativeam/green-chili-stew.html

[c]https://www.allrecipes.com/recipe/187199/blue-corn-cornbread/

[d]https://www.thespruceeats.com/native-american-fry-bread-4045432

[e]https://www.food.com/recipe/native-american-feast-day-cookies-164862

[f]https://www.food.com/recipe/navajo-style-peach-crisp-518055

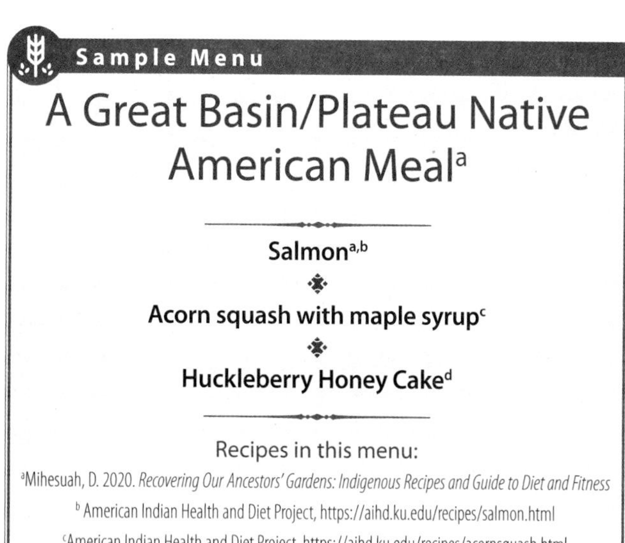

Sample Menu

A Great Basin/Plateau Native American Meal[a]

Salmon[a,b]

Acorn squash with maple syrup[c]

Huckleberry Honey Cake[d]

Recipes in this menu:

[a]Mihesuah, D. 2020. *Recovering Our Ancestors' Gardens: Indigenous Recipes and Guide to Diet and Fitness*

[b] American Indian Health and Diet Project, https://aihd.ku.edu/recipes/salmon.html

[c]American Indian Health and Diet Project, https://aihd.ku.edu/recipes/acornsquash.html

[d]https://tankabar.com/blogs/blog/spirit-of-the-harvest-cherokee-huckleberry-honey-cake

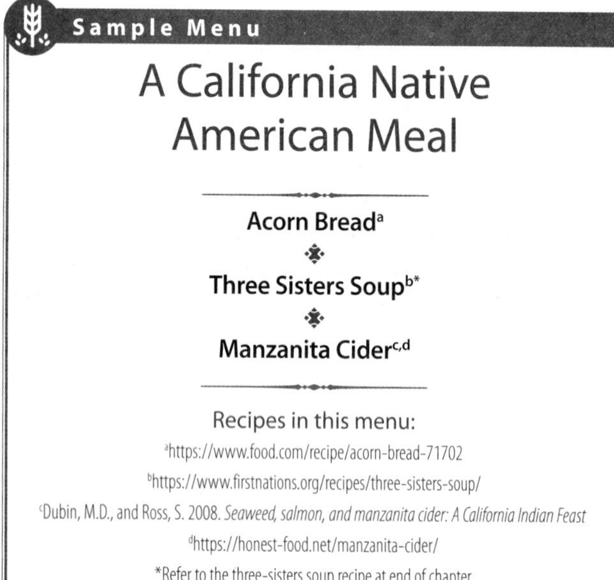

Sample Menu

A California Native American Meal

Acorn Bread[a]

Three Sisters Soup[b]*

Manzanita Cider[c,d]

Recipes in this menu:

[a]https://www.food.com/recipe/acorn-bread-71702

[b]https://www.firstnations.org/recipes/three-sisters-soup/

[c]Dubin, M.D., and Ross, S. 2008. *Seaweed, salmon, and manzanita cider: A California Indian Feast*

[d]https://honest-food.net/manzanita-cider/

*Refer to the three-sisters soup recipe at end of chapter

mountain slopes abound with edible plants and game, and the sea supplies fish, shellfish, and marine mammals. Farther north, in Alaska and Canada, the growing season shortens to only a few summer months, and temperatures in the winter regularly plunge to minus fifty degrees Fahrenheit. Two-thirds of Alaska is affected by permafrost, and the vast stretches of tundra are inhospitable to humans.

The Native American ethnic groups inhabiting this region include the Inuit and the Aleut, known as Alaska Natives. Native American nations such as the Tlingit and Kwakiutl inhabit the northwest coastal area and some interior Alaskan regions. The Aleut live on the thousand-mile-long chain of volcanic islands that arch into the Pacific from Alaska called the Aleutians. The Inuit, including the Yupik and Inupiat, live in the northern and western areas of Alaska, as well as in Canada, Greenland, and Siberia.

The Native Americans of the Northwest Coast did not need agriculture as wild food was plentiful and salmon was their staple. The fish were caught annually in the summer as they swam upstream to spawn. They were roasted over the fire when fresh, and the eggs, known today as red caviar, were a favorite treat when dried in the sun into chewy strips. Extra fish were smoked to preserve them for the winter. In addition, cod, clams, crabs, halibut, herring, shrimp, sole, smelt, sturgeon, and trout were consumed. Ocean mammals such as otters, seals, and whales were also hunted. Bear, deer, elk, and mountain goats were eaten, as were numerous wildfowl and game birds.[55,60]

Even with the abundant fish and game, wild plants made up more than half the diet of the Northwest Coast Native Americans. More than 100 varieties of indigenous fruits, nuts, and vegetables were consumed, including acorns, blackberries, blueberries, chokecherries (*Prunus virginiana*), desert parsley, hazelnuts, huckleberries, mint, raspberries, salal (*Gaultheria shallon*), and strawberries—and even particular varieties of lichen (for some groups this was a delicacy, for others it was only eaten when famine was imminent).[55] Camass roots (*Camassia quamash*), a bulb related to the hyacinth, were roasted or dried by many Indians of the region. Fresh greens were also popular.

In contrast to the plenty of the Northwest Coast, the diet of many Alaska Natives was often more limited in variety. The Inuit and Aleut were usually seminomadic, traveling as necessary to fish and hunt. Fish and sea mammals, such as seals, walruses, and whales, were the staple foods. Arctic hare, caribou, ducks, geese, mountain goats, moose, musk oxen (locally extinct in the Seward Peninsula by 1900 due to climatic conditions and overhunting), polar bears, and mountain sheep were consumed when available. Some items were boiled, but many were eaten raw due to the lack of wood or other fuel. The fat of animals was especially valued as food. Muktuk (also called muntak or onattak), still a commonly consumed item, consists of chunks of meat with a layer of fat and skin attached. Muktuk is typically frozen before use. Walrus or whale muktuk can also be preserved by

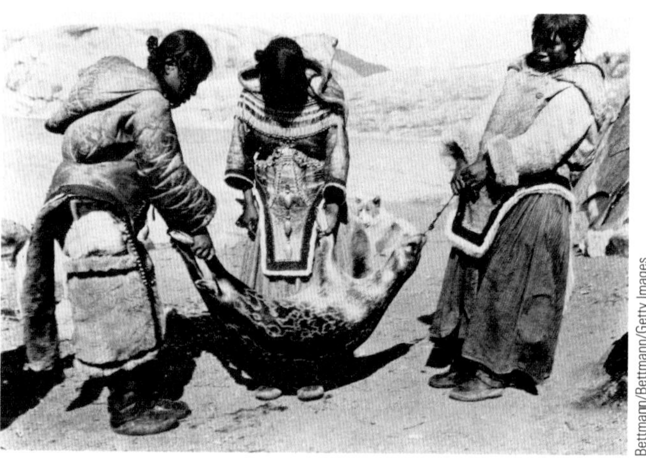

Bettmann/Bettmann/Getty Images

▲ **Inuit women preparing a dead seal for butchering.**

rolling it in herbs (with no salt) and fermenting it in a pit for several months to make a treat known as kopalchen. Akutok, a favored dish, was a mixture of seal oil, berries, and caribou fat. Even the stomachs of certain game were examined for edible undigested foods, such as lichen in elk and clams in walruses. The limited selection of wild plants included willow shrubs, seaweed, mosses, lichen, a few blueberries, salmonberries, and cranberries. Leaves from an aromatic bush known as bog shrub (*Ledum palustre*) were brewed to make tundra tea (also called Hudson Bay tea), a beverage still popular today.[55,63]

Other Native American Cuisines Many traditional Native American diets do not fit conveniently within the five major regional cuisines. Among them was the fare of the population found in what is now Nevada and parts of California, pejoratively called Digger Indians by the first colonizers to encounter them because they subsisted mostly on dug-up roots, such as Indian breadroot, supplemented by small game and insects. In central California, numerous nations, such as the Miwok and Pomo, had an acorn-based diet. Acorns contain tannic acid, a bitter-tasting substance that is toxic in large quantities. To make the acorns edible, Native American women would first crack and remove the hard hull, grind the meat into a meal, add water to make a dough, and then leach the tannic acid from the dough by repeatedly pouring hot water through it. Acorns were sometimes leached in sandy-bottomed streams as well.[56]

In the rugged northern mountains and plains lived nations such as the Blackfeet, Crow, Shoshone, and Dakota, who were nomadic hunters of game. Although many may have hunted bison at one time, they were limited to the local bear, deer, moose, rabbits, wildfowl, and freshwater fish when the expansion of other Native Americans and Whites into the Midwest pushed them northward and westward. Wild plants added variety to their diet. For example, the Nez Percé baked camass roots in a covered pit with heated rocks, which caramelized the starch providing a sweet, onion-like flavor. The cooked roots were made into gruel or dough for bread.

Sample Menu

A Northwest Coast Native American Meal

Pacific Halibut Cakes with Caper Mayonnaise[a]

Wild Rice with Sweet Potatoes[b]

Steamed Fiddlehead Ferns[c]

Whipped Raspberry (Soup)[d]

Recipes in this menu:

[a] Bitsoie, F. and Fraioli, J. 2021. *New Native Kitchen: Celebrating Modern Recipes of the American Indian.*

[b] https://unpeeledjournal.com/recipe-native-american-wild-rice-saute/

[c] https://cookingself.com/steamed-fiddlehead-ferns.html

[d] https://recipegoldmine.com/soupfruit/whipped-raspberry-soup.html

Meal Composition and Cycle

Daily Patterns Traditional meal patterns varied according to ethnic group and locality. In the Northeast, one large, hearty meal was consumed before noon, and snacks, such as soup, were available throughout the day. In some nations, no specific meal time was standard. The men were served first, and women and children ate next.

Serving two meals per day was more common in the Southwest. The women would rise before dawn to prepare breakfast, eaten at sunrise. The afternoon was spent cooking the evening meal, which was eaten before sunset. Two meals per day was also the pattern among the Native Americans of the Pacific Northwest.

In regions with limited resources, meals were often monotonous. The two daily meals of the southwestern Native Americans, for example, regularly consisted of cornmeal gruel or bread and boiled dehydrated vegetables. No distinction was made between morning and evening menus. Other dishes such as game, fresh vegetables, or fruit were included when seasonally available. The single meal of the northeastern Native Americans often included roasted game; the northwest coast Native Americans frequently included some form of salmon twice a day, in addition to the many local edible greens and roots.

Food was simply prepared. It was roasted over the fire or in the ashes or cooked in soups or stews. The northeastern and northwest coast Native Americans steamed seafood in pits; southwestern Native Americans baked cornmeal bread in adobe ovens called hornos. (After the introduction of hogs, flatbreads were commonly fried in lard.) Seasonal items were preserved by drying them in the sun or smoking them over a fire; for meat, fish, and oysters, special wood was often used to impart a distinctive flavor. Other foods were ground into a meal or pounded into a paste. In Alaska, meats, greens, and berries were preserved in fermented (aged) blubber. All nations liked sweets and ate fruits and dishes flavored with maple syrup, honey, or other indigenous sweeteners.

Special Occasions

Many Native American religious ceremonies were accompanied by feasts. Among the northeastern Iroquois, seasonal celebrations were held for planting, and harvests of maple syrup, strawberries, and corn, as well as New Year's festivals. The southern nations held an elaborate Green Corn Festival in thanks for a plentiful summer harvest. No one was allowed to eat any of the new corn until the ceremony was complete. Each home was thoroughly cleaned, the fires were extinguished, and all old pieces of pottery and clothing were replaced with newly made items. The adult men bathed and purged themselves with an emetic. When everything and everyone were thoroughly clean in body and spirit, a central fire was lit by rubbing two sticks together, and each hearth fire was relit with its flames. The feasting on new corn then began. Amnesty was granted for all offenses except murder, and the festival signified the beginning of a new year for marriages, divorces, and periods of mourning.[66]

Role of Food in Native American Culture and Etiquette

Historically, many Native American nations, especially in the inland regions, experienced frequent food shortages. As a result, food is valued as sacred, and, in the holistic worldview of most Native American groups, food is also considered a gift of the natural realm. In some nations, elaborate ceremonies accompanied the cultivation of crops, and prayers were offered for a successful hunt.

The men in many nations were traditionally responsible for hunting or the care of livestock. The job of food gathering, preparation, and storage usually belonged to the women, who also made the cooking utensils, such as watertight baskets or clay pots.[13] In predominantly horticultural societies, both men and women were frequently involved in the cultivation of the crops. Among the nations of the Northeast, the men ate first, followed by women and children. In the Southwest, men prepared the game they caught and served it to the women.

Sharing food is an important aspect of most Native American societies today. Food is usually offered to guests, and in some nations, it is considered rude for a guest to refuse food. It is also impolite to eat in front of others without sharing.[32] Any extra food is often given to members of the extended family. In some nations of the Southwest, meals are prepared and eaten communally. Each woman makes a large amount of one dish and shares it with the other families, who in turn share what they have prepared. Many Native Americans find the idea of selling food inconceivable; it is suggested that this is one reason there are few restaurants featuring Native American specialties.

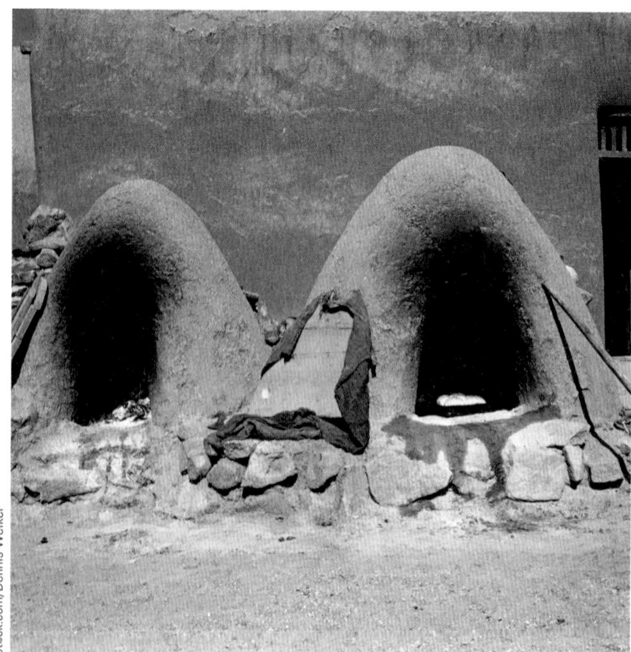

iStock.com/Dennis Welker

▲ Baking bread in a southwestern outdoor oven.

Therapeutic Uses of Food

The role of food in spiritual and physical health is still important for many Native Americans, and many food plants provide medicine in some form. Corn is significant in some healing ceremonies. Cornmeal may be sprinkled around the bed of a patient to protect him or her against further illness. Corn pollen may be used to ease heart palpitations, and fine cornmeal is rubbed on children's rashes. Navajo women drink blue cornmeal gruel to promote the production of milk after childbirth, and Pueblo women use a mixture of water and corn ear smut (*Ustilago maydis*, a kind of fungus) to relieve diarrhea and to cure irregular menstruation. A similar drink was given to Zuni women to speed childbirth and prevent postpartum hemorrhaging. Corn silk tea was used as a diuretic and was prescribed for bladder infections.[68,69]

Numerous other indigenous plants are used by Native Americans for medicinal purposes. For example, agave leaves (from a succulent common in the Southwest) are chewed as a general tonic, and the juice is applied to fresh wounds. Another succulent, yucca, was considered a good laxative by the Hopi. Pumpkin pastes soothe burns. Chili peppers are used in compresses for arthritis and are applied directly to warts. Infusions are used for many remedies, such as wild strawberries or elderberry flowers for diarrhea and mint tea to ease colic, indigestion, and nausea. The Ojibwa boiled blackberry roots to prevent miscarriages and sumac fruit and roots to stop bleeding. Traditionally, maple sugar lozenges were used for sore throats. Bitter purges and emetics are administered because they are distasteful and repugnant to any evil spirits that might cause illness.[69]

Food restrictions are still common during illness. Depending on the nation, many Native Americans believe that cabbage, eggs, fish, meat, milk, onions, or organ meats should be eliminated from a patient's diet. Conversely, some foods may be considered important to maintain strength during sickness, such as meat among the Seminole in Florida, and both meat and blue cornmeal among the Navajo.[70] The Navajo may avoid sweets during pregnancy to prevent having a weak infant.[27] Some foods are prohibited after childbirth, such as cod, halibut, huckleberries, and spring salmon for Nootka women of the Northwest Coast.

Native Americans found many plants had psychotherapeutic properties. They were used to relax and sedate patients, to stupefy enemies, and to induce hypnotic trances during religious ceremonies. The opiates in the roots of California poppies dulled the pain of a toothache, for example. Lobelia was smoked as an antispasmodic for asthma and bronchitis. In the Southwest, knobs from the peyote cactus were used to produce hallucinations, sometimes in combination with other intoxicants. Historically, jimsonweed (*Datura stramonium*) was used to keep boys in a semiconscious state for twenty days so that they could forget their childhood during Algonquin puberty rites.[101] It is still used today by some Native Americans for medicinal and ritual purposes.

Current Medicinal Controversies One of the fastest growing "farm-to-table" crops that Native American farmers are cultivating is hemp and THC-rich cannabis. Native Americans, much like Native Asians, Native Europeans, and Native Africans, used marijuana medicinally for centuries. Hemp and CBD food and beverage manufacturers are working to set up supply-chain partnerships with nations to provide economic impact opportunities in this industry. However, this remains a controversial topic for many tribes based on ethical and moral perspectives. Furthermore, Native American nations receive federal funding that could be in jeopardy as long as cannabis remains federally illegal.[71]

Contemporary Food Habits

The food culture of Native Americans was traditionally passed from older members of a nation to younger members to preserve important knowledge on how to prepare wild game and fish, how to find wild plants, which ones were edible and their names, what plants were medicinal, and how to store key ingredients. Contemporary cuisine weaves this traditional knowledge into new Native American cuisine to help restore and disseminate information and use of precolonial food.[3] Most important Native American food crops included corn, beans, squash, pumpkins, sunflowers, wild rice, sweet potatoes, tomatoes, peppers, peanuts, avocados, papayas, potatoes, and cacao. In 2019, six Native chefs were recognized by the James Beard Foundation as champions of these and other Indigenous foods. The chefs, Sean Sherman (Oglala Lakota), Neftali Duran (Oaxaqueno), Brit Reed (Choctaw), Hillel Echo-Hawk (Pawnee and Athabaskan), Kristina Stanley (Red Cliff Lake Superior Chippewa), and Rich Francis (Tetlit Gwich'in and Tuscarora Nations), work to show how food justice and food sovereignty protect Native food cultures and the health of Native Americans.[72]

Studies have shown that nontraditional processed foods and fast foods contribute to diabetes and other health concerns in Native populations. Cereal grains are usually consumed in a highly refined form in the modern diet, contrasting to traditional Native diets that included grains in whole form, including the fiber, germ, and endosperm.[73] Native lands often are food deserts where little fresh, healthy food is available to buy. To combat this, The National Heart, Lung, and Blood Institute issued a cookbook, *Honoring Traditions with the Heart in Mind—Heart Healthy American Indian Recipes,* to help alleviate health problems through food. More Native cookbooks continually emerge as the foods of a younger North America begin to get their due.

Adaptation of Food Habits

Food habits reflect changes in Native American ethnic identity. Many Native Americans eat a diet that includes few traditional foods. Others are consciously attempting to revive the foods and dishes of their ancestors.[74–76]

Ingredients, Common Foods, and Food Sovereignty When Native Americans were uprooted from their lands and their known food supplies, many immediately became dependent on the foods provided to the reservations. One study evaluating the diets of Havasupai Native Americans living on a reservation in Arizona found that 58 percent of the subjects ate only foods purchased or acquired on the reservation during the 24-hour dietary intake recall period. Food insecurity affects at least 60 reservations in the United States.[77,78] Many reservations are commonly referred to as "food deserts" areas that have little access to fresh fruits and vegetables and other healthful whole foods. Instead, they have access to convenience stores and fast-food restaurants as compared to supermarkets and grocery stores. The combination of food deserts and high poverty rates make many Native American populations at risk for food insecurity.[33,75] Commodity foods currently include items such as canned and chopped meats, poultry, fruit juices, peanut butter, eggs, evaporated and powdered milk, dried beans, instant potatoes, peas, and string beans.[103] Researchers report that many of these foods, such as kidney beans, noodles, and peanut butter, are discarded by the Navajo; powdered milk may also be rejected because it is disliked or is considered a weak food suitable only for infants or older people.[33] On some reservations, large supermarkets provide a selection of foods similar to that found throughout the United States; however, on more remote reservations and in many rural areas access to markets is very limited.[79–81] A new study called THRIVE (Tribal Health and Resilience in Vulnerable Environments) is targeting convenience stores in Chickasaw and Choctaw Nations in Oklahoma to incentivize owners to stock more fruits and vegetables and other healthier foods. The idea is to make these healthy foods easy to access at lower prices. They are also focusing on more culturally appropriate signage written in native languages as well as English. Preliminary study results suggest that the sales of fruits and vegetables are on the rise in these communities.[81,82] Other sources of food include gardening (reportedly practiced by between 43 and 91 percent of rural Native Americans), fishing, hunting, gathering indigenous plants, and raising livestock.

Over the years, traditional foods were lost and substitutions were made. For example, beef is a commonly accepted substitute for game among many Native American ethnic groups. Fry bread is another example. It is a flatbread made from wheat flour typically fried in lard and has been prepared in the Southwest for about one hundred years, and in other regions for even less time. Though made from ingredients introduced by the Europeans, it is one of the items most often identified as "traditional" Native food throughout the nation,[83] and it is often served at Native American festivals.

It has been suggested that the substitution of Western foods, especially commodity items, in the preparation of traditional Indian dishes has adversely affected the nutritional value of these foods.[81,83]

Traditional foods make up less than 25 percent of the daily diet among the Hopi. Older Hopi women lament the fact that younger Hopi are no longer learning how to cook these dishes.[84] In a study of Cherokee women, the degree of Native American heritage of the woman in charge of the food supply in the home directly affected the consumption of traditional foods in that home. Corn and corn products, such as hominy, were among the most popular traditional foods; game meat, hickory nuts, raspberries, and winter squash were the least commonly served. Among Cherokee teenagers, traditional items such as the relatively new wheat-based fry bread, bean bread (cornbread with pinto beans), and chestnut bread (made from chestnuts and cornmeal) were well accepted. Although more than 80 percent of the adolescents were familiar with typical Cherokee dishes, including native greens and game meat (bear, deer, groundhog, rabbit, raccoon, squirrel, and wild boar), these foods were rarely eaten.[85] Pima consume traditional items, such as tepary beans and cactus stew, mostly at community get-togethers.[83] A small sample of children from four different Native American communities recorded that only 7 out of 1,308 items listed in food recalls for the study were traditional.[85–87] California Miwok list mostly southwestern items such as beans, rice, and tortillas as those they most associate with Native American foods and recall numerous items eaten by their grandparents but not consumed now, such as squirrel, rabbit, deer, acorn mush, and certain insects. Access to wild game is limited due to hunting restrictions. Navajo women eat traditional foods infrequently, except fry bread, mutton, and tortillas. Blue cornmeal mush (with ash), hominy, and sumac berry pudding are a few of the native dishes consumed occasionally. Dakota women of all ages take pride in traditional foods but often prepare them only when it is convenient or for special occasions.[32]

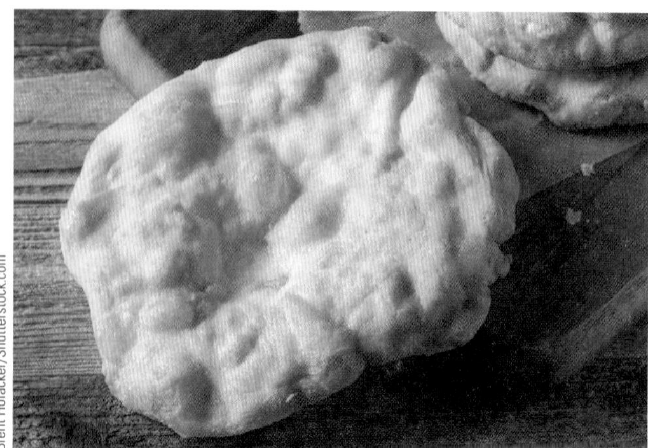

Brent Hofacker/Shutterstock.com

▲ **Indian fry bread has become recognized across the U.S. as "traditional" Native food, even though it is made from wheat flour, a grain introduced by Europeans.**

Broader efforts to preserve traditional and adapted Native American food traditions are also underway. Notably, the group Renewing America's Food Traditions (RAFT), a coalition of organizations dedicated to bringing the foods of the past into the present, has listed over 700 endangered food items, as referenced in Table 5.3. Support of communities attempting to recover and conserve food traditions is their primary goal.[78]

Efforts for Native American food sovereignty are also gaining attention. Food sovereignty aims to counter the rise in heart disease and type 2 diabetes among Native people by linking food policy to local control of the food supply, with the additional goal of restoring and revitalizing community culture through traditional foods. Food sovereignty puts those who produce, distribute, and consume wholesome, local food at the heart of tribal cultural and economic transformation.[88]

Meal Composition and Cycle Little has been reported regarding current Native American meal patterns. It is assumed that three meals per day have become the norm, especially in families without income constraints. Meals consumed by Native Americans vary considerably among regions. In the text *Cultural Food Practices*, the diet for Northern Plains Indians is described as one centered around meats and starches with a limited variety of fruits and vegetables. Access to commodity food supplements also influences food choices.[32] The Navajo still use traditional cooking methods but have also adapted to using more fat and salt in food preparation.[29] Navajo women were found to eat fry bread or tortillas, potatoes, eggs, sugar, and coffee more frequently. Fried foods were preferred for breakfast, and lunch and dinner consisted of one boiled meal and one fried or roasted meal. The Pima in Arizona prefer eggs, bacon or sausage, and fried potatoes for breakfast, while Southwest specialties, such as tacos, tamales, and chili con carne, are common at other meals. A study comparing Indians in New England living on reservations to those living in urban areas found baking and boiling remain favored preparation methods by respondents living on reservations, whereas urban residents were more likely to fry items. Grilled meats and smoked fish were also common ways of cooking.[32,83]

Special Occasions Numerous traditional celebrations are maintained by Native American tribal groups.[22] Among the largest is the five-day Navajo Nation Fair held each Labor Day weekend; the Pawnee Veteran's Day Dance and Gathering where ground meat with pecans and corn with yellow squash are served; the Miccosukee Arts Festival and the Seminole Fair in Miami, where alligator meat is featured; the Iroquois Midwinter Festival held in January to mark the new year; the Upper Mattaponi Spring Festival in Virginia over Memorial Day weekend; the three-day Creek Nation Festival and Rodeo; the Yukon International Storytelling Festival at which wild game such as caribou and musk ox are available; and the Apache Sunrise Ceremony which features gathered

Table 5.3 America's Top Ten Endangered Foods

Chapalote Corn	Considered the original cultivated corn with small ears, coffee-colored kernels, and a flinty flavor
Chiltepin Pepper	Pea-sized, very hot wild chile pepper native to the Southwest considered the ancestor of most varieties used today—drought, diminishing habitat, and unscrupulous harvesting threatens this chile with extinction
Eulachon Smelt	Pacific Northwest source of oil that has suffered serious declines in population—further, traditional methods of processing are gradually being lost
Gulf Coast Sheep	Introduced to the Southeast by the Spanish in the 1500s, this breed adapted well to the humid conditions of the region, providing excellent meat and wool—newer breeds are lessening their popularity
Java Chicken	One of the first chicken breeds introduced to the United States, these birds now number only about one hundred
Marshall Strawberry	An heirloom fruit discovered in Massachusetts in 1890 but grown commercially in the Pacific Northwest—very intense flavor
Native American Sunflowers	Indigenous plants cultivated by the Native Americans for seeds and oil—brought to Europe as an oil source—popularity of the oil led to growing a single "improved" variety, and this one type is now susceptible to numerous rust diseases—few sources of the original seeds remain
Pineywoods Cattle	A foraging breed introduced by the Spanish to Florida, particularly suited to conditions in the South, and popular with early Native American ranchers—approximately 200 animals are left
Seminole Pumpkin	A pear-shaped pumpkin grown on vines that use trees for support—found in the Everglades but rarely cultivated today
White Abalone	The deepest inhabitant of West Coast Abalone, it has neared extinction due to the popularity of its sweet meat—now being bred in a recovery program designed to save it

Source: Nabhan, G.P., & Rood, A. 2004. *Renewing America's Food Traditions (RAFT): Bringing cultural and culinary mainstays of the past into the new millennium.* Flagstaff: Center for Sustainable Agriculture at Northern Arizona University.

foods such as amaranth leaves and the pulp and fruit from the saguaro and prickly pear cacti. More local festivities are also common. Pueblo Feast Days are observed in honor of the Catholic patron saint of each village with a soup of posole (hominy) and beef or pork ribs. Northwest Coast potlatches are common in the spring, featuring herring roe, fish or venison stews, eulachon, salmon, and other traditional foods. In addition, there are all-Indian festivals that draw attendees from throughout the country, such as O'Odham Tash Indian Days in Casa Grande, Arizona; the Red Earth Festival in Oklahoma City; and the Gallup Intertribal Indian Ceremonial in New Mexico. Native Americans may also eat traditional foods on special occasions such as birthdays, but for holidays of the majority culture, other foods are considered appropriate. For example, turkey with all the trimmings is served by many Dakota for Thanksgiving and Christmas.[32]

Nutritional Status

Nutritional Intake Research on the nutritional status of Native Americans is limited. Severe malnutrition was documented in the 1950s and 1960s, including numerous cases of kwashiorkor and marasmus, both malnutrition ailments. In general, however, recent changes in morbidity and mortality figures suggest that Native Americans have transitioned from the conditions associated with underconsumption, such as infectious diseases, to conditions associated with overconsumption, including obesity, type 2 diabetes, and cardiovascular disease.[89–91] One current study outlines a strong demand for increased access to and consumption of Native foods which include plant-based foods such as whole grains, legumes, fruits, and vegetables, and their associated health benefits. Native communities involved in this study were actively engaged in eco-cultural restoration activities to enhance their cultural foodways. They suggest that to understand contributions and solutions to food insecurity in Native American communities, studies must also look at Native foods security. More studies are needed to compare nutritional intakes for those consuming indigenous diets and the effect on chronic diseases, including obesity and diabetes.

Studies of current Alaska Native eating habits suggest that diets high in refined carbohydrates (starchy and sugary foods) and fat, and low in fruits and vegetables, are common. The proteins and nutrients of the Alaska Native diet has declined during the past several decades, as many foods obtained through hunting and gathering were replaced by processed, canned, and packaged items. The estimated carbohydrate content of the Alaska Native diet before contact with Westerners was exceptionally low (3 to 5 percent of daily calories) due to a dependence on sea mammals and fish. Within only a few generations, that figure had increased to 50 percent of total calories, much of it from low-nutrient-density foods.[92,96] Research on Alaska Natives has also shown low intakes of calcium, iron, phosphorus, magnesium, zinc, vitamins A, C, D, and E, riboflavin, and folic acid, as well as fiber, omega-6, and omega-3 fatty acids. Traditional Alaska Native diets have been found lower in fat and carbohydrates, and higher in protein, phosphorus, potassium, iron, zinc, copper, magnesium, manganese, selenium, and several vitamins, including A, D, E, riboflavin, and B_6.[96]

A similar transition occurred in the diets of Native Americans in other parts of the nation; and today, refined carbohydrates are prominent in the diet. Studies have identified white breads, tortillas, potato chips, French fries, sweetened drinks, and candy as the top contributors to energy for many Native Americans. High-fat foods, including fried foods and processed meats and beef dishes, are another significant source of energy.[98–101]

A low intake of fruits and vegetables is prevalent in the diets of both Native American adults and adolescents.[97] The vegetable most often consumed in a study of Native American women in Oklahoma was potatoes in the form of French fries; only tomatoes, tossed salad, green beans, potato salad, and mashed potatoes were also mentioned in the list of the top 53 items most often eaten. Barriers to increased consumption of fruit and vegetables included cost, availability, and quality.[102–104]

Other researchers who investigated rural Native American and White children in Oklahoma suggest that their diets are more influenced by factors such as poverty and living in a rural area than by cultural or structural issues related to race or ethnicity. Nutrient deficiencies in Native American adults and children may occur, most studies suggest, with a dietary adequacy similar to that of the total U.S. population, with the exception of Alaska Natives.[77,78]

As noted from the diagram outlined in Figure 5.3, the traditional plant-based food systems providing ample daily supplies of vegetables and fruits of Native Americans have been disrupted. Many traditional plant-based foods provide a rich source of nutrients and bioactive compounds that benefit health. Strategies to provide a framework for ecological and culturally relevant strategies to restore the traditional plant diversity to Native American diets have been the focus of current studies which can ultimately influence poverty and chronic disease.[78]

Life expectancy has improved over recent years, yet disparities are still found. The average life expectancy is approximately 5.5 years less when compared to the overall U.S. population. According the Indian Health Service (HIS), "American Indians and Alaska Natives continue to die at higher rates than other Americans from a variety of ailments, including chronic liver disease and cirrhosis, diabetes mellitus, unintentional injuries, assault/homicide, intentional self-harm/suicide, and chronic lower respiratory diseases."[106]

The state of maternal and child health among Native American nations is cause for concern. Culturally, pregnancy is considered a natural and healthy state of being by Native American and Alaska Native women, which sometimes leads to little first-trimester prenatal care. Native people are also more likely to lack health insurance and face difficulty accessing care, especially in rural settings. In the overall population, about 700 women die each year in the United States as a result of pregnancy or its complications.[105] Pregnancy outcomes improve for those that receive prenatal care. To protect the lives of Indigenous women and children, researchers recognize that documentation is essential to identify contributing factors. However, data on maternal mortality among Indigenous women are not consistently reported. For instance, data on Indigenous women were not separately described in Centers for Disease Control published 2018 statistics on maternal mortality, which included statistics on racial disparities. In addition, there are limited community-based Indigenous voices in policy discussions on maternal health, and resources and access to local and culturally centered services and supports are limited.[105,107,108] The chronically underfunded Indian Health Service (IHS) often cannot provide obstetric care, and consequentially many Indigenous women give birth outside of IHS facilities or culturally centered health care systems. Adding to this, the pregnancy and childbirth care workforce (physicians, midwives, nurses, social workers, mental health counselors, addiction counselors, lactation consultants, doulas, etc.) does not reflect the demographic characteristics of pregnant patients, and Indigenous people are particularly underrepresented. Finally, recent data from Louisiana showed that mothers were more likely to die of homicide than any specific obstetric cause. Intimate partner violence disproportionately affects rural and Indigenous women, yet many programs designed to address maternal mortality center on clinical risk mitigation.[109]

Sudden Infant Death Syndrome (SIDS), the unexplained death of an infant under one year of age, strikes Native American infants three times more frequently than White infants. Since most SIDS deaths are sleep-related, there are current government campaigns to encourage the placement of infants on their backs to avoid suffocation from sleeping on their stomachs.[111]

Breastfeeding has traditionally been considered the proper way to feed infants among most Native Americans. However, while breastfeeding rates for the U.S. population as a whole have increased from 79.3% to 83.2% from 2011 to 2015, rates for the Native American population have decreased from 77.1% to 66.4% at hospital discharge.[112]

Rates of initial breastfeeding in Native American mothers are higher than average. The Special Supplemental Nutrition Program for Women, Infant, and Children (WIC) has been promoting breastfeeding for over 40 years and operates in 89 WIC state agencies, which include 50 state health departments, 33 Indian Tribal Organizations, the District of Columbia, and 5 territories (Northern Mariana, American Samoa, Guam, Puerto Rico, and the Virgin Islands). The WIC program has been instrumental in promoting baby-friendly tribal hospitals, clinics, and work environments to support an increase in breastfeeding initiation, exclusivity, and duration among Native Americans.[110]

People categorized as overweight or obese are more prevalent among Native Americans than the overall population. National data suggest obesity rates of 48 percent among Native American adults in 2018 compared to 42 percent

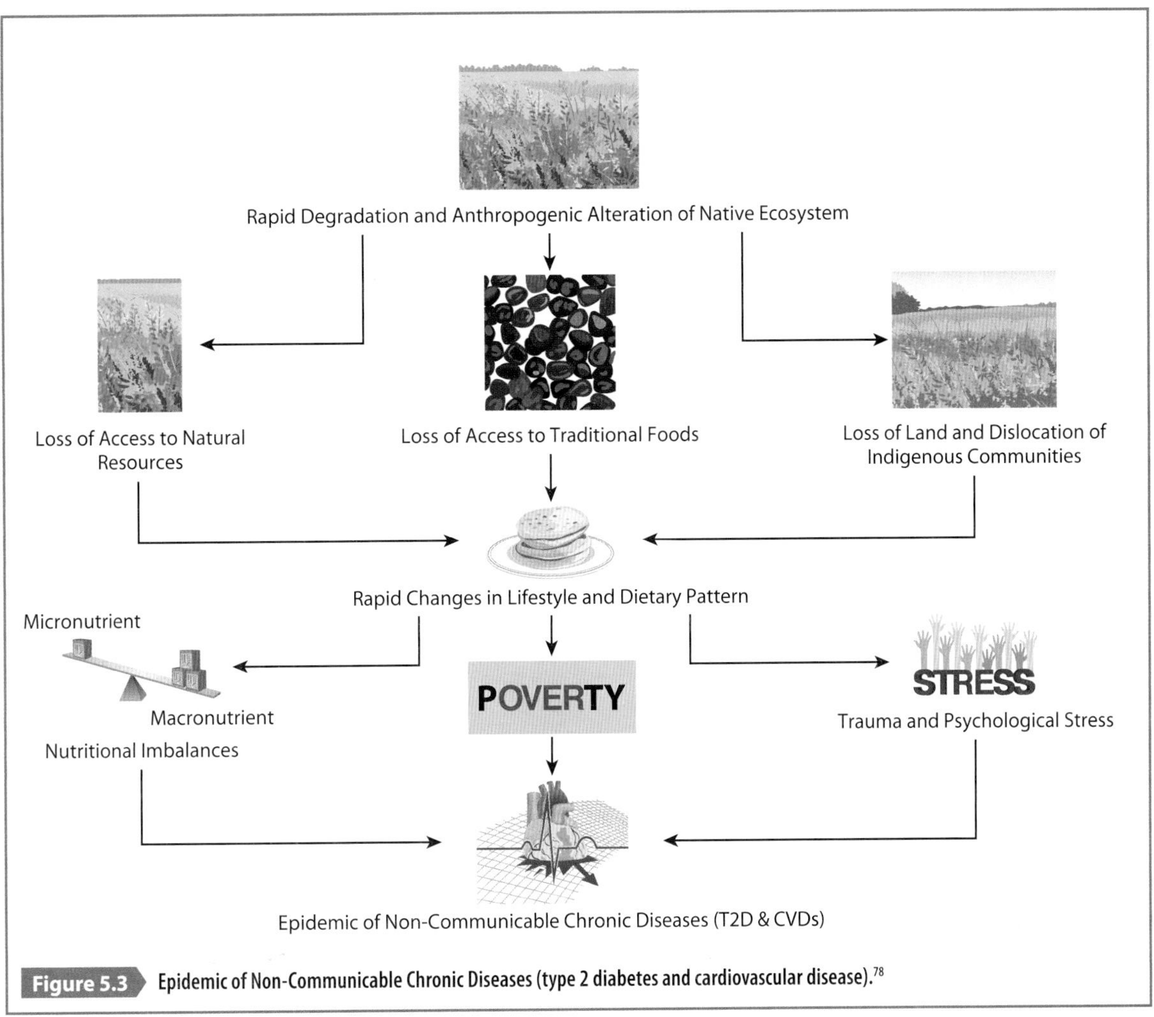

Figure 5.3 Epidemic of Non-Communicable Chronic Diseases (type 2 diabetes and cardiovascular disease).[78]

for the overall population in the U.S. Native American or Alaska Native adults are 50 percent more likely to be obese than non-Hispanic Whites. Native American/Alaska Native adolescents are 30 percent more likely than non-Hispanic White adolescents to be obese which is a serious risk factor for other lifelong diseases and quality of life. Those individuals who are overweight are more likely to suffer from high blood pressure, high levels of blood fats, diabetes, and LDL cholesterol—all risk factors for heart disease and stroke. In another survey, the highest obesity rates were found in Native Americans living in Alaska, and the lowest in the Pacific Northwest.[112]

Native American and Alaska Natives are more likely than the non-Hispanic White population to be overweight and obese. Obesity, as defined earlier in Chapter 3, is having a BMI of 30 or greater. In 2018, Native American adolescents were 30 percent more likely and adults were 50 percent more likely than non-Hispanic White people to be obese.[112]

Figures on obesity contradict some nutritional intake data, which show the caloric intake of many Native Americans to be normal or less than the recommended dietary allowances. Metabolic differences in obese Native Americans may be a factor, or lower rates of energy expenditure through exercise may contribute: Native American and Alaska Natives report a lack of leisure-time physical activity at higher rates than any other U.S. ethnic group.[121] However, a study of Hualapai women of Arizona indicated that the daily caloric intake of women who are obese was significantly higher than for women who are not obese. Sweetened beverages and alcoholic beverages accounted for the differences. Researchers investigating Zuni adolescents suggest that underreporting of foods and/or alcohol may account for low reported energy intakes.[99] Dieting behaviors among adult Native American women mostly involve healthy approaches such as eating more fruits and vegetables and exercising more, according to one study, although skipping meals, fasting, and disordered eating such as self-induced vomiting was also mentioned; 10 percent engaged in binge eating.[100]

As previously discussed in Chapter 3, what is now known as type 1 diabetes results from a complete lack of insulin in the body and is not correlated to lifestyle. Type 2 diabetes is more common; it is associated with normal or reduced levels of insulin and the inability to use insulin efficiently, and it is closely correlated with obesity and limited physical activity. Both types of diabetes result in high levels of blood glucose that over time can cause lifelong disability and death. The incidence of type 2 diabetes, especially among some Native Americans of the plains and southwest, is estimated to be between two and four times that of the general population. More than 23.5 percent of Native Americans and Alaska Natives are estimated to have diabetes, which is the highest rate of any ethnic group in the United States. The U.S. average was 9.1 percent in 2018. Pima Native Americans are believed to have the highest rate of type 2 diabetes in the world, affecting 70 percent of all adults over the age of 45. Rates of the disease among children are also increasing substantially, and it has been noted that acanthosis nigricans (a patchy darkening of the skin) is an independent marker for insulin resistance in Native American youngsters. The death rate from type 2 diabetes is more than three times as high for Native Americans as for the total population. Notably, diabetes was rare among Native Americans 50 years ago.[114–117]

One theory, which sparked controversy and later debunked, speculated that high rates of type 2 diabetes among Native Americans are due to genetic predisposition. The thrifty gene theory proposed that, in the past, populations who have struggled with periods of limited resources and therefore have experienced periods of famine, were more likely to survive if they were metabolically thrifty and stored calories efficiently. Their survival gave a genetic advantage to this characteristic. Based on this hypothesis, however, what had been historically an advantage became detrimental as time elapsed. Through modernization, food has become abundant and continually available. The genetic capacity to store calories efficiently in our current environment becomes a risk factor for type 2 diabetes and obesity. This theory continues to be studied with mixed results. However, a comparison of type 2 diabetes among Pima Native Americans living in Arizona and those living in Mexico found rates in Arizona to be more than five times those found in Mexico, suggesting that genetic predisposition alone does not account for high prevalence in the United States and that a Westernized environment may be a factor.[118,119] Research has shown a significantly lower plasma insulin level in Pima people living in Mexico when compared to the U.S. Pima population even before diabetes is diagnosed. The researchers state: "This finding underscores the importance of lifestyle factors as protecting factors against insulin resistance in individuals with a high propensity to develop diabetes." Higher rates of diabetes are found among Alaska Natives who have significantly increased intake of nonindigenous protein (e.g., beef, chicken), carbohydrates (e.g., white bread, potatoes or rice, soft drinks), and fat (e.g., butter, shortening), combined with a lower intake of native foods such as salmon, caribou, berries, and seal oil; and higher rates are found among Pima people who consume an Anglo diet when compared to Pima who consume a traditional diet. Some researchers suggest the difference is due to the dietary change from indigenous starches to the refined flours and sugars of the adapted diet.[120,121] Traditional starches take longer to digest and absorb, leading to lower blood sugar levels and insulin responses that may be protective in the development of diabetes. Other researchers suggest type 2 diabetes is more complex than initially thought and attributes to the high rates of the complexity of the social determinants of health, one of which is environment (see Cultural Controversy). Rural versus urban living may influence access to healthful food, and diet and may contribute more than once thought (refer to Figure 5.4).[117] Between 2012-2018, the percentage of Native

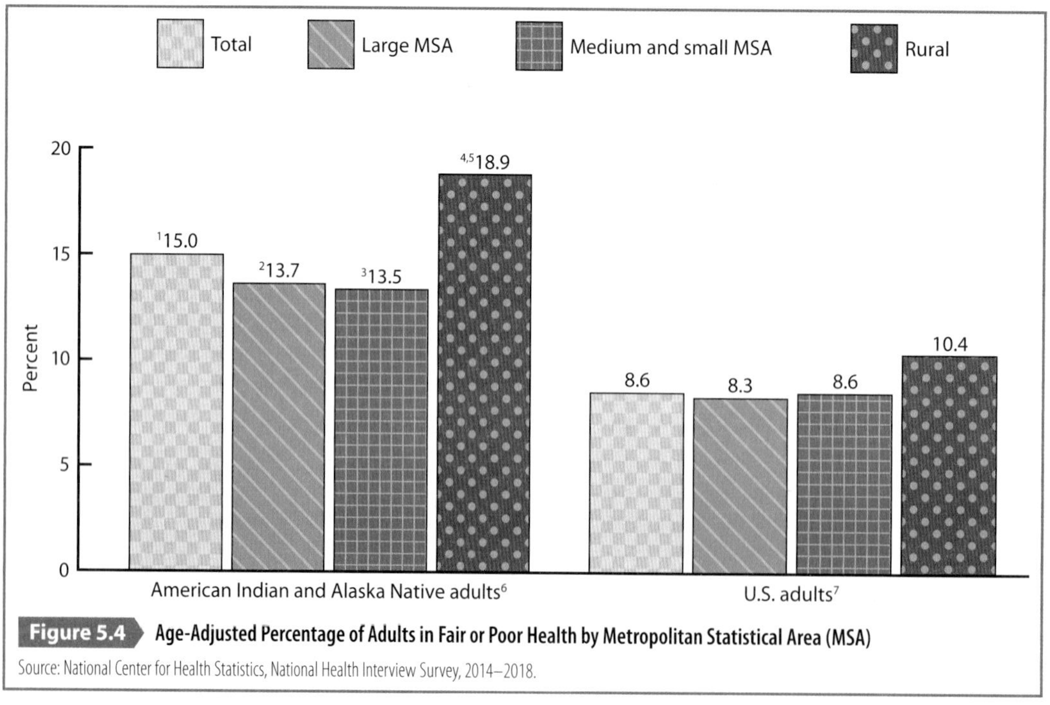

Figure 5.4 Age-Adjusted Percentage of Adults in Fair or Poor Health by Metropolitan Statistical Area (MSA)

Source: National Center for Health Statistics, National Health Interview Survey, 2014–2018.

Americans diagnosed with diabetes was almost twice (15%) as high as all U.S. adults (8.6%) and was highest among those living in rural areas, as seen in Figure 5.4.[117,118]

Associated with obesity and type 2 diabetes is a dramatic increase in the prevalence of heart disease among Native Americans during the last 25 years; heart disease is now the leading cause of death. Rates of cardiovascular disease for Native Americans have surpassed those of the total population in many locations, and are often more fatal. Additional risk factors include high rates of cigarette smoking, alcohol consumption, elevated blood lipid levels, obesity, and hypertension.[114,115]

Chronic kidney disease is also a concern, particularly associated with type 2 diabetes, with incidence up to 20 times higher than in the general population. Native Americans and Alaska Natives die at higher rates than other Americans from tuberculosis, with estimates being up to 600 percent higher.[122,123]

The incidence of alcoholism among Native Americans has decreased in recent years, but it remains a significant medical and social problem. High unemployment rates and loss of tribal integrity, ethnic identity, and self-esteem are frequently cited as reasons for substance abuse among both reservation and urban Native Americans. The rate for alcohol-related deaths is more than eight times that of the general U.S. population.[6]

Health and Longevity Takeaway

Spirituality can have great impacts on health, happiness, stress relief, and longevity. Native American spiritual ceremonies that greet the seasons and the harvests have been used to promote health by living in harmony with the earth. In a recent study, religion, spirituality, and/or belief were found to play a positive role in the everyday lives of older adults. Spirituality can provide strength, comfort and hope in difficult times and provide older adults with a sense of community and belonging. Traditional spiritual ceremonies that promote living in harmony with the earth are being abandoned by younger generations, with a resultant increase in poor health status. Spirituality is seen to be a key factor in the circle of well-being.

Cultural Controversy

Type 2 Diabetes and Social Disparities of Health

Why do some Native Americans develop type 2 diabetes at rates many times above that of the White U.S. population? Current research suggests that the development of type 2 diabetes is much more complex than previously thought, including factors in three domains: political-economic (such as ongoing stress, unavailability of healthy foods, and barriers to health care); ecological (both genetic—thrifty gene theory of adaptation to a history of feast and famine—and non-genetic); and cultural (including traditional health beliefs, values regarding body image, norms about exercise, etc.[124]

What is now known as type 1 diabetes results from a complete lack of insulin in the body and is not correlated to lifestyle. Type 2 diabetes is more common; it is associated with normal or reduced levels of insulin and the inability to use insulin efficiently, and it is closely correlated with obesity and limited physical activity. Both types of diabetes result in high levels of blood glucose that over time can cause lifelong disability and death. Diagnosis of type 2 diabetes has increased by more than 65 percent in the general U.S. adult population over the past ten years. Long considered a disease of middle age, type 2 diabetes was rarely diagnosed in urban pediatric clinics as recently as the early 1990s, but type 2 diabetes is now increasing rapidly as a proportion of all newly diagnosed cases of diabetes in children.[125] Among Native Americans, prevalence rates vary from between 4 and 70 percent of adults over the age of forty-five, depending on the group, with the lowest rates seen in Alaska and the highest found in the Southwest.[126]

Many believe that targeting the social determinants of health and health disparities may be key to reversing these trends. Social determinants of health are the conditions in the environment that affect qualitative life such as:

- Safe housing, transportation, and neighborhoods
- Racism, discrimination, and violence
- Education, job opportunities, and income
- Access to nutritious foods and physical activity opportunities
- Polluted air and water
- Language and literacy skills

For example, many Native Americans live in rural areas without access to grocery stores with healthy foods or without access to health care services. That raises their risk of health conditions like heart disease, diabetes, and obesity—and even lowers life expectancy relative to people who do have access to healthy foods.

Just promoting healthy choices won't eliminate these and other health disparities. Instead, public health organizations and their partners need interventions to address political-economic, ecological, and cultural norms to improve the conditions in people's environments.

A Note to Researchers and Public Health Practitioners

Indigenous people have been studied at great length. To counter deficit-based research that can reinforce stereotypes, the National Aboriginal Health Organization introduced principles of ownership, control, access, and possession (OCAP®) to reduce historical trauma to individuals, families, and communities from research and reporting of findings. A further step in promoting culturally safe and responsible research with Indigenous peoples is to incorporate the Inuit Qaujimajatuqangit, traditional laws and principles that guide a way of life and of knowing.

Based on these two guides, researchers and scholars should be working with Indigenous peoples to co-develop research rather than merely researching Indigenous populations. By working collaboratively with researchers, Indigenous people can provide input to ensure that a project respects Indigenous culture, language, and knowledge and does not re-ignite or exacerbate historical trauma or further current colonial policies that marginalize and oppress Indigenous peoples.

Practitioner Perspectives

Native American

Lorraine Whitehair, RD, MPH, RN, CDE • Worked at Indian Health Services for over ten years, Tribal RD for several years, and currently works for CDC

I was born in Oljato, Utah, a rural Navajo reservation located 150 miles northeast of Farmington, New Mexico. After graduating from high school, I worked as a nurses' aide in a small, 15-bed hospital near my home in Utah. Later, I completed a Bachelor's degree in nutrition science at the University of Utah and a dietetic internship, and a Master's degree in public health at the University of California, Berkeley. As a registered dietitian, I have worked with the Navajo Nation for approximately 12 years.

Briefly, how would you describe the Navajo foods?

Traditionally, during the 50s, 60s, and early 70s, gardening and sheepherding were our livelihood. We hauled all our water and used wood-burning stoves for cooking. My parents told us of Navajo native foods when they were young, some of which I have never seen. My mother told me she spent many days grinding corn for the winter. One stew made by parents was *ad Alth ta' nash besh*, meaning boiled with several mixtures. It had melon seeds, local wild green plants, and a variety of plant seeds, and wild onions, and was thickened with corn meal. When I was young we grew watermelon, cantaloupe, fresh corn, and summer and winter squash. Other favorites included boiled mutton backbone in green chili stew, grilled mutton ribs, liver, and greater omentum (the fatty tissue that covers the stomach) in an open-face sandwich with onions or green chili in a tortilla. We may not have had as much mutton as we wanted, but we had plenty of fruits and vegetables during the summer months.

Traditional food eaten today includes corn prepared many different ways from fresh to dried or ground into meal in varying degrees of texture. One recipe for fresh corn is called "Kneel down Bread" because it is prepared in a sitting position. A one-fourth cup of the ground corn is placed in corn leaves, wrapped and tied together. It is then placed in a large hole that is dug in the ground and is cooked by building a fire on top. All parts of the sheep and goat are used for food. This includes the head, intestine, organs, skin, hoofs, and blood. Blood sausage and liver sausage are very popular. The stuffed intestine is made by wrapping the greater omentum with the intestine. It is then grilled on hot coals until crispy.

Most older people like simple, unmixed foods. Older people dislike marinated meats. They prefer the meats cooked plain. I would say Navajo native food is fairly bland, although men like to eat with very hot chili and raw, fresh onions.

How much has Western food culture influenced the current diet?

In the past three to four decades our diet has changed significantly. Our level of physical activity also decreased at the same time. Popular foods now include spam, canned meat, cold cuts, ramen noodles, chips, candy, sodas, and flavored fruit drinks.

Are there any foods that would be difficult or easy to modify in the diet?

Yes. Fried bread would be hard to modify. People enjoy the texture of bread cooked in hot oil, which makes the recipe difficult to alter. Intestine wrapped in greater omentum (intestinal fat) is the one that could be easy to modify. Replace the intestinal fat with thick sliced vegetables like onions, carrots, cabbage, green peppers, and celery. Ramen noodles, a non-traditional food, are easier to modify as well—I suggest to my clients that they add a variety of vegetables (frozen and fresh) and muscles from beef, chicken, or pork and decrease the serving size, since the noodles contain fat. People seem to like it with fresh ginger as well.

What advice would you give to new Registered Dietitian Nutritionists (RDNs) or other health care professionals working with Native Americans?

Learn about the history of the people. Learn about the way of life then and now. The Navajo people value family and community. There is a saying which states, "Know who you are and where you came from." That is to know your clan system. Introductions are a very important part of interaction with people on the Navajo reservation. As time consuming as it may be, establishing good introductions helps establish trust, kinship, and credibility. Making a good introduction about your family clan (family background) is a cultural practice, and it is believed to help make business meetings successful. For older clients you may address them as your mother (*Shi ma'*) or your father (*Shi yes ah'*) even though they are not related to you.

For the middle-aged and older adult population, living in harmony with the surroundings is important. Parents and grandparents spend a great deal of time talking about being respectful of kinship, older people, and nature, including land and living creatures. We are to look toward living in harmony with our surroundings. Illness is often thought of as a result of an interruption of harmony.

We enjoy laughing. There is great pleasure in tastefully teasing when appropriate. We have many jokes about life on the reservation, our first boarding school experiences, interaction with people in towns, schools, and medical clinics, and meeting with public health officials. We have many animal stories that are funny, and they also teach. For example, I use this story to help teach my clients about diabetes:

Two Birds

Two birds, Jay and Woody, lived near the Interstate 40 highway, 50 miles west of Albuquerque, New Mexico. Jay loves to pick up foods that are left by humans who were traveling back on Interstate 40 highway from Albuquerque, New Mexico. The most common foods that were left along the highway were French fries, hamburgers, shakes, pies, cookies, ice cream, fried chicken, biscuits, potato chips, fried bread, and candy bars. Jay always invited Woody to help him eat the leftover foods that were thrown near the highway. He would tell Woody about the "delicious" food he had for the day. He would say, "You do not have to hunt for your food. It is there along the road." Woody told Jay the food he was eating was not good for him. Woody faithfully hunted for his food supply. He worked to store his food daily so that he would have enough for an emergency during the winter months. Daily, Woody flew long distances to get his food. Meanwhile, Jay had been steadily gaining weight. He also had difficulty flying moderate distances. In the Fall,

(Continued)

Practitioner Perspectives (Continued)

Native American

both birds wanted to visit distant relatives near Albuquerque. Jay was not able to complete the trip to Albuquerque. He experienced shortness of breath and exhaustion halfway to Albuquerque. Jay and Woody decided that Woody should go alone to see their distant relatives. In early Spring, Jay became very ill after the flu he had developed following a large snowstorm. He had frequency of urination, tiredness, sores on his toes not healing, and blurred vision. His doctor told him he had diabetes. Jay took the news very hard. He did not want to change his diet. Woody begged Jay to eat more healthfully. In the end, Jay's diet changed back to eating whole grains, nuts, and seeds to help control his blood sugars. He also had to retrain his wings to fly longer distances daily, which helped bring his good cholesterol (HDL) in excellent ranges. His doctor was very happy to see Jay living more healthfully.

Comfort Food—Choctaw, Native American

D.M.'s Story

Native American comfort foods are as varied as the communities and regions of American in which they originate. But for D.M., one dish is a colorful, healthy reminder that we can be nurtured by what the earth provides in its season.

What is a favorite comfort food that you consider traditional from your home culture?

DM: Many recipes I create use ingredients such as quinoa, squash, lima beans, cranberries, blue corn and more that my Choctaw ancestors might have also enjoyed. I feel it is important in my culture that humans stay in equilibrium with the rest of the world. One step in that direction is to eat seasonally and locally. In the fall I choose pumpkins that Indigenous people from south America to Canada have cultivated for centuries.

Did you eat this food together with community? Where was it eaten?

DM: Pumpkin is typically eaten at dinner time and is eaten in the fall because that is when squash is ready to eat. I most often eat this when a colorful, inviting table is my goal. My recipe uses pre-contact ingredients, but many post-contact spices, meats and cheeses can be added.

Here is DM's family recipe:

Stuffed Squash

Serves 2

- 2 (1)-pound pumpkins or other large winter squash
- 2 yellow squash, chopped
- 2 zucchini, chopped
- 2 cups yellow, orange, and red bell peppers, chopped
- 1 cup mushrooms, sliced
- 2 large tomatoes, chopped
- ½ cup onion, chopped
- Salt, pepper, or other spices to taste
- 1 cup wild rice
- 4 Tbsp. dried cranberries
- Green chilies, jalapenos, ground turkey or venison (optional)

Preheat oven to 350°F. Chose pumpkins or other large winter squashes that weigh approximately 1 lb. Cut the tops off the pumpkins or squash so that you have "lids" that can be replaced when you are ready to serve the finished dish. Scoop out the seeds and the stringy portions. Use a paper towel and lightly coat the insides with vegetable oil. Place the pumpkins on a cookie sheet, scooped-out side down, and cook until the outer skin is slightly tender, about 40-45 minutes. While the pumpkins are in the oven, cook the wild rice and set aside. Remove pumpkins from the oven and set aside. Heat the 2 Tbsp oil in a skillet over medium heat. Add the vegetables to the skillet and sprinkle them with a favored condiment such as pepper, salt, or onion powder, then cook over medium heat. Turn the vegetables after two minutes. Reduce the heat to low, cover and simmer the mixture until the vegetables are tender. Mix in the wild rice and cranberries. Place the mixture into the pumpkin shells and bake at 350°F for 1 hour.

Nutritional Information (per serving):

calories 490; protein 22 g; carbohydrates 105 g; dietary fiber 20 g; sugars 24 g; fat 3 g; saturated fat 0.7 g; cholesterol 0 mg; sodium 65 mg

An Additional Comfort Food RECIPE TO TRY

Three Sisters Soup

Serves 4

Recipe adapted from www.food.com/recipe/three-sisters-soup-410371[63]

- 1 cup dried pinto beans, soaked overnight in 4 cups water
- 1 acorn squash
- 1-2 Tbsp. olive oil
- 2 medium yellow onions, diced
- 2 carrots, sliced
- 5 garlic cloves, minced
- 2 celery stalks, sliced
- 4 cups vegetable stock
- 1 cup corn
- 1 tsp. dried thyme
- Salt and pepper

(Continued)

Comfort Food—Choctaw, Native American (*Continued*)

D.M.'s Story

Drain and rinse the soaked beans. Put them in a large pot and cover with water by an inch. Bring the beans and water to a boil and simmer for about 45 minutes or until the beans are tender but not mushy, adding more water if necessary. While the beans are cooking, cut the squash in half, scoop out the seeds, and bake the halves cut side up in a 375°F oven for about 45 minutes or until tender. Next, add the oil to a large sauce pan with deep sides and heat over medium heat. Add onions and a pinch of salt and sauté, stirring often, for about 10 minutes or until golden brown. Add the carrots, garlic, and celery, and continue to sauté for 5-10 minutes. Scoop cooked squash out of its shell and add it to onion mixture. Mix well, smoothing out any large lumps. Add the vegetable stock and bring to a boil. Turn down the heat and add beans, corn, and thyme. Simmer, covered for 5 minutes, stirring occasionally. Add salt and pepper to taste. Serve hot with bread.

Nutritional information (per serving):
calories 300; carbohydrate 54.8 g; protein 13.2 g; fat: 4.8 g; sodium 29.8 mg

Discussion Starters

Who Are You and what Do You Eat?

After reading about the different regional, traditional Native American diets, decide which one you think would be the healthiest. Why? Then decide which one you think would taste the best to you. Why? Once you've considered the traditional diets, reflect on the differences between the traditional diet you see as the healthiest and the contemporary diet of many Native Americans. Consider the following questions:

- What needs to be done to improve the diets of many Native Americans today?
- What are the major cultural obstacles in improving contemporary Native American diets?

Imagine that you are a member of a research institution that has been asked to recommend dietary policy for a contemporary Native American community. In a small group, compose a list of your major recommendations for such a policy that the majority of your group can agree to. Also provide advice to health care professionals serving that community about how to implement those dietary changes.

Review Questions

1. In Native American culture, what is considered the cause of illness? How may this influence the treatment of a medical disorder such as type 2 diabetes?
2. Pick two regional classifications of traditional Native American cuisine. Describe the similarities and differences between these two classifications in food and their preparation.
3. Describe three therapeutic uses of corn and one therapeutic use of a non-corn item by Native Americans.
4. What is fry bread? Is it a traditional food? Why or why not?
5. What factors may have increased the incidence of type 2 diabetes among Native Americans?

Reflection

1. After reading this chapter, reflect upon what you have learned about this culture. How would you define or change your own communications style to be more sensitive or aware of the preferred conversation norms? Where do storytelling, listening, and using humor play a role in building relations through communication? How will you be more mindful of the values and beliefs of Native American friends, family, and patients?
2. Why is there a difference in type 2 diabetes rates in urban vs. rural areas? What are the contributing factors to this phenomenon?

References

1. Public Information Office. 2021. *Facts for features: American Indian and Alaska Native Heritage Month, November 2021.* Washington, DC: U.S. Census Bureau (accessed November 28, 2022).
2. Treuer, A. 2012. *Everything you wanted to know about Indians but were afraid to ask.* St. Paul, MN: Minnesota Historical Society Press.
3. Frank, L.E. November 11, 2021. History on a plate: How Native American diets shifted after European colonization. Retrieved from https://www.history.com/news/native-american-food-shifts.
4. Mejia, Melissa. n.d. The U.S. history of Native American boarding schools. The Indigenous Foundation. Retrieved from https://www.theindigenousfoundation.org/articles/us-residential-schools
5. Reyhner, Jon. 2018. American Indian boarding schools: what went wrong? What is going right? *Journal of American Indian Education*, 57(1), University of Minnesota Press, 58–78. Retrieved from https://doi.org/10.5749/jamerindieduc.57.1.0058.
6. American Indian/Alaska Native. OMH US Department of Health and Human Services Office of Minority Health. Retrieved from https://www.minorityhealth.hhs.gov/omh/browse.aspx?lvl=3&lvlid=62#:~:text=Economics%3A%20The%20median%20household%20income%20for%20American%20Indian,occupations%2C%20in%20comparison%20to%2044.8%20percent%20of%20whites.(accessed November 26, 2022).
7. Public Information Office. 2021. Facts for features: *American Indian and Alaska Native Heritage Month, November 2021.* Washington, DC: U.S. Census Bureau. Received from https://www2

.census.gov/programs-surveys/sis/resources/aian-ff.pdfandhttps://www.census.gov/newsroom/facts-for-features/2021/aian-month.html (accessed November 28, 2022).

8. Park, S., Hongu, N., & Daily III, J.W. 2016. Native American foods: History, culture, and influence on modern diets. *Journal of Ethnic Foods*, 3(3), 171–177. Retrieved from https://doi.org/10.1016/j.jef.2016.08.001.
9. Historical Newspaper Archives. Library of Congress. Retrieved from https://www.loc.gov/newspapers/?all=true&dates=1800-1899&fa=subject:cherokee+indians (accessed March 21, 2022)
10. Letts, B. 2021. The Cherokee tribal court: Its origins and its place in the American judicial system. *Campbell Law Review*, 43, 47.
11. Starr, Stephen. January 18, 2021. Go inside the close-knit world of Native American Rodeo. *National Geographic*.
12. Birchfield, D.L. 2014. Navajos. In R.V. Dassanowsky & J. Lehman (Eds.), *Gale encyclopedia of multicultural America* (3rd ed.). Farmington Hills, MI: Gale Group.
13. Birchfield, D.L. 2014. Pueblos. In R.V. Dassanowsky & J. Lehman (Eds.), *Gale encyclopedia of multicultural America* (3rd ed.). Farmington Hills, MI: Gale Group.
14. French, E., & Hanes, R.C. 2014. Hopis. In R.V. Dassanowsky & J. Lehman (Eds.), *Gale encyclopedia of multicultural America* (3rd ed.). Farmington Hills, MI: Gale Group.
15. Jones, J.S. 2014. Inuit. In R.V. Dassanowsky & J. Lehman (Eds.), *Gale encyclopedia of multicultural America* (3rd ed.) Farmington Hills, MI: Gale Group.
16. Benson, D.E. 2014. Tlingit. In R.V. Dassanowsky & J. Lehman (Eds.), *Gale encyclopedia of multicultural America* (3rd ed.). Farmington Hills, MI: Gale Group.
17. Kawagley, O. 2014. Yupiat. In R.V. Dassanowsky, & J. Lehman (Eds.), *Gale encyclopedia of multicultural America* (3rd ed.). Farmington Hills, MI: Gale Group.
18. Wien, T., & Gousse, S. Native American. *Britannica*. Retrieved from https://www.britannica.com/topic/Native-American/Reorganization.
19. Whittle, Joe. 2017. Most Native Americans live in cities, not reservations. Here are their stories. *The Guardian*. Retrieved from https://www.theguardian.com/us-news/2017/sep/04/native-americans-stories-california
20. Csaki, S. 2015. Coming around again: Cyclical and circular aspects of Native American thought. Native American Institute, Southeastern Oklahoma State University, Native American Symposium 2015. Retrieved from https://www.se.edu/native-american/2015-native-american-symposium/
21. Hanes, R.C., & Hillstrom, L.C. 2013. Paiutes. In R.V. Dassanowsky & J. Lehman (Eds.), *Gale encyclopedia of multicultural America* (3rd ed.). Farmington Hills, MI: Gale Group.
22. Warren, L.S. 2017. *God's red son: The Ghost Dance religion and the making of modern America*. Hachette UK: Basic Books.
23. Treuer, D. 2019. *The Heartbeat of Wounded Knee: Native America from 1890 to the Present*. New York: Riverhead Books.
24. U.S. Army massacres Sioux Indians at Wounded Knee. January 5, 2022. History.com. Retrieved from https://www.history.com/this-day-in-history/u-s-army-massacres-indians-at-wounded-knee (accessed March 15, 2022).
25. Birchfield, D.L. 2014. Choctaw. In R.V. Dassanowsky & J. Lehman (Eds.), *Gale encyclopedia of multicultural America* (3rd ed.). Farmington Hills, MI: Gale Group.
26. Thomason, T. 2011. Recommendations for counseling Native Americans: Results of a Survey. *Journal of Indigenous Research*, 1(2).
27. Purnell, L.D., Fenkl, E.A., & Paulanka, B.J. 2021. *Textbook for Transcultural health care: A culturally competent approach* (5th ed.). Philadelphia: FA Davis.
28. Connolly, M., & Jacobs, B. 2020. Counting Indigenous American Indians and Alaska Natives in the US census. *Statistical Journal of the IAOS, 36*(1), 201–210.
29. Compton-Dzak, Emily. 2014. *Gale Encyclopedia of Multicultural America. 3rd ed.* Booklist, *111*(3), 10. *Gale Academic OneFile*: link.gale.com/apps/doc/A387347775/AONE?u=anon~9e36c49a&sid=googleScholar&xid=033b3258.(accessedNovember 27, 2022).
30. Matthew, D. 2011. *Seneca Possessed, Indians, Witchcraft, And Power In The Early American republic*. Philadelphia: University of Pennsylvania Press.
31. Goody, C.M., & Drago, L. 2010. *Cultural Food Practices-Diabetes care and education*. Chicago: American Dietetics Association/American Diabetes Association.
32. Brown, T.L., Zephier, E., & Johnson, M.L. 2010. American Indian food practices. In C.M. Goody & L. Drago (Eds.), *Cultural food practices*. Chicago: American Dietetic Association/American Diabetes Association.
33. Kim, K. K., Ngo, V., Gilkison, G., Hillman, L., & Sowerwine, J. 2020. Karuk Youth Leaders. Native American Youth Citizen Scientists Uncovering Community Health and Food Security Priorities. *Health Promotion Practice* 21(1), 80–90.
34. Lewis, Courtney. 2018. Frybread wars: biopolitics and the consequences of selective United States healthcare practices for American Indians. *Food, Culture & Society*, 21(4), 427–448.
35. Calabrese, J.D. 2013 *A different medicine; Postcolonial healing in the Native American Church*. New York: Oxford University Press.
36. Cohen, C. 2018. Bear Hawk. *Honoring the medicine: The essential guide to Native American healing*. New York: Ballantine Books.
37. Heisey, A.W., & Hanes, R.C. 2014. Oneidas. In R.V. Dassanowsky & J. Lehman (Eds.), *Gale encyclopedia of multicultural America*. (3rd ed.). Farmington Hills, MI: Gale Group.
38. Hillstrom, L.C., & Hanes, R.C. 2014. Nez Perce. In R.V. Dassanowsky & J. Lehman (Eds.), *Gale encyclopedia of multicultural America*. (3rd ed.). Farmington Hills, MI: Gale Group.
39. Roy, L. 2014. Ojibwa. In R.V. Dassanowsky & J. Lehman (Eds.), *Gale encyclopedia of multicultural America*. (3rd ed.). Farmington Hills, MI: Gale Group.
40. Deloria, Philip. November 18, 2019. The invention of Thanksgiving. *The New Yorker*.
41. Silverman, David J. 2019. *This land is their land: The Wampanoag Indians, Plymouth Colony, and the troubled history of thanksgiving*. London: Bloomsbury Publishing.
42. Lunsford, L., Arthur, M.L., & Porter, C.M. 2021. African and Native American foodways and resilience: From 1619 to COVID-19. *Journal of Agriculture, Food Systems, and Community Development* 10(4), 241–265.
43. NPR. March 13, 2022. COMIC: One Sioux chef's attempt to reclaim Native American cuisine. Retrieved from https://www.npr.org/2022/05/13/1097955036/comic-one-sioux-chefs-attempt-to-reclaim-native-american-cuisine.
44. Kocher, Taylor. March 3, 2022. Native Chef Pyet DeSpain wants to take indigenous cooking to the next level. *Eater*. Retrieved from https://la.eater.com/2022/3/3/22960250/pyet-despain-next-level-chef-winner-indigenous-native-shkode-pop-up-news.
45. Institute for American Indian Studies.1974. The culture of Corn. *Agricultural History*, 48(1). In Farming in the Midwest, 1840-1900: A Symposium, pp. 94–97.
46. Noble, M. 2018. Bison bars were supposed to restore native communities and grass-based ranches, then came epic provisions. *The Counter*. Retrieved from www.nativeamericanmuseum.com.
47. Rutledge, S. 1847. *The Carolina Housewife, 1782-1855*. Oxford Text Archive. Retrieved from http://hdl.handle.net/20.500.12024/3182 (accessed February 20 2022).
48. https://www.recipezazz.com/recipe/blue-grape-dumplings-native-american-19729
49. https://www.food.com/recipe/buffalo-stew-tanka-me-a-lo-164399
50. Sherman, S. 2017. *The Sioux Chef's Indigenous Kitchen*.
51. https://sweetgrasstradingco.com/recipes/maple-sage-roasted-vegetables/

52. https://recipes.sparkpeople.com/recipe-detail.asp?recipe=1785671
53. Newton, Seth. Pemmican: Recipes, Stories and Stores. Retrieved from https://www.outmoreusa.com/authentic-native-american-pemmican-recipe-and-history/
54. Gunderson, M. 2003. *The food journal of Lewis & Clark: Recipes for an expedition*. Yankton, SD: History Cooks Publishing.
55. Rose, V. J. 2012. Lichens. Washington State University.
56. Editors. 2019. Muskox. National Park Service. Retrieved from nps.gov/bela/learn/nature/muskox.htm (accessed March 15, 2022).
57. Colby, S.E., McDonald, L.R., & Adkison, G. 2012. Traditional Native American foods: stories from northern plains elders. *Journal of Ecological Anthropology*, 15(1), 65–73.
58. Sherman, S. 2019. A dish inspired by a feast for 1,000. *The New York Times*, A2-L.
59. Coastal and Plateau Native Americans. April 27, 2017. Retrieved from https://phdessay.com/coastal-and-plateau-native-americans/(accessed March 22, 2022).
60. Dubin, M.D., and Ross, S. 2008. *Seaweed, salmon, and manzanita cider: A California Indian Feast.*
61. Keegan, M. 1996. *Southwest Indian cookbook*. Santa Fe, NM: Clear Light Publishers.
62. Traditional Native American Recipes. *The Cooking Post*. Retrieved from http://cookingpost.com/recipes.htm.
63. Native American Recipe: Wild Rice with Sweet Potato. Retrieved from https://unpeeledjournal.com/recipe-native-american-wild-rice-saute/.
64. Steamed Fiddlehead Ferns. Retrieved from https://cookingself.com/steamed-fiddlehead-ferns.html.
65. Whipped Raspberry Soup. Retrieved from https://recipegoldmine.com/soupfruit/whipped-raspberry-soup.html
66. Woolf, N., Conti, K.M., Johnson, C., Martinez, V., McCloud, J., & Zephier, E.M. 1999. *Northern Plains Indian food practices, customs, and holidays*. Chicago: American Dietetic Association/American Diabetes Association.
67. Elk Stew with Acorn Dumplings. *Astray Recipes*. Retrieved from https://www.astray.com/recipes/?show=Elk+stew+with+acorn+dumplings
68. Kavasch, E.B., & Baar, K. 1999. *American Indian healing arts*. New York: Bantam.
69. Gonzales, P. 2017. *Traditional Indian medicine: American Indian Wellness*. Dubuque, IA: Kendall Hunt.
70. Moghaddam, J.F., Momper, S.L. & W. Fong, T. 2015 Crystalizing the role of traditional healing in an urban Native American health center. *Community Mental Health Journal*, 51, 305–314.
71. Editors. February 25, 2019. What does the future hold for the CBD industry in Indian Country? *Native American News*. Retrieved from https://www.nativeknot.com/news/Native-American-News/What-Does-the-Future-Hold-for-the-CBD-Industry-in-Indian-Country.html.
72. Concepcion, Mery. 2019. These six chefs are championing Indigenous food. Retrieved from https://www.jamesbeard.org/blog/these-six-chefs-are-championing-indigenous-food (accessed March 21, 2022).
73. Milburn, Michael P. 2004. Indigenous nutrition: Using traditional food knowledge to solve contemporary health problems. *American Indian Quarterly*, 28(3/4), 411–434. Retrieved from http://www.jstor.org/stable/4138925.
74. Beltran, R., Schultz, K., Fernandez, A.R., Walters, K.L., Duran, B., & Evans-Campbell, T. 2018. From ambivalence to revitalization: Negotiating cardiovascular health behaviors related to environmental and historical trauma in a Northwest American Indian community. *American Indian and Alaska Native Mental Health Research: Journal of the National Center*, 25(2), 103–128.
75. Mihesuah, D.A. 2020. *Recovering our ancestors' gardens: Indigenous recipes and guide to diet and fitness*. Lincoln, NE: University of Nebraska Press.
76. Emboden, W.A. 1976. Plant hypnotics among North American Indians. In W.D. Hand (Ed.), *American folk medicine*. Los Angeles: University of California Press.
77. Smith, E., Ahmed, S., Dupuis, V., Running Crane, M., Eggers, M., Pierre, M., Flagg, K., & Byker Shanks, C. 2019. Contribution of wild foods to diet, food security, and cultural values amidst climate change. *Journal of Agriculture, Food Systems, and Community Development*, 9(B), 191–214. Retrieved from https://doi.org/10.5304/jafscd.2019.09B.011
78. Sarkar, D., Walker-Swaney, J., & Shetty, K. 2019. Food diversity and indigenous food systems to combat diet-linked chronic diseases. *Current Developments in Nutrition*, 4, p 3–11.
79. Walch, A., Loring, P., Johnson, R., Tholl, M., & Bersamin, A. 2019 Traditional food practices, attitudes, and beliefs in urban Alaska Native women receiving WIC assistance. *Journal of Nutrition Education and Behavior*, 51(3), 318–325.
80. Keith, J., Stastny, S., Brunt, A., & Agnew, W. 2018. Barriers and strategies for healthy food choices among American Indian tribal college students: A qualitative analysis. *Journal of the Academy of Nutrition and Dietetics*, 118(6).
81. NIH National Heart, Lung and Blood Institute. November 21, 2016. Native American foods, dietary habits take center stage. Retrieved from https://www.nhlbi.nih.gov/news/2016/native-american-foods-dietary-habits-take-center-stage.
82. Love, C.V., Taniguchi, T.E., Williams, M.B., Noonan, C. J., Wetherill, M.S., Salvatore, A.L., Jacob, T. Cannady, T. K., Standridge, J., Spiegel, J., & Jernigan, V.B. 2019. Diabetes and obesity associated with poor food environments in American Indian Communities: The tribal health and resilience in vulnerable environments (THRIVE) study. *Current Developments in Nutrition*, 3(2), 63–68.
83. Williams, D.E., Knowler, W.C., Smith, C.J., Hanson, R.L., Roumain, J., Saremi, A., Kriska, A.M., Bennett, P.H., & Nelson, R.G. 2001. The effect of Indian or Anglo dietary preference on the incidence of diabetes in Pima Indians. *Diabetes Care*, 24, 811–816.
84. Kuhnlein, H.V., Calloway, D.H., & Harland, B.F. 1979. Composition of traditional Hopi foods. *Journal of the American Dietetic Association*, 75, 37–41.
85. Story, M., Bass, M.A., & Wakefield, L.M. 1986. Food preferences of Cherokee teenagers in Cherokee, North Carolina. *Ecology of Food and Nutrition*, 19, 51–59.
86. Story, M., Snyder, P., Anliker, J., Cunningham-Sabo, L., Weber, J.L., Kim, R., Stone, E.J. 2002. Nutrient content of school meals in elementary schools on American Indian reservations. *Journal of the American Dietetic Association*, 102, 253–256.
87. Dennison, M.E., Sisson, S.B., Lora, K., Stephens, L.D., Copeland, K.C., & Caudillo, C. 2015. Assessment of body mass index, sugar sweetened beverage intake spent in physical activity of American Indian children in Oklahoma. *Journal of Community Health*, 40, 808–814.
88. Delormier, T., & Marquis, K. 2019. Building healthy community relationships through food security and food sovereignty. *Current Developments in Nutrition*, 3(Supplement_2), 25–31.
89. Lyttle, L.A., Dixon, L.B., Cunningham-Sabo, L., Evans, M., Gittelsohn, J., Hurley, J., Snyder, P., Stevens, J., Weber, J., Anliker, J. Heller, K., & Story, M. 2002. Dietary intakes of Native American children: Findings from the Pathways Feasibility Study. *Journal of the American Dietetic Association*, 102, 555–558.
90. Bersamin, A., Luick, B.R., Ruppert, E., Stern, J.S., & Zidenberg-Cherr, S. 2006. Diet quality among Yup'ik Eskimos living in rural communities is low: The Center for Alaska Native Health Research Pilot Study. *Journal of the American Dietetic Association*, 106, 1055–1063.
91. Compher, C. 2006. The nutrition transition in American Indians. *Journal of Transcultural Nursing*, 17, 217–223.
92. Risica, P.M., Nobmann, E.D., Caulfield, L.E., Schraer, C., & Ebbesson, S.O. 2005. Springtime macronutrient intake of Alaska Natives

of the Bering Straits region: The Alaska Siberia Project. *International Journal of Circumpolar Health*, 64, 222–233.
93. Kuhnlein, H.V., Receveur, O., Soueida, R., & Egeland, G.M. 2004. Arctic indigenous peoples experience the nutrition transition with changing dietary patterns and obesity. *Journal of Nutrition*, 134, 1447–1453.
94. Nakano, T., Fediuk, K., Kassi, N., & Kuhnlein, H.V. 2005. Dietary nutrients and anthropometry of Dene/Metis and Yukon children. *International Journal of Circumpolar Health*, 64, 147–156.
95. Montgomery, M., Johnson, P., & Ewell, P. 2022. A comparative analysis of rural versus urban preschool children's sugar-sweetened beverage consumption, body mass index and parent's weight status. *SAGE Open Nursing*, 8, 23779608221082962.
96. Nobmann, E.D., & Lanier, A.P. 2001. Dietary intake among Alaska Native women resident of Anchorage, Alaska. *International Journal of Circumpolar Health*, 60, 123–137
97. McLaughlin, 2010. Traditions and diabetes prevention: A healthy path for Native Americans. *Diabetes Spectrum*, 23(4), 272–277.
98. Stroehla, B.C., Malcoe, L.H., & Velie, E.M. 2005. Dietary sources of nutrients among rural Native American and white children. *Journal of the American Dietetic Association*, 105, 1908–1916.
99. Cole, S.M., Teufel-Shone, N.I., Ritenbaugh, C.K., Yzenbaard, R.A., & Cockerham, D.L. 2001. Dietary intake and food patterns of Zuni adolescents. *Journal of the American Dietetic Association*, 101, 802–806.
100. Teufel, N.I., & Dufour, D.L. 1990. Patterns of food use and nutrient intake of obese and non-obese Hualapai Indian women in Arizona. *Journal of the American Dietetic Association*, 90, 1229–1235.
101. Taylor, C.A., Keim, K.S., & Gilmore, A.C. 2005. Impact of core and secondary foods on nutritional composition of diets in Native-American women. *Journal of the American Dietetics Association*, 105, 413–419.
102. Bird Jernigan, V.B., Salvatore, A.L., Williams, M., Wetherill, M., Taniguchi, T., Jacob, T., . . . & Noonan, C. 2019. A healthy retail intervention in Native American convenience stores: the THRIVE community-based participatory research study. *American Journal of Public Health*, 109(1), 132–139.
103. Redmond, L. C., Jock, B., Gadhoke, P., Chiu, D. T., Christiansen, K., Pardilla, M., . . . & Gittelsohn, J. 2019. OPREVENT (Obesity Prevention and Evaluation of InterVention Effectiveness in NaTive North Americans): design of a multilevel, multicomponent obesity intervention for native American adults and households. *Current Developments in Nutrition*, 3(Supplement_2), 81–93.
104. Ornelas, I. J., Osterbauer, K., Woo, L., Bishop, S. K., Deschenie, D., Beresford, S. A., & Lombard, K. 2018. Gardening for health: patterns of gardening and fruit and vegetable consumption among the Navajo. *Journal of Community Health*, 43(6), 1053–1060.
105. Chalouhi, S.E., Tarutis, J., Barros, G., Starke, R.M., & Mozurkewich, E.L. 2015. Risk of postpartum hemorrhage among Native American women. *International Journal of Gynaecology and Obstetrics*, 131(3), 269–272.
106. Indian Health Service. *Facts on Indian health disparities*. 2009–2011. Retrieved from https://www.ihs.gov/newsroom/factsheets/disparities/ (accessed March 17, 2022).
107. Kozhimannil, K.B. 2020. Indigenous maternal health—A crisis demanding attention. *JAMA Health Forum*, 1(5), e200517.
108. Peterson, E.E., Davis, N.L., Goodman, D., Cox, S., Mayes, N., Johnston, E., Syverson, C., Seed, K., Shapiro-Mendoza, C.K., Callaghan, W.M., & Barfield, W. 2019. VitalSigns: Pregnancy-related deaths, United States, 2011-2015, and strategies for prevention, 13 states, 2013-2017. *Morbidity and Mortality Weekly Report*, 68(18), 423–429.
109. Arambula Solomon, T.G., Cordova, F.M., & Garcia, F. 2017. What's killing our children? Child and infant mortality among American Indians and Alaska Natives. National Academy of Medicine.
110. Rates of Any and Exclusive Breastfeeding by Sociodemographics and Children Born in 2018. 2018. National Immunization Survey, Centers for Disease Control and Prevention, Department of Health and Human Services. Retrieved from https://www.cdc.gov/breastfeeding/data/nis_data/rates-any-exclusive-bf-socio-dem-2018.html.
111. Hynes, K. 2020. Culturally Competent Interventions to reduce SIDS rates among Native American/Alaska Native Nations.
112. CDC. 2020. Summary Health Statistics: National Health Interview Survey: 2018. Table A-15a. Retrieved from https://www.cdc.gov/nchs/nhis/shs/tables.htm (accessed March 22, 2022).
113. Poudelk A.M Yi Zhou, J., Story, D., & Li, L. 2018. Diabetes and associated cardiovascular complications in American Indians/Alaskan Natives: A review of risks and prevention strategies. *Journal of Diabetes Research, 2018.*
114. Godfrey, T.M., Cordova-Marks, F.M., Jones, D., Melton, F., & Breathett, K. 2022. Metabolic syndrome among American Indian and Alaska Native populations: Implications for cardiovascular health. *Current Hypertension Report*. Retrieved from https://doi.org/10.1007/s11906-022-01178-5
115. https://www.ncbi.nlm.nih.gov/pmc/articles/PMC4418458/
116. Hegele, R.A. 2001. Genes and environment in type 2 diabetes and atherosclerosis in Aboriginal Canadians. *Current Atherosclerosis Reports*, 3, 216–221.
117. Villarroel, M.A., Clarke, T.C., & Norris, T. 2020. Health of American Indian and Alaska Native Adults, by Urbanization level: United States, 2014-2018. NCHS Data Brief No. 372, August 2020. Retrieved from https://www.cdc.gov/nchs/products/databriefs/db372.htm (accessed March 22, 2022).
118. Schulz, L.O., & Chaudhari, L.S. 2015. High-risk populations: The Pimas of Arizona and Mexico. *Current Obesity Report 4*(1), 92–98.
119. Esparza-Romero, J., Valencia, M.E., Martinez, M.E., Ravussin, E., Schulz, L.O., & Bennett, P.H. 2010. Differences in insulin resistance in Mexican and U.S. Pima Indians with normal glucose tolerance. *Journal of Clinical Endocrinology and Metabolism*, 95(11), E358–362. Epub July 28, 2010.
120. NCHS Data Brief No. 372. August 2020. National Health Interview Survey, 2014–2018. Use this only as a reference to diabetes graphic Age adjusted percentage of those with diabetes.
121. Caring for Native Americans. October 2020. *AMA Journal of Ethics*, *22*(10), E831-905. Retrieved from https://journalofethics.ama-assn.org/sites/journalofethics.ama-assn.org/files/2020-11/joe-2010.pdf
122. Divata Kidney Care. Received from https://www.davita.com/education/kidney-disease/risk-factors/native-americans-and-chronic-kidney-disease-ckd
123. Hill-Briggs, F., Adler, N. E., Berkowitz, S. A., Chin, M. H., Gary-Webb, T. L., Navas-Acien, A., . . . & Haire-Joshu, D. 2021. Social determinants of health and diabetes: a scientific review. *Diabetes Care*, 44(1), 258-279.
124. Hughes, G. J. (2022). The Thrifty Gene Hypothesis: A Total Review. Retrieved from https://repository.arizona.edu/handle/10150/665772
125. Lawrence, J.M., Divers, J., Isom, S., Saydah, S., Imperatore, G., Pihoker, C., . . . & Search for Diabetes in Youth Study Group. 2021. Trends in prevalence of type 1 and type 2 diabetes in children and adolescents in the US, 2001–2017. *JAMA*, 326(8), 717–727.
126. Bullock, A., Sheff, K., Hora, I., Burrows, N.R., Benoit, S.R., Saydah, S.H., . . . & Gregg, E.W. 2020. Prevalence of diagnosed diabetes in American Indian and Alaska Native adults, 2006–2017. *BMJ Open Diabetes Research and Care*, 8(1), e001218.

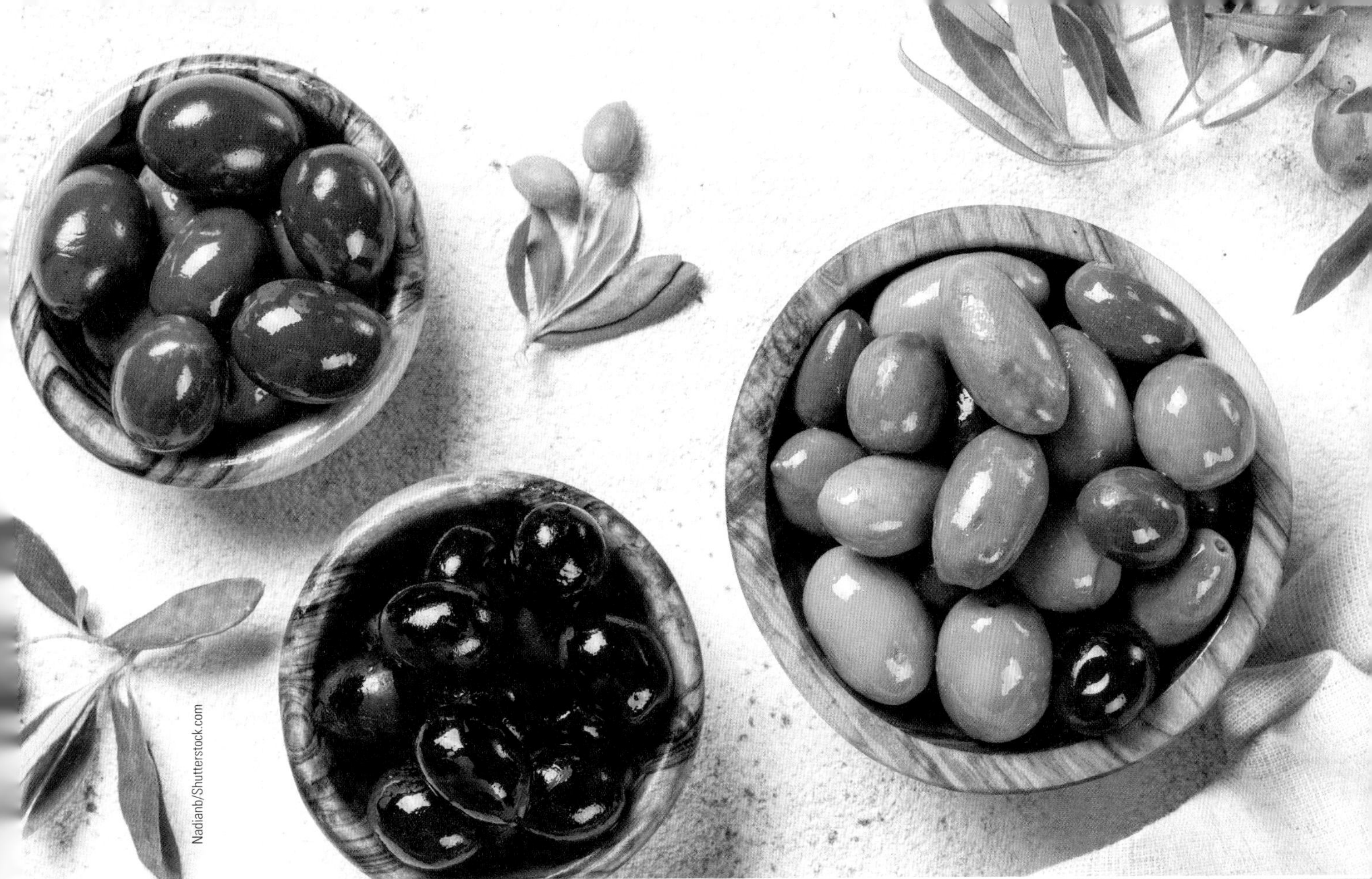

Chapter 6

Northern and Southern Europeans

Learning Objectives

6.1 List the northern and southern European countries.

6.2 State the immigration patterns and historical socioeconomic influences of northern and southern Europeans in America today.

6.3 Differentiate the typical religions, family structures, and traditional health beliefs and practices of northern and southern Europeans before and after immigration to the United States.

6.4 Compare the differences in the staples and regional variations of ingredients from northern and southern Europeans.

6.5 Compare key foods for northern Europeans' food groups to show how these foods have been adapted by U.S. immigrants.

6.6 Identify key foods in each of the food groups of southern Europeans and how they have adapted these foods in the United States.

6.7 Describe regional specialties and dishes these immigrants have contributed to the current American diet.

6.8 Identify health concerns associated with the nutritional intake of northern and southern Europeans.

Some of the largest American subcultures originated in northern and southern Europe, areas noted on the map in Figure 6.1. Immigrants from these regions began appearing in what is now the United States in the sixteenth century and are still arriving, significantly influencing American culture.[1] Many foods and food habits we consider to be American were introduced by these settlers. The northern European idea of a meal, consisting of a large serving of meat, poultry, or fish with smaller side dishes of starch and vegetable, was quickly adopted and expanded in the United States to include even bigger portions of protein foods. Adaptations of some southern European specialties have become commonplace American fare. Each ethnic group from northern and southern Europe has brought a unique cuisine that was combined with indigenous ingredients—blended with the cooking of Native Americans, other Europeans, and Africans, and flavored with the foods of Latinos, Asians, and Middle Easterners—to form the foundational palate of the typical American diet. This chapter discusses the traditional foods and food habits in Great Britain, Ireland, France, Italy, Spain, and Portugal, and examines their contributions to the cooking of the United States.

Northern Europeans

Though Great Britain and the United Kingdom are sometimes used interchangeably, Great Britain comprises England, Scotland, and Wales, whereas the United Kingdom comprises England, Scotland, Wales, as well as Northern Ireland. Although quite northern, the climate is temperate in the United Kingdom (due to the warming influence of the Gulf Stream) and the lowlands are suitable for growing crops. Just across the English Channel is France, regarded for centuries as the center of Western culture politically, as well as in the arts and sciences. Its capital, Paris, is one of the world's most beautiful and famed cities due in part to its leading role during the Age of Enlightenment as a center for Western education and ideas throughout Europe, and more literally because Paris was one of the first European cities to use gas street lighting. The lighting was installed during the reign of Louis XIV on city boulevards, lighting monuments and intricately designed buildings, as well as making the streets safer for citizens. France contains some of the best farmland in Europe, and three-fifths of its land is under cultivation. It is especially well known for premium wine production.

In 1607, people from Great Britain began immigrating to what is now the United States. They brought with them British trade practices and the English language, literature, law, and religion. By the time the United States gained independence from Britain, the British and their descendants constituted one-half of the American population. They produced a culture that remains unmistakably British-flavored, even today, especially in the language people speak, architecture, and legal and political systems. The French came to North America in smaller numbers, at first for the fur trade around 1534, and later for their colonies in Canada, Acadia, the Hudson Bay, Newfoundland, and Louisiana where they made significant contributions. Early leaders such as Thomas Jefferson, a noted Francophile, brought French wines into vogue, as well as dishes he tasted while serving as the American minister to France from 1784 to 1789. James Hemings, enslaved by Jefferson, was trained as a chef during his stay. One dish, pommes de terre frites à cru en petites tranches (potatoes deep-fried while raw, in small cuttings, or known today as "French fries"), was served to Jefferson during a dinner promoting the potato which was new to Europe.[2] The dinner host, Antoine-Augustin Parmentier, was a large proponent of the potato as it is said to have saved him from starvation multiple times while a prisoner of war during the Seven Years' War.[3] However, some stories claim villagers in Belgium are the originators of the French fry, and that American soldiers in World War I brought the idea back with them. Belgium is situated northeast of France and shares many French food habits but may have had little influence on the American diet due to its relatively low number of immigrants to the United States. The traditional foods of northern Europe and their influence on American cuisine are examined in the next section.

Cultural Perspective

History of Northern Europeans in the United States

Immigration Patterns

Great Britain The British who immigrated in the seventeenth century settled primarily in New England, Virginia, and Maryland. Although many originally came to avoid religious persecution, such as the Puritans in New England and the Catholics in Maryland, most later immigrants came for economic gain earning their passage by signing on as indentured servants.[5] Indentured servants were those who traded their labor for a period of time (4–7 years) in exchange for passage to the New World. In the seventeenth century, indentured servants made up the mass of English immigrants and were considered fundamental to the development of the tobacco industry.

By the eighteenth century, British immigration had slowed. After colonial independence, British immigration to the United States further declined due to American hostility and disapproval by the British government. However, reported arrivals of British in the nineteenth century increased substantially. Early in the century, most immigrants were families from rural areas of southern and western England and Wales. In the latter half of the century, the majority of immigrants were from large English towns, and many were seasonal unskilled workers who repeatedly returned to Britain.

It is said there have been Scots in America as long as there have been Europeans on the North American continent. More than 100 towns and cities in the United States bear Scottish names, and it has been estimated that 1.5 million Scots immigrated to America. Although the majority of

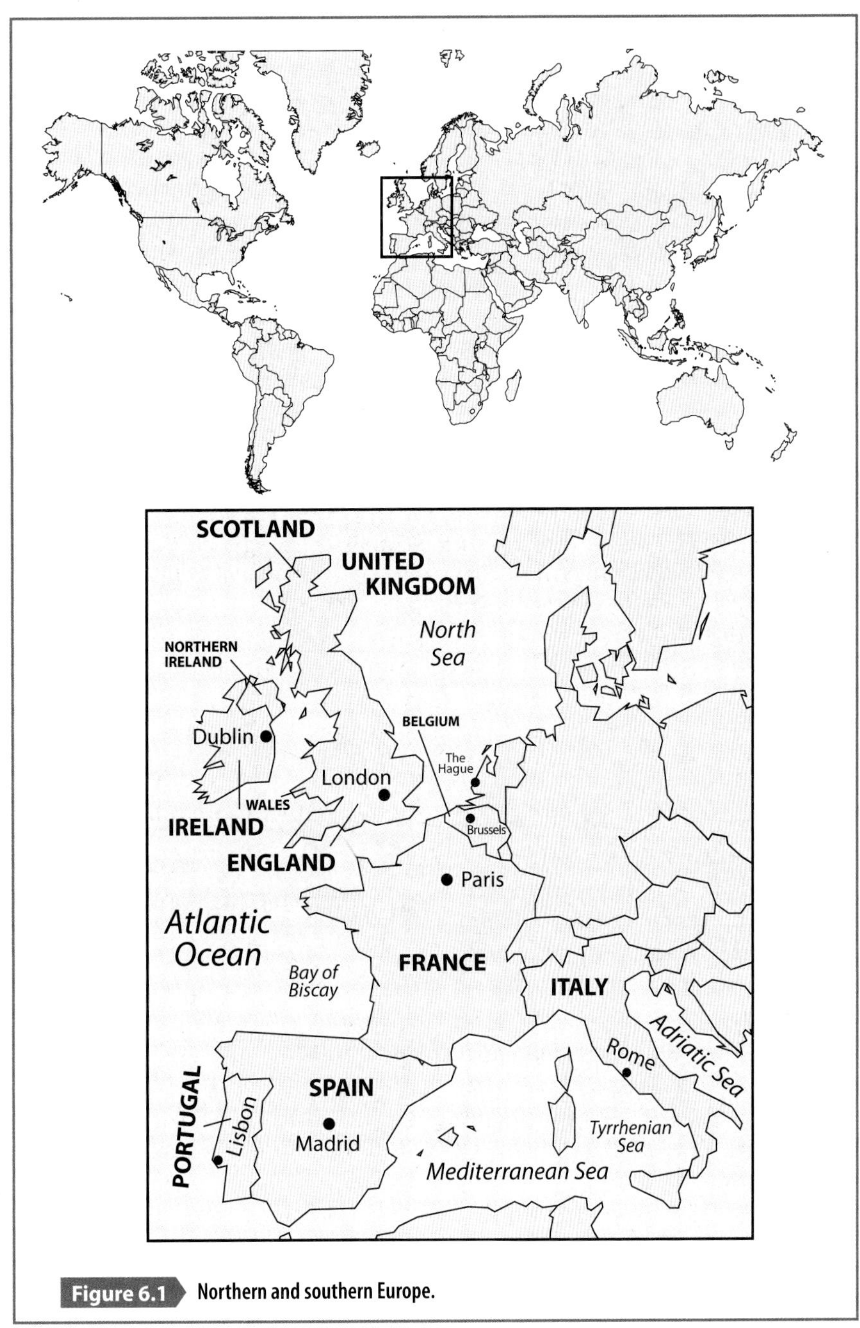

Figure 6.1 Northern and southern Europe.

Scots came during the eighteenth and nineteenth centuries, 400,000 immigrated between 1921 and 1931, when Scotland suffered a severe economic depression. The Scottish settled over most of the United States and were often professionals or skilled laborers.

Although British immigration did not decline in the early twentieth century, the United States was no longer the country of first choice for those leaving Great Britain. During the Great Depression in the 1930s, more British people returned to Britain than came to America. After World War II, increased immigration was attributed to displacement after the war and political tensions. Since the 1970s, British immigration has been constant at about 10,000 to 20,000 persons per year. There are currently more than 2.4 million people of British origin living in the United States (refer to Table 6.1).[4]

Table 6.1 Northern European population in the United States[4]

Country of Origin	U.S. Population as of 2019	Percent
British	2,457,891	<1%
French	7,116,099	<2%
Irish	30,352,567	9%
Total U.S. Population	331,449,281	

Ireland The first Irish people to immigrate in substantial numbers to the United States were the descendants of Scottish Presbyterians who had settled in Northern Ireland in the seventeenth century. Large-scale immigration began in the eighteenth century, and by 1775 there were an estimated 250,000 Scotch Irish living in the American colonies. Most of the immigration was the result of an economic depression brought on by a textile slump in Ireland.

Initially, the Scotch Irish settled in Pennsylvania. Before long, the direction of Scotch-Irish immigration was westward to the frontier, first up the Delaware River and then beyond the Susquehanna into the rich farmlands of the Cumberland Valley. The Scotch Irish played an important role in the settlement of the trans-Allegheny region and eventually clustered around the site of Pittsburgh and in other areas of southwestern Pennsylvania. They also settled in the then-frontier regions of western Maryland, the Shenandoah Valley of Virginia, and the backcountry of Georgia.

Irish Catholics started to arrive in the United States by 1820, and their immigration reached an apex between 1840 and 1860 when approximately 2 million people arrived. The impetus to leave Ireland was not only religious persecution but also repeated crop failures. The potato blight that destroyed the Irish principal crop in 1845 resulted in death by starvation of 1 million Irish people.

The Irish Catholics were one of the first large subcultures in American cities, and their early history set the pattern for later immigrant groups. They settled in the northeastern cities and were at first at the bottom of the socioeconomic ladder. The Scotch Irish, who were often of relatively high economic standing and Protestant, found it fairly easy to move into mainstream American society.

France Immigration directly from France has been the smallest, yet most constant, of that from any European country, but many return. Most of the estimated 1 million persons who have immigrated to the United States from France have been middle-class and skilled and have come for economic opportunity.

Food for Thought

The Scots have been stereotyped as thrifty. "Scotch" tape was so named with the hope it would suggest an economical product.[6]

According to the 2016 Census, English (6.3 million), Scottish (4.8 million), French (4.7 million), and Irish (4.6 million) origins were still among the 20 most common ancestries reported by the Canadian population, either as a single response or in combination with other ancestries (multiple responses).[7]

A smaller number came because of religious persecution. More than 12,000 Huguenots (French Protestants) settled in the American colonies in the eighteenth century. They were considered to be excellent skilled workers. Generally, French people who settled in the United States were eager to assimilate and were aided in doing so because they were economically successful.[8]

Few pockets of French culture remain in the United States, except in southern Louisiana, originally a French holding, northern New England, and in Ste. Genevieve, Missouri, which is now a National Historic Park with the largest collection of French colonial architecture in the United States. However, the Frenchness of these regions is probably due more to the influence of French-Canadian immigration than to direct French immigration. French Canadians are the descendants of explorers and settlers who came from France, primarily Normandy and Brittany, during the seventeenth century. They established New France in what is today known as Canada. When the English gained control of Canada, many French Canadians moved to the United States; in some instances, they were deported from Canada. Most settled in northern New England, especially Maine, and their descendants are known as Franco-Americans. Others from Acadia (Nova Scotia, New Brunswick, Prince Edward Island, and part of Maine) relocated, often not by choice, to central and southern Louisiana; their descendants are known as Cajuns. The Creole people of Louisiana originally were those with French or Spanish parents and born in the colony. Later, Creole came to mean a person of French or other colonial European, African American, and Native ancestry.

Food for Thought

The Welsh honor the patron saint of Wales, St. David, a bishop during the sixth century who founded Christian monasteries and churches and encouraged followers to care for the natural world. To recognize their countrymen in the battle against Saxon invaders, legend has it that St. David asked Welsh soldiers to wear a leek stalk on their helmets. Today, leeks are the national emblem of Wales.

Current Demographics and Socioeconomic Status

British and Irish The British assimilated into American mainstream society easily. Distinct groups from specific regions of Great Britain can still be found, however. For example, Cornish immigrants of the nineteenth century were often

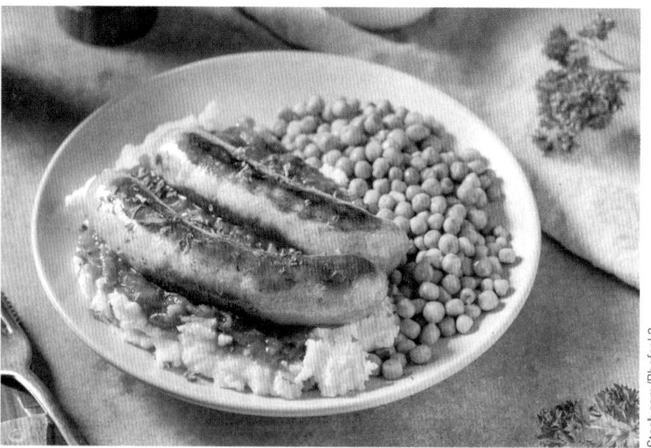

iStock.com/Bhofack2

▲ **Traditional foods of northern Europe. A typical British plate of bangers and mash.**

miners, and their descendants are still living in certain regions known for early mining, such as Grass Valley, California, Butte City, Montana, and areas around Lake Superior. The Welsh who immigrated in the nineteenth century were often miners and mill workers. They settled in the mid-Atlantic and midwestern states, especially Ohio and Pennsylvania; many were Baptist, Calvinist, or Methodist. Remnants of Welsh communities in the United States still celebrate St. David's Day (the feast day of the patron saint of Wales) and the annual festival of the National Gymanfa Ganu Association (an assembly that sings Welsh folk songs).[9] It is estimated that there were nearly 23.59 million Americans of English ancestry in 2019.[10]

Close to 5 million Irish Catholics have immigrated to the United States and as of 2019, there were more than 30 million people of Irish origin living in the United States (Table 6.1). Although they started on a lower economic rung than other immigrant groups that came earlier, they are now scattered throughout the occupational structure.[9]

In the 1950s, the Irish were overrepresented as clergymen, firefighters, and police officers. Today, there are disproportionately more in law, medicine, and the sciences. Although Irish Catholics have often assimilated into mainstream American society, they remain an identifiable ethnic group.

Persons identifying themselves as of Scottish and Scotch-Irish heritage totaled over 5.1 million in the 2019 census estimate.[4] They are well assimilated, though pockets of Scotch-Irish populations can still be found in certain Appalachian communities.

French Over 7 million Americans listed French as their ancestry in the 2019 U.S. census estimate.[8,10] An estimated fewer than 25 percent of French Americans are descended from immigrants who came to the United States directly from France.[4]

More than 2.1 million people of French-Canadian descent live in the United States as of 2005, many of whom make their home in the Northeast.[4] The French Canadians who settled in the New England states worked in factories that processed textiles, lumber, and bricks. Since 1950 there has been an increase in the percentage of Franco-Americans holding white-collar jobs, but they still lag behind other ethnic groups economically. Compared to the French who immigrated directly from France and assimilated rapidly into American culture, the descendants of French Canadians have clung to their heritage, including language, customs, and religious affiliation.

In Louisiana, more than 12 percent of the population has French ancestry. Smaller French populations are located along sections of the Gulf Coast, and one small colony remaining in northeastern Maine.[11] Cajun people, descending from French Canadians who immigrated to Louisiana from Acadia, or what is now Nova Scotia, settled in rural and inaccessible areas of southern Louisiana, the bayous, and along the Mississippi River. Primarily farmers, fishermen, and herders, they were self-sufficient and kept to themselves. Today, they are still rural, but their occupations reflect local economic conditions.

Worldview

Religion

British Nearly all early British immigrants to America were Protestant. Although many came to escape persecution by the Church of England, others maintained this faith and established congregations throughout the American colonies. The Church of England in the United States became the Episcopal Church during the late eighteenth century.

British ethnicity was often expressed through religious affiliation, particularly with the Episcopal, Methodist, Baptist, and Quaker faiths. Many immigrants established distinctively English congregations, but within a generation most became indistinguishable from other American churches. Today, Americans of British descent participate in most U.S. faiths.

Irish Religion is a cornerstone of Irish Catholic society, and in the United States, it is centered on the parish. Over time, the Catholic Church in America came to be dominated by the Irish, often to the resentment of other Catholic immigrants. The church spared no effort to aid its members; it established schools, hospitals, and orphanages across the United States. The church helped to bridge the cultural gap for many Irish immigrants through advice, job placement, savings clubs, and temperance societies. Today, religion plays a less important role in Irish Catholic life, although the role of the Irish in the church is still significant.

French Among French Americans/Franco-Americans, and Acadians, the Catholic Church provided the nucleus of the community, gave it stability, and helped preserve the language and traditions of the people. The church today still plays a central role.

Family

British The immigrant English family formed the model for the typical American family. It included a father, a mother, and their children. This family group sometimes resided near other relatives, but more often established solitary households. The father was in charge of the public and business aspects of the family, while the mother controlled the domestic and social responsibilities. Traditionally, children in the home were well educated and were sent to private schools, if affordable. Such an education was considered an investment in the future, and children were expected to continue the family business and maintain the family's social position. Due to the similarities between the British family and the emerging American family, new immigrants from England assimilated quickly. It was very common for British immigrants to marry non-English spouses.

Irish Many of the characteristics of the Irish family in the nineteenth century persisted into the twentieth century. Irish Catholics tended to marry at a late age, have large families, and divorce rarely. Today, however, many first- and second-generation Irish Catholics marry outside their group and, with increasing frequency, outside Catholicism.

Traditionally, the father was the breadwinner in the Irish Catholic family, but the mother's position was a strong one. Daughters were often as well educated as sons. Irish people have relatively egalitarian attitudes toward gender roles.

French The Franco-Americans in New England maintained many French traditions through their continued contact with French relatives in Quebec and shared ideas of cultural survival. They had little desire to acculturate. While French-speaking people had lived in North America since the 1600s, the French Canadians that crossed into the United States during the late nineteenth century made New Englanders uneasy. Most French Canadians came to work in New England's cotton mills and by 1930 nearly a million had crossed the border. The people of New England little understood their interest in preserving their culture, and the idea of a French Canadian and Catholic "invasion" loomed. In 1885, newspapers were reporting ominous plans to form a New France on U.S. land. As the New England manufacturing base declined, the factory workers that came slowly dispersed, diffusing tensions.[12] Today, the descendants of the French Canadians speak French infrequently and often marry individuals of other nationalities and backgrounds. Family ties are still strong, but, as with Cajuns, family size has decreased.

Food for Thought

Gumbo derives from the African Bantu word, ki ngombo, meaning okra.

The name for the popular Cajun music style, zydeco, is derived from the French term for green bean, *haricot* (pronounced "ar-ee-ko") because it is snappy, like a bean.

Crawfish are also known as crayfish (especially in New Orleans), crawdads, crawdaddy crab (in the Great Lakes area), clawfish, and mudbugs, among other phrases. They are small crustaceans that look like miniature lobsters, found in the fresh waters of Louisiana, Lake Michigan, California, and the Pacific Northwest.

Cajun people originally descended from French Canadians who immigrated to Louisiana from Nova Scotia. Until the twentieth century, most Cajuns lived in rural areas in extended family households with as many as ten or twelve children per couple. The whole family worked as a unit, and decisions that affected the group were made jointly by all the adults. Many Cajuns were functionally illiterate (having literacy skills at the third-grade level) as extended education was thought unnecessary for farming, fishing, ranching, and hunting, their primary occupations. Many spoke only Cajun French. In 1921, the use of Cajun French was prohibited by the public schools and, as a result, many Cajuns today do not speak or understand their cultural language. The average family size today is smaller, and there is more marriage outside the community, but Cajuns still retain strong ties to their families.

Traditional Health Beliefs and Practices Many suggest that American cultural beliefs regarding health originated in northern Europe, although there are similarities in beliefs across the world. For example, when students were surveyed on family home remedies, those of British, Irish, and French descent shared similar health maintenance practices such as a good diet, plentiful sleep, and daily exercise.[13] Fresh air, cleanliness, and keeping warm and dry were also commonly mentioned. The Irish traditionally wear protective religious medallions.

Among the British and the Irish there is the more generalized belief that good health is dependent on a proper attitude (which includes religious faith) and a rigorous lifestyle. Many northern Europeans associate a moderate diet with maintaining bowel regularity, and laxative use is common. Stomach ailments may be explained as due to food that is too spicy, spoiled, or incompatible (causing an allergic reaction).

The traditional French lifestyle, which features leisurely meals and little structured exercise, presents a paradox to researchers. The "French Paradox," a term coined in the 1980s by three French researchers, was essentially that the French consume more total saturated fat and cholesterol than Americans, yet their death rate from heart disease is less than one-half of that in the United States. However, the French had only recently begun to eat unhealthily in the 1980s, and chronic disease takes decades to develop. Scientists now speculate that some other protective factor in the French diet or lifestyle may account for the heart disease discrepancy, such as lifestyle factors. Genetic factors do not appear to be a cause. Studies comparing the French with Americans of French ancestry have not been reported.

The French Canadians who settled in Louisiana brought numerous traditional remedies. Today, Americans of French descent in Louisiana, including Cajuns, rural and urban dwellers in all socioeconomic groups, often use home remedies and consult folk healers. Traditional folk wisdom advises salves of whiskey and camphor or sheep's tallow and turpentine to aid the end of a cold, tobacco smoke blown into the ears to cure earaches, and wearing a red flannel pouch filled with camphor or asafetida to prevent illness. It should be noted that some Americans of French descent living in the region may also consult practitioners of Voodoo for health problems (refer to Chapter 8 for more details). Voodoo has many definitions, but in the case above it is a form of religion developed by West and Central African populations.

Traditional Food Habits

The influence of France on the food habits of Great Britain and Ireland, and vice versa, since the Middle Ages, led to much cross-over in the kitchen. The alimentary raw materials were similar, and after William the Conqueror from France was made King of England, many cooks in aristocratic British households were French. Evidence for the influence in cuisine can be seen in the terms for foods like beef (from boeuf), pork (porc), and venison (venesoun/venaison). Yet the language of the kitchen helpers and farmers remained Anglo-Saxon, and so did the terms used: cow, swine, sheep, pig, hen, and deer. Similarities developed in the cuisines of these countries, although southern French cooking is more like those of Mediterranean countries. The influence of these northern European cuisines on American foods and food habits has been extensive.

Ingredients and Common Foods

Staples and Regional Variations

Great Britain and Ireland Animal products are of key importance in Great Britain and Ireland. Some form of meat, poultry, or fish is present in most meals, in addition to eggs and cheese. In Britain and Ireland, lamb is a commonly eaten meat, as is roast beef, which is often made for Sunday dinner with Yorkshire pudding (a wheat flour popover cooked in meat drippings). Pork is often served as sausages (bangers) and bacon. Various game birds are also eaten. The cultural food groups list (Table 6.2) includes a more complete detailing of ingredients.

The British and Irish diets also contain a variety of seafood. A well-known fast-food item is fish and chips. The fish is battered and deep-fried, served with fried potatoes, and seasoned with salt and malt vinegar. Salt-dried fish, including ling, cod, and pollack, was traditionally served with a white sauce and potatoes for meatless days by Irish Catholics.[14] Preserved fish is also found as an appetizer or at breakfast. Examples are smoked Scottish salmon and kippers, which are salted and smoked fish.

Dairy products and eggs also play an important role in the diet of the British and Irish. Eggs are traditionally served for breakfast, and cheese is the key ingredient in the traditional plowman's lunch served in pubs. It consists of a piece of cheddar cheese, bread, pickled onions, and a pint of beer. Two other popular kinds of cheese produced in England are the tangy, slightly nutty Cheshire, a family of cheeses that are dense and semi-hard, often crumbly, and Stilton, a characteristically strong blue cheese, or less often a white, semi-soft variety. In Ireland, a market for handcrafted farmhouse cheeses has developed in recent years They include both fresh, soft cheeses and aged types (often flavored with herbs or other seasonings), from cow's or goat's milk. One cheese that has gained international acclaim is Cashel blue, which is produced in Tipperary, Ireland.

Food for Thought

Oatcakes, called bannocks, were traditionally eaten to celebrate the pagan Celtic holiday of Beltane on May 1. One section was burnt or covered with ash; the unlucky person who received the marked portion was said to be sacrificed. In more recent times, the person must leap through a small bonfire three times.

Devonshire, England, is known for its rich cream products, such as double cream (which has twice as much butter fat as ordinary cream) and clotted cream, a slightly fermented, thickened cream. It is often spread on scones, which are biscuits made with baking powder.

Though not the main focus of the meal, breads are not overlooked. In Ireland, soda bread, a bread made with baking soda instead of yeast, was traditionally prepared every day to accompany the meal and remains popular today. Another version was made using cornmeal, after corn from the New World became available in the seventeenth century. Wheat flour is commonly used for baking, and oatmeal is eaten as a porridge for breakfast in Scotland or used in making bread and biscuits throughout Britain and Ireland. What is known as a biscuits in England can refer to any hard, thin, bread-like edible such as a cookie in the United States. Scottish shortbread is an example of a sweet, buttery biscuit.

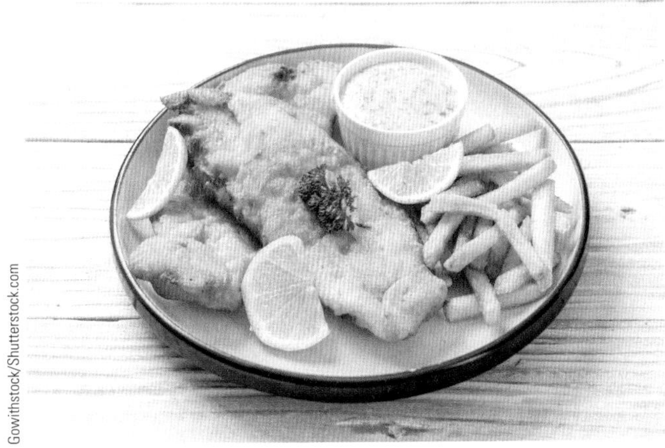

Gowithstock/Shutterstock.com

▲ **Fish and chips are classic pub food in England and Ireland, typically served with malt vinegar.**

Fruits and vegetables are limited to those that grow best in cool climates. Potatoes, brought to Ireland from the New World in the seventeenth century, are the mainstay of the Irish diet and are found in British fare, as well as in most cuisines of the world. Potatoes are found in stews or pies, such as stobhach gaelach, an Irish stew of lamb or mutton that simmers would-be discards such as neck bones, shanks, and other trimmings for hours to make a hearty meal. Another favorite is shepherd's or cottage pie, a meat pie made of ground meat and onions and topped with mashed potatoes. Mashed potatoes are often just referred to as *mash*, as in bangers and mash (sausages and mashed potatoes). Some side dishes made of potatoes are boxty, a type of potato pancake or dumpling; bubble and squeak, a dish made of leftover cabbage and potatoes chopped and fried together; and colcannon, mashed and seasoned boiled white vegetables with onions or leeks. Berries are popular in puddings, pies, and jams. Kitchen gardens are still found in many areas, providing tomatoes, cucumbers, watercress, and other items. Farmers' markets, featuring fresh local produce, are increasingly popular.

Renewed regional interest is growing in seaweeds. In Asian countries such as China, Japan, and Korea, as well as in Polynesia, seaweed has been part of cuisine since ancient times. In contrast, in Europe and the Americas, this tradition has only survived in relatively few places such as Brittany, Ireland, Iceland, Peru, and Chile, where it sometimes evokes memories of shortage and famine. In recent decades, however, seaweed in Ireland has been reinstated as part of trendy and innovative gastronomy.[15] Laver is a purple seaweed (called nori in Japan)

Table 6.2 Cultural Food Groups: Northern European

Group	Comments	Common Foods	Adaptations in the United States
Protein Foods			
Milk/milk products	The English and Irish drink milk as a beverage. Cheese is eaten daily.	Cheese (cow's, sheep's, and goat's milk), cream, milk, sour cream, yogurt	
Meat/poultry/fish/eggs/legumes	Meat, poultry, or fish is usually the centerpiece of the meal. Meats are generally roasted or broiled in Great Britain; also prepared as stews or in pies. Smoked, salted, or dried fish is popular in England.	*Meat:* beef (roasts; variety cuts such as brains, kidneys, liver, sweetbreads, tongue, and tripe), horsemeat, lamb, oxtail, pork, rabbit, snails, veal, venison *Poultry and small birds:* chicken, duck, goose, partridge, pheasant, pigeon, quail, thrush, turkey *Fish and shellfish:* anchovies, bass, clams, cod, crab, crawfish, haddock, herring, lobster, mackerel, mullet, mussels, oysters, perch, pike, pompano, salmon, sardines, scallops, shad, shrimp, skate, sole, sturgeon, trout, whiting *Eggs:* poultry and fish *Legumes:* kidney beans, lentils, lima beans, split peas	The Irish consume more animal protein.
Cereals/Grains	Wheat bread usually accompanies the meal. In Britain and Ireland oatmeal or porridge is common for breakfast.	Barley, hops, oats, rice, rye, wheat	Corn and corn products are consumed more.
Fruits/Vegetables	Potatoes are frequently eaten in Ireland. Arrowroot starch is used as thickener, and tapioca (from cassava tubers) is eaten.	*Fruits:* apples, apricots, cherries, currants, gooseberries, grapes (many varieties), lemons, melons, oranges, peaches, pears, plums, prunes, raisins, raspberries, rhubarb, strawberries *Vegetables:* artichokes, asparagus, beets, brussels sprouts, cabbage, carrots, cauliflower, celery, celery root, cucumbers, eggplant, fennel, green beans, green peppers, kale, lettuce (many varieties), leeks, mushrooms (including chanterelles, cèpes), olives, onions, parsnips, peas, potatoes, radishes, salsify, scallions, sorrel, spinach, tomatoes, turnips, truffles, watercress	Native and transplanted fruits and vegetables, such as bananas, blueberries, okra, and squash, were added to the diet.
Additional Foods			
Seasonings	British and Irish dishes emphasize naturalness of foods with mild seasoning, served with flavorful condiments or sauces used to taste. French dishes are often prepared with complementary sauces or gravies that enhance food flavor.	Angelica (licorice-flavored plant), bay leaf, capers, chile peppers, chives, chocolate, chutney, cinnamon, cloves, coffee, cognac, fennel seeds, garlic, ginger, horseradish, juniper berries, mace, malt vinegar, marjoram, mint, mustard, nutmeg, oregano, paprika, parsley, pepper (black, white, green, and pink), rosemary, saffron, sage, shallots, sweet basil, Tabasco sauce (and other hot sauces), tarragon, thyme, vanilla, Worcestershire sauce	Cajun and Creole cooking are highly spiced. Stews are thickened with filé powder (sassafras).
Nuts/seeds	Nuts especially popular; used primarily in desserts.	*Nuts:* almonds (sweet and bitter), chestnuts, filberts (hazelnuts), pecans, walnuts (including black) *Seeds:* sesame	
Beverages	Alcoholic beverages consumed as part of the meal.	Beer (ale, stout, bitters), black and herbal tea (mint, anise, chamomile, etc.), cider, coffee, gin, hot chocolate, liqueurs, port, sherry, whiskey, wine (red, white, champagne, and fruit/vegetable)	
Fats/oils	Butter used extensively in cooking of northern and central France; olive oil more common in southern regions of the country.	Butter, goose fat, lard, margarine, olive oil, vegetable oil, salt pork	
Sweeteners		Honey, sugar	Molasses and maple syrup are used as sweeteners. Irish Americans use more sugar than members of other groups.

that is a specialty in Wales and parts of northern coastal England. It is customarily boiled into a gelatinous paste, then mixed with oatmeal and formed into patties that are fried. Known as laverbread, these cakes are traditionally served at breakfast with bacon. Dulse, red algae eaten in Ireland, can be consumed fresh but is usually dried, then chewed like beef jerky for a snack, or flaked and added to soups or warm milk.

The most common beverages consumed by adults in Ireland and England are tea, beer, and whiskey. Tea, which has become synonymous with a meal or break in the afternoon, was introduced to England by the British East India Company and made fashionable by the wife of Charles II, Catherine of Braganza, a Portuguese princess. The Portuguese and Dutch were among the earliest Europeans to taste the beverage as their traders brought in regular shipments from the East by 1610. Though England came on the scene later, with Catherine's influence the drink gained popularity quickly. By 1700 over 500 coffee houses in Britain sold the drink. Drunk with most meals and as a refreshment, strong black tea is preferred served with milk and sugar. Frequently consumed alcoholic beverages include beer and whiskey. The British and the Irish do not drink the bottom-fermented style of beer common in the United States. Instead, in Britain the pubs usually serve bitters, an amber-colored, top-fermented beer, strongly flavored with hops, while in Ireland, a favorite is stout, a dark, rich beer that can provide substantial calories to the diet. Both beers are served at cellar temperature and are naturally carbonated.

Whiskey is made in both Ireland and Scotland, but the Irish are usually credited with its invention and name. Generally, both styles are fermented with barley, though Scotch, or Scotch whisky (spelled without an *e*), is often malted (in which the barley is germinated before fermentation) and Irish whiskey is largely un-malted. Scotch is traditionally a much fuller or stronger, smokier-tasting beverage than Irish whiskey, which is said to have superior smoothness due to a triple distilling process. Other alcoholic drinks popular in Britain are gin, port (a brandy-fortified wine made in Portugal), and sherry (a fortified wine from Spain). A less common beverage, but one still popular in some regions. is mead, a type of honey wine made from the fermentation of honey and water. The Welsh prefer a stronger, highly spiced variety called metheglyn.

Sample Menu

An Irish Pub Supper

Steak/Beef and Guinness Pie[a]

Brown Bread[b]

Apple Crumble[c]

Stout

Recipes in this menu:

[a]https://www.food.com/recipe/steak-and-guinness-pie-jamie-oliver-429784#activity-feed

[b]https://www.foodnetwork.com/recipes/ree-drummond/brown-bread-5596230

[c]https://www.thespruceeats.com/easy-traditional-apple-crumble-recipe-435938

Irish Recipes and Baking

Food for Thought

Colcannon was customarily served for the harvest dinner and on Halloween in Ireland. For Halloween, coins were wrapped and buried in the dish so the children could find them as they ate.

The term *honeymoon* originated with the European custom of newlyweds drinking mead for the first lunar month following their wedding.

Tomatoes were introduced to Europe in 1523 from the New World. The reaction was mixed; some people thought they were poisonous, while others believed they brought luck. Tomato-shaped pin cushions developed from the latter superstition.

France The cooking of France has traditionally been divided into classic French cuisine (*haute or grande* cuisine) and provincial or regional cooking.[16] The birth of haute French cuisine, dependent upon trained kitchen staff, quality ingredients, and rigorous attention to detail and presentation, is often credited to George Augustine Escoffier in the mid-nineteenth century, although Chef François-Pierra de La Varenne in the seventeenth century and Marie-Antoine Carême in the late eighteenth century also advanced this approach.[17] Provincial cuisine is simpler fare made at home or in local cafes featuring fresh local ingredients. Broadly speaking, butter and cream enrich many dishes in the northeastern and central regions of the country, while lard, duck fat, and goose fat flavor foods in the northwest and south-central areas.[18] In the southeast, olive oil is prominent. Seafood and lamb are specialties of the north, while pork is common in the regions bordering Belgium and Germany. Beef and veal are favorites in the central areas, and in the southernmost regions near Spain, fish is a specialty. Cold-weather fruits and vegetables are featured in northern dishes, while temperate, Mediterranean produce is the mainstay in southern areas. In the north, foods are subtly seasoned. In the south, garlic flavors many dishes.

The ancestors of most early French Americans came in sporadic waves fleeing religious, political, or economic hardship in France.[19] They brought their particular food preferences with them on the move, depending on their home region.

In Brittany, seafood simply prepared is traditional. Located along the northwest coast with shores washed by the English Channel, the region's delicate Belon oysters are shipped throughout France. Mutton and vegetables from Brittany are said to have a naturally salty taste because of the

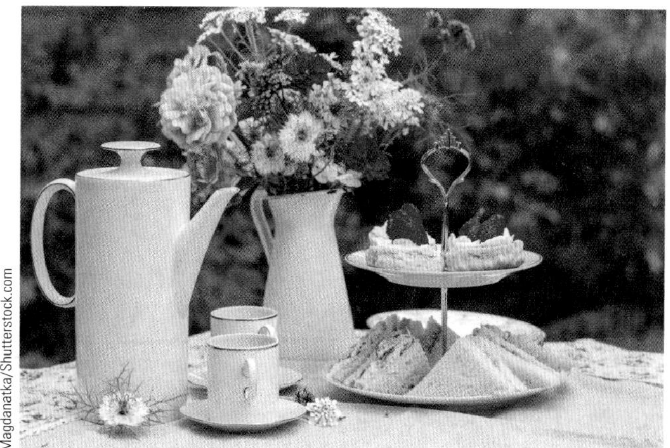
Magdanatka/Shutterstock.com

▲ **Tea time in Great Britain has become an afternoon meal for some, with small sandwiches, scones (on the second rack of the silver tray), and an assortment of cookies and pastries.**

salt spray. Apples are the prevalent fruit, and cider is widely exported.

Normandy, located along the English Channel, east of Brittany, is also known for apples in addition to seafood. Calvados, an apple brandy, is thought to be the mother of applejack, an alcoholic apple drink used to clear the palate during meals in Louisiana. Another alcoholic drink produced in the region is Bénédictine, named after the Roman Catholic monks who still make it at the monastery in Fecamp. Normandy is also renowned for its rich dairy products; its butter is considered one of the best in France. Camembert, a semisoft cheese with a mild flavor, and Pont-l'Évêque, a hearty aromatic cheese, are produced in the area. Dishes from Normandy are often prepared with rich cream sauces. French crêpes, very thin, unleavened pancakes, originated in this region; they are typically served topped with sweet or savory sauces or rolled with meat, poultry, fish or seafood, cheese, or fruit fillings.

Champagne, a region bordered by the English Channel and Belgium, has a cuisine influenced by Germanic cultures. Beer is popular, as are sausages, such as andouille and andouillette, large and small intestinal casings stuffed with pork or lamb stomach. Charcuterie, cold meat dishes such as sausages, pâtés, and terrines, which often are sold in specialty stores, are especially good in this region. Pâté is a spread of finely ground, cooked, seasoned meats. A terrine is commonly made with leftover meats cut into small pieces, mixed with spices and a jelling substance, then baked in a loaf pan. Throughout the world, Champagne is probably best known for its naturally carbonated wines. Only sparkling wines produced in this region can be legally called Champagne after the 2006 trade agreement between the United States and the European Union.

The province that borders Germany, Alsace-Lorraine, has been alternately ruled by France and Germany. One of its principal cities is Strasbourg. Many German foods are favored in the region, such as goose, sausages, and sauerkraut. Goose fat is often used for cooking, and one of the specialties of the area is pâté de fois gras, pâté made from the enlarged livers of force-fed geese, a practice coming under increasing scrutiny for the ethical treatment of animals. Another famous dish is quiche Lorraine, a pie pastry baked with a filling of cream, beaten eggs, and bacon. Alsace-Lorraine is a wine-producing area, as well; its wines are similar to German Rhine wines but are usually not as sweet. Distilled liquors produced in the region are kirsch, a cherry brandy, and the brandy eau de vie de framboise, made from raspberries.

Located south of Normandy and Brittany in the west-central part of France is Touraine, the province that includes the fertile Loire valley. Along the river, chateaux or palaces built by the French nobility dot the banks. Known as the "garden of France," Touraine produces some of the finest fruits and vegetables in the country. A dry white wine produced in the area is Vouvray. The north-central region surrounding the city of Paris, called the Ile-de-France, is the home of classic French cuisine. Some of the finest beef and veal, as well as varieties of fruits and vegetables, are produced in this fertile region. Brie, semisoft and mild flavored, is the best-known cheese in the area. Dishes of the Ile-de-France include lobster à l'américaine, lobster prepared with tomatoes, shallots, herbs, white wine, and brandy; potage St. Germain, pea soup; filet de bœuf béarnaise, filet of beef with a béarnaise sauce (made of herbed emulsified yolk and butter); and tarte tatin, an upside-down apple, and caramel tart.

Located southeast of Paris is Burgundy, one of the foremost wine-producing regions of France. Burgundy's robust dishes contain garlic and are often prepared with olive oil. Dijon, a principal city, is also the name of the mustards of the region, prepared with white wine and herbs. Dishes of the area are escargot, or snails (raised on grape vines) cooked in garlic butter and served in the shell; coq au vin, rooster or chicken cooked in wine; and bœuf bourguignon, a hearty red wine beef stew. In Burgundy, the red wines are primarily made from the pinot noir grape, and the white wines are from the chardonnay grape. The great wines of the area are usually named after the villages in which they are produced; for example, Gevrey-Chambertin, Vosne-Romanée, and Volnay. Cassis, a black currant liquor, is also produced in the region, and brandy from Cognac is a specialty. To the east, along the border with Switzerland, is the mountainous Franche-Comte region, known for its exceptionally tender and flavorful Bresse chicken.

The other major wine-producing region of France is Bordeaux, which is also the name of its principal city. Famous for its hearty dishes, the term *à la bordelaise* can mean (1) prepared in a seasoned sauce containing red or white wine, marrow, tomatoes, butter, and shallots; (2) use of mirepoix, a finely minced mixture of carrots, onions, and celery seasoned with bay leaves and thyme; (3) accompanied by cèpes, large fleshy mushrooms; or (4) accompanied by an artichoke and potato garnish. A red Bordeaux wine is full-bodied and made primarily from the cabernet sauvignon and Merlot grape. (In Great Britain, a Bordeaux wine is called claret.)

Among the wines produced are St. Julien, Margaux, Graves, St. Emilion, Pomerol, and Sauternes, a sweet white dessert wine.

In the south of France is Languedoc, famous for cassoulet, a complex dish containing duck or goose, pork or mutton, sausage, and white beans, among other ingredients. Provence, located on the Mediterranean Sea, is a favorite vacation spot because of its warm Riviera beaches. Provence is also known for the large old port city of Marseilles, its perfumes from the city of Grasse, and the international film festival in Cannes.

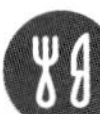

Food for Thought

Belgians are renowned for their beers. One specialty ale is lambic, a fruity brew distinctive for its use of unmalted (raw) wheat and open-tank fermentation with wild yeast.

Fresh cream in France, called fleurette, is often added to sauces or whipped for dessert. Also popular is crème fraîche, a cream that is fermented until it is thickened and slightly tangy.

The first eating chocolate was introduced by the British in 1847, although the Olmec, Mayans, and Aztecs of Mesoamerica had used it as a drink for centuries before. In Europe, too, it was first a luxury drink before it came in bars or small pieces to eat. Europeans now consume 20–25 pounds of chocolate per person each year—twice the amount eaten by U.S. citizens.

The cooking of Provence is similar to that of Italy and Spain. Staple ingredients are tomatoes, garlic, and olive oil; à la Provençal means that a dish contains these three items. Other common food items are seafood from the Mediterranean, artichokes, eggplant, and zucchini. Popular dishes from the region are bouillabaisse, the famed fish stew made with tomatoes, garlic, olive oil, and several types of seafood, seasoned with saffron, and usually served with rouille, a hot red pepper sauce; ratatouille, tomatoes, eggplant, and zucchini cooked in olive oil; salade Niçoise, a salad originating in Nice, containing tuna, tomatoes, olives, lettuce, other raw vegetables, and sometimes hard-boiled eggs; and pan bagna, a French bread sandwich slathered with olive oil and containing a variety of ingredients, such as anchovies, tomatoes, green peppers, onions, olives, hard-boiled eggs, and capers. One unique specialty item in the region associated with haute cuisine is black truffles. This costly, pungent underground fungus flavors or garnishes many classic French dishes.

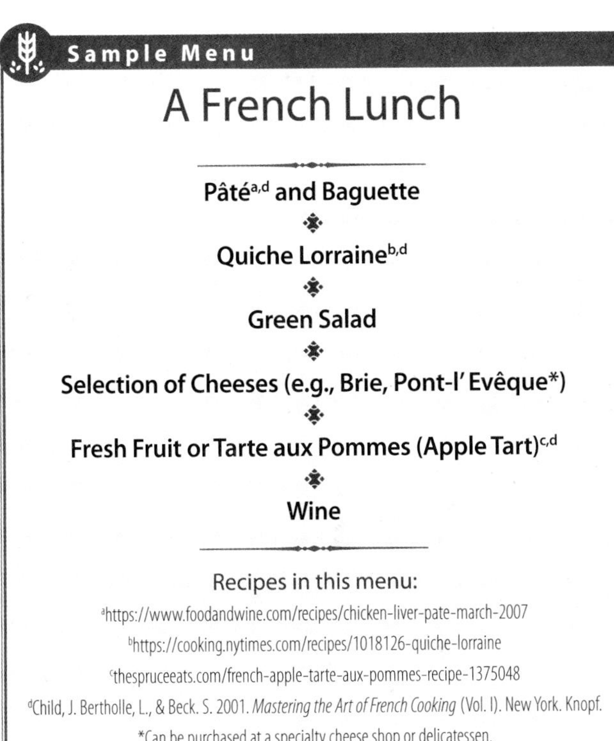

Sample Menu

A French Lunch

Pâté[a,d] and Baguette

Quiche Lorraine[b,d]

Green Salad

Selection of Cheeses (e.g., Brie, Pont-l'Evêque*)

Fresh Fruit or Tarte aux Pommes (Apple Tart)[c,d]

Wine

Recipes in this menu:

[a]https://www.foodandwine.com/recipes/chicken-liver-pate-march-2007

[b]https://cooking.nytimes.com/recipes/1018126-quiche-lorraine

[c]thespruceeats.com/french-apple-tarte-aux-pommes-recipe-1375048

[d]Child, J. Bertholle, L., & Beck. S. 2001. *Mastering the Art of French Cooking* (Vol. I). New York. Knopf.

*Can be purchased at a specialty cheese shop or delicatessen.

Although the ingredients used in the countries on opposite sides of the English Channel are not substantially different, their cooking styles vary greatly. British and Irish food is described as simple and hearty fare that developed out of rural, seasonal traditions, although the wealthy through history ate considerably more diverse meals than the rest of the population.[20,21] French cuisine is admired for its fresh ingredients, attention to detail, and technical proficiency—and has been the public face of French culture around the world.

Both the British and the Irish take pride in the naturalness of their dishes and their ability to cook foods so the flavors are enhanced rather than obscured. In recent years, the eating local movement, as shown in Chapter 15, and government programs promoting regional specialties have led to a renewed interest in traditional fare.[22]

Meat is usually roasted or broiled, depending on the cut, and lightly seasoned with herbs and spices. Strong-flavored condiments such as Worcestershire sauce (flavored with anchovies, vinegar, soy, garlic, and assorted spices) on roast beef or mint jelly on lamb are often served. Chutneys, fruit or vegetable condiments, often spicy and savory or sweet and tart, originally from India, are also popular. Leftover meat is finely chopped, then served in a stew, pie, or pudding. Offal, parts of the animal often discarded, such as lamb's brains, pig's tail, and calf's heart, have become trendy items in England, appreciated for both their traditional heritage and the ecological or ethical value of using the whole animal.

While most Americans think of pies and puddings as being sweet desserts, in Britain and Ireland this is not necessarily the case. A pie is a baked pastry consisting of a mixture of meats, game, fish, vegetables, or fruit, covered with or enclosed in a crust. A Cornish pasty is an individual pillow-shaped pie filled with meat, onions, potatoes, and sometimes fruit. Another well-known British dish is steak and kidney pie.

Pudding is a steamed, boiled, or baked dish that may be based on anything from custards and fruits to meat and vegetables. An example of a sweet pudding is plum pudding, which is served traditionally at Christmas. It is a steamed dish of suet, dried and candied fruit, and other ingredients.

Trifle is a layered dessert made from custard, pound cake, raspberry jam, whipped cream, sherry, and almonds.

Classic French cuisine implies a carefully planned meal that balances the texture, color, and flavor of the dishes, reportedly similar to the harmony found in musical compositions or paintings.[23] The soul of French cooking is its sauces, often painstakingly prepared from stocks simmered for hours to bring out the flavor.

Sauces are subtly flavored with natural ingredients, such as vegetables, wine, and herbs. The aim is to never overwhelm the food, but rather complement it. Five sauces are considered foundational: béchamel (white sauce usually based on milk or cream), velouté (a white stock, traditionally based on chicken but also vegetable or fish), espangnole (a brown sauce, traditionally made from beef or veal), tomato, and hollandaise (egg yolks, clarified butter, and acid such as lemon juice or white wine). In addition, mayonnaise (egg yolks, olive oil, and lemon) is included by many cooks.[24]

Some common rules in preparing French dishes are (1) never mix sweet and sour flavors in the same dish; (2) never serve sweet sauces over fish; (3) do not undercook or overcook food; (4) except salad and fruit, do not serve uncooked food; (5) always use the freshest, best-tasting ingredients; and (6) wine is an integral part of the meal and must complement the food.

French breads and pastries are particularly noteworthy. Breads are typically made with white flour, shaped into long loaves (e.g., thin baguettes), rounds, braids, or rings, then baked in a wood-fired oven. Buttery, flaky croissants or eggy brioche are sweeter and fall between breads and pastries. Specialty doughs, such as cream puff pastry, multilayered puff pastry, and the classic sponge cake génoise, are used to create the numerous desserts of France, such as cakes, petits fours (small, bite-size pastries), and tarts. Chocolate, fresh fruits, and pastry cream thickened with egg yolks enrich these pastries.

In recent years, classic French cuisine has merged with a rediscovery of regional fare to create what is known as nouvelle cuisine (new cuisine). The practice of nouvelle cuisine has influenced the development of local specialties with an emphasis on fresh ingredients. An appreciation for the cooking of other nations, especially those of Asia, has occurred in France, and many dishes now use more varied seasonings and Eastern cooking techniques and presentations.

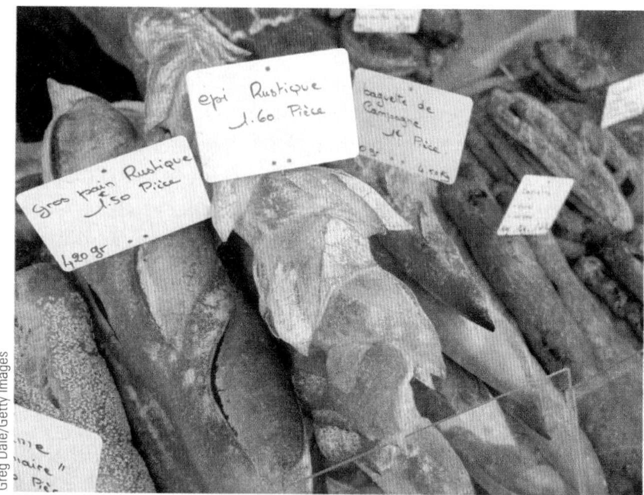

Greg Dale/Getty Images

▲ **French breads are often consumed at every meal, and include baguettes, braids, rings, and sweeter versions such as brioche (with little topknots).**

Meal Composition and Cycle

Daily Pattern

Great Britain and Ireland In Britain, four meals are traditionally served each day—breakfast, lunch, tea, and an evening meal (dinner). In the nineteenth and early twentieth centuries, breakfast was a very substantial meal, consisting of oatmeal; bacon, ham, or sausage; eggs (prepared several ways); bread fried in bacon grease; toast with jam or marmalade; grilled tomatoes or mushrooms; and possibly smoked fish or deviled kidneys. All this was washed down with tea. Today, in Scotland, oatmeal is usually eaten for breakfast, while in England, packaged breakfast cereals are often eaten during the week, and the more extensive breakfast is reserved for weekends and special occasions.

Lunch was originally a hearty meal and often still is on Sundays, but during the week it is squeezed in between work hours. It may include a meat pie, fish and chips, or a light meal at the pub with a pint of bitters or stout. Both Sunday lunch and the weekday dinner are much like a U.S. dinner. The meals consist of meat or fish, vegetable, and starch. The starch is often potatoes or rice, and bread also accompanies the meal. Dessert (often called "pudding") follows the main course.

In the late afternoon in Britain and Ireland, most people take a break and have a pot of tea and a light snack. In some areas, high tea is served. This can be a substantial meal that includes potted meat, fish, shrimp, ham salad, salmon cakes, fruits, and a selection of cakes and pastries. Initially, high tea was the evening meal for the working class during the 18th and 19th centuries, consisting of tea, bread, cheese, vegetables, and meat. It is thought that the upper British classes add the term *high* or *afternoon* to tea as a dinner when it is served occasionally in place of dinner as a novelty, or to children as an informal substitute for dinner. Whether snack or meal, the British often just call it tea.

Food for Thought

Potted is an English term for fish, meat, poultry, or game pounded with lard or butter into a coarse or smooth pâté, then preserved in jars or pots. *Deviled* describes a dish prepared with a spicy hot sauce or seasoning.

In the small town of Palmiers, the city council has banned any ready-made or mass-produced food (e.g., frozen pizza) from the local school cafeteria to "ensure our kids stay healthy, teach them the taste of proper French food, and help keep our small farmers in business."[25]

France The French eat only three meals a day—breakfast, lunch, and dinner. Second helpings are uncommon, and there is very little snacking between meals. Breakfast, in contrast to the British meal, is very light, consisting of a croissant or French bread with butter and jam, and strong coffee with hot milk or hot chocolate. The French breakfast is what is known in the United States as a continental breakfast. Lunch is traditionally the largest meal of the day and, in some regions of France, businesses close at midday for two hours so people can return home to eat. The meal usually starts with an appetizer (hors d'oeuvre) such as pâté. The main course is a meat, fish, or egg dish accompanied by a vegetable and bread. If salad is eaten, it is served after the main course. Dessert at home is usually cheese and fruit. In a restaurant, ice cream (more like a fruit sherbet or sorbet), cakes, custards, and pastries are served in addition to fruit and cheese. Wine is served with the meal and coffee is after the meal. Dinner is similar, but traditionally a lighter meal with a starter course of soup or appetizer, then a main dish, followed by a cheese course. However, meal patterns are changing in France. The popularity of fast foods and shorter lunch periods is resulting in a more American pattern of a smaller lunch followed by a larger dinner.

Food for Thought

In Britain, mincemeat pie is a Christmas tradition stemming from the 16th century. Originally a spiced, sweet meat mixture, they are now commonly made with dried fruits, sugar, spices, and brandy.

Robert Burns once wrote that haggis was the "great chieftain o' the puddin' race." Nevertheless, Scottish government officials recommended in 2006 that haggis be served to children no more than once a week due to its high fat and sodium content.

Etiquette Every culture has its own specific concept and rules of etiquette when it comes to eating. Etiquette is an important social interaction. For example, the fork is not passed from the right hand to the left hand when cutting food in England and Ireland. Instead, the fork remains in the left hand, and the knife in the right. The two are often used together to scoop food onto the fork. All dishes are passed to the left. When not eating, the hands should be placed in one's lap. In Ireland, a small plate to the left of the setting is used for placing potato peelings.[26]

France is similar to Great Britain in the use of forks and knives. For example, lettuce in a salad should not be cut, but folded into a small, easy-to-eat packet. The French also pass dishes to the left. They do not usually use bread plates but place their portions of bread directly on the table. In contrast to England and Ireland, it is considered impolite to put your hands on your lap. The wrists should be rested on the table with the hands in view.[25–27] Chocolates are appropriate gifts to bring to a dinner. In England, a bottle of champagne is appreciated, while in Ireland a bottle of wine to serve with the meal is also common. In France, a dessert-style wine or after-dinner liqueur is the best beverage to give.

Special Occasions Christmas and Easter are the most important Christian holidays celebrated in England, Ireland, and France. Ireland and France are predominantly Catholic countries and tend to observe all the holy days of obligation and patron saints' days. France commemorates the beginning of the French Revolution on July 14, Bastille Day.

Great Britain and Ireland The British celebrate Christmas by serving hot punch or mulled wine; roast beef, goose, turkey, or ham; plum pudding and mincemeat (or just "mince") pies; and, afterward, port with nuts and dried fruit. The plum pudding is traditionally splashed with brandy and then flamed before being served. Mincemeat pies were originally prepared with seasoned, ground meats, suet, and fruit, but today they are usually made with only dried and candied fruit, nuts, and spices. Boxing Day, the day after Christmas, is when friends and relatives visit one another.

Foods served at Easter include hot cross buns and Shrewsbury simnel. In ancient times, the cross on the buns is believed to have symbolized both the sun and fire; the four quarters represented the seasons. Today the cross represents Christ and the resurrection. Shrewsbury simnel is a rich spice cake topped with 12 decorative balls of marzipan originally representing the astrological signs. (It is also served on Mother's Day.) Another holiday celebrated throughout Great Britain is New Year's Day on January 1.

The Scottish traditionally eat haggis on Hogmanay (New Year's Eve). Haggis is a sheep's stomach stuffed with a pudding made of sheep's innards and oatmeal, and is often served with Scotch whisky. It is also the traditional entrée (served with "neeps," mashed turnips, and "tatties," mashed potatoes) on Burns's Night, commemorating the national poet Robert Burns (January 25). St. Patrick's Day began as a religious commemoration for the patron saint of Ireland. The Irish American custom of eating a corned beef and cabbage meal on March 17 is now as popular in Ireland as it is in the United States.[6]

Food for Thought

New England Puritans and English Quakers were among the first in the United States to promote free public education.

Historically in Ireland, *Mac* before a family name meant "son of," whereas *O* signified "descended from."

A "pub," or public house, is a bar that serves beer, wine, hard liquor, and light meals. The British pub is often the place where friends and family meet to socialize.

France In France, the main Christmas meal is served after mass on the night of December 24. Two traditional dishes are a boudin noir and boudin blanc, also known as black pudding and white pudding (dark blood sausage or a light-colored one made from veal, chicken, or pork with milk) and a goose or turkey with chestnuts. In Provence, the Christmas Eve meal is meatless, usually cod, but the highlight is that it is followed by 13 desserts, representing Jesus and his 12 apostles.

On Shrove Tuesday (Mardi Gras), the French feast on pancakes, fritters, waffles, and various biscuits and cakes. During Lent, no eggs, fat, or meat are eaten. Dishes served during Lent often contain cod or herring. Cod is also the traditional dish served on Good Friday; in some regions, lentils are eaten to wash away one's sins. Easter marks the return of the normal diet, and eggs are often served hard-boiled (also colored), in omelets, or in breads and pastries. French toast (croûtes dorée) is a traditional Easter dish. Also common are pies filled with minced meats.

Therapeutic Uses of Food Most northern Europeans share a belief that a good diet is essential to maintaining health. Traditional home remedies for minor illnesses include chicken soup, tea with honey or lemon or whiskey, hot milk, or hot whiskey with cloves. These medicinal foods are still popular in the United States for use during times of illness. Practices less common today are taking sulfur with molasses as a laxative and regular use of cod liver oil. Some Irish Americans may use senna (*Cassia acutifolia*) weekly to cleanse their bowels.[27]

Home remedies popular with Americans of French descent include infusions made from magnolia leaves, elderberry flowers, sassafras, or citronella, which are prescribed for colds. Sore throats are treated by gargling herbal teas or hot water with dissolved honey, salt, and baking soda. Sassafras tea is used to cleanse the blood, and garlic is ingested for worms.[19,27]

Contemporary Food Habits in the United States

Adaptations of Food Habits

Horsemeat is more popular in France (where it is known as chevaline) than in the United Kingdom, though its consumption has been on the decline since 2012. Today, horsemeat consumption in France accounts for just 0.4% of all meat eaten. France legalized the eating of horsemeat in 1866, overruling a 732 Papal ban, so that poor families who could not afford pork or beef could have a source of protein. Approximately 17% of the French population have eaten horse at some time or another and there are approximately 11,000 French farmers who raise horses for the meat trade and 750 horse butchers operating in the country. It is often served as raw tartare or with onions, garlic, and potatoes.[28]

Ingredients and Common Foods

British and Irish Many U.S. dishes have their origins in Great Britain. The Puritans, adapting Native American fare, made a pudding with cornmeal, milk, molasses, and spices. Today, this is called Indian pudding. Pumpkin pie originates from a custard pie to which the Native American squash or pumpkin is added. Apple pie has been so well accepted that we say, "American as apple pie," despite the original birthplace of apples in

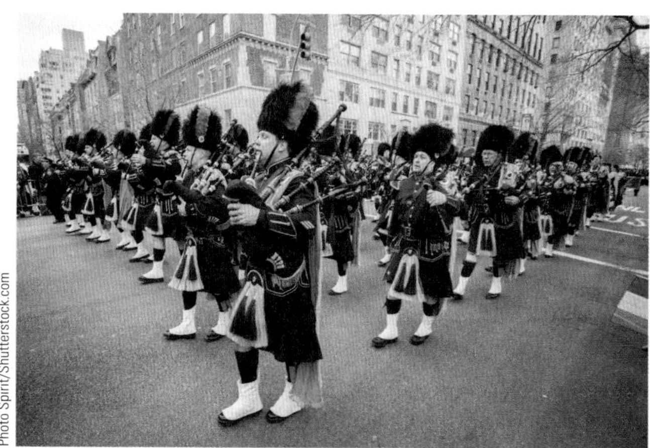
Photo Spirit/Shutterstock.com

▲ St. Patrick's Day in Savannah, Georgia.

Kazakhstan and much later planting by English colonists on U.S. soil. Syllabub, a milk and wine punch drunk in the American South at Christmastime, is also an English recipe, often a dessert when thickened with gelatin or served as a topping.

French French cooking has had less influence on everyday American cooking (except for French fries), but there are probably few large cities that don't have a French restaurant.

French Americans adapted their cuisine to the available ingredients and other ethnic cooking styles. The best example of this is found in Louisiana, where Creole and Cajun cooking developed. Cajun cooking is typically thought more provincial than Creole cooking. Some dishes may sound typically French, such as the fish stew known as bouillabaisse, but is, by virtue of location, made with fish from the Gulf of Mexico, not from the Mediterranean. Even coffee can be slightly different, flavored with the bitter chicory root.

Ingredients for Cajun cooking reflect the environment of Louisiana: Bayou Cajun foods are from lake and swamp areas, whereas prairie Cajun dishes are found in inland areas. Creole foods often use tomatoes, while most Cajun foods do not. Fish and shellfish abound in both cuisines, notably crawfish, crabs, oysters, pompano, redfish, and shrimp, to name just a few. Shellfish is commonly eaten raw on the half-shell (oysters) or boiled in a spicy mixture. Gumbo and jambalaya are often made with seafood. Gumbo, derived from the word "gombo" in West African languages, translates to "okra;" it is an adaptable dish of thick, spicy soup made with a variety of seafood, meat, and vegetables. Contributions from Native American, French, Spanish, and Caribbean people have led to a fusion of culinary creativity in the pot.[29] It is thickened with okra (originating from western Africa and likely brought into the American South by enslaved people), filé powder (dried sassafras, a Native American spice), or roux (a French word for a paste made from oil or other fat and flour), and then ladled over rice. Okra is an affordable source of carbohydrates, minerals and vitamins, dietary fiber, and other phytonutrients with physiological benefits. New Orleans jambalaya, also a highly seasoned stew made with a combination of seafood, meats, and vegetables, was influenced by French, African, and Spanish cooking. The base for these stews and gravies is often roux; Cajun roux is flour and fat (usually vegetable oil) cooked very slowly until the mixture turns dark brown and has a nutlike aroma and taste.

Other key ingredients in Cajun and Creole cooking are rice (which has been grown in Louisiana since the early 1700s), red beans, tomatoes (mostly in Creole foods), chayote squash, eggplant, spicy hot sauce, and a variety of pork products. One of the better-known hot sauces, Tabasco, is produced in the bayous of southern Louisiana from fermented chili peppers, vinegar, and spices. Tasso, a seasoned smoked pork product, is also used to flavor dishes. A deep-fried rice fritter, calas, is the Louisiana version of a doughnut. Other rice dishes are red beans and rice and dirty rice. Dirty rice derives its name from the fact that its ingredients, bits of chicken gizzards, and liver, give the rice a brown appearance. Cajun boudin sausages are a specialty. Boudin blanc is made with pork and rice; boudin rouge has pork blood added to it. Cochon de lait, a suckling pig roasted over a wood fire, is prepared at Cajun festivals in central Louisiana. Fricot is a popular soup made with potatoes and sausage or shredded meat. Cracklings, known as gratons, are bite-size bits of fried pork skin (often with meat attached) popular in some regions.

Pecan pralines are a famous New Orleans candy. Pecans, native to Louisiana, are made into pralines by adding brown sugar, water or cream, and butter and shaping the nutty treat into large flat patties. Another confection eaten often with coffee is beignets, round- or square-puffed French doughnuts dusted with powdered sugar. French toast, or pain perdu, is another French specialty that was transported to New Orleans and is now familiar to many Americans.

The cuisine of French Americans in New England tends to be traditionally French, but it is influenced by common New England foods and food habits, though French Americans typically use more herbs and spices than other New Englanders. Traditional French dishes are pork pâté, called creton by the French, and the traditional Yule log cake (bûche de Noël) served at Christmas. French American cuisine offers numerous soups and stews. One of the most elaborate of the stews, which is also called a pie, is cipate, known as cipaille, si-pallie, six-pates, and sea pie in some areas. A typical recipe calls for chicken, pork, veal, and beef, plus four or five kinds of vegetables layered in a heavy kettle, covered with pie crust. It is slowly cooked after the chicken stock has been added through vents in the crust.

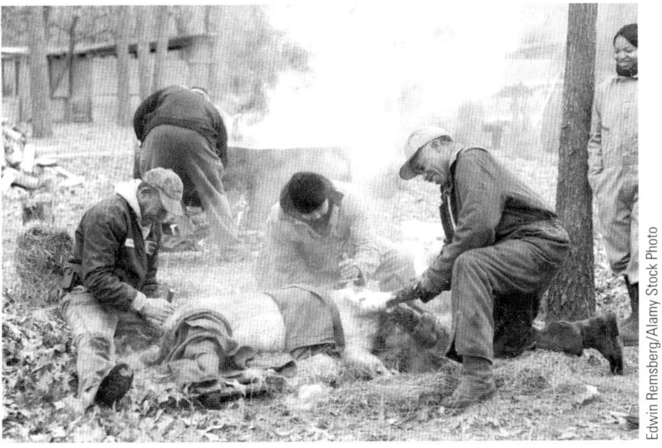

Edwin Remsberg/Alamy Stock Photo

▲ La boucherie: French-speaking Cajuns in Louisiana maintain the hog-butchering traditions of their past. Before the days of refrigeration, everyone in the community helped prepare the meat and lard. Participants went home with fresh pork cuts and spicy sausages called boudin. La boucherie continues today at many Cajun festivals.

Maple syrup is commonly used. One unique breakfast dish is eggs poached in syrup. Maple syrup is also served over bread dumplings or just plain bread. French Americans appreciate wine and distilled spirits. One unusual combination of both is caribou, a mixture of red wine, a spirit (usually rye whiskey), and maple syrup or sugar, which is drunk on festive occasions (also refer to Chapter 15).

Meal Composition and Cycle

British and Irish American food habits have been greatly influenced by British and Irish immigrants. Meal patterns and composition are very similar to those in Great Britain. The typical meal of a meat, poultry, or fish main dish served with vegetable and starch side dishes, and often bread, continues to this day. Though English Americans also consumed a hearty breakfast that often-included ham or bacon and eggs, in more recent years, time constraints and health concerns have changed this pattern on weekdays; weekend breakfast sometimes reverts to the more British-style meal.

Festive meals also reflect British and Irish influence. A traditional Christmas dinner includes roast turkey or ham, stuffing, and mashed vegetables. For dessert, a pie is customary, sometimes mincemeat. Two holidays that Americans think of as being typically American, Thanksgiving and Halloween, have British and Irish influences. In Great Britain and Ireland, Halloween, or All Hallow's Eve, is the night before All Saints' Day honoring all the saints of the Church, which was chosen to be celebrated on the day of the Celtic harvest festival of Samhain, a liminal time when spirits or fairies could more easily come into our world.

French Americans of French descent have adopted the U.S. meal cycle with the main meal in the evening. In Louisiana, a well known celebration tied to food is Mardi Gras, culminating on Shrove Tuesday, just before the beginning of Lent. In New Orleans there are parades, masquerading, and general revelry; the festival reaches its climax at a grand ball before midnight. After this day and night of rich eating and grand merriment, the 40 days of fasting and penitence of Lent begin. In the Cajun countryside, Mardi Gras is celebrated with "run": Men on horseback ride from farmhouse to farmhouse collecting chickens and sausages to add to a community gumbo. Participants enjoy beer, boudin, and faire le maque ("make like a monkey," or clowning around) at each stop. During the rest of the year, Cajuns sponsor many local celebrations, such as the crawfish, rice, and yam festivals.

French Americans, like their French ancestors, serve meat pies on religious holidays. The special pie for Easter has sliced hard-boiled eggs laid down on the bottom crust and then a layer of cooked meat topped with seasoned pork and beef meatballs. For Christmas, tourtière, a pie made with simmered seasoned pork, is eaten cold after midnight Mass.

Food waste is also a focus. France has paved the way for reducing waste, according to the Food Sustainability Index in 2022, which ranks how well countries with the largest global economies are performing with regard to food waste, agricultural sustainability, and nutrition challenges. France received the highest score largely due to public policy shifts. They made it illegal for its supermarkets to throw out food that's nearing its expiration date, instead requiring stores to either compost or donate the groceries. They also banned expiration dates on certain categories of goods such as wine and vinegar which don't necessarily signify food spoilage, and issued incentives for supermarkets to start selling "ugly" produce (those that may be misshaped or bruised) at lower prices. They are also leading the way in using food waste as fuel.[30,31]

Food for Thought

Cornish pasties are still popular in parts of the country where immigrants from Cornwall came to work in the mines, such as the Upper Peninsula in Michigan, where May 24 was declared Pasty Day in 1968.

Nutritional Status

The influence of the British and French on American cuisine is undoubtedly one reason the U.S. diet is high in cholesterol and fat and low in fiber and complex carbohydrates. Current research in Europe suggests continuing similarities. A survey of dietary habits found that consumption of potatoes, animal protein, processed foods, margarine and butter, and sweets is relatively high in the United Kingdom.[24,25] Obesity rates have doubled in France during the last 25 years. In France, the consumption of added animal fats and oils is high.[39,41] The estimated 2020 prevalence of overweight and obese adults in France is 50 percent and 17 percent, respectively, and in the United Kingdom the percentages are 63 percent and 28 percent, respectively.[32,33] More than half of all UK adults (63%) are classified as being overweight or obese, which is over 35 million people.

Parental role modeling was shown to be a predictor for the intake of sweet and fatty foods in children in northern Europe. Parents act as the gatekeepers for home food availability and for European children's eating behaviors and dietary patterns.[35]

Although few studies have been conducted on the nutritional status of Americans who are of French, Irish, and British descent, it is assumed that they have the same nutritional advantages and disadvantages as the general U.S. population. The lifestyle habits of these countries have deteriorated over time. Although there have been interventions to improve blood pressure and lipid management, they are still not optimally controlled despite the use of evidence-based medications (statins). More innovative lifestyle medicine programs would be beneficial to these populations.[36]

Nutritional Intake Very little has been reported on the diets of northern Europeans living in the United States. A classic study to determine differences in mortality from coronary heart disease examined Irish brothers—one group in Ireland, one group living in the United States (Boston)—and a third control group of first-generation Irish Americans in Boston.[37] Although there was no significantly different relative risk for death from heart disease among the three groups, it was found that their diets varied significantly. The Boston brothers and the first-generation Irish Americans had a higher intake (as a percentage of caloric intake) of animal protein, total fat (more vegetable and less animal), sugar, fiber, and cholesterol, and a lower intake of starch. The brothers in Ireland had a higher caloric intake than the Boston brothers and the first-generation Irish Americans, yet their relative weight was significantly lower.

Another concern especially for Northern Europeans is hemochromatosis, an inherited disorder characterized by excessive dietary iron absorption, that can lead to severe iron overload.[38] Prevalence for hereditary hemochromatosis, which may be treated with a low-iron diet (and avoidance of alcohol and foods or supplements high in vitamin C), is higher in northern Europeans. In individuals of Northern European descent, the prevalence is estimated to be as high as 1 in 227 individuals in the general population. Though it is hypothesized that the gene for the disease is Celtic in origin, a study of French Canadians also noted a high prevalence rate.[39] (It should be noted that hemochromatosis is often undetected in these populations, and may not show overt clinical symptoms until middle or late adulthood.)

Another concern was found in a classic study on inherited chylomicronemia which indicates that the frequency of this lipoprotein lipase deficiency is very high among French Canadians.[40] Franco-Americans may also have high rates of this genetic defect, leading to elevated triglycerides and the necessity of a very low-fat diet.

The 2015 National Diet and Nutrition Survey confirms that the UK population continues to consume more than the recommended amount of saturated fat and not enough fruit, vegetables, and fiber:[39]

- average saturated fat intake for adults (19- to 64-year-olds) is 12.5% of daily calorie intake, above the 11% recommended maximum
- adults consume on average 4.2 portions of fruit and vegetables per day, 65- to 74-year-olds consume 4.3 portions and teenagers consume just 2.7 portions per day

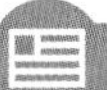

New American Perspectives

Irish

John Casey, Retired

I came to the United States in 1956 from Ireland when I was 26 years old. I first lived in New York City where plenty of other Irish live. When I left Ireland, it wasn't as well-off as it is now, and food was not plentiful, and it was mostly grown locally. You raised pigs and killed two a year, and that provided the bacon for the rest of the year. The foods we ate every day were bread, butter, milk, and eggs. My dad owned a food shop, so we had a bit more of other foods. When I came to America, I was overwhelmed by the amount of food available and all the different types. I had never had juice with breakfast, didn't know what a grapefruit was—thought it was a very big lemon. Other foods that I tried for the first time were watermelon, turkey, hamburgers, corn on the cob, and French fries. I like all of them except the watermelon.

In Ireland the main meal of the day was lunch, and what we usually had was all boiled together, like a New England boiled dinner but without as much meat and usually no meat. On sick days we got toast and tea. But the bread was only toasted on one side. When I first got toast here, it was toasted on both sides, and I wasn't sure if you buttered both sides as well. The three biggest holidays in Ireland are Christmas, Easter, and St. Patrick's Day. Christmas was the biggest feast day—bacon, eggs, and sausage for breakfast, and for the main meal, we had goose with dressing and mashed potatoes, plus custard for dessert. For Easter we often had mutton, and the children—if it was affordable—got chocolate Easter eggs, just like here. St. Patrick's Day wasn't as much fun because it fell during Lent, and the pubs were closed.

I eat a lot of different foods now, more than I did when I was younger, and I like Chinese and German food, but I miss Irish bacon. My grandchildren are still trying to get me to order different flavors of ice cream, but I will only eat vanilla. When I first came to America, Ireland didn't have enough food, and Americans ate too much. Today, both the Irish and Americans eat too much.

- only 31% of adults, 32% of 65- to 74-year-olds, and 8% of teenagers meet the 5 A Day recommendation for fruit and vegetables
- average fiber intake in adults is 19 g per day, well below the recommended 30 g per day.

In France, food and nutrition consumption habits have been changing.[41] In a study on the food consumption and eating habits of the French population (conducted in 2014–2015) noted that French people consume around 2200 kcal, 50% of which comes from beverages. They are consuming more processed foods than in previous years, significantly more food supplements, more salt, and not enough fiber. Physical activity has declined for a large part of the population, and time spent in front of screens every day (outside of working hours) continues to rise, with an average increase over the last seven years of 20 minutes for children, and 1 hour and 20 minutes for adults.

The British, Irish, and French all tend to be more formal than Americans, and politeness is expected. Socioeconomic status and religious practice are likely to have a greater impact on foods and food habits than the country of origin.

Southern Europeans

Southern European countries lie along the Mediterranean Sea and include Italy, southern France, Spain, and Portugal. Italy, shaped like a boot, sticks out into the Mediterranean and includes the island of Sicily, which lies off the boot toe. Italy is separated from the rest of Europe by the Alps, which form its northern border. Spain, located to the west of France (the Pyrenees Mountains form a natural border between the two countries), occupies the majority of the Iberian Peninsula. Portugal sits on the western end of the peninsula and includes the Azore and Madeira Islands located in the Atlantic Ocean (the Cape Verde Islands were formerly Portuguese territory, but they gained independence in 1975). Most of southern Europe enjoys a warm Mediterranean climate except in the cooler mountainous regions.

Immigration to the United States from southern Europe has been considerable, primarily from poorer regions of southern Italy. Many Americans enjoy Italian cuisine in some form. The foods of Spain and Portugal are similar to those of Italy and France due to the shared climate and history of Greek and Roman influence in the region, but their preparations differ. One difference between these world cuisines is the fats used in cooking: historically, the use of butter or oil in cooking is closely linked to the climate. Unclarified butter spoils quickly in warm regions, and is impractical compared to olives, for example, made into oil as a cooking fat. Bread and butter are a classic pairing in the United Kingdom, as bread dipped into extra virgin olive oil is on Italian or Spanish tables (as well as in other countries around the Mediterranean Sea). The following section reviews the traditional diets of Italy, Spain, and Portugal. The influence of these cuisines on U.S. fare is also discussed.

Cultural Perspective

History of Southern Europeans in the United States

Immigration Patterns The majority of immigrants from southern Europe were Italians, who swelled the population of U.S. cities on the Eastern Seaboard during the late nineteenth and early twentieth centuries. Next in number were the Portuguese, primarily from the Azore Islands. Smaller numbers of Spanish immigrants have been reported.

Italians According to immigration records, more than 5 million Italians have settled in the United States. The majority came from the poorer southern Italian provinces between 1880 and 1920. Although earlier immigrants from northern Italy settled on the West Coast of the United States during the gold rush, most of these later immigrants settled in the large industrial cities on the East Coast. Many Italians who arrived faced discrimination and hostility, and, in response, formed concentrated communities within urban centers, often called Little Italies.[42] Several cities still boast Italian neighborhoods such as the North End in Boston and North Beach in San Francisco.

Many Italians came to the United States for economic reasons; more than one-half of the immigrants, mostly men, returned to their homeland after accumulating sufficient money. Italians in the United States often became laborers in skilled or semiskilled professions, especially the building trades and the clothing industry. Immigration from Italy fell sharply after World War I; however, more than 1.6 million Italians have immigrated since World War II.[43,44] The 2019 American Community Survey estimates that over 16.1 million Americans claim Italian descent.[4]

Spaniards More than one-quarter of a million people from Spain have immigrated to the United States since 1820. However, the majority of the Spanish-speaking population in the United States comes from the U.S. acquisition of Spanish territories and the immigration of people from Latin American countries (refer to Chapters 9 and 10 for more detail).

Food for Thought

Among the Basques, it is said that the devil once came to the region to learn their language, Euskera, so that he could entrap the inhabitants. He gave up after seven years when he was able to master only two words: *bai* and *ez* ("yes" and "no").

There are approximately 1.5 million Canadians of Italian ancestry, according to the 2016 Census figures.

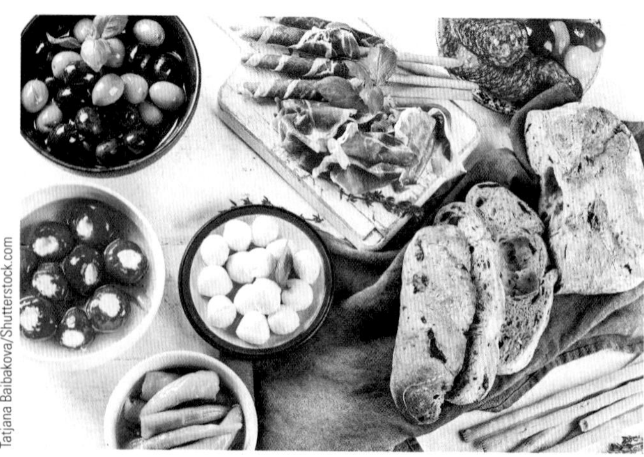

Tatjana Baibakova/Shutterstock.com

▲ Traditional foods of southern Europe particularly Italy include olives, peperoncini, fresh mozzarella balls, artisanal bread, fresh vegetables and salami (cured sliced meats) including proscuitto.

The earliest Spanish settlers arrived during colonial times, establishing populations in what is now Florida, New Mexico, California, Arizona, Texas, and Louisiana. A majority were from the poorest regions of southern Spain and the Canary Islands.[45] Half of all other Spanish immigrants to the United States came later in the nineteenth and early twentieth centuries, due to depressed economic conditions in Spain. In 1939, after the fall of the second Spanish republic, a small number of refugees immigrated for political reasons.

Additional Spanish immigrants were from the Basque region, located in northeastern Spain on the border with France (there are also French Basques). The Basques are thought to be one of the oldest surviving ethnic groups in Europe; they lived in their homeland before the invasion of the Indo-Europeans around 2000 BCE. Their language, Euskera, is not known to be related to any other living language. Though the earliest Basque immigrants to the United States were fishermen and whalers who probably arrived before Columbus, most came in the mid-nineteenth century, arriving first in California for the gold rush, then spreading north and east throughout the West. Many emigrated from South America, where they had first settled, and were listed as Chileans (the umbrella term used for all South Americans at the time). An accurate estimate of their numbers is impossible.[46]

Portuguese Over 1.3 million Portuguese Americans live in the United States.[4,48] Beginning in the early nineteenth century, two waves of Portuguese immigrants arrived in the United States. Early immigrants were primarily from the Azore Islands and Cape Verde Islands, and they were often located in the whaling ports of New England and Hawaii. They were followed in the 1870s by immigrants hoping to escape poverty. They arrived with little education and few skills but were willing to do farm labor in California and Hawaii and work in the service trades of northeastern cities.

After World War II, a small number of Portuguese from Macao, a Portuguese settlement on the coast of China near Hong Kong, settled in California. A much more significant number of Portuguese, more than 150,000, entered the United States after 1958, again mostly from the Azore Islands, following a series of volcanic eruptions that devastated the region. Since 1965 over 210,000 Portuguese have immigrated to the United States.

Current Demographics and Socioeconomic Status

Italians In 2019, there were over 16 million Americans of Italian descent in the United States, most of whom live in or around major cities.[4] Economic conditions improved during the 1980s in Italy, and immigration from the nation slowed significantly.

Economically, Italian Americans shared in the general prosperity after World War II, and today most are employed in white-collar jobs or as skilled laborers. Four generations of Italians living in the United States have been identified. Older adults living in urban Italian neighborhoods are one group; those who are middle-aged and living in either urban or suburban settings are the second group;

the well-educated younger Italian Americans of subsequent generations living mostly in suburban areas are the third group; and the very recent immigrants from Italy are the fourth.[47] These groupings can be expected to change as each group ages and experiences increased assimilation: only 20 percent of Italian Americans born after 1940 married other Italian Americans.

Spaniards People who report Spanish or Spanish American heritage numbered over 1.2 million in the 2010 U.S. Census estimates and are now grouped with Hispanics in the U.S. Census.[4] Seven percent were born in Spain. Most are well integrated into their communities, and larger populations are found in New York and Tampa, Florida. A distinctive group of Isleños, descendants of Canary Island immigrants, is found in southern Louisiana. The Basques settled mostly in the rural regions of California, Nevada, Idaho, Montana, Wyoming, Colorado, New Mexico, and Arizona and became ranchers. Some Basque immigrants, however, were drawn to the mining jobs of West Virginia and the rubber and steel plants of Ohio, Illinois, Michigan, and Pennsylvania.[4] Although the 2008 Census estimates report 58,000 Basque Americans, it is thought that this number may underrepresent the total population, which may be as high as 100,000. Today, most Basque descendants are involved in some aspect of animal husbandry or small business; few have entered other professions. Newer Basque communities now exist in Connecticut and Florida and jai alai (a Basque sport) facilities were established there.

Portuguese As of 2019, over 1.3 million Americans were of Portuguese descent.[4] In 2000, 50,000 claimed Cape Verdean ancestry and 4,000 reported Azore Islands heritage. (Immigrants from the Cape Verde and Azore Islands and those from Madeira may not feel Portuguese. Instead, they identify with their island or city of origin.) Initially, the Portuguese Americans on the West Coast were farmers and ranchers, but eventually, their descendants moved into professional, technical, and administrative positions.[48] On the East Coast, the descendants of the Portuguese who settled in the whaling ports now make up a significant part of the fishing industry, though only 3 percent of all Portuguese Americans work in this occupation. The percentage of Portuguese families living in poverty is half that of the U.S. average.

Worldview

Religion

Italians In Italy, the Roman Catholic Church was traditionally a part of everyday life. Immigrants to the United States, however, found the church to be more remote and puritanical, as well as staffed by the Irish. The church responded by establishing national parishes (parishes geared toward one ethnic group with a priest from that group) that helped immigrants adjust to the United States. Some religious festivals, part of daily spiritual life in Italy, were transferred to the United States and are still celebrated today, such as the Feast of San Gennaro in New York's Little Italy.

Spaniards Most Spaniards are Roman Catholic. The Jesuit Order was founded in Basque country—a region in both Spain and France bordering the Bay of Biscay and encompassing the western foothills of the Pyrenees—and has significantly influenced Basque devotion. Basque Americans, many of whom live in California and Idaho (the largest concentration of Basque Americans live in Boise), are involved in their parishes, and there is the expectation that religion is part of daily life and sacrifice.

Portuguese The Roman Catholic Church also helped the Portuguese ease into the mainstream of U.S. life. Local churches and special parishes often sponsor traditional religious fiestas that include Portuguese foods, dances, and colorful costumes.

Food for Thought

Boise, Idaho is considered the Basque capital of the United States because of its concentration of Basque residents.

Family

Italians The social structure of rural villages in southern Italy was based on the family, whose interests and needs molded each individual's attitudes toward the state, church, and school. The family was self-reliant and distrusted outsiders. Each member was expected to uphold family honor and fulfill familial responsibilities. The father was head of the household; he maintained his authority with strict discipline. The mother, although subordinate, controlled the day-to-day activities in the home and was often responsible for the family budget. Once in the United States, the children broke free of parental control due to economic necessity. Although sons had always been allowed some independence, daughters soon gained freedom, as well, because they were expected to work outside the home like their brothers. Education eventually also changed the family. Early immigrants repeatedly denied their children schooling, sending them to work instead. However, by 1920, education was considered an important stepping-stone for Italian Americans.

Spaniards In the traditional Spanish family, the father spent much of his time working and socializing outside the home, while the mother devoted her life to her children. Typically, one daughter would choose not to marry and would care for her aging parents. In the United States, Spanish American families are usually limited to immediate members, although the obligation to parents remains stronger than for most Americans. An elder may live part of the year with one child, then part of the year with another child. Independent living and retirement homes are also common. The Basque family was customarily an extended one. Basques in Spain are prohibited from marrying non-Basques, but in the United States, many Basques marry other nationalities, who are generally well accepted by the family.

Spanish women hold unique status among southern Europeans. Class distinctions are more important than gender when it comes to educational and professional attainment. Basque women are historically recognized for their equality. Since ancient times, their duties have been as valued as those of men, and jobs are often not gender-specific.

Food for Thought

An Italian proverb states that after age 40, a person can "expect a new pain every morning."

Some Italians believe that wine mixed with milk in the stomach causes too much acid, so milk is avoided at meals and consumed mostly with snacks.

The market for processed pasta sauce in the United States is over $3 billion annually.[49]

The Spanish word tortilla, or "small cake," describes a type of potato omelet. In Mexico and Central America, tortillas made with maize flour are a staple food that has gained popularity in the United States and other places around the world. It is believed that the Spanish called the Mexican bread by that name because of its similar round shape.[50]

Portuguese Like the Italians, the Portuguese have close family solidarity and have had some success in maintaining the traditional family structure. Grown sons and daughters often live near their parents, and family members try to care for the sick at home. Family structure is threatened, however, when women work outside the home and as generational values change. Men tend to dominate the family, and, as a result, some Portuguese American women marry outside the group.

Traditional Health Beliefs and Practices Traditional Italian health beliefs include concepts common in the American majority culture as well as concerns associated with folk medicine. Fresh air is believed necessary to health, and some older Italian Americans maintain that the heavy air—damp, unpleasantly still—of the United States is considered unhealthy compared to the light air—which sailors define as having a wind speed of 1 to 3 miles per hour—of Italy. Well-being is defined as the ability to pursue normal, daily activities. There is the expectation that health declines with age.[47]

Traditional Food Habits

Although the foods of the southern European countries are similar, as detailed in the cultural food groups list in Table 6.3, there are notable differences in preparation and presentation. Many Americans think of Italian cooking as consisting of pizza and spaghetti. In reality, these dishes are only a small part of the regional cuisine of southern Italy, the original homeland of most Italian Americans. Spanish food is sometimes mistakenly equated with the cuisine of Mexico. Although Mexico was a colony of Spain, the foods and food habits of the two countries differ substantially. Portugal and Spain have very similar cuisines, but most of the Portuguese immigrants to the United States are from the Azore Islands and the island of Madeira, with a cuisine focus on seafood, tropical fruit, cheeses, soups, and stews such as cozido, traditionally cooked in holes dug into hot volcanic soil.

Ingredients and Common Foods

The Phoenicians and Greeks, who settled along the Mediterranean coast in ancient times, are believed to have brought olive trees and chickpeas (garbanzo beans) to the region. In addition, fish stew, known as bouillabaisse in France and zuppa di pesce alla marinara in Italy, may be of Greek origin. Arab traders brought eggplants, lemons, oranges, sugarcane, rice, and a variety of sweetmeats and spices to the region from India. Marzipan, a sweetened almond paste used extensively in Italian desserts, and rice flavored with saffron, as in the northern Italian dish risotto alla Milanese, are both believed to have Persian culinary origins, and the word saffron is thought to be Arab, meaning "to turn yellow." The origin of marzipan is disputed and claims on the confection range from China and Persia to Germany, depending on how far back the history is searched. In Spain, the influence of the Persian food exchange is also seen in saffron-seasoned rice and the use of ground nuts in sauces, candies, and other desserts.

Food for Thought

Olive oil is labeled according to the method of processing: extra virgin, virgin, or pure. In the United States, only the oils derived from the first press of the olives can be called virgin or extra virgin depending on their acidity (extra virgin is lower). A blend of olive oil, produced by refining which does not alter its fat structure, as well as virgin olive oils, must be labeled "pure."

Because of its rich source of tocopherols, carotenoids, and polyphenols, which have anti-inflammatory properties, olive oil has been shown to provide cardiovascular and anti-cancer effects. Italy, Spain, and Greece are major producers of olive oil and it is the principal source of dietary fat in these countries. However, not all olives or olive oils are created equally. An olive oil label may say that it is produced in a particular country when, in fact, it was only bottled there. For example, "Product of Italy" does not necessarily indicate that the olives are grown or pressed in Italy—only that it was bottled there. Look for the phrase "Produced and Bottled," which means that the oil is produced and bottled in the place of origin listed on the label. Certain olive varieties — Coratina and Moraiolo from Italy, Cornicabra and Picual from Spain, and Koroneiki from Greece — have the very highest levels of polyphenols. While olive oil is a wonderful source of heart-healthy monounsaturated fats, it does not age well. Antioxidant levels in olive oil may decrease by

Table 6.3 Cultural Food Groups: Southern European

Group	Comments	Common Foods	Adaptations in the United States
Protein Foods			
Milk/milk products	Most adults do not drink milk but do eat cheese. Dairy products are often used in desserts. Many adults suffer from lactose intolerance.	Cheese (cow, sheep, buffalo, goat), milk	It is assumed that second- and third-generation southern Europeans drink more milk into their adulthood than their ancestors did.
Meat/poultry/fish/eggs/legumes	Dried salt cod is eaten frequently. Small fish, such as sardines, are eaten whole, providing substantial dietary calcium.	*Meat:* beef, goat, lamb, pork, veal (and most variety cuts *Poultry:* chicken, duck, goose, pigeon, turkey, woodcock *Fish:* anchovies, bream, cod, haddock, halibut, herring, mullet, salmon, sardines, trout, tuna, turbot, whiting, octopus, squid *Shellfish:* barnacles, clams, conch, crab, lobster, mussels, scallops, shrimp *Eggs:* chicken *Legumes:* chickpeas, fava and kidney beans, lentils, lupine seeds, white beans	More meat and less fish are eaten than in Europe.
Cereals/Grains	Bread, pasta, or grain products usually accompany the meal.	Cornmeal, rice, wheat (bread, farina, a variety of pastas)	
Fruits/Vegetables	Fruit is often eaten as dessert. Fresh fruits and vegetables are preferred.	*Fruit:* apples, apricots, bananas, cherries, citron, dates, figs, grapefruit, grapes, lemons, medlars, peaches, pears, pineapples, plums (prunes), pomegranates, quinces, oranges, raisins, Seville oranges, tangerines *Vegetables*: arugala, artichokes, asparagus, broccoli, cabbage, cardoon, cauliflower, celery, chicory, cucumber, eggplant, endive, escarole, fennel, green beans, lettuce, kale, kohlrabi, mushrooms, mustard greens, olives, parsnips, peas, peppers (green and red), pimentos, potatoes, radicchio, swiss chard, tomatoes, turnips, zucchini	First- and second-generation southern Europeans generally eat only fresh fruits and vegetables. Fruit and vegetable consumption tends to reflect general American food habits by the third generation.
Additional Foods			
Seasonings	Dishes using similar ingredients in Italy, Spain, and Portugal often differentiated by distinctive use of herbs and spices. Seasoning in Azore Islands and Cape Verde Islands is usually very mild.	Basil, bay leaf, black pepper, capers, cayenne pepper, chocolate, chervil, cinnamon, cloves, coriander, cumin, dill, fennel, garlic, leeks, lemon juice, marjoram, mint, mustard, nutmeg, onion, oregano, parsley (Italian and curley leaf), rosemary, saffron, sage, tarragon, thyme, vinegar	
Nuts/seeds	Nuts commonly used in desserts and added to some entrees and side dishes.	Almonds, hazelnuts, pignolis (pine nuts), walnuts, lupine seeds	
Beverages		Coffee, chocolate, liqueurs, port, Madeira, sherry, flavored sodas (e.g., orzata), tea, wine	
Fats/oils	Olive oil flavors numerous dishes; used for deep-frying in Spain.	Butter, lard, olive oil, vegetable oil	Use of olive oil has decreased.
Sweeteners		Honey, sugar	

40 percent after six months of storage. Olive oil does not have a high smoke point, so for cooking foods that require a high amount of heat, another oil with a higher smoke point may be better.[51]

Food for Thought

The Italians eat more rice than any other Europeans. Thomas Jefferson supposedly smuggled rice out of Italy to the United States, where his first attempts to cultivate it were unsuccessful.

Espresso, which comes from the Italian *esprimere*, meaning to express or to press out, is made from finely ground dark roast coffee through which water is forced by steam pressure. Cappuccino is espresso topped with frothy steamed milk.

"Cods' tongues," a delicacy, are an especially succulent strip of meat from inside the fish's mouth; they are not actually tongues.

Fresh pasta can sometimes be found in U.S. grocery stores next to the cold-cut meat and cheese section.

It was the food of the New World colonies, however, that shaped much of Italian, Spanish, and Portuguese cuisine. Chocolate, vanilla, tomatoes, avocados, chili peppers, pineapple, white and sweet potatoes, corn, many varieties of squash, and turkey were brought back from the Americas. The tomato is of particular importance to the character of southern European cooking. Asian ingredients have had a significant impact as well. From India and the Far East came citruses such as lemons and oranges, in addition to coconuts, bananas, mangoes, eggplant, and numerous spices, such as pepper, nutmeg, cinnamon, and cloves.

Staples

Italy Although the cooking styles vary from region to region in Italy, some general statements can be made about ingredients. Pasta, a quintessential dish throughout the nation, is often prepared fresh, from dough made with the addition of eggs, or dried, from a dough usually made without eggs. Increasingly, dried pasta is offered at grocery stores throughout the country. Regardless, fresh or dry pasta is traditionally served three ways: with sauce (asciutta), in soup (en brodo), or baked (al forno). There are hundreds of pasta shapes, such as thin, round strips that include spaghetti (from the Italian word for "string") and capelli d'angelo (angel hair); flat strips such as linguini and fettucini (ribbon); tubular forms, such as macaroni, penne, and the larger manicotti; and sheets such as lasagna and pappardelle. There are additional forms, such as spirals (e.g., fusilli, rotelle), shells (conchiglie), little ears (orechiette), bowties (farfalle), and small barley- or rice-shaped orzo. One of the most common pastas in Italy is tagliatelle, a medium-width flat noodle.[49]

In the north, stuffed pasta made with bits of meat, cheese, and vegetables, such as ravioli, is especially popular. Pasta in the north is also frequently topped with rich cream sauces, due to the high production of dairy products in the region. In the south, pasta is usually served unfilled with a tomato-based sauce.

Other broad differences are that northern fare uses more butter, dairy products, rice, and meat than the south, which is notable for the use of olive oil, more fish, and more beans and vegetables, such as artichokes, eggplants, bell peppers, and tomatoes. Garlic is found throughout the nation, though it is often more popular in the south. Other seasonings common to all of Italy are parsley, basil, and oregano. Anise, cinnamon, nutmeg, mace, and cloves are also used in many dishes.

Spain The rugged terrain in Spain is suitable for raising small animals and crops such as grapes and olives. Spain is the largest producer of olives in the world. Entrées usually feature eggs, lamb, pork, poultry, or dried and salted fish (especially cod, called bacalao). Eggs are consumed day and night. They are enjoyed fried in olive oil, often topped with migas (fried bread crumbs combined with garlic, bacon, and ham). Tortilla española (potato omelet) is perhaps the national dish, eaten as appetizers, entrées, snacks, and as a filling for bocadillos (sandwiches). Sausages, such as the paprika- and garlic-flavored chorizo and the blood sausage called morilla, are common. The acclaimed Serrano (meaning "from the mountains") ham is a salty, dry-cured meat served in paper-thin slices, similar to Italian prosciutto and French jambon de Bayonne, and made from a specific breed of pig. Seafood is popular in coastal regions. Meats are often combined with vegetables in savory stews. Each region has its own recipe for paella, which typically includes saffron-seasoned rice topped with chicken, mussels, shrimp, sausage, tomatoes, and peas, a delicious blend of several cultures. Cocido, a stew of chickpeas, vegetables (e.g., cabbage, carrots, potatoes), and meats (e.g., beef, chicken, pork, meatballs, sausages), also varies from area to area but is always served in three courses. The strained broth with added noodles is eaten first, followed by a plate of boiled vegetables, and concluded with a plate of cooked meats. Crusty bread is served with the meal.

Garlic and tomatoes flavor many Spanish dishes, for example, gazpacho, a refreshing pureed vegetable soup that is usually served cold, and zarzuela (meaning "operetta"), a fresh seafood stew. Olive oil is also a common ingredient used in almost all cooking, even when deep-frying pastries, such as the ridged, cylindrical doughnuts known as churros. Sauces accompany many dishes. Alioli is made from garlic pulverized with olive oil, salt, and a little lemon juice. It is served with grilled or boiled meats and fish. Alioli is not to be confused with aioli (which is a sauce made up of mayonnaise flavored with a generous amount of garlic). Another popular sauce, called romescu, is sometimes mixed with alioli to each diner's taste at the table. Romescu combines pureed almonds, garlic, paprika, and tomatoes with vinegar and olive oil. Fruit, particularly oranges, is popular for dessert, sometimes served in custard. One favorite is membillo, a quince paste served with slices of a salty sheep's-milk cheese known as Manchego. Spain's best-known dessert is flan, a sweet milk-and-egg custard topped with caramel. Wine usually accompanies the

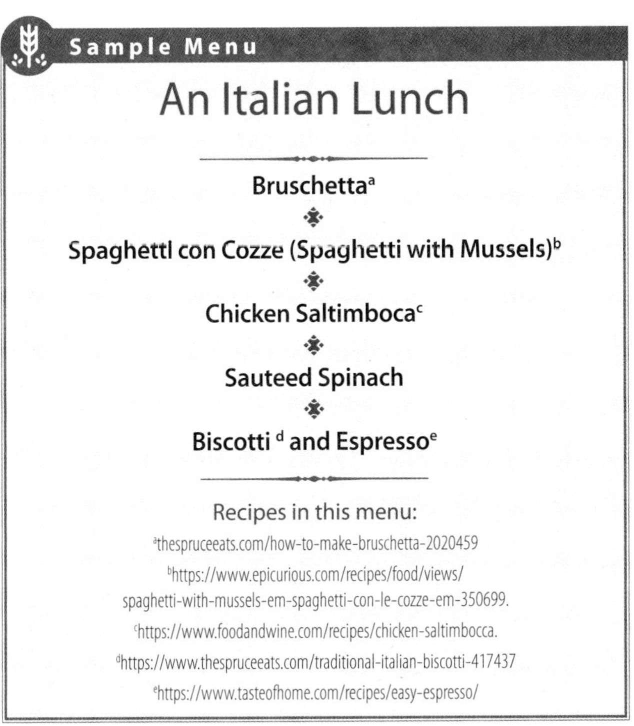

Sample Menu

An Italian Lunch

Bruschetta[a]

Spaghetti con Cozze (Spaghetti with Mussels)[b]

Chicken Saltimboca[c]

Sauteed Spinach

Biscotti [d] **and Espresso**[e]

Recipes in this menu:

[a]thespruceeats.com/how-to-make-bruschetta-2020459

[b]https://www.epicurious.com/recipes/food/views/spaghetti-with-mussels-em-spaghetti-con-le-cozze-em-350699.

[c]https://www.foodandwine.com/recipes/chicken-saltimbocca.

[d]https://www.thespruceeats.com/traditional-italian-biscotti-417437

[e]https://www.tasteofhome.com/recipes/easy-espresso/

meal. Sangria, made with red or white wine and fresh fruit juices, is served chilled in the summer. Spain is probably most famous in the United States for its sherries, which are wines fortified with added brandy. Sherry can be dry or sweet and is categorized by the length of time they are aged. They are often described as having a nutty flavor.

Food for Thought

The word gazpacho may have come from the vinegar, water, and possibly salty herbal drink called posca, reportedly offered to Christ on the cross. The origins of posca might be Greek, but it gained fame from its role as the energy drink of the Roman army. The Roman Republic era (509–27 BCE) rationed posca to its military troops along with grains, and very occasionally, meat and cheese.[52]

Alcohol consumption among the Basques in Spain is high, especially for men.

Portugal Portuguese fare shares some similarities in ingredients with Spanish cuisine, but a more generous addition of herbs and spices, perhaps due to the country's early history in the spice trade from Asia. Particularly, cilantro, mint, and cumin, distinguish the cooking. Fish dominates the diet of the Portuguese; they are said to have as many recipes for bacalao (dried salt cod) as there are days in the year.[53] Sardines are often grilled or cooked in a tomato and vegetable sauce. Lamprey, a cartilaginous fish (having no bones), is a popular food in northern Portugal, where it is often prepared with curry-like seasonings. Shellfish, such as clams, are often combined with pork or other meats in stewed

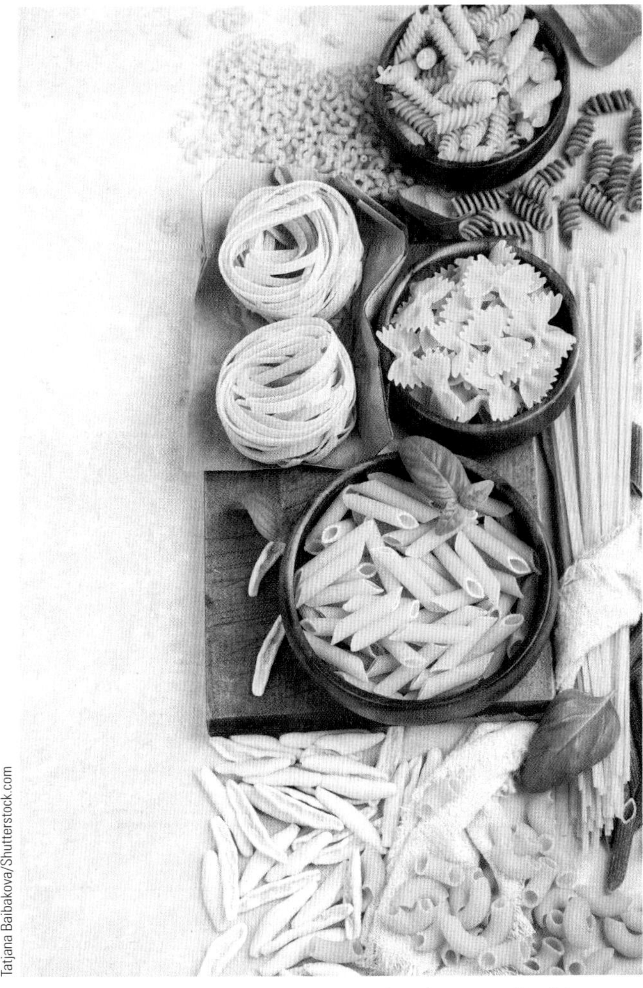

Tatjana Baibakova/Shutterstock.com

▲ **Pasta comes in dozens of forms in Italy, including thin strings, flat ribbons, tubes, spirals, sheets, and shapes that resemble wheels, bowties, little ears, hats, rice, and other shapes.**

dishes. Chouriço, similar to the Spanish pork sausage, chorizo, and linguiça, a pork and garlic sausage, is often eaten at breakfast. Other typical dishes are cacoila, a stew made from pig hearts and liver, then served with beans or potatoes; isca de figado, beef liver seasoned with vinegar, pepper, and garlic, then fried in olive oil or lard; and assada no espeto, meat roasted on a spit. A common soup is caldo verde, or green broth, made from kale or cabbage and potatoes. A unique "dry" soup, açordu, dating to the days of the Moors, is made of bread moistened with oil or vinegar and topped with anything from meat, chicken, or shellfish and vegetables. Fava beans, chickpeas, and lupine seeds (tremocos) are added to some dishes. Rice and fried potatoes are so popular they are often served together. Crusty country bread and, in the north, a cornmeal bread called broa also accompany the meal. Portuguese sweet bread, pan doce, and doughnuts, malassadas, are also specialties. Desserts often feature fruit, such as bananas, grapes, and figs, as well as eggs and almonds. Puddings, custards, and sponge cakes are popular.

Food for Thought

Linguiça comes from the Portuguese word meaning "tongue," a reference to the shape of the sausage.

Sweets were a traditional source of income for Portuguese convents, and the names of many pastries reflect this past, including papas-de-anjo (angel puffs) and gargantas de friera (nun's wattles).[53]

In addition to its culinary uses, basil has a rich history in folklore. In Portugal, basil makes up part of a gift to a sweetheart on certain religious days, for the Greeks and later Romans, basil at one point was associated with hatred; to sow it well required swearing and ranting. Later, basil became a symbol of love in Italy and other nations. In ancient Egypt, basil is found in tombs, evidence it was used as part of the embalming process. It is thought to have originated in India, where it is associated with eternal love and also used in ancient medical practices of Ayurveda, or some feel basil may have come from even farther east, the Hunan province of China.[54]

Forks were originally thought to be the instrument of the devil in Italy when the prevailing etiquette was ritualized hand washing at the table with scented water to eat with clean hands. The first dining forks were used by the ruling class in the Middle East and the Byzantine Empire. When Maria Argyropoulina, niece of the Byzantine emperor, was married to the son of the Doge of Venice in 1004 CE, she brought a small case of two-pronged golden forks to Italy, which she used at her wedding feast. The Venetians, used to eating with their hands, were shocked, and when Maria died two years later of the plague, Saint Peter Damian proclaimed it was God's punishment for using the fork.[55]

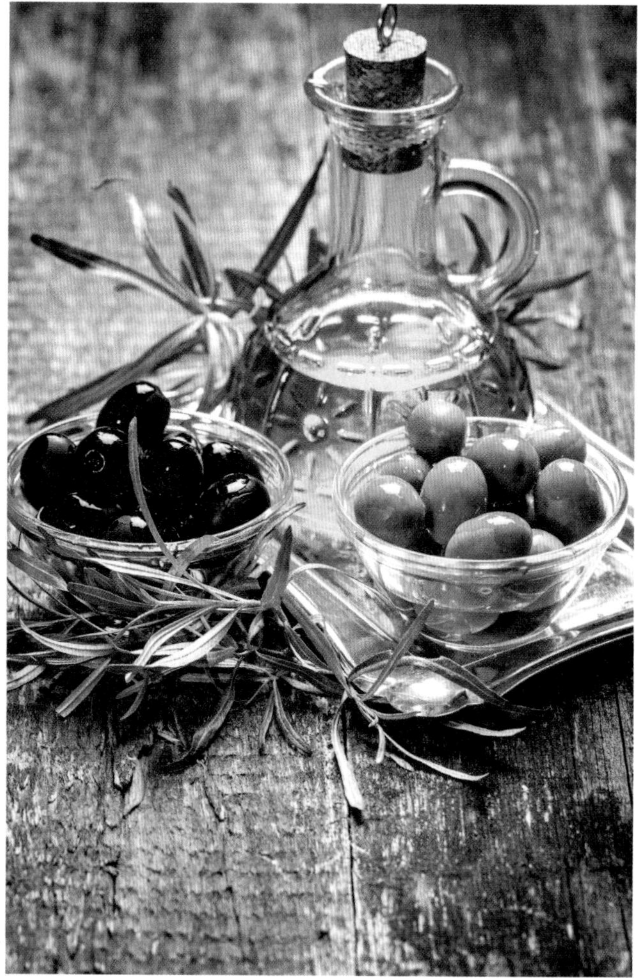

ld-art/Shutterstock.com

▲ Olives and olive oil are found in numerous southern European dishes. Spain is the primary producer of olives worldwide.

Regional Variations

Italy Some of the regional specialties in the northern area of Lombardy, around Milan, are risotto, a creamy rice dish cooked in butter and chicken stock, flavored with Parmesan cheese and saffron; polenta, cornmeal mush (thought to have been made originally from semolina wheat), often served with cheese or sauce; and panettone, a type of fruitcake. Veal is very popular, served in the stew known as osso buco and in veal piccata (chops that are pounded very thin, then breaded and pan-fried, topped with lemon juice, capers, and minced parsley). The cheeses of the region include Gorgonzola, a tangy, blue-veined cheese made from sheep's milk, and bel paese, a soft, mild-flavored cheese. The area is also known for its aperitifs, such as bittersweet vermouth.

Venice, located on the east coast and comprised of about 177 canals and 120 islands, has a cuisine centered on seafood. Its best-known dish is scampi, made from large shrimp seasoned with oil, garlic, parsley, and lemon juice. Inland is Verona, famous for its delicate white wines, such as Soave. Turin, the capital of the western province of Piedmont, is known for its grissini, the slender breadsticks popular throughout Italy, and bagna cauda (meaning "hot bath"), a dip for raw vegetables consisting of anchovies and garlic blended into a paste with olive oil or butter. A summer favorite is vitello tonnato, braised veal served cold with a spicy tuna sauce. Located on the northwest coast of Italy, Genoa is known for its burrida, a fish stew containing octopus and squid, and pesto, a fresh herb, cheese, and nut paste (usually made with basil), which has become popular in the United States.

Moving westward, the city of Bologna is the center of a rich gastronomic region known as Emilia-Romagna. Pasta favorites of the area include lasagne verdi al forno, spinach-flavored lasagna noodles baked in a ragu (a meat sauce typically made with four different types of meat and red wine), and a white sauce, flavored with cheese; and tortellini, egg pasta stuffed with bits of meat, cheese, and eggs, served in soup or a rich cream sauce. A similar stuffed pasta is cappelleti, named for its shape, a little hat. Cured meats are a specialty of the region, including salami and sopressata (dry-cured pork salami); mortadella (pork sausage made of finely hashed meat and small cubes of fat flavored with herbs); pancetta (salt-cured unsmoked pork belly); prosciutto (uncooked, unsmoked, dry-cured ham served thinly sliced); and culatello (an extremely tender deep red center-cut ham also served thinly sliced). Parmesan cheese, a sharply flavored cow's milk cheese with a finely grained texture, also comes from the area, as does aceto balsamico di Modena (or di Reggio Emilia), a vinegar made from white Trebbiano wine grapes. When labeled tradiziolone, it means the vinegar has been fermented and aged in wood casks for at least 12 years, which intensifies and sweetens the flavor, and thickens it into a syrupy consistency. Those labeled condimento are vinegar blends with reduced aging.

Florence, the capital of Tuscany, has a long history of culinary expertise. In 1533, Catherine de' Medici (of the Medici family controlling Florence from 1434 to 1737, with two brief lapses) married into the royal family of France. She is often credited with introducing Italian fare—at the time the most sophisticated cuisine in Europe—to France. The term *alla Fiorentina* refers to a dish garnished with or containing finely chopped spinach. Whole grilled fish and wild game dishes are popular in the region and rosemary flavors many dishes. Tuscany is also famous for its full-bodied red wine, Chianti, and its use of chestnuts, which are featured in a cake eaten at Lent called castagnaccio alla Fiorentina.

Rome, the capital of Italy, has its own regional cooking and is well-known for carbonara, pasta made with eggs, hard cheese such as pecorino Romano, or Parmigiano-Reggiano or both, cured pork and black pepper. Another dish is saltimbocca (meaning "jumps in the mouth")—thin slices of veal rolled with ham and cooked in butter and Marsala wine. Gnocchi, or dumplings typically made with potatoes, flour, and eggs, are eaten throughout Italy, but in Rome, they are made out of semolina and baked in the oven. Fried artichokes are popular at Easter time, as is roast baby lamb or kid. Pecorino Romano is the hard sheep's milk cheese of Rome, similar to Parmesan but with a sharper flavor.

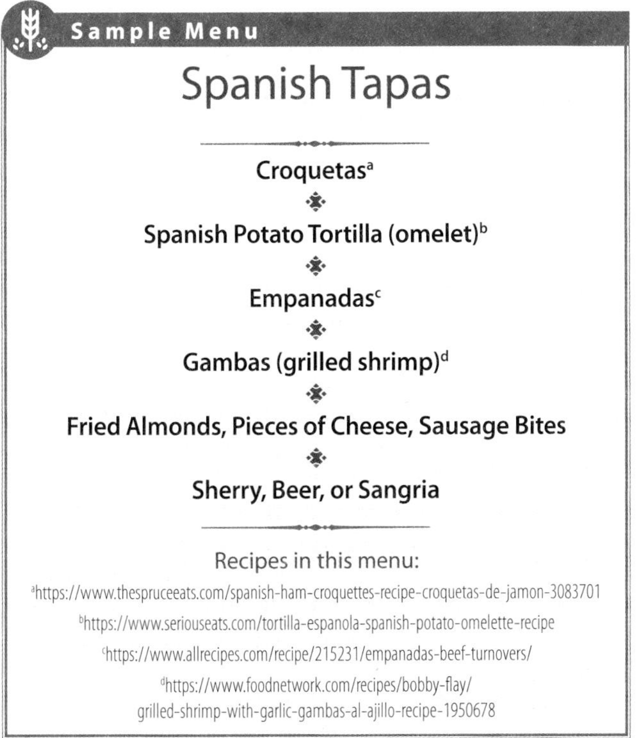

Sample Menu

Spanish Tapas

Croquetas[a]

Spanish Potato Tortilla (omelet)[b]

Empanadas[c]

Gambas (grilled shrimp)[d]

Fried Almonds, Pieces of Cheese, Sausage Bites

Sherry, Beer, or Sangria

Recipes in this menu:

[a]https://www.thespruceeats.com/spanish-ham-croquettes-recipe-croquetas-de-jamon-3083701

[b]https://www.seriouseats.com/tortilla-espanola-spanish-potato-omelette-recipe

[c]https://www.allrecipes.com/recipe/215231/empanadas-beef-turnovers/

[d]https://www.foodnetwork.com/recipes/bobby-flay/grilled-shrimp-with-garlic-gambas-al-ajillo-recipe-1950678

The capital of Campania in southern Italy is Naples, considered the culinary capital of the south. Pasta is the staple food, and a favorite way of serving it is simply with olive oil and garlic, or mixed with beans, in the soup pasta e fagiole. Pizza is native to Naples and is said to date back to the sixteenth century, perhaps originating with toppings for the savory flatbread known as focaccia. Focaccia may have originated in the Etruscan empire before the Roman era. Another form of pizza is calzone, which is pizza dough folded over a filling of cheese, ham, or salami, then baked or fried. The area's best-known cheeses are mozzarella, an elastic white cheese originally made from buffalo milk; provolone, a firm smoked cheese; and ricotta, a soft, white, unsalted cheese made from sheep's milk and often used in desserts. Sicily and other regions of southern Italy use kid and lamb as their principal meats. It is sometimes prepared alla cacciatore (hunter's style), with tomatoes, olives, garlic, wine, or vinegar (and sometimes anchovies)—a method also used with wild boar, venison, and chicken. Along the coast, fresh fish, such as tuna and sardines, are used extensively; baccala, dried salt cod, is often served on fast days. The North African influence shows up in Sicily in the use of couscous, called cuscus in Italy, which is commonly served with fish stews. Southern Italy's cuisine is well known for its desserts. Many examples can be found in Italian American bakeries and espresso bars: cannoli, crisp, deep-fried tubular pastry shells filled with sweetened ricotta cheese, shaved bittersweet chocolate, and citron; cassata, a cake composed of sponge cake layers with a ricotta filling and chocolate- or almond-flavored sugar frosting; gelato, fruit or nut (e.g., black currant or pistachio) ice cream; and granita, intensely flavored ices. Spumoni is chocolate and vanilla ice cream with a layer of rum-flavored whipped cream containing nuts and fruits. Another popular sweet is zeppole, a deep-fried doughnut covered with powdered sugar. The sweet white wine fortified with grape spirits, Marsala, is also a specialty in the region. It develops a deep-tawny color when aged.

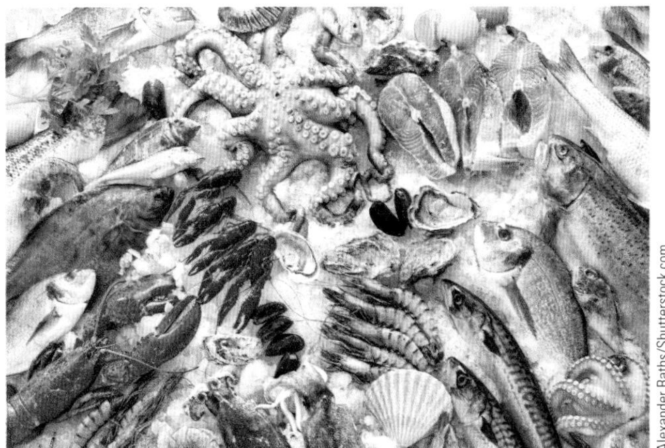

Alexander Raths/Shutterstock.com

▲ **Fish and shellfish are a favorite in Italy, Spain, and Portugal.**

Food for Thought

The art of making ice cream is credited to the Chinese, who brought it to India; from there it spread to the Middle East and eventually to Italy, perhaps when Sicily was an Islamic emirate from 965 to 1072 CE. It was a Sicilian, Francisco Procopio, who introduced ice cream to Paris in the 1660s. The British discovered it soon after and later brought ice cream to America.

During the nineteenth century, Madeira wine from the Portuguese island of the same name was sent to other European nations in the holds of ships where it became very hot. Instead of ruining the wine, it aged it more quickly—Madeira which had circumnavigated the globe twice became popular in England. Today, it is heated during aging to simulate voyage conditions.

Spain The cooking of Spain can be divided broadly by preparation methods. In the north, stewing is most common. In the central regions, roasting is favored. Although deep-fried foods are found in every region of the nation, they are especially popular in the southern regions.[56]

Most Spanish dishes prepared in the United States reflect the cooking of Spain's southern region, with its seafood, abundant fruits and vegetables, and Moorish influence. The Moors, Black Muslims of northwest Africa and the Iberian Penninsula during the medieval era who inhabited present-day Spain, Portugal, the Maghreb, and western Africa, brought many lasting additions to Spanish agriculture and influenced the use of spices, rice, citrus and more in the cuisine. Fried fish, arroz negro (rice blackened with squid ink), and salmorejo (a fresh tomato soup thickened with bread crumbs and garnished with Serrano ham and hard-boiled egg) are popular dishes. In Central Spain, roast suckling pig and baby roast lamb are favorites. Garlic soup starts many meals. In the northwest, fish is common, and often fills empanadas (small pastry turnovers). Octopus flavored with paprika is a specialty. In the Basque provinces, lamb is the primary meat, and charcoal-grilled lamb is a specialty. Seafood, such as bacalao al pil-pil (dried salt cod cooked in olive oil and garlic), bacalao a la vizcaina (dried salt cod cooked in a sauce of onions, garlic, pimento, and tomatoes), and angulas (tiny eel spawn cooked with olive oil, garlic, and red peppers), is a favorite in some Basque areas. Other popular dishes include garlic soup, babarrun gorida (red beans with chorizo), and pipperrada vasca (eggs with peppers). Simple rice puddings or fruit compotes are typical desserts.

Portugal Though Portuguese cuisine varies from north to south, from hearty soups and stews to a lighter style of entrée, the largest regional differences occur between the mainland and the islands. The foods of the Madeiras, Azores, and Cape Verde Islands include tropical ingredients imported from both Africa and the Americas. In Madeira, which attracts many tourists from throughout Europe, avocados, cherimoya, guava, mango, and papaya are featured in its dishes. Corn is common, as is couscous. Honey cakes and puddings reflect the influence of other European nations. In the Azores and Cape Verde Islands, fare varies significantly from island to island and even city to city. Bananas, corn, cherimoya, passion fruit, pineapples, and yams are prominent. Açorda d'azedo is one specialty—a mixture of cornbread, vinegar, onions, garlic, saffron, and a little lard boiled together and eaten for breakfast. Beef is the preferred meat, and seafood, such as cockles, limpets, crab, lobster, and octopus, is eaten in many areas. Little fat or oil is added to dishes; and spicing is mild, often limited to onion, garlic, salt, and pepper. Tea is the preferred beverage. Portugal is famous for its rich sweet wines: Port (from the northern region) and Madeira (from the islands), which are fortified with grape spirits at the start of fermentation. They can be consumed young, or aged for 40 or more years, becoming drier, nuttier, and smoother in flavor. They are popular with dessert or as after-dinner drinks.

Meal Composition and Cycle

Daily Patterns

Italy A traditional Italian breakfast tends to be light, including coffee with milk (caffe latte), tea, or a chocolate drink, accompanied by bread and jam. Lunch is the main meal of the day and may be followed by a rest. It usually starts with an appetizer course of antipasti, such as ham, sausages, pickled vegetables, and olives; or crostini, crispy slices of bread with various toppings, such as tomatoes or cheese. Next, is minestra (wet course), usually soup, or asciutta (dry course) of pasta, risotto, or gnocchi. The main course is fish, meat, or poultry, roasted, grilled, pan-fried, or stewed. It is served with a starchy or green vegetable, followed by a salad. Bread is served with the meal, often with olive oil and balsamic vinegar for dipping. Dessert often consists of fruit and cheese, pastries, or biscotti (crunchy twice-baked cookie slices). Dinner is served at about 7:30 p.m. and is a lighter version of lunch. Wine usually accompanies lunch and dinner. Coffee or espresso is enjoyed after dinner, either at home or in a coffeehouse. Marsala may be served with cheese before the meal for a light appetizer course, or after dinner. It is also often used in the preparation of desserts. One such sweet, now prepared all over Europe, is zabaglione, a wine custard.

Spain By U.S. standards, the Spanish appear to eat all the time. The traditional pattern, four meals plus several snacks, is spread across the day. A light breakfast (desayuno) of coffee or chocolate, bread, or churros is eaten at about 8:00 a.m., followed by a midmorning breakfast around 11:00 a.m. of grilled sausages, fried squid, bread with tomato, or an omelet. A light snack, tapas, is consumed around 1:00 p.m. as a prelude to a three-course lunch (comida) at around 2:00 p.m., consisting of soup or salad, fish or meat, and dessert, which is often followed by fruit and cheese. Many businesses close for several hours in the afternoon to accommodate lunch, the primary meal of the day, and a nap. Tea and pastries (merienda) are eaten between 5:00 and 6:00 p.m. and more tapas are enjoyed at 8:00 or 9:00 p.m. Finally, supper, including three light courses such as soup or omelets and fruit, is consumed between 10:00 p.m. and midnight. Tapas are usually served in bars and cafés and are accompanied by sherry or wine; the variety of tapas is tremendous; it is not unusual for more than twenty kinds to be offered on a menu. They are differentiated from appetizers in Spain in that they are strictly finger foods, such as olives, almonds, croquetas (fried croquettes with fish, ham, cheese, etc.), stuffed mushrooms, shrimp, sausage bits, pieces of cheese, and other small bites. The evening meal may be skipped if a substantial number of tapas are eaten at night.

Portugal Portuguese meal patterns are similar to those of Spain, often starting with the day around 8:00 a.m. with espresso coffee and a roll with marmalade, or pastel de nata, a cinnamon-flavored custard tart in puff pastry. A morning coffee break, including coffee served with hot milk, is followed by lunch in the early afternoon. This is traditionally the largest meal of the day, and even in urban areas often includes several courses. Unlike the Spanish pattern, the evening meal in Portugal is usually eaten earlier. As in Spain, red wine usually accompanies the meal.[48]

Etiquette Italy, Spain, and Portugal share many etiquette rules. The fork remains in the left hand, and the knife remains in the right hand. The knife can be used to help scoop food onto the fork. Bread is not served with butter and should be placed on the edge of the main plate, or next to it on the table. Manners regarding the consumption of pasta include using your fork to twirl the pasta against the edge of the plate or bowl (never use a spoon to help with this) and never slurping. Bread may be used daintily to soak up extra sauce, but should not be used to mop the plate. When not eating, the hands should be kept above the table with the wrists resting on the edge.[55,56]

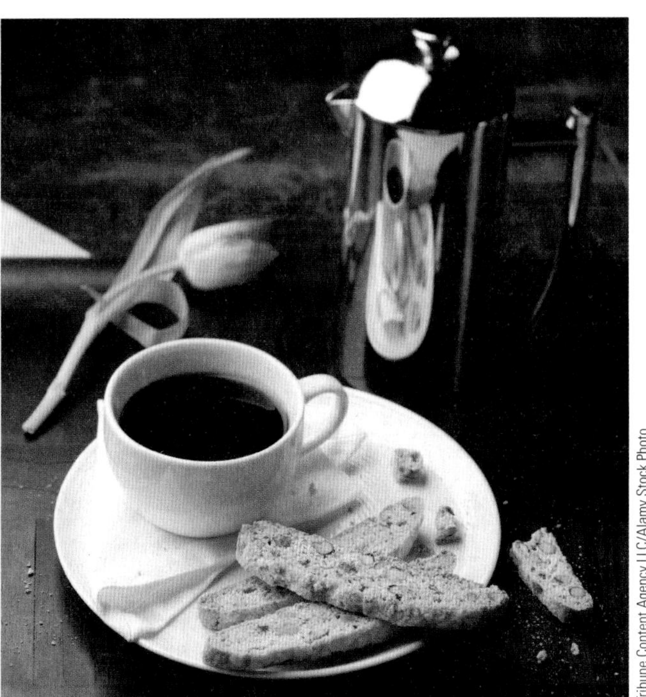

Tribune Content Agency LLC/Alamy Stock Photo

▲ Twice-baked cookies called biscotti are served with coffee or espresso in Italy, often after lunch.

Food for Thought

Legend has it that zabaglione, a custard-like dish made with egg yolks, sugar, and sweet wine and often served with fruit, was created to increase male vigor by a Franciscan monk who tired of hearing the confessional complaints from women about their husbands.

The word tapas comes from the verb *taper,* meaning "to cover" or "lid," and may have first been a simple piece of bread perhaps with a slice of cheese or ham on it used to cover wine glasses to keep out flies. Other accounts say the tradition of small plates originated in the thirteenth century when King Alfonso X insisted that every household in the kingdom should serve a small portion of food alongside alcohol to prevent public drunkenness.

In the 1600s, the Spanish were the first to add sugar to the bitter chocolate beverage native to Mexico. Its popularity spread quickly through Europe, even though certain clerics tried to ban it due to its association with the "heathen" Aztecs. Although the Spanish are fond of chocolate, it is used mostly as a beverage and is rarely added to pastries or confections.

In the Portuguese town Amarante, the Festa de São Gonçalo is held the first weekend in June. Dating back to pre-Christian times, it is traditional for unmarried men and women to exchange phallus-shaped cakes as tokens of their affection for each other.

In rural areas of Portugal, people traditionally collect medicinal plants for home remedies on Quinta-Feira da Espiga (Ear of Wheat Thursday or Ascension Day), the fortieth day after Easter.

When in someone's home, or at a hosted meal, never start eating until the host has said buòn appetito (in Italy), buen apetito (in Spain), or bom appetite (in Portugal). In Italy, when invited to someone's home, it is considered rude to discuss any serious topic before a meal is shared. Chocolates are considered a good hostess gift when invited for dinner in all three nations. In Italy, wine is appreciated if enough is brought for all guests; wine should be avoided as a gift in Spain and Portugal, where hosts have likely chosen favorites to accompany the meal.

Special Occasions

Italy Italy celebrates few national holidays, probably because of its divided history. Most festas are local and honor a patron saint. Other significant religious holidays are usually observed by families at home, although some cities, such as Venice, have a public pre-Lenten carnival. In some areas of the United States where southern Italians predominate, St. Joseph, the patron saint of Sicily, is honored during Lent. Bread in the shape of a cross blessed by the parish priest, pasta with sardines, and other meatless dishes are featured. Among Italian Americans, it is traditional to serve seven seafood dishes on Christmas Eve. During the Easter holidays, Italian American bakeries sell an Easter bread with hard-boiled eggs still in their shells braided into it. Special desserts may accompany the holiday meal, such as panettone, amaretti (almond macaroons), and torrone (nougats) at

Christmastime and cassata (round sponge cake moistened with fruit juice or liqueur and layered with ricotta cheese and candied fruit) at Easter. Colored, sugar-coated Jordan almonds, which the Italians call confetti (meaning "little candies"), are served at weddings.

Spain The most elaborate of Spanish festivals is Holy Week, the week between Palm Sunday and Easter. It is a time of Catholic processions; confections and liqueurs such as coffee, chocolate, and anisette (licorice-flavored) are served. Holiday sweets include tortas de aceite, which are cakes made with olive oil, sesame seeds, and anise; cortados rellenos de cidra, or small rectangular tarts filled with pureed sweetened squash; torteras, or large round cakes made with cinnamon and squash and decorated with powdered sugar; and yemas de San Leandro, which is a sweet made by pouring egg yolks through tiny holes into boiling syrup. It is often served with marzipan.

Special dishes are also prepared for Christmas and Easter. The Basques eat roasted chestnuts and pastel de Navidad, or individual walnut and raisin pies, at Christmas; an orange-flavored doughnut, called causerras, is featured on Easter. At New Year's, it is customary for the Spanish (and the Portuguese) to eat 12 grapes or raisins at the twelve strokes of midnight to bring luck for each month of the coming year.

Portugal Christmas Eve typically features two meals in Portugal: dinner and a post-midnight Mass buffet in the early hours of Christmas morning. Dinner often includes a casserole of bacalhau and potatoes, as well as meringue cookies known as suspiros (sighs). The buffet offers mostly finger foods, such as fried cod puffs and sausages.

In the United States, the Holy Ghost (Spirit) Festival is the most popular and colorful social and religious event in the Portuguese community. It is not widely celebrated in Portugal and probably came to the United States with immigrants from the Azores. Although the origins of the event are obscure, it is believed to date back to Isabel (Elizabeth) of Aragon, wife of Portugal's poet-king Dom Diniz (1326). One story is that the festival derives its character from the belief that because Isabel was particularly devoted to the Holy Ghost, she wanted to give an example of charity in the annual distribution of food to those in need.

The week-long festival is usually scheduled sometime after Easter and before the end of July. It is held at the local church or Hall of the Holy Ghost (also called an IDES Hall, a Portuguese fraternal organization). The main event of the festival takes place on the last day, Sunday, with a procession to the church and the crowning of a queen after the service. The donated food (originally distributed to persons in need on Sunday afternoon but now often served at a free community banquet) is blessed by the priest. The most traditional foods at the feast are a Holy Ghost soup of meat, bread, and potatoes, and a sweet bread called massa sovoda. The bread is sometimes shaped like little doves, called pombas. Also celebrated in the United States is the Feast of the Most Blessed Sacrament, which was started in New Bedford, Massachusetts, by four Madeirans in gratitude for their salvation from a shipwreck en route to the United States in 1915. It attracts over 150,000 visitors on the first weekend in August for music, dancing, and traditional foods such as linguiça, bacalao, fava beans, assada no espeto, and cacoila. The Festa de Sennor da Pedra is held later in the month. This Azore Islands tradition includes a parade and similar traditional foods. Other festivities not mentioned here are associated with the Madeiran cult of Our Lady of the Mount (a shrine on the island of Madeira).

Therapeutic Uses of Food Little has been reported on the therapeutic uses of food by Americans of southern European descent. Some Italians, particularly older immigrants, categorize foods as being heavy or light, wet or dry, and acid or nonacid.[57] Heavy foods, such as fried items and red meats, are considered difficult to digest; light foods, including gelatin, custards, and soups, are regarded as easy to digest and appropriate for people who are ill. Wet and dry refers to how foods are prepared (with or without ample broth or fluid), as well as to their inherent qualities. For example, leafy greens such as escarole, spinach, and cabbage are considered wet. A wet meal is served once a week by some Italian Americans to "cleanse out the system." Wet meals, especially soups, are considered necessary when a person is sick because illness is associated with dryness in the body. Citrus fruits, raw tomatoes, and peaches are thought to be acidic foods that may cause skin ailments and are avoided if such conditions exist.

Other Italian beliefs about foods are that liver, red wine, and leafy vegetables are good for the blood and that too many dairy products make the urine hard (kidney stones). A clove of garlic may be eaten each day to prevent respiratory infections, and raw egg or dandelion greens may be consumed for strength and vitality.[58] Both balsamic vinegar and olive oil, which are served with bread at meals, are believed to be health-promoting foods in Italy.

Contemporary Food Habits in the United States

Adaptations of Food Habits

It is generally assumed that second- and third-generation Americans of southern European descent have adopted the majority American diet and meal patterns, preserving some traditional dishes for special occasions. These assimilated Americans consume more milk and meat but less fish, fresh produce, and legumes than their ancestors. Olive oil is still used often, although not exclusively; pasta remains popular.

Food for Thought

The Spanish American Isleños of Louisiana (an immigrant community from the Canary Islands) marinate shrimp in vinegar with olives and onions, make almond-honey nougat, and use ample olive oil (instead of the butter and lard favored in nearby Cajun cooking).

Descendants of southern Europeans may have a higher incidence of lactose intolerance than other European groups.

Nutritional Status

Nutritional Intake Little research has been conducted on the nutritional intake of southern European Americans. It can be assumed that they suffer from dietary deficiencies and excesses similar to those of the majority of Americans. A study of older Portuguese immigrants in Cambridge, Massachusetts, found that dinner was the main meal of the day, and the subjects had a moderate intake of breads and grains and a low intake of fruits, vegetables, and dairy products. Although dairy intake was low, many of the subjects ate sardines, a rich source of calcium. The subjects reported low consumption of sweets and alcohol, although research indicated that the Americanized Portuguese diet tends to be high in sugar and fat.[34] One study comparing body weights of American and Italian women with polycystic ovary syndrome found that though the BMIs for the American women were significantly higher, the total calorie intake and dietary constituents were similar, suggesting unknown genetic or lifestyle components may play a role.[57]

There are several variations of the Mediterranean diet, depending on the country.[57,60] The term "Mediterranean diet" is a generic term that represents the dietary habits or patterns of the twenty-one countries bordering the Mediterranean Sea, though most people in the United States think of the southern European countries when this term is raised. Each country has different foods consumed as part of its unique culture, but overall, the characteristics of the diet (high consumption of olive oil, vegetables, fruits, fish, poultry, eggs, bread and other grains, nuts, and beans) are shared. The most important part of this diet is the minimum amount of processed foods included. Some have coined these as "real foods," "whole foods," "genuine foods," or "foods from the earth." But some benefits come from what is excluded from the Mediterranean diet. These include highly processed and refined carbohydrates, processed meats, trans fats in processed foods, and sugar-sweetened beverages. Data on the health benefits of this eating pattern is mounting. Emerging research suggests that the Mediterranean diet lowers the risk of stroke, coronary heart disease, cancer, cognitive decline, and other vascular conditions related to inflammation and oxidative stress. The diet is high in monounsaturated fats, low in saturated fats, and high in fiber, mineral, vitamin, and phytochemical levels (refer to Figure 6.2).[60,61]

According to a survey of European dietary habits, a majority of the population in Italy consumes more plant products than protein, and approximately equal amounts of both are consumed in Spain.[61] In addition, meat consumption is highest in the northern regions of these nations, and lowest in the southern areas.[62,63] The greater emphasis on grains, legumes, vegetables, and fruits; lower intakes of meat and dairy foods; and promotion of wine in moderation differentiate the Mediterranean diet from that recommended by U.S. health officials.[64] However, a study by the Italian Association for Cancer Research has found that cancer rates increased as food habits changed in Italy; pasta consumption has fallen, and meat intake has quadrupled since 1950; changes toward a more Westernized diet are found in Spain and Portugal as well.[60,61] Overweight and obesity rates in 2020 in Italy reached

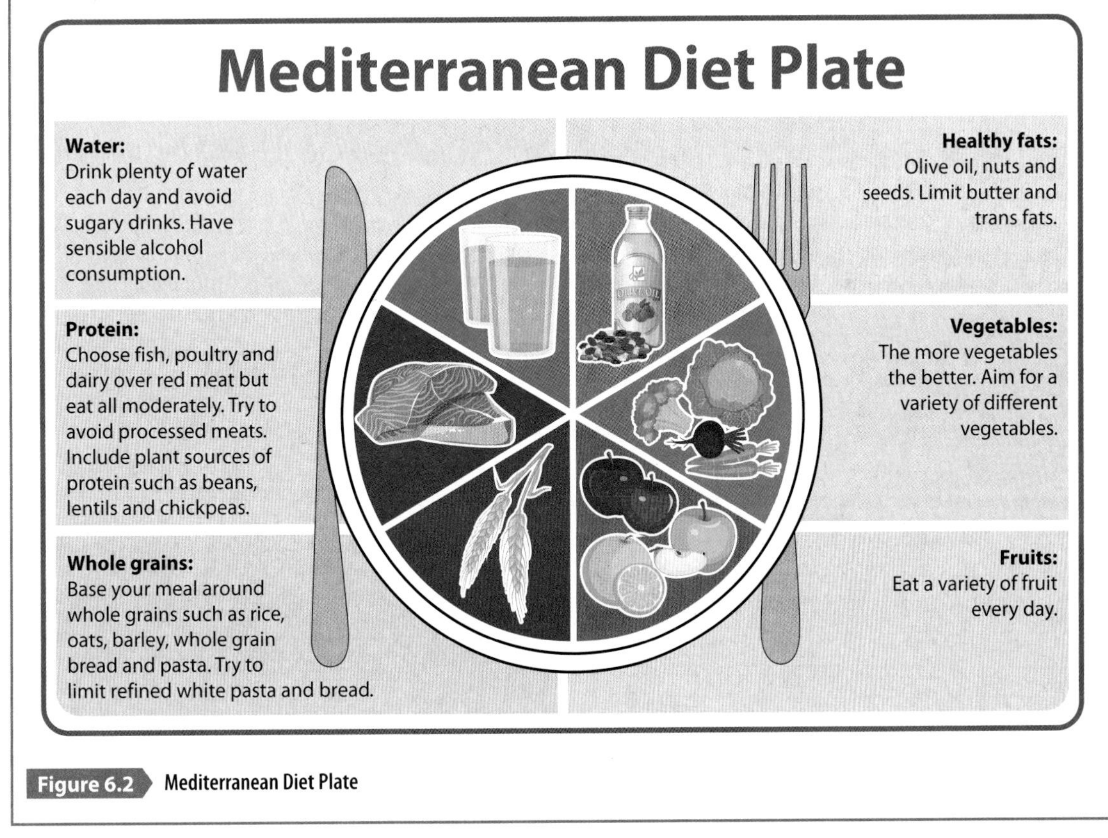

Figure 6.2 Mediterranean Diet Plate

65 percent; in Spain, rates exceed 50 percent; and in Portugal, rates exceed 53 percent.[17]

Health and Longevity Takeaway

What would Ponce de Leon think if we told him the Fountain of Youth was not in the water, but in the love of family and friends? Dr. Antonio Cadoni (age 103) believes that the secret to a long life does not reside in his Sardinian genes, but instead, he contributes his longevity to the importance of his family and friends who visit him daily. People with extensive networks of good friends and confidantes often outlive those with the fewest friends. Friends may encourage older people to take better care of themselves—by cutting down on smoking and drinking, for example, or seeking medical treatment earlier for symptoms that may indicate serious problems.

Cadoni believes that eating as a locavore, from neighboring farms and gardens, is an important part of Italian meals. Minestrone soup in Italy does not follow a precise recipe, rather it is perpetually fresh, depending upon what is being harvested from the garden at that moment. He refers to these foods as "genuine foods," meaning that they are not processed, but come straight from the ground. Cadoni also believes in the 8-8-8 rule: 8 hours of sleeping, 8 hours of working, and 8 hours of family time. He offers a glimpse into the balanced lives that many Italians espouse. These are his secrets to happiness and longevity.

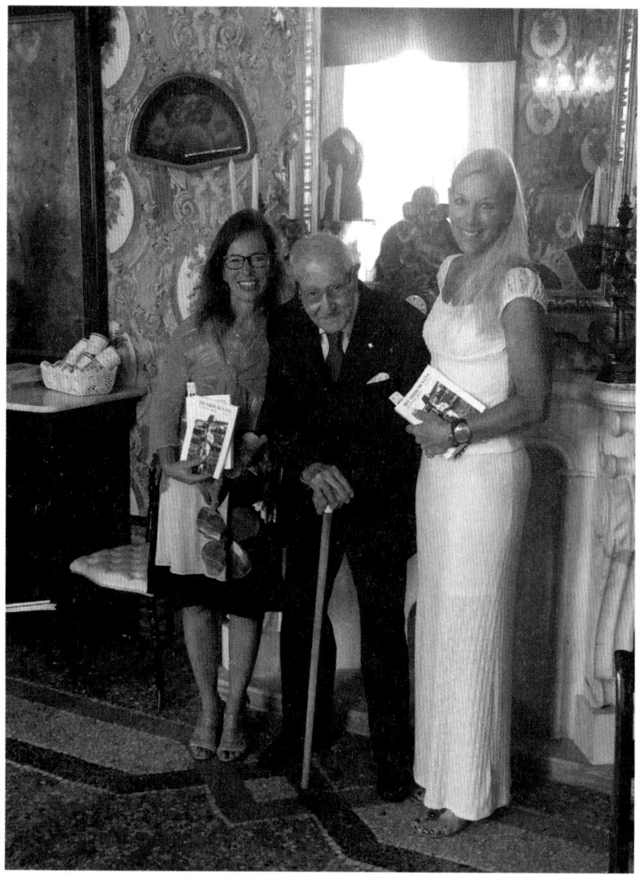

© SeAnne Waite

▲ Dr. Antonio Cadoni at age 103 in Sardinia, Italy, with dietitians Sue Linja (left) and SeAnne Waite (right).

Comfort Food—Sardinia

Michael G. and Michael S.'s story

Michael G. and Michael S., both lifetime residents of Sardinia (a large Italian island in the Mediterranean Sea), are both in their nineties. They spent their lives as goat and sheep herders, climbing the hills of Sardinia with their herds. Often, they would be out with their herds for weeks, running out of food and forging on whatever they could get their hands on to eat. "If the goats wouldn't eat it, I'd be damned if I would eat it," said Michael G. Comfort food takes on a different meaning for these two, it meant survival. So, what do they describe as their comfort foods? Pecorino cheese, which could easily be stashed away in a knapsack for long trips and was often eaten with Italian bread. Upon returning home, it was homemade wine "Vino." As Michael S. stated, "water is for

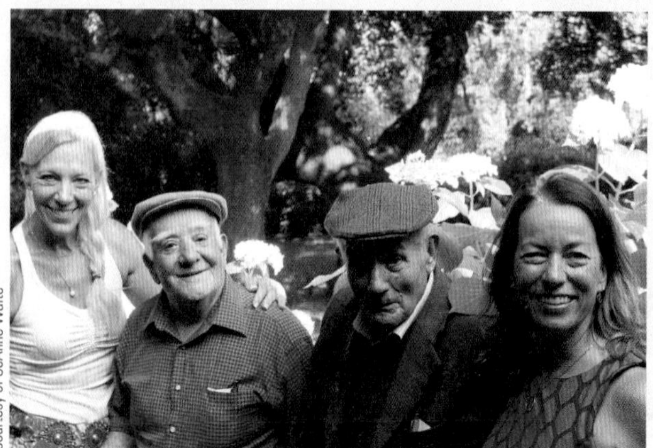

Courtesy of SeAnne Waite

▲ Michael G and Michael S. shepherds of Sardinia.

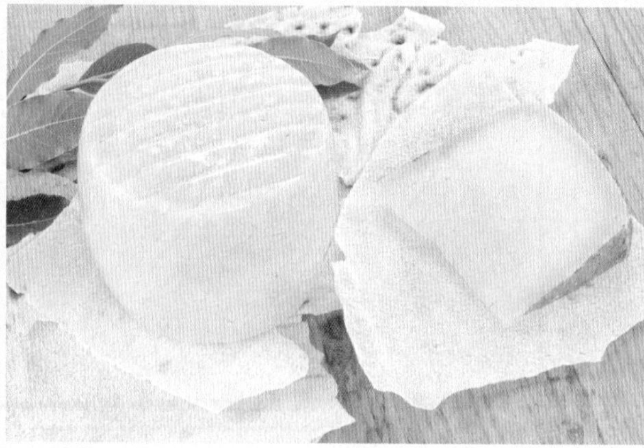

iStock.com/Marmo81

▲ Fresh Pecorino Romano cheese.

(Continued)

Comfort Food—Sardinia (*Continued*)

Michael G. and Michael S.'s story

washing and vino is for drinking." As they are getting older and less active, their memories of pecorino cheese are vivid. Sitting out in the wild, watching over their herds with the Mediterranean Sea in view, sipping "vino" while nibbling on cheese and bread, life is good!

Additional comfort food RECIPE TO TRY

Minestrone Soup

Recipe from Chef Mark Owsley, St. Lukes Hospital Better Cooking at Home[65]
Makes about 4 large servings.
Experiment with different choices of pasta, beans, and vegetables as well.

4 ounces of whole-grain shell pasta or other varieties
2 Tbsp. olive oil
1 medium onion (diced in quarter-inch pieces; you want about 3½ ounces of onion)
2 small carrots (diced in quarter-inch pieces; you want about 3½ ounces of carrot)
3 medium stalks of celery (diced in quarter-inch pieces; you want about 3½ ounces of celery)
1 small fresh zucchini (diced in half-inch pieces; you want about 5 ounces of zucchini)
1½ Tbsp. fresh garlic, minced
2 Tbsp. vegetable base
1 1/3 quarts of water
12 ounces of canned diced tomatoes
3 Tbsp. tomato paste
8 ½ ounces of canned kidney beans, rinsed and drained
Salt and pepper to taste
1 tsp. oregano
1 Tbsp. dried basil
1 tsp. fresh Italian parsley
3 cups of fresh spinach (chopped into 1-inch pieces)
3 Tbsp. cornstarch
1 cup of water

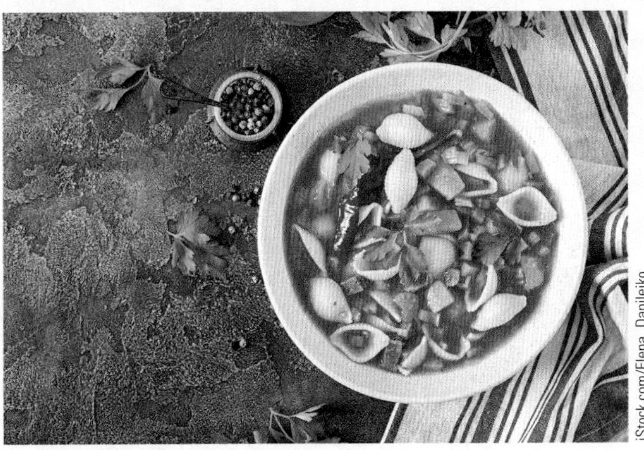
iStock.com/Elena_Danileiko

▲ **Minestrone soup: colorful and ever-changing with seasonal foods.**

Bring 1 quart of water to a boil, add the pasta, reduce the heat, and simmer for 5 to 7 minutes until tender. Drain and "shock" the pasta under cold water to stop the cooking process. When the noodles are cool, drain and set aside.

To make the soup:

In a heavy-bottomed pot, heat the oil over medium heat, and add carrots, celery, and onion. Cook until the vegetables are soft. Add garlic; continue to simmer for 2 minutes. Combine the vegetable base and the 1 1/3 quarts of water. Add to the soup with the tomatoes and tomato paste. Bring this mixture to a boil, and simmer for about 10 minutes. Add kidney beans and continue to simmer for 10 minutes. Add zucchini, spinach, oregano, and basil. (You use fresh basil and oregano if preferred.) Simmer for 10 more minutes. Mix the cornstarch with the 1 cup of water until well mixed. Slowly add this mixture to the soup. (You want to use just enough to slightly thicken the soup. You may not need all the mixture to get the correct thickness.) Add sugar, salt, and pepper to taste. Add pasta shells and parsley and mix. Turn off the heat and ladle into bowls, add your choice of toppers (if desired), and serve.

Nutritional information (per serving):
calories 289, 7.8 g fat (1.0 g saturated fat); 890 mg sodium; 990 mg potassium; 49 g total carbohydrate; 10.8 g fiber; 9.2 g protein

Discussion Starters

Let's Open a Pub!

Americans often have an inaccurate view of British and Irish pubs. Many of us tend to identify these pubs with our American bars but pubs are much more like American "bar and grills," "sports taverns," and restaurants that serve beer and wine. Most British and Irish pubs serve hot lunches and dinners as well as alcoholic beverages. Traditional British pub fare includes fish and chips (what Americans call French fries), shepherd's pie or cottage pie (beef or mutton, mashed potatoes, maybe green peas, and a potato crust on top or cooked in a pie crust), steak or steak and kidney pie, bangers and mash (sausages and mashed potatoes), Yorkshire pudding (a batter such as a pancake batter, covered with beef gravy), Quaker pudding (a grayish spiced pudding), Cornish pasty, and mince pies. The name *pub* is short for *public house* and, historically, these pubs functioned as local meeting places and served to strengthen cultural ties within the community.

Imagine that you plan to open an "authentic" British and Irish pub in your college community. In a small group, decide what your food menu should include. Remember that you will need to balance your effort to be authentic with your need to attract college students and serve students who eat only vegetarian meals.

Review Questions

1. Summarize the immigration patterns of northern and southern Europeans.
2. Describe the dominant cultural beliefs in America regarding health and the origins of these beliefs.
3. Describe the traditional food habits of England, Ireland, and Italy. List five of your favorite foods. Do any of these foods have their roots in Europe? Describe your typical meal cycle and meal composition. Are these similar to those of Europe?
4. What is the difference between Cajun and Creole cooking? What are the origins of both styles of cooking?
5. Compare and contrast the immigrant experiences of the Irish and Italians.
6. How did the New World foods (tomatoes, potatoes, corn, etc.) influence European foodways?
7. Why is the Mediterranean diet considered healthy?

Reflection

1. There is much research on the health benefits of a Mediterranean diet. The diet leaves out such foods as highly processed and refined carbohydrates, processed meats, trans fats in processed foods, and sugar-sweetened beverages. Based upon this information do you believe that the health contributions of the Mediterranean diet are from what is added in or what is taken out?
2. Considering the increasing numbers of overweight people and the low consumption of vegetables and fruit in countries reviewed in this chapter, reflect on your own diet and changes that you can make to move toward a Mediterranean style of eating.

References

1. Zong, J., & Batalova, J. 2015. European immigrants in the United States. *Migration Policy Institute*, 17(2), 1–18.
2. Rupp, Rebecca. 2015. Are French fries truly French? National Geographic. Retrieved from https://www.nationalgeographic.com/culture/article/are-french-fries-truly-french (accessed March 23, 2022).
3. Earle, R. 2017. Promoting potatoes in eighteenth-century europe. *Eighteenth-Century Studies* 51(2), 147–162. doi:10.1353/ecs.2017.0057
4. American Community Survey, BO4006. 2019. People Reporting Ancestry. ACS 1 Year Estimates. Retrieved from https://data.census.gov/cedsci/table?q=B04006&t=Ancestry&tid=ACSDT1Y2019.B04006&hidePreview=false
5. Guasco, M. 2008. From servitude to slavery. *The Atlantic World, 1450–2000*, 69–95.
6. Hess, M.A. 2014. Scottish and Scotch Irish Americans. In R.V. Dassanowsky & J. Lehman (Eds.), *Gale encyclopedia of multicultural America*. Farmington Hills, MI: Gale Group.
7. Statistics Canada. October 25, 2017. Census in brief, ethnic and cultural origins of Canadians: Portrait of a rich heritage. Retrieved from https://www12.statcan.gc.ca/census-recensement/2016/as-sa/98-200-x/2016016/98-200-x2016016-eng.Cfm
8. U.S. Census Bureau. 2021. *Quick Facts-French Valley CDP, California*. July 1.
9. U.S. Census Bureau, Newsroom Archive. 2020. *Facts for features: Irish-American Heritage Month (March) and St. Patrick's Day (March 17): 2020*. Retrieved from http://www.census.gov/newsroom/releases/archives/facts_for_features_special_editions/cb12-ff03.html (accessed February 12, 2015).
10. U.S. Census Bureau. 2019. American community survey 1-year estimates. Retrieved from https://data.census.gov/cedsci/table?q=B04006&t=Ancestry&tid=ACSDT1Y2019.B04006&hidePreview=false (accessed March 20, 2022).
11. French Americans. March 20, 2020. In *Wikipedia*. Retrieved from https://en.wikipedia.org/w/index.php?title=Evolutionary_history_of_life&oldid=983803356 (accessed April 5, 2022).
12. Vermette, D. 2019. When an influx of French-Canadian immigrants struck fear into Americans. *Smithsonian*, 21.
13. Spector, R.E. 2017. *Cultural diversity in health and illness* (9th ed.). Upper Saddle River, NJ: Pearson Education.
14. Gatley, A. 2016. The significance of culinary cultures to diet. *British Food Journal*, 118(1), 40–59. https://doi.org/10.1108/BFJ-06-2015-0228 (accessed March 20, 2022).
15. Mouritsen, O.G., Rhatigan, P., & Pérez-Lloréns, J.L. 2018. World cuisine of seaweeds: Science meets gastronomy. *International Journal of Gastronomy and Food Science*, 14, 55–65.
16. Fisher, M.F.K. 1968. *The cooking of provincial France*. New York: Time-Life.
17. Myhrvold, N. August 16, 2019. Grande cuisine. Encyclopedia Britannica. Retrieved from https://www.britannica.com/topic/grande-cuisine.
18. Zibart, E. 2010. *The ethnic food lovers companion: Understanding the cuisines of the world*. Birmingham, AL: Menasha Ridge Press
19. Mallet, M., & Bastick, Z. 2013. French Americans. In C.E. Cortes & G.J. Geoffrey (Eds.), *Multicultural America*. Thousand Oaks, CA: Sage.
20. Bailey, A. 1969. *The cooking of the British Isles*. New York: Time-Life.
21. Jones, R. 2003. The new look—and taste—of British cuisine. *The Virginia Quarterly Review*, 79(2), 209–231. Retrieved from http://www.jstor.org/stable/26440967
22. French, H.H., & VisitBritain. 2005. United Kingdom: A flavorful adventure. In D. Goldstein & K. Merkle (Eds.), *Culinary cultures of Europe*. Strasbourg, France: Council of Europe Publishing.
23. Poulain, J.P. 2005. French gastronomy, French gastronomies. In D. Goldstein & K. Merkle (Eds.), *Culinary cultures of Europe*. Strasbourg, France: Council of Europe Publishing.
24. Mitchell, Shane. 2021. The mothers of all French sauces. Saveur. Retrieved from https://www.saveur.com/food/the-mothers-of-all-french-sauces/
25. Foster, D. 2000. *The global etiquette guide to Europe*. New York: Wiley.
26. Anonymous. 2016. Ireland guide: A look at Irish language, culture, customs, and etiquette. Cummisceo Global. Retrieved from https://www.commisceo-global.com/resources/country-guides/ireland-guide (accessed March 20, 2022).
27. Purnell L.D., & Fenkl, E.A. 2019. People of Irish heritage. In: *Handbook for Culturally Competent Care*. Cham: Springer (accessed March 20, 2022).
28. Silvius, S. 2015. Horse meat consumption – between scandal and reality. *Procedia Economics and Finance*, 23, 697–703.
29. Williams, Nikesha. 2020. It starts with the roux: Behind every bowl of gumbo, there's a complex history. Eater. Retrieved from https://www.eater.com/2020/1/13/21056973/where-did-gumbo-originate-dish-history-new-orleans
30. Goldberg, E. December 8, 2016. France is doing something amazing with its food. *Huffpost*. Retrieved from https://www.huffpost.com/entry/this-country-wastes-the-least-amount-of-food_n_58485a52e4b08c82e8894c31 (accessed March 21, 2022).
31. The Economist Newspaper Ltd. 2022. Food Sustainability Index. Retrieved from https://foodsustainability.eiu.com/
32. Vauterin, N. July 7, 2021, Obesity is on the rise in France according to the latest epidemiological survey. Retrieved from https://www.c3health.org/blog/obesity-is-on-the-rise-in-france-according-to-the-latest-epidemiological-survey/ (accessed March 21, 2022).

33. FormulateHealth Nutraceutical Supplements. May 28, 2021. Retrieved from https://www.formulatehealth.com/blog/obesity-statistics-uk#:~:text=Today%2C%20around%2063%25%20of%20all%20UK%20adults%20are,obesity.%20Obesity%20and%20Hospital%20Admissions%20-%20the%20Statistics
34. Poe, D. M. (1988). Profile of Portuguese Elderly Nutrition Program Participants: Demographic Characteristics, Nutrition Knowledge, and Practices (Massachusetts).
35. Hebestreit, A., Intemann, T., Siani, A., De Henauw, S., Eiben, G., Kourides, Y.A., Kovacs, E., Moreno, L.A., Veidebaum, T., Krogh, V., Pala, V., Bogl, L.H., Hunsberger, M., Börnhorst, C., & Pigeot, I. 2017. Dietary patterns of European Children and their parents in association with family food environment: Results from the Family Study. *Nutrients,* 9, 126 (accessed March 20, 2022). https://doi.org/10.3390/nu9020126.
36. Kotseva, K., DeBacquer, D., Jennings, C., Gyberg, V., DeBacker, L., Ryden, L., Amouyel, P., Bruthans, J., Cifkova, R., Deckers, J., De Sutter, J., Franz, Z., Graham, I., Keber, I., Lehto, S., Moore, D., Pajak, A., & Wood, D. 2017. Time trends in lifestyle, risk factor control, and use of evidence-based medications in patients with coronary heart disease in Europe: Results from 3 EUROASPIRE surveys, 1999–2013, Global Heart, 12(4), 315–322.e3. Retrieved from https://doi.org/10.1016/j.gheart.2015.11.003 (accessed March 21, 2022).
37. Kushi, L.H., Lew, R.A., Stare, E.J., Curtis, R.E., Lozy, M., Bourke, G., . . ., & Kevaney, J. 1985. Diet and 20-year mortality from coronary heart disease: The Ireland-Boston diet-heart study. *New England Journal of Medicine*, 312, 811–818.
38. Pilling, L.C., Tamosauskaite, J., Jones, G., et al. 2019. Common conditions associated with hereditary haemochromatosis genetic variants: cohort study in UK Biobank. *BMJ*. 364:k5222. Retrieved from https://rarediseases.org/rare-diseases/classic-hereditary-hemochromatosis/ (accessed March 21, 2022).
39. Public Health England. 2018. National Diet and Nutrition Survey. Results from Years 7 and 8 (combined) of the Rolling Programme (2014/2015 to 2015/2016). Food Standards Agency (www.gov.uk/phe). Retrieved from https://assets.publishing.service.gov.uk/government/uploads/system/uploads/attachment_data/file/699241/NDNS_results_years_7_and_8.pdf (accessed March 20, 2022).
40. Ma, Y., Murthy, V., Roderer, G., Monsalve, M.V., Clarke, L.A., Normand, T., . . . Hayden, M.R. 1991 A mutation in the human lipoprotein lipase gene as the most common cause of familial chylomicronemia in French Canadians. *New England Journal of Medicine*, 324, 1761-1766.
41. ANSES. 2017. INCA 3: Changes in consumption habits and patterns, new issues in the areas of food safety and nutrition. Retrieved from https://www.anses.fr/en/content/inca-3-changes-consumption-habits-and-patterns-new-issues-areas-food-safety-and-nutrition
42. Pozzetta, G. 2014. Italian Americans. In R.V. Dassanowsky & J. Lehman (Eds.), *Gale encyclopedia of multicultural America*. Vol 3, (3rd ed.). Farmington Hills, MI: Gale Group.
43. U.S. Census Bureau. 2021. Italian-American heritage and culture month: October 2021. Retrieved from https://www.census.gov/newsroom/stories/italian-american-heritage-culture-month.html (accessed April 5, 2022).
44. Cavaioli, F. 2008. Patterns of Italian immigration to the United States. *The Catholic Social Science Review*, 13, 213–229.
45. Colahan, C. 2014. Spanish Americans. In R.V. Dassanowsky & J. Lehman (Eds.), *Gale encyclopedia of multicultural America*. Farmington Hills, MI: Gale Group.
46. Shostak, E. 2014. Basque Americans. In R.V. Dassanowsky & J. Lehman (Eds.), *Gale encyclopedia of multicultural America*. Farmington Hills, MI: Gale Group.
47. Holtz, C. 2020. *Global Health Care Issues and Policies* (4th ed.). Burlington, MA: Jones and Bartlett Publishing.
48. E.E. 2014. Portuguese Americans. In R.V. Dassanowsky & J. Lehman (Eds.), *Gale encyclopedia of multicultural America*. Farmington Hills, MI: Gale Group.
49. EMR. 2020. Retrieved from https://www.expertmarketresearch.com/reports/pasta-sauce-market.
50. Editors. 2022. Origin and history of the tortilla. *History of Bread*. Retrieved from http://www.historyofbread.com/bread-history/history-of-tortilla/
51. Palmer, S. 2019. Healthful fats: The skinny on unrefined plant oils. *Today's Dietitian*, 21(6), 12.
52. Guilford, Gwynn. September 2, 2018. My favorite beverage is a 2,000-year-old energy drink from ancient Rome. *Quartz*. Retrieved from https://qz.com/quartzy/1372506/posca/
53. Pessoa e Costa, A. 2005. Portugal: A dialogue of cultures. In D. Goldstein & K. Merkle (Eds.), *Culinary cultures of Europe*. Strasbourg, France: Council of Europe Publishing.
54. Filippone, P.F. 2019. The History of Basil: From food to medicine to religion. *The Spruce Eats*. Retrieved from https://www.thespruceeats.com/the-history-of-basil-1807566
55. Azzarito, Amy. March 25, 2020. "A tool of the devil": The dark history of the humble fork. *Fast Company*. Retrieved from https://www.fastcompany.com/90481445/a-tool-of-the-devil-the-dark-history-of-the-humble-for
56. Valverde Villena, D. 2005. Spain: Agape and conviviality at the table. In D. Goldstein & K. Merkle (Eds.), *Culinary cultures of Europe*. Strasbourg, France: Council of Europe Publishing, Norden
57. Dennett, C. 2016. Key ingredients of the Mediterranean diet—The nutritious sum of delicious parts. *Today's Dietitian,* 18(5), 28. Retrieved from https://www.todaysdietitian.com/newarchives/0516p28.shtml
58. Hillman, S.M. 2008. People of Italian heritage. *Cultures Covered in the Text*, 393.
59. Poe, D.M. 1988. Profile of Portuguese elderly nutrition program participants: Demographic characteristics, nutrition knowledge, and practices (Massachusetts).
60. Dernini, S., & Berry, E. 2015. Mediterranean diet: From a healthy diet to a sustainable dietary pattern. *Frontiers in Nutrition*.
61. Aranceta-Bartrina, J., Partearroyo, T., López-Sobaler, A.M., Ortega, R.M., Varela-Moreiras, G., Serra-Majem, L., & Pérez-Rodrigo, C. 2019. Updating the food-based dietary guidelines for the Spanish population: The Spanish Society of Community Nutrition (SENC) proposal. *Nutrients*, 11(11), 2675. Retrieved from https://doi.org/10.3390/nu11112675
62. Visioli, F., Bogani, P., Grande, S., Detopoulou, V., Manios, Y., & Galli, C. 2006. Local food and cardioprotection: The role of phytochemicals. *Local Mediterranean Food Plants and Nutraceuticals*, 59, 116–129.
63. Tomé-Carneiro, J., Crespo, M. C., López de Las Hazas, M. C., Visioli, F., & Dávalos, A. 2020. Olive oil consumption and its repercussions on lipid metabolism. *Nutrition Reviews*, 78(11), 952–968.
64. Delgado-Lista, J., Alcala-Diaz, J. F., Torres-Peña, J. D., Quintana-Navarro, G. M., Fuentes, F., Garcia-Rios, A., . . . & Visioli, F. 2022. Long-term secondary prevention of cardiovascular disease with a Mediterranean diet and a low-fat diet (CORDIOPREV): A randomised controlled trial. *The Lancet*, 399(10338), 1876-1885.
65. Anderson, Holly M. 2020. Hearty minestrone soup warms the soul in challenging times. *Better Cooking at Home*. Retrieved from https://www.stlukesonline.org/blogs/st-lukes/health-and-wellness/2020/mar/minestrone-soup

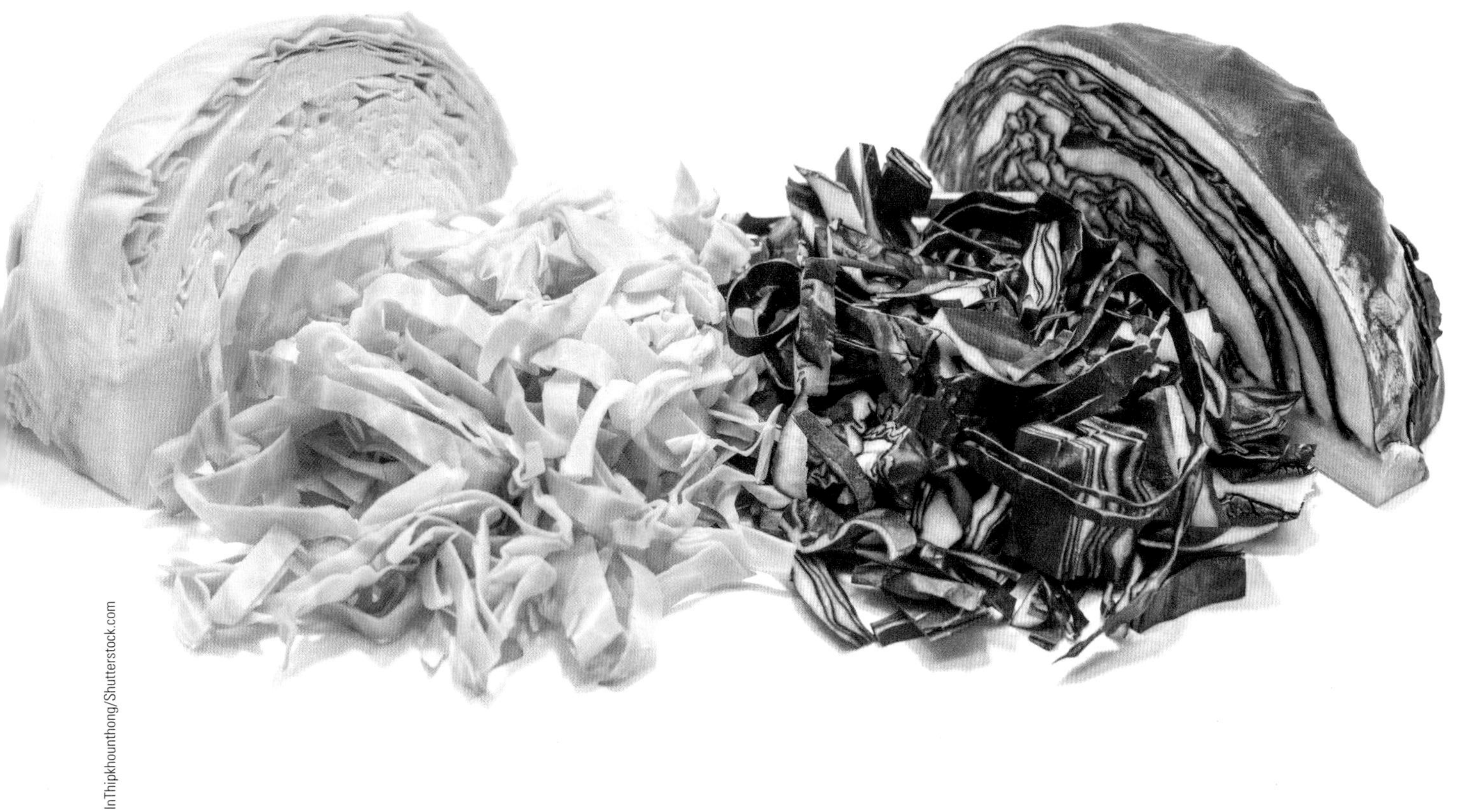
InThipkhounthong/Shutterstock.com

Chapter 7

Central Europeans, People of the Former Soviet Union, and Scandinavians

Learning Objectives

7.1 List the countries that are included as parts of Central Europe, the former Soviet Union (FSU), and Scandinavia.

7.2 Identify the immigration patterns and historical socioeconomic influences of these European, FSU, and Scandinavian groups in America today.

7.3 Differentiate the typical religions, family structures, and traditional health beliefs and practices of these groups before and after immigration to the United States.

7.4 Describe the differences and similarities among staple foods and preparation techniques within and across these countries.

7.5 Compare key foods for each of the food groups for these regions to how these foods have been adapted by immigrants in the U.S.

7.6 Differentiate traditional meal composition and cycles from the meal composition and cycles of these groups living in America today.

7.7 Describe regional specialties and dishes these immigrants have contributed to the current American diet.

7.8 Identify health concerns associated with nutritional intake of these groups.

The European settlers from central Europe, the former Soviet Union (FSU), and Scandinavia were some of the earliest and largest groups to come to the United States. Leif Erikson was a Norse explorer (c.970–c.1020) from Iceland and is thought to have been the first European to have set foot on North American soil in Newfoundland. Though many others arrived as early as the 1600s and most had come before the beginning of the twentieth century, the upheavals of two world wars and the collapse of the Soviet Union have led to continuous immigration from these regions during the last century (refer to the map in Figure 7.1).

The influence of immigrants from central Europe, the FSU (especially Russia), and Scandinavia on American culture, especially in the area of cuisine, is substantial. Bread baking, dairy farming, certain types of meat processing, and beer brewing are just a few of the skills these groups brought with them. Their expertise permitted the expansion of food production and distribution that encouraged nationwide acceptance of their ethnic specialties, leading to the creation of a typical American cuisine for the majority culture. This chapter focuses on the traditional and adapted foods and food habits of people from Germany,

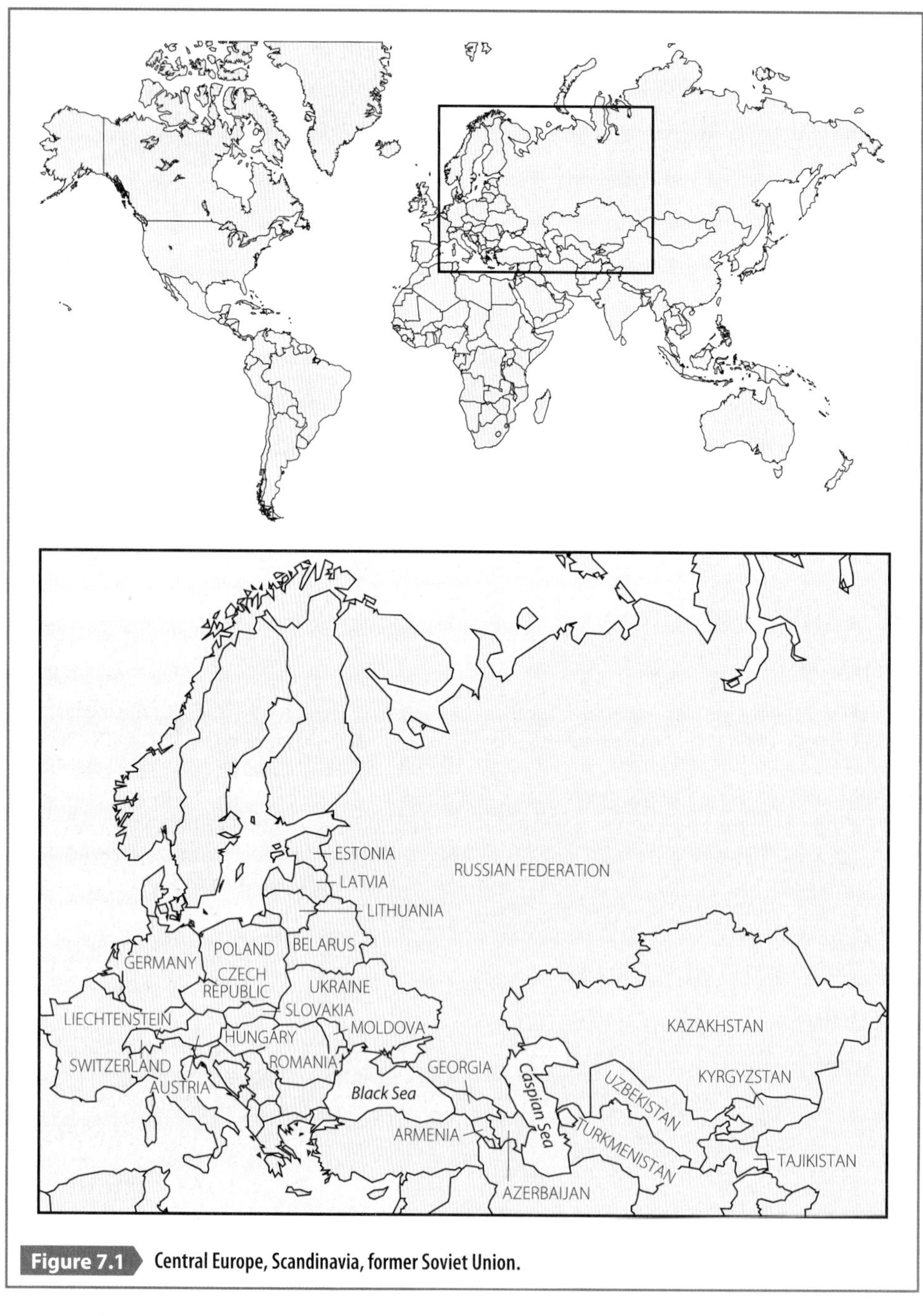

Figure 7.1 Central Europe, Scandinavia, former Soviet Union.

Poland, and other central European countries; Russians and other FSU populations; and people from Denmark, Sweden, and Norway.

Food for Thought

On January 1, 1993, Czechoslovakia separated into two new countries, the Czech Republic and Slovakia in central Europe. In 2016, the Czech Republic adopted "Czechia" as a shortened, informal name. Historically, the region was known as Bohemia and was part of the Holy Roman Empire. The name comes from a Celtic people known as the Boii.[1]

Central Europeans and the People of the FSU

Central Europe stretches from the North and Baltic Seas, south to the Alps, and east to the Baltic states. It includes the nations of Germany, Austria, Hungary, Romania, the Czech Republic, Slovakia, and Poland, as well as Switzerland and Liechtenstein. Most of the countries share common borders; Austria, Hungary, the Czech Republic, Romania, and Slovakia are situated south of Germany and Poland. Switzerland is surrounded by Germany, Austria, France, Italy, and Liechtenstein. The climate of central Europe is harsher and colder than that of southern Europe, and much of the land is fertile.

The FSU includes the Commonwealth of Independent States or CIS (the Russian Federation, Armenia, Azerbaijan, Belarus, Georgia, Kazakhstan, Kyrgyzstan, Republic of Moldavia, Tajikistan, Turkmenistan, Ukraine, and Uzbekistan); the Baltic states (Estonia, Latvia, and Lithuania) declined to join the organization.[2] Its vast geography includes the Arctic and parts of the Middle East. Except in the southern republics, the harsh winters of the region affect agricultural capacity.

The large number of immigrants from central Europe and parts of the FSU made significant contributions to the literature, music, and cuisine of the United States. In fact, many central European foods have become standard American fare. Imagine a baseball game without hot dogs and beer or a picnic without potato salad. This section explores these and other food customs of central Europe and the FSU and their impact on the American diet.

Cultural Perspective

History of Central Europeans and Russians in the United States

Immigration Patterns

Germany For almost three centuries, Germans have been one of the most significant population groups in the United States. According to the 2019 U.S. Census, one in every ten Americans, 40 million, is of German descent, making this the largest ethnic group in the nation.[3] Germans have assimilated into most communities in the United States.[3]

The earliest German settlement in the American colonies was Germantown, Pennsylvania, founded in 1681. By 1709, large-scale immigration began, primarily from the Palatinate region of southwestern Germany. Many of the immigrants, who were mostly of Amish, Mennonite, or other religious faiths seeking freedom from discrimination, settled in Pennsylvania. The majority were farmers who steadily pushed westward searching for new lands for their expanding families. Those in Pennsylvania, Ohio, and Indiana became known as the Pennsylvania Dutch (also called the Pennsylvania Germans or Pennsylvania Deutsch). Immigration dropped off after 1775, but an economic crisis in Europe once again prompted Germans to come to the United States. Approximately 5 million Germans immigrated to the United States between 1820 and 1900. Like the earlier settlers, most were farmers who arrived with their families, although by the end of the century there were increasing numbers of young, single people who were agricultural laborers and servants. Many of these settled in the Mississippi, Ohio, and Missouri River valleys, the Great Lakes area, or other parts of the Midwest. Most Germans avoided the southern United States, but there are sizable German settlements in Texas and New Orleans.

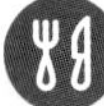

Food for Thought

Small numbers of Schwenkfelders from southern Germany, members of a pacifist religious sect similar to Quakers, settled in Pennsylvania in the mid-1700s. They introduced crocus flowers, the source of the spice saffron.

The word *Dutch* is a corruption of *Deutsch*, meaning "German," and has nothing to do with the Netherlands.

A third significant phase of immigration began after the turn of the twentieth century when approximately 1.5 million Germans arrived. Many were unmarried industrial workers seeking higher pay, and others were the descendants of Germans who had settled in ethnically isolated colonies in Russia as early as the sixteenth century. Discrimination and the revolution of 1917 led to their departure. Most of these third-phase immigrants joined growing numbers of second- and third-generation Germans living in urban areas. Cities with considerable German populations included Cleveland, New York, Toledo, Detroit, Chicago, Milwaukee, and St. Louis. German Russians, however, tended to settle in rural areas, especially in Colorado.

During the 1930s, many of the German immigrants were Jewish refugees. After World War II, displaced persons of German descent and East German refugees made up the sizable German immigrant group who settled in the United States.

Poland People from Poland have arrived in the United States continuously since the 1608 Jamestown colony. The largest wave of immigration occurred between 1860 and 1914, mostly for economic reasons. The early phase was dominated

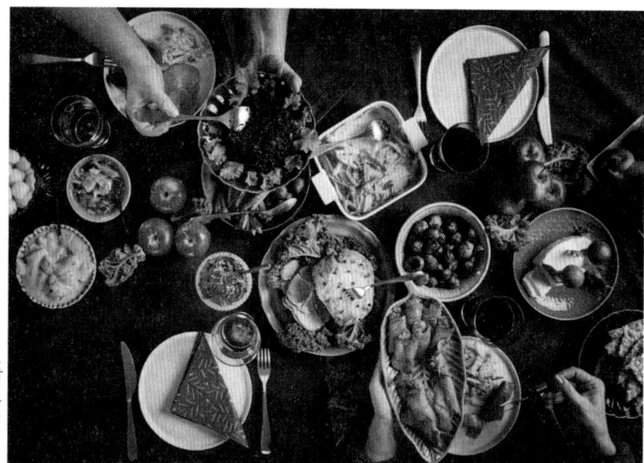
iStock.com/Knape

▲ Traditional foods of central Europe and the FSU. Some typical foods include beets, cabbage, ham, herring, apples, and potatoes.

by the Poles (approximately 500,000) from German-ruled areas of Poland (Pomerania and Poznan) and by those who worked in western Germany. German–Polish immigrants often became part of German or Czech communities or established farming settlements in the Southwest and Midwest.

The number of Polish immigrants from Germany began to decline after 1890 but then increased with the arrival of more than 2 million Polish people from areas under Russian and Austrian rule. The German Poles left their homeland to become permanent settlers, but the Russian and Austrian Polish often came as temporary workers. Although 30 percent returned to Poland, many eventually moved back to the United States permanently. The Austrian and Russian Polish tended to settle in the rapidly developing cities of the Mid-Atlantic and midwestern states, especially Chicago, Buffalo, and Cleveland.

Polish emigration after World War I was usually not for economic reasons. Most (more than 250,000) left because of political dissatisfaction: government instability and dictatorship in the 1920s and 1930s, the German invasion and occupation from 1939 to 1945, and the pro-Soviet communist government after 1945. Many settled in urban areas in which there were substantial existing Polish populations. More recently, small numbers of younger Polish immigrants have taken advantage of the freedom resulting from post-communist rule to come to the United States.

Other Central European Countries Nearly 4 million Austrians, Hungarians, Czechs, Slovakians, and Swiss have come to the United States, primarily during the late nineteenth and early twentieth centuries, for economic and political reasons.

Austrian immigration patterns are not entirely known because Austrians and Hungarians were classified as a single group in U.S. statistics until 1910. More than 2 million Austrians are believed to have come to the United States searching for economic opportunities in the decade following 1900. Most were unskilled, and many were fathers who left families in Austria with the hopes of making their fortune. Many Austrians never found the advancement they were seeking, and approximately 35 percent returned home. A second, smaller wave of immigration occurred in the 1930s when 29,000 well-educated urban Jewish people from Austria fled Hitler's arrival.

The first group of Hungarians arriving in the United States, several thousand political refugees following the revolution of 1848, were mostly men—well-educated, wealthy, and often titled. Later Hungarian immigrants who arrived at the turn of the century were often poor, young, single men who found job opportunities in the expanding industrial workplace. Many worked in eastern Ohio, West Virginia, northern Illinois, and Indiana coal mines. Cities that developed large Hungarian populations were primarily located in the Northeast and Midwest. More than 50,000 additional Hungarians entered the United States as refugees after World War II and the 1956 uprising against the communist government. They first settled in the industrial towns populated by earlier Hungarian immigrants, but many, mostly professionals, soon moved to other cities that offered better jobs.

Immigrants from the Czech Republic initially tended to be farmers or skilled agricultural workers who settled in the states of Nebraska, Wisconsin, Texas, Iowa, and Minnesota, often near German communities. Later Czech immigrants were skilled laborers; they settled in the urban areas of New York, Cleveland, and especially Chicago.

The majority of Slovakian immigrants were young agricultural workers who arrived before World War II. Those who decided to remain in the United States later sent for their wives and families. The majority settled in the industrial Northeast and Midwest; they labored in coal mines, steel mills, and oil refineries.

Most immigrants from Switzerland came to the United States for economic opportunities. The majority arrived before World War I, seeking jobs as artisans or professionals in the urban areas of New York, Philadelphia, Chicago, Cincinnati, St. Louis, San Francisco, and Los Angeles.

Another group found throughout central Europe (as well as in northern and southern Europe) without national boundaries is Roma, also known as Gypsies, a term that can be pejorative. There are an estimated 100,000 to 1,000,000 Roma in the United States, from a variety of communities with different spoken dialects.[4] The Roma were recognized for the first time in the U.S. 2021 Census. Though they originate from numerous European countries, the majority living in the United States are believed to have come from central Europe.

Russia and the FSU Early Russian immigrants originally came to Alaska and the West Coast, rather than to the eastern states. Most of their settlements were forts or outposts used to protect their fur trade and shelter missionaries. When Russia sold Alaska to the United States in 1867, half of the settlers returned home, and many others moved to California. Subsequent immigration was primarily to the East Coast, although some Russians (Molokans, followers of a religion that had rejected the Russian Eastern Orthodox Church) immigrated to the West Coast in the early twentieth century.

Food for Thought

The Rom, or Roma, are an insular ethnic group found throughout the world. Genetic findings suggest their origins are from northern India. When they gradually spread their way across Europe between the eighth and tenth centuries, they were mistaken for Egyptians, and the identifier "Gypsy," often considered a slur, came into use from this error.

People from Russia, mainly impoverished peasants seeking a better life, began to arrive in large numbers during the 1880s. Over 1.5 million were Jewish people seeking freedom from persecution as well as economic opportunity. The second wave of immigrants came after the 1917 revolution when more than 2 million people fled the country, 30,000 of whom settled in the United States. After World War II, only small numbers of Soviet refugees, primarily Jewish people, were allowed to emigrate. Following the breakup of the Soviet Union, nearly 200,000 Russians settled in the United States between 1990 and 1993. The settlement patterns of Russians are similar to those of other immigrants from central Europe. For the later wave of immigrants, the port of entry was New York City. Many remained in New York, and others settled in nearby industrial areas that offered employment in the mines and factories.

The largest populations of immigrants from the FSU are from Ukraine, Lithuania, and Armenia. Lengthy Russian domination of the region hinders estimates of the total numbers in the United States because some settlers were listed as Russians in immigration figures. It is believed that the first significant number of Lithuanians, approximately 300,000, arrived in the United States following the abolition of serfdom (feudal labor) in 1861.[5] Nearly 30,000 refugees fleeing Soviet control came following World War II. The largest influx of Ukrainian immigrants occurred in the 1870s when almost 350,000 men were recruited to work the Pennsylvania mines as strikebreakers. A majority settled in that state, though smaller numbers found factory work in Ohio, New York, and Michigan. Later immigrants, including 80,000 Ukrainians displaced by World War II, favored the urban centers of the Northeast.

Significant Armenian immigration began in 1890 when immigrants came for economic opportunity. The second wave of Armenians from Turkey who were seeking escape from persecution arrived soon after and again following the two world wars. Just before World War I, there were two million Armenians in the declining Ottoman Empire, and by 1922, there were less than 400,000 still living.[6] In 2021, the United States recognized the deaths of those approximately 1.5 million Armenians as genocide.[7] Other waves of Armenian migration into the United States occurred. More than 60,000 Armenian refugees have come since the 1980s, settling primarily in Los Angeles, with fewer joining the older Armenian communities in Boston, New York, Detroit, Chicago, and the agricultural region of Fresno, California.

Current Demographics and Socioeconomic Status

German There are more than 40 million Americans of German heritage in the nation today, according to 2019 Census estimates.[3] Wisconsin-Minnesota-North Dakota-South Dakota-Nebraska-Iowa is considered the German belt; however, only the Pennsylvania Dutch, the rural-dwelling Germans from Russia who settled in the Midwest, and a few concentrated communities in Texas retain some aspects of their cultural heritage.[8]

Germans differ little from the national norms demographically, although they are slightly higher in economic achievement and are generally conservative in attitudinal ratings. The high degree of German acculturation is attributed to their large numbers, occupations, and arrival time in the United States. The entry of the United States into World War I created a storm of anti-German feelings in America even against German Americans. German-composed music was banned, German-named foods were renamed, and German books were burned. As a result, many German Americans rapidly assimilated, abandoning the customs still common in other ethnic groups, such as ethnic associations and the use of their oral and written language.

Polish Polish Americans form one of the largest ethnic groups in the United States today. In 2019, it was estimated that there were over 9 million Americans of Polish descent;[3] many still live in the urban areas of the Northeast and upper Midwest where their ancestors originally settled. Economically, the third-generation Polish American has moved upward, and the majority of Polish Americans live at a solidly middle-class level. Polish immigrants have been active in the formation and leadership of U.S. labor unions. More recent immigrants usually possess higher occupational skills and educational backgrounds than earlier immigrants.[9]

Other Central Europeans It is believed that although only 646,000 Americans identify themselves as being of Austrian descent in the 2019 U.S. Census figures,[3] as many as 4 million U.S. citizens may be of Austrian ancestry.[10] This confusion over Austrian ethnicity dates back to changing national boundaries and names in Europe. Though early immigrants settled mostly in the Northeast, the largest populations of Austrian Americans are now found in New York, California, Pennsylvania, Florida, and New Jersey. At the turn of the century, Austrians were involved in clothing and tailoring, mining, and the food industry, including bakeries, meatpacking operations, and restaurants. Today, Austrians are found in a diverse range of occupations.

In the 2019 U.S. Census figures, 1.3 million Hungarian Americans were estimated to be in the United States.[3] Most settled originally in the Northeast, but younger generations have migrated to California and Texas, while many Hungarian retirees have moved to Florida.[11] Economically, the Hungarians differ little from other central European immigrants. Most live in urban areas and work mostly in white-collar occupations. First- and second-generation Hungarian Americans encouraged their children to become engineers, a science that was respected by the Hungarian aristocracy at the turn of the century.

Nearly 1.5 million Americans of Czech descent were identified in the 2019 U.S. Census estimates.[3] Most of these immigrants now live in cities or rural nonfarm areas[3] and are acculturated. Cities and states with large numbers of people from the Czech Republic are California, Chicago, Iowa, Minnesota, Nebraska, New York City, Texas, and Wisconsin. Occupationally, only a small number of Czech Americans are still farmers; a majority now hold sales, machinist, or white-collar jobs. Many Czech immigrants have been successful in industry, founding businesses that produce cigars, beer, and watches.[12]

There are over 790,000 Americans of Slovakian descent, according to the 2019 U.S. Census figures.[3] Actual numbers may exceed 2 million when those originally misidentified as Czechoslovakian or Hungarian are included.[12] The first two generations of Slovakian immigrants grew up in tightly knit communities anchored by work, church, family, and social activities. The third and fourth generations have sought higher education, work in white-collar jobs, and live in the suburbs; median family income is far above the national average.[12]

There were less than 1 million citizens who declared Swiss ancestry in the 2019 U.S. Census estimates.[3] Most Swiss were multilingual and often multicultural when they arrived, assimilating quickly into U.S. culture. The few Swiss who come to the United States today work mostly in the U.S. branches of Swiss companies.[13]

Russians and People of the FSU In 2019, approximately 2.4 million Russian Americans were living in the United States.[3] They have mostly moved out of city centers and into the suburbs, especially in the Northeast. Figures from the 2019 Census reported close to 1 million Americans of Ukrainian descent, 632,000 of Lithuanian heritage, and 458,000 of Armenian ancestry. In the past decade, one-third of FSU immigrants are from Russia, one-third are from Ukraine, and the remaining third are from all other FSU nations. These recent immigrants have settled in urban areas, including New York, Chicago, Los Angeles, Boston, Detroit, and San Francisco. Today, 40 percent of Ukrainians are found in Pennsylvania, and 60 percent of Armenians are living in California.[14]

Food for Thought

Based on census data, it is estimated that there are over 3.2 million Canadians of German descent and over 1 million of Polish ancestry. In addition, more than 1.3 million Canadians list their heritage as Ukrainian, and over 600,000 report Russian origins.[15–18]

Since World War II, the relations between the Russian American community and American society have largely been dependent on the political relations between the United States and Russia. During the 1950s, anti-Soviet and anticommunist sentiments in the United States caused many Russian Americans to assume a low profile that hastened their acculturation. Since the bulk of Ukrainian and Lithuanian immigration occurred several generations past, most of these populations are assimilated. Armenians, who are typically well-educated and English-speaking on arrival, have also found it easy to adapt to U.S. society.

Immigrants recently arriving from Russia and the FSU have come from relatively advanced educational and professional backgrounds. Estimates are that nearly half of Russian immigrants have a university degree. Most have professional experience, many as engineers, economists, scientists, or physicians.

Food for Thought

Seventy-three percent of the population in Switzerland speaks Swiss German, 20 percent speaks Swiss French, and 5 percent speaks Swiss Italian; in addition, most Swiss speak one or two other languages.

Worldview

Religion

Germans The majority of U.S. German immigrants were Lutheran, though some were Jewish or Roman Catholic. Today many Pennsylvania Dutch (also called the Pennsylvania Germans or Pennsylvania Deutsch) and rural Germans from Russia faithfully maintain their religious heritage. Both groups are primarily Protestant, mostly Lutheran or Mennonite. Mennonites are a religious group derived from the Anabaptist movement, which advocated baptism and church membership for adult believers only. They are noted for their simple lifestyle and rejection of oaths, public office, and pacifism. The Amish, a sect of the Mennonites, more strictly avoid modern technology such as automobiles and electricity, and generally maintain very little contact with the outside world. Their life centers on Gelassenheit, meaning submission to a higher authority through reserved and humble behavior, and placing the needs of others before the needs of the individual. Although there are Amish communities in as many as 31 states, the majority are found in Pennsylvania, Ohio, and Indiana.

Polish Most Polish immigrants were devout Catholics and they quickly established parish churches in the United States. The Catholic Church is still a vital part of the Polish American community, although Polish Americans have been found to marry outside the church more than other Catholics.

Central Europeans Austrians are mostly Roman Catholic and have been actively involved in promoting Catholicism in America. In 1829 the Leopoldine Stiftung was founded in Austria to collect money throughout Europe to introduce religion to the U.S. frontier, resulting in more than 400 Catholic churches established in the East, the Midwest, and in what was traditionally known as "Indian country," lands under the control of Native nations including reservations, trust lands, or more casually, to describe anywhere large numbers of Native Americans lived. There are also small numbers of

Austrian Jews. The majority of Hungarians are Catholic, although, in the United States, nearly 25 percent are Protestant.

In Europe, most Czech people were Roman Catholics, but one-half to two-thirds of nineteenth-century Czech immigrants from rural areas left the church. They were considered free thinkers who believed in a strong separation of church and state. Subsequent generations now belong to a variety of faiths. Religion is still an important factor in the lives of Slovakian immigrants. Most are Roman Catholics who attend services regularly. First- and second-generation Slovakians usually send their children to parochial schools supported by the ethnic parish.

Traditional spirituality for Romans may be derived from Asian Indian religions, such as Hinduism and Zoroastrianism (refer to Chapter 2 regarding Eastern religions, and Chapter 14 for more information on Asian Indian faiths), but many adopted the predominant religion of the regions where they lived. Romani groups today are Catholic, Muslim, Pentecostal, Protestant, Anglican, Baptist, Buddhist, or Hindu.[19] While traditions and customs vary by community group and by the host culture, Romani are thought to be united in their worldview, called romaniya, which is the totality of the Romani spirit, culture, and law. Many believe in God, the devil, and the power of charms and supernatural spirits or ghosts.

Russians and People of the FSU Except for the Soviet Jewish people, the primary organization of the Russian American community today is the Russian Orthodox Church. Religion has always played a central role in the Russian community, and the Orthodox Church has tried to preserve the culture. However, the largest branch of the Eastern church, officially known as the Orthodox Church in America (formerly the Russian Orthodox Church outside Russia), now includes people from other central European and FSU countries, and the Russian traditions have been deemphasized.

Among Ukrainian Americans, more belong to the Roman Catholic Church than to the Eastern Orthodox faith. Lithuanians are also predominantly Roman Catholic; however, there are small numbers of Protestants, Jewish, and Eastern Orthodox followers. Most Armenians are members of the Armenian Apostolic Church (an Eastern Orthodox faith noted for allowing its members to make decisions on issues such as reproductive autonomy and sexual orientation without religious influence), although some Americans of Armenian descent are Protestants or members of the Armenian Rite of the Roman Catholic Church.

Family

Germans The traditional German family was based on an agricultural system that valued large families in which every member worked in the fields to support the household. Even when German immigrants moved to urban areas, family members were expected to help out in the family business. Most German families today are assumed to have adopted the smaller American nuclear configuration. The exception may be among the Pennsylvania Dutch, particularly the Amish, who continue to have large families averaging seven children. It is not unusual for an Amish person to know between 60 and 80 first cousins or for a grandparent to have thirty-five grandchildren.[20] Many Amish families are finding it difficult to maintain traditional values due to growing contact with the American majority culture through suburban sprawl.[21]

Polish Traditionally, the Polish American family was patriarchal, and the father exerted strong control over the children, especially the daughters. The mother took care of the home, and, if the children worked, it was near the home or the father's workplace.

Other Central Europeans Tight nuclear families typify traditional Austrian households. Although the father is in charge of family finances, it is the mother who rules home life. Assimilation in the United States has led to a deterioration of the nuclear family, including an increased divorce rate. Traditional Czechia and Hungarian families were male-dominated and included many relatives. In the United States, participation in church activities, fraternal societies, and political organizations often served to replace the extended family for both men and women. The role of women has become less circumscribed; children are typically encouraged to pursue higher education and professional careers. Family ties are strong among Slovakian immigrants. Parents are respected; they are frequently visited and cared for as they age. Weddings are still a major event, although they are not celebrated for several days, as they once were.

Russians As in many cultures, traditionally, Russians lived in very large family groups with women legally dependent on their husbands. This structure changed, however, with the education and employment opportunities offered to women during the communist rule of the Soviet Union. Most women worked, and families became smaller. Even when employed full-time, however, women remained responsible for all household chores. In the United States, the Russian family structure has shrunk even further. Russian couples have significantly fewer children than the national average for American families. Education is emphasized, especially if it can be obtained at a Russian-language school. Many first-generation immigrants attempted to maintain ethnic identity by restricting their children to spouses from their immediate group, but marriage to non-Russians is now the norm.

Food for Thought

In 301 CE, Armenia became the first nation to adopt Christianity as its state religion through the efforts of Gregory the Illuminator.

Amish and Mennonite people are called the Plain People, a term that reflects their lifestyle based on humility, hard work, and discipline. More traditional Amish groups are called "old-order" Amish.[21]

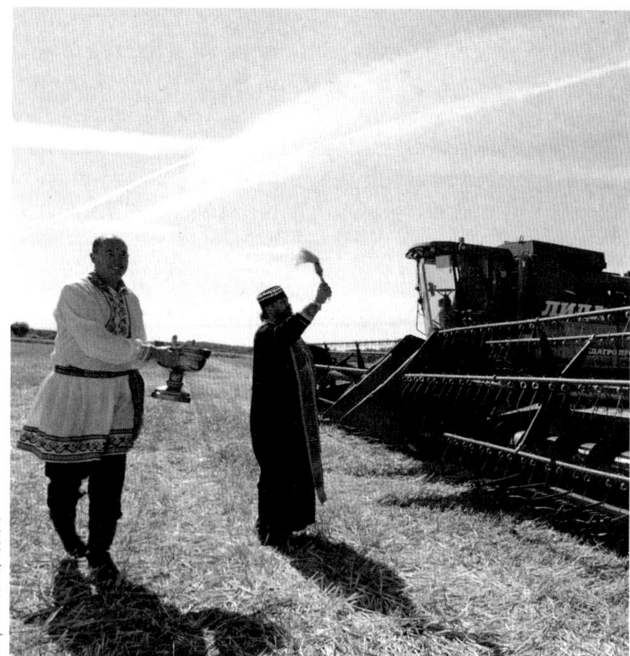
Vasily Fedosenko/Reuters

▲ Eastern Orthodox priest blesses combine harvesters and the drivers during celebrations marking the start of the harvest.

Since many of the Ukrainian and Lithuanian immigrants in the nineteenth century were men, most intermarried with other ethnic groups. The men dominated the household, the women ran the home, and the extended family was the norm. Ukrainian and Lithuanian families have since moved toward a more typically American composition with just two working parents and children. In many ways, Armenian homes are also similar to the average U.S. household. Both parents usually work, and education is a high priority. Nearly 70 percent of second-generation Armenian Americans obtain a college degree.

Traditional Health Beliefs and Practices German biomedicine makes extensive use of botanical remedies, though continued use is not documented in German Americans. A study of older German Americans in Texas showed that many believe illness is caused by infection or stress-related conditions.[22] Some Germans believe sickness is an expected consequence of strenuous labor and that health is maintained by dressing properly, avoiding drafts, breathing fresh air, exercising, doing hard work, and taking cod liver oil. Sneezing also is precarious as the soul can exit the body during a sneeze and the phrase "gesundheit" (good health) or God bless is said to ward off this danger. Numerous home remedies are common (refer to the "Therapeutic Uses of Foods" section for more information).

The Pennsylvania Dutch traditionally believed a hearty diet high in meats, dairy products, and grain foods was important for maintaining good health. Many use home remedies, homeopathic preparations, and healers to treat illness. Sympathy healing is especially well-developed. This traditional folk practice uses charms, spells, and blessings to cure the symptoms of disease. It is called either "powwowing" (not related to Native American beliefs and practices) or by its German name, Brauche or Braucherei. Powwowing is not a gathering as it might be thought of in Native American terms, but a healing practice. There is a strong religious foundation to the practice, and the healer acts as God's instrument, requesting God's direct assistance in treatment. Powwow compendiums still in use today offer everything from household tips to cures for warts, burns, toothache, and the common cold.[23] The Amish in particular subscribe to sympathy healing, the laying on of hands to diagnose illness, and reflexology (foot massage thought to benefit other areas of the body, such as the head, neck, stomach, and back), as well as the use of herbal home cures, especially teas.[24–26]

Polish Americans have reported that a shortage of medical supplies in Poland led to the widespread use of faith healers. The rise in traditional folk medicine was due in large part to the isolation and self-sufficiency of the people of the Polish countryside.[27] Although such healing practices are not documented in the United States, many Polish Americans are deeply religious and believe that faith in God and the wearing of religious medals will help prevent illness. Other health-maintenance beliefs include isolation of people who are sick, a healthy diet, sleep, keeping warm, exercise, a loving home, and avoidance of gossip.

Natural cures and alternative medicine are used extensively in Russia and the nations of the FSU, and they are often integrated with biomedical therapy.[14] For example, cupping is used for respiratory illnesses. Saunas, massage, steam baths, and balneotherapy (bathing in mineral springs) are often prescribed in conjunction with biomedical approaches; mud baths may be used for hypertension and sulfurated hydrogen baths for cardiac ailments. In addition, homeopathic preparations and herbal remedies are popular.[26,28–30] Magic and the occult may be used to cure illnesses due to supernatural causes. Psychics and znakarki (elder women who whisper charms and sprinkle water with magic powers) may be employed for chronic conditions that biomedicine cannot ameliorate. In the Russia's Siberian region, sickness was traditionally attributed to a spiritual crisis, soul loss, evil spirits, breach of taboos, or curses. Treatments used by shamans (magico-religious healers) included realigning life forces or retrieving the soul through visualization techniques, singing, chanting, prognostication, dream analysis, and séances.[31,32] Russians who do not believe in any occult practices may blame illness on other factors outside their control, including social conflict, political problems, war, poor medical care, and starvation.[32]

Traditional Food Habits

Ingredients and Common Foods: Staples and Regional Variations

The regional variations in central European and FSU cuisine are minor. The exceptions are the foods of the southern CIS nations, such as Armenia. (See "Exploring Global Cuisine—Armenia" on page 188.) The temperate climate of the region and proximity to the Arab, Turkish, and Greek cultures have resulted in a cuisine similar to Middle Eastern fare (refer to Chapter 13). Ingredients in traditional central European and FSU dishes were dictated by what could be grown in the cold, often damp climate. Common ingredients are potatoes, beans, cabbage and members of the cabbage family, beets, eggs, dairy products, pork, beef, fish and seafood from the Baltic Sea, freshwater fish from local lakes and rivers, apples, rye, wheat, and barley (refer to Table 7.1 for the cultural food groups). Foods were often dried, pickled, or fermented for preservation—for example, cucumber pickles, sour cream, and sauerkraut.

Bread is a staple item, and there are more than one hundred varieties of bread in the region. Because the climate in central Europe and FSU makes wheat harder to grow, bread is often made with rye and other grains and is often darker in color than bread made solely from wheat flour. Common types, in addition to whole wheat, cracked wheat, and white, are black (made from rye), rye, pumpernickel, caraway, egg, and potato. Cornmeal breads are found in more southern nations such as Romania. Soft pretzels are a favorite in Germany and Switzerland; they are sometimes sliced to make sandwiches. Noodles and dumplings abound and are often served as side dishes. Boiled dumplings (called knedliky in Czechia, Knödel in Germany, and kletski in Russia) can be made with flour or potatoes and with or without yeast. Spätzle are tiny dumplings common in southern Germany. They are made by forcing the dough through a large spoon with small holes into the hot water. Stuffed dumplings, filled with meat, liver, bacon, potatoes, or fruit, are called maultaschen (German), pierogi (Polish), pelmeni (Russian), or varenyky (Ukrainian). Related to the filled dumpling is stuffed pastry dough, which is baked or fried. It is customarily filled with meat or cabbage. Small individual pastries are called pirozhki in Russian, and a large oval pie is known as a pirog (also called a kulebi). One elaborate version, kulebiaka, usually includes a whole fish, such as salmon, with mushroom and rice filling. In Lithuania, lamb-stuffed dumplings served with sour cream are called kulduny. A specialty product of Russia is groats (hulled and crushed grain) of buckwheat (a gluten-free Asian grain with a distinctive, nutty flavor, especially when toasted) prepared in ways similar to rice, often served as a side dish or stuffing.[33] Buckwheat meal is used to make baked goods.

Next to bread, meat is the most important element of the diet. Pork is the most popular. Schnitzel is a meat cutlet, often lightly breaded and then fried. Ham is served fresh or cured. Poland is famous for its smoked ham, and in Germany, Westphalian ham is lightly smoked, cured, and cut into paper-thin slices. Beef is also common. In Germany, sauerbraten, a marinated beef roast, is the national dish. It is also rolled around various fillings, such as bacon, onions, and pickles, to make rouladen. Veal is especially popular in Lithuania. Poultry is well-liked. Germans often eat roast goose stuffed with onions, apples, and herbs on holidays. In Russia, chicken is stewed on special occasions, and breaded chicken cutlets called kotlety are common. A famous dish, chicken Kiev or Kyiv, claimed by both Russia and Ukraine, is made with breaded, fried chicken breasts filled with herb butter. Game meats are a favorite in many areas, especially deer, wild boar, and rabbit. A well-known German dish is hasenpfeffer—hare cooked in red wine with black pepper. In Poland, bigos ("hunter's stew"), made of venison, hare, and vegetables (some form of cabbage is always added), is traditional. Geese and duck are widely eaten, also.

Food for Thought

A Polish saying is, "A doctor's mistakes are covered in earth."

An example of a cultural taboo is that Romini women traditionally do not touch food, water, or utensils intended for other family members during menstruation or following childbirth.

Legend has it that it was people from Central Asia and Mongolia who showed the central Europeans how to broil meat, make yogurt and other fermented dairy products, and preserve cabbage in brine.

Throughout history, meat was often scarce and expensive; thus, many traditional recipes stretched it as far as possible. Dishes common throughout the region consist of seasoned ground meat mixed with a binder such as bread crumbs, milk, or eggs, then formed into patties and fried. In Germany, ground beef (and sometimes pork or veal) is served raw on toast as steak tartare. Ground meat is also used to stuff vegetables (such as cabbage) or pastry, or is cooked as meatballs, such as Königsberger Klopse topped with capers and a white sauce. Cut-up meat is often served in soups, stews, or one-pot dishes. In Germany, a slow-simmered one-pot dish of meat, vegetables, potatoes, or dumplings is called eintopf. Hungary is known for its gulyás, a paprika-spiced stew known as goulash in the United States. Sweet Hungarian paprika is made from ground, dried, mild red chili peppers; the spicier version is known for its smoky flavor. As chili peppers are a New World food, it is thought that the Hungarians used black pepper brought from India along the spice route to season their food before the foods of the Americas were available to Europeans.

Ground meats are also made into sausages. In Germany, there are four basic categories of sausage (wurst). Rohwurst, similar to American-style liverwurst, is cured and smoked by the butcher and can be eaten as is. Examples include teewurst, a raw, spiced pork sausage that is spreadable like pâté, and mettwurst, a mild, sliceable pork sausage. Bruhwurst (the frankfurter or wienerwurst is one type) is smoked and scalded by the butcher; it may be eaten as is or heated by simmering. Knockwurst, which is like a cold cut, may be smoked and fully cooked by the butcher. Leberwurst (liverwurst), blutwurst (blood sausage), and süize (head cheese) are examples. Bratwurst, similar to sausage links, is sold raw by the butcher and must be pan-fried or grilled before eating. The Polish are famous for kielbasa, a garlic-flavored pork sausage. In Austria, some sausages are called wieners. Two popular sausages with both Czech and Slovakian people are jaternice, made from pork, and jelita, a blood sausage, which can be boiled or fried.

Table 7.1 Cultural Food Groups: Central European and Russian/FSU

Group	Comments	Common Foods	Adaptations in the United States
Protein Foods			
Milk/milk products	Dairy items, fresh or fermented, are frequently consumed. Whipped cream is popular in some areas; sour cream popular in other regions.	Milk (cow's, sheep's) fresh and fermented (buttermilk, sour cream, yogurt), cheese, cream	Milk products are still frequently consumed or increased.
Meat/poultry/fish/eggs/legumes	Meats are often extended by grinding and stewing. Russians tend to eat their meat very well done.	*Meat:* beef, boar, hare, lamb, pork (bacon, ham, pig's feet, head cheese), sausage, variety meats, veal, venison *Fish:* carp, flounder, frog, haddock, halibut, herring, mackerel, perch, pike, salmon, sardines, shad, shark, smelts, sturgeon, trout *Shellfish:* crab, crawfish, eel, lobster, oysters, scallops, shrimp, turtle *Poultry and small birds:* chicken, Cornish hen, duck, goose, grouse, partridge, pheasant, quail, squab, turkey *Eggs:* hens, fish (caviar) *Legumes:* kidney beans, lentils, navy beans, split peas (green and yellow)	Consumption of meat and poultry has increased; use of variety meats has decreased. Sausages and other processed meats are often eaten.
Cereals/ Grains	Bread or rolls are commonly served at all meals. Dumplings and kasha are also common. Numerous cakes, cookies, and pastries are popular. Rye flour is commonly used.	Barley, buckwheat, corn, millet, oats, potato starch, rice, rye, wheat	More white bread, less rye and pumpernickel breads are eaten. Breakfast cereals well accepted.
Fruits/ Vegetables	Potatoes are used extensively, as are all the cold-weather vegetables. Cabbage is fermented to make sauerkraut. Fruits and vegetables are often preserved by canning, drying, or pickling. Fruit is often added to meat dishes.	*Fruits:* apples, apricots, blackberries, blueberries, sour cherries, sweet cherries, cranberries, currants, dates, gooseberries, grapefruit, grapes, lemons, lingonberries, melons, oranges, peaches, pears, plums, prunes, quinces, raisins, raspberries, rhubarb, strawberries *Vegetables:* asparagus, beets, broccoli, brussels sprouts, cabbage (red and green), carrots, cauliflower, celery, celery root, chard, cucumbers, eggplant, endive, green beans, kohlrabi, leeks, lettuce, mushrooms (domestic and wild), olives, onions, parsnips, peas, green peppers, potatoes, radishes, sorrel, spinach, tomatoes, turnips	Tropical fruits may be eaten. Greater variety of vegetables consumed; salads popular.
Additional Foods			
Seasonings	Central Europeans tend to season their dishes with sourtasting flavors, such as sour cream and vinegar.	Allspice, anise, basil, bay leaves, borage, capers, caraway, cardamom, chervil, chives, cinnamon, cloves, curry powder, dill, garlic, ginger, horseradish, juniper, lemon, lovage, mace, marjoram, mint, mustard, paprika, parsley, pepper (black and white), poppy seeds, rosemary, rose water, saffron, sage, savory (summer and winter), tarragon, thyme, vanilla, vinegar, woodruff	Saffron is a popular spice in Pennsylvania Dutch fare.
Nuts/seeds	Poppy seeds are often used in pastries; caraway seeds flavor cabbage and bread.	*Nuts:* almonds (sweet and bitter), chestnuts, filberts, pecans, walnuts *Seeds:* poppy seeds, sunflower seeds	
Beverages	Central Europeans drink coffee; Russians drink tea. Many varieties of beer are produced. Hungarians and Austrians tend to drink more wine than other central European people.	Beer, hot chocolate, coffee, syrups and juices, fruit brandies, herbal teas, milk, tea, kvass, vodka, wine	
Fats/oils		Butter, bacon, chicken fat, flaxseed oil, goose fat, lard, olive oil, salt pork, suet, vegetable oil	Soft drinks common.
Sweeteners		Honey, sugar (white and brown), molasses	Commercial salad dressings, nondairy creamers added to diet.

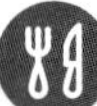 **Food for Thought**

Frankfurter means a sausage from the German city of Frankfurt; wiener means sausage from Vienna. In the United States, the term *hot dog* became popular in the late 1800s because the sausage resembled a dachshund, another import from Germany.

After diners eat smoked eel on pumpernickel bread in some restaurants in northern Germany, the server pours inexpensive Schnapps over their hands to rid them of a fishy odor.[34]

In the 1930s, and again after rationing ended post-World War II, the Swiss Cheese Union promoted fondue (chunks of bread dipped into melted cheese), as the national dish of Switzerland. The Swiss are known for their nutty, buttery cheeses with holes, such as Emmenthal (the original Swiss cheese) and Gruyère.

Freshwater and saltwater fish and seafood are often eaten fresh, smoked, or cured. Trout, carp, and eel are popular throughout much of the region. In Germany herring is commonly pickled and eaten as a snack or at the main meal, sometimes as rollmops, which are herring wrapped around a bit of pickle or onion. In Russia, smoked salmon and sturgeon are considered delicacies, as is caviar, which is the roe of sturgeon. Caviar is classified according to its quality and source. Beluga, the choicest caviar, is taken from the largest fish and has the largest eggs; its color varies from black to gray. Sevruga and osetra, taken from smaller sturgeon, have smaller eggs and are sometimes a lighter color. Sterlet, or imperial caviar, is from a rare sturgeon with golden roe. The finest caviar is sieved by hand to remove membranes and is lightly salted. Less choice roes are more heavily salted and pressed into bricks. In Poland, though some fish is consumed, it is not popular, and in some cases, fish is associated with shortages endured during Soviet rule.[35]

Dairy products are often eaten daily. Cheese may be served at any meal, from the fresh, sweet varieties, such as Lithuanian farmer's cheese, to the strongly flavored aged types like German Limburger. Fresh milk is drunk; butter is the preferred cooking fat. Buttermilk (a thick type called kefir is popular in southern areas of the FSU), sour cream, and fresh cream are also common ingredients in sauces, soups, stews, and baked products. In Austria and Germany, heavy or whipped cream is part of the daily diet, served with coffee or pastries.[36]

Traditionally, cold-weather fruits and vegetables added variety to the diet. Red and green cabbage is ubiquitous—found fried, boiled, fermented as sauerkraut, and added to stuffings, soups, and stews. Potatoes are equally popular. They are most often boiled or roasted and sliced. One German specialty, originating in the eighteenth century after potatoes came to Europe from South America, is called himmel und erde ("heaven and earth"). It's found in the northern area and consists of boiled potatoes and sliced apples topped with fried bacon and onions. Other root crops such as beets and kohlrabi accompany many meals. Cucumbers are frequently pickled or served dressed with vinegar for a salad. Onions and mushrooms flavor numerous dishes. Wild mushrooms are so popular in Poland that they are often used as a meat substitute on religious fast days.[35] Temperate vegetables, including tomatoes and eggplant, are found in the more southern nations of the FSU and are now widely available throughout the region.

In much of central Europe, sweets are enjoyed daily. They are eaten at coffee houses in the morning or afternoon, or bought at the local bakery and served as dessert. There are numerous types, such as cheesecakes, coffee cakes, doughnuts, and nut- or fruit-filled individual pastries. Apple, cherry, raspberry, chocolate, almond, and poppy seed are favorite flavors. Austria is reputed to be the home of apple strudel, though it was likely common to other cultures as well. The thin layers are reminiscent of many Turkish pastry recipes, for instance, and it is frequently mistaken as being German partly due to its German name, according to the Merriam-Webster dictionary. The paper-thin sheets of dough are rolled around cinnamon-spiced apple pieces in a strudel or "swirl" in German. Austria is also known for sachertorte, a chocolate sponge cake with apricot or cream filling. Germany is famous for Schwarzwälder kirschtorte (Black Forest cake), a rich chocolate cake layered with cherries, whipped cream, and kirsch (cherry liqueur). "Branch" cake, gałęziak, which looks similar to a gnarled log, is a popular pastry from Lithuania that is also found in Poland, where it is known as sękacz or "pyramid" cake. Dobosh torte, a multilayered sponge cake with chocolate filling and caramel topping, is a favorite in Hungary. Though fresh fruits are eaten infrequently, cooked fruits, such as the berry pudding called kisel in Russia, are common desserts throughout the region.

In central Europe, the most common hot beverage is coffee. In Russia, strong tea, using water heated in a samovar, is often consumed instead. A samovar is an urn, which may be very ornate brass, heated by charcoal inserted in a vertical tube running through the urn's center. Although southwestern Germany, Austria, and Hungary produce excellent white wine, the most popular alcoholic drink in the region is beer. The Czech Republic is known for pilsner beer, which is bitter tasting but light in color and body. German beers can be sweet, bitter, weak, or strong and are typically bottom-fermented (meaning the yeast sinks during brewing). Lager, a bottom-fermented beer that is aged for about six weeks, is the most common type. Bock beer is the strongest flavor and has a higher-than-average alcohol content. Especially after monks developed an even stronger variant known as doppelbock (meaning double bock), it is sometimes called "liquid bread" because it is so hearty and satiating it could be a meal. Märzenbier, a beer midway between a pilsner and a bock beer, is served at Oktoberfest (refer to the section titled "Special Occasions") in Munich. Weissbier is a light, top-fermented beer brewed from wheat and often mixed with lemon or raspberry fruit syrup for a refreshing summer beverage. In Russia and other FSU nations, a sour beer fermented from rye bread or beets, called kvass, is popular. It is slightly sweet and fizzy and sometimes flavored with black currant leaves, caraway, mint, or lemon. Mead, a beerlike product fermented from honey, is a Polish specialty. Schnapps, a fruit brandy made from fermented fruit, such as cherries, is popular in Germany. Vodka, which is commonly drunk in Poland and Russia, is a distilled spirit made from potatoes. It is served ice cold and often flavored with seasonings, such as lemon or black pepper. In Poland, the vodka goldwasser contains flakes of pure gold.

Meal Composition and Cycle

Daily Patterns

Central Europe In the past, people of this region ate five or six large meals a day, if they could afford it. If they could not afford it, they had fewer meals, which were often meatless. Today, modern work schedules have changed the meal pattern, resulting in three meals with snacks each day.

Food for Thought

Green vegetables as a group are called wloszczyzna in Polish, meaning "Italian commodities," since so many were originally imported from the southern nation.[36]

Sachertorte was the subject of a famous Viennese court battle regarding who had the rights to claim the original cake recipe—it was known as the "Sweet Seven Years War" due to the length of the case.[37]

Sharing food is essential to Roma culture. The harshest punishment that can be imposed on an individual is to be banned from communal meals.[38]

In Germany and the countries of central Europe, the first meal of the day is breakfast, which consists of bread served with butter and jam. Sometimes breakfast is accompanied by soft-boiled eggs, cheese, and ham. In Poland, tea served in glasses is the traditional beverage. Traditionally, tea was sucked through a sugar cube held between the teeth. At midmorning, many people have their second breakfast, which may include coffee, tea, or hot chocolate, and pastries, bread, and fruit, or a small sandwich. Lunch is the main meal of the day. In the past, people ate lunch at home, but today they are more likely to go to a cafeteria or restaurant. A proper lunch begins with soup, followed by a fish course, and then one or two meat dishes served with vegetables, and perhaps stewed fruit. Dessert is the final course, usually served with whipped cream. A quicker and lighter lunch may consist of only a stew or a one-pot meal.

A break is taken at midafternoon if time permits. It typically includes coffee or tea and cake or cookies. The evening meal tends to be light, usually including salads and an assortment of pickled or smoked fish, cheese, ham, and sausages eaten with a selection of bread. In Germany this meal is called Abendbrot, meaning "evening bread." However, Westernization and shorter lunch hours mean that nearly a third of Germans now eat smaller lunches with a larger Abendbrot meal in the evening.[24]

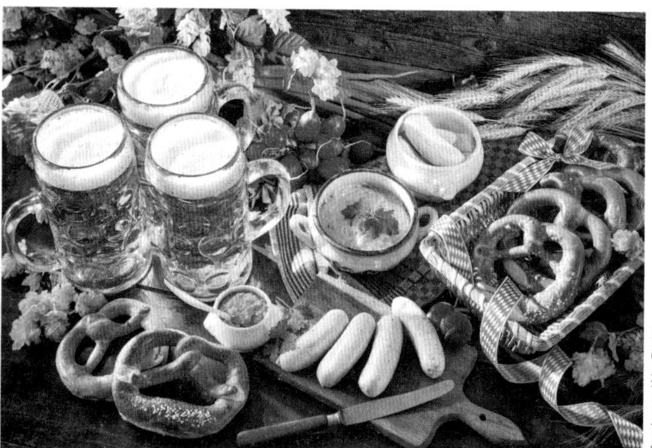

iStock.com/AlexRaths

▲ **Many German foods have been adopted in the United States, including lager-style beer, pork or veal sausages, and pretzels.**

Exploring Global Cuisine

Armenia

A legend in Armenia says that following the flood, Noah's Ark first found land in Armenia and that the nation was founded by his descendants. Armenia has been ruled by a succession of conquerors, from Rome to Russia, and today is surrounded by Muslim nations. Its fare reflects this unique past. Bread is so important that the Armenian word for it is also used colloquially for meals or food in general.[38] Lamb is a staple, though chicken and beef are also popular. Pork is rarely consumed, dating back to pre-Christian prohibitions. Freshwater fish such as trout and sturgeon (including its roe, caviar) are well-liked. Yogurt, known as mahdzoon, is consumed daily in soups, salad dressings, and beverages, as are cheeses such as feta and mozzarella-like string cheese, which are often flavored with spices or herbs. Numerous fruits and vegetables are cultivated, used fresh, dried, and pickled. Apricots, grapes, lemons, persimmons, pomegranates, quince, bell peppers, cabbage, cucumbers, eggplants, okra, squash, and tomatoes are examples. Olives and olive oil are common; however, lamb fat is often preferred for cooking. Dishes are seasoned with onions, garlic, lemon juice, sesame seeds, allspice, basil, cumin, fenugreek, rosemary, and mint. Honey flavors most desserts.[39]

Armenian cuisine has been significantly influenced by neighboring Greeks, Turkish, Persians, Syrians, and other Arabs. Shared dishes include the chickpea puree called hummus, tabouli bulgur salad, grilled kebabs, kufta (meatballs), meat turnovers known as boereg, meat- or grain-stuffed vegetables called dolma, and paklava (baklava). Many dishes have a distinctly Armenian twist. Pilaf, also called plov, is preferred with bulgur and vermicelli instead of rice in many areas. Lahjuman, an Armenian pizza made with lamb, vegetables, and feta cheese, is a favorite, as is keshkeg, a lamb or chicken stew that includes whole hulled wheat kernels called zezads.

Dinner begins with a selection of mezze (appetizers) served with the licorice-tasting aperitif raki, a clear twice-distilled alcoholic drink made from grapes and anise. Soups follow, made with yogurt, eggs, and lemon, or tomatoes, often with added lentils, meatballs, or even fruit. Salads are also served regularly, often with the main course of kebabs, stew, or casserole. Every meal includes bread, such as pita, lavash, or choereg—Armenian yeast rolls. Dessert is usually fruit, with pastries on special occasions. Traditional beverages include coffee, tea, and tahn—yogurt thinned with water and flavored with mint. Armenians are world-acclaimed vintners. Wine and brandy made from grapes, raisins, apricots, or other fruits are frequently consumed.

Russia and the FSU In czarist times, the aristocracy ate four complete meals per day; dinner was the largest. The majority of the population never ate as lavishly or as often. The meal that peasants ate after a long day's work is still the basis of a typical diet in present-day Russia, as well as in some parts of the FSU, including Ukraine. Today, three hearty meals a day are common, with the largest meal consumed at lunch. Snacking is rare. The staples are bread; soup made from beets (borscht, which is of Ukrainian origin), cabbage (shchi), or fish (ukha); and kasha (cooked porridge made from barley, buckwheat, or millet).[40] In Lithuania, soup is often replaced by salads. Tea, kvass, vodka, or beer usually accompanies meals.

One part of the traditional czarist evening meal, zakuski (meaning "small bites"), is still part of dinner in Russia today. This traditional array of appetizers starts the meal and may range from two simple dishes, such as pickled herring and cucumbers in sour cream, to an entire table spread with countless hors d'oeuvres. An assortment of zakuski usually includes a variety of small, open-faced sandwiches topped with cold, smoked fish; anchovies or sardines; cold tongue and pickles; and ham, sausages, or salami. Caviar, the most elegant of zakuski, is served with an accompanying plate of chopped, hard-boiled eggs and finely minced onions. Other zakuski include marinated or pickled vegetables, hot meat dishes, and eggs served in a variety of ways.

Sample Menu

German Abendbrot

A Selection of Sausages, Sliced Ham, and Cheeses (Westphalian Ham, Teewurst, etc.)*

Herring (Salad) in Cream Sauce*,[a]

Pumpernickel Bread, Potato Salad,*,[b] Beet Salad,[c] Pickles
Mohnkuchen (Poppyseed Cake)[d]

Beer or White Wine

Recipes in this menu:

[a]https://www.daringgourmet.com/german-red-herring-salad-roter-heringssalat/
[b]https://www.allrecipes.com/recipe/83097/authentic-german-potato-salad/
[c]https://www.allrecipes.com/recipe/259872/german-beet-salad-with-caraway-seeds/
[d]https://www.thespruceeats.com/german-poppy-seed-cake-1446588
*Can be purchased at German-style delicatessens.

Etiquette Central Europeans tend to be more formal than most Americans. In Germany, guests are generally not invited for dinner but may be asked for dessert and wine later in the evening. If invited for a meal at a home or restaurant, the invitation may indicate "c.t." (cum tempore), meaning guests can arrive up to fifteen minutes late, or "s.t." (sine tempore) meaning to be exactly on time. To begin the meal, the host may say, "*Guten appetit!*" In Poland, people do not begin a meal until everyone is served; the host may say, "*Smacznego!*" In the Czech Republic and Slovakia, the host may say, "*Dobrochot!*" and in Hungary, the phrase is, "*Jo atvadyat!*" In Russia, the host often says, "*Pree yat na vah appeteetah!*" before everyone begins. In Russia, wait for the host to say "pree yat na vah appeteetah." The word for "hospitality" in Russia is *khlebosol'stvo*, meaning "bread" and "salt." Bread is traditionally served with butter and a small bowl of salt for dipping to welcome diners.[41]

Appropriate hostess gifts are good quality dessert wines, candies, or pastries. Do not bring vodka in regions where it is commonly served, because it suggests the host does not have enough on hand. In the Czech Republic, Slovakia, and Hungary, Jack Daniels whiskey may be particularly appreciated.[41]

The continental European style of eating with the fork in the left hand and the knife in the right is common throughout the region. One should avoid switching utensils when eating. In Germany, knives are only used when absolutely necessary. Cutting potatoes, pancakes, or dumplings with a knife is an insult to the cook or host because it suggests that these items are tough. When not eating, guests should keep their hands above the table with their wrists resting on the edge. Pass all dishes to the left. Wine and vodka may be poured into tumblers instead of glasses specific for each beverage, and will usually be refilled as soon as they are emptied. Vodka is traditionally consumed in one shot.

Food for Thought

Fast foods, including U.S. hamburger franchises, are very popular throughout the region. In Germany, street stands offering bratwurst and currywurst (sausage with curry seasoning) and French fries are common. Döner kebabs, Turkish-style lamb in pita bread, are another favorite in Germany and Russia.

Special Occasions The majority of central European holidays have a religious significance, although several traditions date back to pre-Christian times. The two major holidays in the region are Christmas and Easter. Many symbols and activities associated with these holidays in the United States, such as the Christmas tree and the Easter egg hunt, were brought to the United States by central European immigrants.

Germany Germany is a land of popular festivals. Nearly all are accompanied by food and drink. One of the best-known celebrations is Munich's Oktoberfest, which lasts for sixteen days from late September through early October. Founded in 1810 to commemorate the marriage of Prince Ludwig of Bavaria, it is now an annual festival with polka bands and prodigious sausage-eating and beer-drinking. Beer is a major component of German culture. There are as many as 5,500 beer brands created in Germany and it is legal to consume soft alcoholic beverages at 16 years old. Breweries and craft beers have become extremely popular in the United States as well Types of beer can be described by alcohol by volume (ABV) and international bitterness units (IBU) (see Table 7.2).[42]

Table 7.2 Craft Beer Guide[42]

Craft Beer	Color	Calories per 12 fl. Oz.	ABV	IBU	Pairings
Pale Lager	Pale yellow	132	3.2–4.0%	5–15	Chicken, salads, salmon,
Blonde Ale	Light Yellow	124	4.1–5.1%	15–25	Grilled seafood, cobb salad, lobster, mac & cheese, fried chicken
Hefeweizen	Yellow	150	4.9–5.6%	10–15	Tacos, light seafood, salads,
Pale Ale/IPA	Dark Yellow/Golden	170	4.4–7.5%	30–70	Burgers, fish and chips, Cajun shrimp
Amber Ale	Light Brown	190	4.4–6.1%	25–45	Sandwiches, pepperoni pizza, grilled cheese, smoked meat
Irish Red Ale	Reddish Brown	193	4.8–6.6%	5–18	Beef, pork
Brown Ale	Brown	196	4.2–6.3%	25–45	Universal pairing, BBQ, Mac & Cheese
Porter	Dark Brown	210	7.0–12.0%	35–50	Meatloaf, blackened fish, beef, BBQ
Stout	Black/Brown	320	4.0–12.0%	20–80	Beef, BBQ ribs, bacon blue burger, onion rings

Food for Thought

Marzipan, a paste of ground almonds and sugar, is commonly used in desserts and candies throughout central Europe.

In the Polish Easter meal, dairy products, meats, and pastries symbolize the fertility and renewal of springtime, while horseradish is a reminder of the bitterness and disappointments in life.

Advent and Christmas are the holiest seasons in German-speaking countries. The Christmas tree, a remnant of pagan winter solstice rites, is lit on Christmas Eve when the presents, brought not by Santa Claus but by the Christ Child, represented as a golden-haired young girl or female angel, are opened. The Christmas tree is not taken down until Epiphany, January 6. A large festive dinner is served on Christmas Day, and it is customary for families to visit one another. Foods served during the Christmas season include carp on Christmas Eve and roast hare or goose accompanied by apples and nuts on Christmas Day. Brightly colored marzipan candies in the shape of fruits and animals are traditional Christmas sweets. Other desserts prepared during the season are spice cakes and cookies (pfeffernüsse and lebkuchen), fruit cakes (stollen), cakes in the shape of a Christmas tree (baumkuchen), and gingerbread houses.

On Easter Sunday, the Easter bunny hides colored eggs in the house and garden for the children to find. Often, lamb accompanied by spring vegetables and potatoes is served for Easter dinner. Candy Easter eggs and rabbits are also part of the festivities.

Poland Christmas and Easter are the two most important holidays in Poland, a predominantly Catholic country. On Easter, the festive table may feature a roast suckling pig, hams, coils of sausages, and roast veal. Always included are painted hard-boiled eggs, grated horseradish, and a Paschal lamb sculptured from butter or white sugar. Before the feasting begins, one of the eggs is shelled, divided, and reverently eaten. The crowning glory of the meal is the babka, a rich yeast cake. All the foods are blessed by the priest before being served. On Christmas Eve, traditionally a fast day, a meal of soup, fish, noodle dishes, and pastries is served when the first star of the evening emerges in the night sky.[43] One popular soup, barszcz wigilijny, a cousin to Russian boryscht, is made with mushrooms as well as beets. Carp is usually the

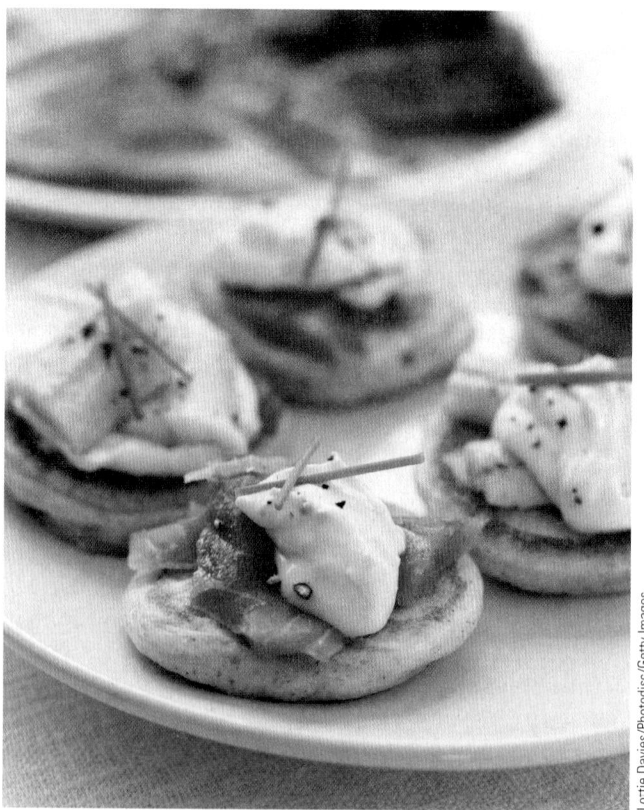

Lottie Davies/Photodisc/Getty Images

▲ Russian appetizers, called zakuski, often feature blini topped with sour cream, smoked salmon or caviar, and chives.

fish served on Christmas Eve. A Christmas cake, makowiec, is shaped like a jelly roll and filled with black poppy seeds, honey, raisins, and almonds. Jelly doughnuts, or paczki, are eaten on New Year's Eve, while on New Year's Day bigos, a hearty stew containing meats, cabbage, and other vegetables plus dried fruit, is washed down with plenty of vodka.

Austria, Hungary, the Czech Republic, and Slovakia At Christmas time, Czechias often prefer carp and prepare it in different ways: breaded and fried, baked with dried prunes, cold in aspic, and a fish soup. The Christmas Eve meal might also include pearl barley soup with mushrooms, as well as fruits and decorated cookies. Christmas dinner might feature giblet soup with noodles, roast goose with dumplings and sauerkraut, braided sweet bread (vanocka or houska), fruits and nuts, and coffee. Kolaches, round yeast buns filled with poppy seeds, dried fruit, or cottage cheese, are served at the Christmas meal and on most festive occasions. For Easter, baked ham or roasted kid is often served with mazanec (vanocka dough with raisins and almonds shaped into a round loaf).

Slovakian people break the Advent fast on Christmas Eve by eating oplatky, or small, wafer-like Communion bread spread with honey. Other items of the meal may be wild mushroom soup, cabbage and potato dumplings, stuffed cabbage (holubjy), and mashed potato dumplings covered with butter and cheese (halusky). A favorite dessert is babalky, pieces of bread that are sliced, scalded, drained, and then rolled in ground poppy seeds, sugar, or honey. Mulled wine usually accompanies this meal, as do assorted poppy seed and nut pastries and a variety of fruits. For Easter, the Slovaks prepare paska, a dessert in the form of a pyramid containing cheese, cream, butter, eggs, sugar, and candied fruits, decorated with a cross. The meal, blessed by the priest on Holy Saturday, includes ham, sausage (klobása), roast duck or goose, horseradish, an Easter cheese called syrek, and an imitation cheese ball made from eggs (hrudka).

In Hungary, the most important religious holiday is Easter. Starting before Lent, pancakes are traditionally eaten on Shrove Tuesday; sour eggs and herring salad are served on Ash Wednesday. During Easter week, new spring vegetables are enjoyed, as well as painted Easter eggs. The Good Friday meal may include a wine-flavored soup, stuffed eggs, and baked fish. On the eve of Easter, the meal might center on chicken soup served with dumplings or noodles, followed by roasted meat (ham, pork, or lamb), then several pickled vegetables, stuffed cabbage rolls, and finally a selection of cakes and pastries served with coffee. The Christmas Eve meal, which is meatless, usually features fish and potatoes. The Christmas Day meal often includes roast turkey, chicken, or goose accompanied by roast potatoes and stuffed cabbage, followed by desserts of brandied fruits or fruit compote and poppy seed and nut cakes.

In addition to Christmas and Easter, the Austrians celebrate Fasching (a holiday also known in southern Germany). Originating as a pagan ceremony to drive out the evil spirits of winter in which a procession would parade down the main street of a town ringing cowbells, it developed into a multi-day carnival associated with Lent. In Vienna, over 300 sumptuous balls are held during the event, including those hosted by the coffee brewers and the confectioners of the city. Doughnuts, fritters, and other sweets are typical festival food.

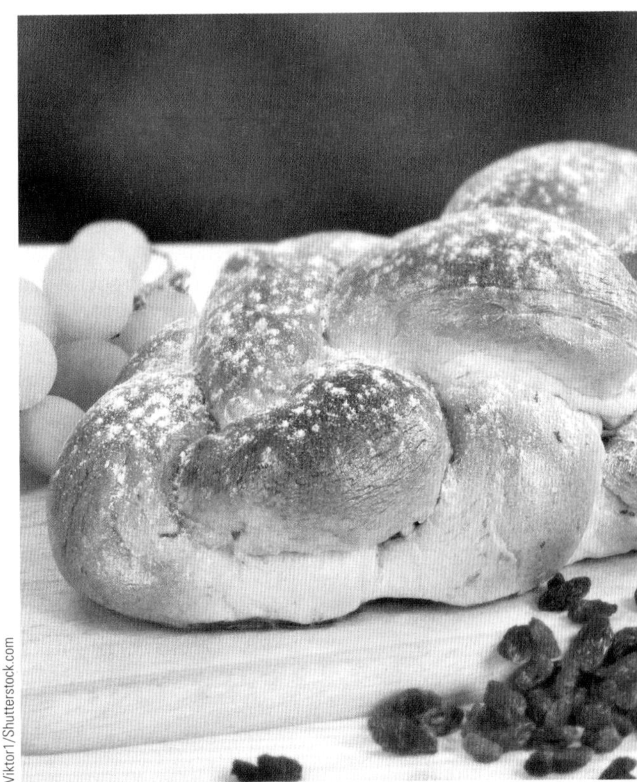

Viktor1/Shutterstock.com

▲ Vanocka, a Christmas bread popular in the Czech Republic.

Food for Thought

One customary Christmas Eve dish in Poland is *karp po zydowsku*, chilled slices of carp in a sweet-and-sour aspic with raisins and almonds. It is of Jewish origin, dating to when Poland was a haven for Jews in the fourteenth century.

Russia and the FSU Before the 1917 revolution, Russians celebrated a full calendar of religious holidays, including 250 fast days.[33] Fish was significant on days when it was allowed, but at other fast meals, mushrooms were so common as entrees that they became known as forest meat.[44] Today, observant people still do not eat any animal products during fasts (refer to Chapter 4 for the fast days in the Eastern Orthodox Church).

The most significant holiday is Easter, which replaced a pre-Christian festival that marked the end of the bleak winter season. The Butter Festival (maslenitsa) precedes the forty days of Lent. One food eaten during this period is blini, raised buckwheat pancakes. Blini can be served with various toppings such as butter, jam, sour cream, smoked salmon, or caviar. Butter is the traditional topping because it cannot be eaten during Lent. Traditional foods served on Easter after midnight Mass are pascha, similar to the Slovakian paska but decorated with the letters *XB* ("Christ is risen"); kulich, a cake made from a very rich, sweet yeast dough baked in a tall, cylindrical mold; and red or hand-decorated hard-boiled eggs. On Pentecost (Trinity) Sunday (fifty days after Easter), kulich left over from Easter is eaten.

Twelve different dishes, representing the twelve apostles, are traditionally served during the Russian and Ukrainian Christmas Eve meal. One of the dishes is kutia, or sochivo, a porridge of wheat grains combined with honey, poppy seeds, and stewed dried fruit consumed when the first stars of Christmas Eve appear. A festive meal is served on Christmas Day. On New Year's Day, children receive gifts, and spicy ginger cakes are eaten. A pretzel-shaped sweet bread, krendel, is eaten on wedding anniversaries and name days (saint's days are celebrated as birthdays in the Eastern Orthodox faith).

Therapeutic Uses of Foods A study of older German Americans found that they sometimes use home remedies to treat minor illnesses. Chicken soup is used for diarrhea, vomiting, or sore throat. Tea is taken for an upset stomach, and milk with honey is commonly used for a cough.[45] Herbal medicine, dietary supplements, and mega vitamins are often used before conventional medicine to treat mild to moderate illnesses.[46] Traditionally, the Pennsylvania Dutch believe cold drinks are unhealthy and that eating meat three times a day is the cornerstone of a good diet. Herbal teas are consumed for a variety of complaints.[46–48]

Food for Thought

A popular Pennsylvania Dutch–Amish "funeral pie," is a raisin pie that is considered a traditional comfort food. This pie would be brought by guests and served at funerals. Fruit for pie making, because of its seasonality, was often hard to come by during certain times of the year so funeral pie is made with staples from the pantry (raisins, sugar, eggs, flour, salt, and lemon). It can be made at a moment's notice, travels well, and offers sweet comfort to bereaved families.[49]

Shoofly pie, made with molasses, emerged out of the Pennsylvania Dutch region of America. It is said its predecessor was a cake created to commemorate the centennial of the signing of the Declaration of Independence at the World's Fair held in 1876 in Philadelphia. Pennsylvania Dutch cooks added the crust. Others say that the sticky and sweet filling bubbling out of the crust caused bakers to have to shoo flies away, hence the name.

Older Polish Americans reportedly believe that sauerkraut is good for colic, as are tea and soda water. Chamomile tea is used for cramps, tea with dried raspberries and wine for colds, cooked garlic for high blood pressure, and warm beverages (milk, tea, or lemonade) for coughs. Tea with honey and alcoholic spirits may be used to help sweat out an illness.[50,51]

Russians and people of the FSU ascribe health benefits to many different foods. Butter is considered good for eyesight, dill for dyspepsia, and honey for flatulence.[29] Interestingly, it is now understood in western medicine that butter is high in beta-carotene which converts to vitamin A in the body which prevents blindness in children and night blindness in adults. Respiratory infections may be treated with gogomul, a mixture of egg yolk, sugar, milk, and baking soda.[29] Teas made from raspberry, chamomile, eucalyptus, and cornsilk are used for numerous complaints. Some alcoholic beverages are of particular therapeutic repute. Kvass, the slightly fermented beverage made from bread, is believed to be good for digestion and to cure hangovers. Kvass may well be very effective because of its probiotic content from fermentation, similar to kombucha.[52,53] Kvass contains a wide range of microbes that produce lactic acid fermentation giving it a different feature from beer. Balsam, flavored vodka, is traditionally used to cure everything from the common cold to alcoholism. More recently, vodka distilled with medicinal herbs, such as ginseng or schizandra berries, has become a favorite supplement consumed as a shot or added to tea or coffee. Full, hearty meals are considered important in maintaining health.[48]

Contemporary Food Habits in the United States

Adaptations of Food Habits

Ingredients and Common Foods The Central European and Russian diet is not significantly different from U.S. fare. Immigrants made few changes in the types of foods they ate after they came to the United States. What *did* change was the quantity of certain foods. Most central European immigrants were not wealthy in their native lands, and their diets included meager amounts of meat. After immigrating to the United States, they increased the quantity of meat they ate considerably.

The people of eastern Pennsylvania, where there is a large concentration of German Americans (many Pennsylvania Dutch were from the Rhine Valley, the Palatinate, and German Switzerland), still eat many traditional German dishes adapted to accommodate available ingredients. Common foods include scrapple (also called ponhaus), a pork and cornmeal sausage flavored with herbs and cooked in a loaf pan, served for breakfast with syrup; sticky buns, little sweet rolls thought to be descended from German cinnamon rolls known as schnecken; *schnitz un knepp* (apples and dumplings), a one-pot dish made from boiled ham, dried apple slices, and brown sugar, topped with a dumpling dough; *boova shenkel*, beef stew with potato dumplings; *hinkel welschkarn suup*, a rich chicken soup brimming with tender kernels of corn; apple butter, a rich fruit spread, very much like a jam; schmierkase, a German cottage cheese; funnel cake, a type of doughnut; shoofly pie, a molasses pie thought to be descended from a German crumb cake called streuselkuchen; fastnachts, doughnuts originally prepared and eaten on Shrove Tuesday to use up the fat that could not be eaten during Lent; and sweets and sours, sweet-and-sour relishes, such as coleslaw, crabapple jelly, pepper relish, apple butter, and bread-and-butter pickles, served with lunch and dinner. Saffron crocuses (an easy-to-grow early spring colorful flower) were cultivated in parts of Pennsylvania, and the seasoning was used to color many dishes dark yellow, from soups to a traditional wedding cake known as Schwenkfelder.

Much of German cooking has been incorporated into U.S. cuisine. In fact, many common American "comfort foods" such as chicken pot pie and potato soup, and preserves such as apple butter, have their roots in Pennsylvania Dutch cookery. Many foods still have German names, although they are so common in the United States that their source is often unrecognized (e.g., sauerkraut, pretzels, pickles). Other foods contributed or greatly influenced by the Germans are hamburgers, frankfurters, braunschweiger (liver sausage), thuringer (summer sausage), liverwurst, jelly doughnuts, and pumpernickel bread. Beer production, especially in Milwaukee, was dominated by the Germans for more than one hundred years. German immigrants created a lager-style beer that is milder, lighter, and less bitter than typical German beer; it can now be described as American-style beer (see also Chapter 15).

Meal Composition and Cycle Third- and fourth-generation central European, Russian, and FSU Americans tend to consume three meals a day (with snacks), and meal composition is similar to that of a typical American meal, although more dairy products and sausages may be eaten. Some traditional foods and ingredients may not be available in areas without large central European or Russian populations.

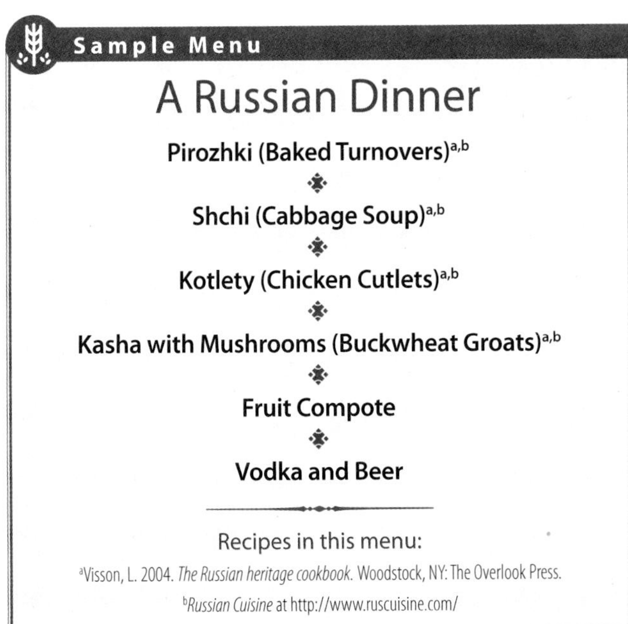
Sample Menu

A Russian Dinner

Pirozhki (Baked Turnovers)[a,b]

Shchi (Cabbage Soup)[a,b]

Kotlety (Chicken Cutlets)[a,b]

Kasha with Mushrooms (Buckwheat Groats)[a,b]

Fruit Compote

Vodka and Beer

Recipes in this menu:

[a]Visson, L. 2004. *The Russian heritage cookbook.* Woodstock, NY: The Overlook Press.

[b]*Russian Cuisine* at http://www.ruscuisine.com/

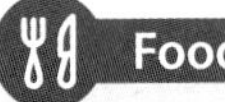
Food for Thought

Some Russian American mothers fear that cold milk may cause illness in their child and leave milk at room temperature for hours to warm it.

On average, Americans drink over 28 gallons of beer per person annually.[42]

Little dietary acculturation was found in a study of recent immigrants from Russia and other FSU countries.[54,55] An increased quantity of familiar foods, particularly soured milk, sour cream, kefir, homemade cheeses, cold cuts, and eggs, and a greater variety of fruits (including citrus, bananas, mangoes, pineapples, kiwis, and fruit juices) and vegetables (especially broccoli, cauliflower, spinach, red cabbage, and mixed salads) are consumed in the United States and are incorporated into traditional dishes and meal patterns. Breakfast cereals are well accepted, and traditional grains such as barley, buckwheat, and millet are consumed less often. Favorite American items include soft drinks, ice cream, yogurt, commercial salad dressings, nondairy cream, and whipping cream. Coffee is consumed more often and soups less often, especially at dinner. Snacking on fruit, milk, bread, pastries, sandwiches, and candy is becoming more common.

Food for Thought

The term pascha, used by the Eastern Orthodox, is closed related to the Hebrew word for Passover, "Pesach."

Most Christmas food traditions in Russia did not survive the Soviet-ruled period when religious ceremonies were discouraged.[44]

Ukrainians set a place at the table for the spirits of dead ancestors at Christmas.

Malzbier is a German beer (1 percent alcohol) that is considered appropriate for young children and nursing mothers.

Many central European and Russian American families serve traditional foods on special occasions. On October 11, Polish Americans celebrate Pulaski Day, a national day of remembrance that features a large parade in traditional apparel down the streets of New York City. The Austrians and Czechs and other pockets of strong Dutch, German, or Ukrainian heritage often observe St. Nicholas Day (December 6), when apples and nuts are put in the stockings of well-behaved children, and coal is given to the naughty ones. Later, St. Nicholas (Sinterklaas in Dutch) evolved into the secular Santa Claus, and the day of gift-giving moved to Christmas Eve. Hungarian Americans observe three unique holidays in the United States with a combination of patriotic and religious activities. The first is March 15, commemorating the revolution of 1848; the second is August 20, St. Stephen's Day, also known as State Foundation Day and Constitution Day; and the third recognizes the attempted revolt known as the Revolution of 1956 on October 23.

Among the Amish, many U.S. national holidays, such as the Fourth of July and Halloween, are not observed. A second day of celebration is added to Christmas, Easter, and Pentecost: the first day is reserved for sacred ceremonies, the second day is for social and recreational activities. Most Amish celebrate all holidays quietly with family.

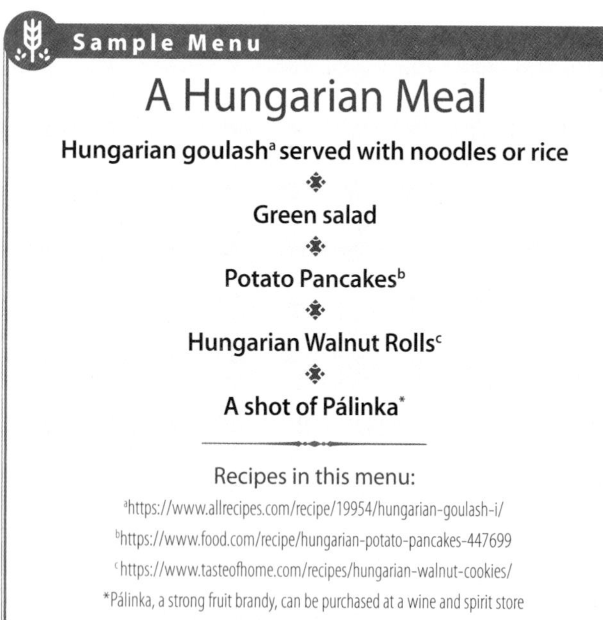

Sample Menu

A Hungarian Meal

Hungarian goulash[a] served with noodles or rice

Green salad

Potato Pancakes[b]

Hungarian Walnut Rolls[c]

A shot of Pálinka[*]

Recipes in this menu:

[a]https://www.allrecipes.com/recipe/19954/hungarian-goulash-i/

[b]https://www.food.com/recipe/hungarian-potato-pancakes-447699

[c]https://www.tasteofhome.com/recipes/hungarian-walnut-cookies/

*Pálinka, a strong fruit brandy, can be purchased at a wine and spirit store

Nutritional Status

Nutritional Intake Very little has been reported on the nutritional intake of acculturated central European or Russian Americans. There are very few dietary surveys assessing food and nutrient intake in many of these countries.[56,57] Recent European-wide studies show the diets of central Europeans are among the highest in animal products, potatoes, sweets, and refined or processed items in Europe.[58] Consumption of fats and oils of animal origin was highest in Germany: the mean daily intake for added fats and oils was 66 grams for men living in Potsdam. In 2019, 27.5 percent of German women self-reported as overweight, and 19 percent as obese. Rates for German men were nearly 41.6 percent overweight and 19 percent obese.[59,60] Slightly lower rates are found in the Czech Republic, Slovakia, and Hungary. Polish men scored higher in the overweight and obese categories than Germans, but Polish women scored lower.[61] Recent immigrants from Russia and other FSU nations were found to consume a diet high in saturated fats, sodium, and sugar.[59] Russia, Ukraine, Romania, Hungary, and the Czech Republic are among the countries with the highest death rates for heart disease, stroke, and high blood pressure. Due to this traditional dietary history, Russian Americans may be at risk of developing cardiovascular disease and other conditions associated with high-fat items (particularly red meats, processed meats, and dairy products) popular both in their traditional cultures and in U.S. fare.[62] Heart disease remains the world's leading cause of death.

Recent immigrants from Russian and FSU nations may suffer some nutritional deficiencies due to inadequate consumption of fruits and vegetables. Low intakes of riboflavin and vitamin C are reported.[61,62,64] In the Chuvash Republic of Russia, significant dietary selenium deficiency and moderate iron and manganese deficiencies have been reported.[58] High rates of diabetes, hypertension, hyperlipidemia, and cardiovascular disease are found in Russian-speaking immigrants. Tuberculosis and HIV incidence has been increasing dramatically in Russia in recent years and is thus a concern for new immigrants. Nearly 80 percent of immigrants from Russia are thought to be from the regions most affected by the Chernobyl nuclear power accident of 1979. Increases in leukemia and thyroid cancer in this population have been noted.[66]

A study of recent immigrant Russian mothers found strong support for breastfeeding. All but one of ninety participants breastfed their infants exclusively or partially for an average of twenty-eight to thirty weeks, regardless of whether the babies had been born in Russia or the United States.[65] Older Russian women use a variety of complementary and alternative medicine. A general distrust of conventional medicine may be associated with the use of alternative medicine and alternative practitioners.[66] Since the Chernobyl nuclear power accident, some Russians may resist having X-rays taken because they fear radiation exposure.[32,62,65,66]

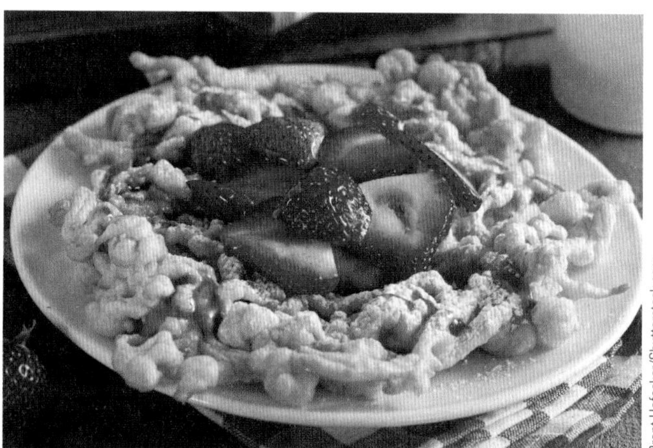

Brent Hofacker/Shutterstock.com

▲ **Pennsylvania Dutch funnel cake is an unusual "doughnut" made by pouring the batter through a funnel or from a pitcher into the hot oil in a swirled pattern.**

Food for Thought

High rates of gastric cancer in Lithuania are believed to be due in part to the high consumption of salted and cured meats and fish.[67]

Eggs are sometimes used raw in uncooked dishes by Russian and FSU Americans, putting them at risk for salmonella poisoning.

Health care providers working with Russians report that some immigrants believe potatoes cause type 2 diabetes.

Scandinavians

The Scandinavian countries of Sweden, Norway, and Denmark are surrounded by the Baltic, the North, and the Norwegian seas. In some parts of the world, the Scandinavian term may be used to include the people and countries of Iceland, the Faroe Islands, and Finland. Scandinavia includes the countries with the highest welfare in the world and are also coined as the happiest countries in the world according to the United Nations World Happiness Report.[68] Their

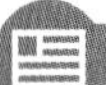

New American Perspectives

Russian

Clara Schmidt

I emigrated from the Moldova Republic (formerly Moldavia in the former Soviet Union), first to Israel in 1988, and then to the United States to be near my son. I was an English professor in the Soviet Union and Israel. My family was originally from Romania.

In the Soviet Union, we had enough food but not in abundance. Food was very important to us because of previous shortages, and as a result, we were forced to finish everything we were served. Food was never thrown away. In the morning we might have tea with a bread sandwich of butter and jam and/or possibly an egg. Snacks were not typical, but it might be a sandwich or fruit. It was something you brought with you if you went out since you couldn't purchase them. Dinner was at lunchtime (1:00–3:00 p.m.) and was the biggest meal of the day. We ate at home, and the meal was served when my father came home. The meal included soup (vegetable, chicken, or beet/cabbage), salad of several types of vegetables, meat, or fish with potatoes/rice, and fruit for dessert. We drank soft drinks with the meal. Supper was from 6:00 to 8:00 p.m. and could include sausage, vegetables, bread, and maybe leftovers, dairy (yogurt, cottage cheese), or cottage cheese pancakes with sour cream.

My diet changed the most after I immigrated to Israel. We ate less soup, less fat, and more fresh fruit and vegetables year-round. We ate much less meat and of course no pork. In Israel, I learned to love avocados and hummus (chickpea dip), and I still eat them here. In the United States, we started to eat the American way. Dinner, now the main meal, was closer to 5:00 or 6:00 p.m. It might include chicken soup with vegetables, lamb, cooked fish (not fried), and vegetables. One thing I love here is barbequed lamb ribs. Breakfast has changed to cereal/oatmeal, yogurt, and fruit. Lunch is now a sandwich or salad. I have switched from tea to coffee, and it is something I can't do without. Other things I couldn't change in my diet would be limiting fruit, vegetables, and dairy products. For special occasions, I still prepare family recipes, like Georgian chicken with walnuts, chicken necks stuffed with chopped liver, and a three-layer sour cream cake with honey and nuts.

My impression of American eating is that some Americans count every calorie they eat but the food they eat is not tasty, and most Americans eat a lot of very tasty but unhealthy food. Fast foods taste good, but the amount of fat is awful—seems like it is all meat and fried food. I prefer plain food made at home.

social welfare system, minimalistic lifestyle, infrastructure, GDP per capita, and work-life balance all contribute to their happiness. In Scandinavian countries, there is less economic inequity than in other European countries. The majority can afford a modest life with clean air, clean tap water, affordable health care, and more free time for exercise. Paid time off for vacation is twice as long as in the United States and parental leave is generous (9–12 months).

Most of the population in Scandinavia is concentrated in the warmer southern regions; the harsher northern areas extend above the Arctic Circle. Norway's weather is more moderate than that of Finland and Sweden because its long western coastline is washed in the temperate North Atlantic Drift. Denmark juts into the North Sea to the north of Germany, and its capital, Copenhagen, is directly opposite from Sweden. Numerous Scandinavians have made their homes in the United States. This section reviews the traditional foods of Scandinavia and the Swedish, Norwegian, and Danish contributions to the U.S. diet.

Cultural Perspective

History of Scandinavians in the United States

Legend says that the Norsemen (ancient Scandinavians), renowned seafarers and explorers, first discovered North America and colonized as far west as Minnesota in the thirteenth and fourteenth centuries. The documented presence of Scandinavians in the United States dates back to the seventeenth century. Jonas Bronck, a Dane, arrived in 1629 and bought a large tract of land from the Native Americans that later became known as the Bronx in New York City.

Immigration Patterns The majority of Scandinavians arrived in the United States in the 1800s, led by the Norwegians and the Swedes. During the nineteenth century, no other country except Ireland contributed as large a proportion of its population to the settlement of North America as Norway. During the 1900s, an additional 363,000 Norwegians, more than 1,250,000 Swedes, 363,000 Danes, and 300,000 Finns entered the United States.

The peak years of Scandinavian immigration to the United States were between 1820 and 1930. The population of all the Scandinavian countries had grown substantially, resulting in economies that could not absorb the unemployed and landless agrarian workers. In Sweden, the problem was magnified by a severe famine in the late 1860s. For the Norwegians, there was the additional lure of religious freedom that the United States offered, and the chance for emancipation for the peasant class. Scandinavian immigrants typically settled in homogeneous communities.

Food for Thought

Few Icelanders have made their home in the United States; the 2019 U.S. Census indicates approximately 49,000 Americans claim Icelandic descent.

Leif Erikson, a Norse explorer from Iceland, was thought to be the first European to set foot on continental North America, about five hundred years before Christopher Columbus. He called the area of coastal North America he explored Vineland for the multitude of grape vines in the area.

Norwegians and Swedes often moved to the homestead states of the Midwest, especially Illinois, Minnesota, Michigan, Iowa, and Wisconsin. One-fifth of all Swedish immigrants settled in Minnesota. Pockets of Finns and Danes also settled in this region, but they were fewer in number. Many Norwegians and Swedes later moved to the Northwest, working in the lumber and fishing industries. The shipping industry attracted some Norwegians to New York City, where they still live in an ethnic enclave in Brooklyn. Although Swedes and Norwegians are often associated with the rural communities of the Midwest, by 1890 one-third of all Swedes lived in cities, and many Norwegians were seeking opportunity in urban areas. Chicago and Minneapolis still have large Scandinavian populations.

Danes, to preserve their ethnicity, developed twenty-four rural communities between 1886 and 1935 in which, for a set number of years, land could be sold only to people of Danish descent. The best-known of these communities are Tyler, Minnesota; Danevang, Texas; Askov, Minnesota; Dagmar, Missouri; and Solvang, California. Today, most Danes live in cities, primarily on the East or West Coasts. The largest concentrations of Danish immigrants are in the Los Angeles area and in Chicago.[71]

Following World War I, U.S. immigration from Finland dropped significantly as Finns chose other countries for emigration. As the Finnish population stagnated, ethnic identity became very difficult to maintain. Second- and third-generation Finns are highly acculturated.[72]

Food for Thought

The Scandinavians introduced the cast-iron stove to the United States in the early 1800s. Cooking was previously done in fireplaces and brick ovens.

Current Demographics and Socioeconomic Status According to the 2019 U.S. Census, there are approximately 1.2 million Danes, 3.5 million Swedes, 4.2 million Norwegians, and 650,000 Finns and their descendants now living in the United States. Most Scandinavians assimilated rapidly into U.S. society, rising from blue-collar to white-collar jobs within a few generations.[3]

A majority of Scandinavian immigrants were literate in their own language and often produced local newspapers, periodicals, and books. Education was valued as a way to improve economic standing. Danish immigrants opened folk schools designed to foster a love of learning in their communities, as well as liberal arts schools. Norwegians and Swedish immigrants established many colleges. The Finns founded summer schools where traditional Finnish culture and religion were taught. Women often had educational opportunities in these schools that were unavailable to them in Scandinavia.[69–72]

Today, many Norwegians and Swedes have continued farming in the Midwest or have taken jobs in the construction industry. However, nearly one-third of Norwegians are employed in management or specialty professions, while many Swedish Americans have moved into engineering, architecture, and education.[69,70] Danes entered a variety of occupations, but they were most prominent in raising livestock and dairying. Urban Danes today are not associated with specific occupations.[73] Finnish-American men have been active in fields such as natural resources management, mining engineering, and geology, while women have been attracted to nursing and home economics.[69]

Worldview

Religion The majority of Scandinavians who immigrated to the United States were Lutheran, though each nationality had its own branch of the church, and within each branch, numerous sects were represented. Factionalism was common until many of the Scandinavian and German Lutheran churches joined together to create the Evangelical Lutheran Church in America (ELCA) in 1987. Those Scandinavians who are not Lutheran often belong to other Protestant churches, including Methodist, Mormon, Seventh-Day Adventist, Baptist, Quaker, and Unitarian.

Family The nuclear Scandinavian family was at the center of rural life. Families were typically large, and the father was head of the household. Kinship ties were strong: families were expected to pay the way for relatives remaining in Scandinavia to come to the United States, where they would be given room, board, and help in finding employment. The power of the father diminished and family size decreased as the Scandinavian Americans became more integrated into mainstream society.

Traditional Health Beliefs and Practices Information on traditional Scandinavian health beliefs and practices is very limited. Fish was considered necessary for good health. In Norway, cough and cold confectionaries (such as lozenges and pastilles) are very popular over-the-counter remedies. A current Norwegian study also found that 56 percent of cancer patients use herbs and dietary supplements primarily to boost immune function.[74] The Finns believe in natural health care, practicing massage, and cupping. Further, the sauna (a traditional steam bath) is reputed to have therapeutic qualities. It is used by Finns when ill and even during childbirth with the assistance of a midwife. It is considered a remedy for colds, respiratory or circulatory problems, and muscular aches and pains.[70,74]

One health practice in Sweden that has been widely adopted in the United States is Swedish massage, also known as therapeutic massage. It is a deep muscle technique that uses five main strokes to provide relaxation, increase circulation, and promote healing. This type of massage is very popular in the United States and is often called a classical massage involving percussion, kneading, vibration, tapping, and rolling. Massage therapy is used for symptoms of depression, stress, anxiety, back pains, headaches, muscle issues, and other chronic pains.

Traditional Food Habits

Scandinavian fare is simple and hearty, featuring the abundant foods of the sea and making the best use of the limited foods produced on land. Scandinavian cooking often reflects the preservation methods of previous centuries. Fish was traditionally dried, smoked, or pickled, and milk was often fermented or allowed to sour before being consumed. Scandinavians still prepare a large variety of preserved foods and prefer their food salty. The basics of the Scandinavian diet are given in the cultural food groups list (Table 7.3).

Ingredients and Common Foods: Staples and Regional Variations

The traditional cooking of Scandinavia is hearty. Spices were expensive in the past, and most dishes feature the natural flavors of ingredients with subtle seasoning. Black pepper, onions, and dill are used in many recipes, and juniper berries add interest to others. Caraway, cloves, nutmeg, and cardamom flavor many baked goods.

Scandinavians are probably best known for their use of fish and shellfish, such as cod, herring, mackerel, pike, salmon, sardines, shrimp, and trout. It is so common that in restaurants the lunch special is often listed simply as dagensratt ("fish of the day").[75] In Norway, the fish-processing industry is believed to date back to the ninth century, and today, Scandinavian dried salt cod is exported all over the world. Popular fish dishes include salmon marinated in dill, called gravlax; smoked salmon, known as lox; and the many varieties of pickled herring. Fish sticks and fish baked with cheese and breadcrumbs are common homestyle dishes.

Cream and butter are used in many dishes, especially in Denmark, which has a slightly warmer climate than the other Scandinavian nations. White sauce made with milk and minced parsley tops many Danish dishes, such as roast bacon, eel, and herring, as well as boiled and cured meats.[76] One Swedish specialty is known as Jansson's frestelse ("temptation") and includes anchovies and grated potatoes baked in a cream and onion sauce. Considerable quantities of fermented dairy products are used throughout the region, such as sour cream, cheese, buttermilk, and yogurt-like products, including filmjölk (Sweden) and skyr (Iceland). Sour cream in particular is added to soups, sauces, and dressings for salads and potatoes. In Norway, it is traditional to prepare an oatmeal porridge known as rømmegrøt with sour cream, and the dish is still found on many festive occasions. Fish, such as fried trout or herring, is also customarily served with a sour cream sauce and boiled potatoes. Denmark is renowned for its cheeses, such as semifirm, mellow, nutty-tasting tybo (usually encased in red wax); firm and bland danbo; semisoft, slightly acidic havarti; rich, soft crèma Dania; and Danish blue cheese. Jarlsberg, a Swiss-style cheese, is a well-known Norwegian product, but brunost, a sweet, brown cheese made from cow's milk mixed with goat's milk and served in thin slices on brown bread, is most popular in the nation.[77] Cheese is eaten daily for breakfast, on sandwiches, and as snacks.

Food for Thought

When Scandinavians toast, they say "skoal," which derives from Danish *skaal*, a toast and literally a bowl/cup, or from Old Norse *skal* meaning bowl/drinking vessel originally a cup made from a shell.

Though fish is popular in many parts of Scandinavia, the more inland areas feature many meat dishes. In the southern regions pork is particularly common. Roast loin stuffed with prunes and apples is a favorite in Denmark, which is also noteworthy for its smoked ham and bacon. Though beef is available, veal is more commonly consumed. Mutton and lamb are used in roasts and stews, such as the Norwegian fårikål (lamb with cabbage), and are also dried or salt-cured, then thinly sliced and used like ham. In the more northern areas reindeer is raised and is a popular meat. Other game meats such as elk, venison, and hare are hunted in the fall and considered a delicacy. Poultry is not especially well-liked; however, pickled goose and stuffed fresh goose are eaten, as are certain game birds, such as grouse.

Historically, meat was in limited supply, so it was stretched by chopping it and combining it with other ingredients, resulting in many traditional dishes. Scandinavians eat many vegetables, such as onions and cabbage, stuffed with ground pork, veal, or beef. The Swedes are known for their meatballs served in cream gravy or brown sauce, though the recipe is actually Turkish. It was brought into Sweden by Charles XII when he returned from five years in Turkey and the Ottoman empire in the early 1700s.[78,79] The Danes are known for frikadeller, which are patties of ground pork and veal, breadcrumbs, and onion fried in butter, and the Norwegians prepare kjøttkaker, minced beefcakes seasoned with a bit of ginger that are pan-fried, then boiled, and served with brown gravy. Beef hash made with beets and onions is another example. Sausages are also very common.

Cold-weather vegetables, including potatoes, cabbage, kale, brussels sprouts, carrots, celery root, cucumber, beets, turnips, onions, and leeks are widely available. Rutabagas, sometimes called "Nordic oranges" or "swedes," are a customary side dish.[57] Yellow and green split pea soups with pieces of ham or pork are a winter specialty throughout Scandinavia, sometimes served with pancakes. Wild mushrooms are a specialty in some areas of Finland and Norway. Though vegetables were traditionally served cooked, fresh salads have become popular in recent years. Apples, cherries, prunes, and several varieties of berries (particularly lingonberries) are typical fruits, often stewed or made into preserves that are sometimes served with meat.

Bread is a staple food item and is often prepared from rye flour, although wheat, barley, and oats are also used. Scandinavian breads may or may not be leavened, vary in size and shape, and may be white, brown, or almost black in color. Some are crisp, such as Norwegian flatbrød Swedish knäckebröd are similar to hardtack or crackers. A thin,

Table 7.3 Cultural Food Groups: Scandinavian

Group	Comments	Common Foods	Adaptations in the United States
Protein Foods			
Milk/milk products	Dairy products, often fermented, are used extensively.	Buttermilk, milk, cream (cow, goat, reindeer); cheese, sour cream, yogurt	
Meat/poultry/fish/eggs/ legumes	Fish is a major source of protein, often preserved by drying, pickling, fermenting, or smoking.	*Meat:* beef, goat, lamb, hare, pork (bacon, ham, sausage), reindeer, veal, venison *Fish and shellfish:* anchovies, bass, carp, cod, crab, crawfish, eel, flounder, grayling, haddock, halibut, herring, lobster, mackerel, mussels, oysters, perch, pike, plaice, roche, salmon (fresh, smoked, pickled), sardines, shrimp, sprat, trout, turbot, whitefish *Poultry and small birds:* chicken, duck, goose, grouse, partridge, pheasant, quail, turkey *Eggs:* chicken, goose, fish *Legumes:* lima beans, split peas (green and yellow)	More meat and less fish are consumed.
Cereals/Grains	Wheat is used less than other grains. Rye is used frequently in breads.	Barley, oats, rice, rye, wheat	More wheat used, fewer other grains.
Fruits/Vegetables	Fruits with cheese are frequently served for dessert. Preserved fruits and pickled vegetables are common. Tapioca (from cassava) is eaten.	*Fruits:* apples, apricots, blueberries, cherries, cloudberries, currants, lingonberries, oranges, pears, plums, prunes, raisins, raspberries, rhubarb, strawberries *Vegetables:* asparagus, beets, cabbage (red and green), carrots, cauliflower, celery, celery root, cucumber, green beans, green peppers, nettles, kohlrabi, leeks, mushrooms (many varieties), onions, parsnips, peas, potatoes, radishes, spinach, tomatoes, yellow and white turnips	A greater variety of fruits and vegetables are obtainable in the United States than in Scandinavia but may not be eaten.
Additional Foods			
Seasonings	Savory herbs and spices preferred. Cardamom is especially associated with Scandinavian sweets.	Allspice, bay leaf, capers, cardamom, chervil, cinnamon, cloves, curry powder, dill, garlic, ginger, horseradish, lemon juice, lemon and orange peel, mace, marjoram, mustard, mustard seed, nutmeg, paprika, parsley, pepper (black, cayenne, white), rose hips, saffron, salt, tarragon, thyme, vanilla, vinegar	
Nuts/seeds	Marzipan (sweetened almond paste) is used in many sweets.	Almonds, chestnuts, walnuts	
Beverages		Coffee, hot chocolate, milk, tea, ale, aquavit, beer, vodka, wine, liqueurs	
Fats/oils	Butter is often used.	Butter, lard, margarine, salt pork	
Sweeteners		Sugar (white and brown), honey, molasses	

round bread called lefse (also known as lompe in Norway) is made with a potato and wheat flour dough, then cooked on an ungreased griddle. It may be used to wrap a sausage, or be eaten with butter and sugar or jam and folded like a handkerchief. In Sweden, a recent innovation is tunnbrød, a very thin, wheat tortilla-like bread that is sold as fast food, rolled around fillings such as mashed potatoes, sausages, or shrimp salad and condiments such as pickles, mustard, and ketchup. Dumplings are a favorite in Norway, often made from potatoes.

Desserts, whether they are served after a meal or at a coffee break, are rich but not overly sweet. Most are made with butter and also contain cream or sweetened cheese and are often spiced with cardamom. Aebleskivers are spherical Danish pancake puffs, sometimes stuffed with fruit preserves. During Advent, they are filled with whole almonds. Another popular dessert is pancakes or crêpes served with preserved berries or jam. The Scandinavians use almonds, almond paste, or marzipan in desserts as often as Americans use chocolate. One regional dessert specialty is kransekake, a stack of progressively smaller frosted almond pastry rings. The Danes are best known for their pastries or, as they call them, Wienerbrød ("Vienna bread"). The pastries were brought to Denmark by Viennese bakers a century ago when the Danish bakers went on strike. When the strike was over, the Danes embellished the buttery yeast dough by adding jam and other fillings. A Finnish specialty is pulla, a braided sweet bread popular at breakfast.

Food for Thought

The cooking of Finland mixes Swedish and Russian elements, such as smörgåsbords, pirozhkis (meat turnovers), and blini (thin buckwheat pancakes).

Whey, a by-product of cheese making, was traditionally mixed with water to make a refreshing beverage in Norway, northern Sweden, and Iceland.

Milk is well-liked as a beverage in Scandinavia. Other common drinks are coffee, tea, beer, wine, and aquavit. *Aquavit*, which means "water of life," is a liquor made from the distillation of potatoes or grain. It may be flavored with an herb such as caraway and is served ice cold in a Y-shaped glass. It is downed like a shot and often followed by a beer chaser.

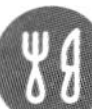

Food for Thought

The word muesli is a Swiss-German variation of the German word "müs" meaning porridge. A Swiss physician, Maximilian Bircher-Benner (1867–1939),[80] formulated the muesli recipe of oat flakes, raw apples, condensed milk, nuts, and lemon juice. Dr. Bircher-Benner would prescribe this food daily to improve the health of many of his patients and saw overwhelming improvements. His aim was to heal and prevent many diet-related diseases through foods rich in raw grains, fruits, and vegetables, and with moderate exercise including walking and gardening daily.

Meal Composition and Cycle

Daily Patterns Scandinavians eat three meals a day, plus a coffee break midmorning, late in the afternoon, or after the evening meal. Breakfast is usually a light meal consisting of bread or oatmeal porridge, cold cereal, eggs, small pastries, cheese, fruit, potatoes, or herring. Sour cream or yogurt-like fermented milk may be served to eat with cereal. Fruit soups may be served in the winter. Milk and coffee or tea accompany the meal.

Traditionally, lunch in Denmark is smørrebrød, which means hors d'oeuvre served on buttered bread as open-faced sandwiches. The buttered bread is topped with anything from smoked salmon to sliced boiled potatoes with bacon, small sausages, and tomato slices. Smørrebrød may also be served as a late afternoon or bedtime snack. Today, Danes are as likely to pick up a quick sandwich made with a bagel or Italian bread as they are to eat smørrebrød.

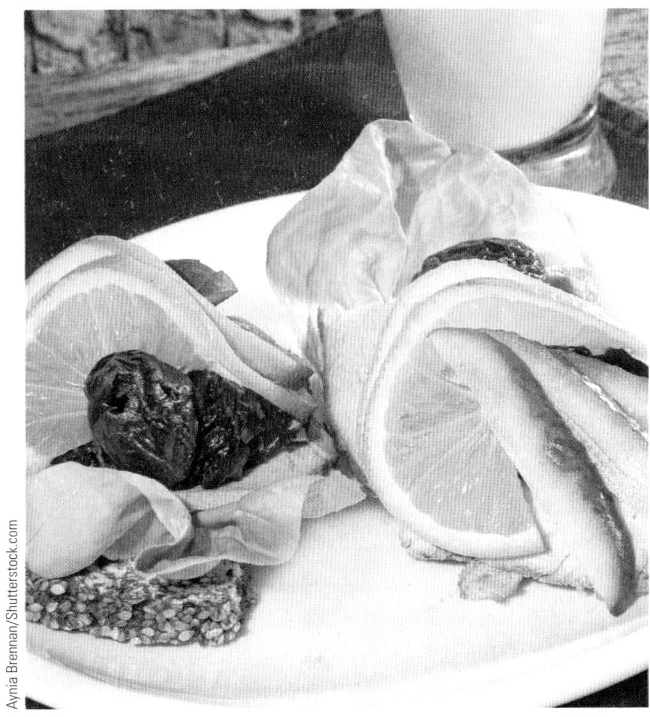

Aynia Brennan/Shutterstock.com

▲ Danish smørrebrød: Danish Fontina and Havarti cheeses, ham, salami, and smoked salmon are a few of the toppings typical of the open-faced sandwiches known in Denmark as smørrebrød.

Food for Thought

Veal Oscar, veal topped with a béarnaise sauce, white asparagus, and lobster or crab, is named after Swedish King Oscar II (1872–1907), a renowned gourmet.

Eating lutefisk has become a symbol of ethnic identity in some Scandinavian-American communities.

A buffet meal in Sweden is the smörgåsbord (bread and butter table), a large variety of hot and cold dishes arrayed on a table and traditionally served with aquavit. Ritual dictates the order in which foods are eaten at a smörgåsbord.[79] The Swedes start with herring, followed by other fish dishes, such as smoked salmon and fried fins. Next are the meats and salads (pâtés and cold cuts), and the final course before dessert is comprised of hot dishes, such as Swedish meatballs and mushroom omelets. Today, the smörgåsbord is rarely served except on special occasions. More typically, Swedes consume a hot lunch that might include pea soup, brisket or hash, and mashed rutabaga at the school or work cafeteria.[81]

If lunch is light sandwiches, dinner often includes an appetizer, soup, entrée, vegetables, and dessert. Potatoes are usually served with the evening meal. If a hot meal is eaten at lunch, a more informal supper with convenience foods is preferred. Italian items are especially popular. For example, the three most common dishes served in Swedish homes today are boiled falun sausage (a Swedish specialty made of beef, veal, and pork), spaghetti with meat sauce, and pizza.[81] Milk, beer, or wine accompanies the meal. Coffee or wine may be served with dessert. If a dessert wine is served, coffee will follow at the end of the meal.

Etiquette As with many other Europeans, the fork remains in the left hand, and the knife remains in the right one. Despite the prevalence of sandwiches in Scandinavian menus, only bread is eaten with the hands at the table; sandwiches are consumed using a fork and knife. Pass dishes to the left. When not eating, keep your hands above the table with your wrists resting on the edge. In Finland, it is important to wait for the host to initiate eating. In Norway, a guest of honor is expected to thank the hosts on behalf of all guests. Wine is expensive throughout Scandinavia, so it is always appreciated as a hostess gift.[41,70]

Special Occasions Social occasions are usually marked with food in Scandinavia. In Sweden, conferences and meetings always offer milk and coffee with sweets, such as cinnamon buns, open-faced sandwiches, or fruit. Sandwich cakes, which are layers of bread with fillings such as pâté, ham, and sliced sausages, garnished with mayonnaise, shrimp, and herbs, are served midafternoon whenever a crowd gathers for an event.

December is the darkest month of the year in Scandinavia, and Christmas celebrations are a welcome diversion. The Christmas season lasts from Advent (four weeks before Christmas) until January 13, Saint Canute's Day. In Sweden, on the morning of December 13, St. Lucia's Day, the eldest daughter in the home, wearing a long white dress and a crown of lingonberry greens studded with lit candles, serves her parents saffron yeast buns and coffee in bed. However, the climax of the season is on Christmas Eve, when the biggest, richest, and most lavish meal of the year is eaten.

In Norway, traditional foods eaten on Christmas Eve begin with rice porridge sprinkled with sugar and cinnamon. Buried in the dish is one blanched almond; the person who receives it will have good fortune in the coming year. Lutefisk, a dried salt cod soaked in lye, then boiled, is customary in the north. In the east, pork ribs and sausages with cabbage are served; in the west, a dried lamb rib specialty with mashed rutabaga is favored, while in the south, cod or halibut served with a white sauce and green peas are preferred. Boiled potatoes are a common side dish at all meals. A selection of cookies and cakes complete the meal. Women traditionally demonstrated their proficiency in the kitchen by offering at least seven types of sweets, a custom still followed in many homes today.[79]

In Sweden, a Christmas smörgasbord with twenty or thirty dishes featuring ham, herring, and other traditional fare is served. In Denmark, roast duck, goose, or pork is served with brown gravy. Typical side dishes are red cabbage and caramelized potatoes. Rice pudding with whipped cream and hot cherry sauce is also traditional. In Finland, the meal starts with pickled herring and salmon, then continues with ham, and vegetable casseroles of potatoes, carrots, or turnips. Prunes are usually featured in one dessert, followed by cookies and pies. In recent years, other European Christmas specialties such as stollen, panettone, and bûche de Noël have also become popular.[81]

Dozens of cookies and cakes are prepared for the Christmas season. The cookies are often flavored with ginger, cardamom, and cloves; the Christmas tree may be hung with gingerbread figures. Deep-fried, brandy-flavored dough, known as klejnerthe, klener, or klenätter, is also popular. The traditional holiday beverage is glögg, a hot alcoholic punch.

Midsummer's Day (June 24) is a popular secular Scandinavian holiday. It features maypoles, bonfires, and feasting. In Sweden, fish accompanied by boiled new potatoes and wild strawberries are eaten; in Norway, rømmegrøt is served; and in Finland, new potatoes with dill and smoked salmon are typical festive fare.

Food for Thought

Midsummer's Day is still observed by many Scandinavian Americans. In some areas of the United States, it has become Svenskarnas Dag (Swede's Day), celebrating Swedish culture and solidarity.

St. Urho's Day (March 16) was invented by Finnish Americans as a spoof on St. Patrick's Day. It commemorates the saints driving out the grasshoppers from Finland.

Contemporary Food Habits in the United States

Adaptations of Food Habits

Scandinavians assimilated quickly into American society, yet their diet did not change significantly because many of their food habits are similar to the diet of the dominant American culture, including three meals per day containing ample dairy products and animal protein. Many Scandinavian foods have been adopted by all Americans (refer to Chapter 15 for more information).

Nutritional Status

Nutritional Intake Very little has been published on the nutritional status of Americans of Scandinavian descent.

In Finland, the estimated overweight and obesity rates are nearly 40 percent for women and almost 60 percent for men. Figures are somewhat lower in Denmark (34 percent overweight and 16 percent obese), Norway (35 percent overweight and 14 percent obese), and Sweden (36 percent overweight and 15 percent obese).[60,76] Because both their traditional diet and the well-accepted typical U.S. diet are high in cholesterol and saturated fat, Scandinavian Americans may be at increased risk of developing cardiovascular disease and other conditions associated with the Westernized diet.

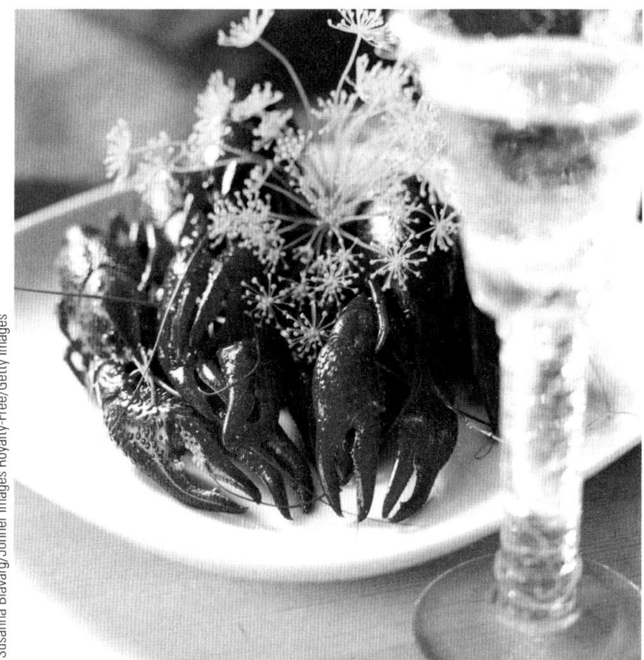

Susanna Blavarg/Johner Images Royalty-Free/Getty Images

▲ **Crawfish are a specialty in Scandinavia, where they are boiled and seasoned with dill, then served chilled at summer festivals with aquavit, vodka, or beer.**

Health and Longevity Takeaway

Fermented foods are in the nutrition spotlight these days and well they should be for their probiotic contribution to the diet. One of the common threads of the countries presented in this chapter is their use of fermented foods. Due to the probiotic content of fermented foods, some recent studies suggest that they may help alleviate gut discomfort from ailments such as diarrhea, irritable bowel syndrome, and Crohn's disease. Though more research is needed to find which strains of probiotics work best for certain conditions, current evidence still gives good reasons for everyone to consider getting a daily dose of probiotics from a fermented food source.

Some fermented foods that seem to be more accepted include yogurt (labeled with live and active cultures), sauerkraut (homemade or found in the refrigerated section of the grocery store—processing destroys bacteria), and miso. Many people already are eating these foods without the full knowledge of their health benefits. Some not-so-widely consumed fermented foods include kvass, kefir milk, kombucha tea, tempeh, kimchi, fermented cheeses, and fermented and pickled fish. These foods, too, are relatively easy to incorporate into the diet. Even some craft beer and wine fall into the fermented food category.

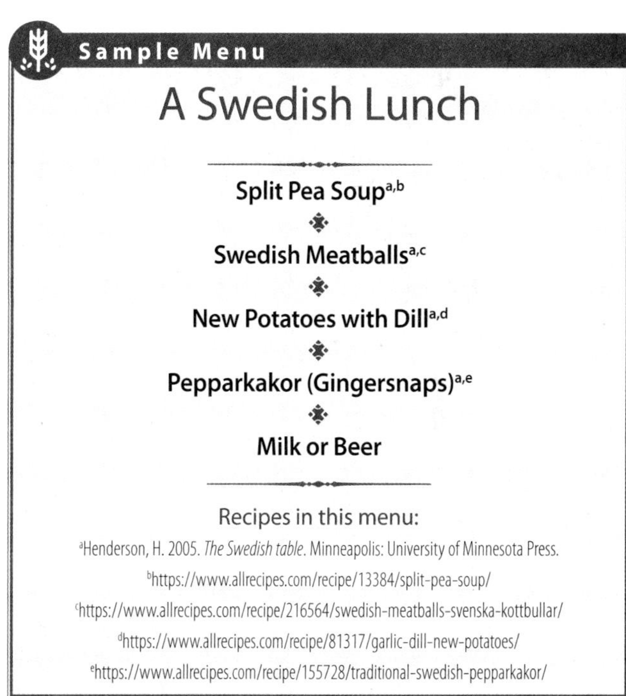

Sample Menu

A Swedish Lunch

Split Pea Soup[a,b]

Swedish Meatballs[a,c]

New Potatoes with Dill[a,d]

Pepparkakor (Gingersnaps)[a,e]

Milk or Beer

Recipes in this menu:

[a]Henderson, H. 2005. *The Swedish table.* Minneapolis: University of Minnesota Press.

[b]https://www.allrecipes.com/recipe/13384/split-pea-soup/

[c]https://www.allrecipes.com/recipe/216564/swedish-meatballs-svenska-kottbullar/

[d]https://www.allrecipes.com/recipe/81317/garlic-dill-new-potatoes/

[e]https://www.allrecipes.com/recipe/155728/traditional-swedish-pepparkakor/

Comfort Food—Armenian

K.I.'s story

Armenia has many traditional ingredients and flavors including eggplant, lamb, and lavash (bread). But for K.I., another dish stands out in family memory.

What is a favorite comfort food that you consider traditional from your home culture?

KI: Kufta is my favorite comfort food. This is a traditional Armenian dish. This is my favorite dish because it brings back memories of my grandmother. She used to make it at home and bring it over to all of us when we were sick to make us feel better. The dish is soup-like, consisting of meatballs made of ground beef or lamb, rice, egg, onions, and parsley rolled into balls and boiled in water and beef broth. Once the meatballs are cooked, lemon and eggs are added to the broth. The broth creates the aroma of beef, onions, and parsley wafting over the stove. It is served hot in a bowl with a piece of toast to soak up the broth. Some people like adding salt to taste, but my mother and others with heart

(*Continued*)

Comfort Food—Armenian (*Continued*)

K.I.'s story

problems prefer kufta just how it is. There was a comfort in knowing that this was a dish that has been passed down through generations and that my ancestors enjoyed it too.

Did you eat this food together with the community? Where was it eaten?

KI: This food is typically eaten at dinner time and is better in the fall and winter because it's a hot soup-like stew that warms you from head to toe. As far as special occasions, we normally cooked it when feeling ill because it can be bland and is easy to eat when sick. My grandmother typically prepared it when I was a child, then once she passed away my mom began to cook it, and now since my mom stopped cooking it, I began to cook it for myself and my family. It is mostly a family dish. We sat together at the dinner table and enjoyed the stew all together.

Here is K.I.'s recipe:

Kufta

Serves: 4-5 people

1 pound hamburger meat
1/2 white onion finely grated
5 eggs
½ cup of rice
3 Tbsp. finely chopped parsley
1 Tbsp. water
1 squeezed lemon
2 beef bouillon cubes
Water

Combine the meat, half the grated onion, one egg, rice, parsley, and water. Mix in a bowl and form into balls. Leave in a container and put into a refrigerator for one hour. Next, take a large pot and fill it ¾ with water, and heat it on the stovetop. Add the beef bouillon cubes. Once the bouillon cubes are melted and the water becomes beef stock, add the meatballs and cook for 45 minutes on medium-to-medium high heat. Be sure the water is covering all the meatballs for them to cook through. After 45 minutes turn the temperature to low. In a separate bowl, add four eggs and a fully squeezed lemon and beat to combine. Add some of the broth to the mixture to temper the eggs and lemon. Once fully mixed, add back into the pot to thicken the broth.

Nutritional Information (per serving):

calories 293; protein 31 gm; carbohydrates 17 gm; dietary fiber 0.4 gm; sugars 2 gm; fat 11 gm; saturated fat 4 gm; cholesterol 233 mg; sodium 368 mg

Additional Comfort Food RECIPE TO TRY

Norwegian Lefse (pronounced Lef Sa)—Bread of the Vikings

This recipe is a great treat for the holidays and a tasty way to use up leftover mashed potatoes. It is often eaten with butter, sugar, and cinnamon.

1 tsp. salt
3 Tbsp. butter
5 large potatoes
½ cup sweet cream
5 Tbsp. (or more) flour

Boil potatoes, mash fine, and add cream, butter, and salt. Beat until light. Cool to room temperature. Stir flour into the potato mixture to make a soft dough. Pull off pieces of the dough and form them into walnut size balls. Lightly flour a pastry cloth and roll pieces of dough as for pie crust, as thin as possible—1/8th inch thickness. Cook on a hot (400°F/200°C griddle or on top of the stove until bubbles form and each side has browned. Place on a damp towel to cool slightly and then cover with a damp towel until ready to serve. Serve with butter, sprinkled cinnamon, and sugar.

Nutrition Information (per serving):

calories 368; protein 7 g; carbohydrates 71 g; fat 6.6 g; sodium 522 g.

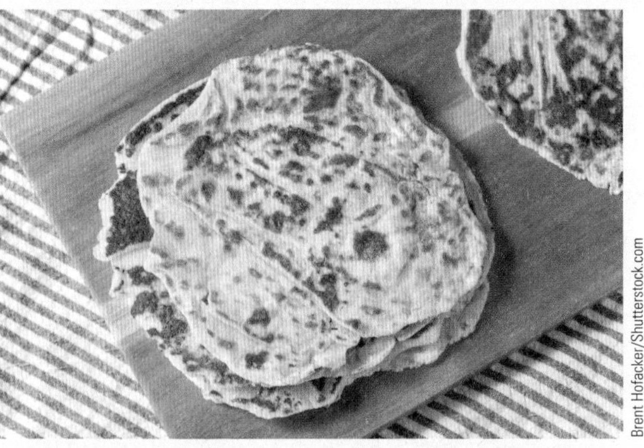

Brent Hofacker/Shutterstock.com

▲ **Norweigian lefse, potato-based breads, are much like pancakes.**

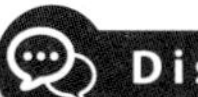

Discussion Starters

Which Cuisines Dominate in U.S. Restaurants?

Often, when Americans go out to eat at a restaurant, they typically end up at an Italian, Asian, or Mexican institution. French restaurants also tend to carry a certain cache with Americans. German and other central European and Scandinavian restaurants are less common, however, and are typically concentrated in areas of the country with a tradition of central European or Scandinavian immigration. Fast-food Italian, Asian, and Mexican restaurants are also widespread in the United States, while there are few fast-food Scandinavian, German, or Russian restaurants.

Individually and then in small groups, brainstorm why restaurant foods are distributed in this way. What possible reasons could explain why central European and Scandinavian restaurants are not more widespread, even though immigration from these countries has been as large historically as that from Italy, Asian countries, and Mexico?

Review Questions

1. Briefly describe the traditional health practices and beliefs of the Russians, Germans, and Scandinavians.
2. What were the common staples of central Europeans, Scandinavians, and people of the former Soviet Union (FSU)? What were their methods of preservation?
3. List two well-known prepared foods associated with Germany, Poland, FSU, one Scandinavian country, and one other central European country. Describe three sausages that can be found in Germany or Poland. List four U.S. foods that are thought to be descended from eastern European countries.
4. What is zakuski in a Russian meal? What foods may be included? What is a smorgasbord in Scandinavian countries? What foods might be included?
5. Describe a traditional Christmas or Easter dessert for three countries in central Europe, FSU, and one Scandinavian country.

Reflection

Given that most of the diets discussed in this chapter are traditionally high in saturated fat, cholesterol, and calories, how might the diets be modified to reduce the risk for cardiovascular disease while still maintaining some of the favorite and traditional foods.

References

1. Pánek, J., & Tůma, O. (Eds.). 2019. *A history of the Czech lands.* Charles University in Prague, Karolinum Press.
2. Britannica, T. Editors of Encyclopaedia. 2018. Commonwealth of Independent States. Encyclopedia Britannica. Retrieved from: https://www.britannica.com/topic/Commonwealth-of-Independent-States.
3. U.S. Census Bureau. n.d. *People reporting ancestry.* 2019 American Community Survey. Retrieved from https://data.census.gov/cedsci/table?q=B04006&t=Ancestry&tid=ACSDT1Y2019.B04006&hidePreview=false (accessed March 25, 2022).
4. Matache, M., Bhabha, J., Alley, I., Barney, M., Peisch, S.F., Lewin, V., Day, K., & Silverman, C. 2020. Romani realities in the United States: Breaking the silence, challenging the stereotypes. Harvard University Voice of Roma, FXB Center for Health and Human Rights. Retrieved from: https://cdn1.sph.harvard.edu/wp-content/uploads/sites/2464/2020/11/Romani-realities-report-final-11.30.2020.pdf
5. Granquist, M.A. 2014. Lithuanian Americans. In R.F. Dassanowsky & J. Lehman (Eds.), *The Gale encyclopedia for multicultural America* (3rd ed.). Cengage Learning.
6. Kifner, J. 2007. Armenian genocide of 1915: an overview. *The New York Times*, 7.
7. Baillie, L. 2021. Why Biden's recognition of the Armenian genocide is significant. United States Institute of Peace. Retrieved from https://www.usip.org/publications/2021/04/why-bidens-recognition-armenian-genocide-significant
8. Rippley, L.V.J. 2014. German Americans. In R.V. Dassanowsky & J. Lehman (Eds.), *Gale encyclopedia of multicultural America*, Vol 2 (3rd ed.) Farmington Hills, MI: Gale Group.
9. Jones, S. 2014. Polish Americans. In R.V. Dassanowsky & J. Lehman (Eds.), *Gale encyclopedia of multicultural America*, Vol 3 (3rd ed.) Farmington Hills, MI: Gale Group.
10. Jones, S. 2014. Austrian Americans. In R.V. Dassanowsky & J. Lehman (Eds.), *Gale encyclopedia of multicultural America*, Vol 1 (3rd ed.). Farmington Hills, MI: Gale Group.
11. Vardy, S.B., & Szendry, T. 2014. Hungarian Americans. In R.V. Dassanowsky & J. Lehman (Eds.), *Gale encyclopedia of multicultural America*, Vol 2 (3rd ed.). Farmington Hills, MI: Gale Group.
12. Alexander, J.G. 2014. Slovak Americans. In R.V. Dassanowsky & J. Lehman (Eds.), *Gale encyclopedia of multicultural America*, Vol 4 (3rd ed.). Farmington Hills, MI: Gale Group.
13. Schelbert, L. 2014. Swiss Americans. In R.V. Dassanowsky & J. Lehman (Eds.), *Gale encyclopedia of multicultural America*, Vol 4 (3rd ed.). Farmington Hills, MI: Gale Group.
14. Magocsi, P.R. 2014. Russian Americans. In R.V. Dassanowsky & J. Lehman (Eds.), *Gale encyclopedia of multicultural America*, Vol 4 (3rd ed.). Farmington Hills, MI: Gale Group.
15. Bassler, G. 2019 updated. German Canadians. *The Canadian Encyclopedia.*
16. Pierce, R. 2021 updated. Russian Canadians. *The Canadian Encyclopedia.*
17. Heydenkorn, B. 2022 updated. Polish Canadians. *The Canadian Encyclopedia.*
18. Swyripa, F. 2021 updated. Ukrainian Canadians. *The Canadian Encyclopedia.*
19. Bradford, A. 2018. Roma culture: Customs, traditions and beliefs. Live Science. Retrieved from https://www.livescience.com/64171-roma-culture.html
20. Kraybill, D.B. 2010. *Concise Encyclopedia of Amish, Brethren, Hutterites, and Mennonites.* JHU Press.
21. Kraybill, D.B., Johnson-Weiner, K.M., & Nolt, S.M. 2013. *The Amish.* JHU Press.
22. Spector, R.E. 2004. *Cultural diversity in health and illness* (6th ed.). Upper Saddle River, NJ: Pearson Education.
23. Donmoyer, P.J. 2018. *Powwowing in Pennsylvania: Braucherei and the ritual of everyday life.* Masthof Press & Pennsylvania German Cultural Heritage Center, Kutztown University.
24. Hirschfelder, G., & Schonberger, G.U. 2005. Germany: Sauerkraut, beer and so much more. In D. Goldstein & K. Merkle (Eds.), *Culinary cultures of Europe.* Strasbourg, France: Council of Europe Publishing.

25. Gruber, L. 2008. Kriebel, David W. Powwowing among the Pennsylvania Dutch: A traditional medical practice in the modern world. *Die Unterrichtspraxis/Teaching German*, 41(2), 219–221.
26. Yehieli, M., & Grey, M.A. 2005. *Health matters: A pocket guide for working with diverse cultures and understanding populations.* Yarmouth, ME: Intercultural Press.
27. Piątkowski, W., & Majchrowska, A. 2015. Unconventional therapists and their patients in Polish traditional folk medicine. *Anthropological Review*, 78(3), 243–250.
28. Lipson, J.G., Weinstein, H.M., Gladstone, E.A., & Sarnoff, R.H. 2003. Bosnian and Soviet refugees' experiences with health care. *Western Journal of Nursing Research*, 25, 854–871
29. Smith, L. 1996. New Russian immigrants: Health problems, practices, and values. *Journal of the American Dietetic Association*, 3, 68–73.
30. Balzer, M.M. 1987. Behind shamanism: Changing voices of Siberian Khanty cosmology and politics. *Social Science and Medicine*, 24, 1085–1093.
31. Grabbe, L. 2000. Understanding patients from the former Soviet Union. *Family Medicine*, 32, 201–206.
32. Brod, M., & Heurtin-Roberts, S. 1992. Older Russian émigrés and medical care. *Western Journal of Medicine*, 157, 333–336.
33. Zibart, E. 2001. *The ethnic food lover's companion: Understanding the cuisines of the world.*
34. Kueppers, A. 2013. Hamburg's slippery specialty: North Sea eels. Deutsche Welle. Retrieved from https://www.dw.com/en/hamburgs--specialty-north-sea-eels/a-16493990
35. Bachórz, A., & Parasecoli, F. 2021. Savoring Polishness: history and tradition in contemporary Polish food media. *East European Politics and Societies*, 08883254211063457
36. Schuhbeck, Alfons. 2018. *The German cookbook* (1st ed.). Phaidon Press.
37. Humble, N. 2010. *Cake: A global history*. Reaktion Books. 68–69.
38. Melikyan, L. 2020. On the material of verbal etiquette. *Cultural, Linguistic and Ethnological Interrelations in and Around Armenia*, 117.
39. Leahy, K. 2019. *Lavash: The bread that launched 1,000 meals, plus salads, stews, and other recipes from Armenia.* Chronicle Books.
40. Morales, B.F. 2017. *Kachka: A return to Russian cooking.* Flatiron Books.
41. Foster, D. 2000. *The global etiquette guide to Europe.* New York: Wiley.
42. Beer Institute. n.d. Beer statistics. Retrieved from http://www.beerinstitute.org/br/beer-statistics/latest-statistics (accessed January 20, 2015).
43. Krzysztofel, K. 2005. Poland: Cuisine, culture and a variety on the Wisla River. In D. Goldstein & K. Merkle (Eds.), *Culinary cultures of Europe.* Strasbourg, France: Council of Europe Publishing.
44. Grigorieva, G. 2005. Russian Federation: Rediscovering classics, enjoying diversity. In D. Goldstein & K. Merkle (Eds.), *Culinary cultures of Europe.* Strasbourg, France: Council of Europe Publishing.
45. Welz, A.N., Emberger-Klein, A., & Menrad, K. Why people use herbal medicine: Insights from a focus-group study in Germany. *BMC Complement Altern Med* 18, 92 (2018). https://doi.org/10.1186/s12906-018-2160-632
46. Anderson, C., & Potts, L. 2021. Physical health conditions of the Amish and intervening social mechanisms: An exhaustive narrative review. *Ethnicity & Health.*
47. Hostetler, J.A. 1976. Folk medicine and sympathy healing among the Amish. In W.D. Hand (Ed.), *American folk medicine.* Berkeley: University of California Press.
48. Romero-Gwynn, E., Nicholson, Y., Gwynn, D., Kors, N., Agron, P., Flemming, J., . . . & Screenivasan, L. 1997. Dietary practices of refugees from the former Soviet Union. *Nutrition Today*, 32, 153–156.
49. Falsetti, J. 2017. Resurrecting funeral pie. The York dispatch. Retrieved from: https://www.yorkdispatch.com/story/life/food/2017/05/16/resurrecting-funeral-pie/101761588
50. From, M.A. 2003. People of Polish heritage. In L.D. Purnell & B.J. Paulanka (Eds.), *Transcultural health care* (2nd ed.). Philadelphia: FA Davis.
51. Purnell, L. D., & Fenkl, E. A. 2019. Transcultural diversity and health care. In *Handbook for culturally competent care* (pp. 1–6). Springer, Cham.
52. Baniwal, P., Mehra, R., Kumar, N., Sharma, S., & Kumar, Shiv. 2021. Cereals: Functional constituents and its health benefits. *The Pharma Innovation Journal*, 10(2): 343–349.
53. Xiong, Y., Zhang, P., Warner, R., Shen, A., & Fang, Z. 2020. Cereal grain-based functional beverages: From cereal grain bioactive phytochemicals to beverage processing technologies, health benefits and product features. *Critical Reviews in Food Science and Nutrition.* Retrieved from https://doi.org/10.1080/10408398.2020.1853037 (accessed March 25, 2022).
54. Rosenthal, T. 2018. Immigration and acculturation: Impact on health and well-being of immigrants. *Current Hypertension Reports*, 20(8), 1–8.
55. Knaifel, E. 2022. Acculturation as a two-way process: Immigrants from the Former Soviet Union in Israel. *Routledge Handbook on Contemporary Israel*, 323–336.
56. Rippin, H. L., Hutchinson, J., Evans, C., Jewell, J., Breda, J. J., & Cade, J. E. 2018. National nutrition surveys in Europe: A review on the current status in the 53 countries of the WHO European region. *Food & Nutrition Research*, 62. Retrieved from https://doi.org/10.29219/fnr.v62.1362 (accessed on March 25, 2022).
57. Rippin, H., Hutchinson, J., Jewell, J., Breda, J., & Cade, J. 2017. Adult nutrient intakes from current national dietary surveys of European populations. *Nutrients*, 9(12), 1288. Retrieved from https://doi.org/10.3390/nu9121288 (accessed on March 25, 2022).
58. Slimani, N., Fahey, M., Welch, A.A., Wirfalt, E., Stripp, C., Bergstrom, E., . . . & Riboli, E. 2002. Diversity of dietary patterns observed in the European Prospective Investigation into Cancer and Nutrition (EPIC) project. *Public Health Nutrition*, 5, 1311–1328.
59. Arbel, Y., Fialkoff, C., & Kerner, A. 2020. Migration and food consumption: The impact of culture and country of origin on obesity as an indicator of human health. *Sustainability*, 12(18), 7567.
60. Global Obesity Observatory. Prevalence of adult overweight & obesity (%) Data Tables. (2022). Retrieved from https://data.worldobesity.org/tables/prevalence-of-adult-overweight-obesity-2/ (accessed March 27, 2022).
61. Buranbaeva, O. 2016. Chapter seven access to health services by indigenous peoples in the Russian Federation. *State of the world's indigenous peoples*, 159.
62. Tagaeva, T. O., & Kazantseva, L.K. 2017. Public health and medical care in Russia: Status and problems. *International Journal of Economic Research*, 14(7), 165–177.
63. Rabotaev, E.F., & Khokhlova, E.A. 2009. January–February. Topical problems of micronutrients deficiency in the Chuvash Republic. *Gigiena i sanitaria*, 1, 36–38.
64. Ackerman, L.K. 1997. Health problems of refugees. *Journal of the American Board of Family Practice*, 10, 337–348.
65. Rito AI, Buoncristiano M, Spinelli A, et al. 2020. Association between characteristics at birth, breastfeeding and obesity in 22 countries: The WHO European Childhood Obesity Surveillance Initiative. *Obesity Facts* 12, 226–243.
66. Van Son, C.R., & Stasyuk, O. 2014. Older immigrants from the former Soviet Union and their use of complementary and alternative medicine. *Geriatric Nursing*, 35(2 Suppl.), S45–S48.
67. Strumylaite, L., Zickeute, J., Dudzevicius, J., & Dregval, L. 2006. Salt-preserved foods and risk of gastric cancer. *Medicina (Kaunas, Lithuania)*, 42, 164–170.

68. https://worldhappiness.report/ed/2017
69. Granquist, M.A. 2014. Swedish Americans. In R.V. Dassanowsky & J. Lehman (Eds.), *Gale encyclopedia of multicultural America,* Vol 4 (3rd ed.). Farmington Hills, MI: Gale Group.
70. Lovoll, O.S. 2014. Norwegian Americans. In R.V. Dassanowsky & J. Lehman (Eds.), *Gale encyclopedia of multicultural America,* Vol 3 (3rd ed.). Farmington Hills, MI: Gale Group.
71. Nielsen, J.M., & Petersen, P.L. 2014. Danish Americans. In R.V. Dassanowsky & J. Lehman (Eds.), *Gale encyclopedia of multicultural America,* Vol 2 (3rd ed.). Farmington Hills, MI: Gale Group.
72. Wargelin, M. 2014. Finnish Americans. In R.V. Dassanowsky & J. Lehman (Eds.), *Gale encyclopedia of multicultural America,* Vol 2 (3rd ed.). Farmington Hills, MI: Gale Group.
73. Nielsen, J.M., & Petersen, P.L. 2000. Danish Americans. In R.V. Dassanowsky & J. Lehman (Eds.), *Gale encyclopedia of multicultural America*. Farmington Hills, MI: Gale Group.
74. Johansen, R., & Toverud, E.L. 2006. Norwegian cancer patients and the health food market—What is used and why? *Tidsskrift for den Norske Laegeforening,* 126, 773–775.
75. Nilsson, Magnus. 2015. *The Nordic cookbook*. Phaidon Press.
76. Boyhus, E.M. 2005. Denmark: Nation-building and cuisine. In D. Goldstein & K. Merkle (Eds.), *Culinary cultures of Europe*. Strasbourg, France: Council of Europe Publishing.
77. Roos, G.M., Hansen, K.V., & Skuland, A. V. (2016). Consumers, Norwegian food and belonging: a qualitative study. *British Food Journal.*
78. Rasch, D. 2018. A meatball by any other name. *Journal of the International Ombudsman Association.*
79. Brown, D. 1968. *The cooking of Scandinavia*. New York: Time-Life.
80. Medical Centre Bircher-Benner, Dorfstrasse 12, 8784 Braunwald, Switzerland Retrieved from http://www.bircher-benner.com/index.php?id=24&l=en
81. Tellstrom, R. 2005. Sweden: From crispbread to ciabatta. In D. Goldstein & K. Merkle (Eds.), *Culinary cultures of Europe*. Strasbourg, France: Council of Europe Publishing.

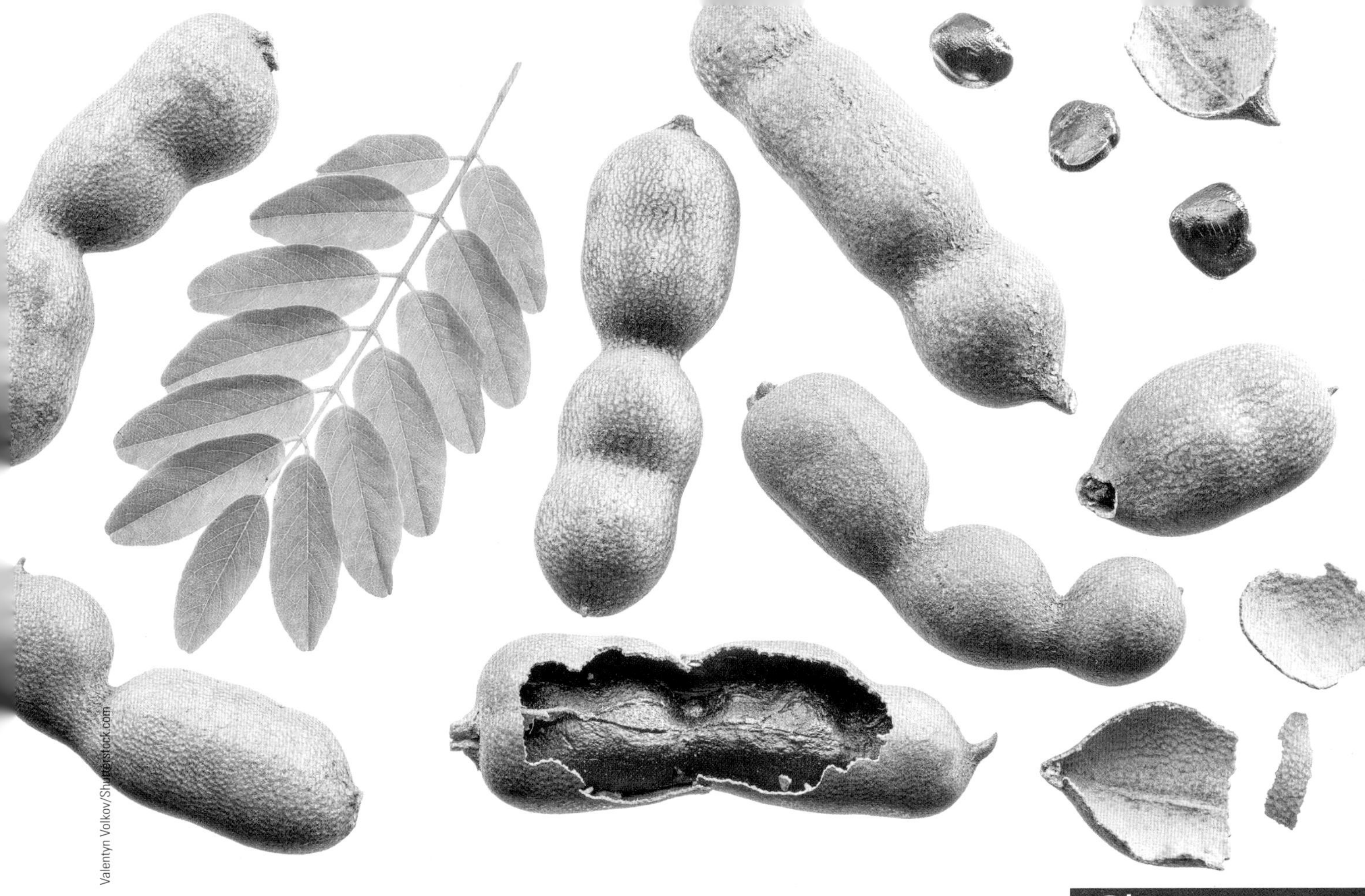

Chapter 8

Africans, African Americans, and Black Americans

Learning Objectives

8.1 List the regions of Africa that are reviewed as well as current locations of African Americans and Black Americans in America today.

8.2 Differentiate the religions, family structures, and traditional health beliefs and practices of Africans and African Americans.

8.3 Compare the differences between staple foods, foodways, and preparation techniques within and across the regions of Africa and for African Americans.

8.4 Compare key foods and foodways in African regions, to how these foods have been adapted by immigrants in the United States.

8.5 Compare the traditional meal composition and cycles to the meal composition and cycles of those who live in American today.

8.6 Describe regional specialties and dishes of African Americans.

8.7 Describe the importance of sharing food and eating as a social activity for these populations.

8.8 Identify health concerns associated with nutritional intake of Africans and Black Americans.

Black Americans are one of the largest cultural groups in the United States, comprising nearly 46.9 million people in 2020, more than 14 percent of the total American population.[1,2] The majority are originally from West Africa, although some arrived from the Caribbean, Central America, and East African nations. A small number of Americans of African heritage are White, primarily immigrants from the nation of South Africa. Others from North Africa carry Arab and Berber ancestry.

Food for Thought

The terms *African American, Black,* and *Black American* are used interchangeably in the research literature. African American has often been a preferred term to emphasize cultural heritage. However, Black is increasingly used by many African Americans who feel this term more accurately reflects their current identity. Some consider African American to be too limiting for the current population as the percentage of Black Americans who are direct descendants of enslaved Africans is decreasing. Also, there are Black Americans who are from countries other than Africa. The U.S. Black population is growing to include 46.8 million that identify as Black, either alone or as part of a multiracial or ethnic background.[3,4]

Africans and Black Americans

Most Black Americans are the only U.S. citizens whose ancestors came by force, not choice. Their long history in America has been characterized by persecution and segregation. At the same time, Black people have contributed greatly to the development of American culture. The languages, music, arts, and cuisine of Africa have mingled with European and Native American influences, among others, since the beginning of the nation to create a uniquely American cultural mix.

Black Americans live with this difficult dichotomy. They are in many ways a part of the majority culture because of their early arrival, their large population, and their role in the development of the country. Much of their native African heritage has been assimilated, and their cultural identity originates more from their residence in the United States than from their countries of origin. However, Black people are often more alienated than other ethnic groups from the dominant American society. This chapter discusses sub-Saharan African cuisines, touches on North African cuisine (refer to Chapter 13 for ways in which North African culture and fare align more closely with that of the Middle East), and their contributions to U.S. foods and food habits. The historical influence of West African Blacks on southern foodways in current American cuisine is examined.

Cultural Perspective

Africa is the second largest continent in the world and has a population estimated in 2020 at more than 1.3 billion people.[5] It straddles the equator, and much of its climate is tropical, yet rainfall varies tremendously (refer to Figure 8.1). Rain forests, grassland savannas, high mountain forests, and temperate zones are found in the far south and along the Mediterranean. Most of the world's unexploited arable land is in Africa, making its potential for agriculture to feed the world critical.[6]

In the north, the Sahara, the largest desert in the world, stretches from the Atlantic to the Red Sea, separating the Arabic northern African nations (Morocco, Algeria, Tunisia, Libya, and Egypt) from the sub-Saharan western, eastern, and southern regions. Numerous ethnic groups have evolved in Africa, and it is estimated that between 800 and 1,700 distinct languages are spoken. Cultural identity is strong. The long history of conflict and conquest on the continent has never completely eliminated tribal affinity; often, destabilization in individual nations today arises over ethnic issues. African cuisine is as diverse as the many cultures that exist on the continent, and its food flavorfully reflects this diversity.

History of Africans in the United States

The arrival of West Africans who were taken forcefully preceded the arrival of the *Mayflower* in America. Though historians sometimes point to 1619 when Dutch traders sold about twenty West Africans to colonists in Jamestown as the beginning of the slave trade to America, the story is more complex than that. The selling of African people (as well as Native Americans and others) by Europeans has roots nearly 100 years before Jamestown.[7] Between 1525 and 1866, the Trans-Atlantic Slave Trade Database estimates that 12.5 million Africans were shipped to the New World due to the efforts of the Portuguese, Spanish, English, French, Dutch, and others. Of that number, 388,000 went directly to North America. These Africans are the ancestors of the majority of Black Americans residing in the United States today.

Slavery was prevalent in many West and Central African societies before and during the trans-Atlantic slave trade. When conflict for various political and economic reasons occurred, individuals from one African group regularly enslaved captives from another group. These slaveholding societies could then use their captives as prisoners of war, for labor needs, to expand their kinship group or nation, to influence and disseminate spiritual beliefs, or as a potential trade for economic gain.[8]

Food for Thought

The word Creole has numerous definitions, mostly describing Africans and Europeans who moved to the U.S. South and Latin America during the colonial period. Commonly today, Creole refers to people of mixed French, African, Spanish, and Native American ancestry, and many reside in or have familial ties to Louisiana.

African country borders are relatively recent, due to how colonizers divided the continent politically. Traditionally, Africans most often identified with their kin-groups, such as Ashanti, Bambara, Fulani, Ibo, Malinke, or Yoruba, rather than with a specific country or Africa as a whole. The villages of West Africa were predominantly horticultural. Individuals viewed their existence in relation to the physical and social needs of the group. The extended family and religion were the foundations of community culture. It was especially difficult for individuals to be separated from their community because

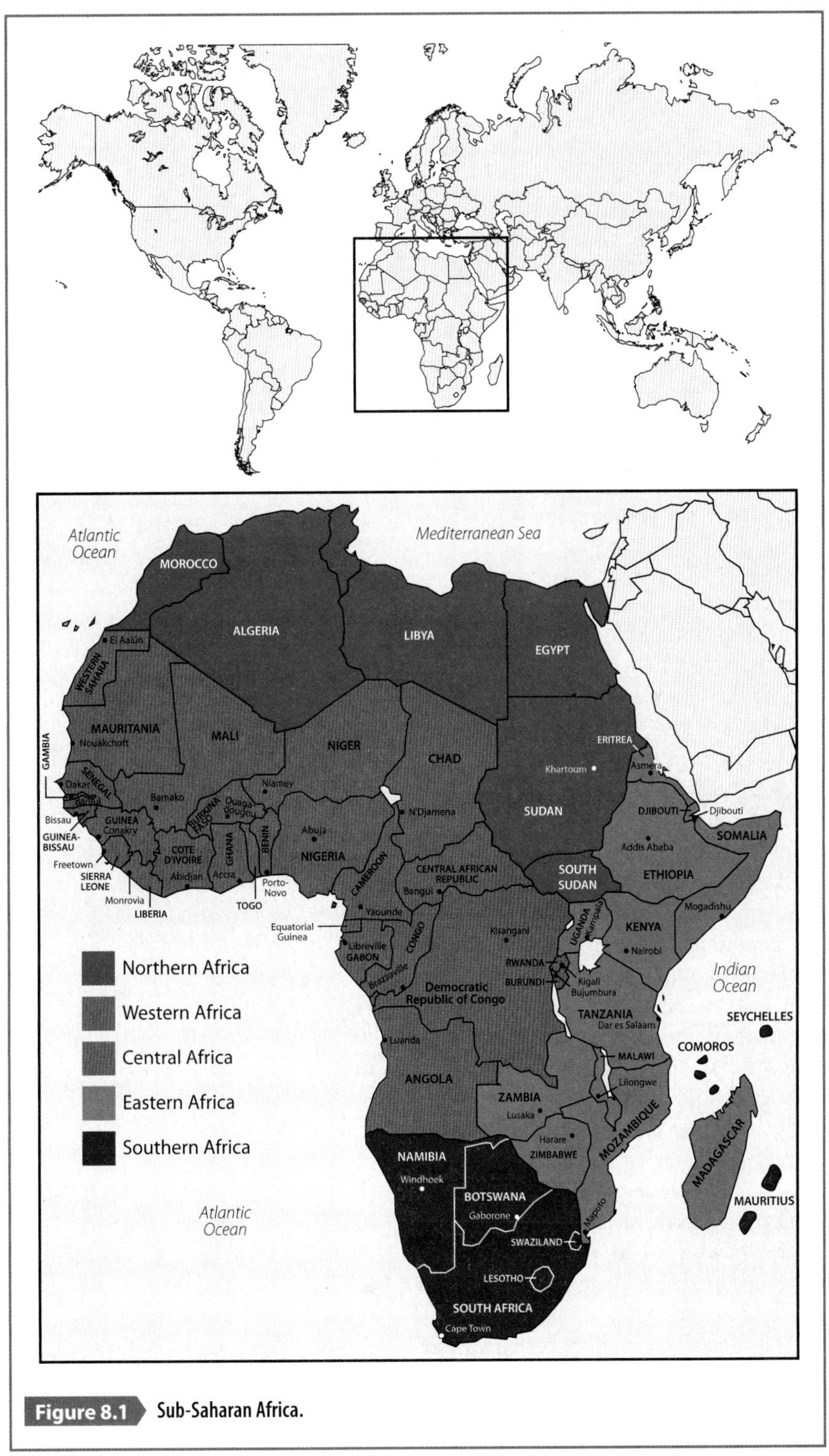

Figure 8.1 Sub-Saharan Africa.

identity was so closely associated with the group. It is perhaps for this reason that Africans in America held on tenaciously to their African traditions even though African language, ornamentation, and other customs were threatening to colonizers. Africans, usually in small groups from eight to thirty, were often housed at the perimeter of plantations until they became acclimated. Often, they learned English in two or three years through contact with Native Americans or White indentured servants. When they became sufficiently acculturated, they would be allowed to work in positions closer to the main plantation house.

This initial period of separation allowed Africans to maintain many cultural values despite exposure to people from other African communities, indentured servants of different ethnic groups, and the dominant culture of the White owners. At the same time, frontier farming was sufficiently difficult that farm owners were quite willing to learn from the Africans' agricultural expertise; therefore, intercultural communication was inevitable. Instead of becoming acculturated to the ways of the White farmers, Africans and others developed a Black Creole, native-born culture during the early slave period, combining both White and West African influences. The term Black Creole was used to distinguish between those born in the colonies from those directly from Africa. Later, it came to mean those of mixed French, African, Spanish, and Native American ancestry.

After the end of slave importation in 1808, the Black Creole population swelled. By law, slavery was a generational condition; children of people were also enslaved. Although most people worked on farms and on cotton, tobacco, sugar, rice, and hemp plantations, many others worked in mines and on the railroads. A large number of African people worked in the cities doing manual labor and service jobs.

Migration Patterns and Emancipation The earliest African migrations—both forced and voluntary—to North America forever changed history. Between 1500 and the 1860s, millions of Africans were forcibly taken to the "New World" of the Americas. The majority went to South America and the Caribbean.[9] Movements to free enslaved people in America intensified with the 1775 American Revolution. In 1862, President Abraham Lincoln signed the Emancipation Proclamation. Union victory over the Confederacy in 1865 and the subsequent ratification of the Thirteenth Amendment gave all enslaved people living in the United States their freedom. Then, by the turn of the twentieth century, depressed conditions and racial injustice in the South, coupled with industrial job opportunities in the northern states, prompted nearly six million Black Americans to settle in the Northeast and Midwest between the 1910s and 1970s.[10] Most moved to large metropolitan areas, such as New York, Boston, Detroit, Chicago, and Philadelphia. The movement, known as the Great Migration, flanked by the 1861–1865 Civil War and the 1960s civil rights movement, dynamically impacted history. Laws that established racial segregation were enacted for the first time in the early 1900s, resulting in inner-city tensions. "Sundown towns" developed throughout the country. These were so named because some all-White municipalities marked city limits with placards warning specific groups of people to stay away after the sun went down. This allowed needed unskilled laborers to work during the day, but banned the workers from the city limits, if they were Black Americans, after dark.[11] Restrictive covenants were written into deeds outlawing Black people from leasing or living in properties in White neighborhoods, except servants, and more. Even so, the many arrivals of the Great Migration and their descendants, people such as James Earl Jones, Miles Davis, Ralph Ellison, Toni Morrison, Diana Ross, Tupac Shakur, Prince, Michael Jackson, Shonda Rhimes, Venus and Serena Williams, Jackie Robinson, and countless others, reshaped the American landscape. In professions from sports and music to literature and art, the children of the Great Migration, freed from more limiting choices, made history.[12]

Because of poor economic conditions throughout the country, there was a pause in African American migration north during the Great Depression. The flow increased in the 1940s, and in the following 30 years, more than 4 million Black Americans left the South to settle in other regions of the country. When the migration began, 90 percent of all Black Americans were living in the South. By the time it was over in the 1970s, 47 percent of all Black Americans were living in the North and West. This migration resulted in more than a change in regional demographics. It meant a change from a slow-paced rural lifestyle to a fast-paced, high-pressured, urban industrial existence.[13]

In the 1960s, a movement began against the injustices of "separate but equal" laws (which permitted segregation as long as comparable facilities, such as schools, were provided for Black American students). Often, the facilities were never truly comparable. The movement gained momentum under the leadership of Black Americans such as Martin Luther King Jr. Violent riots in inner cities underscored the need for social reform. Civil rights activism resulted in the repeal of many overtly racist practices and the passage of compensatory laws and regulations meant to reverse past discrimination, as typified by federal affirmative action requirements.

Current Demographics Today, slightly more than one-half of Black Americans live in the U.S. South (55 percent), most in suburban areas. Since 1988, more Blacks have been moving to the South than to the northern states, reversing the demographic trend northward established in 1900. The remaining Black American population is found predominantly in northeastern and midwestern urban areas.[14] The most recent Census data indicate that most Black Americans live in geographic areas that are predominantly Black American or Hispanic.

As of 2020, approximately 5.4 percent of immigrants to the United States were of African descent. About 29 percent of African immigrants in the United States are from West Africa, including the countries Nigeria and Ghana. Approximately 17 percent are from East Africa, including the countries Kenya, Ethiopia, and Somalia. Less than 1 percent of the Black population is of Caribbean or Central American descent.

Socioeconomic Status Black Americans continue to suffer from the discriminatory practices that began with their enslavement, yet it is estimated that 70 percent are making steady economic progress. The Black middle class is growing, and the economic gap between Black and White people is narrowing as Black Americans increasingly enter fields such as business, health care, and law. Nevertheless, according to 2020 Census data, the poverty rate for Black Americans was 16.8 percent, more than twice the rate for non-Hispanic White families (5.8 percent) nationally. According to 2020

Census data, high school graduation rates were close to 88 percent, just below the national average of 90 percent.[15,16] The Black American unemployment rate is more than double that of White Americans, and median income is lower. In 2020, nearly one in every four Black households (27.6 percent) lived below the poverty line, which is double the national average of 12.3 percent.

Many Black Americans believe they are not completely accepted in U.S. society. Black people isolated in depressed inner cities frequently experience alienation. At the same time, discrimination has promoted ethnic identity among Black Americans, due in part to a shared history of persecution. Although Americans of African descent are geographically, politically, and socioeconomically diverse, there is a strong feeling of ethnic unity.

The socioeconomic status of recent immigrants from Africa tells a different story, as they are among the most educated groups in the United States. An estimated 49 percent of all African immigrants hold a college diploma. Nigerians often come to the United States for educational opportunities, and 61 percent have advanced college degrees.[15,16]

Worldview

Religion Spirituality was integral to African society, and indigenous religious affiliations were maintained by most early Africans in America, despite attempts to convert them to Christianity. Although the first Black church, a Baptist congregation, was founded in the 1770s in South Carolina, it was only after U.S. religious groups became involved in the antislavery movement that the Black Creole community responded with large numbers of conversions. The majority of Black Protestants (81 percent) credit church for moving Black Americans towards equality, and almost 7 in 10 (69 percent) of non-Christians credit Black Muslim organizations. About three-quarters of Black adults say that opposing racism is essential to their faith.[17,18]

Religion is as essential to Black American culture today as it was to African society. For many Black Americans, the church represents a sanctuary from the trials of daily life. It is a place to meet with others in the community, and to share fellowship and hope. More than 75 percent of Black Americans belong to a church. Seven major Black Protestant denominations make up the majority of "the Black church," a term that evolved from a pioneering sociological study by W.E.B. Dubois (who called it "the Negro church") at the turn of the twentieth century. These denominations are the National Baptist Convention, the National Baptist Convention of America, the Progressive National Convention, the African Methodist Episcopal Church, the African Methodist Episcopal Zion Church, the Christian Methodist Episcopal Church, and the Church of God in Christ. The Black Americans who are Muslim are often members of either the World Community of All Islam or the Nation of Islam (refer to Chapter 4 for more information about this religion).

Sixty percent of Black Americans who attend religious services go to Black congregations, though this pattern appears to be changing in younger generations. The broad consensus, among Black Americans of all faiths, values the role that Black churches have played in the struggle for racial equality in U.S. society. The majority view (61 percent) of those that attend historically Black congregations and those who do not, however, say their congregations should become more racially and ethnically diverse. Overall, Black Americans are more religious than the American public, based on a whole range of measures of religious commitment. For example, they are more likely to say they believe in God or a higher power (97 percent versus 90 percent for the majority culture), and to report that they attend religious services regularly (44 percent versus 29 percent).[20]

Recent immigrants from Africa adhere to a variety of faiths. While there are many different traditional African religions like Yoruba (where all things are connected and energized by one supreme god call Olorun with many Orishas that control parts of nature), most people in Africa today practice either Christianity or Islam. Both of these religions emerged out of Africa and spread throughout the continent. Many in Africa may continue to practice traditional religions in tandem with both Christianity and Islam and combine elements of several faiths. Those who immigrated from northern Africa or the northeast coast, where 93 percent of residents follow Islam, are more likely to be Muslim.[21] Those from sub-Saharan Africa are more likely to be Christian and primarily Protestant.[17,18,20,21] Many Ethiopians and Eritreans follow an Eastern Orthodox faith that is similar to, but separate from, the Egyptian Coptic Church.

Family The importance of the extended family to Black Americans has been maintained since pre-enslavement times. It was kinship that defined the form of African societies. During the early slave period, the proportion of men to women was two to one, and the family structure included many unrelated members.

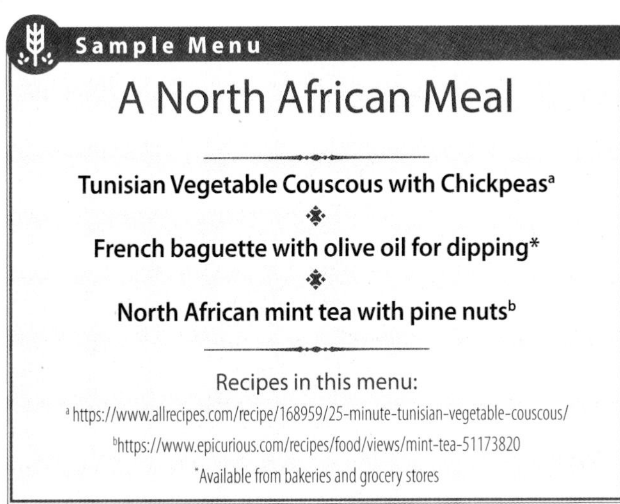
Sample Menu

A North African Meal

Tunisian Vegetable Couscous with Chickpeas[a]

French baguette with olive oil for dipping*

North African mint tea with pine nuts[b]

Recipes in this menu:

[a] https://www.allrecipes.com/recipe/168959/25-minute-tunisian-vegetable-couscous/

[b] https://www.epicurious.com/recipes/food/views/mint-tea-51173820

*Available from bakeries and grocery stores

In 2020, 50 percent of Black American families were headed by single women[22] within a family network often including grandparents, aunts, uncles, sisters, brothers, deacons or preachers, and friends. Such extended kinship still supports and protects individuals, especially children, from the problems of a discriminatory society. The extended family is equally valued by both wealthy and less wealthy Black Americans.

Family patterns typical in sub-Saharan Africa are altering due to movement from rural to urban areas throughout the continent. Despite this, family remains a prominent nexus of the social life of Africans. Respect for elders and ancestors is strong, and communities are characterized by the prevalence of collectivism as opposed to individuality.

In the North African Maghreb countries (Morocco, Algeria, Tunisia, Libya, and Mauritania), family relationships are the most important component of social life, and extended family members typically live together. As in many traditional cultures, the bond between parents and children is revered and it is considered polite to show respect to elders.

Food for Thought

The region of North Africa—Morocco, Algeria, Tunisia, Libya, and some also include Mauritania—collectively are called the Maghreb or Maghrib. The word maghreb is an Arabic term meaning "place of setting (of the sun)" and hence, "west." It lies west of the Arabian Peninsula and was the Africa Minor of ancient times. At one time, it included Moorish Spain and the majority of the people are of Arab and Berber heritage.[19]

The Phoenicians created the port of Carthage in Tunisia, and the historic city now lies partially excavated under the capital city of Tunis.

Traditional Health Beliefs and Practices Many sub-Saharan Africans view life as energy rather than matter. A person lives transitionally on earth, interacting with all environmental forces, from those of the gods and nature to those exerted by the living and dead. Life events can be influenced by these forces, and a person can, in turn, influence these forces toward good or evil.

Health is maintained through harmony. Disharmony and illness occur when someone (living or dead), the gods, or nature is intentionally malevolent. One traditional example of how a person may become ill is the evil eye, whereby one person causes illness and misfortune by sending negative energy through an evil gaze. A traditional African healer must first diagnose the illness, determine the supernatural cause of the illness, then dislodge the evil and take measures to prevent reoccurrence. The healer often uses herbs and other natural prescriptions to treat the symptoms and may depend on the spirits of the ancestors to transmit medical knowledge. Bleeding, massage, dietary restrictions, chants, and charms may complete the cure.[20]

The health beliefs and practices of some Black Americans reflect traditional African concepts as well as those encountered through early contact with both Native Americans and Whites, though it is often difficult to determine the origins of a specific practice. Some Americans of African heritage maintain health by eating three meals each day, including a hot breakfast. Laxatives may be used regularly, and cod liver oil may be taken to prevent colds. In folklore, a copper or silver bracelet is sometimes worn for protection; if it is removed, harm will occur. If the skin darkens around the bracelet, illness is impending and precautions, such as more rest and a better diet, should be undertaken.[23,24]

One study of Black men found that they defined health as more than simply a lack of illness. The ability to support their family, fulfill social obligations, and maintain emotional and spiritual well-being was also important. Self-empowerment was one method used to combat the difficulties of racism and poverty thought to undermine good health. Prayer for health is common and practiced by a significant amount of this population. Some Black Americans believe that illness is a punishment from God, and many feel that God acts through physicians to heal patients. Stress is frequently cited as the cause of poor health. It is considered by some Black Americans to be the source of hypertension; likewise, "worriation" results in diabetes.[25] Others, especially in the rural South, believe that illness is due to evil spirits or witchcraft. A person may be "hexed," "fixed," "mojoed," or "rooted" by someone with supernatural skills. Healers and conjurers are needed to "fix" or "trick" the evil. The resulting illness can be cured by herbal treatments, incantations, or magical transference. For example, a toad is placed on the head of someone with a headache, and when the toad later dies, the headache will disappear.[25]

The best-known traditional healers in the United States are the practitioners of Voodoo, also called Hoo-doo. This combination of African and Catholic beliefs is thought to have originated in the Caribbean (see Chapter 10); where it is still practiced in the South, it was also likely influenced by European witchcraft.[26] The men and women practitioners can use Voodoo use magic sympathetically. They cure unnatural illnesses (those of supernatural cause) through casting spells, the use of magic powders and gris-gris, bags worn around the neck with powders, animal bones or teeth, stones, and/or herbs. Other healers include traditional herbalists or root doctors, and spiritual, sympathy, or faith healers who derive their powers from God. A patient may choose to use one or all such healers to treat an illness, and the specialty of one may overlap with another. In most cases, healers of all kinds use a holistic approach and spend a great deal of time with a patient, providing a feeling of spiritual as well as physical well-being.[27,28]

Few Black Americans today believe in African witchcraft. However, the influence of traditional healing practices is still found in the idea that ill health is due to bad luck or fate, in the frequent use of home remedies, and in a preference for natural therapies, such as the use of garlic pills found in one study, by some Black people.[29]

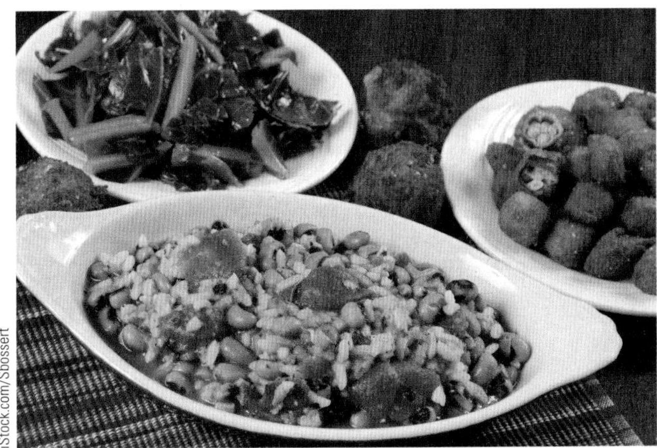

iStock.com/Sbossert

▲ Some typical foods of the southern Black diet include okra, black-eyed peas, greens, and hush puppies (fried corn bread).

Traditional Food Habits

Ingredients and Common Foods

Historical Influences Black American foods offer a unique glimpse into the development of a cuisine. Even before West Africans were brought to North America, their food habits had changed significantly due to the introduction of New World foods such as cassava (*Manihot esculenta*, a tuber that is also called manioc), corn (best known as maize in Africa), chilies, peanuts, pumpkins, and tomatoes during the fifteenth and sixteenth centuries. African Americans brought a diet based on these new foods and native West African foods, such as watermelon, black-eyed peas, okra, sesame, and taro. Adaptations and substitutions were made based on available foods. Black cooks added their West African preparation methods to British, French, Spanish, Latinx, and Native American techniques to produce American southern cuisine, emphasizing fried, boiled, and roasted dishes using pork, pork fat, corn, sweet potatoes, and local green leafy vegetables. The cuisines of other African regions have had little impact at this point on the typical U.S. diet, although recent immigrants may continue to prepare and consume traditional fare.

African Fare

West African Knowledge of West African food habits before the nineteenth century is mostly based on the records of North African, European, and U.S. traders. Most West Africans during the seventeenth and eighteenth centuries lived in preliterate, horticulturally based groups.[30] Researchers found communities with more slave trade engagement had lower literacy. The loss of the millions of people in West and Central Africa over nearly 400 years of the trans Atlantic slave trade fundamentally altered African economies by discouraging state-building and the cultivation of citizenry for taxation, and encouraging raiding and capture. The relationship between slave intensity and literacy, researchers say, affected basic levels of society: families, informal institutions of villages, towns, and ethnic groups.[30]

Throughout this time and historically, West African staple foods varied in each locality. Locally grown foods were pivotal, although some items, such as salt and fish (usually salt-cured), could be traded at the daily markets held throughout each region.

Corn, millet, and rice were used in the coastal areas and Sierra Leone. Yams were popular in Nigeria. Cassava (often roasted and ground into a flour known as gari) and plantains formed the dietary foundation of the more southern regions, including the Congo and Angola. The arid savanna region of West Africa bordering the Sahara Desert was too dry for cultivation, so most tribes were pastoral, herding camels, sheep, goats, and cattle. In the north, these animals were eaten; in other regions, local fish and game were consumed. Insects such as termites and locusts were consumed in many regions of Africa and are considered a treat in some areas. Chickens were also raised, though in many tribes the eggs were frequently traded, not eaten, and the chicken itself was served mostly as a special dish for guests. Chicken remains a prestigious meat in many regions today.

There were many similarities in cuisine throughout West Africa. Most foods were boiled or fried, and then small chunks were dipped in a sauce and eaten by hand. Starchy vegetables including yams, plantains, cassava, sweet potatoes, and potatoes were and still are often boiled, then pounded into a paste (called fufu). Each diner formed the dough into bite-size scoops used like spoons to eat stew. Palm oil was the predominant fat used in cooking, giving many dishes a red hue. Peanut oil, shea oil (from the nuts of the African shea tree), and occasionally coconut oil were used in some regions. The addition of tomatoes, chili peppers, and onions as seasoning was so common that these items were simply referred to as "the ingredients." Most dishes were preferred spicy, thick, and sticky.

Legumes were popular throughout West Africa. Peanuts (a non-indigenous legume in the same family as peas and lentils) were especially valued and were eaten raw, boiled, roasted, or ground into meal, flour, or paste. Cowpeas (*Vigna unguiculata*, neither a standard pea nor a bean—black-eyed peas are one type of cowpea) were eaten as a substitute for meat, often combined with a staple starch such as corn, yams, or rice. Bambara groundnuts, similar in some ways to peanuts but indigenous to Africa and cultivated there many years before the peanut arrived from South America, were also common. Nuts and seeds were frequently used to flavor and thicken sauces. Mango seeds (called agobono, og bono, or apon), cashews, egusi (watermelon seeds, usually dried and ground), kola nuts, and sesame seeds were popular.

Many varieties of tropical and subtropical fruits and vegetables were available to West Africans, but only a few were widely eaten. Ackee apples, baobab (both the pulp and seeds from the fruit of the baobab tree), guava, lemon, papaya (commonly called pawpaw in Africa, though it is not the same as the North American fruit also called pawpaw), pineapple, and watermelon were the most common fruits. Many dishes included coconut milk. In addition to starchy staple roots and the flavoring ingredients of onions, chili peppers, and tomatoes, the most popular vegetables were eggplant, okra, pumpkin, and the leaves from plants such as cassava, sweet potato, and taro (also called callaloo or cocoyam).

West African cuisine today remains very similar to that of the past. Fish is favored, and little meat is consumed. A mostly vegetarian fare has developed based on regional staples such as beans, yams, and cassava. Gari foto is a popular Ghanaian specialty that combines gari (cassava meal), onions, chilies, and tomatoes and is sometimes served with beans. Stews featuring root vegetables, okra, or peanuts and flavored with small amounts of fish, chicken, or beef are common. Saucy dishes with distinctive East Indian flavors are popular in Nigeria, often served with dozens of condiments and garnishes such as coconut, raisins, chopped dates, peanuts, dried shrimp, and diced fruits. Pili-pili, a sauce made from small, orange scotch bonnet or habanero peppers, salt, and often tomatoes, onion, and garlic, is often offered at the table so that each diner may spice dishes to taste. Ghana's pepper sauce is similar. In other regions of Africa, the sauce, called piri piri or peri peri, is made from African bird's eye chili peppers and garlic, lemon juice, or vinegar among other ingredients.

Deep-fried fish, fried plantain chips, and balls made from steamed rice, black-eyed peas, yams, or peanuts are snack foods available at street stalls in urban areas. A favorite West African sweet is kanya, a peanut candy. Chin-chins, sweet fried pastries topped with sugar and flavoring such as cinnamon or orange zest, are also popular. Bananas are commonly baked and flavored with sugar, honey, or coconut for dessert. Fried dough balls much like a round donut (see the Togbei/Bofrot/Puff Puff recipe at the end of the chapter) prepared from millet or wheat flour are a specialty in many areas; in Ghana, they are called togbei, bofrot, or puff puff, and are deep fried in vegetable oil to a golden-brown color and can be eaten plain, sprinkled with powdered sugar, or with fruit jams or other toppings.

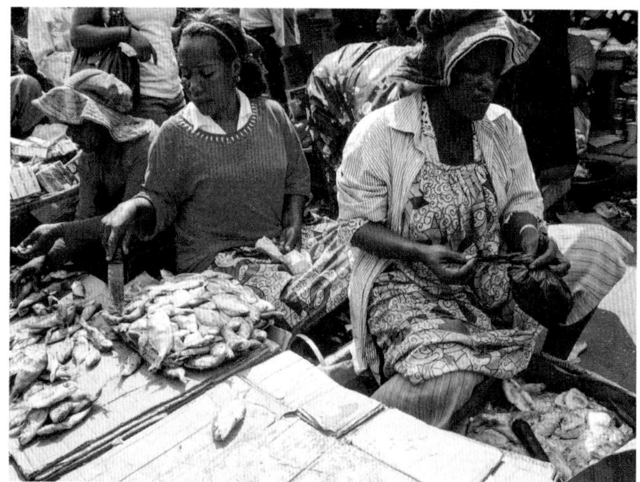

iStock.com/Sanjeri

▲ Market scene in Ghana, West Africa.

Sample Menu

A West African Meal

Spicy Fried Plantains[a,b]

Groundnut Chop/Stew over Rice[b,c]

Ginger Beer[b] or Green Tea with Mint

Tropical Fruit Salad[b]

Recipes in this menu:

[a]https://www.allrecipes.com/recipe/215278/kelewele-spicy-fried-plantains/

[b]http://www.congocookbook.com

[c]https://www.allrecipes.com/recipe/217952/west-african-peanut-stew/

Ethiopian, Eritrean, Somali, and Sudanese Mountainous terrain and lowland valleys cover much of Ethiopia, Eritrea, and Somalia, and the climate is mostly arid. Though Ethiopia is landlocked, Eritrea and Somalia have lengthy coastal access along the horn of Africa. Millet (including a variety unique to the region called teff), sorghum, and plantains are the staple foods produced, and coffee is the leading export crop. All coffee, in fact, can trace its heritage to the Ethiopian plateau.[31] Other foods common to the region include barley, wheat, corn, cabbage, collards, onions, kale, and potatoes, as well as peanuts and other legumes. Enset, a plantain-like plant, is a staple in the high mountainous regions of Ethiopia. Some chicken, fish, mutton, goat, and beef are available.

Historically, Ethiopian cuisine had minimal outside influences, though a large number of Muslims now living in the nation have introduced certain halal dietary practices in some regions (refer to Chapter 4 for more information on religious dietary practices). More significant has been the Ethiopian Eastern Orthodox religion, which has encouraged a diet based on vegetables, legumes, fruit, cereals, bread, and olive oil with periodic abstinence from meat and other animal products during fasting periods. Food examples include yataklete kilkil, a garlic- and ginger-flavored casserole, and yemiser selatta, a lentil salad. A mixture of ground legumes called mitin shiro is added to most vegetarian stews. Wat, meaning stew, is the national dish of Ethiopia. Typically, wat is thick and spicy and may include legumes, meats, poultry, or fish. Milder versions are known as alechas, and most stews can be prepared either in mild or spicy versions.[32,33] Doro wat is one popular example, featuring chicken and whole hard-boiled eggs. Yemiser wat is made with red lentils, sega wat with beef, and yebeg wat with lamb. Wat is served with rice or the traditional Ethiopian flat bread called injera. Injera is prepared with a spongy, fermented dough made from teff cooked in a very large circular loaf on a griddle. (Sometimes wat is prepared with added pieces of injera in the stew, known as fitfit.) Another variation of this flatbread, known as kocho, is made with enset.

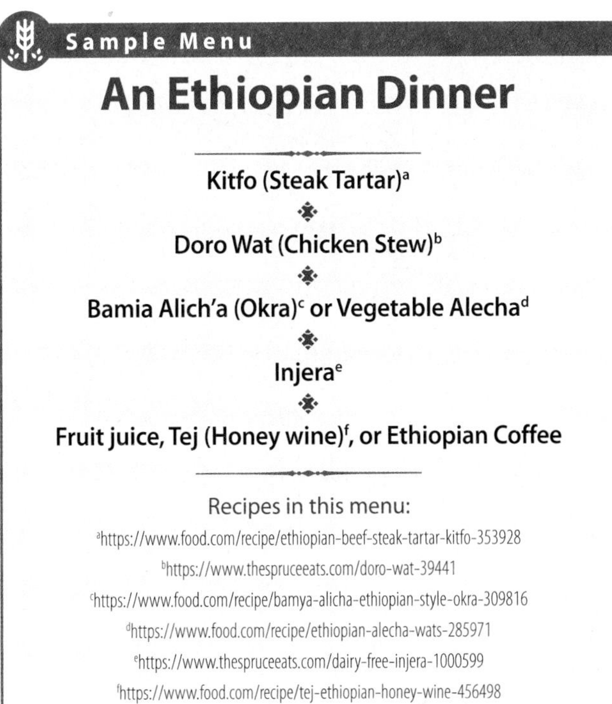
Sample Menu

An Ethiopian Dinner

Kitfo (Steak Tartar)[a]

Doro Wat (Chicken Stew)[b]

Bamia Alich'a (Okra)[c] or Vegetable Alecha[d]

Injera[e]

Fruit juice, Tej (Honey wine)[f], or Ethiopian Coffee

Recipes in this menu:

[a]https://www.food.com/recipe/ethiopian-beef-steak-tartar-kitfo-353928
[b]https://www.thespruceeats.com/doro-wat-39441
[c]https://www.food.com/recipe/bamya-alicha-ethiopian-style-okra-309816
[d]https://www.food.com/recipe/ethiopian-alecha-wats-285971
[e]https://www.thespruceeats.com/dairy-free-injera-1000599
[f]https://www.food.com/recipe/tej-ethiopian-honey-wine-456498

Ethiopian foods are frequently flavored with a hot spice mixture known as berbere, which includes allspice, cardamom, cayenne, cinnamon, cloves, coriander, cumin, fenugreek, ginger, nutmeg, and black pepper, proof that early spice traders bringing spices from the East stopped in this region. Niter kebbeh, clarified butter with onions, garlic, ginger, and other spices, is added to many dishes, including kitfo, a raw ground beef specialty. Salted and sweet cheeses are common. Honey (sometimes consumed with the bee grubs) is especially popular as a sweetener and is used in savory dishes such as alechas, and desserts such as baklava, a drier version of the Greek pastry.[34] It is also fermented to make tej, a mead-like beverage. Tella, home-brewed millet or corn beer, is commonly consumed, as is coffee, especially espresso (introduced by the Italians).

Eritrean and Somali food is very similar to Ethiopian, except for more the frequent use of seafood. For example, a typical meal includes a spicy stew, often with beef, lamb, kid, or fish, eaten with injera-like breads, known in Somalia as anjeero. The Eritreans often consume their bread with shuro, a thick paste made from chickpeas, onions, tomatoes, and a touch of berbere, similar to Ethiopian mitin shiro. Of note: many Eritreans belong to the Coptic Eastern Orthodox faith and adhere to the proscriptions on meat, and nearly all Somalis are Muslim and follow halal dietary practices. Camel milk is consumed in some areas, and in Somalia, sweetened tea is consumed frequently. In Eritrea, coffee is preferred, and a bitter, fermented barley beverage called sowa is served at most meals. On special occasions a wine similar to tej, called mez, is popular.

Former forced Italian occupation of the region introduced dishes that were adapted to local tastes, including spaghetti, lasagna, pasta, and frittata, a scrambled egg dish made with green peppers and onions, among ingredients.[34] In some parts of Ethiopia and Eritrea and throughout Somalia, Asian Indian–influenced saucy main dishes, unleavened breads such as roti and chapati, and vegetable- or meat-stuffed fritters known as sambosa are also common.[34]

The Sudan, which bridges the desert regions of North Africa and the tropical forests of West and East Africa, has a cuisine reflecting both Middle Eastern and African influences. For example, fava beans or a salad of cucumber and yogurt might be served at the same meal as an okra stew and kisra, the Sudanese staple bread similar to injera.

East African The climate and topography of Kenya, Tanzania, and Uganda are well suited to farming and ranching. Cassava, corn, millet, sorghum, peanuts, and plantains combine to form the foundation of the diet. Crops grown for export include coffee, tea, cashews, and cloves. Cattle are raised in the northern plateaus of Kenya; they are considered a gift of the gods (especially among the Maasai tribe), and they indicate wealth. Abundant game animals are also often considered sacred, although specific taboos vary from region to region. Eating fish and seafood is common along the coast.

The cuisines of East Africa are predominantly vegetarian, influenced in part by Arab, Asian Indian, and British fare. Breads are common at every meal, including chapatis, kitumbua, a rice fritter, and mandazi, a slightly sweetened doughnut-like bread. In Kenya, the national dish is ugali, a very thick, doughy cornmeal porridge. Ugali is also found in Tanzania. Mashed beans, lentils, corn, plantains, and potatoes are also popular. Coconut milk, chili peppers, and curry spice blends flavor in many dishes. In Uganda, which is inland and less influenced by foreign cuisines, peanuts are a staple food used in everything from stews—such as beef, tomato, and onion stew with peanut sauce—to desserts. Plantains are the core food of Tanzania. They are used in soups (with or without beef), stews, fritters, custards, and even wine. Coconut milk is a frequent flavoring, as is curry powder. Throughout the region, dishes made with taro greens or other leafy vegetables and side dishes of local grains and produce, such as eggplant and papaya, round out the cuisine.

South African South Africa has a very temperate climate favorable to many fruits and vegetables uncommon in the rest of the continent, such as cucumbers, carrots, apricots, tangerines, grapefruit, quinces, and grapes. The Dutch, French, German, English, Malay, and East Asian influence on food culture is visible on the plate. The food is often spiced variations of European fish, meat, and game dishes. Malay people, who had a great deal of influence on the seasonings in South African food, were enslaved by the Dutch and brought to South Africa from Java, Sumatra, Bengal, Madagascar, and Indonesia. Long, slow, moist heat and skillful use of ingredients are the marks of what is called Cape Malay cooking. Mutton, beef, pork, fish, and seafood are popular.

South African meat specialties include sosaties, or skewered, curried mutton; bredie, a mutton stew that may include onions, chilies, tomatoes, potatoes, or pumpkin; frikkadels,

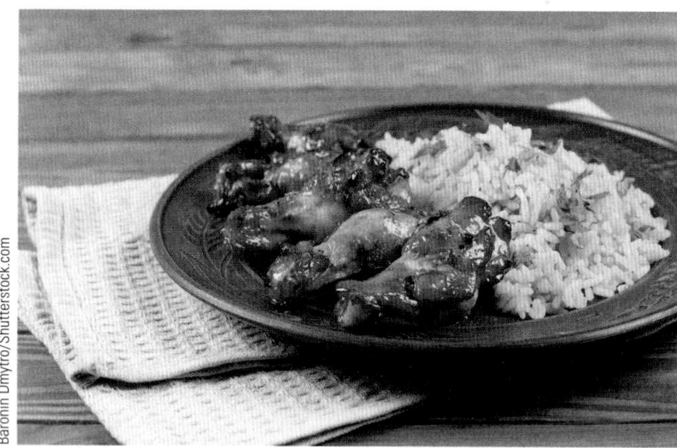
Baronin Dmytro/Shutterstock.com

▲ **Many traditional southern foods reflect West African influences.**

braised meat patties; bobotie, a meatloaf flavored with curry seasoning and topped with a custard mixture when baked; and biltong, meat strips dried and preserved over smoke. Grape-stuffed chicken or suckling pig is sometimes served for special occasions. Spicy fruit or vegetable relishes called chutney (for more information see Chapter 14); atjar, fruit or vegetables preserved in fish or vegetable oil with spices like turmeric and dried chilies; and fresh grated fruit or vegetable salads flavored with lemon juice or vinegar and chilies accompany the dishes.

Sweets are very common. Dried fruits, fruit leathers called planked fruit, and fruit preserves or jams are popular. Many pastries are available, too, such as tarts made with raisins, sweet potatoes, coconut, or custard. Cookies are a favorite. Koeksister are braided crullers that are deep-fried and dipped in cinnamon syrup, and soetkoekies are spice cookies flavored with the sweet wine Madeira.

The Traditional African Diet in the United States When West Africans were forcefully taken from their communities, they were not immediately separated from their accustomed foods. Conditions on the slave ships were appalling, but most slave traders did provide a traditional diet for the people on board as that was the food readily available to stock the ship. The basic staples of each region, plus dried salt cod (which was familiar to most West Africans), were fed to the Africans in minimal quantities. Chili peppers and the native West African malagueta peppercorns were used for seasoning because they were believed to prevent dysentery. It wasn't until the Africans were sold in the United States that significant changes in their cuisine occurred.

The diet of field workers was largely dependent on whatever foods the slave owners provided. Salt pork and corn were the most common items. Since many West Africans were purchased because of their expertise in growing African indigenous rice (to help bolster commerce of the American South), sometimes rice instead of corn was included in their provisions, along with salted fish, and molasses. Greens, legumes, milk, and sweet potatoes were occasionally added. The foods provided, as well as their amount, were usually contingent on local availability and agricultural surplus.

Many Africans maintained garden plots to plant additional vegetables around the periphery of the cotton or tobacco fields to supplement their food supplies. Okra and cowpeas from Africa were favored, as well as American cabbage, collard and mustard greens, sweet potatoes, and turnips. Herbs were collected from the surrounding woodlands, and small animals such as opossums, rabbits, raccoons, squirrels, and an occasional wild pig were trapped for supplementary meat. Children would often catch catfish and other freshwater fish.

During the hog-slaughtering season in the fall, variety pork cuts, such as chitterlings (intestines, pronounced *chitlins*), maw (stomach lining), tail, and hocks, would sometimes be available. Some were encouraged to raise hogs and chickens. The eggs and the primary pork cuts were usually sold to raise cash for the purchase of luxury foods. Chickens, a prestigious food in West Africa, continued to be reserved for special occasions.

West African cooking methods were adapted to surrounding conditions. Boiling and frying remained the most popular ways to prepare not only meats but also vegetables and legumes. Bean stews maintained their popularity as main dishes. Corn was substituted for most West African regional staple starches and was prepared in many forms, primarily as cornmeal pudding, cornmeal breads known as pone or spoon bread, grits (coarsely ground cornmeal), and hominy (hulled, dried corn kernels with the bran and germ removed). Pork fat (lard) replaced palm oil in cooking and was used to fry or flavor everything from breads to greens. Hot pepper sauces were used for seasoning. No substitutions were available for many of the nuts and seeds used in West African recipes, although peanuts and sesame seeds remained popular.

Food for the field workers had to be portable. One-dish vegetable stews were common, as were fried cakes, such as hush puppies (perhaps named because they were used to quiet whining dogs), and the cornmeal cakes baked in the fire on the back of a hoe, called hoecakes. Meals prepared at home after a full day of labor were usually simple. Often, these foods of scarcity, made tasty by ingenuity, are now identified with U.S. Southern foodways.

Cooks in plantation houses are credited with popularizing fried chicken and fried fish. They more widely introduced the sticky vegetable-based stews (thickened with African okra, or Native American sassafras, which when ground is called filé powder), such as the southern specialty gumbo z'herbes, or green gumbo. This style of stew, familiar to West Africans, is much like stews made by the Choctaw and Apache. Green leafy vegetables (simply called greens) became a separate dish instead of being added to stews, but they were still cooked for hours and flavored with meat. Ingredients familiar to West Africans, such as nuts, beans, and squash, were used for pie fillings.

Foods after the Abolition of Slavery The food traditions of Black Americans did not change significantly after emancipation, and they differed little from those of White farmers of similar socioeconomic status. One exception was that pork variety cuts and salt pork remained the primary meats for Black people, while White people often switched to beef during the post-Civil War period.

Black American Southern Staples The traditional Southern American cuisine that evolved from Native, European, West African, and post-abolition fare greatly emphasizes texture—the West African preference for sticky food, crispy fried chicken, and flaky biscuits continues, as a few examples—before flavor. Pork, pork products, corn, and greens still form the foundation of the diet. The cultural food groups list (Table 8.1) includes other common southern Black foods. (For information about the food habits of Black people from the Caribbean, refer to Chapter 10; for more information on foods of the American South, refer to Chapter 15.)

Table 8.1 Cultural Food Groups: African American (Southern United States)

Group	Comments	Common Foods	Adaptations in the United States
Protein Foods			
Milk/milk products	Dairy products are uncommon in diet (incidence of lactose intolerance estimated at 60–95 percent of the population). Milk is widely disliked in some studies; well accepted in others. Few cheese or fermented dairy products are eaten.	Milk (consumed mostly in desserts, such as puddings and ice cream), some buttermilk; cheese	Blacks in urban areas may drink milk more often than rural blacks.
Meat/poultry/fish/eggs/legumes	Pork is most popular, especially variety cuts; fish, small game, poultry also common; veal and lamb are infrequently eaten. Bean dishes are popular. Frying, boiling are most common preparation methods; stewed dishes preferred thick and sticky. Protein intake is high.	*Meat:* beef, pork (including chitterlings, ham hocks, sausages, variety cuts) *Poultry:* chicken, turkey *Fish and shellfish:* catfish, crab, crawfish, perch, red snapper, salmon, sardines, shrimp, tuna *Small game:* frogs, opossum, raccoon, squirrel, turtle *Eggs:* chicken *Legumes:* black-eyed peas, kidney beans, peanuts (and peanut butter), pinto beans, red beans	Pork remains primary protein source; prepackaged sausages and lunch meats are popular. Small game is rarely consumed. Variety cuts are considered to be "soul food" and eaten regardless of socioeconomic status or region. Frying is still popular, but more often at evening meal; boiling and baking are second most common preparation methods.
Cereals/Grains	Corn is primary grain product; wheat flour is used in many baked goods. Rice is used in stew-type dishes.	Biscuits; corn (corn breads, grits, hominy); pasta; rice	Store-bought breads often replace biscuits (toasted at breakfast, used for sandwiches at lunch).
Fruits/Vegetables	Green leafy vegetables are most popular, cooked with ham, salt pork, or bacon, lemon and hot sauce; broth is also eaten. Intake of fresh fruits and vegetables is low.	*Fruits:* apples, bananas, berries, peaches, watermelon *Vegetables:* beets, broccoli, cabbage, corn, greens (chard, collard, kale, mustard, pokeweed, turnip, etc.), green peas, okra, potatoes, spinach, squash, sweet potatoes, tomatoes, yams	Fruits are eaten according to availability and preference; intake remains low. Green leafy vegetables ("greens") are popular in all regions; other vegetables are eaten according to availability and preference; intake remains low.
Additional Foods			
Seasonings	Dishes are frequently seasoned with hot-pepper sauces. Onions and green pepper are common flavoring ingredients.	Filé (sassafras powder), garlic, green peppers, hot-pepper sauce, ham hocks, salt pork or bacon (added to vegetables and stews), lemon juice, onions, salt, pepper	
Nuts/seeds	Nuts often used in ways similar to traditional West African dishes, such as nut- or seed-based desserts.	Peanuts, pecans, sesame seeds, walnuts	
Beverages		Coffee, fruit drinks, fruit juice, fruit wine, soft drinks, tea	
Fats/oils		Butter, lard, meat drippings, vegetable shortening	
Sweeteners		Honey, molasses, sugar	Cookies (and candy) are preferred snacks

Pork variety cuts of all types are used. Pig's feet (or knuckles) are eaten roasted or pickled; pig's ears are slowly cooked in water seasoned with herbs and vinegar and then served with gravy. Bits of pork skin (with meat or fat attached) are fried to make cracklings. Chitterlings also are usually fried, sometimes boiled. Sausages and head cheese (a seasoned loaf of meat from the pig's head) make use of smaller pork pieces. Barbecued pork is also common. A whole pig (or just the ribs) is slowly roasted over the fire. Each family has its own recipe for spicy sauce, and each has its opinion about whether the pork should be basted in the sauce or the sauce should be ladled over the cooked meat. Other meats, such as poultry, are also popular.

Occasionally, the small game that was prevalent during the seventeenth and eighteenth centuries, such as opossum and raccoon, is eaten. More often the meal includes local fish and shellfish, such as catfish, crab, or crawfish. Frog legs and turtle are popular in some areas. Meats, poultry, and fish are often combined in thick stews and soups, such as gumbos (still made sticky with okra or filé powder) that are eaten with rice. They may also be coated with cornmeal and deep-fried, as in southern-fried chicken and catfish.

The vegetables most characteristic of Southern Black American cuisine are the many varieties of greens. Food was scarce during the Civil War, and most Southerners were forced to experiment with indigenous vegetation, in addition to cultivated greens such as chard, collard greens, kale, mustard greens, spinach, and turnip greens. Dockweed, dandelion greens, lamb's quarter, marsh marigold leaves, milkweed, pigweed, pokeweed, and purslane were added as acceptable vegetables. Traditionally, greens are cooked in water flavored with salt pork, fatback, bacon, or ham, plus hot chili peppers (or hot-pepper sauce) and lemon. As the water evaporates, the flavors intensify, resulting in a broth called "pot likker." Both the greens and the liquid are served; hot sauce is offered for those who prefer a spicier dish. Other common vegetables include black-eyed peas, okra, peas, and tomatoes. Onions and green peppers are frequently used for flavoring.

Corn and corn products are as popular in southern Black cuisine today as they were during the seventeenth and eighteenth centuries. Cornbread and fried hominy are served sliced with butter. Wheat flour biscuits are also served with butter or, in some regions, gravy. Dumplings are sometimes added to stews and greens.

Squash is eaten as a vegetable (sometimes stuffed) and as a dessert pie sweetened with molasses. Sweet potatoes are also used both ways. Other common desserts include bread pie (bread pudding), crumb cake, chocolate or caramel cake, fruit cobblers, puddings, and shortcakes, as well as sesame seed cookies and candies.

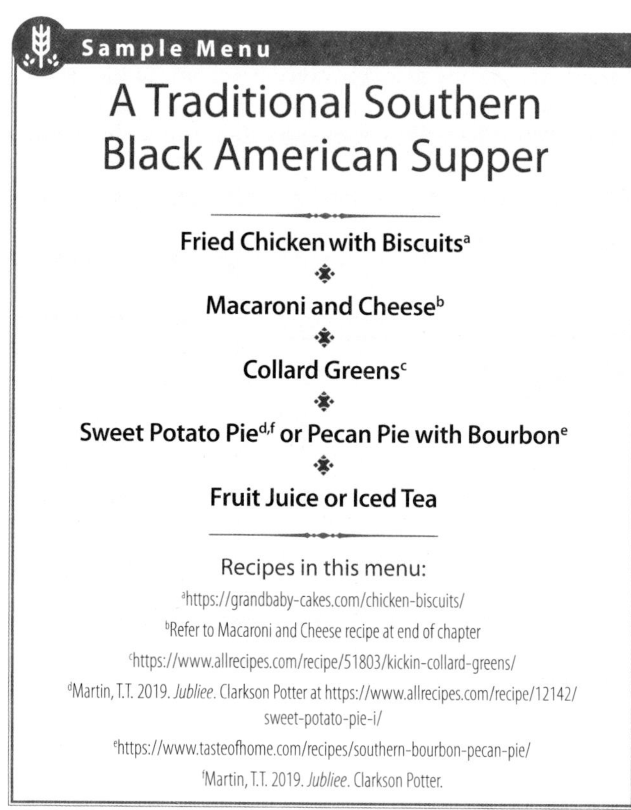
Sample Menu

A Traditional Southern Black American Supper

Fried Chicken with Biscuits[a]

Macaroni and Cheese[b]

Collard Greens[c]

Sweet Potato Pie[d,f] **or Pecan Pie with Bourbon**[e]

Fruit Juice or Iced Tea

Recipes in this menu:

[a]https://grandbaby-cakes.com/chicken-biscuits/

[b]Refer to Macaroni and Cheese recipe at end of chapter

[c]https://www.allrecipes.com/recipe/51803/kickin-collard-greens/

[d]Martin, T.T. 2019. *Jubliee*. Clarkson Potter at https://www.allrecipes.com/recipe/12142/sweet-potato-pie-i/

[e]https://www.tasteofhome.com/recipes/southern-bourbon-pecan-pie/

[f]Martin, T.T. 2019. *Jubliee*. Clarkson Potter.

Meal Composition and Cycle

Daily Patterns Historically, two meals a day were typical in West Africa, one late in the morning and one in the evening. Snacking was common; for the less wealthy, snacks would replace the morning meal and only dinner would be served. Food was eaten family style or, more formally, the men were served first, then the boys, then the girls, and last the women. Sometimes men gathered together for a meal without women. Mealtimes often were solemn, people concentrated on the attributes of the food, and conversation was minimal.

Throughout Africa, lunch is considered the main meal of the day. It consists of vegetables, legumes, and sometimes meat. Unlike meals in the United States, meat and fish are not the focus of the meal. They are considered accompaniments to the meal which is focused on stews made with vegetables, legumes, and grains. The West African tradition of frequent snacking continued through emancipation. Meals were often irregular, perhaps due to the variable hours of agricultural labor. The traditional southern-style meal pattern was adopted as economic conditions for both Blacks and Whites improved. Breakfast was typically large and leisurely, almost always including boiled grits and homemade biscuits. In addition, eggs, ham or bacon, and even fried sweet potatoes would be served. Coffee and tea were more common beverages than milk or juice.

Since lunch, called dinner, was the main meal of the day, it was eaten at midafternoon and featured a boiled entrée, such as legumes or greens with ham, or another stew-type dish. Additional vegetables or a salad may have been served, as well as potatoes and bread or biscuits. Dessert was mandatory and was usually a baked item, not simply fruit. In some homes, a full supper of meat, vegetables, and potatoes was served in the evening. Less wealthy agricultural families often ate only two of these hearty meals a day. Today, few Southerners continue this traditional meal pattern in full. The southern-style breakfast might be served just on weekends or holidays, for example. As in the rest of the country, a light lunch has replaced the large dinner on most days, and supper has become the main meal.

Common foods eaten in North Africa are quite different from other African cuisines and tend to resemble Middle Eastern meals. Goat, lamb, beef, and seafood are available and these foods are often combined into vegetable stews. Dates, almonds, and fruits are also consumed daily. One of the most popular foods in the United States coming from North Africa is couscous, which is small wheat kernels that resemble round rice when cooked. Very little pork is consumed due to a large number of practicing Muslims[35] in the North African region.

Traditions vary for recent African immigrants to the United States today. Throughout West Africa, three meals a day are typical, though, in some areas, only two meals are consumed especially in times of scarcity before the season's harvest.[36] Ethiopians, Eritreans, and Somalis usually eat one or two meals a day, snacking in between. In Eritrea and Somalia, fool, which is a puree made from chickpeas in Eritrea, and pinto beans in Somalia, is a popular breakfast item. Food is typically offered on a communal plate, and individuals use bread to scoop up what is desired. Meals are often joyous and noisy. Three meals each day are common in East Africa, and in Kenya many people also stop for British-style tea in the afternoon. However, in many areas, meals are limited to two daily when food is in short supply. Traditionally, men were served first, followed by women, and then children dined. In South Africa, a Westernized pattern of three meals, with dinner being the largest, is usually followed.

Special Occasions Sunday dinner became a large family meal for people who were enslaved as most were allowed the day off for personal work, and it continued to be the main meal of the week after emancipation. It was a time to eat and share favorite foods with friends and relatives, a time to extend hospitality to neighbors.

Many Southern Black Americans still enjoy a large Sunday dinner, usually prepared by the mother of the house, who begins cooking in the early morning. The menu might include fried chicken, spare ribs, chitterlings, pig's feet (or ears or tail), black-eyed peas or okra, corn, cornbread, greens, potato salad, rice, and sweet potato pie. Homemade fruit wines, such as strawberry wine, might also be offered.

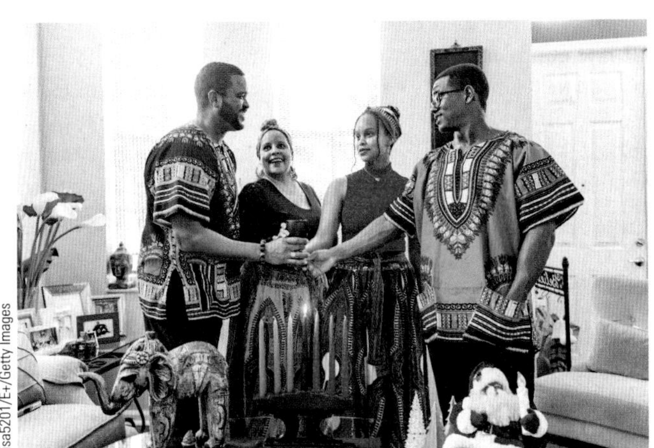

Lisa5201/E+/Getty Images

▲ Kwanzaa, the African American holiday celebrated from December 26 through January 1 each year, culminates with a feast featuring dishes from throughout Africa, the Caribbean, the U.S. South, and other regions where Africans now live.

Other holiday meals, especially Christmas, feature menus similar to the Sunday meal, but with added dishes and even greater amounts of food. Turkey with cornbread stuffing and baked ham are often the entrees; other vegetable dishes, such as corn pudding, sweet peas, and salads, are typical accompaniments. A profusion of baked goods, including yeast rolls, fruit cakes, and cobblers, custard or cream pies, and chocolate, caramel, and coconut cake, round out the meal. Some Black Americans eat symbolic foods on New Year's Eve, such as fish for motivation, greens for money, black-eyed peas for good luck, and rice for prosperity.[37]

Southern Black cuisine is particularly well suited to buffet meals and parties. A pot of gumbo, a pot of beans, or a side of barbecued ribs can be stretched to feed many people on festive occasions. Informal parties to celebrate a birthday, or just the fact that it's Saturday night, are still common. Traditional southern food is also served at Juneteenth celebrations held in many American communities to commemorate the emancipation of the enslaved.

Celebrating the Kwanzaa holiday has gained popularity in recent years. Created in Southern California in 1966, Kwanzaa recognizes the African diaspora and celebrates the unity of all people of African heritage. It begins on December 26th and runs through New Year's Day. Each day, a new candle is lit to symbolize one of seven principles: unity, self-determination, collective work and responsibility, cooperative economics, purpose, creativity, and faith. The holiday culminates with a feast featuring dishes from throughout Africa, the Caribbean, the U.S. South, and any other region where Africans were transported.

Recent African immigrants may celebrate many religious holidays, especially those associated with the Eastern Orthodox and Islamic faiths. In Nigeria, child-naming ceremonies are particularly important celebrations.[37,38] A grandmother performs the ritual, offering symbolic foods to the infant, including water (purity), oil (power and health), alcohol (wealth and prosperity), honey (happiness), kola nuts (good fortune), and salt (intelligence and wisdom). Following the tasting, the name is whispered to the child, then announced aloud to the attendees. The family and guests then enjoy a meal together. Many Nigerian Americans continue the custom in the United States.

Role of Food in African American Society and Etiquette

In the American South, food has traditionally been a catalyst for social interaction, and southern hospitality is renowned. For some Black Americans, eating is an intimate or spiritual experience that is shared with others in social church networks.[38,39] Food is lovingly prepared for family and friends and is considered an important factor in the cohesiveness of Black society.

In Africa today, sharing food is still an important social activity, often accompanied by loud conversation and gaiety. Food is offered to anyone who is in the home, and in some nations, such as Nigeria, it is common for extended family members to drop by unannounced for a meal.[40] In many urban areas, Western styles of dining are practiced. However, in rural regions meals are often served communally and consumed with the hands. Only the right hand may be used for eating, and the left hand should not touch anything on the table. Although it is usually a sign of respect or affection to feed a bite of food directly into another person's mouth, it is considered exceptionally rude to pass food from one person's hand to another person's hand.[41] In Uganda, diners stay seated until all people have finished eating, and sticking one's legs out or leaning on an elbow is not acceptable. In Eritrea, an invitation to coffee means a visit of over an hour, with a minimum of three cups consumed in a ritual that includes the burning of incense.

Therapeutic Uses of Food Many Black Americans maintain health by eating three hearty meals each day, including a hot breakfast. Numerous other beliefs about food and health are noted among small numbers of Black Americans living in the rural South. Some of these dietary concepts were brought to other regions of the country during the great migrations and may be found among older Black adults. The conditions known as "high blood" and "low blood" are one example. High blood (often confused with high blood pressure and high blood sugar levels) is most prevalent and thought to be caused by excess blood migrating to one part of the body, typically the head. High blood is caused by eating excessive amounts of rich foods, sweet foods, or red-colored foods (beets, carrots, grape juice, red wine, and red meat, especially pork). Low blood, associated with anemia, is believed to be caused by eating too many astringent and acidic foods (vinegar, lemon juice, garlic, and pickled foods) and not enough red meat. Other blood complaints include "thin blood" which cannot nourish the body, causing a person to feel chilly; "bad blood," due to hereditary, natural, or supernatural contamination; "unclean blood" when impurities collect over the winter months and the blood carries more heat; and "clots," when the blood thickens and settles in one area, associated with menstruation or stomach and leg cramps.[42,43]

Tea made from the yellowroot shrub (*Xanthorhiza simplicissima*) is thought to cure stomachache and fever and is used to treat diabetes. Some Black Americans also believe peppermint candies are helpful in diabetes. Sassafras tea or hot lemon-flavored water with honey is considered good for colds, and raw onion helps break a fever. Turpentine sweetened with sugar reputedly cures intestinal worms when consumed orally, while a mixture of figs and honey will eliminate ringworm. Goat's milk with cabbage juice is used to cure a stomach infection. In some areas, eggs and milk may be withheld from sick children to aid in their recovery.[44-47]

Pica, the practice of eating nonnutritive substances such as clay, chalk, and laundry starch, one of the most perplexing of all food habits practiced by many communities and ethnicities and is often associated with iron deficiency. Studies have determined that Black women most often practice pica during pregnancy and the postpartum period and that rates are unchanged since the 1970s (information on pica among other ethnic groups or age groups in the United States is limited). It is common in the South, where anywhere from 16 to 57 percent of pregnant Black American women admit to pica. But pica is also found in other areas of the country where large populations of Black Americans reside. In rural regions, the substance ingested is usually clay. In urban areas, laundry starch is often the first choice, though instances of women who ate large amounts of milk of magnesia, coffee grounds, plaster, ice, and paraffin have also been reported. Many causes for pica have been postulated—a nutritional need for minerals, hunger or nausea, a desire for special treatment, and cultural tradition are the most common hypotheses. One study found pica was more common among women with limited social support. Another theory suggests it may be related to obsessive-compulsive disorder (OCD). Reasons for pica reported by women include flavor, anxiety relief, texture, and the belief that clay prevents birthmarks or that starch makes the skin of the baby lighter and helps the baby slip out during delivery.[48,49]

Recent immigrants from Africa may hold traditional beliefs about maintaining health through a balance of proper diet, exercise, good relations with family and community, emotional well-being, and spirituality. Poor diet is identified as a tangible cause of some conditions, and being overweight is often valued as a sign of health. Meat consumption may be associated with longevity. Many people in Africa have limited access to biomedical care and make extensive use of botanical home remedies. In Nigeria, for example, unripe plantains and dried soursop (a tropical fruit) are two treatments used for diabetes.[50] In a 2015 study conducted, the use of home remedies for self-management of health revealed many food-related therapies for Black American adults. Vinegar was used by over half of the participants for high blood pressure. Swallowing a teaspoonful mixed with some water is often consumed daily. Baking soda and water is often used to relieve stomachache or heartburn. Baking soda is often made into a paste and placed on insect bites, burns, and rashes. Lemon is used in tea for colds, sore throats, and digestive problems. Salt is used as a topical remedy to treat tissues in the mouth, throat, and sinuses, although sometimes it is ingested for muscle cramps. Honey is used to treat cold symptoms, arthritis pain, and lower blood pressure. This is also added to tea with lemon.[40,50,51]

Contemporary Food Habits in the United States

Researchers have noted that the food habits of Black Americans today, like many in the United States, usually reflect their current socioeconomic status, geographic location, and work schedule more than their earlier African or southern heritage. Even in the South, many traditional foods and meal patterns have changed due to the pressures of a fast-paced society. Nevertheless, the same foods consumed by Black people and by White people are likely to have different meanings within each cultural context. Like the Native American and other diets, the African diet was predominantly vegetarian, centered around staple foods such as rice, millet, field peas, okra, hot peppers, and yams. Cooking was done largely with leafy greens, grains, legumes, and onions and contained far more vegetables and legumes than the Europeans typically consumed. Once forced to migrate to North America, Black diets changed. Often, plantation owners provided salt pork and cornmeal, which Black families made tasty in many ways. Today, plant-based eating is returning to modern Black American life, as communities begin to reclaim their food heritage.[52]

Adaptations of Food Habits

Ingredients and Common Foods Food preferences do not vary greatly between Black and White people in similar socio-economic groups living in the same region of the United States. One study shows that Black women in the United States aged 65 and older often shopped less frequently, traveled a longer time from home to their grocery store, and ate out at restaurants somewhat less frequently than their White counterparts.[53] Under-resourced Black American neighborhoods, as well as Hispanic ones, have notably fewer large supermarkets than their White neighborhood counterparts, resulting in food deserts that lead to a dependence on convenience stores selling poor quality food and fast food options.[54,55] Black American households purchase fewer fruits and vegetables, fewer dairy products, less cereal and baked goods, fewer snack foods (such as potato chips), and less coffee than any other households.[56] One study determined that there are nearly 60 percent more fast-food restaurants in predominantly Black neighborhoods than in mainly White neighborhoods.[57,58]

The popularity of *soul food*—a term coined in the 1960s for traditional southern Black cuisine—is notable. It is associated with fresh meats and vegetables made from scratch and thoroughly cooked. Items are preferred well spiced.[59] Many Black Americans have adopted this cuisine as a symbol of ethnic solidarity, regardless of region or social class. Today, soul food serves as an emblem of identity and a recognition of history for many Black Americans.

Meal Composition and Cycle While the common foods that Black Americans eat reflect their geographic location and socioeconomic status, meal composition and cycle have changed more in response to work habits than to other lifestyle considerations. The traditional southern meal pattern of a substantial breakfast, followed by a large dinner with boiled foods and a hearty supper, has given way to the pressures of contemporary industrial job schedules.[60]

Earlier research indicated that some Black Americans no longer identified certain foods or preparation methods, such as okra and yams, and one-pot meals, as African in origin, though greens were understood to be traditional. Items such as pig's feet and chitterlings were not often eaten.[61,62] A resurgence in interest in Black American food history can be seen in the many cookbooks and food histories held up to acclaim such as *Jubilee: Two Centuries of African American Cooking* by Toni Tipton Martin, *The Cooking Gene* by Michael W. Twitty, *In Pursuit of Flavor* by Edna Lewis, *High on the Hog: A Culinary Journey from Africa to America* by Jessica B. Harris. These books and others reveal a growing interest in the preservation of this food history.

Black Americans throughout the country, like other Americans, now eat lighter breakfasts and often consume sandwiches at a noontime lunch. Dinner is served after work, and it has become the biggest meal of the day. Snacking throughout the day is still typical among most Black Americans. In many households, meal schedules are irregular, and family members eat when convenient. It is not unusual for snacks to replace a full meal.

Frying is still one of the most popular methods of preparing food. An increase in the consumption of fried dinner items suggests that the customary method of making breakfast foods has been transferred to evening foods (which were traditionally boiled) when time constraints prevent a large morning meal. Boiling and baking are second to frying in popularity as it is perceived that frying provides more flavor. One study on the effect of adding spices and herbs to vegetables in school meals revealed increased vegetable intake at an urban, economically underserved predominantly Black school.[63]

Research is limited to the food habits of more recent African immigrants. It has been noted that among Somalis, cheese, sodas, and sweetened fruit drinks are very popular, as they are with many groups. Traditional recipes are being adapted to available ingredients. For example, wheat flour or pancake mix is now used to make anjeero (a thin pancake created from fermented batter).[64] A study of Sudanese Americans found that foods typically consumed at breakfast and lunch included fava or lentil beans made with feta cheese, vegetables, and sesame oil; eggs, fried liver, meat and vegetable stews, bread, salad, fresh fruit, yogurt, custard, Jell-O, and highly sweetened tea. Frying, stewing, sautéing in sesame oil (which was called "boiling"), fermenting, and grilling were the most common methods of preparation. Baking and steaming were extremely rare.[65]

Nutritional Status

The nutritional status of Black Americans is difficult to fully characterize because a limited number of studies have addressed this population, and conflicting data exist. In general, however, research has shown that Black Americans' nutritional intake is similar to that of the general population and varies more by socioeconomic status than by ethnicity. However, the traditional African diet is more plant-based than the standard American diet. The health consequences of an American diet higher in processed foods, higher in fat and saturated fat, and lower in fiber have placed Black Americans at higher risk for cardiovascular diseases, cancer, hypertension, diabetes, and obesity. Dietary preferences for particular types of cuisine referred to as soul food has contributed to these problems. Soul food is typically high in fat—fried foods, fatty meats, and rich gravies. These types of foods have a deep history and are symbolically associated with the history of slavery. Efforts to change these foods to healthier versions are often met with resistance because it can be associated with trying to eradicate Black culture.[66]

Nutritional Intake As previously mentioned, a larger percentage of Black Americans have poor diets compared to the total population, with low intakes of dairy products, vegetables, whole fruit, and total grains.[64,67] Black Americans have also been reported to have diets high in fat—similar to that of the typical U.S. diet—associated with high meat intake, the popularity of frying, and fast food consumption.[52] The percentage of calories from animal proteins for Black Americans is often greater than for White Americans, due in part to a high intake of fatty meats, such as bacon and sausage. A DASH-style diet high in intake of whole grains and low in consumption of red meat is associated with reduced mortality rates in healthy African-American women.[68] Engagement with plant-based diets has become popular among all ethnic groups often for health reasons. The available data suggests that following a plant-based diet may be beneficial to reduce the risk of heart disease and some cancers in the Black American population, but more research is needed.[70] However, it is noteworthy that many dietary comparisons use food frequency data without defined portion sizes. A study of rural Blacks found that when portion size was explained, it was found participants ate on average larger portions of fruits and most vegetables than standard definitions, increasing their daily intake of fruits and vegetables by a significant two-thirds serving.[71,72]

Approximately 20 percent of adult Americans of African descent are lactose intolerant. Some studies show that milk is widely disliked and avoided; others indicate milk is consumed as often by Black people as it is by White people. Many Black Americans avoid dairy products when in fact they could have a role in reducing the risk of heart disease, hypertension, and type 2 diabetes.[69]

According to a 2016 report from the Pew Research center, more women than men report food allergies, and Black Americans are more likely to say they have food allergies (27 percent) than either White Americans (13 percent) or Hispanics (11 percent). Those with food allergies are more likely to be vegan or vegetarian. For those adults with food allergies, 21 percent identify as strictly or mostly following vegan or vegetarian diets.[73]

When comparing life expectancy in the United States by race and ethnicity, Hispanic people have the longest expectancy at 82 years, White people at 78.5 years, and Black people have the lowest at 75 years. However, the gap in life expectancy is far greater for certain subpopulations. Black men living in high-risk inner-city neighborhoods are likely to die earlier than other races.[74] From 2019 to 2020, Hispanic and Black Americans suffered a far steeper drop in life expectancy than White Americans due to the coronavirus pandemic. In the steepest decline in the United States since World War II, Hispanic life expectancy dropped three years and Black Americans dropped 2.9 years on average, while White people experienced the smallest decline of 0.5 years. These declines were mainly attributed to racial and ethnic inequities in access to health care.[74,75]

Morbidity and mortality rates for Black American mothers and their infants are also disproportionately high. Maternal deaths are over three times higher for Black mothers than for White mothers, and infant deaths are more than two times higher.[76] Once again the social disparities of health factors may come into play here. Dietary factors, a large number of teenage pregnancies, and inadequate prenatal care for Black Americans all contribute to a higher incidence of low-birth-weight infants (14.5 percent, over double the rate for White infants which was 6.8 percent) in 2019.[76] Black American mothers are also more likely (14.4 percent) than non-Hispanic White mothers (9.2 percent) to have preterm births, and the rate for sudden infant death syndrome mortality is twice that of non-Hispanic White mothers.

In 2018, 75 percent of Black American mothers breastfeed their infants, compared to 83 percent of all races of U.S. mothers, but only 50 percent continued to breastfeed past six months postpartum.[77] Black Americans reported concerns about breast milk quality—if their diet wasn't healthy or if they become sick, the illness would be passed to the infant. In addition, they also indicated that they are reluctant to breastfeed in public.[78] Some Black Americans differ somewhat from White Americans regarding which solid foods they feed their infants and how soon after birth these are introduced. While obesity rates have historically been quite low in Africa, they are steadily on the rise. Those countries with the highest rates of obesity include Libya (32.5 percent), Egypt (32 percent), and South Africa (28 percent). This has mainly been attributed to a lack of physical activity and higher meat, fat, and sugar consumption. Being overweight is a common problem for adult Americans of African descent. Black American women have the highest overweight and obesity rates in the United States—about four out of five women. In 2020, all Black Americans were 1.4 times more likely to be obese than non-Hispanic White Americans. Adolescents and children are also at risk, especially girls, who are 80 percent more likely to be obese compared to non-Hispanic White girls. Fat patterning has also been shown to differ between Black Americans and White Americans. Black Americans may have more upper-body and deep-fat depositions than White Americans.[79]

Table 8.2 Obesity Rates in the U.S. by race.

Characteristic	Obesity Rate
White	30.2%
Black	42.4%
Hispanic	35.9%
Asian/Pacific Islander	13.2%
American Indian/Alaska Native	37.1%
Other	30.5%

Excess weight gain may be attributed to many factors, including differences in body-size ideal and a more permissive attitude regarding obesity.[80] Though some research suggests income and education levels are inversely associated with the risk for obesity, especially among children, one large study of adolescents found that the prevalence of being overweight remained elevated or even increased with socioeconomic status among Black American girls. An environment that promotes a high intake of fast foods and limits access to healthy items may be another factor. Food choice barriers are often linked to poverty as foods high in fat, salt, and carbohydrates are often less expensive. Fruits, vegetables, lean meats, and fish are often more expensive.[81] A sedentary lifestyle is also more prevalent among Black Americans and is not associated with income, education, occupation, marital status, poverty levels, or other indicators of social class. Data from one study found families living in low-income areas and those with higher percentages of minority residents were significantly less likely to have access to recreational facilities. In addition, a desire to consume traditional Black American foods and to care for others through cooking, as well as a lack of family support were barriers to weight loss cited in studies.[82,83]

Some researchers have suggested that standard anthropometric measures may be inappropriate for Black Americans. One study found that when body mass index (BMI) values were compared to body fatness, Black women had lower body fatness than did White women with identical BMI numbers.[82] BMI does not account for differences in fat-free mass, such as muscle and bone, which accounts for the discrepancy between measures. Weight-for-height growth charts as indicators of the percentage of body fat and the use of waist-to-hip ratios in defining heart disease risk have also been found misleading in some studies (refer to Table 8.2).[81,83]

Studies propose that Black American women do not necessarily equate being overweight with being unattractive and that they are less preoccupied with dieting than White women. Research on disordered eating in Black Americans has been limited and contradictory. Some studies suggest Black Women have lower rates of dieting and are protected from eating disorders due to a collective acceptance of larger body size.[82–84] More current pooled epidemiological data suggest more similarities than differences in the rate of disordered eating among different race/ethnic groups. However, men and ethnic/racial minorities are significantly less likely to seek help than non-Hispanic White women.[84]

Table 8.3 Percentage of Diagnosed Cases of Diabetes in the U.S. of Adults 18 years and over.

	Age-adjusted percentage of persons 18 years of age and over with diabetes, 2018		
	Non-Hispanic Black	Non-Hispanic White	Non-Hispanic Black / Non-Hispanic White Ratio
Men	13.4	8.7	1.5
Women	12.7	7.5	1.7
Total	13.0	8.0	1.6

Source: CDC 2021. Summary Health Statistics: National Health Interview Survey: 2018. Table A-4a. Retrieved from: http://www.cdc.gov/nchs/nhis/shs/tables.htm[86]

Concurrent with obesity is a disproportionately high rate of type 2 diabetes among Black Americans—almost twice the rate of diabetes and twice the number of incidents of complications compared to Whites.[85] There is a genetic predisposition for type 2 diabetes, but also a significant relationship with lifestyle factors such as obesity, sedentary lifestyle, and westernized dietary habits (refer to Table 8.3).

Hypertension is a significant health problem for Black Americans. In 2017, the prevalence of high blood pressure was more common in non-Hispanic Black adults (56 percent) than non-Hispanic White adults (48 percent), non-Hispanic Asian adults (46 percent), or Hispanic adults (39 percent). Hypertension is a potent risk factor for coronary heart disease (CHD) in Black Americans, especially women (whereas having diabetes was not predictive for CHD). Black American adults are twice as likely to have a stroke than their White counterparts. Further, Black men are 60 percent more likely to die from a stroke than their White counterparts.[81,86,87]

Rates of iron-deficiency anemia among Black Americans are higher than for White Americans at every age, regardless of sex or income level. This incidence remains excessive even after adjustments for differences in hemoglobin distributions are made using reference standards appropriate for Black Americans. Hookworm can be a cause in the rural South. Other blood disorders resulting in anemias prevalent in Black Americans include alpha-thalassemia, sickle-cell disease, and glucose-6-phosphate dehydrogenase deficiency. Researchers have also suggested that undiagnosed celiac disease in Black Americans may underlie some cases of iron-deficiency anemia.[88,89]

Little has been reported on the nutritional adequacy of the traditional diet of recent African immigrants. Studies in Israel of Ethiopian immigrants found deficiencies in vitamin D (resulting in rickets in children), iodine (due in part to food goitrogens), and calcium. Vitamin A deficiency has led to xerophthalmia and blindness in many regions. Consumption of foods made from enset, a banana leaf plant, common in many parts of Ethiopia, is associated with esophageal cancer.[90–92] Among Sudanese immigrants in the United States, blindness due to trachoma is also common. High rates of extreme malnutrition, malaria, typhoid, hepatitis B, HIV infection, dengue fever, tuberculosis, syphilis, dental problems, diabetes, and parasitic infection have also been reported.[93,94]

Dietary changes of Ethiopians in Israel are marked. A survey of teens found that within eighteen months of arrival into the United States only 30 percent maintained a traditional diet, 60 percent consumed a mixed diet, and 15 percent ate only Israeli foods.[94,95] More than half of the daily calories came from snacks and fast foods, especially sweets and soft drinks. Most milk products were disliked, except hot chocolate, a favorite with youth. Fat intake increased, while fruit and vegetable intake decreased. Though obesity is unusual, glucose intolerance is common, and the prevalence rate of type 2 diabetes increased from 0.4 percent to between 5 and 8 percent within a few years. Over 20 percent of men also developed hypertension after immigration.[94,95] In Australia, immigrants from Ghana experienced similar changes in diet and health status. Fat intake accounted for 33 to 35 percent of total calories, and overweight was observed in 71 percent of men and 66 percent of women. High rates of diabetes, hypertension, and dyslipidemia were reported.[95,96,97]

In Nigeria, some women believe that edema during pregnancy is an indication that the infant is male, and treatment may not be sought for the condition.[98] Studies of Ethiopian mothers in the United States found that most breastfed their infants on average of four months, and breastfeeding is acceptable in public. Going back to work and reduction in mother's milk were the primary reasons given for cessation. Somali immigrants often associate fatness with health and may overfeed their children. The Somali Bantus are often in particularly poor health due to acute or chronic malnutrition when living in African refugee camps before arriving in the United States. Most have little knowledge of American foods. The prevalence of low-birth-weight infants is high, and weaning often occurs before six months due to subsequent pregnancy. Diarrheal diseases and infections are common. Posttraumatic stress syndrome is also frequently found.[98]

Health and Longevity Takeaway

Beans are a regular staple of the Black American diet. Dried beans, an inexpensive, protein-rich legume, are a great source of fiber, folate, magnesium, and potassium. Colored beans possess greater antioxidant properties than white beans. Beans also contain choline, a vitamin-like compound essential for brain development, which may potentially improve communication in the brain and prevent age-related memory loss.

Comfort Food—Black American

L. Hudson's Story

Le Greta Hudson, a registered dietician, grew up with large family gatherings, Sunday dinners, and food as comfort. She had a lot of choices when it came to her favorite comfort food.

What is one of your favorite comfort foods that you consider traditional from your home culture?

LH: One of my favorite comfort foods is macaroni and cheese. It was never served by itself but always part of the meal that included greens and cornbread. You could always count on it for Sunday dinner, which is important in all my memories, and it made a nice trio to add to pot roast or fried chicken. But the greens (most often collards), cornbread, and macaroni and cheese were key. We don't eat this way often anymore, but as we gather as a family, these foods are still very much a part of what appears on the table.

Did you eat this food together with community? Where was it eaten? Who prepared it?

LH: We had an eat-in kitchen. Even at my aunt's house with all the festivities going on, she put her dining room furniture in the kitchen where you could see and smell the foods being cooked. When you go to any kind of special occasion with Black families, there are at least two meats most of the time, or three. Maybe there'll be a pot of neck bones or some fried chicken, smoked turkey on the grill, and everybody is involved (in preparing the meal).

At my parents' parties, I can remember the kitchen full of flavors, aromas, and when the adults would sit on the patio, us kids would peek out at them. I tease my mother's family, "you all will drive 2,000 miles just to get a meal." At our family occasions there's always commentary about the food, even at a funeral—who makes the best macaroni and cheese, the best fried chicken. My aunt in Chicago made the best fried chicken and collard greens, flavored with salt pork (fat back), smoked neck bones, and smoked ham hocks. The cornbread she made was amazing: it tasted like cake but wasn't that sweet; it was rich and moist and always cooked in a cast iron pan and never put in the refrigerator.

Because my family traveled as part of the military, to Alaska, to Japan, when we ate these foods, it felt like we were back in the States, back

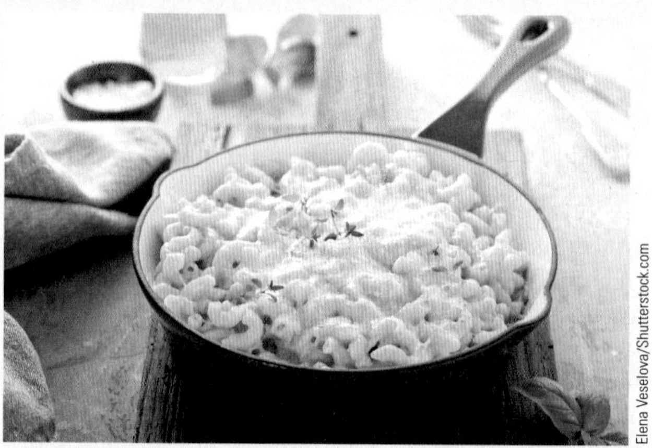

Elena Veselova/Shutterstock.com

▲ Baked Macaroni and Cheese

(Continued)

Comfort Food—Black American (*Continued*)

L. Hudson's Story

home. In Japan, my mother was always big on inviting Black military airmen there without their families to our home for a meal. Our comfort foods were extended to our wider culture even though we were in a foreign land.

Here is L. Hudson's Favorite Recipe:

Macaroni and Cheese

Recipe courtesy of Joann McMillian of Palm Bay, Florida
Serves 8

- 8 ounces elbow macaroni
- 1 egg
- ½ cup evaporated milk or half and half
- 8 ounces cheddar cheese + 4 ounces
- 1 cup sour cream
- 1 cup cottage cheese
- Dash sugar
- Salt to taste

In a deep pot, bring 4 cups of lightly salted water to a boil, then add noodles and cook for 5-10 minutes until the noodles are a little less than al dente. Drain the noodles and pour them into a 9 x 9 square or 9-inch round baking dish. In a small bowl, beat the egg slightly and add the evaporated milk or half and half. Mix well, then add the sour cream, cottage cheese, and 8 ounces of the cheddar cheese. Add a dash of sugar. If adding salt, so do at this time. Mix well and add this mixture to the macaroni in the baking dish. Sprinkle remaining 4 ounces of cheese on top and bake at 350 F until heated through, about 20 minutes.

Nutrition information (per serving):

calories 386; carbohydrates: 26 g; fat: 23 g; protein: 20 g; sodium: 376 mg

An Additional Comfort Food RECIPE TO TRY

West African Togbei/Bofrot/Puff Puff Recipe (sweet fried dough similar to a donut)

Recipe from Sweet Adjeley
Serves 4

- 1 cup warm water + ¾ cup water
- 1 tablespoon sugar + 1 cup sugar
- 2 teaspoon active dry yeast mix
- 4 cups all-purpose flour
- 1 cup sugar
- 1 tsp. nutmeg
- 1 tsp. salt

Vegetable oil, enough to deep fry puff puffs

Add 1 Tbsp. sugar and active dry yeast to 1 cup warm water, cover, and set aside for 5 minutes. In a separate bowl, add flour, the remaining 1 cup sugar, nutmeg, and salt. Mix well. After the 5 minutes, add the activated yeast in the warm water to the dry ingredients. Add in the remaining ¾ cup water, mixing until the batter is light (3 to 5 minutes by hand). Cover the bowl and set the mixture aside to rise for 2 hours in a warm place. Next, add oil to a deep-sided small pot, and heat. Mix the batter vigorously to get some of the air out. Once the oil is hot, scoop a large spoonful of the dough and drop it into the oil. Add as many dollops as will fit without crowding. Decrease the heat to medium, and simmer the puff puffs until uniformly brown and cooked through. Serve with powdered sugar, fruit jam, chocolate syrup, or plain.

Nutrition information (per serving):

calories 397; carbohydrates: 72 g; protein: 10 g; fat: 6 g; sodium: 9 mg

Discussion Starters

Health Risk Factors of Black Americans

Black Americans today often suffer from obesity, diabetes, hypertension, infant and maternal morbidity and mortality, and depression in greater numbers than other American races. Make a list of all the possible reasons for this phenomenon. Don't limit yourself to just one or two, and look back at the diet and culture of the geographical area from which the ancestors of most modern Black Americans came. In a small group, share your lists of reasons and come up with one group list. Again, your task is to list all the possible reasons that you can.

After making this group list, individually take a blank sheet of paper and cluster the items on that list. That is, look at the listed items and identify reasons that you see as possibly being somehow linked. On the blank sheet of paper, rewrite the reasons on the group list but locate them as best you can near other reasons that you somehow related. Circle each reason and draw lines between the ones that you believe are connected.

Finally, imagine that you have been hired by a local health department in an area of the country with a large Black population to write a brief (one-page) resource handout for local health professionals on the reasons why many of their clients may have the above health problems. As you plan this short paper, consider whether—or not—it might have made a difference had the slave trade focused on East Africa instead of West Africa.

Review Questions

1. Describe the cuisine that West African people brought to America, and one American food recipe that has its origins in Africa. What traditional food might be served on Juneteenth?
2. Compare similarities and differences in West and East African traditional cuisines. What countries have influenced East African cuisine?
3. Name the presented symbolic foods used in the Nigerian child-naming ceremonies, and explain what they symbolize.
4. Describe three therapeutic uses of food among Black Americans. What is pica and why is it practiced?
5. For Black Americans, how might diet affect the incidence and treatment of hypertension and type 2 diabetes mellitus?

Reflection

How might some traditional soul foods be modified with heart health in mind while honoring African American culinary heritage? Keep in mind that nutrient-rich dishes and leafy green vegetables can play a role in maintaining food culture while promoting health. How might the comfort food recipe of macaroni and cheese in this chapter be modified to have less fat?

References

1. U.S. Census Bureau, Newsroom. 2022. Facts for features: Black (African-American) history month: January 20, 2022. Retrieved from: https://www.census.gov/newsroom/facts-for-features/2022/black-history-month.html (accessed March 29, 2022).
2. U.S. Department of Health and Human Services, Office of Minority Health. 2019. Profile: Black/African Americans. Retrieved from: https://www.minorityhealth.hhs.gov/omh/browse.aspx?lvl=3&lvlid=61 (accessed March 29, 2022).
3. Tamir, Christine. 2021. The growing diversity of Black America. Pew Research. March 25, 2021. Retrieved from: https://www.pewresearch.org/social-trends/2021/03/25/the-growing-diversity-of-black-america/
4. U.S. Census Bureau. 2011–2015. American Community Survey five year estimates. Retrieved from: http://www.census.gov/acs (accessed March 29, 2022).
5. Worldometer. Retrieved from: https://www.worldometers.info/world-population/africa-population/ (accessed on March 29, 2022).
6. Bruinsma, Jelle. 2009. The Resource Outlook to 2050. Food and Agriculture Association of the United Nations (FAO). Retrieved from: https://www.fao.org/3/ak971e/ak971e.pdf.
7. Guasco, Michael. 2017. The misguided focus on 1619 as the beginning of slavery in the US damages our understanding of American history. *Smithsonian Magazine*. Retrieved from: https://www.smithsonianmag.com/history/misguided-focus-1619-beginning-slavery-us-damages-our-understanding-american-history-180964873/
8. The Lowcountry Digital History Initiative. African passages, low country adaptations. Retrieved from: https://ldhi.library.cofc.edu/exhibits/show/africanpassageslowcountryadapt/introductionatlanticworld/slaverybeforetrade
9. Gates, H.L. 2013. The African-American migration story. *The African American, Many*. Retrieved from: https://www.pbs.org/wnet/african-americans-many-rivers-to-cross/history/on-african-american-migrations/
10. National Archives. African American heritage: The Great Migration (1910–1970). Retrieved from: https://www.archives.gov/research/african-americans/migrations/great-migration#:~:text=The%20Great%20Migration%20was%20one,the%201910s%20until%20the%201970s.
11. Unitarian Universalist Association. Sundown Towns. Retrieved from: https://www.uua.org/multiculturalism/racial-justice/history/engaging/sundown-towns
12. Wilkerson, I. 2016. The long-lasting legacy of the Great Migration. *Smithsonian Magazine*.
13. Collins, W.J. 2021. The Great Migration of Black Americans from the US South: A guide and interpretation. *Explorations in Economic History*, 80, 101382.
14. U.S. Department of Health and Human Services, Office of Minority Health. 2019. Profile: Black/African Americans. Retrieved from https://www.minorityhealth.hhs.gov/omh/browse.aspx?lvl=3&lvlid=61 (accessed March 29, 2022).
15. U.S. Census Bureau, Newsroom. 2022. Facts for features: Black (African-American) history month: January 20, 2022. Retrieved from: https://www.census.gov/newsroom/facts-for-features/2022/black-history-month.html (accessed on March 29, 2022).
16. Cheesman Day, J. 2020, 88% of Blacks have a high school diploma, 26% a Bachelor's degree. United States Census Bureau. Retrieved from: https://www.census.gov/library/stories/2020/06/black-high-school-attainment-nearly-on-par-with-national-average.html (accessed June 7, 2022).
17. Banks, Adelle M. 2021. Exploring faith and black churches in America. *Pew Trust Magazine*. Retrieved from: https://www.pewtrusts.org/en/trust/archive/fall-2021/exploring-faith-and-black-churches-in-america
18. Pew Research Center. 2013. The religious affiliation of U.S. immigrants: Majority Christian, rising share of other faiths. Retrieved from: http://www.pewforum.org/2013/05/17/the-religious-affiliation-of-us-immigrants/ (accessed February 18, 2015).
19. Encyclopedia Britannica. Maghreb region, North Africa. Retrieved from: https://www.britannica.com/place/Maghreb
20. Mohamed B., Cox, K., Diamant, J., & Gecewicz, C. 2021. Faith among Black Americans.
21. Pew Research Center. 2015. The future of world religions: Population growth projections, 2010–2050. Pew Research Center. Retrieved from: https://www.pewforum.org/2015/04/02/middle-east-north-africa/
22. U.S. Census Bureau. 2016–2020. American Community Survey five year estimates. Retrieved from: https://data.census.gov/cedsci/table?q=S0201%3A%20SELECTED%20POPULATION%20PROFILE%20IN%20THE%20UNITED%20STATES&t=004%20-%20Black%20or%20African%20American%20alone&tid=ACSSPP1Y2019.S0201&hidePreview=true (accessed March 29, 2022).
23. Wallace, S.A., Strike, K.S., Glasgow, Y.M., Lynch, K., & Fullilove, R.E. 2016.' Other than that, I'm good: formerly incarcerated young Black men's self-perceptions of health status. *Journal of Health Care for the Poor and Underserved*, 27(2), 163–180.
24. Shikany, J.M., Schoenberger, Y.M.M., Konety, B.R., & Vickers, S.M. 2018. African American men's health: Research, practice, and policy. *American Journal of Preventive Medicine*, 55(5), S1–S4.
25. Carter-Edwards, L., Lindquist, R., Redmond, N., Turner, C.M., Harding, C., Oliver, J., ... & Shikany, J.M. 2018. Designing faith-based blood pressure interventions to reach young Black men. *American Journal of Preventive Medicine*, 55(5), S49–S58.
26. Brandon, E. 1976. Folk medicine in French Louisiana. In W.D. Hand (Ed.), *American folk medicine*. Berkeley: University of California Press.
27. Purnell, L.D., & Fenkl, E.A. 2019. The Purnell model for cultural competence. In *Handbook for Culturally Competent Care* (pp. 7–18). Springer, Cham.

28. Novotna, B., Polesny, Z., Pinto-Basto, M.F., Van Damme, P., Pudil, P., Mazancova, J., & Duarte, M.C. 2020. Medicinal plants used by "root doctors", local traditional healers in Bié province, Angola. *Journal of Ethnopharmacology*, 260, 112662.
29. Lewis, C.S. 2018. Conjure women, root men, and normative visions of freedom in antebellum slave narratives. *Arizona Quarterly: A Journal of American Literature, Culture, and Theory*, 74(2), 113–141.
30. Obikili, N. 2016. The impact of the slave trade on literacy in West Africa: Evidence from the colonial era. *Journal of African Economies*, 25(1), 1–27. Retrieved from: https://doi.org/10.1093/jae/ejv018
31. Mehrabi, Z., & Lashermes, P. 2017. Protecting the origins of coffee to safeguard its future. *Nature Plants*, 3(1), 1–3.
32. Seleshe, S., Jo, C., & Lee, M. 2014. Meat consumption culture in Ethiopia. *Korean journal for Food Science of Animal Resources*, 34(1), 7–13.
33. Gebreyesus, Yohanis. 2019. *Ethiopia: Recipes and traditions from the Horn of Africa*. Interlink Books.
34. Riggs, T. 2014. *The Gale encyclopedia of multicultural America*.
35. Spices Inc., n.d. The culinary Regions of African Cuisine. Retrieved from: https://www.spicesinc.com/p-3808-the-culinary-regions-of-african-cuisine.aspx#:~:text=Despite%20these%20differences%2C%20the%20spices%20used%20in%20each,also%20popular%20spices%20in%20Northern%20Africa.%20Southern%20Africa (accessed March 29, 2022).
36. Thurow, R. 2013. *The last hunger season: a year in an African farm community on the brink of change*. Hachette UK.
37. Crowder, A. 2018. *Community through consumption: The role of food in African American cultural formation in the 18th century Chesapeake*. University of Massachusetts Boston.
38. Talleyrand, R.M., Gordon, A.D., Daquin, J.V., & Johnson, A.J. 2017. Expanding our understanding of eating practices, body image, and appearance in African American women: A qualitative study. *Journal of Black Psychology*, 43(5), 464–492.
39. Collins, W.L. 2015. The role of African American churches in promoting health among congregations. *Social Work & Christianity*, 42(2).
40. Sarkodie-Mensah, K. 2014. Nigerian Americans. In R.V. Dassanowsky & J. Lehman (Eds.), *Gale encyclopedia of multicultural America*. Farmington Hills, MI: Gale Group.
41. Miller, O. 2014. Ugandan Americans. In R.V. Dassanowsky & J. Lehman (Eds.), *Gale encyclopedia of multicultural America*. Farmington Hills, MI: Gale Group.
42. Weatherspoon, L., Chester, D., & Kidd, T. 2010. African American food practices. In C.M. Goody & L. Drago (Eds.), *Cultural food practice*. Chicago: American Dietetic Association.
43. Jackson, J.J. 1981. Urban black Americans. In A. Harwood (Ed.), *Ethnicity and medical care*. Cambridge, MA: Harvard University Press.
44. Jackson, B. 1976. The other kind of doctor: Conjure and magic in black American folk medicine. In W.D. Hand (Ed.), *American folk medicine*. Berkeley: University of California Press.
45. Brandon, E. 1976. Folk medicine in French Louisiana. In W.D. Hand (Ed.), *American folk medicine*. Berkeley: University of California Press.
46. Glanville, C.L. 2003. People of African American heritage. In L.D. Purnell & B.J. Paulanka (Eds.), *Transcultural health care* (2nd ed.). Philadelphia: FA Davis.
47. Boyd, E.L., Taylor, S.D., Shimp, L.A., & Semier, C.R. 2000. An assessment of home remedy use by African Americans. *Journal of the National Medical Association*, 92, 341–353.
48. Borgna-Pignatti, C., & Zanella, S. 2016. Pica as a manifestation of iron deficiency. *Expert Review of Hematology*, 9(11), 1075–1080.
49. Jackson, M.S., Adedoyin, A.C., Winnick, S.N. 2020. Pica disorder among African American women: A call for action and further research. *Social Work in Public Health*, 35(5), 261–270.
50. Olawale, F., Olofinsan, K., Iwaloye, O., & Ologuntere, T.E. 2021. Phytochemicals from Nigerian medicinal plants modulate therapeutically-relevant diabetes targets: Insight from computational direction. *Advances in Traditional Medicine*, 1–15.
51. Quandt, S.A., Sandberg, J.C., Grzywacz, J.G., Altizer, K.P., & Arcury, T.A. 2015. Home remedy use among African American and White older adults. *Journal of the National Medical Association*, 107(2), 121–129. https://doi.org/10.1016/S0027-9684(15)30036-5
52. Mercer, A. 2021. A homecoming. Eater Longform. Retrieved from: https://www.eater.com/22229322/black-veganism-history-black-panthers-dick-gregory-nation-of-islam-alvenia-fulton.
53. Li, W., Youssef, G., Procter-Gray, E., Olendzki, B., Cornish, T., Hayes, R., Churchill, L., Kane, K., Brown, K., & Magee, M.F. 2017. Racial differences in eating patterns and food purchasing behaviors among urban older women. *The Journal of Nutrition, Health & Aging*, 21(10), 1190–1199. https://doi.org/10.1007/s12603-016-0834-7
54. Brooks, Kelly. 2014. Research shows food deserts more abundant in minority neighborhoods. *Johns Hopkins Magazine*. Retrieved from: https://hub.jhu.edu/magazine/2014/spring/racial-food-deserts/
55. Eckert, J., & Vojnovic, I. 2017. Fast food landscapes: Exploring restaurant choice and travel behavior for residents living in lower eastside Detroit neighborhoods. *Applied Geography*, 89, 41–51.
56. Kwate, N.O.A., & Loh, J.M. 2016. Fast food and liquor store density, co-tenancy, and turnover: Vice store operations in Chicago, 1995–2008. *Applied Geography*, 67, 1–13.
57. James, P., Arcaya, M.C., Parker, D.M., Tucker-Seeley, R.D., & Subramanian, S.V. 2014. Do minority and poor neighborhoods have higher access to fast-food restaurants in the United States? *Health & Place*, 29, 10–17.
58. Ohri-Vachaspati, P., Isgor, Z., Rimkus, L., Powell, L.M., Barker, D.C., & Chaloupka, F.J. 2015. Child-directed marketing inside and on the exterior of fast food restaurants. *American Journal of Preventive Medicine*, 48(1), 22–30.
59. Weatherspoon, L., Chester, D., & Kidd, T. 2010. African American food practices. In C.M. Goody & L. Drago (Eds.), *Cultural food practice*. Chicago: American Dietetic Association.
60. Jarrett, R.L., Bahar, O.S., & Kersh, R.T. 2016. When we do sit down together: Family meal times in low-income African American families with preschoolers. *Journal of Family Issues*, 37(11), 1483–1513.
61. Varghese, H.T. 2019. The Unpopular History of the Black Food: African-American Food Stereotypes in Popular Media.
62. Garth, H., & Reese, A.M. (Eds.). 2020. *Black food matters: Racial justice in the wake of food justice*. University of Minnesota Press.
63. D'Adamo,C.R.,Parker,E.A.,McArdle,P.F.,Trilling,A.,Bowden,B.,Bahr-Robertson, M.K., Keller, K.L., & Berman, B.M. 2021. The addition of spices and herbs to vegetables in the National School Lunch Program increased vegetable intake at an urban, economically-underserved, and predominantly African-American high school. *Food Quality and Preference*, 88, 104076.
64. Othman, S.I., Fertig, A., Trofholz, A., & Berge, J.M. 2022. How time in the US and race/ethnicity shape food parenting practices and child diet quality. *Appetite*, 171, 105870.
65. Youfa Wang, Jungwon Min, Kisa Harris, Jacob Khuri, Laura M Anderson, A Systematic Examination of Food Intake and Adaptation to the Food Environment by Refugees Settled in the United States, Advances in Nutrition, Volume 7, Issue 6, November 2016, Pages 1066–1079.
66. Lee, L. 2022. Nutrition and the African-American diet. *The Sampson Independent*. Retrieved from: https://www.clintonnc.com/features/lifestyle/27515/nutrition-and-the-african-american-diet.
67. Kirkpatrick, S., Dodd, KW., Reedy, J., & Krebs-Smith, S.M. 2012. Income and race/ethnicity are associated with adherence to food-based dietary guidance among US adults and children. *Journal of the Academy of Nutrition and Dietetics*, 112(5), 624–635.

68. Boggs, D.A., Ban, Y., Palmer, J.R., & Rosenberg, L. 2015. Higher diet quality is inversely associated with mortality in African-American women. *The Journal of Nutrition*, 145(3), 547–554.
69. Brown-Riggs, C. 2014 Lactose intolerance: Dispelling myths and helping minorities enjoy dairy. *AADE in Practice*, 3(10), 32–36.
70. Sterling, S.R., & Bowen, S.A. 2019. The potential for plant-based diets to promote health among blacks living in the United States. *Nutrients*, 11(12), 2915.
71. Chan, Q., Stamler, J., & Elliott, P. 2015. Dietary factors and higher blood pressure in African-Americans. *Current Hypertension Reports*, 17(2), 1–8.
72. Saab, K.R., Kendrick, J., Yracheta, J.M., Lanaspa, M.A., Pollard, M., & Johnson, R.J. 2015. New insights on the risk for cardiovascular disease in African Americans: the role of added sugars. *Journal of the American Society of Nephrology*, 26(2), 247–257.
73. Funk, C., & Kennedy, B. 2016. The new food fights: US public divides over food science. *Pew Research Center*, 1–100.
74. USA Facts. August 27, 2020. Retrieved from: https://usafacts.org/articles/health-by-race-asthma-obesity-vaccination-life-expectancy-black-hispanic-white/?utm_source=bing&utm_medium=cpc&utm_campaign=ND-Race&msclkid=c7d3ae9f5a5518e87571cc00ea386169 (accessed June 7, 2022).
75. New York Times. n.d. U.S> Life Expectancy Plunged in 2020, Especially for Black and Hispanic Americans. Retrieved from: https://www.nytimes.com/2021/07/21/us/american-life-expectancy-report.html (accessed June 7, 2022).
76. National Vital Statistics Reports. 2019. Births: Final Data for 2019. 70(2). Retrieved from: cdc.gov.
77. Centers for Disease Control and Prevention. 2020. Breastfeeding Report Card. Retrieved from: https://www.cdc.gov/breastfeeding/data/reportcard.htm (accessed on March 29, 2022).
78. Reeves, E.A., & Woods-Giscombé, C.L. 2014. Infant-feeding practices among African American women: Social-ecological analysis and implications for practice. *Journal of Transcultural Nursing*. Published online printed May 8, 2014.
79. https://www.statista.com/statistics/207436/overweight-and-obesity-rates-for-adults-by-ethnicity/
80. Kelly, N.R, Bulik, C.M., & Mazzeo, S.E. 2011. An exploration of body dissatisfaction and perceptions of black and white girls enrolled in an intervention for overweight children. *Body Image*, 8(4), 379–384.
81. Vance, K.E. 2018. *Culture, food and racism: The effects on African American Health*. University of Tennessee at Chattanooga.
82. Evans, E.M., Rowe, D.A., Racette, S.B., Ross, K.M., & McAuley, E. 2006. Is the current BMI obesity classification appropriate for black and white post menopausal women? *International Journal of Obesity*, 30, 837–843.
83. Katzmarzyk, P.T., Bray, G.A., Greenway, F.L., Johnson, W.D., Newton, R.L., Ravussin, E., Ryan, D.H., & Bouchard, C. 2011. ethnic-specific BMI and waist circumference thresholds. *Obesity*, 19(6), 1272–1278. Retrieved from: https://doi.org/10.1038/oby.2010.319.
84. Sim, L. 2019. Our eating disorders blind spot: Sex and ethnic/racial disparities in help-seeking for eating disorders. *Mayo Clinic Proceedings*, 94(8), 1398–1400.
85. Khosla, L., Bhat, S., Fullington, L.A., & Horlyck-Romanovsky, M.F. 2021. HbA1c performance in African descent populations in the United States with normal glucose tolerance, prediabetes, or diabetes: A scoping review. *Preventing chronic disease*, 18, E22.
86. CDC. 2021. Summary Health Statistics: National Health Interview Survey: 2018. Table A-4a. Retrieved from: http://www.cdc.gov/nchs/nhis/shs/tables.htm
87. Centers for Disease Control and Prevention. 2018. Age-adjusted percentages of selected circulatory diseases among adults aged 18 and over, by selected characteristics: United States, 2018, Table 2. *Summary Health Statistics for U.S. Adults: 2018*. Retrieved from: https://ftp.cdc.gov/pub/Health_Statistics/NCHS/NHIS/SHS/2018_SHS_Table_A-1.pdf
88. Zakai, N.A., McClure, L.A., Prineas, R., Howard, G., McClellan, W., Holmes, C.E., Newsome, B.B., Warnock, D.G., Audhya, P., & Cushman, M. 2009. Correlates of anemia in American blacks and whites: The REGARDS Renal Ancillary Study. *American Journal of Epidemiology*, 169(3), 355–364. Retrieved from: https://doi.org/10.1093/aje/kwn355
89. Le, C.H.H. 2016. The prevalence of anemia and moderate-severe anemia in the US population (NHANES 2003-2012). *PloS One*, 11(11), e0166635.
90. Belachew, T., Nida, H., Getaneh, T., Woldemariam, D., & Getinet, W. 2005. Calcium deficiency and causation of rickets in Ethiopian children. *East African Medical Journal*, 82, 153–159.
92. Fogelman, Y., Rakover, Y., & Luboshitzky, R. 1995. High prevalence of vitamin D deficiency among Ethiopian women immigrants to Israel: Exacerbation during pregnancy and lactation. *Israeli Journal of Medical Sciences*, 31, 221–224.
92. Mengesha, B., & Ergete, W. 2005. Staple Ethiopian diet and cancer of the oesophagus. *East African Medical Journal*, 82, 353–356.
93. Pfortmueller, C.A., Graf, F., Tabarra, M., Lindner, G., Zimmermann, H., & Exadaktylos, A.K. 2012. Acute health problems in African refugees. *Wiener klinische Wochenschrift*, 124(17), 647–652.
94. Hamid, S., Groot, W., & Pavlova, M. (2019). Trends in cardiovascular diseases and associated risks in sub-Saharan Africa: a review of the evidence for Ghana, Nigeria, South Africa, Sudan and Tanzania. *The aging male*, 22(3), 169–176.
95. Rasbridge, L.A. 2006. Sudanese. Refugee health—Immigrant health. Baylor University. Retrieved from: http://www3.baylor.edu/~Charles_Kemp/refugees.htm (accessed February 21, 2015).
96. Salah, A., Amanatidis, S., & Samman, S. 2002. Cross-sectional study of diet and risk factors for metabolic diseases in a Ghanaian population of Sydney, Australia. *Asia Pacific Journal of Clinical Nutrition*, 11, 210–216.
97. Okafor, C.B. 2000. Folklore linked to pregnancy and birth in Nigeria. *Western Journal of Nursing Research*, 22, 189–202.

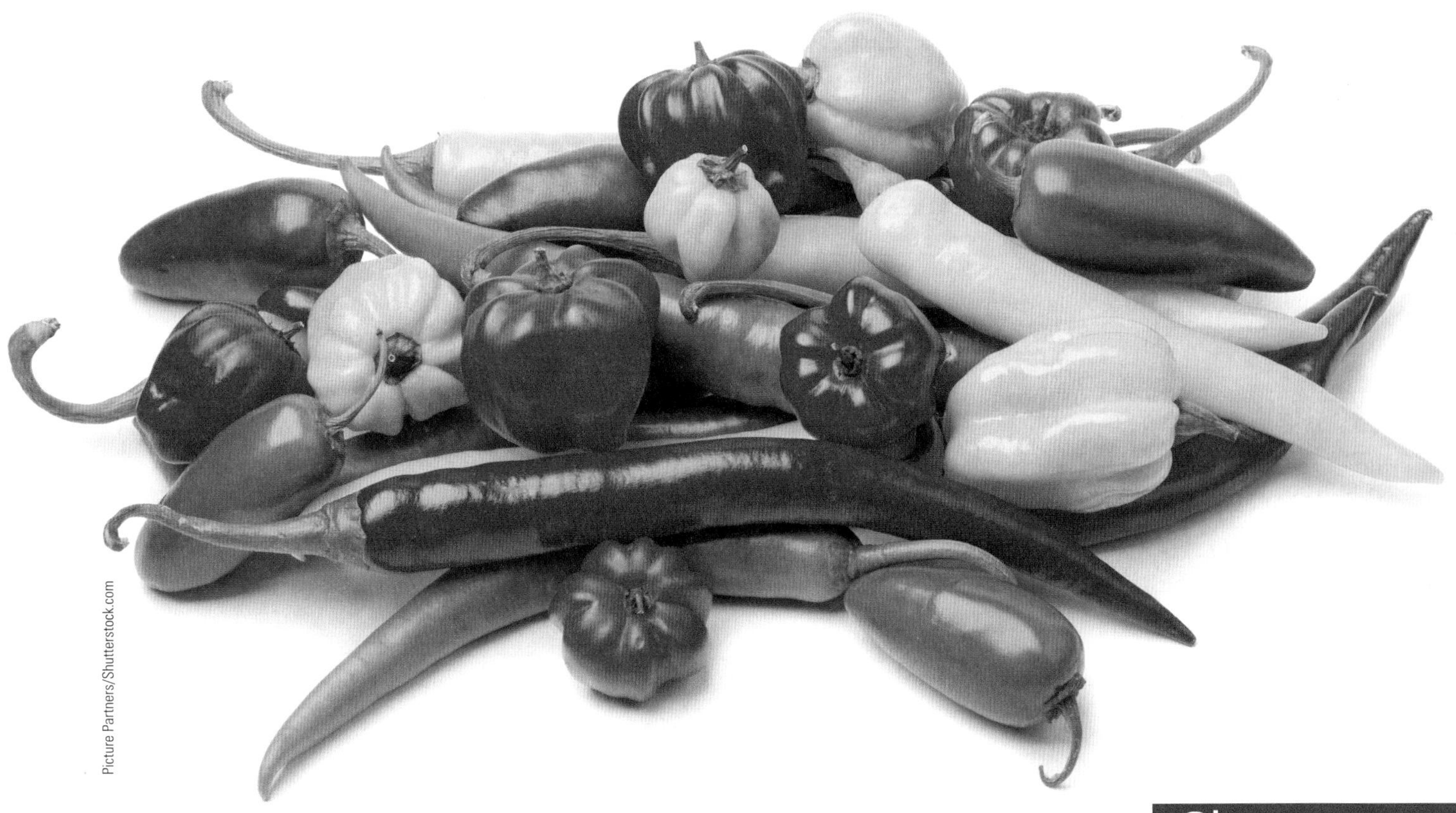
Picture Partners/Shutterstock.com

Chapter 9

Mexicans and Central Americans

Learning Objectives

9.1 List the regions of Mexico and the countries of Central America that are reviewed.

9.2 Discuss the immigration patterns, historical socioeconomic influences, and current locations of Mexicans and Central Americans in America today.

9.3 Differentiate the religions, family structures, and traditional health beliefs and practices of Mexicans and Central Americans before and after immigration to the United States.

9.4 Compare the differences and similarities among staple foods and preparation techniques within and across Mexico and the Central American countries.

9.5 Compare key foods for each of the food groups for both Mexico and Central America to how these foods have been adapted by immigrants in the United States.

9.6 Compare the traditional meal composition and cycles and compare these to the meal composition and cycles of Mexicans, Mexican Americans, and Central Americans living in America today.

9.7 Describe regional specialties and dishes of Mexico and Central America.

9.8 Identify health concerns associated with nutritional intake of Mexicans, Mexican Americans, and Central Americans.

Latinx people are the largest non-European ethnic group in the United States, representing 18.5 percent of the total population or 61.4 million in 2021.[1,2] They are not a single cultural group. Latinx people come from more than twenty-five Latin American nations with diverse ethnic populations. Though a majority share Spanish as a common language of origin, others speak English, French, Portuguese, or an indigenous dialect as their mother tongue.

Immigrants from Mexico and the countries of Central America bring a rich cultural history (refer to Figure 9.1). The Olmec culture, known for its sophisticated sculpture, existed in southeastern Mexico as early as 1200 BCE. The great Aztec, Mayan, and Toltec civilizations thrived while Europe was in its Dark Ages. Their independent mastery of astronomy, architecture, agriculture, and art astonished later explorers. Spanish occupation of Mexico and Central America introduced new ideas and traditions, most notably Roman Catholicism. Foods from the British, French, and Austrian intrusions also provided contributions. The foods of Mexico and Central America, which traveled with Spaniards returning to Europe, embodied the Indigenous heritage of the region. Today, the mix of Indigenous and European history of the region is reflected on the plate not only in Mexico and Central America but in the regional foods of the United States and across the globe. The Indigenous inhabitants of the Americas domesticated three productive nutritious staples: corn, potatoes, and manioc (also known as cassava, yuca, arrowroot, or tapioca), now widely eaten around the world. Foundational foods in U.S. diets, such as corn, beans, potatoes, and squash prepared in many ways, in addition to chili pepper and much more, reflect the diversity from Latin America's history of settlement and intermarriage.[3] This chapter examines Mexican cuisine and the food habits of Americans of Mexican descent. An overview of recent immigration from Central America and its traditional fare is also included. The following chapter reviews Latinx cultures from the Caribbean Islands and South America.

Food for Thought

The terms Latino and Latina describe men and women, respectively, who are originally from Mexico, the Caribbean, and Central and South America. It suggests the culture of Latin heritage, not exclusively of Spanish background. The word "Latin@" which means both Latino and Latina is also widely accepted. A rising term for people of various backgrounds linked to Central and South American cultures is Latinx. "Latinx" is used as a gender-neutral or nonbinary term inclusive of all genders. In this book, the term Latinx is used. Hispanic is preferred by some, though there is no clear definition of this term as it can mean people born in Latin America, people whose ancestors were born in Latin America, people with Spanish surnames, or those that are Spanish speaking.

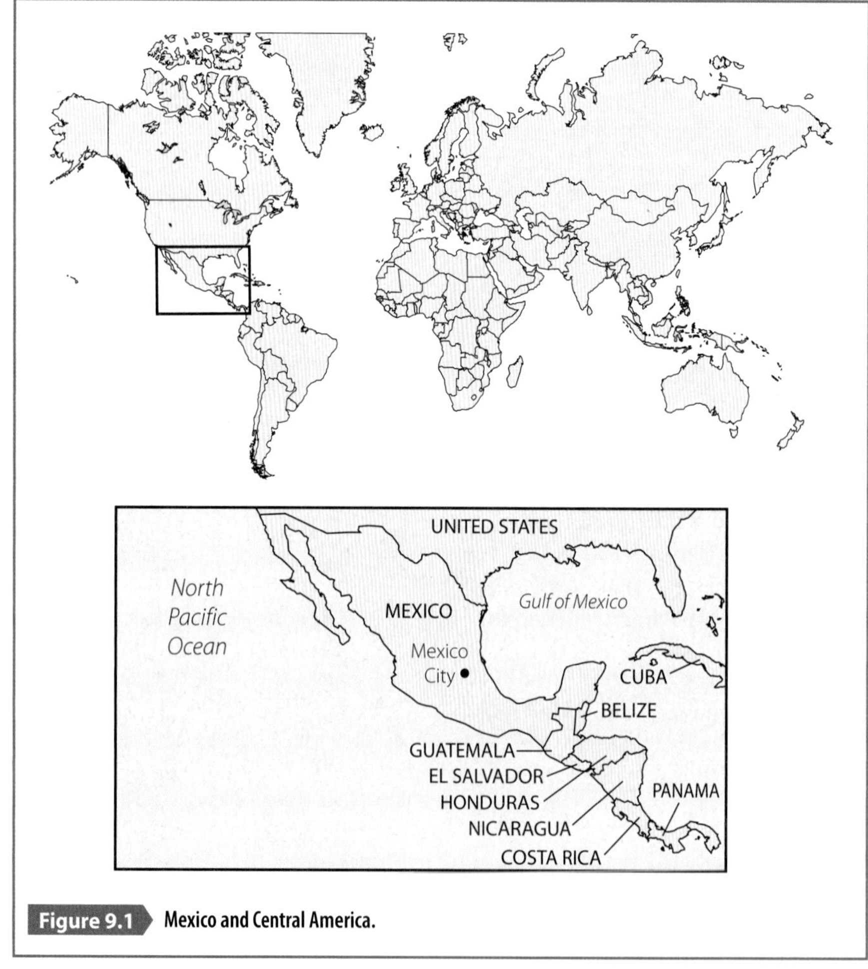

Figure 9.1 Mexico and Central America.

Mexicans

Estados Unidos Mexicanos, the United Mexican States, is the northernmost Latin American country. Though Mexico can seem a part of Central America, it is geographically a part of North America. It is more than one-fourth the size of the United States, with 756,065 square miles of territory. The varied geography includes a large central plateau surrounded by mountains except to the north. Coastal plains edge the country along the Gulf of Mexico and the Pacific. The separate Baja peninsula is found in the west, and the Yucatán peninsula juts out in the southeast. Snow-capped volcanoes, such as Orizaba, Popocatépetl, Ixtacchiuatl, and El Chichón, and frequent earthquakes also affect the landscape. The climate ranges from arid desert in the northern plains to tropical lowlands in the south.

Over 80 percent of Mexicans are mestizos—people of mixed Indigenous and Spanish ancestry based on genomics, while European and Indigenous ancestry is approximately even. Spanish is the official language. Indigenous language-only speakers, primarily speaking Nahuatl, make up 1.5 percent of Mexicans.[4]

Cultural Perspective

History of Mexicans in the United States

Immigration Patterns Mexican immigration patterns have changed over the years since the Mexican-American War defined the United States–Mexican border. Mexicans lived in what is now the American Southwest for hundreds of years before the United States declared its independence in 1776. Although they welcomed American settlers, they soon found themselves outnumbered, and their economic and political control of the region weakened. At the end of the Mexican-American War in 1848, the 75,000 Mexicans living in the ceded territories became U.S. citizens.

Between 1900 and 1935, it is estimated that 10 percent of the Mexican population, approximately 1 million people, emigrated north to the United States. Then, during the Great Depression, tens of thousands of unauthorized migrants, plus those admitted legally under the 1917 contract labor laws, were repatriated and sent back to Mexico.

After the Great Depression, there were labor shortages. The Bracero program was created to meet this shortage and was composed of those who legally worked in the United States but remained Mexican citizens. Thousands of Mexicans were offered jobs in agriculture and on the railroads. Following World War II, the continued need for farm workers encouraged additional immigration, resulting in a total of over 4.5 million contracts (some individuals obtained multiple contracts over several years) issued to Mexican nationals between 1942 and 1964. In the past thirty-five years, Mexicans have been the largest single group of legal immigrants to the United States.[5]

Current Demographics More than half of the growth in the total population of the United States between 2010 and 2020 was due to the increase in the Latinx population. Population estimates from 2019 show Mexican Americans in the United States accounting for 62 percent of the Latinx population.[6] The majority of Mexican Americans live in California, Texas, and Arizona. However, the settlement pattern for new immigrants has changed since the 1990s, becoming more nationwide as evidenced by Illinois having over 1.5 million Mexican American residents.[7] Eighty percent of the immigrants from Mexico settle in U.S. cities such as San Diego, Los Angeles, San Antonio, and Chicago—and more recently, Dallas, Houston, Las Vegas, Minneapolis, New York City, and Phoenix.[8] Many recent immigrants settle in the urban Latinx neighborhoods called barrios.

Socioeconomic Status Mexican Americans primarily occupy three main socioeconomic groups: migrant farmworkers, who maintain a culturally isolated community; residents of the urban barrios, who also are segregated from much of American society; and a growing number of acculturated middle-class Mexican Americans. Undocumented people tend to move in with family members who already reside in the United States. Usually, this is in a predominantly Latinx neighborhood where they can live comfortably among the residents while becoming familiar with the American social and economic systems. Specific data on Mexican Americans are limited because they are often grouped with data from all Latinx communities.

Approximately 20 percent of Latinx people in the United States hold professional or managerial positions. By 2030, one out of five workers will be Latinx. The skill level for the Latinx working population is rising with increasing education throughout Latinx communities. Today, 80 percent of Mexican Americans graduate from high school, compared to 60 percent of adults who were born in Mexico. Despite the rapidly growing Mexican American middle to upper class, others in this community fall below the poverty level (15 percent of Mexican American families in 2019 compared to a national average of 10.5 percent). Forty-three percent are employed in agricultural, fishing, and forestry jobs, and, 27 percent, work in manufacturing or service occupations.[5]

Food for Thought

The terms Chicano and Chicana, for men and women, respectively, came from the Aztec word for Mexicans, Meshicano.

The 2016 Canadian Census listed more than 674,640 residents of Latin American heritage.

Some immigrants from Mexico seeking migrant agricultural jobs are from Indigenous groups or people from Mexico (mostly mixtecos from Oaxaca), who speak neither English nor Spanish.

When a girl turns fifteen years old, her family often hosts a quinceañera, an elaborate coming-out party with music, feasting, and dancing. With the conquest by the Spanish, European elements were introduced to the Aztec tradition including the opening waltz, the girl's tiara, and a court of attendants.[9,10]

Worldview

Mexican immigrants frequently live in culturally homogeneous communities. Many proudly maintain their ethnic identity, speaking Spanish and enjoying Mexican music and food. The concept of la raza (meaning "the people") was first promoted in the 1960s as a pride and solidarity movement for all persons of Latin American heritage.

When exposed to the majority American society, however, immigrants from Mexico can be highly adaptive. Some (those born in the United States) are completely assimilated and may speak no Spanish. Others are completely bicultural. The number of undocumented people from Mexico is declining. This group in 2017 made up less than half, or 47 percent (4.9 million), of the total 10.5 million undocumented people from all countries such as El Salvador, Guatemala, and Honduras, as well as Asia, in the United States.[11] Cross-cultural marriages are becoming more common, especially in the northern regions of the United States.

Religion Approximately 55 percent of Americans of Mexican descent are Roman Catholics, which is less than the percentage found in Mexico (81 percent). Traditional religious ceremonies, such as baptism, communion, confirmation, marriage, and the novenas (nine days of prayer for the deceased), are important family events (refer to Chapter 4).[12]

A strong faith in the will of God influences how many immigrants from Mexico perceive their world. Many believe that events and circumstances are predetermined and that an individual is powerless in the face of luck, fate, and destiny. This fatalistic approach to life can affect how people manage health issues.[13] Most Mexican Americans who are not Catholic practice Protestant faiths (22 percent) or are unaffiliated (18 percent).[12] Evangelical churches are particularly popular in urban areas.

The Mexican American Family The family is the most important social unit in this community. In contrast to the dominant society in America, the well-being of the family comes before the needs of the individual.

The father (or eldest male relative) is typically the head of the household. He is the primary decision-maker and wage earner. Machismo, roughly translated as "manhood," is the traditional word for the pride and self-worth a man feels when fulfilling his obligations and duties to his family and community. In usage today, machismo can be described as aggressive masculinity with very strict ideas of how men and women should behave. In traditional Mexican culture, the wife is a homemaker, the person who provides all child care and holds the family together. Women are expected to defer to their husbands. In America, however, this role is changing. One-half of Mexican American women work outside the home, are responsible for household management, and are likely to be involved in family decisions. Men rarely increase involvement in chores as women increase their hours of employment. Some women find that their new roles can conflict with their self-concept as mothers and caregivers.

Food for Thought

Aztec medicine was a highly developed system featuring an elite group of certified practitioners with access to a zoo and herbarium for research. It was abolished during the Spanish conquest.

Children are cherished in the Mexican American family. Families are typically large among new immigrants and first-generation families, but research suggests lower rates of marriage and improvements in educational attainment and socioeconomic status for women of subsequent generations result in the birth of fewer children and smaller families. Children are taught to share and to work together; sibling rivalry is minimal. When possible, an extended family is the preferred living arrangement for many Mexican Americans.

Grandparents are honored and are often involved in child care. Because of space limitations in the United States, however, many elders live in separate apartments. During periods of hardship, other relatives such as aunts, uncles, and godparents willingly accept the care of children. Girls were traditionally raised differently from boys and were kept at home to learn household skills; they were carefully chaperoned in public. Family expectations sometimes limited education and professional attainments for young women, although such strict supervision diminishes with successive generations born in the United States.

Traditional Health Beliefs and Practices Traditional health care in Mexico includes elements of Indigenous supernatural rituals combined with European folk medicine introduced from Spain. Beliefs and practices are closely interrelated with the culture, resulting in a health system widely shared throughout Latin America. Most Mexican Americans are familiar with the conditions specific to the culture and may use traditional cures.

Health is seen as a gift from God, and illness is almost always due to outside forces (unless one is being punished by God for one's sins). An individual must endure illness as inevitable. Prayer is appropriate for all illnesses and beseeching the saints for intervention through the lighting of candles on behalf of a sick person is common. Pilgrimages may be made to religious shrines, especially those devoted to the Virgin Mary or St. Francis.

Health care is traditionally sought from a hierarchy of healers.[14,15] Treatment is first discussed with *señoras* or *abuelas*—mothers, grandmothers, wives, or older female neighbors who are the health experts in each family. Home remedies, especially teas and over-the-counter remedies such as Pepto Bismol®, Alka Seltzer®, and Vicks Vapo-Rub®, are nearly always tried first before outside help is sought.[14] Laxatives and enemas are common. If a cure is not found, a yerbero (herbalist), sobador (massage therapist or occupational therapist), or a patera (midwife who also specializes in the care of small children) may be consulted. Traditional herbal remedies, homeopathic cures, and amulets are available at pharmacies called botánicas.[16] Therapeutic items may also be sold at religious fiestas.

When an ailment is unresponsive to these cures, the services of a healer known as a curandero (or curandera if the healer is female) are sought. Curanderos are esteemed members of each community who see patients and customarily do not charge for their services, though they may accept gratuities.[17,18] Their healing powers may be God-given at birth, learned, or received through a calling.[19] Curanderos are sought for a broad range of complaints, such as marital problems, infertility, alcoholism, and business failure, as well as for specific illnesses, including diabetes and cancer. They are sought after in diagnosing the underlying causes of a condition, which may be natural or supernatural in nature. Thus, diabetes in a client may be due to lifestyle and diet and amenable to biomedicine, or it may be considered to be due to evil spirits or witchcraft, in which case biomedicine is ineffective and a curandero is sought.[16,17] Curanderos specialize in somatic ailments and are essential to curing illnesses due to supernatural causes. In regions where witchcraft is practiced, a curandero can counteract the hexes or spells of a brujo (a person who works on behalf of the devil). Faith is crucial to the success of a curandero. Prayer is their primary treatment; the lighting of candles or the use of wood or metal effigies formed in the shape of the afflicted body part (called milagros or exvoto) may also be used. Cleansing rituals are applied in certain conditions. For many, illness is believed to be due to supernatural influencers such as (1) excessive emotion, (2) dislocation of organs, (3) magic, (4) an imbalance in hot or cold, or (5) an Anglo disease, such as pneumonia and appendicitis.[16] Preferred treatment is based on the cause of the disorder.

Susto is perceived to be an ailment due to excessive emotion—such as smoldering anger or shame—usually associated with a specific event. The response may be physical, physiological, or psychological, and symptoms include anxiety, depression or sadness, lack of appetite, paleness, shaking, headaches, bad dreams and too much sleep, and ennui.[16,20,21] A type of susto known as espanto, which occurs when an individual is so frightened by a ghost that the soul leaves the body, is the most typical form of the disorder. Susto is considered a serious condition, associated with other illnesses such as epilepsy and infectious diseases. Mild susto is sometimes treated at home with sugar or sugar water. More serious susto, particularly when the soul is involved, must be cured by a curandero and may require lengthy treatment. Susto is also believed to be a cause of nervios, a condition affecting primarily adult women (nervios may also cause susto). Symptoms include crying attacks, sleep problems, headache, trembling, sadness or hopelessness, ill-temper, lack of appetite, stomachache, feeling of choking, chills, itching, and general body ache. Nervios responds best to sedatives (provided by a biomedical physician), prayer, or massage. Unlike susto, nervios cannot be cured by a traditional healer. Nervios is often a chronic condition in response to poor diet, alcoholism, drug use, or other underlying health behaviors. Some Mexicans believe that nervios can cause diabetes if not cured.

Food for Thought

Aztec pharmacology included over 1,200 medicinal herbs.

The treatments by a curandero (healer) include help for arthritis, gastrointestinal ills, hepatitis, and more. The three levels of knowledge needed by a curandero are the material (essences of herbs, animals, etc.), spiritual (a healer as medium), and mental (a curandero as a channeler of mental healing vibrations to the patient).

Feeling too much rage and suffering from revenge fantasies can result in bilis, a condition where excess bile is thought to spill into the blood, causing symptoms such as loss of appetite, vomiting, headaches, nightmares, and inability to urinate. Envidia is another ailment taking the form of various illnesses (some terminal) caused by the emotion of envy among one's friends and neighbors. A person's success may be tempered by the misfortune of envidia.

A problem caused by the displacement of organs in infants is *caida de la mollera*, or fallen fontanel. It occurs from a fall, yanking the nipple out of a baby's mouth too quickly, or holding a baby vertically when it is too young. The fontanel appears depressed, and the palate is believed to drop, preventing the infant from feeding. The inability to suckle and a change in stools are symptoms, and serious weight loss may occur. Tight caps on the infant is believed to help prevent the condition, and the application of salt poultices or olive oil (followed by a dip in water accompanied by prayers) may be used to treat it. The baby may be held upside down and shaken gently, the hair pulled, the fontanel sucked, or the palate pressed up with a finger or thumb to reposition the fontanel.

Food for Thought

One researcher has shown that some Mexican dishes reflect Islamic culinary traditions (which arrived via Spain and stem from the years that the Moors ruled Andalusia), such as aromatic nut-thickened sauces, fruit pastes, and sugar figurines (refer to Chapters 6 and 13).[22]

Chili or chile (with an *e*) comes from the Nahuatl word chili. Foods like powders, sauces, and stews made with chili peppers are conventionally called chili (with an *i*).

The scientific name for the cacao tree is *Theobroma cacao*, meaning "food of the gods."

Mal de ojo (evil eye) is a condition with supernatural origins. Children are considered especially vulnerable to the ailment, which has flu-like symptoms, including fever and headache. It is caused when one person casts an admiring or envious stare sending the receiver negative energy that can lead to illness or misfortune. A curandero is required for treatment. A cleansing ritual is performed that includes sweeping over the ill individual with an egg, then breaking the egg into a saucer. The egg is read to see whether the cure has been effective. It may be read immediately or left under

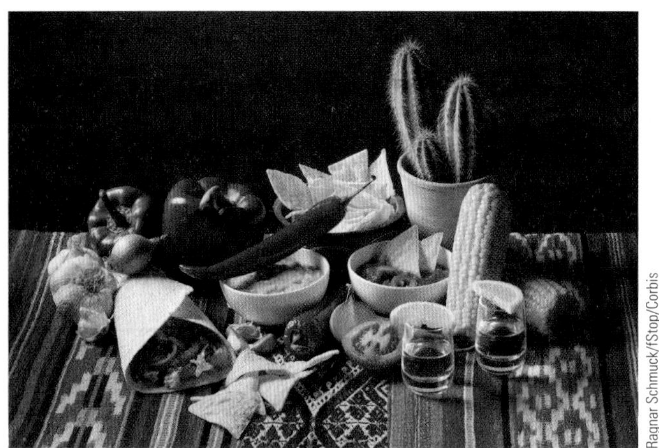

▲ Traditional Latin American foods include avocado, chili peppers, sweet peppers, corn tortillas/corn, and tomatoes, with the prevalent use of onion, garlic, and lime/lemon.

the bed overnight before examination. Prayers, herb teas, and sweeping with herb bundles may also be part of the treatment. Mal aire (bad air or wind) may cause headaches and colds,[16] and mal puesto (witchcraft) accounts for certain other disorders, such as swelling, trembling, or paralytic twitching.

Empacho, a digestive ailment characterized by nausea, gas, and weakness, is widely known throughout Latin America. Empacho is sometimes classified as an illness due to eating too many hot or cold foods, or a hot–cold imbalance in the stomach due to emotional upset (refer to the "Therapeutic Uses of Food" section in this chapter). The direct cause is believed to be a ball or wad of food adhered to the stomach. Herb teas are administered at home, and if they are ineffective, a curandero is employed. Treatment consists of prayer, pinching the spine, and a stomach massage to restore a proper hot–cold balance.

Traditional Food Habits

Mexicans are very proud of their culinary heritage, which is a unique blend of Native and European foods prepared with Indigenous (mostly Aztec) and Spanish cooking techniques. There are even some French and Viennese influences from the Maximilian reign. The resulting cuisine is both flavorful and sophisticated.

Ingredients and Common Foods

Many people associate the cooking of Mexico with chili peppers. Although chili peppers are used frequently, not all Mexican dishes are hot and spicy. Other New World foods such as beans, drinkable cocoa (from the Aztec word, xocatl, or "bitter water"), corn, and tomatoes are equally important to the cuisine. These indigenous ingredients were the basis of fare throughout Mexico before the arrival of the Spanish.

Aztec Foods The Aztec social hierarchy consisted of nobles (about 5 percent of the population), commoners, serfs, and enslaved people. The enslaved people were mostly in that position due to economic reasons or failure to pay tax to the nobles resulting in debt, or as punishment for certain other crimes; they could marry and have children and generally could not be resold. Slave owners were responsible for housing and feeding their enslaved people who were released upon the death of the owner. Aztec enslaved people were also able to purchase their freedom from this arrangement.[23] The capital city of Tenochtitlán was surrounded by lakes on which were built chinampas (floating gardens). These rich agricultural fields of mud scooped from the lake bottoms and made into raised beds for food crops were drought-resistant and are believed to have produced enough food to feed 180,000 people annually. The monarchy stored surplus crops, as well, to protect against famine. The Aztecs were also known for their animal husbandry and game protection laws.

Documents from early Spanish expeditions recorded in glowing terms the enormous variety of foods enjoyed by the Aztec nobility.[24] More than 1,000 dishes are described. Montezuma II reportedly ate up to thirty different items per meal, each kept warm on a pottery brazier. These items included roast turkey, quail, and duck; fish, crab, lobster, frog, turtle, newt, and insect dishes garnished with red, green, or yellow chilies; squash blossoms; and sauces of chilies, tomatoes, squash seeds, or green plums.[25-27] Chocolātl, or xhocolātl, pulverized toasted native cacao beans and water made into a unsweetened frothy and slightly bitterdrink , was the most popular beverage.

Corn was the staple grain. Legumes, fruits, and vegetables were plentiful; turkeys and dogs were domesticated for meat; and some game was available, including deer, peccary, and rabbits. The notable deficiency of the Aztec diet was a consistent source of fat or oil, and the average Native ate a mostly vegetarian diet of corn and beans.[24]

Pulque, a frothy drink made from the naturally fermented sap of the maguey (agave) plant, is said to have been popular in Mexico at least 1,500 years before the Spanish arrival. The drink is the ancestor of mescal and tequila, and all three drinks come from the same family of plants.[28]

Spanish Contributions The Spanish arrived in Mexico with Asian cinnamon, garlic, onions, rice, and sugarcane, made familiar to the Spanish by the Moors and earlier trade routes. They also brought wheat and, most importantly, hogs, which added a reliable source of domesticated protein and lard to the native diet. These additions combined with Indigenous ingredients produce the classic flavors and foods of Mexican cuisine, such as corn tortillas with pork filling; tomato, chili, and onion sauces, or salsas; rice and beans; and panfried boiled beans, known as frijoles refritos, or refried beans in English. The Spanish also introduced the distillation of alcohol to native Mexican fermented beverages such as pulque, creating tequila and mescal.

Staples The cuisine of Mexico is very diverse, and many inaccessible regions have retained their native diets. Others have held on to traditional foods and food habits despite Aztec or Spanish domination. The diets of still other areas differ because of the availability of local fruits, vegetables, or meats. Those with lower incomes in Mexico, as in most areas of the world, have little variety in their diet; some subsist almost entirely on corn, beans, and squash. This divergence makes it difficult to typify Mexican foods in general (Table 9.1). Nevertheless, some foods are found, in varying forms, throughout Mexico.

Table 9.1 Cultural Food Groups: Mexican

Group	Comments	Common Foods	Adaptations in the United States
Protein Foods			
Milk/milk products	Few dairy products are used (incidence of lactose intolerance estimated at two-thirds of the population). Dairy products are used more in northern Mexico than in other regions.	Milk (cow, goat), evaporated milk, *café con lèche*, hot chocolate; *atole*; cheese	Aged cheese is used in place of fresh cheese; more milk (usually whole) is consumed; ice cream is popular.
Meat/poultry/fish/ eggs/legumes	Vegetable protein is the primary source for majority of rural and urban poor. Pork, goat, poultry are common meats. Beef is preferred in northern areas and seafood in coastal regions. Meat is usually tough, prepared by marinating, chopping, grinding (sausages are popular), or slicing thinly. It is cooked by grilling, frying, stewing, or steaming, and is usually mixed with vegetables and cereals.	*Meats:* beef, goat, pork (including *chicharrónes* and variety cuts) *Poultry:* chicken, turkey *Fish and seafood: camarónes* (shrimp), *huachinango* (red snapper), other firm-fleshed fish *Eggs:* chicken *Legumes:* black beans, chickpeas (garbanzo beans), kidney beans, pinto beans	Traditional entrées remain popular. Fewer variety cuts are used. Protein intake may decline in second-generation Mexican Americans. Beans are eaten less frequently.
Cereals/Grains	Corn and rice products are used throughout the country; wheat products are more common in the north. Principal bread is tortilla; European-style breads and rolls are also popular.	Corn (*masa harina, pozole*, tortillas); wheat (breads, rolls, *pan dulce*, pasta); rice	Wheat tortillas are used more than corn tortillas; convenience breads are used. Increased consumption of baked sweets, such as doughnuts, cake, and cookies, is noted. Increased consumption has occurred of sugared breakfast cereals.
Fruits/Vegetables	Vegetables are usually served as part of a dish, not separately. Semitropical and tropical fruits are popular in most regions (limited availability in north).	*Fruits:* bananas, *carambola, casimiroa, cherimoya*, coconut, custard apple, *granadilla* (passion fruit), *guanábana*, guava, lemons, limes, *mamey*, mangoes, melon, oranges, papaya, pineapple, strawberries, sugarcane, sweet sop, *tuna* (cactus fruit), *zapote* *Vegetables:* avocados, cactus (*nopales* or *nopalitos*), *calabaza criolla* (green pumpkin), chile peppers, corn, *jícama*, lettuce, onions, peas, plantains, potatoes, squashes (*chayote*, pumpkin, summer, etc.), squash blossoms, sweet potatoes, *tomatillos*, tomatoes, yams, *yuca* (cassava)	Fruit remains popular as dessert and snack item; apples and grapes are accepted after familiarization.
Additional Foods			
Seasonings	Food is often heavily spiced; 92 varieties of chiles are used. Regional sauces are typical.	Anise, *achiote* (annatto), chiles, cilantro (coriander leaves), cinnamon, cocoa, cumin, *epazote*, garlic, *hoja santa*, mace, onions, vanilla	Use of spices depends on availability.
Nuts/seeds	Seeds are often used in flavoring.	*Piñons* (pine nuts), *pepitas* (pumpkin seeds), sesame seeds	
Beverages		*Atole*, beer, coffee (*café con lèche*), hot chocolate, soft drinks, *pulque*, mescal, tequila, whiskey, wine	Noted are increased consumption of fruit juices, Kool-aid, soft drinks, and beverages with caffeine; and decrease in use of hard spirits.
Fats/oils	Traditional diet is relatively low in fat.	Butter, *manteca* (lard)	Fat intake increases, including use of mayonnaise and salad dressings.
Sweeteners	Spanish-influenced pastries, candies, and custards and puddings are popular.	Sugar, *panocha* (raw brown cane sugar)	

Tortillas are the flatbread of Mexico. Traditionally, they are made by hand. Corn kernels are heated in lime solution until the skins break and separate. The treated kernels, called nixtamal, are then pulverized on a stone slab (metate). The resulting flour, masa harina, is combined with water to make the tortilla dough. Small balls of the dough are patted into round, flat circles, about six to eight inches across. The tortillas are cooked on a griddle (often with a little lard) until soft or crisp, depending on the recipe.[29]

Beans are ubiquitous in Mexican meals. They are served in some form at nearly every lunch and dinner and are frequently found at breakfast, too. They are often the filling in stuffed foods and are common in side dishes, such as simmered frijoles de olla ("out of the pot") and frijoles refritos.

One-dish meals are typical, almost always served with warm tortillas. Hearty soups or stews called caldos are favorite family dinner entrées. Casseroles known as sopas-secas, using stale tortilla pieces, rice, or macaroni, are eaten as main dishes. Stale tortillas can also be broken up and softened in a sauce to make chilaquiles, which are served as a side dish or light entrée. They can also be soaked in milk overnight, and then pureed to make a thick dough. This dough is used to prepare gordos, which are fat-fried cakes, or bolitos, which are added to soup and are similar to dumplings.

Meats are normally prepared over high heat. They are typically grilled, as in carne asada (beef strips), or fried, as in chicharrónes (fried pork rind). Slow, moist cooking (stewing, braising, etc.) may also be used. These techniques help tenderize the tough cuts that are generally available, as does marinating, another common preparation method. Nearly all parts of the animal are used, including a variety of cuts and organs. Sausage, such as spicy pork or beef chorizo, is especially popular.

Mexico is famous for its stuffed foods, such as tacos, flautas, enchiladas, tamales, quesadillas, and burritos. These are found throughout the country, with regional variations. Tacos are the Mexican equivalent of sandwiches. Tortillas, either soft or crisply fried, are filled with anything from just salsa to meat, vegetables, and sauce. Flautas ("flutes") are a variation on the taco, with tortillas tightly rolled around the filling, then fried until crispy. They may be served with a red or green chili sauce or guacamole. Enchiladas are tortillas softened in lard or sauce and then filled with meat, poultry, seafood, cheese, or egg mixtures. The tortilla rolls are then baked while covered with sauce. Tamales are one of the oldest Mexican foods, dating back at least to the Aztec period. Dough made with either masa harina or leftover pozole (hominy) is placed in corn husks (in the north) or young leaves of avocados or bananas (in the south). The leaves are folded and then baked in hot ashes or steamed over boiling water. The tamale may be plain, filled with a meat or vegetable mixture, or sweetened for a dessert (tamales dulce). After cooking, the husk or leaf is unfolded, revealing the aromatic tamale. Quesadillas are tortillas filled with a little cheese, leftover meat, sausage, or vegetable, then folded in half and heated or crisply fried. Burritos are popular in northern Mexico. They are similar to tacos, but large, thin, wheat flour tortillas—instead of corn tortillas—are folded around a filling such as beans with salsa.

Food for Thought

Corn (*Zea mays* L.) is believed to have been domesticated from extinct wild varieties in southern Mexico about 10,000 years ago. It spread south into Central America and north into what is now the United States. In just a couple of centuries, native Mesoamerican farmers transformed the ancestors of corn into the genetic source for all varieties today.[29]

Vegetables are usually part of the main dish or served as a substantial garnish. Potatoes, greens, tomatoes, and onions are the most common. Chili peppers are used extensively in seasonings and sauces and are stuffed, as in chiles rellenos and the Independence Day dish *chiles en nogada*, garnished

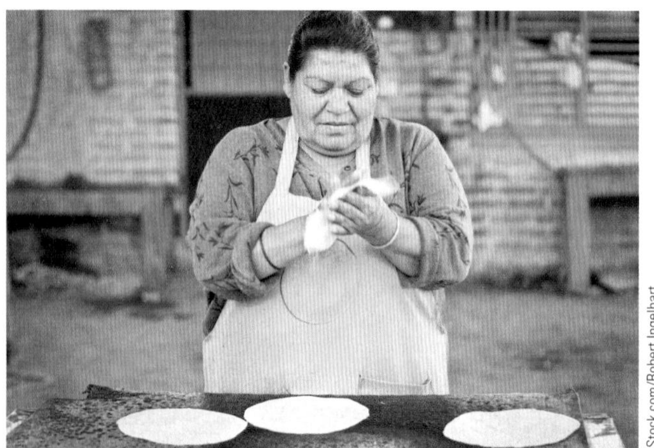

iStock.com/Robert Ingelhart

▲ **Handmade tortillas, made from masa harina (a type of cornmeal) or wheat flour, are the staple bread of Mexico. In this photograph, a tortilla is patted into a flat circle by hand.**

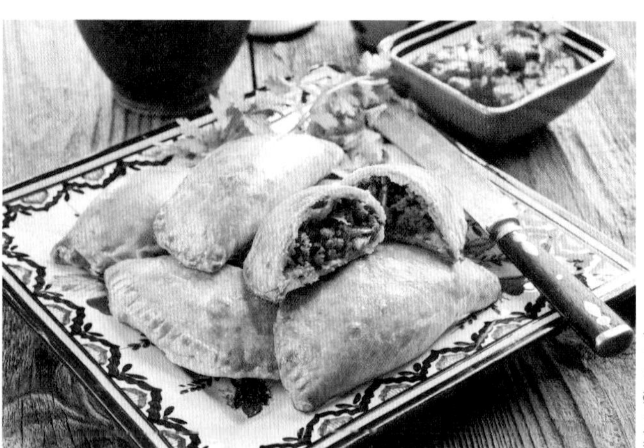

Hlpf oto/Shutterstock.com

▲ **Each region in Mexico and across Latin America has a version of the empanada, made by folding dough around a stuffing of meat, vegetables, or even fruit.**

with the colors of the Mexican flag—white sauce, green cilantro, and red pomegranate seeds.

Sugarcane grows well in Mexico, and sweets of all kinds are popular. Dried fruits and vegetables, candied fruits and vegetables, and sugared fruit or nut pastes are eaten alone and used in more complex desserts. The Spanish make many desserts with eggs, and some of these recipes have been adopted in Mexico. Flan, a sweetened egg custard topped with caramelized sugar, is the most common. Huevos reales is another popular dessert, made with egg yolks, sugar, sherry, cinnamon, pine nuts, and raisins. *Dulce de leche* is made by boiling condensed milk down until the sugars caramelize and it thickens. It is used as a spread or hardened to make candy. A similar, distinctive, Mexican specialty is cajeta, made like dulce de leche but using goat's milk flavored with cinnamon. It is eaten by itself as a pudding or used to top fresh fruit or ice cream.

Food for Thought

Epazote, a pungent herb (wormseed) with minty overtones, is added to many dishes, especially those with beans because it is thought to reduce flatulence.

Menudo is a tripe and hominy soup believed to have curative properties, particularly for hangovers. It is a popular weekend breakfast dish.

Placement of a worm (actually a larva of a moth or beetle) from the maguey plant in a bottle of mescal—supposedly a sign of authenticity—may have begun as a marketing gimmick.

The most common beverage in Mexico is coffee, which began to be grown in the south in the late 1700s. Soft drinks and fresh fruit blended with water and sugar, called aguas naturales, are also favored. Adults drink milk infrequently, except in sweetened, flavored beverages such as hot chocolate with cinnamon, or café con leche (coffee with milk). The most popular alcoholic beverage in Mexico is beer. The Mexican wine industry is also developing rapidly.

Regional Variations

Mexican Plains The northern and central regions of Mexico, nearly half the nation, consist of mostly arid plains and high mountain valleys. The Indigenous people who originally inhabited the area were called Chichimecs, translated as "sons of the dog" and used much like the pejorative "barbarian" was first used, by the Aztecs. The Chichimecs were actually several ethnic cultural groups with a seminomadic lifestyle grouped together. Their diet probably consisted of corn, beans, squash, greens, cactus fruit (tuna), and young cactus leaves (nopales). They also hunted small game and ate domesticated poultry, such as turkey. When the Indigenous peoples of Mexico and the American Southwest mixed, they were introduced to piñons (also called pine nuts or pignolis), pumpkin, and plums. Some specialties of the region, such as hominy-based

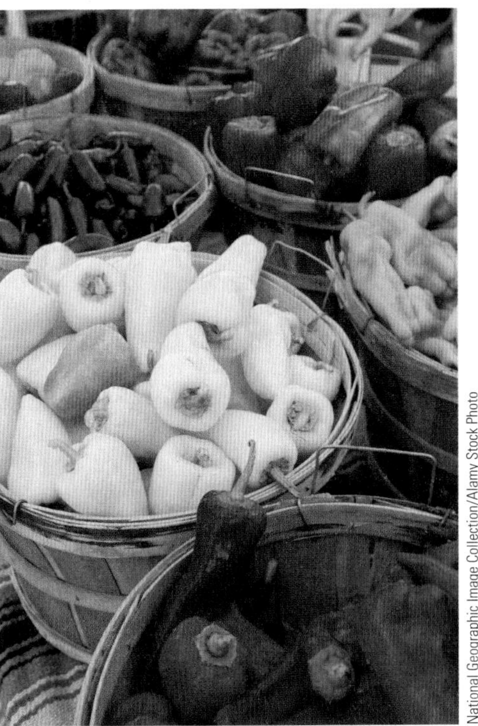

National Geographic Image Collection/Alamy Stock Photo

▲ **A large variety of chili peppers are used in Mexican cuisine, providing complexity of flavor, heat (very mild to incendiary), and color (yellow, orange, red, green, brown, and black).**

stews known as pozoles and salads made with sliced, cooked nopales, reflect this history. Traditional preparations emphasize the natural flavors of the ingredients, and sauces, when used, feature simple seasoning.

The Spanish introduced longhorn cattle to the northern plains, as well as dairy cows and wheat. It is the only area in Mexico where beef is frequently consumed, often served as steaks or in stews. Another favorite way to prepare beef is to air-dry it in thin slices called cecinas. Cecinas can be used in stews or soups; they can be fried or used as fillings for other foods. In Chihuahua, beef is shredded and then fried to make a snack known as móchomos. Goats and sheep are also raised. Spit-roasted kid, cabrito al pastor, is served in the Monterrey area, and birria—kid or lamb stewed in a sauce flavored with roasted chilies and vinegar—is a specialty in Guadalajara. This area is also known for barbacoa, a method of pit-roasting meats that are first wrapped in maguey leaves. Cow cheeks (or more traditionally, the whole head) and kid are commonly prepared this way in the more northern areas, while in the more central regions lamb is preferred.[30,31]

In the Baja peninsula and along the Gulf of California and Gulf of Mexico coasts, fish is important in the diet. Huachinango, red snapper, is a specialty, cooked in orange sauce, used as a filling in tacos, or served chilled, marinated in vinegar with onions and chilies. Shark is found on the eastern coast, shredded and layered between tortillas and beans in a dish from Campeche known as pan de cazón.[19,31] Shrimp and clams are other favorites. In the more inland areas, fish from freshwater lakes are available, such as pescado blanco, a small whitefish that is popularly served fried or added to soups.

Cheese (refer to Table 9.2) is more common in the north than in other parts of Mexico, and one specialty is queso flameado (called queso fundido in the Guadalajara area), which is a fondue-like dish sometimes topped with chorizo crumbles and served with fresh tortillas and salsa. Wheat products are more popular as well, particularly wheat tortillas.

A very popular dessert of northern Mexico is buñuelos, which may be made at home or purchased at street stands. Circles of sweet pastry dough are fried until they slightly puff. They are eaten fresh, sprinkled with sugar and cinnamon, or broken up and added to hot cinnamon-laced syrup. *Cafe con leche*, coffee with milk, is a common accompaniment to buñuelos.

The sap of the maguey cactus (century plant) is credited with being a reliable substitute for fresh water in the arid countryside; it is called aguamiel or "honey water." Tequila is probably the best-known beverage of the region, made from the distillation pulque (fermented aguamiel). Tequila is the more refined, twice-distilled version of mescal. It is produced in the central-western state of Jalisco around the towns of Tequila and Tepatitlan from the maguey subspecies *Agave tequiliana*.

Tropical Mexico The southern coastal areas of eastern Mexico include hot lowlands and tropical forests. Seafood and freshwater fish are prominent in the cuisine. Red snapper with a Spanish-influenced sauce of tomatoes, garlic, onions, olives, capers, and chilies, called huachinango a la Veracruzana (Veracruz-style red snapper), is a specialty. Arroz a la Tumbada, rice cooked and seasoned with tomatoes and garlic, topped with fresh fish, shrimp, octopus, crabs, and clams, is another favorite. It is often served in individual clay pots. Tamales and tostadas stuffed with shrimp are also popular. One unusual food enjoyed in some areas is black iguana.[31,32]

Food for Thought

The word avocado comes from the Nahuatl word for the fruit, ahuactl, meaning "testicle," which avocados resemble while hanging from the tree.

The chemical heat of chilies comes from the alkaloid capsaicin, found mostly in the fleshy ribs and seeds inside the fruit. One theory as to why eating chilies is pleasurable is that capsaicin may cause the body to release pain-killing endorphins in reaction to the irritation, creating a comfortable, gratified feeling.

Achiote, a spice and coloring agent, is called annatto in the United States. Made from the seeds of the achiote tropical tree (*Bixa orellana*), annatto is reddish-orange and sometimes used to color cheddar-style cheeses, ice creams, margarine, and some baked goods.

Table 9.2 Traditional Mexican Cheeses

Fresh: Unripened cheeses that do not melt, but soften when heated. Often used in stuffed foods and as a garnish on top of dishes.	
Queso blanco	Crumbly cow's milk cheese similar to a soft, dry, fresh mozzarella. Sometimes made by using lemon juice to coagulate the milk, providing a distinctive flavor. Sold commercially in blocks.
Queso fresca	A fine-grained, creamy farmer's cheese or pot cheese. Sometimes called *queso metate* when formed in a traditional stone grinder. Often made daily in homes; sold commercially in small rounds.
Queso panela	A salty, semisoft white cheese formed in small baskets that leave an imprint. Is often served cubed or sliced with chorizo sausage or guava paste.
Ranchero seco	Drier version of queso fresco with much stronger flavor (similar to Romano); curds are broken apart and remolded during processing. Used grated over foods.
Requesón	Milky, ricotta-like cheese good for fillings, spreads, and desserts.
Soft: Smooth, aged cheeses that melt well when heated, often used for baked dishes.	
Queso añejo	Aged queso fresco that is firm and salty, similar to feta.
Queso asadero	Buttery, mild cheese that tastes like Provolone but with the slightly stringy texture of aged Mozzarella; used in *queso flameado*.
Queso Chihuahua	Mild, cheddar-like yellow cheese formed in large wheels, introduced by Mennonites in the farming communities of Chihuahua.
Queso Oaxaca	Tangy string cheese from the city of Oaxaca. Sold in balls.
Firm: Semihard or hard aged cheeses, often eaten thinly sliced or added for flavoring to dishes.	
Queso añejo enchilada	Strong, salty cheese made from longer-aged *añejo*, coated with spicy ground chiles.
Queso Cotija	Sharp goat's milk cheese that is crumbled over beans or salads, sometimes called "Mexican Parmesan." From the Michoacan city of Cotija.
Queso Manchego	Spanish-style, full-bodied, hard cheese that is served shaved with fruit or eaten with snacks, beer, or other drinks.

Tomatoes, green tomato-like tomatillos, chayote squash, onions, jícama (a sweet, crispy root), bananas and starchy plantains, carambola (star fruit), cherimoya (custard apple), guanábana (soursop), guava, mamey (a type of plum), mango, pineapple, yucca (a tuber also called cassava or manioc), and zapote (the fruit of the sapodilla tree) are just a small sampling of the produce available in this area. Avocados are also cultivated. They vary in size from two to eight inches across, in skin color from light green to black, and in flavor from bland to bitter. Their succulent, smooth flesh is added to soups, stews, and salads. They are most popular in guacamole—mashed avocado with onions, tomatoes, chili peppers, and cilantro, the pungent leaf of the coriander plant. Guacamole is used as a side dish, a topping, or a filling for tortillas.

More than ninety varieties of chili peppers are found in the region, varying enormously in the degree of hotness (refer to Figure 9.2). In general, the smaller the chili the hotter it is, and each variety develops more heat as it ripens. The heat also intensifies when it is dried. Most believe all chilies in the world traveled from Latin America after the start of the Columbian Exchange, the dynamic biological globalization that occurred after 1492 (though there could be exceptions, such as a the bhut jolokia or ghost pepper cultivated in northeastern India). Some of the more common varieties include ancho (dried, red-ripened poblano chilies), chilaca (thin, ribbed, dark green chilies which are often cut into very thin strips after roasting), chipotle (dried, smoked jalapeño chilies), de arbol (long, very thin, curved green or red chili used fresh and dried), guajillo (long, thin, dark red chili used primarily dried), habañero (lantern-shaped, yellow, orange, or dark red, added fresh to sauces but removed before serving, or roasted and chopped into dishes), pasilla (dried chilaca chilies), jalapeño (short, three-inch chiles with smooth green or red skin and blunt end, used fresh in salsas and sauces, or sliced and pickled), mulato (dried chili with very dark brown, wrinkled skin, and sweet overtones, often used to make moles), pequin (tiny, oval chilies used whole in stews, added pureed in sauces, soups, salsas, or pickled as a table condiment), poblano (large, heart-shaped, black-green chilies that are often stuffed), and serrano (small, two-inch dark green or red, torpedo-shaped chilies that are often chopped to add zest to salsa and cooked dishes or sliced and pickled, known as escabeche).

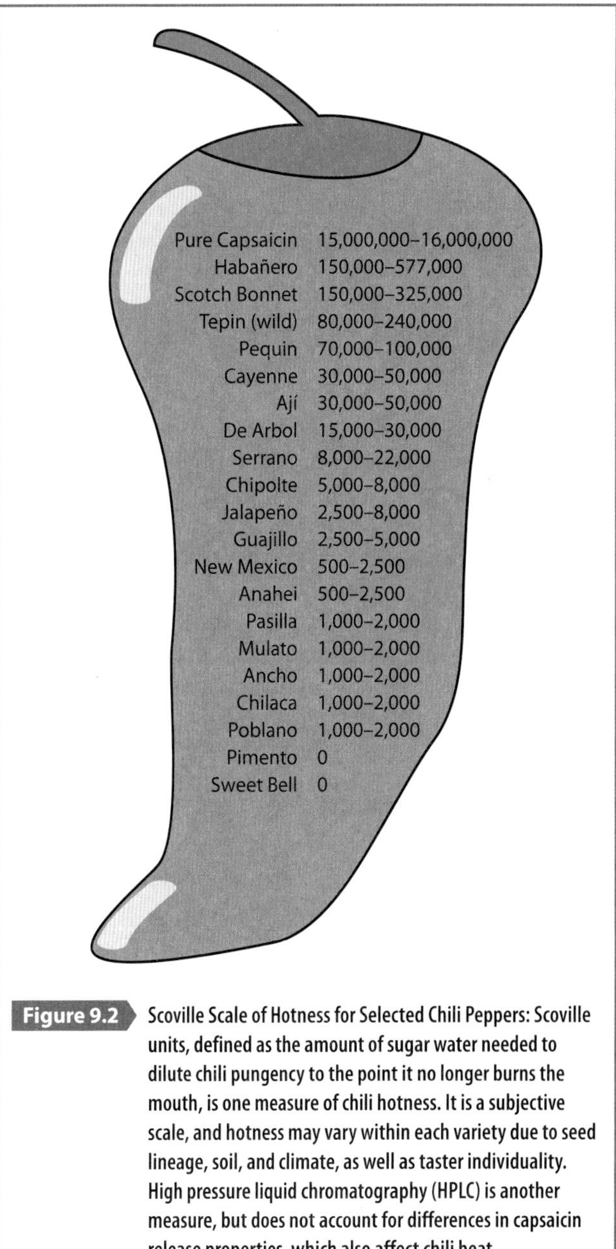

Figure 9.2 Scoville Scale of Hotness for Selected Chili Peppers: Scoville units, defined as the amount of sugar water needed to dilute chili pungency to the point it no longer burns the mouth, is one measure of chili hotness. It is a subjective scale, and hotness may vary within each variety due to seed lineage, soil, and climate, as well as taster individuality. High pressure liquid chromatography (HPLC) is another measure, but does not account for differences in capsaicin release properties, which also affect chili heat.

Yucatán The cuisine of the Yucatán peninsula reflects its unique history. It was isolated from the rest of the country by dense, mountainous jungles until modern times. Many of the residents are descendants of the Mayans, the early dynasty of the region. Some regional favorites date from this time. For example, one popular preparation method is to steam foods wrapped in banana leaves, called píbil. Traditionally, food was cooked this way in an outdoor pit, but today it is prepared more often in a covered pot. Salbutes, small corn tortillas (some made with black bean paste so that they are black in color), are often fried until they puff, then layered with lettuce or cabbage, tomato, onion, bell pepper, and píbil-cooked meats. In some versions, the black beans are stuffed inside the pocket of the puffed tortilla, in which case the treat is known as panucho.

Citrus fruits flavor some dishes of the region. For example, in the recipe for chicken píbil, the poultry is marinated in sour orange juice, garlic, and cumin before steaming. A popular sliced pork dish, poc chuc, also uses sour orange juice to tenderize the meat before grilling. Bitter lime juice is featured in a specialty of the area called sopa de lima, a chicken and vegetable soup made with bits of fried tortillas. Lime juice is also found in *frijoles con puerco*, a traditional dish of black beans with pork served weekly in most homes of the region. Some foods are pickled in citrus juice, including vegetables such as onions, and other items, including fish and oysters.

Achiote is the other hallmark seasoning of the region, a bright red, nutty-flavored seed mixed with sour orange juice and mild spices to make a flavorful paste called recado colorado, used to coat foods before cooking.

Shrimp are a local specialty; the long coastline of the Yucatán along the Gulf of Mexico provides ample seafood. Grouper with recado baked in banana leaves is one example, and fish soups are also common. Eggs are prominent, served with tortillas, black beans, cheese, tomato sauce, and fried plantains, or wrapped in tortillas and served with a pumpkin seed sauce. Sauces of the region are often thickened with toasted squash seeds.

Southern Mexico The foods of southern Mexico are similar to those of the Yucatán in that they are more tropical and more influenced by Indigenous flavors and cooking techniques than the foods of other regions. Cacao trees are cultivated in this area and chocolate flavors both savory and sweet dishes. In particular, the renowned sauces of the region, moles (probably from the Nahuatl word "molli," or sauce or concoctione), sometimes include unsweetened chocolate. Chilies, tomatoes, nuts, raisins, sesame seeds, avocado leaves, and seasonings are other typical ingredients. The complex, spicy sauces are the base for thick stews with added pork, beef, poultry, or game, though some recipes call for the mole to be poured over the top of the meat. In Oaxaca, mole manchamanteles (meaning "stew that stains the tablecloth") is a deep-red sauce with yams, pineapple, plantains, and chicken or pork. Mole negro, another Oaxacan specialty, includes dark-roasted chilies, blackened tortillas, and chicken. The best-known mole in Puebla is poblano de guajolote, a rich brown sauce served with turkey. Other variations include mole amarillo (an orange-colored sauce) and mole coloradito (a brick-red version also known as mole roja). Mole verde is yet another example, popular along the coast, made with green chilies and tomatillos. Hoja santa (*Piper sanctum*), an herb with a peppery, anise flavor, seasons the sauce—the large leaves of the herb are also used to wrap steamed and grilled foods in the region.

Poultry, goat, and pork are the most popular meats in the region. One favorite is pork cut into thin strips and coated with ground chilies to make cecina enchilada (a version of the northern recipe above). It is frequently served as a topping on crunchy, platter-sized baked tortillas called tlayuda, which also include layers of black beans (more popular in the south than pintos), cabbage, salsa, tesajo (thinly sliced beef), asiento (bits of pork skin fried in lard), chorizo, and cheese. Game, such as venison and quail, are eaten in some areas. One delicacy of the region is chapulines, a grasshopper found in the cornfields. They are pan-fried with chilies, garlic, salt, and lemon juice and traditionally served with beer or mescal.[33–35]

Hot chocolate, coffee, atole (a warm beverage of thin cornmeal and milk gruel), and horchata, a sweetened rice-based drink, are favorite beverages. Ice creams, including those made with fresh vanilla bean, and fruit ices are popular, as is chocolate flan.

Meal Composition and Cycle

Daily Patterns In families where income is not limited, the preferred meal pattern is four to five daily meals: desayuno (breakfast), almuerzo (coffee break), comida or almuerzo (lunch), merienda (late afternoon snack), and cena (dinner). Most meals are eaten at home and served family style. If there are too many people to sit at the table along with platters of food, each person is served individually from the stove.

Desayuno is a quick, early breakfast, which features pan dulce (sweet bread, pastry, or cake) or fresh fruit, served with café con lèche. Late morning is when almuerzo (similar to brunch) is eaten, often including tortillas, eggs, meat, beans left over from the previous night, bolillos (wheat rolls), pan dulce, and fruit. Coffee and hot chocolate are the preferred beverages.

Comida is traditionally the largest meal of the day, traditionally eaten in the early afternoon. A complete comida includes several courses, individually served. Customarily this would include a soup, a sopa-seca (including items such as seasoned rice), a main course, beans, salad, and dessert. Today, the courses may be combined or, often, fewer are served. For example, soup, a sopa-seca, or a vegetable dish may precede the entrée. When possible, an afternoon rest period (siesta) follows this meal. Merienda is a light meal of sweet rolls, cake, or cookies eaten around 6:00 p.m. Coffee, hot chocolate, or atole (a hot corn and masa-based beverage) accompanies the sweets. Cena, a light supper (often leftovers), follows between 8:00 and 10:00 p.m. This meal may be skipped entirely or expanded into a substantial feast on holidays or other formal occasions. Recently, many Mexicans have adopted the American habit of eating a light lunch (sometimes called almuerzo) and a heavy supper, eliminating merienda altogether.

Snacking is frequent in urban Mexico; munching occurs from morning to midnight. Antojitos, or "little whims," include foods made with masa, such as tostadas (called chalupas in northern Mexico), fried tortillas topped with shredded lettuce, cheese, or meat. These may be eaten as a snack or served for a light supper. Nearly every block offers street-side food vendors, providing everything from fresh fruits to grilled meats. Pastelerías offer coffee, chocolates, and pastries. In addition, many neighborhoods feature an open-air market that also sells ready-to-eat foods. Cantinas are popular gathering places. They were originally male-only drinking establishments, but now many welcome women and families. Botanas, roughly translated as "cocktail foods," are small plates of items that go well with alcoholic beverages (especially beer), such as cheese, sausages, fritters, tortillas with beans or salsa, and sometimes Anglicized Mexican dishes such as guacamole with tortilla chips, or other non-Mexican items, such as hummus. The term is often used for appetizers of any kind.

Special Occasions Sundays, family celebrations (such as weddings, baptisms, and quinceañeras), and holidays are typically times when more difficult preparations are served. For example, homemade tamales or moles are labor intensive and may require numerous ingredients, so these foods are often reserved for special occasions.[36] Turkey, arroz con leche (rice pudding), and pastel de tres leches, a rich sponge cake lightly soaked in three types of milk (whole or cream, condensed milk, and evaporated milk) and then topped with whipped cream, are other festive foods eaten throughout the year.

Many foods are associated with specific holidays. For example, Día de los Santos Reyes (also called Día de los Reyes Magos, or Three Kings Day) on January 6 is customarily celebrated with rosca de reyes, a raisin-studded, ring-shaped loaf of bread. Baked inside the bread is a figurine of the infant Jesus, and the person who receives it is obligated to give a party on Candelaria Day (February 2). Candelaria Day includes a mass, followed by games and sweets such as tamales dulce, and pink-tinted atole.[37]

During Lent, capirotada is a traditional dessert. Many families have their own recipe for this holiday bread pudding, often made with honey or brown sugar, cinnamon, nuts, raisins, and cheese. Another holiday food is pan de muerto, bread decorated with a skull and crossbones, eaten on Días de los Muertos (Days of the Dead, November 1 and 2) as part of a large feast honoring the deceased (the first day for children, the second for adults—additional days, for deaths due to certain causes, such as accidents, are identified in some regions). Sugar paste is used to mold skulls and skeletons of the dead, known as alfeñique (a word of Arab origin meaning sugar candy), which are colorfully decorated with icing. Altars for the dead are set up in homes with a bowl of water to quench the thirst of the spirit, his or her favorite foods, pan de muerto, sugar skulls, fruit pastes, and dulce de calabaza (pumpkin cooked with brown sugar). Coffee, chocolate, atole, soft drinks, and preferred alcoholic beverages are offered as well.[38] After the departed soul has absorbed the essence of the meal through the aromas, the family eats the remaining food.

Christmas festivities, called posadas, frequently feature piñatas, or brightly decorated papier-mâché animals and figures that are filled with sweets. Blindfolded children take turns swinging a large stick at the hanging piñata until it breaks and candies fly everywhere. In some regions, buñuelos are a Christmastime treat, drenched in syrup and served in pottery bowls that, when empty, are smashed on the street for good luck. On Christmas Eve a salad of fruits, nuts, and beets is served.

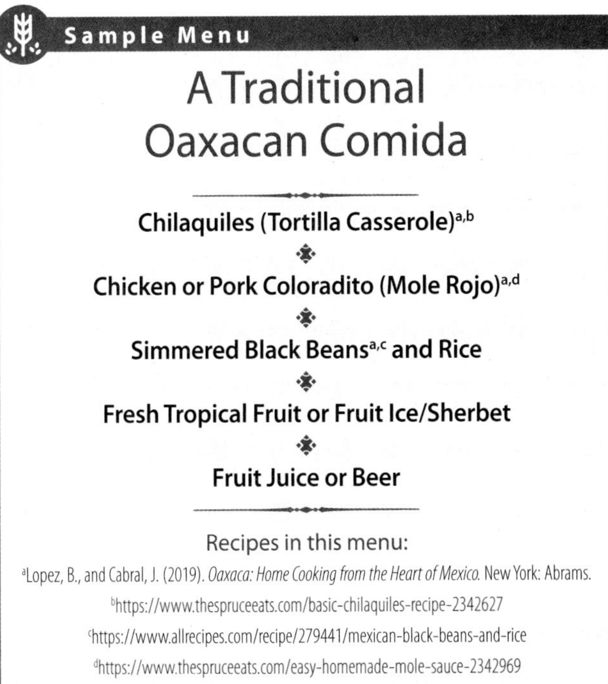
Sample Menu

A Traditional Oaxacan Comida

Chilaquiles (Tortilla Casserole)[a,b]

Chicken or Pork Coloradito (Mole Rojo)[a,d]

Simmered Black Beans[a,c] and Rice

Fresh Tropical Fruit or Fruit Ice/Sherbet

Fruit Juice or Beer

Recipes in this menu:

[a]Lopez, B., and Cabral, J. (2019). *Oaxaca: Home Cooking from the Heart of Mexico.* New York: Abrams.

[b]https://www.thespruceeats.com/basic-chilaquiles-recipe-2342627

[c]https://www.allrecipes.com/recipe/279441/mexican-black-beans-and-rice

[d]https://www.thespruceeats.com/easy-homemade-mole-sauce-2342969

Role of Food and Etiquette in Mexican Society

In family-centered Mexican society, food-related activities facilitate interactions between family members and help delineate family roles. Meal planning is usually the wife's responsibility. Depending on economic status, food is prepared by the wife or, because Mexican foods can be laborious to prepare, by workers supervised by her.[25] The final dishes are greatly appreciated by all who partake in the meal, and it is considered an insult not to eat everything that is served. In rural areas, food sharing is an important social activity, reflecting the Indigenous worldview. To reject offered food or drink is a severe breach of social conduct. Even refusal of an invitation to dine may be considered rude, though not attending an agreed-upon event is often completely acceptable.[39]

Guests often wait to begin eating a Mexican meal until after the host says "¡*Buen provecho*!,"[40] which translates to "Enjoy your meal!" Mexicans share many dining rules with Europeans. The fork remains in the left hand and the knife in the right one. No switching is done when cutting food. When not eating, the hands should remain above the table, with the wrists resting on the edge. Dishes are passed to the left. Portions are usually large. Leaving the table for any reason before others are finished with the meal is impolite.

Therapeutic Uses of Food

Some Native Mexicans and those living in rural communities practice a hot–cold system of diet and health. It is believed to have derived from the Arab system of humoral medicine brought to Mexico by the Spanish, combined with the Native worldview. Although it has parallels with other classification systems, such as the South Asian Ayurvedic goal of balance (refer to Chapter 14 for details) and the East Asian practice of yin–yang (refer to Chapter 11 for details), the Mexican system is applied only to foods and to the prevention and treatment of illness.

The Mexican hot–cold theory is based on the concept that the world's resources are limited and must remain in balance. People must stay in harmony with the environment. Hot has the connotation of strength; cold, of weakness. When the theory is applied to foods, items can be classified according to proximity to the sun, method of preparation, or how the food is thought to affect the body. Meals balanced between hot and cold foods are considered to be health-promoting.

Food for Thought

Early researchers were perplexed by the absence of the niacin-deficiency disease, pellagra, in Mexicans who consumed a corn-based diet. Pellagra was common in Europe after corn was introduced and in the southern non-Native populations of the United States, where corn was also a staple. It was found that when Mexican cooks prepared the corn kernels for *masa harina* (corn flour), the alkaline lime solution used to soften them released the niacin that was bound to a protein, thus preventing the disease.[41] Native Americans also achieved this result through their preparation techniques.

Some Mexicans avoid cold air and drafts after eating chilies (which are classified as hot) to avoid causing a sudden imbalance in their bodies.

Unbalanced meals may cause illness. Thus, a typical comida in a rural village would consist of rice (hot), soup (made with hot and cold ingredients), and beans (cold).

Although the hot–cold classification of foods does vary, items generally considered hot are alcohol, aromatic beverages, beef, chilies, corn husks, oils, onions, pork, radishes, and tamales. Cold foods include citrus fruits, dairy products, most fresh vegetables, goat, and tropical fruits. Some foods, such as beans, corn products, rice products, sugary foods, and wheat products, can be classified as either hot or cold depending on how they are prepared.

Illnesses are also believed to be hot or cold and are usually treated with a diet rich in foods of the opposite classification. Examples of hot conditions include pregnancy, hypertension, diabetes, indigestion, susto, bilis, and mal de ojo.[9] In particular, many Mexican women increase their intake of cooling fruits, such as melons, mangoes, and bananas, and avoid hot, spicy foods and chilies during pregnancy. Some also believe that very cold foods, including cucumbers, tomatoes, and watermelon, can create a sudden imbalance. Examples of cold conditions are pneumonia, colic, and empacho. Sour foods are thought by some to thin the blood and are avoided by menstruating women because they are thought to increase blood flow; acidic foods may also be avoided because they are said to cause menstrual cramps (menstruation is considered a hot condition by some, and a cold condition by others).

Though the hot–cold system of food classification is practiced by small numbers of Mexicans, one study reported that Latinos are more likely than non-Latinos to consider certain foods as herbal medicines, and other research suggests home remedies are common.[39,42,43] For example, chamomile is believed by many to cure colic, menstrual cramps, anxiety, insomnia, and itching eyes. Mint and anise tea are also prepared for nausea, gas, diarrhea, and colic. Garlic is chewed for yeast infections in the mouth, toothache pain, and stomach disorders; boiled peanut broth is used to cure diarrhea; boiled corn silk is taken for kidney pain; honey and water are given to infants for colic; oregano is used for fever, dry cough, asthma, and amenorrhea; and papaya is thought to help cure digestive ailments, asthma, tuberculosis, and intestinal parasites.[15,19]

Of particular interest are remedies for hypertension and diabetes. Hypertension may be treated with garlic, passion flower, or linden flowers. The leaves of the sapodilla tree, known as zapote blanco, which act as a strong sedative, are also used in tea to lower blood pressure.[15,39] For diabetes, several botanical remedies are used. Sage tea is common, as are infusions made from tronadora root (trumpet flower) and prodigiosa leaves and flowers (bricklebush). Preparations made with matarique (a plantain variant), papayas, bitter gourds, aloe vera juice, and prickly pear cactus (both the tuna and nopales) are also popular.[39] Several of these remedies have been shown to have potent diuretic or hypoglycemic properties.

Contemporary Food Habits in the United States

The foods of Mexico have significantly influenced cooking in regions of the United States bordering the nation. It is generally recognized that seven distinct Mexican cuisine regions exist, and four regional variations are prominent in U.S. bordering states (see Chapter 15 on regional U.S. foods for more information).[44] In Texas, for instance, Mexican food has often been modified into distinct foods, such as tamale pie and nachos, and called Tex-Mex. Other foods retain slightly more of their Mexican heritage, such as chili con carne, which was developed just after the Mexican-American War in the 1850s. The recipe probably began as chile colorado (colorado is Spanish for red, and chile colorado is red chili stew), but was tamed and extended to feed more people by adding beans to the traditional meat dish and reducing the spicing. Barbecued chili-spiced meat kebobs called anacuchos and capriotada with whiskey sauce known as "drunken pudding" are other examples of Tex-Mex creativity. The most commonly used chilies in Tex-Mex cooking are anchos and jalapeños, though pequins are also popular in some dishes, and a favorite seasoning is cumin. Beef is commonly ground rather than shredded for stuffed dishes.[45] The Mexican restaurant staple in the United States—known as a combo plate, featuring a selection of enchiladas, tacos, and other stuffed items served with rice and beans all at one time—is also thought to be a Texas invention.[46]

The second region in the United States that showcases Mexican flavors is New Mexico, where a single chili pepper developed for the region, the New Mexico chili, or hatch chili, dominates seasoning. It is mildly pungent, used green in chile verde and red in chile colorado. Unlike the complex sauces of southern Mexico that include numerous types of ground chilies and different seasonings, these northern-Mexico-influenced sauces are often made simply with ground red chili pepper, water, garlic, oregano, and salt to taste. Pork replaces beef, kid, and lamb in many dishes.

The third region is Sonora, encompassing both the Mexican state and southern Arizona. As in New Mexico, milder chilies are preferred (in this case, Anaheims), and in some recipes, the seasoning is so tepid that "chili" has been dropped from the name, resulting in "carnore verde," for example.[46] Beef is the favored meat, and a traditional dried beef jerky,

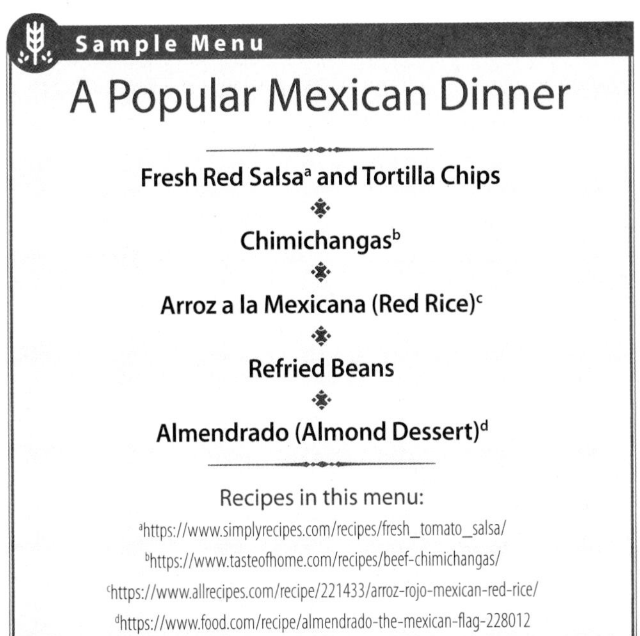

Sample Menu

A Popular Mexican Dinner

Fresh Red Salsa[a] and Tortilla Chips

Chimichangas[b]

Arroz a la Mexicana (Red Rice)[c]

Refried Beans

Almendrado (Almond Dessert)[d]

Recipes in this menu:

[a]https://www.simplyrecipes.com/recipes/fresh_tomato_salsa/

[b]https://www.tasteofhome.com/recipes/beef-chimichangas/

[c]https://www.allrecipes.com/recipe/221433/arroz-rojo-mexican-red-rice/

[d]https://www.food.com/recipe/almendrado-the-mexican-flag-228012

machaca, is still used and shredded for stuffed foods. Large, finely textured wheat tortillas are a specialty, and this region may be the original home of burritos and their deep-fried version, chimichangas.

The fourth region in the United States strongly influenced by the foods of Mexico is along the California border, where the fluid movement of people back and forth between the nations has resulted in fare that cannot be claimed by either nation as its own, or as a cuisine unique to the area.[47,48] Numerous American fast-food franchises are established in Mexico, and on the U.S. side, taco shops and Latinx grocery stores offer Mexican dishes. However, most businesses, including franchise restaurants, provide a mix of products. For example, Mexicans can purchase hamburgers and fries with jalapeños on the side, and diners in the United States can order "American burritos" filled with refried beans, carne asada, and French fries.

Food for Thought

In the late nineteenth and early twentieth century, chili con carne stands were common in San Antonio, offering a spicier version of the Texas stew. Made by Latinx women in the community, and known as the "Chili Queens," they were shut down in the 1930s due to supposed health concerns.[45]

The market for Latinx foods throughout the United States has grown dramatically since the 1980s, when the fare of Texas, New Mexico, and Arizona gained national recognition. It was predicted to be a $10 billion-a-year industry in 2014.[50] But in 2020, the sales of these foods in the U.S. market were over 21 billion.[49] In the 1990s, sales of salsa surpassed those of ketchup for the first time, and salsa has continued to dominate the condiment market. Tortillas and tortilla chips are also selling well. At the same time that Americanized Mexican foods, such as tacos in hard shells and fajitas, are spreading throughout the country, an appreciation of authentic regional Mexican fare is also increasing. Two things have influenced the food market in Mexico: increased demand for year-round fruit (berries, citrus, avocados) and increase demand for plant-based protein foods such as dried peas, lentils, beans, quinoa, etc. In 2020, over 237 million Americans used Mexican food and ingredients.[49] Mexico tends to follow food consumption patterns of the United States and, consequently, there has recently been an increased demand for plant-based proteins in Mexico. Plant-based manufacturing businesses are on the rise to try to meet this demand.[58,59]

Adaptations of Food Habits

Ingredients and Common Foods Many Mexicans in the United States eat a diet similar to that of their homeland which is often heavy in beef and chicken, though portions of these proteins remain small. Recent immigrants, those who live near the U.S.–Mexican border, and migrant workers are most likely to continue traditional food habits. In a comprehensive review of published research on the effect of acculturation on the diet of Latinx in the United States, no relationship between acculturation and dietary fat intake or percentage of energy from fat was evident. However, the source of the fat differed depending on acculturation. Less acculturated fat sources were from the consumption of whole milk and fat added during food preparation, whereas among the more acculturated Latinx, fat sources were fast food, snacks, and added fats. In addition, the less acculturated individuals consumed more fruit, rice, and beans and fewer sugar and sugar-sweetened beverages than the more acculturated Latinx.[51,52]

Mexican people who are well-established in the United States often become quite acculturated. Immigration has influenced dietary habits and behaviors. Mexican immigrants living in the southwestern United States are more likely to eat a diet with a high intake of red meats, lower in fiber, fruits, and vegetables, and higher in fat, white bread, and sugar-sweetened beverages than their socioeconomic

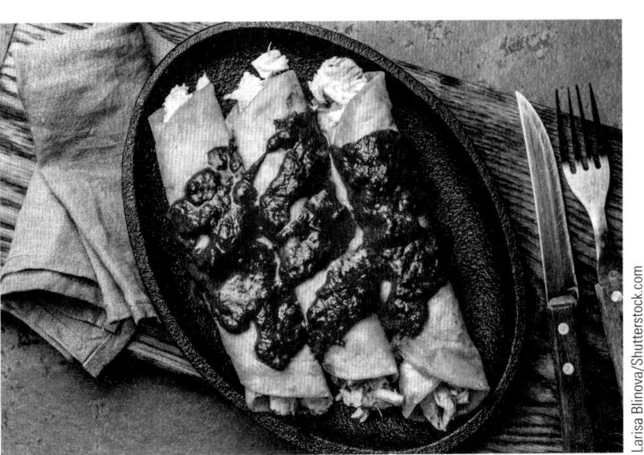

Larisa Blinova/Shutterstock.com

▲ **Stuffed Tortillas with Mole Sauce.**

counterparts in Mexico. This suggests that, rather than adopting a diet that falls somewhere between the food habits of Mexico and those of the United States, the Mexican immigrants in the survey accepted the stereotypical American consumption patterns of the 1950s through 1970s. Other studies have offered confirmation of these data. Studies on Latinx in Southern California (who would be predominantly Mexican American) and Mexican Americans living in Washington have found higher intakes of fast foods, convenience items, salty snacks, chocolate, and added fat at the table with bread and potatoes, combined with lower intakes of beans, peas, fruits, and vegetables associated with acculturation.[53]

School-age children from immigrant families are often exposed to an "Americanized Diet" like hamburgers, macaroni and cheese, and fried potatoes at school. Shopping for food can be complex for immigrant families, and they prefer Hispanic specialty stores rather than big chain grocery stores. However, not all communities have these specialty stores.

A preference for sweet or carbonated beverages usually increases in the United States. Soft drinks, Kool-Aid®, and juices are popular with meals and as snacks. More acculturated Mexican Americans buy many prepared and convenient foods. Baked goods are usually purchased, including tortillas (often wheat tortillas are chosen over corn), breads, pan dulce, and even special desserts like flan. Extra income is usually spent on meats, especially more expensive cuts such as steaks and pork chops, and processed meats, such as hot dogs and bologna.[53,54]

Meal Composition and Cycle

Daily Patterns Few current data on the meal patterns of Mexican migrant farmworkers have been reported, but older data indicate that traditional foods are preferred for most meals. These include eggs, beans or meat, and tortillas or pan dulce for breakfast; a large lunch of beans, tortillas, and meat, or a soup or stew; and a lighter dinner of tortillas, beans or meat, and rice or potatoes. As in Mexico, vegetables tend to be served as part of a soup or stew. Fruit remains a typical snack and dessert. Food insecurity among Mexican farm workers ranges between 20 and 93 percent. As more and more migrant farm workers are female, the impact on family food intake changes, as women remain responsible for providing food for the family even when working long hours.[55] Mexican people more often adopt the American meal pattern of small breakfast, small lunch, and large dinner; and meal-skipping may occur. As tortilla consumption declines, breads and breakfast cereals have become popular with all family members, and sandwiches are a common lunch item. Meats and cheese become more prevalent at meals, beans are eaten less frequently, and vegetables are served as side dishes. Snacking has been found to increase, especially in the evenings. Acculturation, sex, and age are often significantly related to healthy and unhealthy food choices. One recent study reported that Mexican Americans who are less acculturated in the United States tend to prepare and eat healthier foods. Age was also associated with healthier dietary patterns, as older individuals demonstrated a greater likelihood of consuming healthier foods.[56]

Changes in preparation methods may also occur. Recent immigrants may not know how to use the baking and broiling apparatus in an oven and may continue to fry and grill foods outdoors. Newer immigrants sometimes avoid canned and frozen foods because they do not know how to prepare them. Soup is prepared at home three times more often by Latinx than by non-Latinx people, according to one marketing survey, but this rate drops significantly with acculturation.[57] General spending patterns, however, suggest that cooking at home is still common: Latinx spend more than double the average for flour and 166 percent more on dried beans.[50] Single women, those with larger families to feed, and those who identify more strongly with their Mexican heritage have been found more likely to shop at small ethnic groceries or convenience stores that often have fewer healthy food options and may charge more for items such as low-fat milk compared to whole milk.[58]

Food for Thought

In Mexico, the prevalence of malnutrition resulting in stunting/short stature, anemia, and overweight status of children varies by wealth, education, and ethnicity and has been estimated to range between 10 and 35 percent depending on the region.[59]

Latinx people frequent restaurants more than any other ethnic group in the United States. Among Mexican Americans' favorite types of establishments (in order of popularity) are fast food, pizza, Mexican fast food, Chinese, coffee shops, and full-service Mexican.[60] One study of Latinx women in the Los Angeles area found that younger, employed women with lower incomes who had lived more years in the United States preferred fast-food restaurants, stating that distance, price, and a child-friendly environment were deciding factors in the choice of establishment. A report from the CDC indicates that over one-third of Black and Latinx children ate fast food on any given day.[61]

Special Occasions The Mexican custom of reserving foods requiring extensive preparation, such as tamales and enchiladas, for Sunday and holiday meals is continued in the United States.[37,58] Even if such dishes are served only occasionally at family celebrations, Mexican Americans reconnect with their heritage through the preparation and consumption of these traditional items.[29] In one study that included holiday practices of migrant workers,[62] no main dish preferences were found for Easter, and tamales were favored for Christmas. Turkey with mashed potatoes was the most popular Thanksgiving entrée, indicating that this American holiday was adopted along with its traditional foods.

In addition to religious holidays, two secular celebrations are significant in the Mexican American community. The first is Mexican Independence Day on September 16th, commemorating the war of liberation from Spain. Observations emphasize ethnic unity with mariachi music and traditional clothing. Foods the color of the Mexican flag, such as white rice, green avocado, and red or green chili peppers, are eaten. Cinco de Mayo (May 5), the second secular holiday celebrated, is more widely recognized by all ethnic groups throughout the United States even though the meaning of the event (remembrance of a historic victory over France) is often forgotten amid the parades, piñatas, and Aztec dancing that typify the day.

More recently, Aztec Mexica New Year's Day has emerged as a celebration in some Mexican American communities. It welcomes the beginning of the Aztec solar year, comprised of eighteen periods of twenty days each, plus several separate days of reflection. Four signs—"rabbit," "reed," "flint," and "house"—are used to designate each year, along with a number between one and thirteen, resulting in a 52-year cycle. Each new cycle begins with an elaborate New Fire Ceremony that involves fasting and sacrifice. The annual event emphasizes Indigenous identity, as opposed to the Latinx or Hispanic ethnicity that incorporates aspects of European culture, such as the use of the Spanish language.[63]

Nutritional Status

Nutritional Intake It can be difficult to determine health statistics for Chicanos, Braceros, and unauthorized migrants because they are often grouped with Whites or other Latinx in collected data. Information from research on Latinx should be used cautiously since Mexicans comprise a majority of the total Latinx population of the United States. Nevertheless, some nutritional problems have been identified in both new and acculturated immigrants from Mexico through studies of Spanish-surnamed patients, especially those residing in Texas, the southwest, and California.

Life expectancy for Mexican Americans is similar to that of Whites in the United States despite disadvantages such as higher rates of poverty, lower levels of educational achievement, and reduced access to health care. Overall mortality rates as well as cause-specific mortality rates are lower for Mexican Americans compared to White Americans when controlled for gender, age, nativity, marital status, socioeconomic status, and demographic variables. (One notable exception is mortality among younger Mexican Americans, aged 18 to 44, who have elevated mortality risks, mostly due to external causes of death).[64–66] Researchers propose several reasons for the lower-than-expected mortality rates in Mexican Americans. Some report that nativity outside the United States is a factor, accounting for health-promoting lifestyle differences.[67] Another theory is that the selective return migration to Mexico among less healthy migrants, often referred to as "salmon bias," is what causes the Mexican health outcome advantage.[68,69]

Similar trends are seen in infant mortality statistics. Overall, birthrates in the United States have declined from 2019 to 2020 by about 3 percent. However, birth rates continue to be highest for Latinx women followed by non-Latinx Black and non-Latinx White women. Nearly 8.2 percent of Mexican American women receive no prenatal care during the first trimester of pregnancy compared to 4.5 percent of White women.[70] This number is even higher (11.3 percent) for women with Central and South American backgrounds.[71,72] Despite these risk factors, rates for low birth-weight infants and infant mortality are lower for Mexican Americans than for the total population (refer to Cultural Controversy: Breaking the Mold).

The World Health Organization and the American Academy of Pediatrics recommend breastfeeding exclusively for the first six months of life, if possible, and continued breastfeeding until the infant reaches one year of age and is on solid foods. In 2017, 85 percent of Latinx mothers breastfed their newborn babies. However, rates of exclusive breastfeeding at three months (42 percent) and six months (23 percent) are lower than the national average.[71] Latinx are more likely than any other racial/ethnic group to supplement with formula before two days of life, which is associated with shorter breastfeeding duration rates overall. In Mexico, breastfed babies are often given other fluids, including Brotanekformula, water, and sweetened herbal teas to reduce colic or cure diarrhea,[72,73] a practice that may continue in the United States. Babies are usually weaned from the breast to the bottle. Long-term use of the bottle or sleeping with one at night, with milk or sweetened liquids (e.g., fruit-flavored drinks, fruit juice, tea), is sometimes a problem, resulting in iron-deficiency anemia and tooth decay among toddlers (baby-bottle tooth decay).[73,74]

One recent study conducted using focus groups reported that Latinx women were motivated to breastfeed because of their knowledge of the benefits, observations, and support from other Latinx and family members. However, they were often embarrassed about breastfeeding in the United States, due to non-supportive public environments, and chose to initiate bottle feeding as a complement to avoid feelings of shame.[75]

Food for Thought

A study on the prevalence of iron overload disorders in Latinx populations suggests the rate may be slightly higher than non-Latinx populations. Nutritional inadequacies may contribute to other diseases.[76]

Obesity has become a large risk factor among the Latinx community in the United States. More than 78 percent of Latinx women were overweight or obese, compared to 64 percent of non-Latinx White women in 2018. Latinx adults of all sexes were 1.2 times more likely to be obese than non-Hispanic White adults. From 2013 to 2016, Latinx children were 1.8 times more likely to be obese as compared to non-Hispanic White children.

Low socioeconomic status, increased screen time, and less leisure-time physical activity are thought to be factored into high rates of being overweight. Cultural ideal weight may be greater for some Mexicans than for other Americans and, traditionally, Latinx women believed it was normal to gain weight after marriage. Extra weight may indicate health

Cultural Controversy

Breaking the Mold: The Mexican American Immigrant Experience

A previously held assumption regarding assimilation is that health improves continually for immigrants the longer they reside in the United States. Yet recent studies of the largest immigrant population contradict this model. Foreign-born Mexican Americans are found to be healthier overall, eat slightly better diets, and have lower rates of infant mortality than U.S.-born Mexican Americans with foreign-born parents and U.S.-born Mexican Americans with U.S.-born parents—despite higher rates of poverty and less access to medical care.[77–79]

The scientific community expressed little interest in differences in immigrant health status associated with place of birth until researchers in the late 1980s discovered a startling trend. Economically disadvantaged women who had immigrated from Mexico were giving birth to babies who were as healthy as those of White U.S. women with overall higher levels of income and education. Rates of premature births, low birth-weight rates, and newborn death rates among immigrant women were equal to or less than those for Whites.[80,81] The foreign-born women also demonstrated better birth outcomes and fewer maternal disorders than Mexican American women who were born in the United States.[82–84] A comprehensive review of statistics on adolescents was even more revealing. The longer a subject's family had lived in the United States, the poorer the subject's health and the more likely the subject was to engage in risky behaviors, even after controlling for the neighborhood, family, education, and income variables. Mexican Americans who were born in the United States with U.S. parents had significantly higher rates of health problems (including obesity, asthma, and missing school due to illness) compared to those who were born in Mexico. Health risk behaviors, determined by sexual experience, delinquency, violent behavior, and use of controlled substances, were more than double in U.S.-born Mexican American adolescents with U.S. parents than in Mexican American youth born in Mexico.[79]

Suddenly, the assimilation model of health was in question. What accounts for such significant differences? Most hypotheses have addressed the disparities in birth outcomes, suggesting that selective migration occurs (only healthy women come to the United States), that deaths during pregnancy may be greater (thus skewing the data), or that infant deaths are underreported in the foreign-born Mexican American community (which may include high numbers of unauthorized residents). Other theories emphasize the protective factors of the Mexican culture.[84] Research suggests that pregnant, foreign-born Mexican American women behave in ways different from those who are born in the United States. Intake of nutrients, including protein, folate, vitamin C, iron, and zinc is better; smoking and alcohol consumption rates are substantially lower.[82,86] Other factors considered important to positive pregnancy outcomes, such as adequate weight gain and prenatal care, are less likely in foreign-born Mexican Americans. Researchers suggest these negatives may be compensated for by greater community, family, and spousal support, and less accumulative acculturation stress.[70,79,86,87] Determining the reasons that place of birth is so significant will help researchers devise a new assimilation model and suggest approaches for improving the diet, pregnancy, and health outcomes for all Mexican Americans.

and well-being, not only for adults but also for children, and some parents may not recognize that their children are overweight.[88] However, research suggests that many Latinx adults and children perceive themselves as being overweight and are dissatisfied with their body image.[89–91] Unhealthy dieting practices are prevalent in some Latinx groups, and it is believed that Latinx teens are at high risk for developing eating disorders.[92,93]

Latinx Americans are at high risk of developing prediabetes and type 2 diabetes. Generally, U.S. adults have a 40 percent likelihood of developing type 2 diabetes, but for a Latinx American adult, the chance is 50 percent. This high rate is not explained by the incidence of obesity, age, or education, but may be related to the individual's percentage of Indigenous heritage.[94,95] Research suggests that Latinx have greater insulin resistance than non-Latinx Americans, and their lower sensitivity may be due to a higher intake of carbohydrates.[96] Many Mexican Americans live several years undiagnosed and lack of health insurance contributes to this. Type 2 diabetes in Latinx adolescents is three times that of White adolescents.[96] Complications from diabetes, including kidney failure and diabetic retinopathy, are also more prevalent.[97,98] Death rates from diabetes are estimated to be over 50 percent higher for Latinx than for non-Latinx White people, and this difference is even greater in the counties along the Mexican border. Further, diabetes mortality rates are higher for Mexican Americans than for any other Latinx group.[97,98] The main cause of death for Mexican Americans with diabetes is cardiovascular disease. Equally alarming is the increase in the prevalence of overweight in Latinx youth. The results from NHANES cross-sectional data indicate that Mexican American children 8 to 11 years old had the highest percentages (>21 percent for overweight and >21 percent for obesity) than other ethnic groups. Type 2 diabetes is more common in Latinx youth.[98]

Latinx Americans have very high rates of metabolic syndrome, a clustering of conditions related to type 2 diabetes and heart disease, including insulin resistance, hypertension, and dyslipidemia.[99] Interestingly, Mexican Americans have similar rates of hypertension to that of non-Latinx White Americans, but data on dyslipidemia show higher prevalence in Mexican Americans than in non-Latinx White Americans and Black Americans. The incidence of cardiovascular disease in Latinx Americans is lower than the incidence in non-Latinx White Americans, and they are less likely to have heart disease but are 30 percent more likely to have a stroke.[100] Researchers have noted the heart-healthy elements of the traditional Mexican diet. Though studies on cardiovascular mortality risk relative to non-Latinx White Americans are contradictory, and subpopulation risk varies, cardiovascular diseases are the number one cause of death in Latinx adults. A higher prevalence of gallbladder disease has been found in Mexican Americans, and a higher rate is found in those born in the United States, compared to those born in Mexico. Diet may be involved in some cases, but more recent research suggests a genetic vulnerability may be a more important factor.[92,93]

Knowledge of osteoporosis and risk-reducing behavior was low among Latinx women in Chicago, in an earlier study.[103] Cavities are common among Americans of Mexican descent, as is gingivitis. Studies show that nearly one-third of all immigrants from Mexico never receive any dental care. Migrant workers and their children are especially at risk.[101,102]

Mexican American men drink large quantities of alcoholic beverages less often and have lower rates of dependency than non-Latinx men, and Mexican American women have low alcohol consumption rates that increase with acculturation.[103]

Food for Thought

In an early study of Tarahumara people in Mexico, the effects of a high-calorie, high-fat, low-fiber diet on a population that traditionally consumes a low-fat, high-fiber diet were observed. After five weeks, blood cholesterol levels increased by 31 percent, and triglyceride levels increased by 18 percent; all subjects also gained weight.[104]

Licorice root, known as yerba dulce or orozús, may be used in the Mexican American community as a general tonic or for infections, coughs, ulcers, and menstruation problems. It can be toxic in large quantities or taken over long periods and may potentiate the effects of hypotensive drugs.[105]

Studies suggest that anywhere from 20 to 81 percent of Mexican Americans use folk remedies, and Latinx in one survey used the services offered at their local botánica interchangeably with those offered by their biomedical provider.[16] Another study found that increased use of herbal remedies by Mexican American women corresponded with fewer visits to biomedical practitioners. This association may be related to the lack of medical insurance, which was also found to be a factor in the use of traditional medicines.[105] Sixty-one percent of surveyed Latinx elders in New Mexico reported drinking herbal teas to maintain health, alleviate stress, and cure minor ailments.[2] The most commonly consumed infusions included peppermint (called both yerba buena and poleo), chamomile (manzanilla), lavender (alhucema), and osha (related to parsley). However, it is important not to assume adherence to certain folk beliefs, such as the hot–cold classification of foods and illness. Though prevalent among some people in Mexico, these traditional practices may be limited in the United States (even among healers), and younger, urban clients may be offended by the use of such theories. Traditional healers, such as curanderos, are consulted by anywhere from 4 to 21 percent of the Mexican American population.[106] Those who consult curanderos often believe that healers are most effective for symptoms caused by folk illnesses. In one small sample, nearly 26 percent of Mexican American women had personally used the services of a curandero; however, even larger numbers (almost 39 percent) had seen a sabadores (therapists that use massage to care for muscles and injured joints as well as to move internal organs).[16] However, it should be noted that the use of traditional healers does not prevent a client from also seeking biomedical care concurrently.[107] Although traditional practices are most common in poor, rural regions, most Mexican Americans are knowledgeable about folk conditions.

Most traditional health beliefs and practices among Mexican Americans support the emotional well-being of a client and do not interfere with other therapy. Many researchers have suggested that folk conditions provide an important release valve in Latinx cultures, especially for men who are expected to endure pain. Disorders due to outside causes are not blamed on an individual, and the resulting irrational behavior or lethargy is excused.

Several potentially harmful situations are noteworthy. Suboptimal medication use has been noted, especially in diabetes treatment where intake is inconsistent, and in situations where prescription drugs are mixed with home remedies.[108–110] For example, diabetes and hypertension may be treated with botanical remedies in addition to prescribed oral medications, risking excessive hypoglycemic and hypotensive activity, respectively. Clients consult friends and neighbors about effective treatments and are unlikely to disclose home remedies to their physicians.[110] Digestive complaints such as empacho are sometimes treated with toxic lead- or mercury-based medications, such as greta, azarcón, and healing attributed to asogue (destiny or luck).[112] Failure to thrive syndrome may also be a concern. Providers should be aware of these possibilities when presented with this disorder. In some regions, a tea made from psychoactive wormwood (the toxic ingredient formerly found in the alcoholic beverage absinthe) is used for diarrhea. Finally, babies may be given home remedies made with honey, a known cause of infant botulism. In one study, Latinx were the ethnic group least likely to discuss the use of alternative and complementary therapies with their biomedical care providers.[112,113]

Family participation in health care is common, and members should be consulted in both making a diagnosis and prescribing treatment. They may have specific ideas about the cause of an illness and the best approach for a cure; their confidence and cooperation can help ensure client compliance. One study found that family involvement in serious choices about issues such as life support is more important to Mexican Americans than patient autonomy.[114] Dietary changes may affect family members and social interactions; thus, gaining family support has also been suggested to increase compliance.[112,115]

Latinx families face greater barriers to making healthy eating changes due to resistance from older family members, and they are more likely to eat at fast-food restaurants, eat more

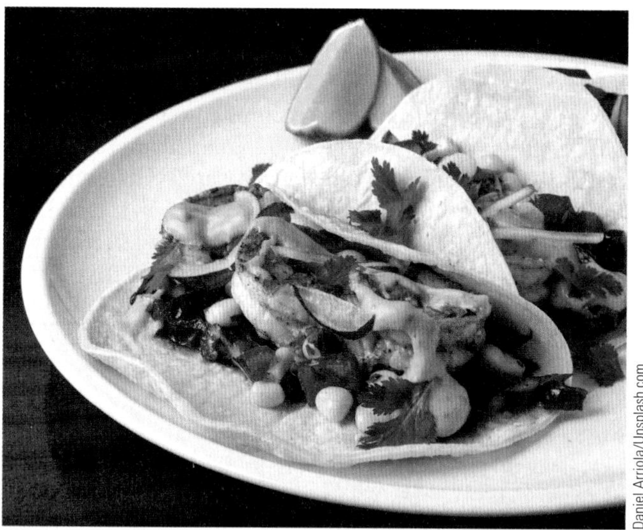

Daniel Arriola/Unsplash.com

▲ Spicy shrimp tacos with creamy cilantro sauce.

saturated fat, and make fewer efforts to increase fiber intake. Traditional meal preparation avoids some of these pitfalls.[117]

Children are also an important influence on food habits in some households. Those raised in the United States may be the only English-speaking members of the family and may be responsible for translating in the market. These children have been found to prefer foods that they have seen advertised on television. The adoption of new foods is influenced by the presence of bilingual children in the family. Researchers studied newly immigrated Latinx in the San Francisco area and found that the importance of the family unit can be used to motivate changes in food habits. Adults unwilling to make changes that would benefit their own health may make those same changes to improve the well-being of their children.

As with all clients, an in-depth interview is crucial in effective nutrition counseling. Experts in the health care of Latinx people recommend that health professionals who work often with Latinx people learn Spanish or work with a translator. Familiarity with Spanish medical terminology is the minimum proficiency needed for meaningful communication. Further, interventions should be tailored to account for differences in acculturation.[115–117]

Central Americans

The seven nations of Belize, Guatemala, El Salvador, Honduras, Nicaragua, Costa Rica, and Panama make up Central America, an isthmus between North America and South America. The eastern coastal region edges the Caribbean Sea. An 800-mile chain of active volcanoes and mountains, beginning at the Mexican border in the north and continuing with only one break into central Panama in the south, forms the temperate backbone of the region. Central America is similar to the rest of Latin America in history of foreign intervention and heterogeneous culture.

Cultural Perspective

History of Central Americans in the United States

Immigration Patterns Central American immigrants to the United States arrived in two distinct waves, though early records are inexact because separate statistics on Central Americans were not kept by the U.S. Census Bureau until the 1960s. Until the early 1980s, immigrants to the United States were of two groups. The first were well-educated professional men who arrived in search of employment opportunities. The second were women, who often outnumbered the men two to one, coming in search of temporary domestic jobs. These Central American immigrants were largely urban residents and settled mostly in New York, Los Angeles, San Francisco, Miami, and Chicago, where they blended into existing Latinx communities.

The second major wave began in the late 1970s and early 1980s, with the exodus of refugees from the brutal civil wars in El Salvador, Guatemala, and Nicaragua. Millions of residents are estimated to have been displaced in these countries, about one-third of whom have emigrated. Many moved to Mexico, and a substantial number continued to the United States.

 **Food for Thought**

Tamales, a dough-wrapped bundle of meat and vegetables steamed in corn husks or banana leaves, are among the oldest of Mesoamerican foods. The "tamal" was eaten by the Mayans and Aztecs, as well as the Olmecs and Toltecs before them, perhaps as early as 8,000 BCE. The "packaging" of corn husks made them perfect as travel food, for hunting trips, or just to take over to the neighbors for dinner.

There are three different colors of corn tortilla: yellow, red, and blue.

Mole is a sweet and savory Mexican sauce made with many ingredients. While there are several varieties, traditional mole is made sweet from the addition of chocolate, or blended dried fruit/nuts, or both, mixed with several types of dried chilies.

Queso fresco, like other cheeses traditionally made from raw milk, is responsible for more food-borne illnesses than any other cheese in the United States.[118]

The number of immigrants in the United States from the Northern Triangle countries of Central America, El Salvador, Guatemala, and Honduras, rose by 25 percent from 2007 to 2015.[119]

Current Demographics and Socioeconomic Status The Central American-born population living in the United States was 3.8 million in 2019, which makes up 8 percent of the U.S. foreign-born population. The U.S. Latinx population is primarily from six nations of Central America. The largest populations are the 1.4 million Salvadorans, 1.1 million Guatemalans, 746,000 Hondurans, and 257,000 Nicaraguans. Immigration from Costa Rica, Belize, and Panama is minimal, comprising about 150,000, or 4 percent, of the total Latinx people in the United States.[120]

Central American descendants, even those from the first wave, are slow to become naturalized citizens, and only 31 percent of Central Americans in the United States have

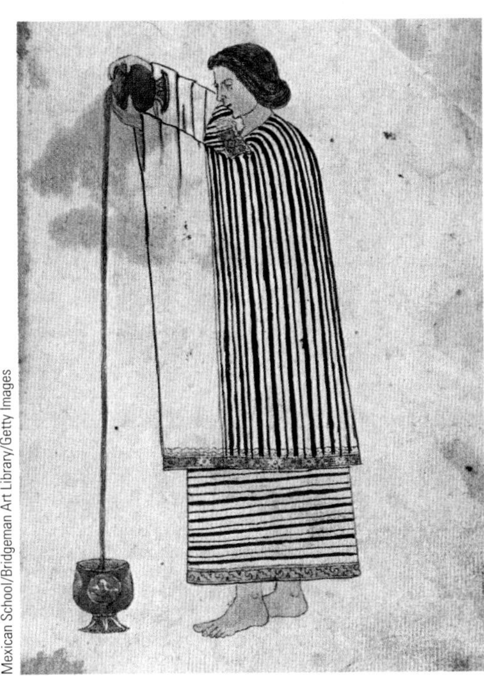
Mexican School/Bridgeman Art Library/Getty Images

▲ A Mayan chocolate container.

obtained citizenship.[121] Those who are not refugees often return to Central America for visits and maintain active contact with their homeland.

An estimated 16 percent of Central Americans live in Los Angeles, 11 percent in New York, 9 percent in Washington, DC, 7 percent in Houston, and 7 percent in Miami. Central Americans are a very heterogeneous population, however, and it is a mistake to assume similar settlement patterns for each group. Identity is sometimes more related to race and class than to the country of origin. Even among recent immigrants, differences in associations are found. Guatemalans, for example, may assimilate into the broader Latinx community, while Mayan Guatemalans, some of whom do not speak Spanish, often establish ethnic enclaves.[120]

Of the Central American immigrants, about one-third work in service and personal care occupations. Roughly 50 percent have graduated from high school. Central American immigrants are more likely to live in poverty (19 percent) than those born in the United States (12 percent) or foreign-born people in the United States overall (14 percent).[120]

Information on unauthorized residents is scarce. It is thought that they often face difficulties in obtaining employment and education opportunities. In addition, disposable family income may be impacted by money sent to support relatives still living in the homeland.

Worldview

The large numbers of recent immigrants from Central America suggest that ethnic identity can be preserved by many new residents. For example, Salvadorans often establish highly insular neighborhoods within the larger Latinx community, where an immigrant can live and conduct business exclusively with other Salvadorans.[121] Guatemalans are a more diverse population of immigrants, and it is their Mayan communities that are most likely to keep traditional beliefs and practices.[122] In contrast, and broadly speaking, Nicaraguans disperse among other Latinx and adapt more to the pan-Latinx community rather than retain their own heritage exclusively.[122]

One unique Central American population in the United States is the Garifuna, also called Black Caribs. Garifuna people are descendants of the African-Caribbean-Arawak people originally from Saint Vincent Island in the West Indies forcibly deported by the British to the Bay Islands in 1797, with later migrations to Honduras.[123] Traditionally, men traveled great distances for work, leaving the women to farm and raise children. Today, their way of life is threatened by coastal development for tourism and lack of government support. Garifuna men often come to the United States for employment, sending much of their earnings home to save their culture.[123]

Religion Most Central Americans are Roman Catholic. Some Guatemalans observe Catholic practices while adhering to Mayan religious beliefs; participation in native religions decline in the United States because they are usually dependent on sacred locations in Guatemala. Evangelical and fundamentalist denominations, such as the Pentecostal Church, have attracted many Central Americans after they arrive in the United States. Small storefront congregations that involve active participation and those churches that offer traditional Central American social activities in addition to worship have been especially successful.

Family Central Americans highly value family and extended kinship. It has been noted that some apartment buildings in Latinx neighborhoods are rented entirely to several families from the same village in Central America. The father is traditionally the undisputed head of the household and provider. Many Costa Ricans define the term family as having both a father and mother in the home.[122] However, some studies suggest this dominance is changing, and shared decision-making between men and women is becoming more common. Children are often carefully controlled, especially daughters.

The roles of men and women often change even further in the United States, where women are sometimes more easily employed, and husbands must take on some domestic responsibilities. Family disintegration has taken place in some refugee camps, where overcrowding and unemployment led to intergenerational conflict before immigration to the United States.[124] In other situations, family members were forced to immigrate separately. Some married outside the Central American community for immigration benefits; others found that when their families were reunited, children had become more independent.[123]

Food for Thought

As in many cultures, the staple grain of the region is woven into creation mythology. Myths of the Maya describe how humans were improved over time: first made of mud, then wood, and finally perfected when their flesh was made from corn dough. In European cultures, often wheat-based bread is considered the "staff of life" in religious contexts. In many Asian cultures, rice is a gift from the gods.

Traditional Health Beliefs and Practices A good diet, especially the consumption of fruits and vegetables, fresh air, and regular hours are thought necessary to preserve health by many Central Americans.[125] Exercise is considered important by some Guatemalans and Panamanians, although the concept of structured exercise is unfamiliar to some Central Americans.[124,126] Salvadorans believe that being too thin can cause sickness, and Americans are considered at risk for ill health because they are so thin.

Some Central Americans view health as a balance between the spiritual and social worlds. For most, health is a gift of God, and prayer is often used to restore harmony during illness.[126,127] Some Nicaraguans believe in witchcraft, practiced by brujos or brujas who can assume the shapes of animals and have the power to cure illness. Guatemalans consider outside forces to be the cause of some illnesses, which include diseases sent by Satan to punish unbelievers and sickness due to witchcraft. Traditional healers include curanderos and sabadores, as well as jeberos (herbalists) and espiritistas who treat witchcraft with prayer. Naturalist doctors (sometimes called naturopaths) who work in association with naturalist shops that provide botanical remedies may be used by some Guatemalans.[128] Priests may also be sought to help with prayers for health.

A balance of hot and cold is also necessary for health and can be disrupted by sudden exposure to extremes in temperature or strong emotions. In addition to susto and mal de ojo, other folk conditions include bilis and cólera, which in extreme cases are associated with anger and general distress and precipitate stroke. In a survey of Latinx immigrants (with a large sampling of Central Americans) regarding beliefs about hypertension, respondents reported that cólera and susto may lead to high blood pressure, as may living at too high an altitude or having too much blood.[124,129]

In the culturally diverse region of Nicaragua's east coast, more than 200 plants with traditional medicinal uses have been identified. One older study reported rural ethnic groups in Nicaragua were found to use traditional healing practices more often than urban residents of mixed heritage.[130] Another survey, however, found that more than three-quarters of respondents in an urban barrio used herbal remedies.[130]

Food for Thought

The Mayan word for corn, *wah*, also means "food."

In Guatemala, refried black beans (fríjoles volteados) are fondly called "Guatemalan caviar."

Guatemalans believe that strength is maintained through the quantity and quality of a person's blood. In urban regions of Guatemala, researchers have noticed the emergence of new categories of food items, deemed "strong" or "health promoting" foods, perhaps due to the influence of modern health promotion concepts.[124]

Over-the-counter remedies, such as analgesics and cough suppressants, are commonly used by Guatemalan Americans, although they are considered weak by Guatemalan standards. Medications (including antibiotics) and herbs, such as chamomile, are sometimes brought to immigrant families by new arrivals from Guatemala.

Traditional Food Habits

Ingredients and Common Foods

Central American cuisine offers many of the foods common throughout Latin America. Native dishes remain prominent in the highland areas, Spanish influences are found in the lowland regions, and the cooking of the multicultural eastern coast shares many similarities with Caribbean Islander fare. The northern nations have foods similar to those of southern Mexico; the southern countries have been more greatly influenced by European and African cuisines.

Staples Early Mayan records indicate that the foundation of their diet was corn and beans, supplemented with squash, tomatoes, chilies, tropical fruit, cocoa, and some game. Indigenous foods were particularly important in the development of Guatemalan cuisine but gradually become less significant in the south of Central America. Rice, introduced by the Spanish, has become a staple in most regions. (Refer to the cultural food groups listed in Table 9.3.)

Beans are eaten daily. Black beans are especially popular in Guatemala, while red beans are common in other nations. Beans are served simmered with spices (called frijoles sancochadas in El Salvador), pureed, or fried, and are often paired with rice. In Nicaragua, red beans and rice fried with onions are called gallo pinto ("painted rooster") due to the colors of the dish.

Corn is eaten mostly made into tortillas. Enchiladas in Central America are open-faced sandwiches similar to Mexican tostadas. They typically feature meat covered with pickled vegetables such as cabbage, beets, and carrots. They are known as mixtas in Guatemala, and here the tortilla is spread first with guacamole, then topped with sausage and pickled cabbage. In El Salvador, a stuffed specialty is called pupusas. A thick tortilla is filled with chicharrónes (deep-fried pork rind or pork belly or both), cheese, or black beans and then completed with another tortilla; the edges are sealed and the pupusa is then fried. They are traditionally served with pickled cabbage. Tamales are also common, often stuffed with poultry or pork. They are called nactamal in Nicaragua, where the dough is flavored with sour orange juice, and the filling includes meat, potatoes, rice, tomatoes, onions, sweet peppers, and mint. Black tamales are served on special occasions in Guatemala, stuffed with a mixture of chicken, chocolate, spices, prunes, and raisins. Empanadas, small turnovers made with wheat flour dough and filled with a savory meat mixture, are popular.

French bread, introduced from Mexico, is eaten regularly in the form of small rolls in Honduras and Guatemala. In El Salvador, French bread is used with native turkey and pickled vegetables to make sandwiches. Coconut bread is a specialty on the Caribbean seacoast. Rice is often stir-fried before boiling, cooked with coconut milk, or, in Costa Rica, served as pancakes.

Table 9.3 Cultural Food Groups: Central Americans

Group	Comments	Common Foods	Adaptations in the United States
Protein Foods			
Milk/milk products	Milk is not widely consumed as a beverage, but evaporated milk and cream are popular in some regions.	Milk (evaporated), cream; cheese (aged and fresh—crumbly farmer's cheese type)	Milk and hard cheese may be disliked by Guatemalans, but increased intake reported for Salvadorans.
Meat/poultry/fish/eggs/legumes	Legumes are important in the cuisine and are often served with rice. All types of meat/poultry are eaten, but pork is popular throughout the region. Eggs are commonly served. Fish and shellfish are consumed in the coastal regions. Sea turtle eggs are popular.	*Meat:* beef, iguana, lizards, pork (all parts, including knuckles, tripe, and skin), venison *Poultry:* chicken, duck, turkey *Fish and shellfish:* clams, conch, flounder, mackerel, mussels, sea snail, shark, shrimp, sole, tarpon, turtle *Eggs:* poultry, turtle *Legumes:* beans—black, chickpeas, fava, kidney, red, white	Bean dishes remain popular.
Cereals/Grains	Rice and corn are the predominant grains of the region. Wheat flour breads are common.	Corn (tamales, tortillas), rice, wheat (bread, rolls)	Tortillas may be replaced by breads.
Fruits/Vegetables	Tropical fruits are abundant. Some temperate fruits such as grapes and apples are also available. Salads and pickled vegetables are popular.	*Fruits:* apples, bananas, breadfruit, cherimoya, coconut, custard apple, grapes as well as raisins, guava, mameys, mangoes, nances, oranges (sweet and sour types), papaya, passion fruit, pejihaye, pineapples, prunes, sour-sop, sweetsop, tamarind, tangerines, zapote (sapodilla) *Vegetables:* asparagus, avocados, beets, cabbage, calabaza (green pumpkin), carrots, cauliflower, chayote, chile peppers, corn, cucumbers, eggplant, green beans, hearts of palm, leeks, lettuce, loroco flowers, onions, pacaya buds (palm flowers), peas, plantains, potatoes, pumpkin (ayote), spinach, sweet peppers, tomatillos, tomatoes, watercress, yams, yuca (cassava), yucca flowers (izote)	Increased intake of potato chips has been reported. Increased consumption of vegetable salads.
Additional Foods			
Seasonings	Cilantro (fresh coriander) and *epazote* are important herbs. Sour orange juice gives a tang to some food; coconut milk flavors others. *Achiote* is used to color foods orange.	*Achiote* (annatto), chile peppers, cilantro, cinnamon, cloves, cocoa, *epazote*, garlic, onions, mint, nutmeg, thyme, vanilla, Worcestershire sauce	
Nuts/seeds		Palm tree nuts, *pepitoria* (toasted squash seeds)	
Beverages	Hot chocolate and coffee, grown in the region, are favorite hot beverages. *Refrescas*, cold drinks, are made with tropical fruit flavors. *Boj*, *chicha*, and *venado* are locally made alcoholic beverages.	Coffee, chocolate, tropical fruit drinks, alcoholic beverages (rum, beer, and fermented or distilled fruit, sugarcane, and grain drinks)	Increased intake of soft drinks.
Fats/oils	Lard is the most commonly used fat.	Butter, lard, vegetable oils, shortening	Lard and shortening use may decrease; vegetable oils and mayonnaise may increase.
Sweeteners	Honey and sugar are used as sweeteners.	Honey, sugar, sugar syrup	Increased intake of candy is noted.

Soups and stews are popular throughout Central America, often including fruit or fruit juices. Beef, plantains, and cassava in coconut milk, spicy beef stew, beef in sour orange juice, pork and white bean stew, chicken cooked in fruit wine; mondongo (Nicaraguan tripe soup), sopa de hombre ("a man's soup") made with seafood, and plantains in coconut milk are a few specialties. In Guatemala, the stews of meat and poultry, such as pepián and jocon, are thickened with toasted squash seeds. Meat, poultry, and fish are frequently roasted as well.

Fruits and vegetables are numerous. Although bananas, coconut, oranges, and mangoes all arrived from Asia at various points in history, they became staples in Central America. Plantains, yucca (cassava), tomatoes, sweet peppers, cabbage, chayote squash (known as huisquil in Guatemala), and avocado predominate, cauliflower, carrots, beets, radishes, green beans, lettuce, spinach, pumpkin, breadfruit, passion fruit (granadilla), pineapples, mameys, and nances (similar to yellow cherries) are also common. Flowers from yucca, palms (pacaya buds), and loroco (Fernandia pandurata) are eaten as vegetables throughout the region.[131] Starchy fruit from the peach palm (pejibaye) and spiny palm (coyoles) are especially popular in Costa Rica and Honduras. Onions and garlic (originally from Asia) flavor many dishes. Salads and pickled vegetables are common as appetizers, as side dishes, and on sandwiches.

Food for Thought

Although iguana is eaten throughout Central America and parts of Mexico, South America, and the Caribbean, it is especially popular with Indigenous people in Nicaragua.

Chocolate was so prized in Mayan culture that cacao beans were used as currency.

Coffee, originally from Ethiopia, was brought into Latin America in the early 18th century and is grown throughout the region, and usually consumed heavily sweetened. Hot chocolate is another favorite. Refrescas, cold beverages, are made in tropical fruit flavors, such as mango and pineapple. Tiste, a Nicaraguan favorite, is made with roasted corn, cocoa powder, sugar, cold water, and cracked ice. Beer is widely available. Fermented beverages such as boj (from sugarcane) and chicha (a wine made from fruit or grain, fortified with rum) are consumed. Venado is a common distilled drink made from sugarcane. Sweets, such as the praline-like candy called nogada, sweetened baked plantains, ices made with fruit syrups, custards, rice puddings, and cakes or fritters flavored with coconut or rum, are eaten as snacks and for dessert.

Regional Variations Although many foods across Central America are similar, they are often flavored with local ingredients for a unique taste. Coconut milk flavors many dishes in Belize and Honduras; seafood specialties include conch and sea turtle. The foods of El Salvador are often fried and feature many indigenous flavors including corn, beans, tomatoes, chilies, and turkey. Achiote is common in mild seasoned Guatemalan fare. The juice of sour oranges is mixed with sweet peppers or mint in many Nicaraguan recipes. Costa Ricans prefer foods simmered with herbs and seasonings such as cilantro, thyme, oregano, onion, garlic, and pimento; rice is also frequently consumed. Panamanian fare incorporates more flavors from afar; one specialty is sancocho, a stew of pork, beef, ham, sausage, tomato, potato, squash, and plantains.

Meal Composition and Cycle

Daily Patterns As in other Latin American regions, beans and corn are the cornerstones of the daily diet, eaten at every meal by the most economically disadvantaged. Rice is also common. Queso blanco (a fresh cheese) or meat is added whenever resources permit. Dinner in wealthier areas usually includes soup, meat or poultry (sometimes fish), tortillas or bread, and substantial garnishes such as avocado salad, fried plantains, and pickled vegetables. Appetizers, such as slivers of broiled beef, bites of meat- or cheese-filled pastry, and soft-boiled turtle eggs, are eaten in some urban regions before dinner; dessert may also be served, typically including custards, ice creams, cakes, or fritters.

Special Occasions Celebrations in Central America are focused on Catholic religious days. Christmas, Easter, and Lent, saints' days (including All Saints' Day), and even Sundays may mean a change in fare. Special dishes include the cheese-flavored batter bread called quesadilla that is served in El Salvador on Sundays; sopa de rosquillas, a soup made with ring-shaped corn dumplings traditionally eaten on the Fridays of Lent in Nicaragua; gallina rellena Navidena, a Nicaraguan Christmas dish of chicken stuffed with papaya, chayote squash, capers, raisins, olives, onions, and tomatoes; and plantains served in chocolate sauce during Semana Santa (the Holy Week before Easter) in Guatemala.

Chicken in tomato sauce (guisado), chicken served with cornmeal porridge, or stews thickened with masa harina are Indigenous specialties eaten at ceremonial occasions. In some areas, the stews are provided by the village leader to serve the community. In Guatemala, All Saints' Day is celebrated with a unique salad called fiambre. These enormous salads involve a family social event at which as many as fifty friends and relatives share the creation.[132] They feature vegetables (e.g., green beans, peas, carrots, cauliflower, beets, radishes, cabbage) mixed with chicken, beef, pork, and sausages and then artfully garnished with salami, mortadella, cheese, asparagus, pacaya buds, and hard-boiled eggs. The dressing is either a vinaigrette or a sweet-and-sour sauce.

Etiquette Dining customs in Central America are often similar to those of Mexico. For example, guests often wait to begin eating a meal until after the host says "¡Buen provecho!"[40] Most Central Americans eat European-style, with the fork remaining in the left hand and the knife in the right one. However, certain more Americanized groups, such as some Nicaraguans,

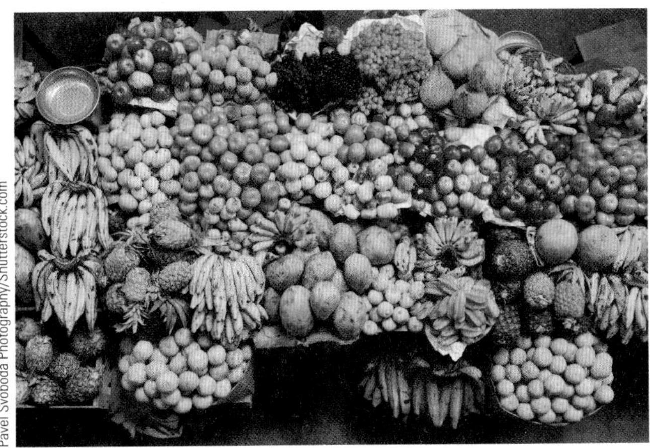
Pavel Svoboda Photography/Shutterstock.com

▲ Tropical fruit from Latin America.

may eat in the American fashion of using the fork in the right hand, switching to the left when cutting food. When not eating, the hands should remain above the table, with the wrists resting on the edge. Bread or tortillas may be served (typically without butter) and should be placed on the side of the plate. It is acceptable to scoop up small bits of food with pieces of tortilla. Dishes are passed to the left. Diners are expected to clean their plates, so taking small portions is appropriate. Asking for seconds is considered a compliment.

Food for Thought

In Guatemala, eggs poached and served with a seasoned broth are used to treat hangovers.

Sample Menu

A Guatemalan Dinner

Chicken Jocon[a,b] or Pollo en Pipian

(Chicken in Tomato-Pumpkin Seed Sauce)[b]

Rice

Frijoles Volteados (Refried Black Beans)[a,b]

Radish Salad[a,b]

Plátanos al Horno (Baked Sweet Plantains) or Coconut Candy[a]

Hot Chocolate or Coffee

Recipes in this menu:

[a]Marks, C. 2014. *False tongues and Sunday bread: A Guatemalan and Mayan cookbook*. M. Evans & Company.

[b]*Guatemalan Cuisine & Recipes* at http://www.whats4eats.com/central-america/guatemala-cuisine

Therapeutic Uses of Foods Some Central Americans follow the hot–cold theory of health and illness, and some also go by the need to balance wet–dry. Guatemalan Americans commonly believe that diarrhea is caused by hot weather and can be alleviated by consuming cold drinks, such as Kool-Aid or Gatorade.[124] However, ice cubes may be avoided during hot weather. Panamanians may avoid cold foods when sick, but in one sample, none applied hot–cold principles to daily meals.[124] Guatemalans also appeared not to balance hot and cold foods; however, it has been suggested that the practice is so enculturated that it is done without conscious effort.[124] Fatty foods and highly spiced dishes may also be avoided by both Guatemalans and Panamanians when ill.

Herbal remedies are popular throughout Central America, especially teas. Studies of Guatemalans and Panamanians found that the teas were consumed to maintain health, and even more often, to cure minor illnesses.[116,133] Examples include teas such as manzanilla (chamomile) for improving circulation, menstrual cramps, and flu or colds; banana leaf and hierbabuena (mint) for good digestion and regularity; and lemon for general health. Rosa de jamaica (hibiscus) was used for respiratory illness, diarrhea, and urinary tract infections, while papaya-leaf tea was considered good for gastritis and as a laxative. Lime, fig leaf, and grapefruit teas were consumed for anxiety and alleviation of stress. Notably, avocado, garlic, ginseng, and valleriana were mentioned as remedies for hypertension and diabetes among Panamanians. Coca leaves, the source of cocaine, are also reported to be used medicinally in some areas.[132,133]

Contemporary Food Habits in the United States

Adaptations of Food Habits

There is scant information on the Central American diet in the United States. Low rates of assimilation among many Central American immigrants are assumed to result in the preservation of traditional food habits. Most Central American ingredients are available in the Latino communities where they settle. One older study found that more than half of Honduran women living in New Orleans continued to consume a diet very similar to what they ate in their homeland.[134] Rice, beans, fruit juices, tortillas, cheese, bananas or plantains, beef, and eggs were the items eaten most often. Few new foods were added by a small number of women, and only kiwi fruit, plums, canned vegetables, and olive oil were used by more than 10 percent of the sample. Prepared items, especially hamburgers (eaten by 30 percent of respondents), fried chicken, pizza, and regional dishes, such as jambalaya and Cajun foods (13 percent for each dish), were other new items consumed by a few of the Honduran women. Some also reported baking more foods, frying less, and using more vegetable oil instead of lard or coconut oil in cooking. A meal was defined as having courses, including meat of some sort, and requiring the diner to sit down. Though the women reported skipping meals, this sometimes meant that they ate a sandwich for lunch, which was not considered a meal.

Older studies of Salvadoran refugees report, in general, the quality of their diet declined since arriving in the United States. Salvadorans stated that in El Salvador more foods were made at home from fresh ingredients; they believed that in the United States more processed items and junk foods were eaten, and some nutritious foods were too costly to consume.[127,135,136] However, findings from another older study of Salvadorans found that there were some beneficial dietary changes after immigration to the United States. Though intake of high-sugar and high-fat foods such as jams or jellies, soft drinks, ice cream, mayonnaise, and vegetable oil increased, consumption of lard, shortening, and fatty meats, including chicharrones and sausage, decreased. Bean dishes, such as frijoles sancochados, remained popular, although other traditional items including pupusas, tamales, and plantain empanadas were eaten significantly less often. Although milk, fruit juice, and fresh salad intake increased, some Salvadorans sampled consumed inadequate servings of dairy products, fruits, and vegetables.[127,135] A recently published study found that fruit and vegetable intake among all Latinx subgroups in California, including Central Americans, were higher when compared to non-Latinx ethnic groups.[137]

Health workers in Florida report that Guatemalan refugees believe that if a food is tasty and does not cause stomach discomfort, it must be good to eat. A high intake of candy, soft drinks, and potato chips has been noted. Milk, which is often not well tolerated, may be avoided. WIC (Supplemental Food Program for Women, Infants, and Children) nutritionists found that some food supplements, including milk and cheese, are disliked because of their taste or texture and are sometimes discarded.[136]

Nutritional Status

Nutritional Intake Limited data on the nutritional status of Central American immigrants have been published. Those who arrive after spending time in refugee camps may suffer high rates of malnutrition resulting in diseases such as beriberi, pellagra, scurvy, and vitamin A deficiency problems, especially in children younger than the age of five. Infectious diseases often follow; tuberculosis and parasites are common.[137] Endemic infections may cause problems as well. Chagas heart disease, resulting from infections with *Trypanosoma cruzi* (found in most of Central America), presents symptoms similar to other coronary artery conditions. Rates of sickle-cell anemia were found to be high (5.7 percent) among mostly Central American adolescents in Los Angeles, and the disease appears to be associated with this population independent of African heritage.[138]

Infant mortality rates for Central Americans in the United States are below the average for Whites.[140] Low-birth-weight infants were not found to be a problem among Central Americans in a Chicago study. Even those at significant personal or environmental risk (i.e., living in low-income, urban neighborhoods) did not show excessive rates of low birth weight. Researchers report that Guatemalans consider breastfeeding healthy for infants but impractical. Breastfeeding often is used as supplementation to formula and solid foods for the first two to three years of a child's life.[140,141]

Food for Thought

Lactose intolerance may be prevalent among Central Americans.

Pupusas, tortillas, or flatbreads made from corn or rice flour stuffed with flavorful ingredients such as cheese, fried beans, pork, spinach, or loroco, a native flower, are among Salvadoran breakfast foods. They also make an easy-to-carry meal on the go.

A study of Salvadoran American youth aged six to eighteen years in Washington, DC, found the rate of youth considered overweight double that of the national average and 1.7 times higher than that of Mexican American children in national surveys. Thirty-eight percent were overweight (BMI 95th percentile), and another 22 percent were at risk for being overweight. Being overweight in this sample was associated with elevated blood pressure, body fat percentage over 30 percent, and early puberty.[142]

An occupational hazard for many Central Americans employed as U.S. farm-workers is pesticide or herbicide poisoning. Exposure occurs when labor codes are unenforced or through worker mishandling of dangerous products.

Health and Longevity Takeaway

In Nicoya, Costa Rica residents are known for their longevity. Their diets are rich in fiber from whole-grain rice and beans. They get plenty of vitamin D from sunshine and they eat fewer calories than most other Central American countries. Eating fewer calories appears to be one of the surest ways to add years to your life. Most Nicoyans eat a light dinner early in the evening.

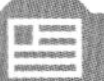

New American Perspectives

Latinx

Margaret K. Ward, MS, RD, LD/N

I have worked with Hispanic clients, primarily Mexican Americans, since 1990 when I returned to the western states after living eight years in the Midwest. In my experience, many of the clients/patients tend to cook without recipes. The less acculturated client/patient tends to use many more "basic" or less processed foods. They may or may not have been influenced by American food practices to the extent that they use less lard *(manteca)* and more oil (though the vegetable oils chosen are not necessarily the "best/healthiest" choices). I would say it's dependent upon the length of time the person has been in the United States and his or her level of acculturation. If he or she has been here awhile and is learning English, the person tends to acquire more of the Western food culture. Also, the number and age of children can have an effect. Families with older, school-aged children tend to acculturate more because of the influences of school and interaction with "American" children.

My advice to new health care professionals working in this community is to acquire Spanish language skills as soon as possible. I began my learning in the clinic; then in desperation, I took two semesters of Spanish in the community college to acquire the grammatical background that the clinic wasn't providing. Facility in the language is critical to communication. I'm a teacher of nutrition; if I can't communicate with my student, I'm not able to do my job very well. Having good Spanish skills made working with clients on modifying their diet much easier, and most Mexican foods can be modified to meet nutritional needs.

Don't be afraid to make mistakes with Spanish language speakers. I have found that my Hispanic patients have almost always been extremely forgiving of my horrible Spanish. They seem to appreciate any attempt that one makes to communicate with them in their language. The worst that will happen if you do make an error is that you'll both laugh. I have several Spanish error stories. One took place in the Women, Infant, and Children (WIC) clinic when a postpartum patient returned for a follow-up hemoglobin determination, which was low again the second time. We reviewed the foods to include in her diet to increase her hemoglobin, and I again encouraged her to continue her prenatal vitamin use. At the end of my spiel, I told her that if she took her vitamins and ate well that she would "*sentarse bien*." Unfortunately, I told her that she would sit well, rather than feel well (which is *sentirse bien*).

Comfort Food—Mexico

A Father's Story

My father grew up in Jalisco, Mexico and migrated to the United States when he was six years old. He lives in a Latinx community in downtown Kansas City.

What is a favorite comfort food that you consider traditional from your home culture?

My father's comfort food was and still is fideo with pinto beans. He specifically liked it when the fideo was soupy and nearly scalding hot. He says that his family did not normally eat any meat with it, especially if they were just eating it for lunch or as a snack, and he ate it often both in Mexico and in the United States. It was relatively inexpensive to make and the ingredients were always something that they had in the house. My dad is the oldest of three so he would often be in charge of his siblings when my grandmother was at work. Fideo was the easiest dish for him to make and everyone liked it.

Did you eat this food together with community? Where was it eaten?

Though this was an everyday, quick food for my dad and his siblings, often eaten for lunch and sometimes in larger portions for dinner, large batches were made for family gatherings. It seems it was a fan favorite for the entire family, even for my dad's tias, tios, and primos (aunts, uncles, and cousins). My dad made fideo sound like a staple, eaten at all times in any situation. When they first immigrated, my family had little money, so it was an inexpensive way to get a lot of nutrients. Now that my dad has a career and can provide for his family, he still makes this for us. Most often, he uses the entire package of noodles because leftover fideo is delicious. Like many traditional cooks, my father prides himself in not taking measurements so I do not have any to provide from him, but the recipe to follow is close.

Fideo (Bean and pasta soup from Mexico)

7-ounce package Fideo noodles (vermicelli, or angel hair pasta, can be substituted)

2 Tbsp. oil

Water to desired consistency, for "soupy" fideo, add enough to cover the pasta

1 cube chicken bouillon

1 can (8 ounces) tomato sauce

1 cup Pinto beans, soaked and cooked (canned pinto beans also work)

Break the angel hair pasta into small pieces, approximately ½–1 inch long. After the angel hair is broken up, put about 2 Tbsp. of oil in a pan. When hot, add the noodles and stir until the pasta just begins to brown, being careful

(*Continued*)

Comfort Food—Mexico (*Continued*)

A Father's Story

to not burn it. After the pasta is brown, add water to the pan. The amount of water you add depends on how soupy you want the finished fideo. My dad likes his soupy so he adds enough water until the pasta is completely covered, plus some. After about 15 minutes, the pasta should have soaked up the water, then add a chicken bouyon cube for seasoning and a can of tomato sauce and stir it all in. Finally, scoop the fideo into a bowl, add however many beans you prefer and the dish is done. (More embellished fideo recipes are available that include chopped onions, cumin, coriander, chili peppers, plus queso fresco, and cilantro for serving.)

Note: How you cook the beans is dependent on the kind of beans you have, dried or from the can. Growing up, my dad always used dry beans which took a lot of preparation to make, although, there were usually always soaked and ready-to-cook beans in his house. After the beans soak in water for at least a day, they would be put in a pot and boiled for about an hour. Nothing is added to the beans.

Nutritional Information (per serving):

Calories 375; protein 16 g; carbohydrates 58 g; fat 8 g; sodium 98 mg.

Additioinal RECIPE TO TRY

Mexican Skillet Quiona

Recipe adapted from *Eating Well* magazine

Serves 4

Ingredients

1 peeled sweet potato, cut into ⅓-inch pieces (about 1 cup)
½ cup water
1 Tbsp. olive oil
1 cup chopped medium yellow onion
1 Tbsp. minced garlic
1 tsp. ground cumin
1 tsp. ground coriander
½ tsp. chili powder
½ tsp. dried oregano
1 (15 oz can) black beans, drained and rinsed
1 (15 oz can) fire-roasted tomatoes, undrained
1¼ cups vegetable broth
1 cup frozen corn
1 cup uncooked quinoa
1 tsp. salt
½ cup fresh cilantro leaves
½ cup light sour cream

Combine sweet potato and water in a large skillet; bring to a boil over high and cook, stirring occasionally, until sweet potato is mostly tender and water is completely evaporated, about 3 minutes. Reduce heat to medium-high and add oil and onion; cook, stirring often, until onion is softened, about 3 more minutes. Add garlic, cumin, coriander, chili powder, and oregano, and cook, stirring constantly, until fragrant, about 1 minute. Add beans, tomatoes, broth, corn, quinoa, and salt, and stir to combine. Bring to a boil. Reduce heat to medium; cover and cook until quinoa is tender and liquid has been completely absorbed, about 20 minutes. Remove from heat; uncover and top with cilantro, plain non-fat yogurt, or reduced-fat sour cream.

Nutritional Information (per serving):

calories 421; protein 16 g; carbohydrates 65 g; fat 11 g; sodium 739 mg

Discussion Starters

Comic Books as Nutrition Education

In a story on helping migrant workers in the United States improve their diets, Evelyn Theiss, a medical writer for the Cleveland, Ohio, newspaper *The Plain Dealer* (http://www.cleveland.com/healthfit/index.ssf/2010/07/comic_book_helps_families_in_m.html) tells how Jill Kilanowski, an assistant professor at Case Western Reserve University, developed a comic book for migrant worker mothers and their young children. Kilanowski explains, "The mothers told me they wanted reading materials with primary colors to use as a teaching tool for their small children, as well as a storyline and pictures." It turns out that comic books are very popular in Mexican and Mexican American cultures. The major focus of this comic book story is on limiting portion sizes because Mexican American immigrants often suffer from obesity, diabetes, and hypertension.

Imagine that you have been hired to write another comic book for Mexican American migrant workers on making some changes to their dietary or health habits to improve their health. Because limiting portion sizes has been covered in Evelyn Theiss's book, what other change might you focus on? Outline the storyline, if you can. Consider a comic book for Central American immigrants. Would the same themes and storylines work for them? In small groups, share your themes and storylines, get feedback from your group members, and then revise your ideas for your comic books.

Review Questions

1. Compare and contrast the staple foods of Mexico's different regions.
2. Describe the hot–cold system of diet and health practiced traditionally by Mexicans.
3. List two regional U.S. foods that are modifications of Mexican recipes. First, describe the possible original dish, and then explain how it is modified.
4. Which countries make up Central America? Roughly, what are the demographics of immigrants in the United States from Central America?
5. Compare the traditional health beliefs and practices of Mexicans and Central Americans.
6. Describe the food staples of Central America.
7. What are the most common health problems of Mexicans and Central Americans and their descendants living in the United States? How may acculturation to the American diet contribute to these problems?

Reflection

1. How might present-day Mexican food be modified for someone with metabolic syndrome? How could the diet be modified toward a lower fat and lower carbohydrate intake without compromising traditional foods?

References

1. U.S. Census Bureau. n.d. Selected population profile in the U.S. 2016–2020. *American Community Survey 1-5-Year Estimates.* Retrieved from https://data.census.gov/cedsci/table?q=hispanic&tid=ACSDT5Y2020.B01001I
2. U.S. Census Bureau. 2019. Hispanic *alone or in combination with one or more other races.* Retrieved from https://www.census.gov/data/tables/2019/demo/hispanic-origin/2019-cps.html
3. Pilcher, J. n.d. American Latino theme study: food. National Park Service. Retrieved from https://www.nps.gov/articles/latinotheme-food.htm
4. Silva-Zolezzi, I., Hidalgo-Miranda, A., Estrada-Gil, J., Fernandez-Lopez, J.C., Uribe-Figueroa, L., Contreras, A., . . . & Jimenez-Sanchez, G. 2009, May 26. Analysis of genomic diversity in Mexican Mestizo populations to develop genomic medicine in Mexico. *Proceedings of the National Academy of Sciences,* 106(21), 861–916.
5. U.S. Census Bureau. 2020. This Hispanic population. Retrieved from https://www.census.gov/search-results.html?q=this+hispanic+population&page=1&stateGeo=none&searchtype=web&cssp=SERP&_charset_=UTF-8
6. Passel, J., & Cohn, D'Vera. n.d. *Mexican immigrants: How many come? How many leave?* Retrieved from http://pewhispanic.org/reports/report.php?ReportID5112 (accessed February 11, 2011).
7. Mexican Americans. n.d. In Wikipedia. U.S. Census Bureau: Table QT-P10 Hispanic or Latino by Type: 2010. Retrieved from http://en.wikipedia.org/wiki/ (accessed February 26, 2015).
8. Peri, G., & Rutledge, Z. 2020. Revisiting economic assimilation of Mexican and Central American Immigrants in the U.S. *Social Science Quarterly,* 81, 1–15.
9. Alvarez, J. 2018. What quinceaneras can teach adults—as well as young girls—about values. Zocalo. Retrieved from https://www.zocalopublicsquare.org/2018/05/09/quinceaneras-can-teach-adults-well-young-girls-values/ideas/essay/.
10. Simon, Y. 2017. Meet 5 of the Tejana teems who made this quinceanera-themed protest a success. REMezcla. Retrieved from https://remezcla.com/features/culture/meet-the-quinceaneras-at-the-capitol/
11. Krogstad, J.M., Jeffrey S. Passel, & D'vera C. 2019. Five facts about illegal immigration in the U.S. Pew Research Center. Retrieved from https://www.pewresearch.org/fact-tank/2019/06/12/5-facts-about-illegal-immigration-in-the-u-s/
12. Pew Research Center. 2014. The shifting religious identity of Latinos in the United States. Retrieved from https://www.pewforum.org/2014/05/07/chapter-1-religious-affiliation-of-hispanics/
13. Salazar-Collier, C.L., Reininger, B.M., Wilkinson, A.V., & Kelder, S.H. 2021. Exploration of fatalism and religiosity by gender and varying levels of engagement among Mexican-American adults of a Type 2 diabetes management program. *Frontiers in Public Health,* 1414.
14. Hill, L.E., & Johnson, H.P. 2002. *Understanding the future of Californians' fertility: The role of immigrants.* San Francisco: The Public Policy Institute of California.
15. Neff, N. 1998. *Folk medicine in Hispanics in the southwestern United States.* Retrieved from http://www.rice.edu/projects/Hispanic Health/Courses/mod7/mod7.html (accessed February 13, 2011).
16. Lopez, R.A. 2005. Use of alternative folk medicine by Mexican American women. *Journal of Immigrant Health,* 7, 23–31.
17. Trotter, R.T., & Chavira, J.A. 1997. *Curanderismo: Mexican American folk healing.* Athens: University of Georgia Press.
18. Mikhail, B.I. 1994. Hispanic mothers' beliefs and practices regarding selected children's health problems. *Western Journal of Nursing Research,* 16, 623–638.
19. Spector, R.E. 2004. *Cultural diversity in health and illness* (6th ed.). Upper Saddle River, NJ: Pearson Education.
20. Baer, R.D., Weller, S.C., De Alba Garcia, J.G., Glazer, M., Trotter, R., Pachter, L., & Klein, R.E. 2003. A cross-cultural approach to the study of the folk illness nervios. *Culture, Medicine, and Psychiatry,* 27, 315–337.
21. Zoucha, R., & Purnell, L.D. 2003. People of Mexican heritage. In L.D. Purnell & B.J. Paulanka (Eds.), *Transcultural health care: A culturally competent approach* (2nd ed.). Philadelphia: F.A. Davis.
22. Laudan, R. 2004. The Mexican's kitchen's Islamic connection. *Saudi Aramco World,* 55, 32–39.
23. Monson, A., & Scheidel, W., eds. (2015). *Fiscal regimes and the political economy of premodern states.* Cambridge University Press.
24. Morán, E. 2016. *Sacred consumption: Food and ritual in Aztec art and culture.* University of Texas Press.
25. Leonard, J.N. 1968. *Latin American cooking.* New York: Time-Life Books.
26. Abarca, M. E. 2013. Moctezuma's table: Rolando Briseño's Mexican and Chicano tablescapes edited by Norma E. Cantú.
27. Keen, B. 2019. *Latin American civilization: History and society, 1492 to the present.* Routledge.
28. Cohen, B. 2014. Mexico's ancient drink makes a comeback. BBC. Retrieved from https://www.bbc.com/travel/article/20141125-mexicos-ancient-drink-makes-a-comeback
29. García-Lara, S., & Serna-Saldivar, S.O. 2019. Corn history and culture. *Corn,* 1–18.
30. Bendele, M. 2021. Barbacoa?: The curious case of a word. In *Republic of Barbecue: Stories Beyond the Brisket* (pp. 88–90). New York: University of Texas Press. Retrieved from https://doi.org/10.7560/719989-026.
31. Kennedy, D. 2021. My Mexico. In *My Mexico.* University of Texas Press.
32. Pilcher, J.M. 2016. Taste, smell, and flavor in Mexico. *Oxford Research Encyclopedia of Latin American History.*
33. Gates, S. 2017. *Insects: an edible field guide.* Random House.
34. Reyes-Prado, H., & Moreno, J.P. 2020. Insects used as foodstuff by indigenous groups in Morelos, Mexico. *Journal of Insects as Food and Feed,* 6(5), 499–505.

35. Menzel, P., & D'Aluisio, F. 1998. *Man eating bugs: The art and science of eating insects*. Berkeley, CA: Ten Speed Press.
36. Pew Research Center. 2014. *Religion in Latin America*. Pew Research Center's Religion and Public Life. Retrieved from http://www.pewforum.org/2014/11/13/religion-in-latin-america/ (accessed April 15, 2015).
37. Romero-Gwynn, E., & Gwynn, D. 1994. Food and dietary adaptation among Hispanics in the United States. In T. Weaver, N. Kanellos, & C. Esteva-Fabregat (Eds.), *Handbook of Hispanic cultures in the United States: Anthropology*. Houston, TX: Arte Publico Press.
38. Carmichael, E., & Sayer, C. 2005. Feasting with dead souls. In C. Korsmeyer (Ed.), *The taste culture reader*. Gordonsville, VA: Berg Publishers.
39. Davidow, J. 1999. *Infusions of healing: A treasury of Mexican American herbal remedies*. New York: Simon & Schuster.
40. Foster, D. 2002. *The global etiquette guide to Mexico and Latin America*. New York: Wiley.
41. Berdanier, C.D. 2019. Corn, niacin, and the history of pellagra. *Nutrition Today*, 54(6), 283–288.
42. Bharucha, D.X., Morling, B.A., & Niesenbaum, R.A. 2003. Use and definition of herbal medicines differ by ethnicity. *Annals of Pharmacotherapy*, 37, 1409–1413.
43. Dole, E.J., Rhyne, R.I., Zeilmann, C.A., Skipper, B.J., McCabe, M.L., & Low Dog, T. 2000. The influence of ethnicity on use of herbal remedies in elderly Hispanic and non-Hispanic whites. *Journal of the American Pharmaceutical Association*, 40, 359–365.
44. Pilcher, J.M. 2001. Tex-Mex, Cal-Mex, New Mex, or whose Mex? Notes on the historical geography of southwestern cuisine. *Journal of the Southwest*, 43, 659–680.
45. Pilcher, J. M. 2017. *Planet taco: a global history of Mexican food*. Oxford University Press.
46. Martynuska, M. 2017. Cultural hybridity in the USA exemplified by Tex-Mex cuisine. *International Review of Social Research*, 7(2), 90–98.
47. Seasons, F.G. 2021. The evolution of Mexican cuisine. *Food, Texts, and Cultures in Latin America and Spain*. Vanderbilt University Press.
48. Aburto, D. 2019. From "Unfit for Human Consumption" to Taco Tuesday: Mexican food in Los Angeles from the Early 1900s. Doctoral dissertation, California State University, Northridge.
49. CISION PR Newswire. April 7, 2017. United States Hispanic foods and beverages market, 2020 - research and markets. Retrieved from https://www.prnewswire.com/news-releases/united-states-hispanic-foods-and-beverages-market-2020---research-and-markets-300436479.html
50. *Hispanic food and beverages in the U.S.: Market and consumer trends in Latino cuisine* (5th ed.). July 2012. Rockville, MD: Packaged Facts.
51. Torres-Aguilar, P., Teran-Garcia, M., Wiley, A. et al. 2016. Factors correlated to protective and risk dietary patterns in immigrant Latino mothers in non-metropolitan rural communities. *Journal of Immigrant Minority Health* 18, 652–659. Retrieved from https://doi.org/10.1007/s10903-015-0212-2
52. Ayala, G.X., Baquero, B., & Klinger, S. 2008. A systematic review of the relationship between acculturation and diet among Latinos in the United States: Implications for future research. *Journal of the American Dietetic*, 108, 1330–1344.
53. Villegas, E., Coba-Rodriguez, S., & Wiley, A.R. 2018. Continued barriers affecting Hispanic families' dietary patterns. *Family and Consumer Science Research Journal*, 46, 363–380. Retrieved from https://doi.org/10.1111/fcsr.12262
54. Russo, R.G., Northridge, M.E., Wu, B. et al. 2020. Characterizing sugar-sweetened beverage consumption for US children and adolescents by race/ethnicity. *Journal of Racial and Ethnic Health Disparities*, 7, 1100–1116. Retrieved from https://doi.org/10.1007/s40615-020-00733-7
55. Castañeda, J., Caire-Juvera, G., Sandoval, S., Castañeda, P.A., Contreras, A.D., Portillo, G.E., &Ortega-Vélez, M.I. 2019. Food security and obesity among Mexican agricultural migrant workers. *International Journal of Environmental Research and Public Health*, 16(21), 4171. Retrieved from https://doi.org/10.3390/ijerph16214171
56. Reininger, B., Lee, M., Jennings, R., Evans, A., & Vidoni, M. (2017). Healthy eating patterns associated with acculturation, sex and BMI among Mexican Americans. *Public Health Nutrition*, 20(7), 1267–1278. doi:10.1017/S1368980016003311
57. NPD Group. 2005. *At the table with Hispanic families across America*. Port Washington, NY: Author
58. Lisabeth, L.D., Sánchez, B.N., Escobar, J., Hughes, R., Meurer, W.J., Zuniga, B., . . . Morgenstern, L.B. 2010, May. The food environment in an urban Mexican American community. *Health Place*, 16(3), 598–605. Epub February 2, 2010.
59. Batis, C., Denova-Gutiérrez, E., Estrada-Velasco, B.I., & Rivera, J. 2020. Malnutrition prevalence among children and women of reproductive age in Mexico by wealth, education level, urban/rural area and indigenous ethnicity. *Public Health Nutrition*, 23(S1), s77–s88.
60. Elder, J., Sallis, J.F., Zive, M.M., Hoy, P., McKenzie, T.L., Nader, P.R., & Berry, C.C. 1999. Factors affecting selection of restaurants by Anglo- and Mexican-American families. *Journal of the American Dietetic Association*, 99, 856–857.
61. Fryer, C.D., Carroll, M.D., Ahluwalia, N., & Ogden, C. 2020. Fast food intake among children and adolescents in the United States, 2015–2018. NCHS Data Brief No. 375. Retrieved from https://www.cdc.gov/nchs/products/databriefs/db375.htm
62. Martinez, A. (2019). Latino studies celebrates winter holidays with tamales, storytelling at Merry Merienda. *UWIRE Text*, 1-1.
63. Normand, V. 2005. *Montezuma's revenge*. Metro, July 13–19. Retrieved from http://www.metroactive.com/papers/metro/07.13.05/aztecs-0528.html (accessed February 14, 2011).
64. MacDorman, M.F., & Mathews, T.J. 2011. *Understanding racial and ethnic disparities in U.S. infant mortality rates*. NCHS data brief, no 74. Hyattsville, MD: National Center for Health Statistics.
65. National Center for Health Statistics. 2013. Deaths: Final data for 2010. *National Vital Statistics Report*, 61(4), Table 7.
66. Xu, J.Q., Kochanek, K.D., Murphy, S.L., & Tejada-Vera, B. 2010. Deaths: Final data for 2007. *National Vital Statistics Reports*, 58(19). Hyattsville, MD: National Center for Health Statistics.
67. Hummer, R.A., Rogers, R.G., Nam, C.B., & LeClere, F.B. 1999. Race/ethnicity, nativity, and U.S. adult mortality. *Social Science Quarterly*, 80, 1083–1118.
68. Markides, K.S., & Eschbach, K. 2005. Aging, migration, and mortality: Current status of research on the Hispanic paradox. *Journals of Gerontology, Series B, Psychological Sciences and Social Sciences*, 60, 68–75.
69. Palloni, A., & Arias, E. 2004. Paradox lost: Explaining the Hispanic adult mortality advantage. *Demography*, 41, 385–415.
70. Paz, K., & Massey, K.P. 2016. Health Disparity among Latina Women: Comparison with Non-Latina Women: Supplementary Issue: Health Disparities in Women. *Clinical Medicine Insights: Women's Health*, 9, CMWH-S38488.
71. National Immunization Survey. 2018. Centers for Disease Control and Prevention, Department of Health and Human Services. Retrieved from https://www.cdc.gov/breastfeeding/data/nis_data/rates-any-exclusive-bf-socio-dem-2018.html
72. Mathews, T.J., & MacDorman, M.F. 2010. Infant mortality statistics from the 2006. *National Vital Statistics Reports*, 58(17). Hyattsville, MD: National Center for Health Statistics. 2010.
73. Brotanek, J.M., Schroer, D., Valentyn, L., Tomany-Korman, S., & Flores, G. January–February 2009. Reasons for prolonged bottle-feeding and iron deficiency among Mexican-American toddlers: An ethnographic study. *Academic Pediatrics*, 9(1), 17–25.
74. Huntingdon, N.L., Kim, I.J., & Hughes, C.V. 2002. Caries-risk factors for Hispanic children affected by early childhood caries. *Pediatric Dentistry*, 24, 536–542.
75. Chiang, K.F., Li, R., Anstey, E.H., & Perrine, C.G. 2021. Racial and ethnic disparities in breastfeeding initiation - United States, 2019.

MMWR, 70(21), 769–774. Retrieved from https://www.cdc.gov/mmwr/volumes/70/wr/mm7021a1.htm.

76. Raffield, L.M., Louie, T., Sofer, T., Jain, D., Ipp, E., Taylor, K.D., Papanicolaou, G.P., Avilés-Santa, L., Lange, L.A., Laurie, C.C., Conomos, M.P., Thornton, T.A., Chen, Y., Qi, O., Cotler, S., Thyagarajan, B., Schneiderman, N., Rotter, J.I., Reiner, A.P., Lin, H.J., (2017) Genome-wide association study of iron traits and relation to diabetes in the Hispanic Community Health Study/Study of Latinos (HCHS/SOL): potential genomic intersection of iron and glucose regulation?, Human Molecular Genetics, Volume 26, Issue 10, 15 Pages 1966–1978, https://doi.org/10.1093/hmg/ddx082
77. Basiotis, P.P., Carlson, A., Gerrior, S.A., Juan, W.Y., & Lino, M. 2002. *The Healthy Eating Index: 1999–2000*. Washington, DC: U.S. Department of Agriculture, Center for Nutrition Policy and Promotion. CNPP-12.
78. Harris, K.M. 2000. The health status and risk behaviors of adolescents in immigrant families. In D.J. Hernandez (Ed.), *Children of immigrants: Health adjustment and public assistance*. Washington, DC: National Research Council.
79. Landale, N.S., Oropesa, R.S., & Gorman, B.K. 1999. Immigration and infant health: Birth outcomes of immigrant and native-born women. In D.J. Hernandez (Ed.), *Children of immigrants: Health, adjustment, and public assistance*. Washington, DC: National Academy Press.
80. Franzini, L., & Fernandez-Esquer, M.E. 2004. Socioeconomic, cultural, and personal influences on health outcomes in low-income Mexican-origin individuals in Texas. *Social Science & Medicine*, 59, 1629–1646.
81. Gould, J.B., Madan, A., Qin, C., & Chavez, G. 2003. Perinatal outcomes in two dissimilar immigrant populations in the United States. *Pediatrics*, 111, e676–e682.
82. Page, R.L. 2004. Positive pregnancy outcomes in Mexican immigrants: What can we learn? *Journal of Obstetrical and Gynecological Nursing*, 33, 783–790.
83. Jenny, A.M., Schoendorf, K.C., & Parker, J.D. 2001. The association between community context and mortality among Mexican-American infants. *Ethnicity & Disease*, 11, 722–731.
84. Wingate, M.S., & Alexander, G.R. 2006. The healthy migrant theory: Variations in pregnancy outcomes among US-born migrants. *Social Science & Medicine*, 62, 491–498.
85. Guendelman, S., Thornton, D., Gould, J., & Hosang, N. 2006. Mexican women in California: Differentials in maternal morbidity between foreign and US-born populations. *Paediatrics and Perinatal Epidemiology*, 20, 471–481.
86. Acevedo, M.C. 2000. The role of acculturation in explaining ethnic differences in the prenatal health-risk behaviors, mental health, and parenting beliefs of Mexican-American and European American at risk women. *Child Abuse and Neglect*, 24, 111–127.
87. Collins, Jr. J.W., & Shay, D.K. 1994. Prevalence of low birth weight among Hispanic infants with United States–born and foreign-born mothers: The effect of urban poverty. *American Journal of Epidemiology*, 139, 184–192.
88. Eckstein, K.C., Mikhail, L.M., Ariza, A.J., Thomson, J.S., Millard, S.C., & Binns, H.J. 2006. Parents' perceptions of their child's weight and health. *Pediatrics*, 11, 681–690.
89. Robinson, T.N., Chang, J.Y., Haydel, K.F., & Killen, J.D. 2001. Overweight concerns and body image dissatisfaction among third-grade children: The impacts of ethnicity and socioeconomic status. *Journal of Pediatrics*, 138, 181–187.
90. Sanchez-Johnsen, L.A., Fitzgibbon, M.L., Martinovich, Z., Stolley, M.R., Dyer, A.R., & Van Horn, L. 2004. Ethnic differences in correlates of obesity between Latin-American and black women. *Obesity Research*, 12, 652–660.
91. Talamayan, K.S., Springer, A.E., Kelder, S.H., Gorospe, E.C., & Joye, K.A. 2006. Prevalence of overweight and weight control behaviors among normal weight adolescents in the United States. *Scientific World Journal*, 26, 365–373.
92. U.S. Department of Health and Human Services, Office of Minority Health. n.d. *Profile: Hispanic/Latino Americans*. Retrieved from http://minorityhealth.hhs.gov/omh/browse.aspx?lvl53&lvlid564 (accessed March 31, 2020).
93. A Pathfinder to Resources-Hispanic/Latino Health in the United States. 2019. Office of Minority Health. Retrieved from https://minorityhealth.hhs.gov/Assets/PDF/pathfinders/Hispanic%20Latino%20Pathfinder%20September%202021%20final_508.pdf
94. Burke, J.P., Williams, K., Gaskill, S.P., Hazuda, H.P., Haffner, S.M., & Stern, M.P. 1999. Rapid rise in the incidence of type 2 diabetes from 1987 to 1996: Results from the San Antonio Heart Study. *Archives of Internal Medicine*, 159, 1450–1456.
95. Grant, R.W., Moore, A.F., & Florez, J.C. 2009. Genetic architecture of type 2 diabetes: Recent progress and clinical implications. *Diabetes Care*, 32(6), 1107–1114.
96. Centers for Disease Control and Prevention. n.d. 2011 *national diabetes fact sheet*. Retrieved from http://www.cdc.gov/diabetes/pubs/-figuretext11.htm#fig4 (accessed February 15, 2011).
97. Fisher-Hoch, S.P., Vatcheva, K.P., Rahbar, M.H., & McCormick, J.B. (2015) Undiagnosed diabetes and pre-diabetes in health disparities. *PLOS ONE 10*(7), e0133135. Retrieved from https://doi.org/10.1371/journal.pone.0133135
98. Aguayo-Mazzucato, C., Diaque, P., Hernandez, S., Rosas, S., Kostic, A., & Caballero, A.E. 2019. Understanding the growing epidemic of type 2 diabetes in the Hispanic population living in the United States. *Diabetes/Metabolism Research and Reviews*, 35, e3097. Retrieved from https://doi.org/10.1002/dmrr.3097.
99. Quezada, A. 2019. Examining the association between acculturation indicators and metabolic syndrome among Hispanic adults. Texas Woman's University.
100. Arispe, I. E., Gindi, R. M., & Madans, J. H. (2021). Health, United States, 2019.
101. Lukes, S.M., & Simon, B. 2005. Dental decay in southern Illinois migrant and seasonal farmworkers: An analysis of clinical data. *Journal of Rural Health*, 21, 254–258.
102. Aguila, Andrea, 2016. Prevalence of dental caries in Mexican-American children and adolescents attending Rawlings Pediatric Dental Clinic in El Paso, Texas. Open Access Theses & Dissertations. 589. Retrieved from https://digitalcommons.utep.edu/open_etd/589
103. Chartier, K., & Caetano, R. 2010. Ethnicity and health disparities in alcohol research. *Alcohol Research & Health*, 33(1 and 2), 154.
104. McMurray, M.P., Ceriqueira, M.T., Conner, S.L., & Conner, W.E. 1991. Changes in lipid and lipoprotein levels and body weight in Tarahumara Indians after consumption of an affluent diet. *New England Journal of Medicine*, 325, 1704–1708.
105. Green, R.R., Santoro, N., Allshous, A., Neal-Perry, G., & Derby, C. 2017. Prevalence of complementary and alternative medicine and herbal remedy use in Hispanic and Non-Hispanic White Women: Results from the Study of Women's Health Across the Nation. *Journal of Alternative and Complementary Medicine*, 23(10), 805–811. Retrieved from https://www.liebertpub.com/doi/full/10.1089/acm.2017.0080
106. Hendrickson, B. 2015. Neo-shamans, curanderismo and scholars: Metaphysical blending in contemporary Mexican American folk healing. *Nova Religio 1*, 19(1), 25–44. Retrieved from https://doi.org/10.1525/nr.2015.19.1.25.
107. Yehieli, M., & Grey, M.A. 2005. *Health matters: A pocket guide for working with diverse cultures and underserved populations*. Boston: Intercultural Press.
108. Espino, D.V., Bazaldua, O.V., Palmer, R.F., Mouton, C.P., Parchman, M.L., Miles, T.P., & Markides, K. 2006. Suboptimal medication use and mortality in an older adult community-based cohort: results from the Hispanic EPESE Study. *Journal of Gerontology, Series A, Biological Sciences and Medical Sciences*, 61, 170–175.
109. Kuo, Y.F., Raji, M.A., Markides, K.S., Ray, L.A., Espino, D.V., & Goodwin, J.S. 2003. Inconsistent use of diabetes complications, and mortality in older Mexican Americans over a 7-year period: Data from the Hispanic established population for the epidemiologic study of the elderly. *Diabetes Care*, 26, 3054–3060.

110. Poss, J., Jezewski, M.A., & Stuart, A.G. 2003. Home remedies for type 2 diabetes used by Mexican Americans in El Paso, Texas. *Clinical Nursing Research*, 12, 304–323.
111. Galanti, G. 2014. *Caring for Patients from Different Cultures: Case Studies from American Hospitals* (5th ed.). Philadelphia: University of Pennsylvania Press.
112. Graham, R.E., Ahn, A.C., Davis, R.B., O'Conner, B.B., Eisenber, D.M., & Phillips, R.S. 2005. Use of complementary and alternative medical therapies among racial and ethnic minority adults: Results from the 2002 National Health Interview Survey. *Journal of the National Medical Association*, 97, 535–545.
113. Juckett, G. 2013. Caring for Latino Patients. American Academy of Family Physicians. Retrieved from https://www.aafp.org/afp/2013/0101/afp20130101p48.pdf
114. Blackhall, L.J., Murphy, S.T., Frank, G., Michel, V., & Azen, S. 1995. Ethnicity and attitudes toward patient autonomy. *Journal of the American Medical Association*, 274, 820–825.
115. Purnell, L., & Fenkl, E. 2019. *Handbook for Culturally Competent Care.* Springer International Publishing.
116. Purnell, L., & Fenkl, A. 2020. *Textbook for Transcultural Health Care: A population Approach* (5th ed.). Springer International Publishing.
117. Hammons, A., Olvera, N., Teran-Garcia, M., Villegas, E., & Fiese, B. 2021. Mealtime resistance: Hispanic mothers' perspectives on making healthy eating changes within the family. Appetite.
118. Centers for Disease Control and Prevention. 2013. Listeria and food. Retrieved from http://www.CDC.gov/foodsafety/specific-foods/listeria-and-food.html (accessed February 27, 2015).
119. Pew Research Center. 2017. Rise in U.S. immigrants From El Salvador, Guatemala and Honduras outpaces growth from elsewhere. Retrieved from https://www.pewresearch.org/hispanic/2017/12/07/rise-in-u-s-immigrants-from-el-salvador-guatemala-and-honduras-outpaces-growth-from-elsewhere/.
120. Babich, E., & Batalove, J. 2021. Central American Immigrants in the United States. Migration Policy Institute. Retrieved from https://www.migrationpolicy.org/article/central-american-immigrants-united-states/#:~:text=The%20total%20Central%20American-born%20population%20in%20the%20United,of%2044.9%20million%20%28see%20Figure%201%29.%20Figure%201.
121. International Migration Institute. n.d. *Central American immigrants in the United States.* Retrieved from http://www.migrationinstitute.org (accessed February 26, 2015).
122. Riggs, T. (Ed.). 2014. Nicaraguan Americans. *Gale Encyclopedia for Multicultural America.*
123. Crawford, M.H. 1983. The anthropological genetics of the Black Caribs "Garifuna" of Central America and the Caribbean. Wiley Online Library. Retrieved from https://onlinelibrary.wiley.com/doi/abs/10.1002/ajpa.1330260508
124. Ellis, T.A., & Purnell, L.D. 2021. People of Guatemalan heritage. In *Textbook for transcultural health care: A population approach* (pp. 445–467). Springer, Cham.
125. Leonard, J.N. 1968. *Latin American cooking.* New York: Time-Life Books.
126. Boyle, J.S. 1991, April–May. Transcultural nursing care of Central American refugees. *National Student Nurses Association, Inc./Imprint*, 73–77.
127. Rutherford, M.S., & Roux, G.M. 2002. Health beliefs and practices in rural El Salvador: An ethnographic study. *Journal of Cultural Diversity*, 9, 3–11.
128. Zapata, J. 1999. The use of folk healing and healers by six Latinos living in New England: A preliminary study. *Journal of Transcultural Nursing*, 136–142.
129. Ailinger, R.L., Molloy, S., Zamora, L., & Benavides, C. 2004. Herbal remedies in a Nicaraguan barrio. *Journal of Transcultural Nursing*, 15, 278–282.
130. Barrett, B. 1995. Ethnomedical interactions: Health and identity on Nicaragua's Atlantic coast. *Social Science and Medicine*, 40, 1611–1621.
131. Fedick, S.L., Mathews, J.P., & Guderjan, T.H. 2017. Plant-food commodities of the Maya Lowlands. *The Value of Things: Prehistoric to Contemporary Commodities in the Maya Region*, 163–172.
132. Marks, C. 2004. *False tongues and Sunday bread: A Guatemalan and Mayan cookbook.* Takoma Park, MD: Takoma Books.
133. Figueroa, J. C., Paniagua-Avila, A., Sub Cuc, I., Cardona, S., Ramirez-Zea, M., Irazola, V., & Fort, M. P. (2022). Explanatory models of hypertension in Guatemala: Recognizing the perspectives of patients, family members, health care providers and administrators, and national-level health system stakeholders. *BMC Public Health*, 22(1), 1–14.
134. Edmonds, V.M. 2005. The nutritional patterns of recently immigrated Honduran women. *Journal of Transcultural Nursing*, 16, 226–235.
135. Mumford, J. 2014. Salvadoran Americans. In R.V. Dassanowsky & J. Lehman (Eds.), *Gale encyclopedia of multicultural America.* Farmington Hills, MI: Gale Group.
136. Fuster, M., & Colón-Ramos, U. 2018. Changing places, changing plates? A binational comparison of barriers and facilitators to healthful eating among central American communities. *Journal of Immigrant and Minority Health*, 20(3), 705–710.
137. Abbas, M., Aloudat, T., Bartolomei, J., Carballo, M., Durieux-Paillard, S., Gabus, L., . . . & Pittet, D. 2018. Migrant and refugee populations: a public health and policy perspective on a continuing global crisis. *Antimicrobial Resistance & Infection Control*, 7(1), 1–11.
138. Ablard, J.D. 2021. Framing the Latin American nutrition transition in a historical perspective, 1850 to the present. *História, Ciências, Saúde-Manguinhos*, 28, 233–253.
139. Wali, Y., Kini, V., & Yassin, M.A. 2020. Distribution of sickle cell disease and assessment of risk factors based on transcranial Doppler values in the Gulf region. *Hematology*, 25(1), 55–62.
140. Mathews, T.J, & MacDorman, M.F. 2010. Infant mortality statistics from the 2006 period linked birth/infant death data set. *National Vital Statistics Reports*, 58(17). Hyattsville, MD: National Center for Health Statistics.
141. Little, E.E., Polanco, M.A., Baldizon, S.R., Wagner, P., & Shakya, H. 2019. Breastfeeding knowledge and health behavior among Mayan women in rural Guatemala. *Social Science & Medicine*, 242, 112565.
142. Mirza, N.M., Kadow, K., Palmer, M., Solano, H., Rosche, C., & Yanovski, J.A. 2004. Prevalence of overweight among inner city Hispanic-American children and adolescents. *Obesity Research*, 12, 1298–1310.

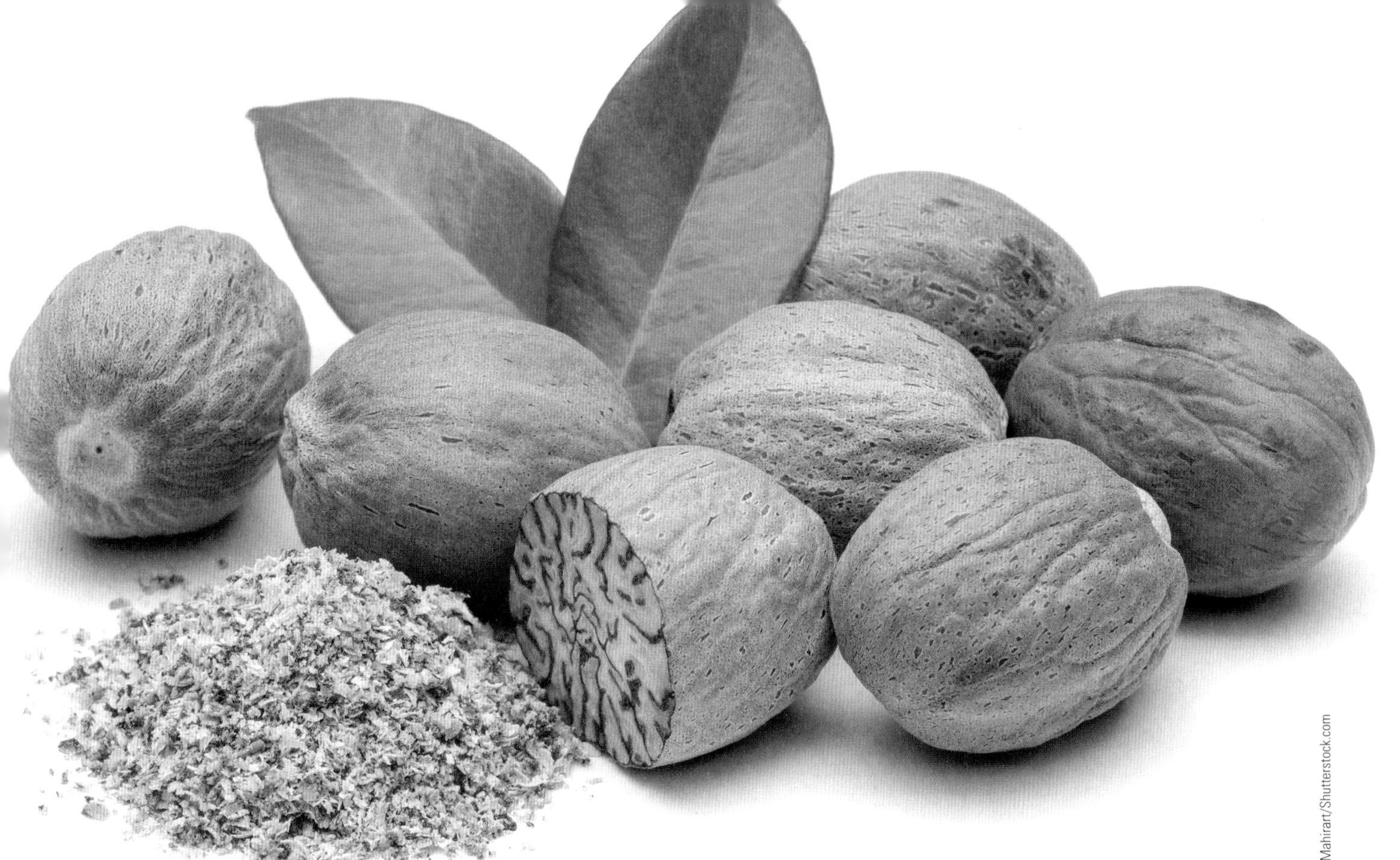

Chapter 10

Caribbean Islanders and South Americans

Learning Objectives

10.1 List the nations that are reviewed as part of the Caribbean Islands and South America.

10.2 Describe the immigration patterns, historical socioeconomic influences, and current locations of Caribbean Islanders and South Americans in America today.

10.3 Differentiate the religions, family structures, and traditional health beliefs and practices of the people of the Caribbean Islands and of South America before and after immigration to the United States.

10.4 Compare the differences and similarities among staple foods and preparation techniques within and across the Caribbean Islands and South America.

10.5 Compare key foods for each of the food groups for the Caribbean Islands and South America to how these foods have been adapted by immigrants in the United States.

10.6 Compare traditional meal composition and cycles to the meal composition and cycles of Caribbean Islanders and South Americans living in America today.

10.7 Describe regional specialties and dishes in the Caribbean Islands and South America.

10.8 Identify health concerns associated with the nutritional intake of people from the Caribbean Islands and South America.

Latinx people from the Caribbean islands and South America often seem disparate rather than similar to each other. Their homelands vary from the tropics of the islands and northern Brazil to the highland plains of Argentina and the snow-topped mountains of Peru. Their ethnic backgrounds include Indigenous, Spanish, Portuguese, French, British, Danish, Dutch, African, Asian Indian, Chinese, Italian, German, and Japanese. And although Roman Catholicism is practiced by a majority, many others follow Protestant faiths, Judaism, and numerous indigenous Afro-European religions including Voodoo (also Vodou, Vodú), Santería, and Candomblé.

Food for Thought

When Columbus landed in the Bahamas in 1492, he believed he had discovered a new route to the "Indies" (Asia) and called the native people "Indians." The Caribbean islands later became known as the West Indies often referred to in historical accounts and literature.

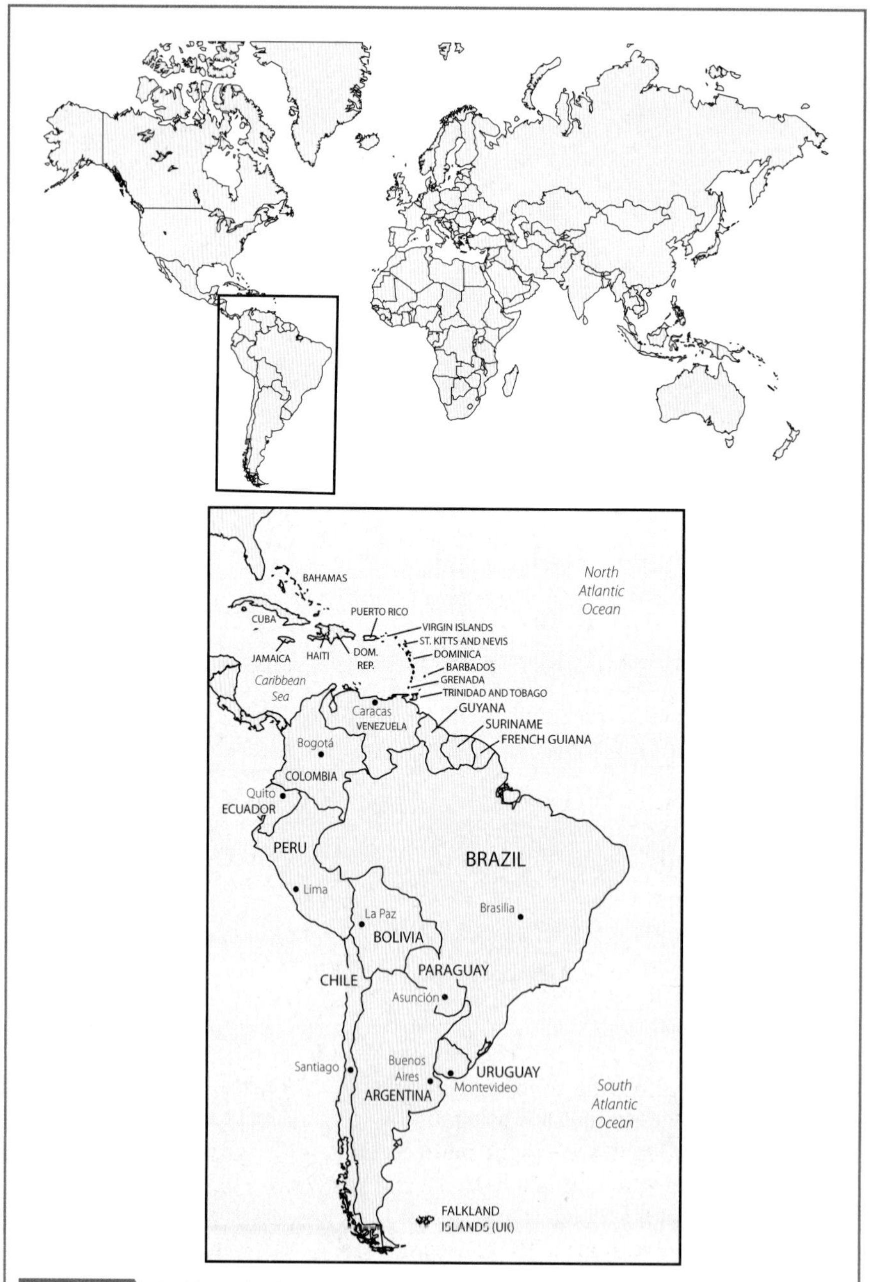

One commonality between Caribbean Islanders and South Americans is a variety of regional fares with few national cuisines. Dishes typically combine native ingredients with foods introduced from Africa, Asia, and Europe, with a broad preference for strong, spicy flavors. This chapter reviews Caribbean Islanders and their fare, focusing on Puerto Ricans, Cubans, and Dominicans. A summary of South Americans is also presented (refer to Figure 10.1). Other Latinx people are covered in Chapter 9.

Figure 10.1 Caribbean islands and South America.

Caribbean Islanders

More than 1,000 tropical islands in the Caribbean stretch from Florida to Venezuela. They include the Bahamas, the Greater Antilles (Jamaica, Cuba, Hispaniola, and Puerto Rico), and the Lesser Antilles. The largest island is Cuba, and the smallest islands are barely more than exposed rocks. In addition, the independent nations of Antigua/Barbuda, the Bahamas, Barbados, Cuba, Dominica, Dominican Republic, Grenada, Haiti, Jamaica, St. Christopher/Nevis, St. Lucia, St. Vincent/Grenadines, and Trinidad and Tobago, as well as the U.S. territory of Puerto Rico, are included in this classification, with many islands, such as the Virgin Islands (U.S.) and Martinique (France), still under foreign control.

The islands have lush plant cover that includes numerous indigenous fruits and vegetables. The tropical climate gives rise to stunning scenery, as well as torrential rains. Indigenous people, Europeans, Africans, and Asians have intermarried over the centuries to produce an extremely diverse population across all the islands.

Food for Thought

Bob Marley, one of Jamaica's greatest musicians, was responsible for reggae and Rastafarian music that continues today worldwide.

Cultural Perspective

History of Caribbean Islanders in the United States

Immigration Patterns It is estimated that the Latinx population was 61.4 million, or 18.5 percent, of the United States' total population in 2021. For Latinx people from the Caribbean, residents from Puerto Rico constituted the largest group, followed by those from Cuba and the Dominican Republic. In addition, there were small groups of immigrants from other Caribbean nations, most significantly from Jamaica and Haiti.[1,2]

Puerto Ricans Puerto Ricans differ from most other people who come to the United States in that they are technically not immigrants. They come to the mainland as U.S. citizens and are free to travel to and from Puerto Rico without restriction. Over half of all Puerto Rican people reside on the mainland of the United States, and the number of Puerto Ricans who live in New York City is almost double the number living in San Juan, the largest city in Puerto Rico.

Small numbers of political exiles from Puerto Rico arrived in America in the 1800s, but most returned home when Puerto Rico became a U.S. territory. Others arrived when unemployment increased in the depressed agricultural economy of the island during the 1920s and 1930s. The largest numbers of Puerto Ricans moved to the mainland after World War II. Unlike other immigrants, the Puerto Rican population in the United States is in continual flux and many Puerto Ricans live alternately between the mainland and the island, depending on economic conditions.[3]

Food for Thought

Terms of identity vary for Puerto Ricans, including Puerto Rican American, Borrinqueño or Boricua (used by those who prefer the native Taíno name for the island), and Nuyorican (used by second-generation Puerto Ricans living in New York City), among others.

Cubans Cuban people have immigrated to the United States since the early nineteenth century. In the early years, the majority were those who found economic conditions disadvantageous or who were politically out of favor with the government.

The majority of Cubans came to the United States after Fidel Castro overthrew the dictatorship of Fulgencio Batista in 1959. In the three years following the revolution, more than 150,000 Cubans arrived in America. Most of these were families from the upper socioeconomic group fleeing the restraints of communism. Commercial air travel between Cuba and the United States was suspended after the Cuban missile crisis in 1962. Airlifts of immigrants from 1965 to 1973 increased the total number of Cubans in the United States to nearly 700,000. Due to the political differences between the two countries, most Cubans have not been subject to the usual immigration quotas.

Immigration from Cuba slowed with the end of the airlifts. In 1980, another large group of 110,000 Cubans arrived in Florida in private boats (the Mariel boatlift) seeking asylum. After four decades of few immigrants coming to the U.S. from Cuba, in 2022 numbers soared to 220,000 migrants.

Dominicans Information on early immigrants from the Dominican Republic is limited because, before 1990, Dominicans were counted within the broader Latinx category in the U.S. Census data (in 1990 "Dominican" was a write-in category; in 2000 it became a check-off category).[1] Four immigration groups have been identified.[2] The first

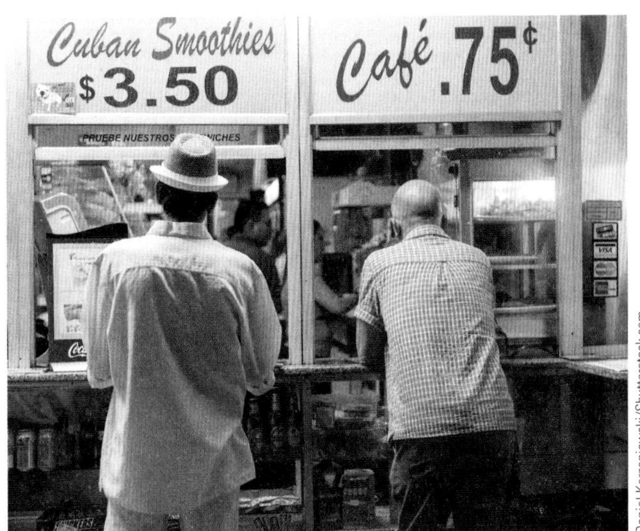

Daniel Korzeniewski/Shutterstock.com

▲ Cuban cafeteria with ventanitas (windows where you can order from the counter and go), Miami, Florida.

was during the Trujillo era (1930–1960) when political dissidents came to the United States to escape the regime of President Rafael L. Trujillo. The second group came during the post-Trujillo era (1961–1981) when improved social and economic conditions slowed emigration to a trickle. The third group (1982–1986) left the country by boat, seeking escape from oppressive poverty and hoping for a new start in the United States. The fourth group includes those who have left since the early 1980s, many of whom are urban Dominicans better educated than those they leave behind, seeking employment opportunities. Some Dominicans enter the U.S. mainland after making Puerto Rico their home. The numbers of Dominicans who are undocumented, or those who return to the island, are unknown.[2,4]

Current Demographics

Puerto Ricans The number of Puerto Ricans living on the U.S. mainland reached over 5 million in the 2020 Census estimates.[3] They are the second largest Latinx subgroup in the United States after Mexicans, making up 9.5 percent of the total U.S. Latinx population. Over 25 percent of Puerto Ricans make New York State their home, with most living in New York City.[4] In the 1930s, Puerto Ricans began moving into East Harlem, which became known both as El Barrio and as "Spanish Harlem."

Cubans In 2019, the U.S. Census estimated that the number of Americans of Cuban descent was under 2 million.[5] Most Cubans live in urban areas, but the largest number live in the Miami area, which is sometimes called "Little Havana," where the climate is similar to that of their homeland.[3]

Dominicans Approximately 2 million individuals of Dominican descent are living in the United States.[6–8] The majority live in the urban areas of New York, New Jersey, Massachusetts, and Florida.[4]

Other Caribbean Islanders Steady immigration to the United States during the 1990s increased the numbers of other Caribbean Islanders in 2017 to over 745,000 Jamaicans and nearly 680,000 residents from Haiti.[5] Many Jamaicans have settled in the cities of the Northeast and South.

Socioeconomic Status Immigrants from the Caribbean vary in both economic and educational attainment. More than 28 percent of Puerto Ricans live in poverty, which is higher than the rate for both the general U.S. population (24 percent) and Latinx people in the United States overall (18 percent). However, it should be noted that second-generation mainland Puerto Ricans living in regions outside New York may have a different socioeconomic profile, with significantly higher rates of college graduation and white-collar employment.[6] Economically, U.S. Cubans have a higher median income than non-Latinx Whites in the United States.[7] Dominicans have the same median earnings similar to other Latinx, but less than the U.S. population.[8]

Educational rates for first-generation immigrants from the Caribbean are very similar to those of other Latinx people. Figures from 2018 show that for adults, both Puerto Ricans and Cuban Americans graduate from high school at rates of 76 and 81 percent, respectively, which are somewhat below that of the general population. However, rates of high school attendance are lower for those who were born in Puerto Rico or Cuba. The percentage of Puerto Ricans and Cubans who have college degrees was 18 and 26 percent, while the total number of Americans with degrees was 30 percent.[9] Post-secondary education has increased with about 42 percent of U.S. Latinx adults having some college experience in 2019, up from 36 percent in 2010. Eighteen percent of Latinx people in the U.S. hold a bachelor's or higher degree.[6]

Many factors influence socioeconomic differences among Latinx groups from the Caribbean. Puerto Ricans living on the mainland are free to travel between the United States and their homeland, and the frequent changes in residence may hamper socioeconomic improvement. Many Puerto Ricans have chosen to reside in New York City, as a new community.

Furthermore, some Puerto Rican, Dominican, Jamaican, and Haitian people face biases similar to that experienced by those of African heritage. Racial distinctions are not as significant in the Caribbean islands, and more overt discrimination is a new challenge for some immigrants.[7] In contrast, Cubans in the United States are historically political refugees who emigrated out of necessity, not choice. There are a disproportionate number of Cubans in the United States from the upper socioeconomic levels, although many lost all their material possessions when they emigrated. Those from a lower socioeconomic status seek education and financial success but are often faced with historical discrimination and decreased access. Circumstances surrounding their immigration have influenced the general socioeconomic status of both groups in general.

Worldview

Ethnic identity is strongly maintained in the Puerto Rican, Cuban, and Dominican communities in the United States. Often, Puerto Rican Americans continue close ties with the island, frequently returning to visit family and friends. Many Cuban Americans believe it is important to retain their heritage because they cannot return. Dominican Americans sometimes consider their stay in the United States temporary and may resist acculturation to maintain their identity. In all three groups, Spanish may be spoken at home, but Caribbean Islanders were more likely to use English at home (32 percent) than those from South America (15 percent), Central America (7 percent), or Mexico (3 percent).[4,8–10]

Religion A majority of Caribbean Islanders remain Roman Catholics, although the church's historically dominant position has declined in recent decades. For example, although 73 percent of Puerto Ricans living on the mainland were raised Catholic, only 56 percent remain so.[11] Other Caribbean Islander groups who have been in the United States for shorter periods, such as Dominicans, are 95 percent Christian, of which 53 percent are Catholic.[11,12]

Several other religions are practiced on the islands, including Protestantism and Judaism. For example, a majority of Jamaicans, who at one time lived under British rule, belong to Protestant congregations, such as the Church of God and Seventh-Day Adventists. Folk religions are found as well. The best known of these is Voodoo (also Vodou, Vodún), a unique combination of West African tribal rituals syncretized with Catholic symbols and local customs. It was developed by descendants of the Dahomean, Kongo, Yoruba, and other enslaved ethnic groups transported to Saint-Domingue (Haiti today). To avoid persecution, Catholic saints were often placed on altars although to those followers they represented older customs from Africa: St. Patrick is associated with the African snake spirit Damballah, for example, and St. Christopher is identified with Bacoso, the god responsible for infectious illness. Certain rites, such as repeating the Hail Mary, making the sign of the cross, and baptism, are practiced in conjunction with ancestor worship, drums, and African dancing. Worship is family-based, and there is no central leadership or organization of activities. Typically, ceremonies are conducted for annual events such as Christmas and the harvest as well as for funerals.

Voodoo originated in Haiti and is called Vodou there. Other similar Afro-Catholic belief systems are found on other islands, such as Santería in Cuba and Puerto Rico. Many followers of Voodoo and Santería are also members of Christian faiths and do not believe there is any contradiction in practicing both religions simultaneously.[13] Rastafari is a Afro-Caribbean faith and political movement that began in Jamaica in the 1930s. Rastas practice a natural, simple lifestyle combined with Protestant Christianity, mysticism, and pan-African political consciousness.

Family The Puerto Rican family is based on the concept of compadrazgo, which means co-parenting. Grandparents, aunts and uncles, cousins, and godparents are all considered part of the immediate family, and responsible for the care of children.[14] Traditionally, men are the heads of households as well as being in charge of community matters. The oldest boys in the family are expected to help with the supervision of younger siblings, particularly daughters. Women maintain the home and are reserved in manner. As in most Latinx cultures, age is respected and elders are honored. Younger children are taught to defer even to older children. Duty to family is extremely important.[17]

Traditional Cuban families are also patriarchal and extend to include relatives. Godparents are significant in child-rearing. Children are deferential to elders and well-chaperoned in public.

Caribbean Islander family dynamics often change in the United States as work situations shift. Women who work, and who may make a higher income than the men in the family, often gain greater authority within the home. Caribbean Islander children also gain greater autonomy in the United States. Economic pressures, American values of individualism and equality, and intergenerational stress are often cited as the reason for nontraditional adaptations. Studies of early immigrants have shown that one-third of Dominican people, for example, lived in nuclear family groupings in the United States even though only 1 percent did so in the Dominican Republic. Dominican women in the United States also had fewer children than those on the island.[14]

Among the rural population of Haiti, common-law marriage is frequent, and it is acceptable for a man to maintain several different households as long as he supports each wife and their children. This system is believed to be a remnant of the polygamous societies found in parts of West Africa.[15] Gender roles are inflexible, with men responsible for farming and providing for the family, and women in charge of the household budget, marketing, and child care. Haitians have maintained more traditional families than some other Caribbean groups living in the United States. Typically, men still head the family, although Haitian American women often insist on a greater role in making decisions than is customary in Haiti. Haitian children are still expected to obey their parents, bring honor to their family, and reside at home until marriage. Haitian Americans establish a close network with other Haitian immigrants and often keep in touch with family and friends remaining in Haiti. Those who are unable to return for political reasons may sponsor voodoo ceremonies on their behalf.[7,15,16]

Traditional Health Beliefs and Practices Many Caribbean Islanders hold health beliefs similar to those of other Latin American cultures. For example, Puerto Rican, Cuban, Dominican, and Haitian people often believe that illness is a punishment from God, or that fate determines life and death. Prayer, the lighting of candles to saints, and the laying on of hands are important ways of maintaining health and curing disease.[17–19] In addition, some believe that all individuals have a guardian angel who protects them from evil. Some, especially Dominican and Haitian people, also believe illness can be caused by evil spirits or the devil.[20–22]

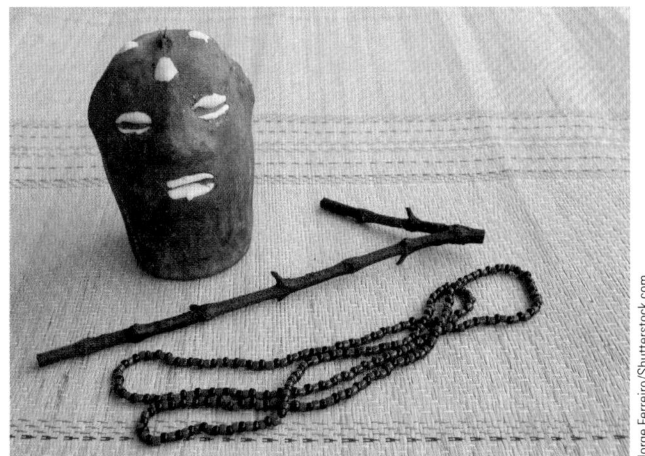

Jorge Ferreiro/Shutterstock.com

▲ **Serious conditions, such as sickness due to supernatural causes may be thought to require the cures associated with the healing practice of Santería.**

Nervios, a health condition, is recognized by many Puerto Ricans, but not by all. It can take several forms including crying bouts, headaches, stomach maladies, and sometimes causes a tendency toward violence.[23,24] This condition can be tempered by the use of herbal teas and talking with family members, religious advisers, or mental health professionals. Padecer de los nervios is a mental illness associated with depression that develops in adults. It is treated with the help of psychologists or psychiatrists. Ataques de nervios, also known as ataques, is a hysterical reaction to stressful events. It may include acute breathing difficulties, frenzy, or the sudden onset of illness. Nervios is a problem found more often in women than men, and it is associated with a weak character.[21] In general, nervios is helped by prayer, massage, sedatives, and herbal teas. Physicians and mental health specialists are also useful. Other folk conditions reported by Puerto Ricans include pasmo, a type of paralysis due to an imbalance of hot and cold, fatigue, and acute breathing difficulties.

Haitian people are especially concerned with the flow of blood, considered essential to balance health. Foods are placed in hot–cold categories depending on how they are digested. For example, a common belief is that after vigorous activity, people should not consume "cold" foods such as avocado, lime, and mango. Warm foods include eggs, raw rum, and nutmeg, among others. Many blood irregularities are recognized and classified as hot, cold, weak, thin, thick, dirty, and yellow.[15,17] Febles (general weakness) occurs when there is insufficient blood or anemia due to poor diet. The condition is cured by eating items such as liver, red meat, pigeon meat, cow's feet, or leafy green vegetables. Sezisman is a disruption of normal blood flow, due to sudden emotional trauma or chronic ill-treatment by others. It can cause vision loss, headaches, high blood pressure, or stroke. It is treated with relaxation, cold compresses, sipping cool water, or drinking coffee mixed with rum.[27] Haitian women may be encouraged to eat red fruits and vegetables (such as beets or pomegranates) to strengthen their blood.[19]

Gaz (gas) is another common condition for some Haitians. Gaz may settle between the ears, causing headache; in the stomach, causing indigestion; or in other parts of the body, where it causes pain. Eating leftovers (especially beans) is one cause of gaz. A nursing mother may undergo a thickening of her milk, which causes headaches or depression in the woman and impetigo in her baby. "Bad blood" (move san) is a more serious condition in which a nursing mother experiences fright or negative emotions, causing her milk to spoil, resulting in diarrhea and failure to thrive syndrome in her infant.[26] Some Haitian people believe mal dyok (evil eye) can also cause illness.

The traditional healing practices common in the Caribbean are more closely related to African beliefs than the Arab Spanish humoral system used in hot–cold applications. Mild conditions are treated through an informal system of older women (mothers, grandmothers, or neighbors) who are knowledgeable about the use of teas, herbs, amulets, and charms.[22,23] A study of Dominican healers found that the women learned their skills from relatives or through spiritual guidance.[28,29] When at home in the Dominican Republic, they treated only clients they knew personally from within their communities. In the United States, healers expanded their practice to include strangers and clients of all ethnicities. They typically accepted a wide variety of physical and psychological cases. When possible, the healers preferred to consult with the entire family in full support for recommended treatment.

More serious conditions, such as those that are thought to be due to supernatural causes, particularly witchcraft, require the cures associated with Voodoo and Santería. Voodoo priests (hougans or bokors), priestesses (mambos), or spiritualist healers (espiritos and santeros) intervene with the saints on behalf of a bewitched person (also noted in practices related to those of the American South; refer to Chapter 8). Santeros specialize in soul possession and mental disorders. Dreams may play an important role in health care because they are a connection with the supernatural world. Ancestors provide instructions to an individual regarding health behaviors through dreams. Brujos (witches) and curanderos (healers) (refer to Chapter 9 for more information) may also be sought for medical care.[24]

Dominicans often believe the best way to treat illness is to use a traditional healer who will consult with Catholic saints about which home remedies are appropriate for the symptoms.[25] This allows believers to address the spiritual and emotional aspects of physical problems as well as seek symptom relief. Many Haitian people recognize two types of illness. The first is a natural illness, due to a poor diet, blood conditions, bone displacement, or cold drafts and other environmental factors. These can be cured by home remedies or visits to biomedical practitioners. The second is a supernatural illness due to angry spirits. These can only be treated by a Voodoo feast for the dead (manger mort) ceremony.[26] Cubans often consider Santería a link to their past and while they use a biomedical provider for relief of physical symptoms, they may employ a santero to help them restore balance or counteract the circumstances that led to their illnesses.[27]

Good hygiene, especially daily bathing, is done to promote health among Puerto Ricans. Some Puerto Rican, Dominican, and other Caribbean people practice a modified version of the hot–cold classification system in their diet, and some use it for categorizing illness (refer to the "Therapeutic Uses of Food" section in this chapter).[21,28] Dominican healers may consider junk food, red meat, lack of exercise, emotional distress, contact with negative people, and environmental stresses as some contributing factors to health problems.[28] Haitians consider eating well, cleanliness, and regular sleep essential to health. Laxatives or enemas may be used to refresh the bowel, remove impurities, and prevent acne in children.[29]

Most Caribbean people use herbal teas, and over-the-counter medications are often used to relieve symptoms—Dominican people may also take baths with herbs or flowers. Many Americans of Caribbean Island heritage are also likely to use home remedies or visit bontánicas (herbal pharmacy) or a bodega (small market) to purchase cures (including antibiotics obtained without a prescription) as a first step in treating symptoms.[29,30] One study notes that some Dominican people refer to home remedies of all types as zumos, a word that, strictly translated, means "juices."[32]

Traditional Food Habits

Ingredients and Common Foods

Caribbean food habits across the region are remarkably similar for an area influenced by so many outside cultures. Indigenous people, as well as the Spanish, French, British, Dutch, Dane, African, Asian Indian, and Chinese, have all had an impact on the cuisine. Even so, the basic diet is similar throughout the region, with regional variations found on each island. In recent years, tourism has helped spread specialties from one nation to another to meet visitor expectations about what dishes are available, and the global economy has furthered the development of pan-Caribbean cuisine.[31,32]

Indigenous Foods The islands are naturally laden with fresh fruits and vegetables originally from Central or South America, including the staple cassava (two varieties of tuber, bitter and sweet, also known as manioc and yuca with tapioca a starch product of manioc), acerola (Barbados cherry, a small, sour fruit with exceptionally high vitamin C content), avocados, bananas and plantains, some varieties of beans, calabaza (a type of pumpkin), cashew apples (fruit of the cashew nut), cocoa, coconuts, corn, guavas, malanga (a mild yam-like tuber sometimes called cocoyam, yautia, tannier, or tannia), mammee apples (a small green fruit with flesh reminiscent of apricots), papayas (sometimes called pawpaws), pineapple, sapodilla or naseberry (a small fruit with aromatic flesh that has a gritty texture similar to pears), soursop (a fruit with a cotton-like consistency), several types of squash (including chayote, called chocho or christophene in the islands), sweet potatoes, and tomatoes. Fish and small birds are also plentiful.

As in Latin American areas, chili peppers grow profusely in the West Indies. Extremely hot varieties are favored, including Scotch bonnet and bird peppers (also called tepins—refer to Chapter 9, for more information on chilies). Native cuisine makes frequent use of these for flavoring, especially in pepper sauces, such as mixtures of cassava juice and chilies. Other native seasoning includes allspice, recao (*Eryngium foetidum*, a pungent herb also known as culantro, long cilantro, or shandon beni), and annatto (achiote).

Because of the abundance of fresh fruits and vegetables year-round, traditionally there was little need for complicated preparations or preservation of foods. Consequently, some cooking techniques were not as developed in native populations. Cassava was baked most often in a kind of bread, made from pressed, dried, grated cassava that was fried in a flat loaf. Fish and game were either covered with mud, baked in a pit, or grilled over an open fire.

Food for Thought

Cassava contains hydrocyanic acid, which is toxic in large amounts. The acid must be leached out and the tuber cooked before it can be eaten safely.

Foreign Influence Despite the abundant supply of native fruits and vegetables, Europeans who settled in the Caribbean longed for the accustomed tastes of home and began raising familiar comfort foods where they lived. The Spanish brought cattle, goats, hogs, and sheep to the islands, in addition to introducing rice. Plants introduced for trade by the Europeans included breadfruit, coffee, limes, mangoes, oranges (both sweet and sour varieties), and spices such as ginger, nutmeg, and mace. Africans influenced food history by cultivating akee (a mild, apple-sized fruit), yams, okra, and taro (also called eddo or dasheen; both the roots and the leaves are eaten). The demand for Asian ingredients by later immigrants resulted in the introduction of soybean products, Asian greens, lentils, and tamarind to the Caribbean.

Food for Thought

Nearly all parts of the akee fruit (that grows on evergreen trees most abundantly in Jamaica) contain hypoglycins, which can cause severe hypoglycemia if eaten when unripe. Because of this toxicity, most akee products are banned in the United States. However, Jamaican cooks with knowledge on how to handle the fruit often use the slightly bitter and nutty-tasting ackee as a vegetable with onions, tomatoes, sweet peppers, chilies, allspice, and salt fish.

Staples Legumes are often eaten throughout the Caribbean in the dish "rice and peas." Rice with red (kidney) beans is popular in Puerto Rico and is also found in the Dominican Republic and Jamaica (where the dish is nicknamed "coat of arms"). Black beans with rice, called Moros y Cristianos ("Moors and Christians," in a reference to Spanish history), are preferred in Cuba. In Haiti, black-eyed peas (a type of cowpea from Africa) are combined with rice. The legumes in all countries are prepared similarly, flavored with lard and salt. Onions, sweet peppers, and tomatoes or coconut milk are added in some variations. Other popular legumes include pigeon peas, popularly known as gungo (originally from Africa, often cooked with rice, also), lentils (from India), chickpeas (also known as garbanzo beans, introduced from Europe and originally from the Middle East and Mediterranean region), and bodi beans (another variety of cowpea eaten as a green bean, also called Chinese long beans).

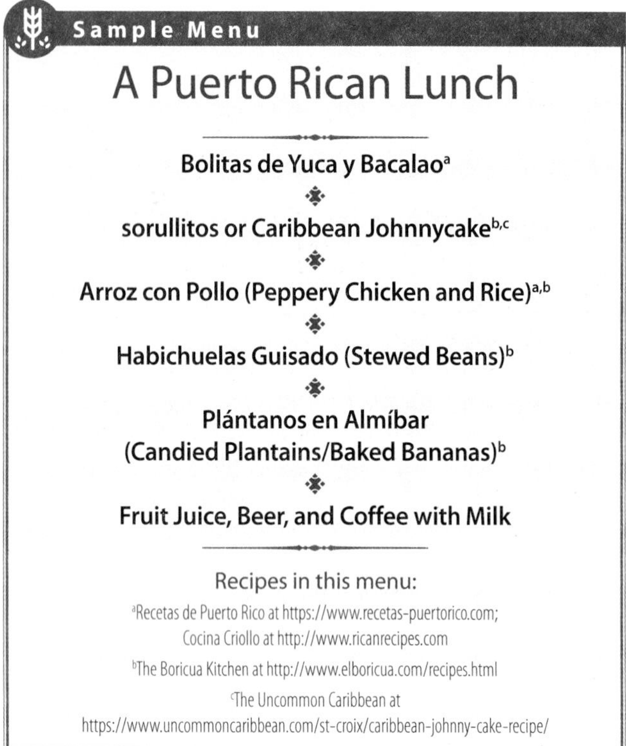

Sample Menu

A Puerto Rican Lunch

Bolitas de Yuca y Bacalao[a]

sorullitos or Caribbean Johnnycake[b,c]

Arroz con Pollo (Peppery Chicken and Rice)[a,b]

Habichuelas Guisado (Stewed Beans)[b]

Plántanos en Almíbar (Candied Plantains/Baked Bananas)[b]

Fruit Juice, Beer, and Coffee with Milk

Recipes in this menu:

[a]Recetas de Puerto Rico at https://www.recetas-puertorico.com; Cocina Criollo at http://www.ricanrecipes.com

[b]The Boricua Kitchen at http://www.elboricua.com/recipes.html

[c]The Uncommon Caribbean at https://www.uncommoncaribbean.com/st-croix/caribbean-johnny-cake-recipe/

Examples of other foods common throughout the West Indies are found in the cultural food groups list (Table 10.1). They include Native foods such as cassava bread, chili sauces, and pepper pot (a meat stew made with the boiled juice of the cassava, called cassareep). Tamales and pasteles are steamed cornmeal, cassava, or plantain dough packets with savory (such as meat, seafood, or cheese) or sweet (including coconut or guava) fillings. European-influenced items popular in many Caribbean countries include escabeche (fried, marinated seafood or poultry), asopao (a thick rice soup with chicken, pork, or seafood, often garnished with Parmesan cheese in Puerto Rico and slices of avocado or fried plantains in the Dominican Republic), morcillas (a type of blood sausage), flaky pastry turnovers with meat, poultry, seafood, or fruit fillings, and fried corn cakes (known as sorullitos in Puerto Rico). Foods from Africa found throughout the region include callaloo (taro or malanga greens cooked with okra), dried salt cod fritters which have a different name on nearly every island (bacalaitos in Puerto Rico, accras de morue in several islands, Jamaica's "stamp and go"), foofoo made from plaintain or cassava or a mixture, and cou-cou, a cornmeal-okra bread. Dishes from India and Asia are also common on many islands, although they are better known in the areas where cheap labor was most needed: the islands dominated by the French, British, and Dutch (few Asians immigrated to Puerto Rico, Cuba, or the Dominican Republic). Curried dishes, called kerry on the Dutch-influenced islands, and colombo on the French-influenced islands, and variations of pilaf are considered Caribbean foods. Chinese cuisine is also popular and Chinese-owned restaurants are omnipresent.

Food for Thought

The Indies refers to a collection of islands in the Caribbean Sea and the Atlantic Ocean that have nothing to do with India but were misnamed when Christopher Columbus arrived in Hispaniola in 1492. The region was renamed the West Indies after it was realized that the islands were not, in fact, the Indian subcontinent, and to distinguish them from the Southeast Asian East Timor, India, Indonesia, and the Malay Archipelago.

The most popular beverage in the Caribbean is coffee. It is often mixed with milk and is consumed at meals, as a snack, and even as dessert, flavored with orange rind, cinnamon, whipped cream, coconut cream, or rum. Some of the most expensive coffee in the world is produced in the Blue Mountains of Jamaica, where the cool, moderately rainy climate is ideal for coffee cultivation. Most of the rich beans are exported to England and Italy, although small amounts can be found in the United States.

The most important beverage in the Caribbean, at least historically, is the spirit distilled from fermented molasses—rum. This alcoholic drink is believed to have originated on the island of Barbados in the early 1600s as a by-product of sugarcane processing. Molasses is the liquid that remains after the syrup from the sugarcane has been crystallized to make sugar. It is fermented, naturally or with the addition of yeast, and then distilled to make a clear, high-proof alcoholic beverage. Rum can be bottled immediately or aged in oak casks from a few months to 25 years. Caramel is added to achieve the desired color. Nearly every island produces its own variety of rum.

The molasses produced in the West Indies was crucial to the development of the region during the seventeenth and eighteenth centuries. The Caribbean islands were one part of the infamous route formed when molasses was shipped to New England for distillation into rum, then shipped to Africa in exchange for enslaved people.

Juices made from tropical fruits such as lime, otaheite apple (also called ambarella, originally from Polynesia), pineapple, roselle (also known as "Jamaican sorrel," brought from Africa), soursop, and tamarind are common. Ginger often spices the juice mixtures, and coconut milk or condensed milk may also be added.

Regional Variations Despite the similarities in foods throughout the Caribbean, some regional differences are notable. Same-named dishes prepared on one island may not taste the same on another island due to variations in ingredients and seasoning. For example, butter is the preferred cooking fat in French-influenced countries, whereas lard is more popular in Spanish-influenced nations. Coconut oil is common in Jamaica. In British-influenced countries, dishes often include scallions, parsley or cilantro, and thyme. On French-influenced islands roux (flour blended with butter or oil, then cooked until browned) is used to

Table 10.1 Cultural Food Groups: Caribbean Islands

Group	Comments	Common Foods	Adaptations in the United States
Protein Foods			
Milk/milk products	Few dairy products are used; incidence of lactose intolerance is assumed to be high. Infants are given whole, evaporated, or condensed milk.	Cow's milk (fresh, condensed, evaporated), *café con leche, café latte*; aged cheeses	More milk and cheese are consumed.
Meat/poultry/fish/ eggs/legumes	Traditional diet is high in vegetable protein, especially rice and legumes; red and kidney beans are used by Puerto Ricans, black beans by Cubans. Pork and beef are used more in Spanish-influenced countries. Dried salt cod is preferred over fresh fish; some seafood specialties. Eggs are a common protein source, especially among the poor. Entrées are often fried in lard or olive oil.	*Meats*: beef, pork (including intestines, organs, variety cuts), goat *Poultry*: chicken, turkey *Fish and shellfish*: *bacalao* (dried salt cod), barracuda, bonito, butterfish, crab, dolphin fish (*dorado*), flying fish, gar, grouper, grunts, land crabs, mackerel, mullets, *ostiones* (tree oysters), porgie, salmon, snapper, tarpon, turtle, tuna *Eggs*: chicken *Legumes*: black beans, black-eyed peas, chick-peas (garbanzo beans), kidney beans, lima beans, peas, red beans, soybeans	More beef and poultry are eaten as income increases, though pork intake may decline. Less fresh fish is consumed. Traditional entrées remain popular.
Cereals/Grains	Breads of other countries are well accepted. Fried breads are popular.	Cassava bread; cornmeal (fried breads, *sorullitos*, puddings); oatmeal; rice (short-grain); wheat (Asian Indian breads, European breads, pasta)	Short-grain rice is still preferred. More wheat breads are eaten.
Fruits/Vegetables	Starchy fruits and vegetables are eaten daily; leafy vegetables are consumed infrequently. Great diversity of tropical fruits is available, eaten mostly as snacks or dessert. Lime juice is used to "cook" (a marinating method called escabeche or ceviche) meats and fish.	*Fruits*: acerola cherries, akee, avocados, bananas and plantains, breadfruit, *caimito* (star apple), cashew apple, *cherimoya*, citron, coconut, cocoplum, custard apple, gooseberries, *granadilla* (passion fruit), grapefruit, guava, *guanábana* (soursop), jackfruit, kumquats, lemons, limes, *mamey*, mangoes, oranges, papayas, pineapple, pomegranates, raisins, *sapodilla*, sugarcane, sweetsop, tamarind *Vegetables*: *arracacha*, arrowroot, black-eyed peas, broccoli, cabbage, *calabaza* (green pumpkin), *callaloo* (malanga or taro leaves), cassava (*yuca*, manioc), chiles, corn, cucumbers, eggplant, green beans, lettuce, *malan-gas*, okra, onions, palm hearts, peppers, potatoes, radishes, spinach, squashes (chayote, summer, and winter), sweet potatoes, taro (*eddo, dasheen*), tomatoes, yams	Temperate fruits are substituted for tropical fruits when latter are unavailable. More fresh fruit is eaten. Starchy fruits and vegetables are still frequently consumed. Low intake of leafy vegetables is often continued.
Additional Foods			
Seasonings	Aromatic, piquant sauces are often used to flavor foods. Very hot chiles popular in some regions.	Anise, annatto, bay leaf, chiles, chives, cilantro (coriander leaves), cinnamon, *coui* (chiles mixed with cassava juice), garlic, mace, nutmeg, onions, parsley, *pimento* (allspice), *recao* (culantro), scallions, thyme	
Beverages	Teas of all sorts are common and are often thought to have therapeutic value. Rum is especially popular and is often added for flavoring to foods and beverages.	Beer, coffee (*café con leche*), teas, soft drinks, milk, rum, Irish moss (seaweed extract), sorrel	Fruit juice and soft drink consumption may increase.
Fats/oils		Butter in French-influenced countries; coconut oil; *ghee* (Asian Indian clarified butter); lard in Spanish-influenced countries; olive oil	
Sweeteners		Sugarcane products, such as raw and unrefined sugar and molasses	

thicken stews and sauces, and sauce chien ("dog sauce") is a popular fresh condiment served with pork, chicken, and seafood, made with olive oil and lime juice often seasoned with ginger, garlic, scallions, parsley, chilies, allspice, and thyme. A similar preparation known as sauce ti-malice is found in Haiti. Spanish-influenced islands use seasonings with less heat, including greater use of tomatoes, onions, annatto (a red coloring made from the seeds of the achiote tree), and sweet bell peppers.

Each island is also known for its specialties. In addition to rice and red beans, Puerto Rican fare is notable for its use of distinctive flavorings, such as alcaparrado, a pickle mix of capers, olives, and pimento, and recaito, an aromatic blend of recao, onions, garlic, and bell peppers. Sofrito, an all-purpose sauce that is the foundation for many Puerto Rican dishes, combines alcaparrado and recaito with tomatoes. Some foods are seasoned with adobo, a mixture of lemon, garlic, salt, pepper, and other spices. Ajilimojili sauce is a puree of bell peppers, garlic, olive oil, and lemon juice. Sazón, a commercial spice blend that is a mix of monosodium glutamate (MSG, used to enhance flavors), salt, garlic, cumin, coriander, and coloring agents is a popular seasoning as well, though in recent years, making home blends are encouraged to avoid the MSG version.[29,31,32]

Starchy foods have a central role in Puerto Rican cuisine, traditionally consumed at nearly every meal as a side dish or in soups and stews. They are known as viandas and include bland-tasting, white- or creamy-colored roots, tubers, and fruits that must be cooked, such as cassava, malanga, potatoes, sweet potatoes (white or yellow are preferred), yams, celery root, breadfruit (and breadfruit seeds), underripe bananas, and plantains.[19,31,33] One especially popular preparation is mofongo, fried and mashed plantains flavored with either pork cracklings or bacon. Calabaza (winter squash) and carrots are significant sources of vitamins.

Pork is a favorite meat in Puerto Rico, especially roast pork adobo. It is also used frequently for added flavor in the form of salt pork, ham, cracklings, or bacon. Beef and goat are also consumed. One very popular stew is sancocho, which includes beef short ribs, calabaza, malanga, yams, and corn. Chicken is frequently prepared with rice as arroz con pollo and served with stewed beans (known as habichuelas guisada), or in asopao. Land crabs and ostiones, a type of oyster that grows on the roots of mangrove trees, are eaten, as is some seafood, including shrimp, lobster, and conch, often prepared as soups or stews. Fresh fish is not consumed frequently (though a few dishes, such as escabeche, are popular), but dried salt cod, called bacalao, is used in many dishes. It is soaked and drained before being used to remove some of the salt and then added to numerous dishes including serenata, a mixture of cod and potatoes. Variety meats are featured in several national dishes, such as mondongo (tripe soup), lengua relleno (stuffed tongue), rinones guisados (calf kidneys), and sesos empanados (calf brains).[31]

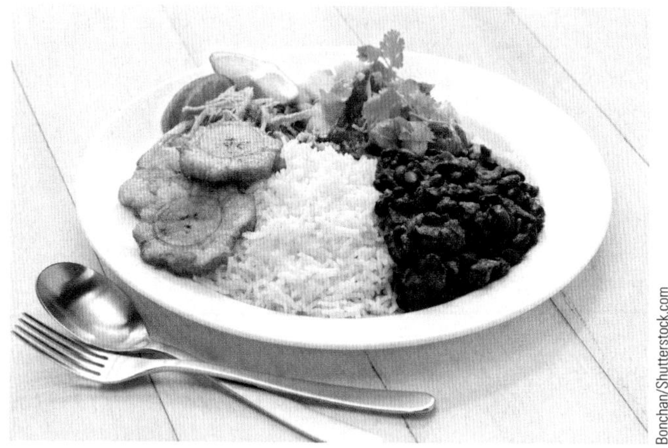
Bonchan/Shutterstock.com

▲ A Cuban meal with black beans, rice, and tostones (twice-fried plantains).

Fritturas, or finger foods, are also a specialty, consumed as snacks or appetizers or added to meals. They include simple fritters (e.g., banana, squash, or bacalaitos); alcapurrias (starchy vegetable dough stuffed with spicy beef, pork rind, poultry, or seafood and then fried); piñones (plantain strips wrapped around sausage, poultry, or seafood fillings and fried); pastelillos (fried meat or cheese turnovers); and cuchifritos (deep-fried chitterlings or variety meats). Empanadillas, small baked turnovers typically filled with ham, beef, lobster, conch, or cheese, are also a favorite. Sweets including cakes, pastries, puddings, and cookies are popular for desserts and snacks. One specialty is tembleque, the Puerto Rican version of Spanish-style flan. Flans are also flavored with chocolate, coconut, pineapple, pumpkin, or rum. Candied ripe plantains and baked bananas are common fruit-based sweets in Puerto Rico, also found throughout the Caribbean.

Though changing, over 80 percent of the food in Puerto Rico is imported from the mainland. Early priorities of colonizers (where sugar production, not food production, was encouraged or demanded), and other factors such as natural disasters, economic crises, and mismanagement, led to most foods coming from outside the island.[34] American dishes are common, especially among younger diners. Pizza, canned spaghetti, hot dogs, canned soups, and cold cereals have become favorites.[33,35] Empanadillas (savory pastries), rellenos de papa (potato croquettes stuffed with ground beef hash), and tostones (crispy, salty, fried green plantain slices that have been pressed flat) are among the local foods that are well-liked.

Cuba is noted for the prominent use of black beans in its cuisine. In addition to black beans and rice, spicy black bean soup is very popular. As in Puerto Rico, viandas, tropical root vegetables often served like a potato with meat or fish, are standard fare, especially in the more rural eastern sections of the island where Indigenous heritage is prominent. Favorites include foofoo (cassava balls) and tostones. Meats and viandas are often served with mojito, a sauce of olive oil, juice from limes or sour oranges, onions, and garlic.[36]

The western parts of the island are more urban and cosmopolitan, especially around Havana, where Spanish and Asian culinary influences are evident. Picadillo is a type of beef hash flavored with the traditional Spanish ingredients featured in alcaparrado (the same mix of olives, raisins, and capers used in Puerto Rico), as well as Caribbean tomatoes and chili peppers. Picadillo is served with fried plantains or boiled rice, or topped with fried eggs. Other Spanish-influenced beef dishes are ropa vieja ("old clothes"), made of spicy beef strips cooked until they begin to shred, and brazo gitano, a cassava dough pastry filled with corned beef. Roast pork is popular, and eggs are often prepared as Spanish-style potato omelets. Of note: rice and beans are usually served separately in this region. Asian ingredients are less prominent but notable. *Chicharrónes de pollo* is prepared with small pieces of chicken marinated in lime juice and soy sauce, breaded, and then fried in lard. Another example is arroz salteado, a fried rice dish made with eggs, shrimp, and vegetables cooked in olive oil and seasoned with soy sauce. Fish are eaten in western coastal areas, and one specialty is grilled or stewed crocodile.[31,33,34] Fruit pastes, such as those made from guava, are typical desserts, sometimes served with a slice of salty cheese. Spanish-style egg desserts are also found, especially custards, flans, and puddings. Turrones, a nougat candy made with peanuts, is a Cuban favorite.

Stews are a specialty in the Dominican Republic. Examples include pollo guisado (chicken with bell peppers, tomatoes, onions, and olives, seasoned with oregano), mondongo (similar to the Puerto Rican tripe soup), and stews made with fish or seafood, such as shrimp, conch, or herring. Best known is the Dominican version of sancocho made with several kinds of meats (including pork, chicken, beef, and Spanish-style longaniza pork sausage), plus numerous starchy vegetables cooked in sour orange juice. On special occasions, additional types of meats (e.g., goat, ham) are added to make sancocho prieto. Stews are often served with rice and red beans, and cassava bread.

Locrio is another Dominican favorite—a rice dish that has its origins in Spanish paella (see Chapter 6 for more information), but differs in that only a single item, such as chicken, shrimp, or sardines, distinguishes each version. Other common dishes include chicharrónes de pollo (prepared like the Cuban recipe), rice with chicken and pigeon peas, and mangu (mashed plantains topped with olive oil-fried onions). Salads are especially popular in the Dominican Republic. A few salads feature lettuce and tomatoes, but, more often, cooked vegetables such as okra, potatoes, chayote squash, or cabbage are cooled and dressed with oil and vinegar. Avocado and hearts of palm (a specialty of the island) are featured in other versions. Habichuelas con dulce is a unique Dominican dish served as a side dish or as a dessert, combining red beans, coconut milk, evaporated milk, whole milk, sugar, and butter.[30,37] Desserts include fruit compotes, Spanish-style flan, plantains or guavas with caramel sauce, coconut biscuits, or sweet potato or squash puddings.

Jamaica specialties include akee fruit and salt cod, curried goat, bammies, a type of cassava bread, mackerel rundown, cooked in coconut milk with vegetables, and jerked foods (see the Exploring Global Cuisine box for more information). Haiti is known for its banana-stuffed chicken dish called *poulet rôti à la créole* and barbecued goat with chile peppers (kabrit boukannen ak bon piman). Griot is another popular dish made with pork that is first marinated in seasoned sour orange juice, then boiled, and then fried. Patties, a curried meat turnover, are a Haitian specialty now served throughout the Caribbean. Common Haitian side dishes include cornmeal mush and *diri ak djon djon* (also called riz noir, or black rice, this is rice cooked in a broth made by boiling dried mushrooms native to the island called djon djon—the mushrooms themselves are not consumed). Curaçao is famous for its orange-flavored liqueur of the same name, and, in Dominica, crapaud, or "mountain chicken," a large, tasty frog, is considered a delicacy. In Barbados, many more unusual seafood dishes are popular, including those made with flying fish, green turtles, and sea urchins.

Meal Composition and Cycle

The most typical aspect of a Caribbean meal is its emphasis on starchy vegetables with some meat, poultry, or fish served with rice and beans. Bread of all sorts is now common in many areas. Meats are frequently fried or grilled. Sometimes before the meat is added to mixed dishes it is cooked first with sugar to caramelize it (a technique thought to have been brought by Africans).[38] Soups and stews are also popular. Soups are sometimes served in two courses—the strained broth first, followed by the cooked meats and vegetables. Leafy vegetables are sometimes ingredients in soups, stews, and stuffed foods, are and only served uncooked as part of the lettuce and tomato salads found in many regions, including Puerto Rico, Cuba, and the Dominican Republic. Fruits are eaten infrequently in many areas but are found fresh in some desserts and as snacks.

As in most countries, ethnic heritage and social class determine which dishes are served.[38] An Indigenous person without means may eat mostly cassava, tomatoes, and chilies with a bit of salted fish at every meal. An Asian Indian may serve typically Asian Indian meals adapted to Caribbean ingredients, such as a curried dish garnished with coconut, fried plantains, and pineapple. Most menus, however, consist of a multicultural mix, such as European blood sausage and accra, West African-style fritters made from the meal of soybeans or black-eyed peas. More meats and foreign dishes are consumed by wealthy Caribbean Islanders and some reportedly visit the United States weekly to shop for groceries.[30] American fast foods have become popular throughout the region at all economic levels.

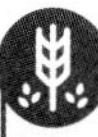

Sample Menu

A Caribbean Sampler

Patties (Haiti, Jamaica)[a]

Fritters-Black-Eyed Pea, Salt-Cod, or Conch (Pan-Island)[a,b]

Callaloo Soup (Pan-Island)[a]

Puerco Asado (Cuban Pork Roast)[a,b]

Mangú (Dominican Republic)[c]

Black Cake/Rum Cake (Pan-Island)[d]

Recipes in this menu:

[a]Caribbean Recipes at http://www.recipezaar.com/recipes/caribbean

[b]Cuban Recipes at http://www.recipehound.com/Recipes/cuba.html

[c]Aunt Clara's Kitchen Dominican Cooking at http://www.dominicancooking.com/dominican-recipes/

[d]Food 52 at https://food52.com/recipes/78421-black-cake

Daily Patterns Meal patterns vary somewhat throughout the region. Three meals each day, with lunch being the largest meal, is typical in most regions. In Haiti, however, two meals a day is not uncommon.

In Puerto Rico, the traditionally large lunch and smaller dinners are gradually changing to a dining schedule similar to that on the mainland, especially in urban areas. Toast and coffee are a common breakfast, though eggs are popular as well, often served as a Spanish-style omelet. Lunch and dinner menus may be similar, starting with soup (such as black bean soup or chicken with rice soup), followed by a stew served with rice and beans, fried plantains, and chayote squash. Quick lunches, such as fast-food fare, may replace the full meal. Dessert is usually eaten daily, following whichever meal is largest, lunch or dinner. Bread puddings with rum sauce are favored. Soda, fruit juice, beer, or rum accompany the meal. Restaurants are widely available in the cities, serving traditional Puerto Rican cuisine, as well as international fares, such as Spanish, Italian, and Japanese. Snacking is prevalent, particularly on fried items, such as bacalaitos, sorullitos, and cuchifritos.

Toast and coffee is a customary breakfast in Cuba, often followed by a midmorning coffee break with pastries or cakes. Lunch and dinner menus are similar, with meat, poultry, or

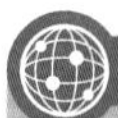

Exploring Global Cuisine

Specialty Cooking of Jamaica

The nearly half million Americans of Jamaican ancestry have had a significant impact on U.S. pop culture. Calypso, reggae, the Rastafari religion, and locs are among the many cultural additions. Locs (often the preferred to the outdated term, dreadlocks or dreds, used by colonizers to mean the style was dreadful) is hair sculpted into ropes. They are created by coiling, braiding, twisting, or allowing to hair to "lock" naturally by not combing it and allowing it to take on rope-like forms over time. Locs are generally considered a style particularly connected to the people across the African diaspora. In cuisine, two regional specialties have piqued American interest: jerk and i-tal foods.

The jerk cooking technique is believed to have been developed by the Jamaican Taino, an Arawak people greatly decimated by European discovery, and the Maroons (from the Spanish word for "mountaineer" referring to Africans who escaped from Spanish slave traders into the mountains of Jamaica in the seventeenth century). The Maroons and Tanio shared culinary traditions to survive enemies. The result was a technique to transform tough cuts of meat (traditionally wild boar) into tender dishes. The Maroons and Tanio used available spices (traditionally allspice berries, salt, and bird peppers), pepper elder leaves to wrap the meat in, and an underground smokeless pit method of cooking to evade discovery.[39] This history gives jerk cooking a deeper connection to Jamaican culture and can connote freedom. Today, the word jerk is used to identify the wet spice mixture used as a barbecue seasoning. It includes allspice, black pepper, cinnamon, ginger, nutmeg, thyme, scallions, and extremely hot Scotch bonnet chili peppers—some recipes also call for garlic, onions, ground coriander, bay leaves, brown sugar, or other seasonings. The spices are moistened with a little oil, lime juice, or soy sauce to make a paste. Traditionally, the meat is rubbed with the jerk blend and marinated for several hours. It is then grilled in a pit over Jamaican pimento (allspice) wood, covered with banana leaves, typically for one to four hours, depending on the meat. Though pork and chicken are found at every street jerk stand in Jamaica, more recently the cooking technique has been applied to turkey, fish, seafood, and even vegetables. Jerk pork is used to make jerk sausage in some parts of Jamaica. For a complete meal, rice and peas, cassava bread, or cornsticks accompany the meat.[40]

I-tal, meaning "vital," is the Rasta way of life. Applied to food it emphasizes simple, unprocessed vegetarian fare. Fruit, vegetables, and grains are permitted, while pork, red meat, salt, and artificial additives are prohibited. This way of eating is similar to plant-based or whole-food diets in the United States. Some Rastas will eat chicken or fish (but shun bottom feeders such as shrimp and lobster, scaleless fish such as shark, and any fish more than twelve inches long). In general, milk, coffee, soft drinks, and alcohol are not consumed. I-tal foods are ideally eaten raw or cooked over a fire (microwave ovens are avoided by many Rastas), prepared and served using pots, dishes, and utensils made from natural products, such as wood or earthenware. Typical i-tal dishes include rice and peas, cassava bread, baked yams, vegetable stews, cornmeal porridge, sautéed plantains, and freshly squeezed juices. Thyme, cinnamon, allspice, coconut, and reputedly marijuana are used to flavor foods.[41,42]

fish served with fried plantains, rice and black beans, and often cassava. Custards and puddings (bread or rice) are typical desserts. Coffee is served after the meal. Lunch is typically the largest meal of the day, even in urban areas, and dinner is often leisurely, and may include beer, rum, or wine. Snacking on fruit, fruit juices, batidas (fruit juice blended with milk and ice), or ice cream is frequent.

In the Dominican Republic, breakfast may be just bread and coffee, but more often it is larger, including eggs, cheese, and salami or longaniza sausage (scrambled together, or each fried separately), fried or mashed plantains, and espresso or hot chocolate. Lunch is usually the biggest meal of the day, traditionally served between noon and 2 p.m. La Bandera ("the flag") Dominicana is a lunch consisting of red beans and rice often with meat (pork, chicken, beef, or fish), and salad, incorporating the colors similar to national banner.[10] Plantains or other starchy vegetables may also accompany lunch. Dessert always follows, and espresso or sweetened coffee with milk ends the meal. American meal patterns are influencing many Dominicans, and abbreviated lunches are becoming more common, including only a main dish, dessert, and coffee. When lunch is the main meal of the day, dinner is light, consisting of scrambled eggs or soup, and fried plantains or cassava bread. But when lunch is light, dinner is more substantial, similar to the traditional lunch.

Jamaicans often include fish at breakfast, including sardines, mackerel, herring, or salt cod. Other common items are eggs, fried plantains, cornmeal porridge, and bammies. On the weekends, liver with bananas is a breakfast specialty. Lunches and dinners are similar to those of other Caribbean Islanders, including soups, rice, and peas with added beef, chicken, or curried goat, pork stews, fish dishes, and tossed salad or sweet potatoes on the side.[10]

Special Occasions Early European dominance in the West Indies resulted in an emphasis on Christian holidays. Christmas is important, especially in the Spanish-influenced islands that are predominantly Catholic. In Puerto Rico, pasteles are prepared to celebrate Christmas. Similar to Mexican tamales, pasteles are a savory meat mixture surrounded by cornmeal or mashed plantains, wrapped in plantain leaves, and steamed. Carolers traditionally stop at houses late at night to request hot pasteles from the occupants. Christmas Eve, or Noche Buena, includes Mass and a feast with lechón asado (spit-roasted pig), morcillas, rice with pigeon peas, coquito (rum and coconut milk), and special desserts such as rice pudding and coconut custard. In the Dominican Republic, a whole-roasted pig is also customary, served with rice and peas, and a salad. Cubans associate pasteles with large turnovers or pastelitos (smaller turnovers) at the holidays as well and make them with a dough that is similar to French puff-pastry, stuffed with spicy meat or cheese fillings, or sweet fillings, such as guava, mango, or coconut.[10]

Other holidays reflect the multicultural history of the islands. Carnival is celebrated in some Caribbean countries such as Trinidad and Tobago and is similar to Mardi Gras in the United States. The pre-Lenten festivities feature parades of dancing celebrants; many are elaborately costumed as traditional European or African figures. Food booths that line the parade route provide a day-and-night supply of carnival treats. Fried Asian Indian fritters are particularly popular.

Examples of nonreligious events include the day-long birthday open house for friends, relatives, and acquaintances. Thanksgiving is observed in Puerto Rico, but it has little to do with Pilgrims and Native Americans. This holiday began in 1898 when the island was invaded by the United States and the people of Puerto Rico adopted this ritual, which is mainly celebrated as a day for sharing and preparing for the Christmas season.[43] Turkey, stuffed with a Spanish-style meat filling, is the main course. Rum cake (also known as black cake) is a fruitcake specialty of the Caribbean, especially in Jamaica, where it is served at weddings, Christmas, and other special occasions. Dominican cake, a citrus-flavored cake with a cooked pineapple filling or mashed green plantains or casaba (winter melon), topped with a caramelized sugar meringue, is popular in that nation for all holidays and events.

Traditionally, Sunday meals emphasize fresh meats when available, especially beef or pork roasts. In the Dominican Republic lunch on Sunday is very large and may last into the early evening. On many islands, Sundays are also times when picnics are enjoyed, called día del campo ("field day") in Spanish-speaking nations. One dish often served is carne fiambre, a selection of cold cuts served with pickles, olives, and green salad.[43]

Etiquette In Puerto Rico, forks and knives are held European style—the fork in the left hand and the knife in the right hand with no switching hands for cutting food. This pattern is also the norm in Cuba, though in the Dominican Republic both European-style and American-style use of utensils is accepted. In these nations, dishes are passed to the left, and when not eating, hands should be kept visible, with the wrists resting on the edge of the table. In Puerto Rico, it is impolite to start eating until a host says "*Bon appetite*!" whereas in Cuba and the Dominican Republic the host may say, "¡*Buen provecho*!"[28]

Food may be in short supply in some parts of the Caribbean, and respectful behavior is expected when eating. For example, in Cuba vegetables and fruits should not be consumed with the hands. In Puerto Rico, food should not be wasted, and one should not take more than one can eat.

Therapeutic Uses of Food Some Caribbean Islanders adhere to a hot–cold classification system of diet and health similar to that found in Mexico (refer to Chapter 9). In addition to the categories of hot and cold, Puerto Ricans add cool. Imbalances in hot and cold—for example, sitting in the shade of a tree after being out in the sun—can cause illness even years after the imbalance has occurred. Haitians believe that women are warmer than men and that a person cools as he or she ages.[44,45] Among Caribbean Islanders, it is mostly Puerto Ricans, Dominicans, and Haitians who follow dietary and disease hot–cold classifications, and only small numbers are strict adherents.[46,47]

The hot–cold theory of foods practiced in the Caribbean sometimes includes not only the category of cool foods but also those considered heavy or light. A balance of hot–cold elements is attempted at meals, and heavy foods, such as starches, are consumed during the day, whereas light foods, such as soup, are eaten in the evening. Although the specific classification of items varies from person to person, one guideline for Puerto Ricans indicates bananas, coconuts, and most vegetables are cold; chilies, garlic, chocolate, coffee, evaporated milk and infant formula, and alcoholic beverages are hot. Cool foods include fruit, chicken, bacalao, whole milk, honey, onions, peas, and wheat. Excessive intake of cool or cold foods can make a cold condition, such as a cough, develop into a chronic illness, such as asthma.

Pregnancy, defined as a hot condition by most Puerto Ricans, is a time when a hot–cold balance is practiced carefully, and hot foods are avoided. When infants suffer from hot ailments, including diarrhea or rash, infant formula may be replaced with whole milk, or cooling ingredients such as barley water, mannitol, or magnesium carbonate may be added to the formula. High-calorie tonics (eggnogs and malts are popular types) are taken by some Puerto Ricans to stimulate the appetite and provide strength or energy. These are considered especially appropriate for pale children and for pregnant or postpartum women.[55]

Research with Dominican Americans suggests the use of hot–cold classifications for numerous conditions. Examples cited are excessive cold causing asthma and fibroids, whereas perimenopausal hot flashes are a hot problem.[17] Home remedies given to children for asthma include warming foods, such as oils (whale, cod liver, almond, and castor), honey or royal jelly (bee-larva food), onion, garlic, oregano, lemon, and aloe vera juice. Beets combined with molasses are used by traditional Dominican healers to treat fibroids (and may be used by some Caribbean Islanders to lower blood pressure or treat arthritis and ulcers). Research on Dominican mothers suggests that nutritional practices during lactation may sometimes include avoidance of certain protein foods and increased intake of fluids such as malt beer, milk, orange juice, chocolate milk, and noodle soup. Formula may be withheld from sick infants and tea provided instead.[29,45–47]

Haitians apply the hot–cold theory, including the heavy-light categories, to a broader number of conditions impacting health. A person's life cycle, a woman's reproductive cycle, the climate, and the time of day are categorized, and they must be balanced to maintain health. For example, heavy foods should be eaten in the morning and light foods in the evening. Environmental forces (such as wind, or seeing a lightning strike) and social interactions can disrupt equilibrium and result in illness. Women and their newborn infants may spend the first month after birth in seclusion to avoid excessive chilling.[48,49]

Therapeutic use of food is not limited to balancing hot–cold conditions. Some Haitians believe that certain illnesses in infants can be caused if a nursing mother's milk is too thick or too thin. Further, if a woman is frightened while breastfeeding, it is believed by some that her milk goes to her head, causing a headache in her and diarrhea in the baby. Gaz, another condition, causes pain in the shoulders, back, legs, or appendix, and headaches, stomachaches, or anemia. Foods such as corn or a tea made from garlic, cloves, and mint are home remedies for gaz.[16]

Other Caribbean Islanders, including Cubans, do not generally subscribe to the hot–cold theory but often use food-based home remedies. One study of Latinx people in the Miami area reported 75 percent had used herbal cures during the previous twelve months. Cubans reportedly use grapefruit and garlic for hypertension, chayote to calm nerves, and beets to treat anemia and flu. Star anise tea is consumed to relieve intestinal pain and flatulence in adults and colic in infants. Other teas used for stomach aches include those made with aloe vera or spearmint. Teas with cinnamon, sour orange, or honey and lemon are used for colds and coughs. Cinnamon tea is also believed useful for menstrual cramps. Gastrointestinal parasites are treated with pumpkin seed tea. Linden leaf, also popular, is used for anxiety.[46,47,50]

Some non-Hispanic Caribbean Islanders believe cassava helps prevent heart disease and cancer. Plantains are also used to decrease the risk of heart disease, as well as for treating hypertension, ulcers, and constipation. Teas are used for many ailments, including lemon-grass tea for fever, and ginger tea for indigestion and flatulence (ginger may also be added to rum for diabetes). Cerasse tea, made from Asian bitter melon (which has hypotensive properties), may be consumed to lower blood sugar levels, and wild sage tea is also used to treat diabetes.[50]

Contemporary Food Habits in the United States

Adaptations of Food Habits

Traditional food habits are often maintained in the self-sustaining immigrant communities of Spanish Harlem in New York City and Little Havana in Miami. Ingredients for Caribbean cuisine are readily available through Puerto Rican and Cuban American markets. Cubans, for example, may consider drinking strong coffee a way to maintain their ethnic identity; by comparison, Americans drink "weak" coffee. Changes do occur, however, as immigrants settle into culturally mixed communities and children grow up as Americans.[51,52]

Food habit changes for immigrants are affected by several factors, and often, there are health consequences for these shifts. Factors such as a busier lifestyle, lack of social relations, higher level of stress, children's preferences, taste, food insecurity lack of traditional foods, and others can be problematic for health. These pressures can result in high fat and sugar diets, low consumption of fruits/vegetables, bigger portions, consumption of convenience food, and inactivity. In turn, these habit changes can cause chronic diseases such as cardiovascular, hypertension, type 2 diabetes, and others. The impact of these negative outcomes increases with time spent in a foreign country, especially in the United States and

Canada. Interestingly, in Europe, immigrants show minor negative or even positive impacts on their health. There is little recent data specifically on Caribbean Islander food habits in the United States. One older study compared the diet of three groups of women from Puerto Rico: (1) those living in New York (forward migrants), (2) those who had lived on the mainland but later returned to the island (return migrants), and (3) those who never lived on the mainland (non-migrants). It was found that non-migrants and return migrants ate more starchy vegetables, sugar, and sweetened foods than did forward migrants. Forward migrants ate a greater variety of foods, including more beef, eggs, bread, fresh fruit, and leafy green vegetables. Puerto Rican women who had lived on the mainland quickly reverted to their traditional food habits when they returned to the island.[52]

Research shows a shift in diets for Afro-Caribbean adults born in Great Britain or those with prolonged residence. Earlier research found that traditional items such as fish (boiled, baked, or fried), chicken (fried, roast, or curried), homemade soups, rice and peas, plain rice, and boiled potatoes were consumed by respondents several times each week. Few Western foods were popular: Eighty-three percent ate hamburgers less than once a month, and similar numbers reported rarely eating pizza, pasta, butter, and margarine.[53,54] But many traditional Caribbean foods that featured in the earlier research (curried mutton, homemade West Indian soup, and hard dough bread), are no longer eaten—replaced by Westernized food. Sweet and salty snacks, processed meats, breakfast cereals, sugar-sweetened beverages, and foods such as hamburgers and soda are increasingly eaten with acculturation. There is very little reliance on traditional foods. Compared with the general UK population, the risk of chronic diseases such as obesity, hypertension, type 2 diabetes, and stroke, all linked to dietary patterns, is much greater for people of Black African and Caribbean ethnicity, with diseases developing earlier and having poorer outcomes. The fact of increases in fat and saturated fat suggests the impact of migration and residence on dietary intake.[54]

Ingredients and Common Foods Research on the food habits of Caribbean immigrants in the United States is limited. It is thought that rice, beans, starchy vegetables, sofrito (a fresh mixture often of onions, chilies, garlic, cilantro, tomatoes, and red pepper), and bacalao (dried, salted codfish) remains the basis of the daily diet of many Puerto Ricans who live on the mainland. Poultry is used when possible, and egg intake decreases. When there is greater discretionary income, Cuban American diet usually includes more pork and beef.

Caribbean Islanders accept some American foods, especially convenience items, and purchase frozen and dehydrated products when they can afford to do so. The proportion of meat in the diet often increases on the mainland, as does the consumption of milk (and other dairy foods) and soft drinks. One study showed that in Puerto Rican adults, with more Spanish use, there is a stronger orientation psychologically to Puerto Rico. The shorter length of mainland-U.S. residency was associated with traditional dietary patterns. Higher income and stronger psychological association with the United States were linked to higher diet quality. Intake of leafy vegetables continues to be low. Local fruits often replace the tropical fruits of Puerto Rico.[30,55]

Data regarding Dominicans in the United States indicate that only small changes have occurred in consumption patterns. Protein and fat intake has increased slightly, mostly due to eating more meat, while carbohydrate intake has decreased. Dominican women reported that their diet was more varied and abundant than in their homeland.[30,60]

A study of foreign-born adult immigrants in the United States showed they consumed less ultra-processed foods than U.S.-born adults (45 vs. 58 percent). Within foreign-born adult participants, ultra-processed food consumption increased when English was spoken at home (increasing from 40 percent among individuals speaking non-English languages only, to 50 percent among those speaking English only). In addition, ultra-processed food consumption increased from 41 percent among foreign-born adults who spent less than 30 percent of their life in the United States to 48 percent among those who lived in the United States for more than 50 percent of their lives.[56]

Meal Composition and Cycle The meals of Puerto Ricans residing on the mainland are similar to those of people on the island, with a few changes. A light breakfast of bread and coffee may be followed by a light lunch of rice and beans or a starchy vegetable, with or without bacalao (salted cod). Often, this traditional midday meal becomes a sandwich and soft drink, however. A late dinner consists of rice, beans, starchy vegetable, meat if available, or soup. Salad is included in some homes. Many researchers have reported an increase in the amount of snacking between meals, mostly on high-calorie foods with little nutritional value.[57–59]

In Dominica, breakfast and lunch are the larger meals and may include salt fish and bakes. Meals often feature root crops such as yams and tannias. Common drinks include fresh juices, coconut water, and fresh water. Hot drinks include coffee, cocoa, tea, and local bush teas.[50] Interviews with Haitians living in New York City suggest that some traditional dietary practices are discontinued; for example, the main meal is eaten in the evening instead of at noon. Although some Haitians adhere to hot–cold classifications of food, they may differ from those used in Haiti.[28]

 **Food for Thought**

In Haiti, protein foods are usually served first to the father in the household, then to the wife and children. This pattern is believed to continue in Haitian American homes.

Practicing Voodoo (also Vodou, Vodún) in the United States is no longer stereotyped as secretive and shameful by many younger Haitians and other newcomers to the religion. Many invite friends to Voodoo ceremonies and have visible altars in their homes.

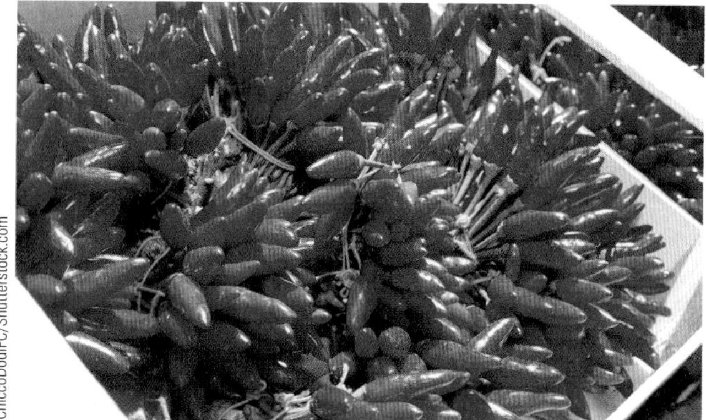

ChiccoDodiFC/Shutterstock.com

▲ **Bright chilies are often offered in markets throughout South America and the Caribbean.**

One older study reported that many low-income Latina women living in New York did not plan menus far in advance and that this hampered their ability to add variety to their diets. It was found that food shopping serves as a social occasion for many women and is one of the few opportunities they have to get out of the house; thus, they may go to the grocery store more often than is necessary. The investigators reported that nearly half of the women questioned preferred to fry main dishes. Boiling was the second choice, baking third. Broiling food was a distant fourth choice. The researchers noted that in many low-income households the oven or broiler element may not work, restricting food preparation methods to frying and boiling.[58]

Special Occasions It is assumed that many Caribbean Islander holiday food traditions are retained after immigration to the United States. Several events have been added to the annual calendar, however, often featuring traditional foods and music of the region. One of the largest is the West Indian Carnival which has been held annually for over sixty-five years in New York City. The carnival celebrates the cultures of the Caribbean, featuring an enormous parade, music competitions, and street vendors selling items such as curried goat and Jamaican jerk barbecue. In June, cities with large Puerto Rican populations often host Puerto Rican Day parades. The Dominican Day Parade is held every August in New York City. Major reggae music festivals with ample Caribbean food are held throughout the United States on February 6—reggae artist Bob Marley's birthday.

Nutritional Status

Nutritional Intake There is limited information on the nutritional status of Caribbean American immigrants to the United States. The few studies available suggest several health trends in these immigrants that have important nutritional implications. Health disparities for Latinx people compared to the general population have been reported, including lower rates of preventive care (such as inoculations and screenings) health care insurance coverage, and higher rates of risk factors.[61] Differences among Puerto Ricans have been reported between those living on the mainland and those living in Puerto Rico, with those living on the mainland experiencing more physical illness and having less access to health care.[65] Low socioeconomic and education levels are often associated with some disparities. Ten percent of Latinx report having fair or poor health compared to 8.3 percent of Whites [61,62] One study showed that some chronic health conditions, such as disability and diabetes, are more prevalent among Puerto Rican elders than in white elders living in the same neighborhoods.[70]

Mortality data suggest that although Puerto Rican and Cuban men have lower overall rates compared to Whites, younger men die in disproportionately higher numbers (often due to preventable causes). Among Puerto Ricans, those who are born in Puerto Rico have lower mortality rates than those born on the mainland.[63,64]

Preterm birth and low birthweight rates are disproportionately higher in Puerto Rican infants born on the mainland as compared to other infants. These factors contribute to a high infant mortality rate. Nearly 8.3 percent of Puerto Rican infants born on the mainland are of low birth weight. Elevated levels of mid-pregnancy stress are predictors of preterm birth and low birthrate. High rates of low-birth-weight infants have also been reported in the Haitian American community, associated with hypertension and preeclampsia. In contrast, the infant mortality rate of Cuban American babies is below the national average.[60–63]

Recent data on breastfeeding practices are limited. One older anecdotal report on Puerto Rican women states that breastfeeding is common.[64–67] However, earlier studies found breastfeeding infrequent among women in the United States, and in another study, overweight Latinx women in New York were found to be less likely to initiate and more likely to discontinue breastfeeding than lower-weight women. A CDC survey of maternity practices in Puerto Rico reported that 69 percent of infants were initially breastfed and that rate dropped to 39 percent for those infants born by Cesarean. This finding is significant when obesity rates in this population are considered (see Overweight/Obesity Rates by Ethnicity below). Those few who started breastfeeding often switched to bottle feeding after two to four weeks. Whole milk, condensed milk, and evaporated milk were frequently fed to infants, as were juices. Solid food typically was introduced at a young age.[67]

Dietary intake data from the largest population-based cohort of Latinx populations of diverse origins identified these dietary patterns: Burgers, fries, and soft drinks; white rice, beans, and red meats; fish; egg and cheese; and alcohol. Fewer years living in the United States was associated with more rice and bean consumption, which are traditional foods. There was an insufficient intake of vegetables and fruits. These dietary patterns have led to obesity and chronic health conditions.[68–70]

Several studies suggest that rates of overweight and obese people are higher than national or state averages for many U.S. Latinx populations (refer to Table 10.2). Data from 2020

Table 10.2 Overweight and Obesity by Race/Ethnicity 2019–2020*

2019	Non-Hispanic White	Non-Hispanic Black	Hispanic	Asian	Hawaiian / Pacific Islander	American Indian / Alaska Native	2 or more races
Overweight Adolescents							
Percent	14.6	16.4	19.6	11.0	-	27.4	18.5
Obese Adolescents							
Percent	13.1	21.1	19.2	6.5	-	21.3	15.6
Overweight Adults							
Percent	35.4	32.6	35.7	31.0	34.3	31.4	32.3
Obese Adults							
Percent	30.4	40.7	34.7	11.4	42.8	37.9	33.9

- Data not available because the sample size is insufficient or data is not reported.

† Overweight is defined as body mass index (BMI)-for-age and ≥85th percentile but <95th percentile based on the 2000 CDC growth chart; BMI was calculated from self-reported weight and height (weight [kg]/ height [m^2]).

Data Source: CDC

*This text uses Latinx for cross-Latin American people. This CDC information uses the term Hispanic and non-Hispanic for the same populations.

indicate that Latinx have a higher rate of obesity than Whites, but they rank about the same in the overweight category. However, for adolescents, rates for both overweight (19.6 percent) and obese (19.2 percent) are much higher than non-Latinx Whites (14.6 and 13.1 percent, respectively).[71,75]

Low levels of physical activity and cultural norms regarding weight and health may be significant factors in being overweight among Caribbean Islanders.[72] Puerto Rican, Cuban, and Haitian people often associate well-being with being gordita, or a little fat. This is particularly true for children, even when a thinner body ideal is desired by mothers. Thinness is thought by some Caribbean people to be indicative of poor health due to emotional or psychological conditions.[72–74]

Research has established a genetic contribution to the development of the clustering of health characteristics (including obesity/waist circumference, insulin resistance, hypertension, and dyslipidemia) known as metabolic syndrome in Caribbean Latinx families.[76,77] The prevalence of hypercholesterolemia was 52 percent among men and ranged from 48 percent (Dominican and Puerto Rican men) to 55 percent (Central American men). In women, the prevalence of hypercholesterolemia was 37 percent and ranged from 31 percent (South American women) to 41 percent (Puerto Rican women). Overall, 25 percent of men had hypertension; hypertension prevalence was highest among Dominican men. Hypertension prevalence overall among women was 24 percent. The prevalence of hypertension ranged from 16 percent (South American women) to 29 percent (Puerto Rican women). Overall, 17 percent of men and women had diabetes; prevalence ranged from 10 percent in South American men 7and women to 19 percent in Mexican men and women and Puerto Rican women.[78,79]

Persons with metabolic syndrome are at increased risk for type 2 diabetes and cardiovascular disease. Health statistics in 2019 estimated that 11.8 percent of Hispanics had been diagnosed with diabetes. In one study, the Hispanic Community Health Study/Study of Latinos (HCHS/SOL), determined the prevalence of diabetes and rates of awareness and control among adults from diverse Latinx backgrounds in the U.S. Hispanic Community. The rate of type 2 diabetes among the participants in the study was 10.2 percent in South Americans and 13.4 percent in Cubans to 17.7 percent in Central Americans, 18.0 percent in Dominican and Puerto Rican, and 18.3 percent in Mexican people, and the prevalence increased with length of residence in the United States. Hispanics are about 50 percent more likely to die from diabetes or liver disease than White people.[82,83]

The prevalence of hypertension is slightly lower in Latinx than in Whites.[80,81] Rates of mortality due to hypertension, heart disease, and stroke, however, vary between groups. Puerto Rican people have the highest rates of all Latinx, approximately 13 percent above White people. Higher rates of diabetes, which is a risk factor for high blood pressure, may be one reason for the discrepancy. In comparison, Cuban Americans have the lowest rates, 39 percent below those of White people. Deaths from hypertension are higher for men than for women in all Latinx populations. Although Latinx experience cardiovascular disease at rates lower than the national average, there is some evidence that it may be higher than average among some subpopulations, such as in Latinx women living in New York City. Heart disease is still the leading cause of death among Latinx populations.[82,83] Rates of renal failure due to diabetes among Latinx are approximately 1.7 times higher than in Whites. Death rates associated with diabetes are also 1.5 times higher in Latinx.[84]

Chronic liver disease and cirrhosis are ranked as the sixth leading cause of death among Latinx.[61,83,84] Dental health is also problematic for Latinx. Data indicate that Latinx preschool children have a high rate of dental caries. Latinx adults have a larger proportion of untreated caries than whites.[62] Smoking overall among Latinx (14 percent) is less common than among Whites (24 percent) but is high among Puerto Rican males (26 percent) and Cuban males (22 percent).

New American Perspectives

Puerto Rican

Paula Velazquez

I was born and raised in Puerto Rico and came to the United States when I was thirteen years old. In Puerto Rico, I grew up on a farm, and my diet included rice and beans and products that we grew, such as fresh green bananas, sweet potatoes, and plantains. When my parents went to town to shop, that was when we ate meat and bread. Once a year we had pork for Christmas and turkey for Thanksgiving because these animals were raised by my parents for the holidays. My sister still owns the farm, and I try to get back for visits.

Here in the United States, I live with my aunt and uncle, and their diet is high in meat, vegetables, and "healthy" foods. They are in their eighties and still very healthy. The food that made the biggest impression on me when I came to the United States was mashed potatoes. I had never seen or eaten mashed potatoes, and it took me a while before I would even try them. The second thing was having meat every day—that was really a treat. However, my favorite foods are bread and then vegetables. I like all kinds of seafood. I will eat seafood rather than meat. Meat I could give up but not bread and vegetables.

Whether a Latinx person was born in the United States makes a difference. Cancers related to infections (cervical, stomach, and liver) are more common among Latinx born in other countries. However, compared with United States-born Latinx, foreign-born Latinx have half as much heart disease, 48 percent less cancer, and 29 percent less high blood pressure.[84]

Food for Thought

Lactose intolerance is thought to be a problem among many Caribbean people, although an estimated incidence has not been reported.[85]

South Americans

South America is a vast land that features the rugged ridge of the Andes Mountains stretching from north to south. Highland plains, tropical rain forests, temperate valleys, and desert dunes extend from where the mountain peaks slope toward the coastal edges of the continent. Extremes in terrain and climate limit agriculture in many areas. The continent contains 12 independent nations: Argentina, Brazil, Bolivia, Chile, Colombia, Ecuador, Guyana, Paraguay, Peru, Suriname, Uruguay, and Venezuela. In addition, France retains control of the territory called French Guyana, and Great Britain claims the Falkland Islands.

Numerous Native groups populated the continent before settlement by Europeans. Although the Spanish were the first to arrive, significant numbers of Portuguese, Italians, and Germans also settled in South America. Forced labor from West Africa introduced Africans to the continent, followed by Asian Indian workers after slavery was outlawed. Native and mixed Native-European populations live in the tropical highlands; Creoles (in South America, Creole typically denotes descendants of the Europeans) have concentrated in the southern, temperate regions of the continent; and parts of northeastern Brazil are populated primarily by Black and mixed Black Europeans. In more recent times, Japanese immigration to South America has become notable.

Cultural Perspective

History of South Americans in the United States

Immigration Patterns Chileans were among the first South Americans to immigrate to the United States for the California gold rush. It is believed that several thousand worked in the mines. Approximately half returned to Chile and those who remained quickly intermarried and were absorbed into the general population. Before the 1960s, all South American immigrants were counted as Other Latinx people in the U.S. Census. Specific figures regarding the individual nations before this time are uncertain but are thought to be minimal. Most South American immigration has occurred in the past twenty years during periods of land reform, economic hardship, or political repression. Jobs and educational opportunities are the primary attractions for the majority of immigrants, although significant numbers of political exiles have come from Argentina and Chile.

Current

Demographics Over 1.8 million Americans of South American descent are living in the United States.[96] There are approximately 639,000 million Americans of Colombian ancestry; 398,000 from Ecuador; 396,000 from Peru; 3,000 from Guyana; 2,000 from Brazil; 152,000 from Argentina; 84,000 from Chile; 183,000 from Venezuela; and 69,000 from Bolivia.[86]

Most South Americans settle in the Northeast, especially New York and New Jersey. In New York City, Colombians, Ecuadorians, and Peruvians have established ethnic enclaves in Queens, and "Little Brazils" are found in both Queens and Manhattan. Miami and Los Angeles also host large South American populations from most nations. In addition, Brazilians are found in Pennsylvania and Washington, DC; Many Chileans have settled in Texas; Colombians have clustered in Stamford, Connecticut, the urban areas of Illinois, and California; and Peruvian neighborhoods have developed in Houston, Chicago, and Washington, DC.

Most South American immigrants are proud of their heritage and differentiate themselves from Americans of Mexican, Caribbean, or Central American background. Brazilians in particular may dislike being mistaken as Latinx who speak Spanish (Portuguese is their official language). Some South Americans suffer from discrimination directed toward Mexican Americans or Latinx people in general. Others, who are mostly of European heritage, are not recognized as Latinx people but may continue the prejudices among some South Americans. Second- and third-generation South Americans often leave homogeneous neighborhoods and relocate into mixed communities.

Socioeconomic Status Few data are available on the socioeconomic status of Americans of South American descent who have lived in the United States for extended periods. Most data are related to foreign-born immigrants who have come in the past 25 years. Regardless of arrival date, a majority of immigrants from South America come to the United States in search of employment opportunities. Many are well-educated professionals; however, they sometimes find that their credentials are not accepted after arrival, forcing them to accept positions in the sales, service, trade, and labor fields, such as restaurant work, construction, child care, or textile and garment industry jobs.

Foreign-born Colombians arrive in the United States with overall education levels slightly lower than the U.S. average, although some are professionals with college degrees who hope to find employment commensurate with their skills. Most Ecuadorans are better educated than other Latinx Americans, but still less than the total U.S. population.[87]

Peruvians generally have higher levels of education than the U.S. population and Argentineans have the highest levels of education among the Latin population overall.[92] Of the Brazilian population in the United States aged 25 and older, 20 percent have a high school diploma and 22 percent have a Bachelor's degree, which is higher than the U.S. population.[87,88]

Worldview

Religion South Americans are mostly Roman Catholic, a legacy of European conquest. In most nations approximately 42 to 89 percent of adults are Catholic, reflecting a decline from the 90 percent affiliation with the Catholic Church from 1900–1960.[89] In some regions, the Christian religion is often blended with other belief systems. In Peru, Incan gods may be included in Catholic rites, for example, and the Venezuelan religion, the cult of Maria Lionza, mixes Indigenous, Catholic, and African practices. Religious syncretism is the greatest in Brazil. Spiritism imported from France, is based on the belief that spirits of the dead exist, can communicate with the living, and can provide useful knowledge. It combines Christian precepts with scientific principles. Popular with the upper-middle class of the country, adherents communicate with the dead through spiritual mediums. Umbanda is very common in rural areas and among the urban poor, combining several Afro-Brazilian faiths with spiritism and the idea of Christian charity. Candomblé is probably the best known of the mixed religions, and is an Afro-Brazilian faith founded by Blacks in the Bahia region and is now practiced nationwide by followers of all ethnicities.[90,91] African-derived beliefs dealing with earthly matters such as health and wealth are combined with Catholic cosmology. Yoruba deities called orixá or orisha are venerated with rites of worship that include animal sacrifice, feasting, and dancing. Over 20 orixás are recognized in Brazil and most are correlated with a Catholic entity: Oxalá, god of creation, with Jesus Christ; Exú, the messenger god, with the devil; Ogun, god of war and iron craft, with St. Anthony or St. George; Oxóssi, god of affluence, with St. Sebastian; Omolu, god of plagues and illness, with St. Lazarus; and Oxum, the fertility goddess (also called the goddess of vanity), with the Virgin Mary. Each orixá is associated with certain personality traits, day of the week, color, plants, animals, foods, and drinks; and each person has an orixá owner of his or her head who influences individual temperament and behavior.

Protestant missionaries were active in South America starting in the twentieth century and were especially successful in Honduras and Uruguay where Catholics are 42 and 46 percent, respectively, of the population.[89] In Brazil, the Baptist, Pentecostal, Seventh-Day Adventist, and Universalist denominations are the most popular. Chilean Protestants are usually members of the Pentecostal or Seventh-Day Adventist churches, though those of German ancestry often follow the Lutheran or Baptist faiths. Small numbers of Jewish people and Buddhists are also found in South America, in total less than 1 percent of the population together.

Most South Americans who emigrate to the United States are Roman Catholic and very involved with their local parish. A majority of Guyanese Americans belong to Guyanese-led Episcopal churches and often also send their children to church-run schools with Guyanese teachers. In addition, some Guyanese Americans frequent "Unity Centers," which function as community centers and promote spirituality but are not affiliated with any organized religion.[92,93]

Family Family life is important in all South American societies. In Argentina, Spanish and Italian traditions have shaped family structure. The extended family usually gathers together at least once a week and on holidays as well. Grandparents are involved in most family decisions, and children often stay at home until marriage. In Brazil, extended family members typically live close to one another, and daily visits are common. Relatives mentor children through rites of passage such as confirmation, graduation, the start of a career, and marriage.

Traditionally, the father is the head of the household in Chilean homes. In Colombia, the father holds all authority, and children are taught to obey their parents. Ecuadoran families follow two models: Spanish-influenced families are ruled by the father, who has few responsibilities to the home other than financial support; and Indigenous-influenced families, where the father and mother share more power and household responsibilities. In Peru, extended families typically include godparents, who sponsor baptisms and provide both social and economic assistance. Families are predominantly patriarchal, though more so in the Spanish-speaking upper and middle classes than in less affluent, rural Indigenous homes. In contrast to most of South America, the Venezuelan family weathered severe changes in the economy, first due to increased national prosperity and then to its rapid decline since the country's dependence on oil as a major resource. Since 2014, nearly six million Venezuelans have relocated to neighboring countries and beyond. Many of those who remained, relocated to urban centers. Many families have declined in size, and the extended family is less common.

In many areas of South America, it is unacceptable for women to work outside the home. Even those with a profession traditionally stay at home after marriage. Among some Indigenous groups, however, women contribute to the well-being of the family through farm work, and in the urban areas of Venezuela, many women have outside jobs but remain responsible for household chores. In Chile, women are often involved in local social and political issues.

Most South Americans prefer to immigrate as family groups, although financial pressures often demand that a single family member become established in the United States before the rest of the family follows. Individual immigrants commonly move to neighborhoods where relatives, godparents, or friends have settled. They depend on these contacts for housing and support. This system of mutual assistance is maintained after the immediate family arrives, bringing more relatives into the extended family. Colombians and Ecuadorians often broaden their relationships beyond national boundaries to form strong bonds with other Latinos.

Many families suffer from the stresses of American informality and freedom. Men lose some authority over wives and children, and women find it difficult to adjust to working outside the home. Furthermore, many upper- and middle-class women, who had paid help with the housework in South America, must learn to balance a job with the responsibility of running a home.

Traditional Health Beliefs and Practices There are few sources available on how Americans of South American heritage maintain health or how they approach illness. Brazilians often attribute bad health to liver problems or an imbalance between hot and cold, such as drinking a glass of cold water on a hot day or taking a cool shower after eating a hot meal. Many South Americans self-diagnose or seek health advice from their mothers or friends. They then visit a pharmacist where they can purchase many medications, such as antibiotics, by the pill.

Most Brazilians associate faith with health. Catholics may believe in fate and seek intervention from patron saints when ill. Spiritists employ homeopathy, exorcism, past-lives therapy, acupuncture, yoga therapy, and chromotherapy to cure sickness.[92,93] Followers of Candomblé, a mixture of traditional Yoruba, Fon, and Bantu African faiths, believe that health is maintained by achieving a balance between the earthly and spiritual spheres. The pain-de-Santo or babalorixá (high priest) or the mäe-de-Santo or ialorixá (high priestess) may be hired to read the oracle of a personal orixá, for example, so that an individual can improve his or her relationship with the deity.[94] Harmonious relations with one's orixá can maximize axé (vital force). Spiritual equilibrium is maintained by observing the preferences and prohibitions of one's orixá, including certain food and beverages, colors, therapeutic herbs, beaded necklaces, and other limitations. The priest or priestess also serves as the local curendiero, diagnosing physical and spiritual problems, prescribing healing herbal baths or botanicals, and manipulating occult forces. In Ecuador, either a healer, called a curandero, or a witch doctor, called a brujo, treats many illnesses in small villages. In Peru, urban residents typically obtain biomedical health care, but in rural regions, home remedies and ritual magic are often preferred.[94]

Herbal teas are a favorite remedy throughout most of South America, where street stands and small markets called yerbeterías sell medicinal botanicals for home use.[95] Numerous plants, many unfamiliar in the United States, are used therapeutically. Soursop leaves are used to treat diabetes, and the seeds of the guaraná are thought to relieve fatigue and help with weight loss. Papaya leaves are considered useful in getting rid of intestinal worms. Rue is taken for uterine pain and as an abortive, and black nightshade is used for coughs. Pau d'arco, the bark of a tree native to Brazil, is widely used to treat rheumatism, diabetes, venereal diseases, yeast infections, enlarged prostate, and several cancers.[93,94]

Traditional Food Habits

Ingredients and Common Foods

Staples The cooking of South America is similar to that of other Latin American regions in that it combines some native ingredients and preparation techniques with the foods of colonial Europeans. The diet is largely corn-based and spiced with chili pepper (refer to Table 10.3). Tomatoes are common, and in tropical areas cassava (called yuca) is a popular tuber. Pumpkins, bananas, and plantains are consumed often. Beef, rice, onions, and olive oil, introduced by the Spanish and the Portuguese, are eaten regularly. Tropical fruits, such as those found in the Caribbean (Table 10.3), are plentiful in many regions. However, South American fare also features several ingredients used infrequently in the dishes of other Latin American areas. Potatoes, which were first cultivated by the

Table 10.3 Cultural Food Groups: South Americans

Group	Comments	Common Foods	Adaptations in the United States
Protein Foods			
Milk/milk products	Milk is not usually consumed as a beverage but used in fruit-based drinks and added to coffee. Many milk-based desserts are enjoyed.	Cow's, goat's milk; evaporated milk; fresh and aged cheeses	Available cheeses are sometimes substituted for unavailable traditional cheeses.
Meat/poultry/fish/eggs/legumes	Beef is a foundation of the diet in parts of Argentina, Brazil, Paraguay, and Uruguay. Some game meats are consumed. Fish and seafood are significant in coastal regions, popular as *ceviche* in Ecuador and Peru. Beans are commonly consumed.	*Meat:* alligator, armadillo, beef (including variety cuts), capybara, frog, goat, guinea pig (*cuy*), iguana, llama, mutton, pork, rabbit, tapir *Poultry:* chicken, duck, turkey *Fish and shellfish:* abalone, bass, catfish, cod (including dried salt cod), crab, eel, haddock, lobster, oysters, scallops, shrimp, squid, trout, tuna *Eggs:* chicken, quail, turtle *Legumes:* beans (black, cranberry, kidney), black-eyed peas	Less acceptable meats such as guinea pig may no longer be eaten.
Cereals/Grains	*Cuzcuz*, made from cornmeal, is prepared in parts of Brazil; *arepa*, cornmeal bread, is staple in some areas. Pasta is popular in Argentina, Paraguay, and Uruguay. Rice and corn puddings are a favorite.	Amaranth, corn, rice, quinoa, wheat	
Fruits/Vegetables	Tropical and temperate fruits are plentiful and popular, added to savory and sweet dishes. Fruit compotes and fruit pastes are enjoyed. Potatoes are a staple in the Andes. Cassava flour and meal are common in many areas; tapioca is used in desserts.	*Fruits: Abiu, acerola*, apples, banana/plantains, cashew apple (*cajú*), *caimito, casimiroa*, cherimoya, custard apple, *feijoa*, guava, grapes, jackfruit, *jabuticaba*, lemons, limes, *lulo (naranjillo)*, mammea, mango, melon, olives, oranges (sweet and sour), palm fruits, papaya, passion fruit, peaches, pineapple, *pitango*, quince, raisins, roseapple, *sapote*, soursop, sweetsop, strawberries, sugarcane *Vegetables: abipa (jicama), arracacha (apio)*, avocado, *calabaza* (green pumpkin), cassava (*mandioca; yuca*), green peppers, hearts of palm, kale, okra, *oca*, onions, *roselle*, squash (chayote, winter), sweet potatoes, tomatoes, *yacón*, yams	
Additional Foods			
Seasonings	Toasted cassava meal, *farinha*, is sprinkled over foods in Brazil. Spicy hot foods are preferred in many areas; salsas are common.	*Achiote*, allspice, chiles (*aji*, malagueta, pimento), cilantro, cinnamon, citrus juices (lemon, lime, and sour orange), garlic, ginger root, oregano, paprika, parsley, scallions, thyme, vinegar	
Nuts/seeds	Coconut and coconut milk are added to numerous dishes. Peanut sauces flavored with chiles are common in the Andes.	Brazil nuts, cashews, coconut, peanuts, pumpkin seeds	
Beverages	Coffee is often served concentrated, then diluted with evaporated milk or water. *Maté* is more popular than coffee or tea in parts of Argentina, Brazil, and Paraguay.	*Batidas* (tropical fruit juices, sometimes made with alcoholic beverages), coffee, *guaraná*, soft drinks, sugarcane juice, tea, *yerba maté* and alcoholic beverages: beer, *cachaça* (sugarcane brandy), *pisco* (grape brandy), *chicha* (distilled corn liquor), wine	
Fats/oils	Dendê oil flavors and colors many dishes in the Bahia region of Brazil.	Dendê (palm) oil, olive oil, butter	Vegetable or peanut oil is substituted for dendê oil.
Sweeteners		Sugarcane, brown sugar, honey	

Incas on mountain terraces, are particularly important in the highlands of Peru and Ecuador. Sweet potatoes (the orange-fleshed root vegetable sometimes mistaken for African yams in the United States) are also native to the region. A white root similar to a mild carrot, known as apio or arracacha, is found in Colombia, Peru, and Venezuela; oca (a tuber similar to the potato in appearance but with leaves like clover) and yacón (an elongated tuber that has the taste and texture of a sweet turnip) are commonly eaten raw and cooked in Bolivia, Brazil, Colombia, Ecuador, and Peru; and the tuber known as ahipa (called jicama in the United States and Mexico) is native to the Amazon River basin.

Beans, a foundation food in many Latin American regions, are common in most South American countries yet not eaten at every meal. Other legumes and nuts, such as peanuts and cashews, are used often in dishes. Indigenous meats, including llama, deer, rabbit, wild pig, capybara, tapir, and cuy (guinea pigs who are raised for consumption), are consumed in some areas. Fish, such as anchovies and tuna, and shellfish, particularly shrimp, crab, spiny lobster, oysters, clams, giant sea urchins (evisos), and giant abalone (locos), are significant foods in the extensive coastal regions. Iguana is consumed occasionally, and alligator is a specialty in some areas.

A favorite way to prepare meats in South America is grilling. Traditionally, sides of beef, whole lambs, hogs, and kids (young goats) are hung over smoldering wood to slowly cook for hours in a method called asado. Today, a grill is used more often. Steaks and marinated kebobs (which often include organ meats) are favorites. Another, even older cooking tradition is to steam foods in a pit oven. In Peru, this method is called a pachamanca and typically includes a young pig or goat with guinea pigs, chickens, tamales, potatoes, and corn tucked around layers of hot stones and aromatic leaves and herbs.[106] In Chile, a curanto is closer to an elaborate coastal clambake, including shellfish, suckling pig, sausages, potato patties, peas, and beans layered with seaweed.

Stuffed foods are also common, including pastry turnovers filled with savory meat, fish, or cheese fillings. Empanadas, a turnover with a flaky, Spanish-style dough enriched with indigenous ingredients such as mashed potatoes, cassava, or corn, are made into many popular varieties throughout South America. The turnovers are usually baked, but sometimes they are fried. Fillings are as many as there are cooks; Argentina offers special variations from each region. Chopped meat, olives, raisins, and onions are popular, which point to the origins of empanadas as emanating from the Moorish invasions of Spain or perhaps from even earlier in Persia. In Chile, the turnovers may be filled with abalone, and in Brazil, where they are known as empadinhas, a spicy shrimp mixture is traditional. In Bolivia, where they are called salteñas, the turnovers are filled with cheese. Tamale-like steamed packets of dough-wrapped fillings are also popular throughout South America. In Peru, chapanas are made with cassava dough, while in Ecuador bollos are formed around cooked chicken meat with plantain dough. In Brazil, a freshly grated corn kernel dough is mixed with coconut and cassava (and no filling) to prepare pamonhas. Ground cornmeal dough flavored with annatto and tomatoes is preferred for Venezuelan hallacas. A favorite in Argentina, Bolivia, Brazil, Chile, and Ecuador are humitas, which feature fresh kernel or ground cornmeal dough wrapped around a variety of savory or sweet meat, fish, or vegetable fillings.

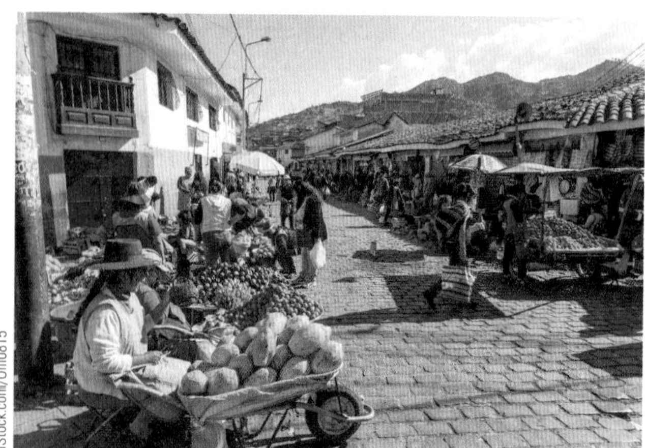

iStock.com/Olli0815

▲ A market in Pisaq, Peru.

Regional Variations National differences exist, although there are few clearly distinctive divisions in South American fare. Several countries share similar dishes.

Peru and Ecuador The cooking of Peru and Ecuador is divided into the highland fare of the Andes and the lowland dishes of the coastal regions. The cuisine of the mountain areas is among the most unique in South America, preserving many ingredients and dishes of the Inca people. Potatoes are eaten at nearly every meal and often for snacks. Over one hundred varieties are cultivated. Ocopa, boiled potatoes topped with cheese sauce and chili peppers or peanuts, is a typical dish in Peru. In Ecuador fried potato and cheese patties, called llapingachos, and potato cheese soup served with slices of avocado, known as locro, are common. Traditionally, the tubers are preserved by freezing in the cold night air and then drying in the hot daytime sun. Papa seca, a staple in Peru, are boiled, diced potatoes, dried in the sun and rehydrated before consumption; chuño, uncooked potatoes soaked in icy water for days and sun dried for a long shelf life are rich in calcium, phosphorus and iron. Corn is also grown in the mountains. Some varieties have kernels the size of small strawberries that when prepared as hominy are known as mote and are a popular snack item. Bananas and plantains are cooked as savory chips and made into flour for breads and pastries.

The foods of Peru and Ecuador are often served with a picante condiment for diners interested in adding spicy-heat to their dishes. One example is salsa de ají, a combination of freshly chopped chili, onion, and salt, appearing at most meals. Orange- or yellow-hued dishes are favored; along the coast, annatto colors foods, and in the Peruvian highlands an herb known as palillo is used. Charqui, dried strips of llama meat, is a specialty of the Andes. Anticuchos, chunks of beef heart marinated in vinegar with chilies and cilantro, then skewered

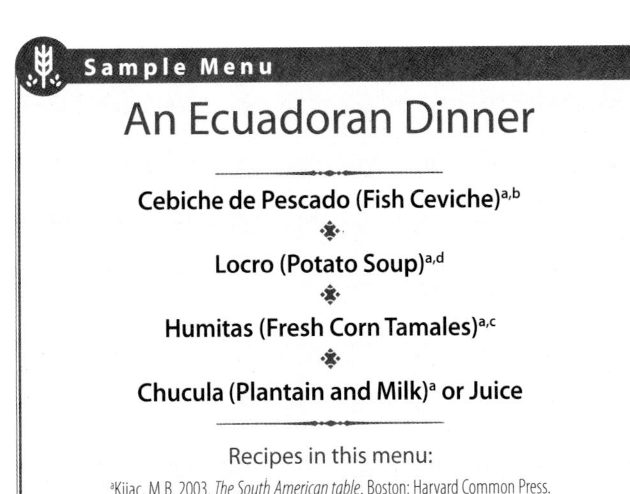
Sample Menu

An Ecuadoran Dinner

Cebiche de Pescado (Fish Ceviche)[a,b]

Locro (Potato Soup)[a,d]

Humitas (Fresh Corn Tamales)[a,c]

Chucula (Plantain and Milk)[a] or Juice

Recipes in this menu:

[a]Kijac, M.B. 2003. *The South American table*. Boston: Harvard Common Press.

[b]https://www.laylita.com/recipes/ecuadorian-fish-ceviche/

[c]https://www.laylita.com/recipes/humitas/

[d]https://www.whats4eats.com/south-america/ecuador-cuisine

and grilled, are a spicy Peruvian favorite also from the Andes. Rabbit dishes are also found in the region. Along the coast, seafood dominates the diet. The region is famous for its ceviches (also spelled cebiche), a method of preparing fresh fish, shrimp, scallops, or crab by marinating small raw chunks in citrus juice. The acidity of the juice cooks the fish and turns it opaque. At many beaches, cevicherias offer the dish as a snack or light meal with beer. Chopped onion, tomato, avocado, and cilantro are often added. In Peru, ceviche is typically garnished with sliced sweet potato. Chucula is a thick plantain and milk beverage flavored with cinnamon popular along the coastal regions of Ecuador.[107] Pisco, a grape brandy that originated in Peru, is a national favorite, often mixed with orange juice to make the refreshing drink called yugeno.

Argentina, Chile, Bolivia, Uruguay, and Paraguay Hearty, ample fare with an emphasis on beef exemplifies the cooking of these southern nations. Argentina is a major beef-producing region, and its people eat more beef per capita than in any other country worldwide. The temperate weather permits the cultivation of numerous fruits and vegetables, notably strawberries, grapes, and Jerusalem artichokes (known as topinambur in Chile). The cooking of Argentina, Chile, Paraguay, and Uruguay has been influenced more by their immigrant populations than by the numerous small Indigenous groups native to the area. The Spanish introduced cattle, and the Italians brought pasta. Smaller numbers of Germans, Hungarians, and other central Europeans have added their foods as well.

A celebrated dish of Argentina is matambre, which means "to kill hunger." A special cut of flank steak is seasoned with herbs, then traditionally rolled in pinwheel fashion around a filling of spinach, whole hard-boiled eggs, and whole or sliced carrots, and then tied with a string and poached in broth or baked. Matambre can be served as a main course, but it is often chilled first and offered as a cold appetizer. Grilled steaks are particularly popular in Argentina and surrounding nations. In Paraguay, steaks are typically served with sopa Paraguaya, a cornmeal, cheese and onion bread. In Uruguay, beef is eaten nearly as often as in Argentina, although mutton and lamb are also common.

Robust soups and stews are everyday fare. In Bolivia, beef stew is made with carrots, onions, hominy, and chuño. The stews of Argentina often pair meat with fruits as well as vegetables, such as carbonada criolla (beef cooked with squash, corn, and peaches) or carbonada en zapallo (veal stew cooked in a pumpkin). In Paraguay, soups reveal European origins combined with Indigenous ingredients, such as bori-bori, beef with cornmeal and cheese dumplings, and so' o-yosopy, beef soup with bell peppers, tomatoes, and vermicelli or rice, topped with Parmesan cheese. Fish soups and stews are popular in Chile, which has an extensive coastline and plentiful seafood. A specialty is clam or abalone chowder with beans (chupe de loco) and congrio (an elongated, firm-fleshed fish that looks a little like an eel) cooked with potatoes, onions, garlic, and white wine.

National favorites include pasta (e.g., spaghetti, ravioli, and lasagna), which is served in many homes on Sundays in Argentina. It is considered lucky to eat gnocchi on the twenty-ninth of every month as well. In Chile, beans are especially popular, and seafood is eaten regularly. Wines from the temperate midlands of the country are considered some of the best on the continent. Pisco, a type of brandy distilled from wine or fermented fruit juice, is consumed in both Bolivia and Chile, where it is mixed with lemon juice, sugar, and egg whites to make a pisco sour. In Bolivia, legs from the giant frogs found in the Andean Lake Titicaca are a specialty, and chicha, a distilled corn liquor, is popular.

Although coffee is consumed throughout the area, another caffeinated beverage is equally popular in some regions. Called maté, it is an infusion made from the leaves of a plant (*Ilex paraguariensis*) in the holly family native to Paraguay. Served hot or chilled, maté is consumed nearly every afternoon with small snacks in Paraguay and parts of Argentina. The dried, powdered leaves are called yerba and are traditionally mixed in a gourd with boiling water. A special metal straw is inserted to drink the brew.

Colombia and Venezuela The fare found in Colombia and Venezuela often is colonial Spanish in character, cooked with olive oil, cream, or cheese and flavored with ground cumin, annatto, parsley, cilantro, and chopped onions, tomatoes, and garlic. Yet native tastes are still evident. Guascas, or huascas (*Galinsoga parviflora*), an herb native to Colombia, provides a flavor similar to boiled peanuts in soups and stews. Hot chili pepper sauces are served on the side of most dishes. Tropical fruits and vegetables, including avocados, bananas and plantains, naranjillo (a small, orange fruit related to tomatoes used for its tart juice), pineapple, and coconut milk or cream are other common regional ingredients.

In Colombia, Bogatá chicken stew (made with chicken, two types of potatoes, and cream) and sancocho (a boiled dinner traditionally made with beef brisket or another roast, and ample starchy vegetables such as potatoes, sweet potatoes, plantains, or cassava) are typical Spanish-influenced

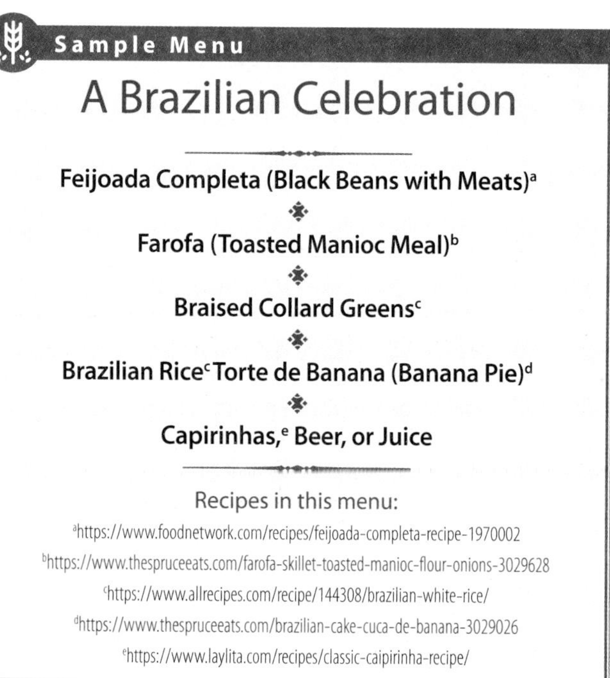

Sample Menu

A Brazilian Celebration

Feijoada Completa (Black Beans with Meats)[a]

Farofa (Toasted Manioc Meal)[b]

Braised Collard Greens[c]

Brazilian Rice[c] Torte de Banana (Banana Pie)[d]

Capirinhas,[e] Beer, or Juice

Recipes in this menu:

[a]https://www.foodnetwork.com/recipes/feijoada-completa-recipe-1970002

[b]https://www.thespruceeats.com/farofa-skillet-toasted-manioc-flour-onions-3029628

[c]https://www.allrecipes.com/recipe/144308/brazilian-white-rice/

[d]https://www.thespruceeats.com/brazilian-cake-cuca-de-banana-3029026

[e]https://www.laylita.com/recipes/classic-caipirinha-recipe/

dishes. Examples in Venezuela include ropa vieja, shredded flank steak served in a sauce made with tomatoes, onions, and olive oil; and pabellón caraqueño, flank steak served on rice with black beans, topped with fried eggs, and garnished with fried plantain chips. Dishes with more indigenous flavors include arepa, the staple cornmeal bread of Venezuela that is formed into one-inch-thick patties and cooked on a griddle (it is sometimes stuffed with meat or cheese before it is fried), cachapas, tender cornmeal crepes, and mashed black beans, known as caviar criollo or "native caviar." Tropical fruits, such as guavas and pineapple, are often sweetened and dried to make favorite snacks of fruit leathers and fruit pastes.

Guyana Guyana has a cuisine widely influenced by its proximity to the Caribbean, as well as by the many immigrants from throughout the world who have called Latin America home. For example, one national favorite is pepper pot, a stew made with a variety of meats and onions and flavored with the Caribbean cassava-based sauce cassareep (refer to Chapter 9). Other common dishes similar to those in the Caribbean include salt-fish cakes, blood pudding, cou-cou (cornmeal and okra bread), cookup rice (rice with black-eyed peas or split peas), bammies, and ginger beer. Caribbean desserts are common, such as the dense fruitcake known as black cake, and konkee, a tamale made from sweetened cornmeal, coconut milk, and raisins wrapped in banana leaves, then boiled. African influence is found in foofoo, a pounded plantain, yam, or cassava paste made into a dough, boiled, and pinched into small balls for dipping into soup or sauce, and stews made with fish or meat, plantains, onions, and okra (refer to Chapter 8). Dumplings are often added to metegmgee, a thick vegetable soup cooked in coconut milk broth. Asian foods include Indian curries, roti (flatbread), the use of dal (a type of legume; refer to Chapter 14), and Chinese noodle dishes. One national specialty is Portuguese garlic pork, which is marinated in vinegar, then fried. The country is famous for Demerara sugar, a very rich, brown-colored, and crumbly raw cane sugar named for a region in Guyana. It is the source of Demerara rum, a Guyanese specialty.

Brazil The cooking of Brazil is very different from that of other South American countries due to Portuguese and African influences. The Portuguese arrived in the sixteenth century, looking for land on which to cultivate sugarcane. They contributed dried salt cod and linguiça (sausage) to the diet, stews known as cozidos made with many different types of meat and vegetables (known as cocido in Portugal), and a variety of exceptionally sweet desserts based on sugar and egg yolks, such as caramel custards and corn (canjica) or rice (pirão de arroz) puddings flavored with coconut. Enslaved Africans put to work on the sugar plantations brought foods unknown in nearby countries, such as dendê oil (a type of palm oil) and okra. Spicy dishes were preferred. In West Africa, malagueta peppercorn, a small, hot grain, was used to season foods; in Brazil, Africans adopted a very small, mouth-searing chili pepper indigenous to the area and also called it malagueta. It is typically minced and added to dendê oil, often with dried shrimp and grated ginger root, to make a hot sauce.

Although Indigeneous, Portuguese, and African tastes and textures have influenced cooking throughout Brazil, nowhere are they more prominent than in the state of Bahia. Known as Afro-Brazilian fare, or cozinha baiana, this cuisine is famous for fritters made from dried shrimp, dried salt cod, yams, black-eyed peas, mashed beans, peanuts, and ripe plantains fried in dendê oil. Vatapá, another specialty, is a paste made with smoked dried shrimp, peanuts, cashews, coconut milk, and malagueta chilies. It is used as a filling for black-eyed pea fritters called acarajé and sometimes served with rice as an entree.

The national dish of Brazil is feijoda completa, which originated in Rio. Black beans cooked with smoked meats and sausages are served with rice, sliced oranges, boiled greens, and a hot sauce mixed with lemon or lime juice. Toasted cassava meal, called farinha, is sprinkled over the top like Parmesan cheese. Farinha is served with many dishes and is often mixed with butter and other ingredients, such as bits of meat, pumpkin, plantains, or coconut milk to create crunchy side dishes called farofa. Rice or cornmeal porridge, called pirão, is another type of side dish. Middle Easterners who immigrated to the southeastern areas of Brazil brought the concept of couscous to the country and adapted the dish to native ingredients. Cuzcuz paulista is prepared with cornmeal in a cuscuzeiro/a, which looks like a colander on legs that is inserted over a pot of boiling water to steam. The basket of the cuscuzeiro/a is first lined with seafood or poultry and vegetables, which flavors the cornmeal as it cooks and looks decorative when the cuzcuz cake is inverted.

In the far south, the cuisine has been influenced by the foods of Argentina. Grilled meats are a favorite in Brazil, especially in the south, home of the frontiersmen known as gauchos, who herded cattle on the grassland plains. Sides of beef were traditionally staked at the edges of a bonfire for slow cooking in a method called churrasco. The popularity of the outdoor barbecue led to *churrascaria rodizio*, restaurants located in cities throughout the nation that specialize in spit-roasted beef, pork, lamb, and sausages brought to the table on large skewers and carved to taste. Specialties include picanha (rump roast) and beef heart. Assorted side dishes such as salads, potatoes, condiments, and desserts round out the meal. Brazilians in the South also drink maté, which they call chimmarão. Coffee, rum, and beer are common beverages in Brazil, but several other drinks are also popular. Guaraná is a delicious, stimulating carbonated soft drink made from the seeds of the native guaraná fruit, which contain caffeine. Cachaça (called aguardiente in other South American nations) is an alcoholic beverage, often compared to brandy, distilled from sugarcane. It is used to make batidas, a refreshing punch with fruit juice, or caipirinhas, mixed with a little lime juice, sugar and mint, then consumed over ice.

Meal Composition and Cycle

Daily Pattern Three meals a day are traditional among middle-class and affluent South Americans, with an afternoon snack often added. Lower-income households, especially those in rural areas, are often limited to an early breakfast with a large dinner around 6:00 p.m.[95]

For those who can afford more than two meals daily, breakfast is typically light, often bread or a roll with jam and a cup of coffee, served black or with milk. A more complete meal features fresh fruit or pastries and occasionally ham or cheese. Lunch is usually the main meal, consumed in a leisurely manner with family or friends. Appetizers such as fritters, humitas, or empanadas may start the meal, followed by a meat or seafood stew or a grilled meat dish. Side dishes may include rice, beans, farofa, fried potatoes, and greens such as kale. Salads, typically featuring cooked vegetables, are popular in some areas, including Brazil, and are served with the meal. Dessert, most often flan or another sweet custard or pudding, is usually served. In Argentina, the time spent relaxing and socializing after lunch is called la sobremesa and sometimes includes a nap. Dinner is traditionally lighter, sometimes just cold cuts, a seafood salad, or a serving of soup or stew, and usually eaten around 9:00 each evening, often continuing past midnight. Beer, wine, fruit juice, and soft drinks are beverages commonly consumed at meals.

An afternoon break is enjoyed in much of South America: coffee is typically consumed in Argentina, Colombia, Ecuador, and Brazil; tea is served in the late afternoon in Chile and Uruguay; and maté is popular in parts of Argentina, Paraguay, Uruguay, and Brazil. Snacks eaten with the beverage are often fruit, cachapas or arepa, sandwiches, or a pastry. Street vendors offering coffee, fruit juice, and snacks throughout the day are common in urban areas. Unlike wealthier South Americans, the less affluent often skip lunch and eat a large dinner. The meal may consist of soup or a serving of stew with a side dish of potatoes, plantains, cassava, corn, or rice and beans, depending on the region.

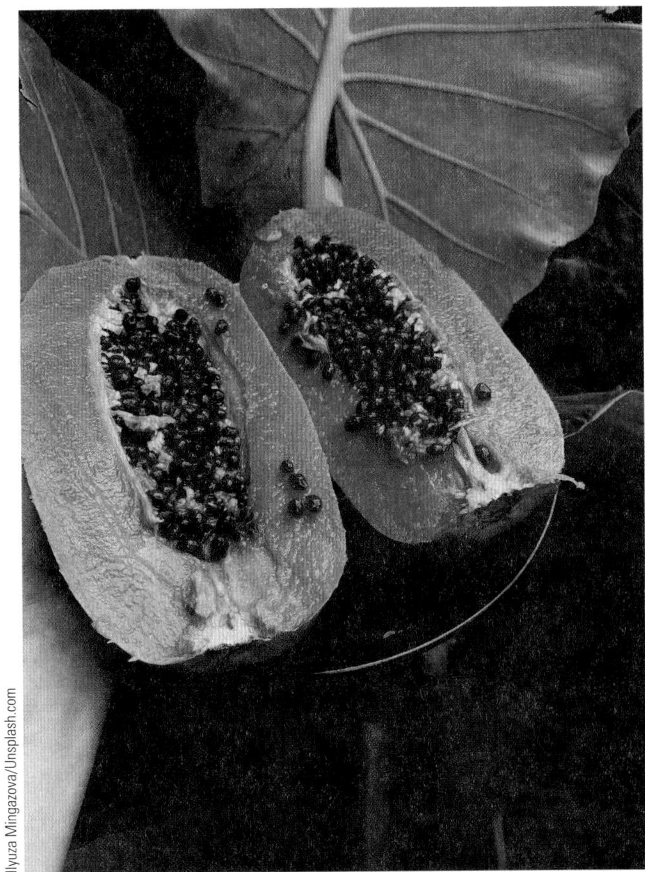
Ilyuza Mingazova/Unsplash.com

▲ Papaya is one of many temperate and tropical fruits in the region.

Special Occasions Catholic traditions have influenced many South American holidays. A rich Christmas Eve dinner is traditional in most nations, often with a roast, such as lechón (suckling pig) in Brazil and cuy or lechón in Ecuador. Italian specialties including torrone and panettone are Christmas items in Argentina, where Epiphany is another significant religious holiday (refer to Chapter 6).

Easter is important in many homes, and Carnaval festivities featuring dancing, parties, and traditional fare are popular in Brazil, Ecuador, Peru, and Uruguay. Americans from these countries sometimes celebrate with parties during the three days before Lent. During the time of Lent, animals associated with water habits, such as alligators, armadillos, capybaras, iguanas, and turtles, were traditionally classified as fish; thus, the Catholic Church permitted their consumption on meatless days.[96,97] These game meats are still considered Lent specialties in some regions.

St. John's Day is a favorite in Brazil, featuring foods made with corn and pumpkin, and it is also celebrated by the citizens of Otavalo, Ecuador with all-night feasting and dancing. In Peru, All Soul's Day on November 2 includes gifts of food and family picnics at the gravesites of deceased kin. Also significant for many Americans of South American descent are the independence days observed in various nations. Brazilian Americans commemorate their independence on September 7 with day-long festivities in Boston, New York, and Newark, New Jersey. Americans from Chile sponsor traditional food and craft booths for fairs to celebrate their Independence on September 18. Many Colombian Americans consume tamales, empanadas, arepas, and other specialties on their Independence Day, July 20. In Ecuador, the primer grito ("first cry" of independence) is held on August 10 and is officially marked as Ecuador Day in New York City. Independence Day in Peru is July 28. The Day of Tradition is popular in the Argentinian American community, with customary foods, folk music, and equestrian displays by men dressed as gauchos.

Etiquette European-style dining is common in most of South America. The fork is kept in the left hand, and the knife in the right, with no switching for cutting food. Bread is often served without butter and placed on the side of the plate. It is the only food that should be eaten with the hands. All other items, including fruit, require cutlery. Salads, however, should not be cut. Instead, the lettuce should be folded into bite-size packets with a fork. In Brazil, even sandwiches are eaten with a knife and fork. All items are passed to the left. The hands should remain above the table when a person is not eating, with wrists resting on the table edge. In Colombia, the host may start a meal with the phrase, "¡Buen provecho!" In Bolivia, it is an insult to pour wine with your left hand or to hold the bottle at the base when pouring, which is interpreted to mean you dislike the person for whom the glass is intended.[98,99]

Therapeutic Uses of Foods A hot–cold system of medicine, most likely introduced by European immigrants, has also been adopted by Candomblé healers, treating hot conditions associated with hot orixás with cool prescriptions associated with cool orixás. Classification is inconsistent, however, and cold conditions are rarely treated with hot remedies.[98,99]

Some South Americans may adhere to more general hot–cold classifications not associated with Candomblé.[98,99] Foods that are hot in temperature, or irritating to the stomach, may be avoided during fevers, for example. Conditions such as menstruation, pregnancy, and lactation also require specific foods. In addition, some people believe that certain foods should be eaten at specific times of the day, such as fruit, which is considered wholesome in the morning but harmful in the evening. Some South Americans avoid combinations of some foods, such as eating acidic fruits at the same time as drinking milk.

Contemporary Food Habits in the United States

Adaptations of Food Habits

Very little has been reported on the adapted food habits of South Americans living in the United States. Many continue cooking their favorites from home, although recipes are often adapted to accommodate U.S. ingredients or to improve acceptability (e.g., cuy is not often prepared). Substitutions for unavailable ingredients, such as feta cheese for fresh farmer's cheese or peanut oil for dênde oil, are common. Sometimes the fact that certain customary ingredients are unobtainable makes other dishes that can be prepared traditionally more popular in the United States than these dishes are in their countries of origin. For instance, llapingachos (crisp potato patties or potato pancakes stuffed with cheese) are probably eaten more often by Ecuadorian Americans than by Ecuadorians. Among Chileans, many find it difficult to adapt to typical American schedules with a work day that begins earlier than in Chile (difficult after a late dinner) and has a short lunch period precluding a leisurely meal.

Food for Thought

Chileans and most Latin American people, commonly use both their paternal and maternal surnames.

Nutritional Status

Nutritional Intake There are minimal data on the nutritional status of Americans of South American descent.

Parasitic infection, iron-deficiency anemia, and protein-calorie malnutrition are common in many rural areas of South America and some crowded urban neighborhoods as well. Chronic Chagas, an inflammatory, infectious disease caused by the parasite *Trypanosoma cruziis*, is endemic in some regions and may be a risk factor for cardiovascular disease.[100]

Studies in South America reveal trends that may apply to the population in the United States, particularly recent immigrants. Overweight and obesity rates are prevalent in some regions, with overall reported rates in 2018 of overweight adults at 36 percent, and obese adults at 21 percent. Overweight and obesity rates in Chile are 40 percent and 34 percent, respectively.[101] In Ecuador, 41 percent of adults are overweight and 23 percent are obese. In Brazil, 35 percent of adults are overweight and 20 percent are obese. The prevalence of high blood pressure in South American Countries ranges from 23 to 46 percent.[101]

Among Brazilians, traditional diets low in calorie density and high in fiber were associated with lower BMI whereas more Westernized diets with foods high in added fats (especially butter, margarine, and fried snacks) and sugars (particularly soft drinks) were associated with a higher BMI. The cost of balanced, healthier diets is an issue and studies are underway to make lower-cost diets culturally acceptable.[102–107]

Type 2 diabetes rates in South American countries are one of the lowest at 10.1 percent in men and 9.8 percent in women. However, 24 percent of the adult cases with diabetes are undiagnosed.[102–104] Research in Venezuela estimated that one-third of the adult population in the region had metabolic syndrome associated with dyslipidemia. Among men, rates varied widely by ethnicity and were highest in those of mixed heritage (37 percent), followed by whites and blacks. The lowest rates (17 percent) were found in the Native group.[102–104]

Health and Longevity Take Away

Rastafarianism is often described as an Afro-Jamaican religion. The average lifespan of Rastafarians is 86.9 years, which is quite a bit longer than that of the United States. The Rastafarian diet is known as "Ital," a words that comes from the English word "vital." Diet is seen as a key factor in longevity and should have good vibrations and promote life. The Ital diet is primarily a whole foods vegan diet that is organic, chemical-free, and uses unprocessed foods. Only clay pots are used for making food because of the belief that aluminum pots and pans transfer traces of metal into the food. The diet is based on vegetables, fruits, legumes, and lentils, some fish, herbal tea, plant-based milk, coconuts, and cooking herbs. Alcohol, coffee, tea, and soda are avoided. While adhering to this strict diet may be difficult, its healthy components may be worth giving a try.

Comfort Food—Brazil

Angela Badham's story

Brazil may not come to mind first when you think of rice, but this descendant, Angel Badham, of the country has strong ties to rice and its aroma and texture—as well as to the tropical fruit added to make Brazilian rice pudding.

What is a favorite comfort food that you consider traditional from your home culture?

AB: Rice was always in my mom's pantry. It's easy to make and doesn't require a trip to the market. I love its soft, smooth, soothing texture and the aroma of rice cooking in our kitchen.

Did you eat this food together with community? Where was it eaten?

AB: Rice pudding is served as a special dessert that we often had at home on the weekend, especially after Sunday lunch. Tropical ingredients, like mango and pineapple, were always in our orchard at my father's farm in Brazil. Rice was a staple and we could combine it with lots of different organic fruits.

Angel shares her family recipe here:

Rice Pudding

Serves 4-6

1 cup any kind of rice (even brown rice)
2 cups room-temperature water
Pinch of salt
2 14-ounce cans unsweetened coconut milk (preferably full fat)
½ cup sugar
1 tsp. vanilla extract
1 mango, peeled and sliced
1 banana, peeled and sliced
Toasted slivered coconut (to garnish)

Place rice, water, and salt in a heavy, deep pan and bring to a boil. Reduce the heat and simmer, covered, for about 40 minutes. (Do not open the pan while the rice is cooking.) Remove cooked rice from heat and uncover. Let it cool. Stir one can of coconut milk and sugar into the rice and bring to a boil, uncovered. Reduce heat and simmer, stirring frequently, for about 5 minutes. Remove from heat. Add vanilla extract and let cool to room temperature; refrigerate rice.

Remove the cream from the top of the second can of coconut milk; reserve the coconut milk for another purpose. To serve, spoon the rice pudding into individual bowls. Arrange the mango, banana, and pineapple slices the around rice and drizzle with the reserved coconut cream from the top of the second can. Garnish with toasted coconut.

Nutritional Information (per serving):
calories 530; protein 6 g; carbohydrates 62 g; fat 32 g; sodium 22 mg

Additional RECIPE TO TRY

Cinnamon-Scented Rice Milk

Serves 12

2 cups long-grain white rice
1 cup sugar
4 tsp. vanilla
1½ tsp. ground cinnamon

In a bowl, combine rice and 10 cups of water. Cover and chill until grains break easily when squeezed, about 24 hours, or up to 2 days. In a blender, whirl about 2 cups of the rice and water mixture with the sugar, vanilla, and cinnamon until sugar is dissolved and the mixture is smooth. Pour into a large bowl or pitcher (at least 3 ½ qt.). Blend the remaining rice and water mixture without seasonings, in batches if necessary; add to the bowl and stir until well blended with the flavored batch. Taste, and add more sugar if desired. Just before serving, stir the mixture (ground rice will have settled to the bottom). Fill glasses with ice cubes, then horchata.

*Recipe courtesy of https://www.myrecipes.com/recipe/cinnamon-scented-rice-milk

Nutritional Information (per serving):
calories 182; protein 2.2 g; carbohydrates 42 g; fat 0.2 g; sodium 1.9 mg

Discussion Starters

Understanding Cultural Differences

This chapter covers many cultures. Some share traits; others do not. Cultural differences can be subtle. It's easy to stereotype people from unfamiliar cultures, but doing so can cause poor outcomes for U.S. health care professionals trying to counsel immigrant patients. Below are examples of two matrixes, intended to help us differentiate between immigrants from various Carib-bean Island and South American cultures. Your task is to create two tables using the following models, each with two rows: Caribbean Islands and South America. The first table lists health issues, and the second lists cultural issues for the two groups. Place a plus sign in the squares where the features are present for the immigrants in each row.

In the first matrix, identify which of the immigrant groups have been generally recognized as suffering from which diseases. This is an example of how you can organize your information:

	Obesity	Hypertension	Diabetes	Liver Disease	Parasitic Disease
List the country in this column					

In small groups, share your completed matrix. Within your group, come to a consensus on your identifications and discuss the implications this information might have for training health professionals. Are there categories shared by several immigrant groups? Do the matrixes suggest some general guidelines for addressing the dietary needs of immigrants from the Caribbean Islands and South America?

Review Questions

1. Choose one Caribbean country and summarize the worldview of its immigrants living in the United States. Include an example of the use of the hot–cold system for the cause or treatment of an illness. Describe the types of traditional healers used in this region.
2. Select one indigenous food found in the Caribbean. Describe its taste and use in recipes from the region. Next, select a foreign food that was brought to the region and is still commonly consumed—provide a recipe. Which foods are now the staples of the diet? Describe a holiday meal in one Caribbean country plus the specialties of the island.
3. What health problems have become common for people from the Caribbean living in the United States? If you were a nutritionist, how would you modify the diet in the treatment of these disorders?

Reflection

Most traditional meal patterns in the Caribbean and South America revolve around the noon meal being the largest, with a smaller meal for dinner. This meal pattern changes when coming to the United States where a lighter lunch and larger dinner are adopted. How might the change in traditional meal pattern behavior have contributed to overweight and obesity patterns for this population when living in the United States? What are some ways the rates might be turned around?

References

1. U.S. Census Bureau. n.d. Quick Facts—Population Estimates, July 1, 2021. Retrieved from https://www.census.gov/quickfacts/fact/table/US/PST045221.
2. U.S. Census Bureau. n.d. Selected population profile in the U.S. *2020 American Community Survey 1-Year Estimates*. Table S0201. Accessed from https://data.census.gov/cedsci/table?t=400%20%20Hispanic%20or%20Latino%20%28of%20any%20race%29&tid=ACSSPP1Y2019.S0201. (Retrieved April 4, 2022).
3. U.S. Census Bureau. n.d. Selected characteristics of the foreign-born population by region of birth. *2016–2020 American Community Survey 5-Year Estimates*. Table S0506. Retrieved from https://www2.census.gov/programs-surveys/acs/data/pums/2020/ (accessed March 1, 2022).
4. Buffington, S.T. 2014. Dominican Americans. In R.V. Dassanowsky & J. Lehman (Eds.), *Gale encyclopedia of multicultural America*. Farmington Hills, MI: Gale Group.
5. Noe-Bustamante, L. April 7, 2020. Education levels of recent Latino Immigrants in the U.S. Reached New Highs as of 2018. Pew Research Center, Hispanic Trends. Retrieved from https://www.pewresearch.org/fact-tank/2020/04/07/education-levels-of-recent-latino-immigrants-in-the-u-s-reached-new-highs-as-of-2018 (accessed March 30, 2022).
6. Krogstad, J.M., Noe-Bustamante, L., September 9, 2021. Key facts about US Latinos for National Hispanic Heritage Month. Retrieved from https://www.pewresearch.org/fact-tank/2021/09/09/key-facts-about-u-s-latinos-for-national-hispanic-heritage-month/
7. Unaeze, F.E., & Perrin, R.E. 2014. Haitian Americans. In R.V. Dassanowsky & J. Lehman (Eds.), *Gale encyclopedia of multicultural America*. Farmington Hills, MI: Gale Group.

8. Zong, J., & Batalova, J. 2019. Caribbean immigrants in the United States. Migration Policy Institute. Retrieved from https://www.migrationpolicy.org/article/caribbean-immigrants-united-states-2017
9. U.S. Census Bureau, Immigration Statistics Staff. 2013. *Foreign-born profiles* (ACS-19). American Community Survey Reports 2013. Retrieved from http://www.census.gov/acs/www/
10. Murrell, N.S. 2014. Jamaican Americans. In R.V. Dassanowsky & J. Lehman (Eds.), *Gale encyclopedia of multicultural America*. Farmington Hills, MI: Gale Group.
11. Romero, T. 2021. Religion affiliation in the Dominican Republic as of 2020, by type. Statista. Retrieved from https://www.statista.com/statistics/1067044/religious-affiliation-in-the-dominican-republic/
12. Romero, T. 2021. Religion affiliation in selected countries in Latin America and the Caribbean in 2020. Statista. Retrieved from https://www.statista.com/statistics/1261540/religion-affiliation-selected-countries-in-lac/
13. Taylor, P., & Case, F.I. (Eds.). 2013. *The Encyclopedia of Caribbean Religions: Volume 1: A-L; Volume 2: M-Z*. University of Illinois Press.
14. Menjívar, C., Abrego, L.J., & Schmalzbauer, L.C. 2016. *Immigrant families*. John Wiley & Son.
15. Colin, J.M. 2021. People of Haitian heritage. In *Textbook for Transcultural Health Care: A Population Approach*. Springer, Cham, pp. 469–495.
16. Unaeze, F.E., & Perrin, R.E. 2014. Haitian Americans. In R.V. Dassanowsky and J. Lehman (Eds.), *Gale encyclopedia of multicultural America*. Farmington Hills, MI: Gale Group.
17. Purnell, L.D., & Fenkl, E.A. 2019. People of Puerto Rican heritage. In *Handbook for Culturally Competent Care*. Springer, Cham, pp. 283–298.
18. Sutherland, P. 2014. The history, philosophy, and transformation of Caribbean healing traditions. *Caribbean healing traditions: Implications for health and mental health*, pp. 153–163.
19. Raghunandan, S., & Moodley, R. 2020. Caribbean healing. In *The Routledge International Handbook of Race, Culture and Mental Health*, Routledge, pp. 517–529.
20. Quinlan, M.B. 2022. Ethnomedicines: Traditions of medical knowledge. *A Companion to Medical Anthropology*, pp. 315–341.
21. Fernandes, B., Hashmi, S.I., & Essau, C.A. 2014. Ataque de nervios. *The Encyclopedia of Clinical Psychology*, pp. 1–3.
22. Sutherland, P., Moodley, R., & Chevannes, P. 2013. *Caribbean healing traditions: Implications for health and mental health*. Routledge.
23. Gómez, P.F. 2017. *The experiential Caribbean: Creating knowledge and healing in the early modern Atlantic*. UNC Press Books.
24. Moreno-Walton, L., Martin, M.L., Walker, L.U., Wong-Pérez, R.E., & Klein, J.H. 2016. Case 12: spiritualism in the Latino Community. In *Diversity and inclusion in quality patient care*. Springer, Cham, pp. 263–269.
25. García, W.C.G., & Núñez, M.R.T. 2022. Cultural-Spiritual Guidance in Caring for Cancer Patients in the Dominican Republic, Dominican Republic. *Global Perspectives in Cancer Care: Religion, Spirituality, and Cultural Diversity in Health and Healing*, p. 446.
26. George, N. 2020. Understanding Haitian Immigrant's Health Practices.
27. Valdes, J.A., & Delgado, V. 2021. People of Cuban Heritage. In *Textbook for Transcultural Health Care: A Population Approach*. Springer, Cham, pp. 321–341.
28. Pesoutova, J. 2019. *Indigenous ancestors and healing landscapes: cultural memory and intercultural communication in the Dominican Republic and Cuba* (Doctoral dissertation, Leiden University).
29. Goucher, C. 2014. *Congotay! Congotay! A global history of Caribbean food*. Routledge.
30. Beushausen, W., Commichau, A.S., Helber, P., Brüske, A., & Kloss, S. 2014. *Caribbean Food Cultures*. Transcript Verlag.
31. Chabrán, R. 2015. Eating Puerto Rico: A History of Food, Culture, and Identity. *Diálogo*, 18(1), 23.
32. Trinidad, C. 2020. The ugly truth about sazon. *Latin Trends*. Retrieved from https://latintrends.com/the-ugly-truth-about-sazon/.
33. García-Quijano, C.G., Poggie, J.J., Pitchon, A., & Del Pozo, M.H. 2015. Coastal resource foraging, life satisfaction, and well-being in southeastern Puerto Rico. *Journal of Anthropological Research*, 71(2), 145–167.
34. Gould, W.A., Wadsworth, F.H., Quiñones, M., Fain, S.J., & Álvarez-Berríos, N.L. 2017. Land use, conservation, forestry, and agriculture in Puerto Rico. *Forests*, 8(7), 242.
35. Ginzburg, S.L. 2021. Colonial comida: the colonization of food insecurity in Puerto Rico. *Food, Culture & Society*, 1–14.
36. Pelaez, A.S. 2014. The Cuban Table: A Celebration of Food, Flavors, and History. St. Martin's Press.
37. Garcia Polanco, V. 2017. "Transnational" Eating: The Food Culture of Dominican Immigrants in RI.
38. Picking, D., & Vandebroek, I. 2019. Traditional and local knowledge systems in the Caribbean: Jamaica as a case study. In *Traditional and indigenous knowledge for the modern era: A natural and applied science perspective*. Boca Raton: CFC Press, pp. 89–116.
39. Gray, Vaugh Stafford. December 22, 2020. A brief history of Jamaican Jerk. Smithsonian. https://www.smithsonianmag.com/arts-culture/brief-history-jamaican-jerk-180976597/
40. DeMers, J. 2012. *Authentic recipes from Jamaica*. Tuttle Publishing.
41. Croxford, S. and Itsiopoulos, C. 2020. Cultures, beliefs and food habits. *Food and Nutrition Throughout Life: A comprehensive overview of food and nutrition in all stages of life*.
42. Rousseau, M. and Rousseau, S. 2018. *Provisions: The Roots of Caribbean Cooking—150 Vegetarian Recipes*. Hachette UK.
43. Captain Tim, November 15, 2018. Thanksgiving Traditions in Puerto Rico. Caribbean Trading Post. Retrieved at https://caribbeantrading.com/thanksgiving-traditions-in-puerto-rico/
44. Colin, J.M. 2021. People of Haitian heritage. In *Textbook for Transcultural Health Care: A Population Approach*. Springer, Cham, pp. 469–495.
45. Fugh-Berman, A., Balick, M.J., Kronenberg, F., Oroski, A.L., O'Conner, B., Reiff, M., . . . Lee, R. 2004. Treatment of fibroids: The use of beets (*Beta vulgaris*) and molasses (*Saccharum officinarum*) as an herbal therapy by Dominican healers in New York City. *Journal of Ethnopharmacology*, 92, 337–339.
46. Raghunandan, S., & Moodley, R. 2020. Caribbean healing. In *The Routledge International Handbook of Race, Culture and Mental Health*. Routledge, pp. 517–529.
47. Joseph, M.A. 2020. The lived experiences of folklore healing practices as a health patterning modality. *Journal of Holistic Nursing*, 38(3), 263–277.
48. Fuster, M., & González, E. 2019. Traditional diets in everyday life: Perspectives from Hispanic Caribbean communities in New York City. *Food and Foodways*, 27(4), 316–337.
49. Vardeman, E., & Vandebroek, I. 2021. Caribbean women's health and transnational ethnobotany. *Economic Botany*, 1–22.
50. Abrons, J.P., Andreas, E., Jolly, O., Parishi-Mercado, M., Daly, A., and Carr, I. 2019. Cultural Sensitivity and global pharmacy engagement in the Caribbean: Dominica, Jamaica, Puerto Rico, and St. Kitts. *American Journal of Pharmaceutical Education*, 83(4), 7219.
51. Popovic-Lipovac, A., & Strasser, B. 2015. A review on changes in food habits among immigrant women and implications for health. *Journal of Immigrant and Minority Health*, 17(2), 582–590.
52. Immink, M.D.C., Sanjur, D., & Burgos, M. 1983. Nutritional consequences of U.S. migration patterns among Puerto Rican women. *Ecology of Food and Nutrition*, 13, 139–148.

53. Sharma, S., Cade, J., Landman, J., & Cruickshank, J.K. 2002. Assessing the diet of the British African-Caribbean population: Frequency of consumption of foods and food portion sizes. *International Journal of Food Sciences and Nutrition*, 53, 439.
54. Goff, L.M., Timbers, L., Style, H., & Knight, A. 2015. Dietary intake in Black British adults; an observational assessment of nutritional composition and the role of traditional foods in UK Caribbean and West African diets. *Public Health Nutrition*, 18(12), 2191–2201.
55. Mattei, J., McClain, A.C., Falcón, L.M., Noel, S.E., & Tucker, K.L. (2018). Dietary acculturation among Puerto Rican adults varies by acculturation construct and dietary measure. *The Journal of Nutrition*, 148(11), 1804–1813.
56. Steele, E.M., Khandpur, N., Sun, Q., & Monteiro, C. A. 2020. The impact of acculturation to the US environment on the dietary share of ultra-processed foods among US adults. *Preventive Medicine*, 141, 106261.
57. Joyce, B.T., Wu, D., Hou, L., Dai, Q., Castaneda, S.F., Gallo, L.C., Talavera, G.A., Sotres-Alvarez, D., Van Horn, L., Beasley, J.M., Khambaty, T., Elfassy, T., Zeng, T., Mattei, J., Corsino, I., & Daviglus, M.I. 2019. DASH diet and prevalent metabolic syndrome in the Hispanic Community Health Study/Study of Latinos, *Preventive Medicine Reports*, 15.
58. Bermudez, O.I., Falcon, L.M., & Tucker K.L. 2000. Intake and food sources of macronutrients among older Hispanic adults: Association with ethnicity, acculturation, and length of residence in the United States. *Journal of the American Dietetic Association*, 100, 665–673.
59. Centers for Disease Control and Prevention. 2011. *Fact sheet: CDC health disparities and inequalities report—US 2011*. Retrieved from http://www.cdc.gov/minorityhealth/reports/CHDIR11/FactSheet.pdf (accessed March 5, 2015).
60. Fuster, M. 2017. "We like fried things"; negotiating health and taste among Hispanic Caribbean communities in New Your City. *Ecology of Food and Nutrition*, 5(2), 124–138.
61. Fact Sheet. May 7 2020 Health Disparities by Race and Ethnicity CAP. Retrieved from https://www.americanprogress.org/article/health-disparities-race-ethnicity/
62. U.S. Department of Health and Human Services. 2019. Profile: Hispanic/Latino Americans. Retrieved from https://www.minorityhealth.hhs.gov/omh/browse.aspx?lvl=3&lvlid=64
63. Szegda,K.,Bertone-Johnson,E.R.,Pekow,P.,Powers,S.,Markenson,G., Dole, N., & Chasan-Taber, L. Prenatal Perceived Stress and Adverse Birth Outcomes Among Puerto Rican Women. J Womens Health (Larchmt). 2018 May;27(5):699-708. doi: 10.1089/jwh.2016.6118. Epub 2017 Dec 7. PMID: 29215314; PMCID: PMC5962329.
64. Schuurmans, J., Borgundvaag, E., Finaldi, P., Senat-Delva, R., Desauguste, F., Badjo, C., Lekkerkerker, M., Grandpierre, R., Lerebours, G., Ariti, C., & Lenglet, A. 2021. Risk factors for adverse outcomes in women with high-risk pregnancy and their neonates, Haiti. *Revista Panamericana de Salud Publica = Pan American Journal of Public Health*, 45, e147. Retrieved from https://doi.org/10.26633/RPSP.2021.147
65. Dahl, M. 2004. Working with Puerto Rican clients. *Health Care Food & Nutrition Focus*, 21, 10–12.
66. Kugyelka, J.G., Rasmussen, K.M., & Frongillo, E.A. 2004. Maternal obesity is negatively associated with breastfeeding success among Hispanic but not black women. *Journal of Nutrition*, 134, 1746–1753.
67. Puerto Rico Results Report. 2013 Survey. CDC Survey of Maternity Practices in Infant Nutrition and Care. Retrieved from https://www.cdc.gov/breastfeeding/pdf/mpinc/states/2013/puertoricompinc13_508tagged.pdf
68. Tucker, K.L. 2021. Dietary patterns in Latinx groups. *The Journal of Nutrition, 151*(9), 2505–2506, https://doi.org/10.1093/jn/nxab225
69. Food Policy And Obesity. October 11, 2021. Concerning dietary patterns among Latinx Linked to years living in the US. Retrieved from https://www.publichealth.columbia.edu/public-health-now/news/concerning-dietary-patterns-among-latinx-linked-years-living-us#:~:text=Using%20data%20from%20the%20Hispanic%20Community%20Health%20Study%2FStudy,Red%20Meats%3B%20Fish%3B%20Egg%20and%20Cheese%3B%20and%20Alcohol.
70. Maldonado, L.E., Adair, L.S., Sotres-Alvarez, D., Mattei, J., Mossavar-Rahmani, Y., Perreira, K.M., Daviglus, M.L., Van Horn, L.V., Gallo, L.C., Isasi, C.R., & Albrecht, S.S. 2021. Dietary patterns and years living in the United States by Hispanic/Latino heritage in the Hispanic Community Health Study/Study of Latinos (HCHS/SOL). *Journal of Nutrition, 151*(9), 2749–2759.
71. Centers for Disease Control and Prevention. 2020. *Summary health statistics for U.S. adults: 2020*. Retrieved from https://www.cdc.gov/obesity/data/prevalence-maps.html#race
72. Liao, Y., Tucker, P., Okoro, C.A., Giles, W.H., Mokdad, A.H., & Harris, V.B. 2004. REACH 2009 surveillance for health status in minority communities—United States, 2011. *Morbidity and Mortality Weekly Report*, 60(6), 1–36.
73. Mojica, C.M., Liang, Y., Foster, B.A., & Parra-Medina, D. 2019. The association between acculturation and parental feeding practices in families with overweight and obese Hispanic/Latino children. *Family & Community Health*, 42(3), 180–188. Retrieved from https://pubmed.ncbi.nlm.nih.gov/31107728
74. Paz, K., & Massey, K.P. 2016. Health disparity among Latina Women: comparison with Non-Latina women. *Clinical Medicine Insights: Women's Health*, 9(1), 71–74. Retrieved from https://pubmed.ncbi.nlm.nih.gov/27478393
75. Toward a more equitable future: The trends and challenges facing america's Latino Children. Washington, DC: National Council of La Raza, 2016. Retrieved from http://publications.unidosus.org/bitstream/handle/123456789/1627/towardamoreequitablefuture_9291 6.pdf W
76. Arias-Gastélum, M., Lindberg, N.M., Leo, M.C., Bruening, M., Whisner, C. M., et al. 2021. Dietary patterns with healthy and unhealthy traits among overweight/obese Hispanic women with or at high risk for type 2 diabetes. *Journal of Racial & Ethnic Health Disparities*, 8(2), 293–303. https://pubmed.ncbi.nlm.nih.gov/32495304
77. Kim, J.H., Lee, C., & Sohn, W. 2016. Urban natural environments, obesity, and health-related quality of life among Hispanic children living in inner-city neighborhoods. *International Journal of Environmental Research and Public Health, 13*(1). Retrieved from http://www.ncbi.nlm.nih.gov/pubmed/26771623
78. Daviglus, M.L., Talavera, G.A., Avilés-Santa, M., Allison, M., Cai, J., Criqui, M.H., . . . Stamler, J. 2012. Prevalence of major cardiovascular risk factors and cardiovascular diseases among Hispanic/Latino individuals of diverse backgrounds in the United States. *Journal of the American Medical Association*, 308(17), 1775–1784. doi:10.1001/jama.2012.14517
79. Schneiderman, N., Llabre, M., Cowie, C.C., Barnhart, J., Carnethon, M., Gallo, L.C., . . . Avilés-Santa, M.L. 2014. Prevalence of diabetes among Hispanics/Latinos from diverse backgrounds: The Hispanic Community Health Study/Study of Latinos (HCHS/SOL). *Diabetes Care*, 37, 2233–2239.
80. Your Heart, Your Life: A Community Health Worker's Manual for the Hispanic Community. Bethesda, MD: U.S. Department of Health and Human Service (HHS), National Institutes of Health (NIH), 2008. https://www.nhlbi.nih.gov/files/docs/resources/heart/lat_mnl_en.pdf
81. Hernandez, R., Carnethon, M., Giachello, A.L., Penedo, F.J., Wu, D., et al. 2018. Structural social support and cardiovascular disease risk factors in Hispanic/Latino adults with diabetes: Results from the Hispanic Community Health Study/Study of Latinos (HCHS/SOL). *Ethnicity & Health*, 23(7), 737–751. Retrieved from https://pubmed.ncbi.nlm.nih.gov/28277024
82. Centers for Disease Control and Prevention n.d. Hispanic or Latino People and Type 2 Diabetes. Retrieved from https://www.cdc.gov/diabetes/library/features/hispanic-diabetes.html#:~:text=Over%20their%20lifetime%2C%20US%20adults%20

overall%20have%20a,harder%3A%20Hispanics%2FLatinos%20have%20higher%20rates%20of%20kidney%20failure

83. U.S. Department of Health and Human Services Office of Minority Health. 2021. Diabetes and Hispanic Americans. Retrieved from https://www.minorityhealth.hhs.gov/omh/browse.aspx?lvl=4&lvlid=63
84. CDC Vital Signs, May 2015, Hispanic Health. Retrieved from https://www.cdc.gov/vitalsigns/hispanic-health/index.html#:~:text=Hispanics%20are%20about%2050%25%20more%20likely%20to%20die,deaths%2C%20which%20is%20about%20the%20same%20for%20whites.
85. Thompson, M.S. 2020. Milk and the motherland? Colonial legacies of taste and the law in the Anglophone Caribbean. *Journal of Food Law & Policy*, 16, 135.
86. U.S. Census Bureau. 2015. Place of birth for the foreign-born population in the United States. ACS 5-Year Estimates selected population detailed tables B05006. Retrieved from https://data.census.gov/cedsci/table?q=south%20american%20&tid=ACSDT5YSPT2015.B05006
87. Noe-Bustamante, L., Flores, A., & Shah, S. September 16, 2019. *Facts on Hispanics of Colombian origin in the United States, 2017.* Retrieved from https://www.pewresearch.org/hispanic/fact-sheet/u-s-hispanics-facts-on-colombian-origin-latinos (accessed April 5, 2022).
88. Lopez, G. September 15, 2015 *Hispanics of Argentinean origin in the United States, 2013.* Retrieved from https://www.pewresearch.org/hispanic/2015/09/15/hispanics-of-argentinean-origin-in-the-united-states-2013/ (accessed April 5, 2022).
89. Wormald, B. 2014. Religion in Latin America: Widespread Change in a Historically Catholic Region. Pew Research Center. Retrieved from https://www.pewforum.org/2014/11/13/religion-in-latin-america/
90. Cruz, S. 2018. Syncretic Brazil: The Beginnings.
91. Wright, R.M. 2017. The state of the arts of the study of Indigenous religious traditions in South America. *International Journal of Latin American Religions*, 1(1), 42–56.
92. Packel, J. 2014. Peruvian Americans. In R.V. Dassonowsky & J. Lehman (Eds.), *Gale encyclopedia of multicultural America*. Farmington Hills, MI: Gale Group.
93. Cañigueral, S., & Sanz-Biset, J. (2015). Ethnopharmacology in Central and South America. *Ethnopharmacology*, 379.
94. Chevallier, A. 2016. *Encyclopedia of Herbal Medicine: 550 Herbs and Remedies for Common Ailments*. Penguin.
95. Lovera, J.R. 2005. *Food culture in South America*. Westport, CT: Greenwood Press.
96. Jefferson, A.W. 2014. Brazilian Americans. In R.V. Dassanowsky & J. Lehman (Eds.), *Gale encyclopedia of multicultural America*. Farmington Hills, MI: Gale Group.
97. Packel, J. 2014. Peruvian Americans. In R.V. Dassanowsky & J. Lehman (Eds.), *Gale encyclopedia of multicultural America*. Farmington Hills, MI: Gale Group.
98. Albuquerque, U.P. 2014. A little bit of Africa in Brazil: Ethnobiology experiences in the field of Afro-Brazilian religions. *Journal of Ethnobiology and Ethnomedicine*, 10(1), 1–7.
99. Voeks, R.A. 2018. *The Ethnobotany of Eden*. University of Chicago Press.
100. Mayo Clinic n.d. Chagas Disease. Retrieved from https://www.mayoclinic.org/diseases-conditions/chagas-disease/symptoms-causes/syc-20356212 (accessed 4-5-2022)
101. World Obesity - Chile. Obesity Prevalence Adults, 2016–2017. Retrieved from https://data.worldobesity.org/country/chile-4/#data_prevalence (accessed April 5, 2022).
102. Verly, E., Darmon, N., Sichieri, R., & Sarti, F. 2020. Reaching culturally acceptable and adequate diets at the lowest cost increment according to income level in Brazilian households. *PLoS ONE*. Retrieved from https://journals.plos.org/plosone/article?id=10.1371/journal.pone.0229439 (accessed April 4, 2022).
103. Spanakis, E.K., & Golden, S.H. 2013. Race/ethnic difference in diabetes and diabetic complications. *Current Diabetes Reports*, *13*(6), 814–823. Retrieved from https://doi.org/10.1007/s11892-013-0421-9
104. Aschner, P., Aguilar-Salinas, C., Aguirre, L., Franco, L., Gagliardino, J.J., de Lapertosa, S.G., Seclen, S., & Vinocour, M. 2014. Diabetes in South and Central America: An update. *Diabetes Research and Clinical Practice, 103*(2), 238–243. Retrieved from https://pubmed.ncbi.nlm.nih.gov/24439209/
105. Aballay, L.R., Eynard, A.R., Díaz Mdel, P., Navarro, A., & Muñoz, S.E. 2013. Overweight and obesity: A review of their relationship to metabolic syndrome, cardiovascular disease, and cancer in South America. *Nutrition Reviews*, 71(3), 168–179.
106. ChavezBush, L. 2022. Pachamanca: In Peru, layers of potatoes, meat, and sweets are steamed in a pit filled with volcanic rocks. *Gastro Obscura*. Retrieved from https://www.atlasobscura.com/foods/pachamanca
107. Sotelo-Díaz, L. I., Ramírez, B., García-Segovia, P., Igual, M., Martínez-Monzó, J., & Filomena-Ambrosio, A. 2022. Cricket flour in a traditional beverage (chucula): Emotions and perceptions of Colombian consumers. *Journal of Insects as Food and Feed*, 8(6), 659–671.

New Africa/Shutterstock.com

Chapter 11

East Asians

Learning Objectives

11.1 List the regions of agriculture and geography in China, Japan, and Korea that affect food production and regional patterns of intake.

11.2 Describe immigration patterns, historical socioeconomic influences, and current locations of Chinese, Japanese, and Koreans in the United States today.

11.3 Differentiate the religions, family structures, and traditional health beliefs and practices of the people of China, Japan, and Korea before and after immigration to the United States.

11.4 Compare the differences and similarities among staple foods and preparation techniques within and across China, Japan, and Korea.

11.5 Compare key foods of each of the food groups for people living in China, Japan, and Korea with foods that have been adapted by immigrants from those countries in the United States.

11.6 Describe the traditional meal composition and cycles of China, Japan, and Korea and compare them to those of Chinese, Japanese, and Korean people living in the United States today.

11.7 Describe the regional specialties and dishes of those in China, Japan, and Korea.

11.8 Identify health concerns associated with the nutritional intake of those from China, Japan, and Korea.

Asia is the world's largest continent, stretching from the Ural Mountains and Suez Canal in the east and the Arctic Circle in the north, to the tropical peninsulas of India and Southeast Asia. It encompasses almost one-third of the world's landmass and nearly two-thirds of the global population. Asia is divided into the regions of East Asia, Southeast Asia, and South Asia. Though the continent has historically included parts of Russia and several nations of the former Soviet Union (sometimes known as Central Asia) and the Middle East (sometimes known as Asia Minor), the people of these countries are culturally distinct from the rest of Asia and are covered in Chapters 7 and 13, respectively.

The diverse ethnic and national origins of Asian Americans mean numerous cultures and religious backgrounds, just as the term *Native American* encompasses people from many nations. The first Asian Americans, perhaps of varied races, may have migrated from North and East Asia into North America before there was an Asia or an America. When these people settled, they were likely the ancestors of Native Americans.[1]

East Asia is defined as China (the People's Republic of China), Taiwan, Japan, the Democratic People's Republic of Korea (North Korea), the Republic of Korea (South Korea), and the Mongolian People's Republic (refer to Figure 11.1). Immigrants from these nations, particularly

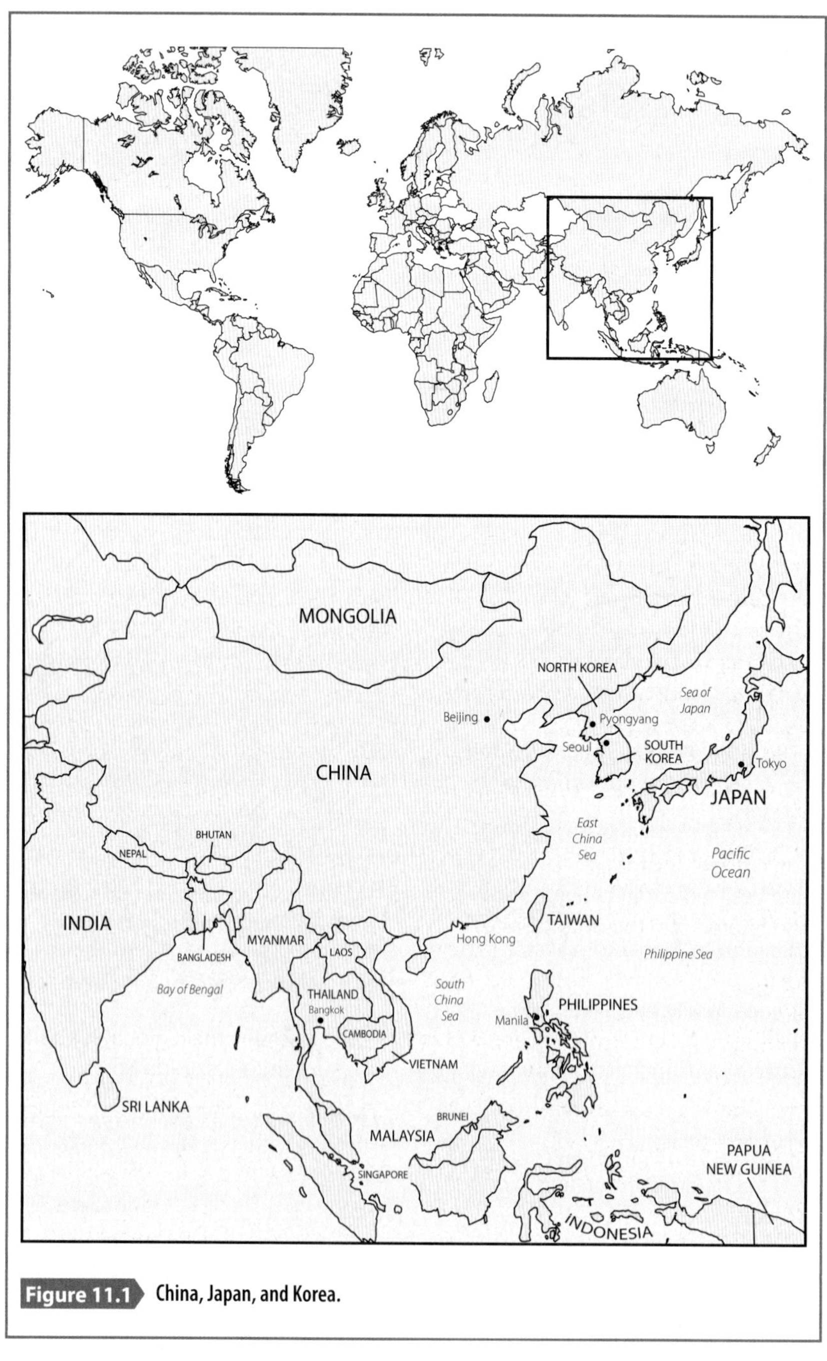

Figure 11.1 China, Japan, and Korea.

China and Japan, have been coming to the United States since the 1800s. Many settled on the West Coast, where the majority of their descendants still live. In recent years, large numbers from throughout the region have arrived in the United States; many are refugees from political oppression, whereas others seek education and employment opportunities. This chapter introduces the people and cuisines of China, Japan, and Korea. Southeast Asians are discussed in Chapter 12 and South Asians are considered in Chapter 14.

Food for Thought

Although the origin of pasta is debated, the first historical evidence of pasta-like food was excavated in Lajia in Northern China in 2005. The 4,000 year-old noodle remains were made of two types of millet flour. Theories claim nomadic Arabs are responsible for bringing early Chinese forms of pasta westward. After noodles reached the Mediterranean, durum wheat became the ingredient of choice for pasta flour.[4]

Chinese

Chinese civilization is more than 4,000 years old and is the world's oldest continuing civilization.[2] Chinese culture and people have made numerous significant contributions to agriculture, the arts, religion, philosophy, and warfare. Silk and embroidered brocade cloth, intricate jade sculpture, Chinese porcelain and lacquerware, book printing, Confucianism, Taoism, and gunpowder are just a few examples. An early name for China was Zhongguo, meaning "middle kingdom" or center of the world. The word China is believed to have come into use as trade along the Silk Road became popular with the West and derives from the Sanskrit *Cina* (from the name of the Chinese Quin Dynasty, pronounced "Chin"). The Romans and Greeks knew the country as Seres, the land where silk comes from. In the thirteenth century CE, Marco Polo referred to the land as Cathay. It wasn't until 1516 that the word China appeared in print in the West.[3]

Geographically, China is an isolated civilization. It is bound on the east and south by the Pacific Ocean, the southwest and west by the Himalayan and Pamir mountains, and the north by steppe lands and harshly cold Siberia.[2] This landscape did not cut off contact with the rest of the world, however. People could and did travel to China via overland routes such as the Silk Road, and by sea. China's landscape is dominated by the valleys of two great rivers, the Huang (Yellow) River in the north, which gets its name from the rich, yellowish-brown soil sediment it carries,[2] and the Chang Jiang ("Long River" as it is known in China, Yangtze in West) in the south. In the north, the climate is blazingly hot in the summer and sometimes bitterly cold in the winter, much like the Utah and Nevada Great Basin in the United States.[2] The north is relatively dry compared to the south and dryland crops grow best, such as barley, millet, and wheat. There is usually only one crop per year and a growing season of four to six months.[2] In the south, the climate is warm and humid, and rainfall is abundant. The southern countryside can be lush, with green rice paddies, picturesque mountains, and tea bushes.[2] The Chang Jiang River starts in Tibet, traverses the southern provinces, and eventually empties into the China Sea near the city of Shanghai. South of the mouth of the Chang Jiang delta is a rugged and mountainous coastline off which are located the islands of Hong Kong and Taiwan. The southern provinces are warmer and wetter and have a longer (six to nine months) growing season than the north.

The population of China is estimated to exceed 1.4 billion people, nearly four and a half times as large as the population of the United States.[5,6] The Chinese have a heterogeneous society with numerous ethnic and racial groups. The Chinese language is equally diverse, with many dialects, some of which are little understood by people of other Chinese regions.

Cultural Perspective

History of Chinese in the United States

Immigration Patterns The first major surge in Chinese immigration to the United States occurred in the early 1850s when the Chinese joined in the gold rush to California; some Chinese still refer to America as the "Land of the Golden Mountain." As mining became less lucrative, the Chinese opened their own businesses, such as laundries and restaurants, but also found employment in other occupations. The Central Pacific Railroad, which joined the Union Pacific as the first cross-country line, was built primarily by 10,000 Chinese workers.

By 1870, there were 63,000 Chinese in the United States, nearly all on the West Coast. Another 120,000 Chinese people are estimated to have entered the United States during the following decade. Racial discrimination against Asians increased as their numbers swelled. By 1880, Chinese immigration slowed to a trickle due to exclusion laws directed against Asians. The Chinese also immigrated to Hawaii, and when the islands were annexed by the United States in 1898, approximately 25,000 Chinese were living there.

Most early Chinese immigrants were from the southeastern Guangdong province of China, formerly referred to as Canton. Most were young men with no intention of staying—they came to make their fortune and then return to China and their families. Many married before coming to the United States, and more than half returned to China. By the 1920s the Chinese population in the United States had dropped to 1870 levels.

In each city where the Chinese settled, they usually lived within a small geographic area known as "Chinatown." Large Chinatowns evolved in San Francisco, New York, Boston, Chicago, Philadelphia, Los Angeles, and Oakland, California. These neighborhoods offered protection against a sometimes hostile social and economic environment. Conditions were often crowded and unusual in the predominance of men but were tolerated with the expectation of eventual return to China. It was not until 1943 that the Chinese could become naturalized U.S. citizens.

Current Demographics and Socioeconomic Status When the exclusion laws were repealed in 1943, people from many Asian countries once again entered the United States. Chinese immigrants who arrived after World War II are usually not from Guangdong but urban dwellers from other regions.

Chinese immigrants account for 5 percent of the 45.3 million immigrants in the United States as of 2021. Following the pro-democracy uprising in Tiananmen Square in 1989, U.S. immigration laws were changed with the Chinese Student Protection Act of 1992. More than 41,000 Chinese residents were granted visas and are eligible for citizenship under the provision. Furthermore, the return of Hong Kong to mainland China and the uncertainty about Taiwan's future have led to increased immigration from these islands.

Food for Thought

The first Chinese restaurants in the United States opened in San Francisco in 1849. Today, virtually every American community has Chinese restaurants. This may be due in part to a 1915 court case that granted special immigration privileges to Chinese restaurant owners, steering newcomers from China into the restaurant industry. By 1920, New York Chinese restaurants generated \$77.9 million in annual sales.[7] In 2023, some estimate that the Chinese restaurant market size nationwide is nearly \$21 billion.[8]

In 2019, the U.S. Census estimated that the fastest-growing racial or ethnic group in the United States was Asian Americans. Between 2000 and 2019, the Asian population grew 81 percent, from 10.5 million to 18.9 million. Of this group, Chinese Americans, largely residing in California and New York, make up the largest at 5.4 million (24 percent) people.[9–11] Other cities with large numbers of Chinese Americans are Boston, Washington, DC, Chicago, Seattle, Honolulu, and Houston.[12] Figure 11.2 illustrates the population concentrations of Asian Americans by each origin group.[9–13]

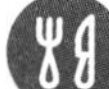

Food for Thought

The number of Chinese American women in the United States did not equal men until the 1970s.

As of 2019, it is estimated that there are over 226,000 people from Taiwan living in the United States.[12] Sizable populations are found in California, New York, and Texas.

WA Chinese
OR Chinese
CA Chinese
ID Filipino
NV Filipino
MT Filipino
WY Chinese
UT Chinese
CO Chinese
AZ Indian
NM Filipino
ND Filipino
SD Filipino
NE Vietnamese
KS Indian
OK Vietnamese
TX Indian
MN Hmong
IA Indian
MO Chinese
AR Indian
LA Vietnamese
WI Hmong
IL Indian
MS Vietnamese
MI Indian
IN Indian
OH Indian
KY Indian
TN Indian
AL Korean
GA Indian
FL Indian
SC Indian
NC Indian
VA Indian
WV Filipino
PA Indian
NY Chinese
VT Chinese
NH Indian
ME Chinese
MA Chinese
RI Chinese
CT Indian
NJ Indian
MD Indian
DE Indian
DC Chinese
AK Filipino
HI Filipino
Indian
Filipino
Hmong
Chinese
Vietnamese
Korean

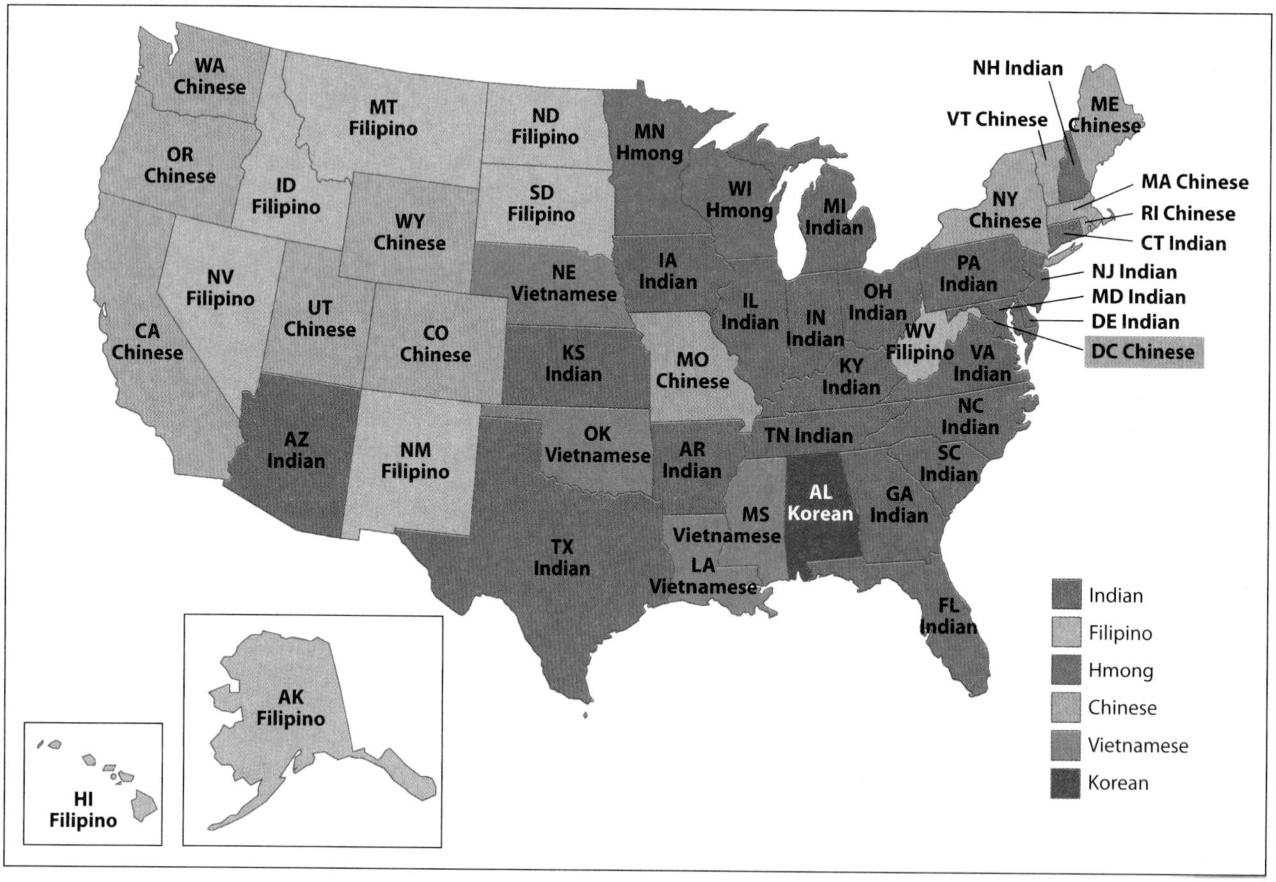

Figure 11.2 Largest Asian Origin Groups by State, 2019.

Food for Thought

In general, the 300-plus Chinese dialects can be classified into one of seven major language groups. Seventy percent of Chinese people speak Mandarin (Putonghua). Other major languages are Hakka (Kejia), Cantonese (Yue), Hunanese (Xiang), Min, Gan, and Wu. As most early Chinese immigrants to the United States came from southern China, as well as the many current immigrants from Hong Kong, their native language is Cantonese.[8]

2016 Census data reports 1.8 million Canadians of Chinese heritage.[9]

Over 1.5 million people of Chinese heritage in the United States live in California, more than any other region. New York has the next largest population with about 865,000 residents with this heritage.[11]

Chinese Americans value education, and there are disproportionately large numbers of them (over 50 percent according to 2019 Census figures) holding college and graduate degrees.[13] Fewer than 18 percent of foreign-born Chinese in the United States do not have a high school diploma.[9] High levels of educational attainment often translate into well-compensated professional employment. Though many Chinese Americans are in the upper and middle classes, immigrants who came before the 1950s were often poorly educated, and many found work in sweatshops. Even those who had college degrees were sometimes unable to find jobs suitable to their skills due to discrimination.[14]

Worldview

Religion A little over half (52 percent) of Americans of Chinese descent are not affiliated with a specific church. Others are Protestant (22 percent), Buddhist (15 percent), and Catholic (8 percent).[15] Religious practices can include a combination of ancestor worship, Confucianism, Taoism, and Buddhism. Many early Chinese immigrants learned about beliefs and practices orally, with traditional knowledge passed from generation to generation as it has been throughout history in Asia. Spirituality is integrated into family and community life. Daily living includes avoiding any actions that might offend the gods, nature, or ancestors.

Early Religion The word "religion" (zongjiao) did not exist in China until the nineteenth century, yet a complex belief system greatly impacted life and is critical to understanding Chinese culture.[16] The ancient faith of China was probably a mixture of ancestor worship and respect for the forces of nature and the heavenly bodies. The supreme power was either Tien (heaven) or Shang Ti (the Supreme Ruler or the Ruler Above). One gained favor with the spirits through the correct performance of ceremonies. These beliefs and practices were later incorporated into subsequent Chinese traditions. One example of ancient influence in Chinese thought is the ceremonies for the dead which are a prominent Chinese religious practice. The dead depend on the living for the conditions of their existence after death. In turn, the dead can influence the lives of the living.

Confucianism Confucius was a sage, one of many who gave order to Chinese society by defining how people should live and work together. Confucianism incorporated the ceremonies of earlier religions, with the following cornerstones:

1. Fatherly love and filial piety in the son (i.e., children are expected to obey their parents, and adults are expected to take care of their children)
2. Tolerance in the eldest brother and humility in the younger
3. Proper behavior by the husband and submission by the wife
4. Respect for those older than yourself and compassion in adults
5. Allegiance to rulers and benevolence by leaders

Inherent in these relationships is the ideal of social reciprocity, which means that one should treat others as one would like to be treated. To enhance harmony in the family and society as a whole, one must exercise self-restraint. An individual must never lose face—meaning a person's favorable name and position in society—because that would defame the whole family. Many of these values influence Chinese behavior today.

Taoism The Taoist, like the Confucianist, believes that heaven and humanity function in unison and can achieve harmony, but under Taoism people are subordinate to nature's way. There is a fundamental duality within the universe of interacting, opposite principles or forces which are interconnected: yin and yang. Yin and yang elements can be observed in pairs—such as the moon and sun: female and male, dark and bright, cold and hot, passive and active, steadfast and mysterious, and so on. Everything in nature contains both yin and yang, and a balanced unity between them is necessary for harmony. This balance is important. For example, yang will be weaker if yin is stronger, and vice versa. Yang is also sometimes referred to as *shen;* yang as *kwei.* (Figure 11.3). It is believed that for human health,

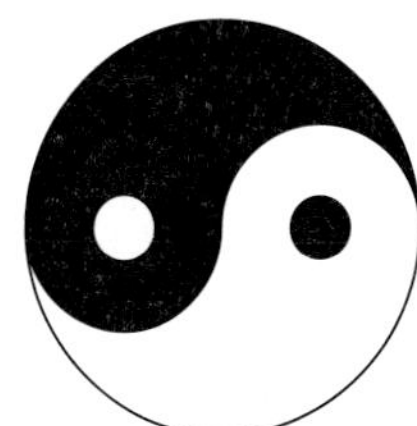

Figure 11.3 Yin–yang symbol. This symbol represents the fundamental duality of the universe and the balance between the forces of yang (light) and yin (dark), male and female. Each force has a little of the other in it (indicated by the dot of the opposite color).

one needs balance between yin and yang forces within the body as well as the outside environment. This balance occurs when Tao, the way of nature, is allowed to take its course unimpeded by human willfulness. Taoism advocates a simple life, communion with nature, and the avoidance of extremes.

Buddhism Buddhism took root in China in part because native language was used to explain its concepts to Chinese people, and also because it was linked with familiar and deeply magical Taoist ideas.[17] Both Taoism and Buddhism benefited. Even so, it took over a century to assimilate Buddhism into the Chinese culture, after which it flourished as a state religion from 581 CE to 618 CE. Buddhism is based on principles of compassion and non-attachment that originated in the sixth century BCE. It was most likely brought to China by monks from India, and by trade routes from Central Asia.[16] Buddhism grew during the T'ang Dynasty but then suffered major persecution under the emperor Wuzong in 845 CE, and again during the Cultural Revolution (1966–76). At its height, the two schools of Buddhism that had the greatest vitality in China were the Chan school (better known in the West by its Japanese name, Zen) and Pure Land (refer to Chapter 2 for more information). After the end of the Cultural Revolution, the Chinese government initiated more regulations and became more tolerant of religious expression. Buddhism in China is remerging.[17]

Chinese American Spirituality Both Catholic and Protestant churches were established in early Chinatown neighborhoods, usually organized by the Chinese dialect spoken in the area. Few first-generation Chinese Americans joined Christian religions, but converts were found in subsequent generations. Others maintain aspects of Buddhism, Taoism, or spirit and ancestor worship in their daily lives, keeping small altars at home in which to offer respect and perform the rites that will preserve good relations with the gods and bring good fortune.

Only a minority of Taiwanese belong to Protestant faiths in their homeland; however, Baptist, Presbyterian, and several evangelical churches have found Taiwanese followers in the United States. Services are conducted in Mandarin or Taiwanese dialects, and the church serves as a social network for the immigrant community. Taiwanese Buddhism, adapted to life in the United States, is also practiced.[18]

Family Confucian teachings about correct relationships are still important for many Chinese American families, even if they practice Christianity. Chinese American families are usually patriarchal. In traditional Confucian teaching, women should be unassuming and yielding. Children are expected to be quiet, acquiescent, honor the family, and be deferential to older family members.

Harmony in the family is the ideal, so children are taught not to fight or cry. Showing emotion is discouraged.

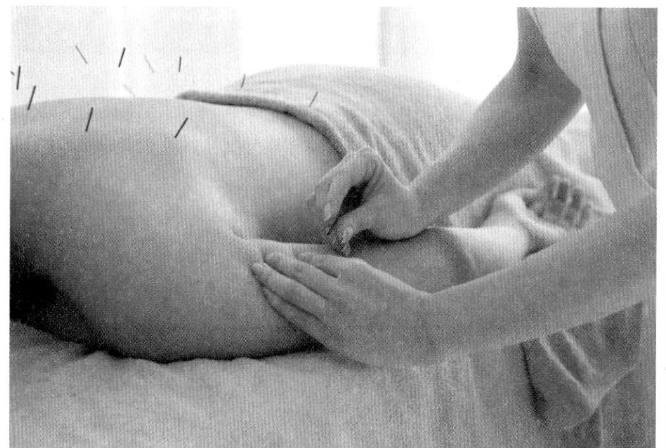

Leonardo da/Shutterstock.com

▲ One form of Traditional Chinese Medicine (TCM) is acupuncture. Exceptionally thin metal needles are inserted along meridians to facilitate balanced flow of qi (chi) and restore harmony to the afflicted organ.

Chinese parents may be very strict. Sometimes family teachings conflict with American ideals of equal rights and freedom of speech and may lead to intergenerational conflict in the Chinese American home.

Traditional Health Beliefs and Practices Chinese medicine includes a complex humoral system of professional practice by physicians, known as Traditional Chinese Medicine (TCM), as well as correlated folk remedies used by laypersons at home. Health beliefs and practices have developed over generations, incorporating Confucian, Taoist, and Buddhist concepts regarding the interdependencies of humans and nature and the need for balance and moderation in life.

Food for Thought

Most Chinese believe in feng shui, the way in which a home should be situated and its furnishings arranged to promote the optimal flow of energy and personal well-being.

Chinese physicians were traditionally paid for their services when the client was healthy. Payment stopped if the client became ill.

Jade charms are worn to keep children safe and to bestow health, fertility, long life, power, and wisdom on adults. From the earliest times, jade seems to have been credited with medicinal qualities.

TCM follows texts prepared between approximately 2500 BCE and the third century BCE, outlining the dynamic equilibrium of forces necessary for health. These include the five elements, or five evolving phases, of fire, earth, metal, water, and wood, each of which may become unbalanced, much as fire consumes wood or wood (as a tree) absorbs the earth. These elements correspond with five organs: the heart, spleen, lungs, kidneys, and gallbladder, respectively. Associations with secretions (perspiration, saliva, mucous, spit, and tears); the seasons (summer, late summer, autumn, winter, and spring); colors (red, yellow, white, blue, and green); tastes (bitter, sweet, pungent, salty, and sour); and directions (south, center, west, north, and east); as well as times of day may also occur. A TCM practitioner may use smell, hearing, voice vibration, touch, and pulse diagnosis to discover the source of an unbalanced health condition, which organ it is related to, and which meridians in the body are affected.[19,20]

This system was further elaborated somewhere between the third and sixth centuries by the adoption of Buddhist principles of hot and cold humoral medicine, which were congruent with the Taoist system of yin and yang.[21,22] The concept of harmony was refined to include a balance of these opposites; illness develops when disequilibrium occurs. Organs such as the liver, heart, spleen, kidneys, and lungs are yin, as are the outside and the front of the body. The gallbladder, stomach, intestines, and bladder are yang, as well as the body surface and the back. Outside forces, such as the seasons, are also defined as yin (winter/spring) and yang (summer/fall), and illnesses associated with these times may fall into corresponding categories.

Symptoms of disease usually reflect an imbalance between yin and yang. When there is an excess of yang, acne, rashes, conjunctivitis, hemorrhoids, constipation, diarrhea, coughing, sore throat, ear infections, fever, or hypertension may occur. Anemia, colds, flu, frequent urination, nausea, shortness of breath, weakness, and weight loss suggest that an excess of yin is the problem. Also associated with yin and yang is the condition of the blood. Weak blood (yin) may develop during growth or pregnancy, postpartum, and in old age. Treatment includes yang therapies, particularly the intake of herbs and certain foods.

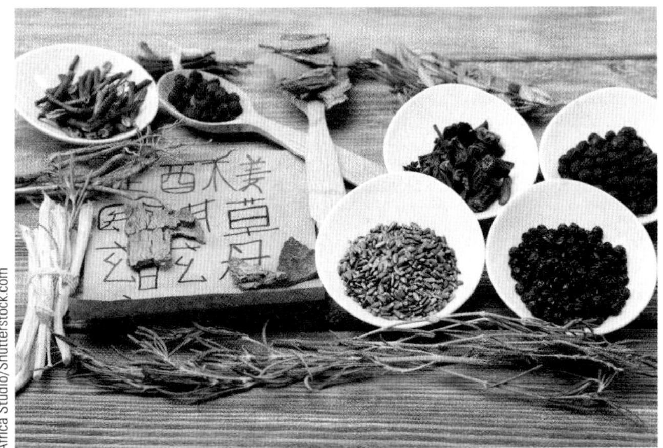

Africa Studio/Shutterstock.com

▲ **Botanical remedies are usually combined in formulary mixtures in traditional Chinese medicine.**

The vital force of life is qi (also written as chi and pronounced "chee") and is equated with energy, air, and breath. Qi flows along twelve defined meridians in the body, and some conditions are related to the disruption of qi or excessive qi. Other types of energy that must be balanced for health include jing, sexual or primordial energy, and sheng, spiritual energy, or the essence of consciousness.[19,20,22]

Other lesser forces that may influence health include wind (including natural drafts and those resulting from fans, air conditioners, or exposure); poison, which is somewhat related to the Western concept of allergies; and fright, when the soul is believed to be scattered, a condition in children that includes listlessness, anorexia, low fever, and crying.

A major difference between TCM and U.S. biomedicine is the idea that the body and mind are unified, governed by the heart. There is no English word to describe the concept. TCM also understands the human body as a whole system and disease from a systemic point of view. Because early Confucian dogma was against mutilation of the human body, medicine and diagnosis were far more important than surgery in Chinese history. Although early doctors examined many factors of the patient such as the color of the patient's skin, and other external signs, the pulse and its variations of sounds and rhythms are central.[20,23]

Herbs are classified according to their flavors (sour, salty, sweet, bitter, and pungent), the properties of herbs are characterized according to their effects (cold, hot, warm, cool, and even), and the target organs of herbs are defined by meridian tropisms (lung meridian, liver meridian, etc.).[19,22]

Emotions are often somaticized, meaning that feelings are related to specific conditions. More than 500 symptoms corresponding to emotions have been identified, each characteristic of one or more organs. For example, tou yun (or tou hun) is vertigo, the most common complaint made by Chinese patients worldwide. Dizziness or a confused state of mind indicates significant imbalance and serious illness. It is a nonspecific condition thought to originate from anger or anxiety manifested in liver, heart, or kidney dysfunction (if the patient is a young man, too much sexual intercourse or masturbation may be believed to be the cause). Liver disorders develop from suppressed hostility. Anger is discouraged in Chinese culture and is thought to accumulate in the liver, causing it to expand and attack other organs. This diagnosis is common for many gastrointestinal complaints. Generalized stomachaches are believed to be due to eating bitterness in life, often including an inadequate diet when one is young. Anxiety, nervousness, or the stronger emotion of fear results in heart palpitations. According to an earlier study, many Chinese prefer this integrated approach to health.[24]

Many Chinese maintain health through a properly balanced diet, moderation in activities and sleep, and avoidance of sudden imbalance caused by forces such as wind. Qi must flow freely and blood must be strengthened through nourishment. When home cures are ineffective, advice from a TCM physician may be sought. Diagnosis is made through taking an extensive history, and examination of the client, particularly palpitation of pulses and evaluation of the tongue. Through this process, a medical pattern is detected, in contrast to determining a specific disease or condition based on symptoms or laboratory testing. It is the medical pattern that determines the appropriate intervention, not the illness.

Treatment for nearly all illnesses involves the restoration of harmony. Therapy may emphasize dietary and lifestyle changes, or attempt to balance the organs so that emotional balance results. Nearly every visit to the doctor results in a botanical remedy, and most medicinal herbs are only available through prescription. For instance, ginseng may be used to fortify qi and aid in acute respiratory tract infection.[25,26] and antelope horn is thought to be cooling for excess yang in the liver. Formulary mixtures of five to ten substances are common. Most TCM remedies are prepared as decoctions, taken in a single dose. The client owns the prescription and can reuse it when symptoms occur or share it with family and friends.

Acupuncture is another traditional Chinese treatment. It involves the use of nine types of exceptionally thin metal needles inserted at various points on the body where the qi meridians surface. Meridians are considered yin or yang and correspond with specific organs. The needles are placed to facilitate a balanced flow of qi, restoring harmony to the afflicted organ, mostly for symptoms of excess yang. Acupuncture may be performed by a TCM physician or by a specialist. Another therapy is moxibustion, a treatment that burns mugwort leaves to strengthen the blood and stimulate the flow of qi. Small bundles of this spongy herb are heated and carefully applied to certain meridians. Massage, therapeutic exercise, and breathing exercises are also treatment options in TCM.

National board certification for TCM practitioners, which requires three to four years of full-time, postgraduate study at an accredited educational institution, is required in most states. Word-of-mouth recommendations are common within the Chinese community. TCM practitioners may use first aid on injuries or broken bones, prescribe herbs, perform acupuncture or moxibustion, or they may diagnose the condition and provide a recommended course of therapy by a specialist in one of these practices. Asians concerned with humoral conditions use TCM (often concurrently with biomedical therapies), and in recent years these practitioners have attracted a growing multiethnic clientele. More and more, integrated treatments using Western biomedicine and TMC are available.

Traditional Food Habits

The Chinese eat a wide variety of foods and avoid very few. This may have developed out of necessity, as China has long been plagued with recurrent famine caused by too much or too little rainfall. Chinese cuisine largely reflects the food habits and preferences of the Han people, the largest ethnic group in China, but not to the exclusion of other ethnic groups' cuisines. For example, Beijing has a large Muslim population whose halal restaurants serve lamb and kid, but no pork. Foreigners have also introduced ingredients that have been incorporated into local cuisines. Some foods now common in China, but not indigenous, are watermelon, tomatoes, bananas, peanuts, and chili peppers.

Ingredients and Common Foods

Staples Traditional Chinese foods are listed in Table 11.1. In China, numerous fruits, vegetables, and protein items are consumed but few dairy products, whether fresh or fermented, are eaten. Grains are the foundation of the diet.

Rice, the world's largest food crop, is essential in the cuisine of southern China. It is believed to have been first cultivated in the lower Yangtze River Valley and in India around 4000 BCE, though evidence of rice and human settlement dates much earlier. It is so commonly eaten in southern China, much like in northeastern India, that people greet each other by asking, "Have you had rice today?" There are many different forms of rice, but the Chinese prefer a polished, white, long-grain variety that is not sticky and remains firm after cooking. Short, sticky, glutinous rice is used occasionally, mainly in sweet dishes. Although it is usually steamed, rice can also be made into a porridge called congee, eaten for breakfast or as a late-night snack, with vegetables, meat, or fish added for flavor. Congee is also fed to people who are ill. Rice flour is used to make rice sticks, which can be boiled or fried in hot oil.

Food for Thought

Congee, rice porridge, may be eaten at any meal in Hong Kong, where a family version topped with lobster is popular. In Taiwan, congee is also consumed throughout the day. One variety served in Chinese American restaurants is "sizzling rice soup."

Wheat is also common throughout China, although it is used more often in the north than in the south. It is popular as noodles, thin wrappers, dumplings, pancakes, and steamed bread. Noodles are popular in soups or pan-fried, then topped with meats and vegetables that have been stir-fried separately. Thin, square wheat-flour wrappers are used to make steamed or fried egg rolls with a meat, vegetable, or mixed filling and wontons (in which the wrapper is folded

Table 11.1 Cultural Food Groups: Chinese

Group	Comments	Common Foods	Adaptations in the United States
Protein Foods			
Milk/milk products	Dairy products are not routinely used in China. Many Chinese are lactose intolerant. Traditional alternative sources of calcium are tofu, calcium-fortified soy milk, small bones in fish and poultry, and dishes in which bones have been dissolved.	Cow's milk, buffalo milk	Many Chinese consume dairy products, especially milk and ice cream, some cheese. Some alternative sources of calcium may no longer be used.
Meat/poultry/fish/eggs/legumes	Mostly protein-rich foods are eaten. Beef and pork are usually cut into bite-size pieces before cooking. Fish is preferred fresh and is often prepared whole and divided into portions at the table. Preservation by salting and drying is common. Shrimp and legumes are made into pastes.	*Meat*: beef and lamb (brains, heart, kidneys, liver, tongue, tripe, oxtails); pork (bacon, ham, roasts, pig's feet, sausage, ears); game meats (e.g., bear, moose) *Poultry*: chicken, duck, quail, rice birds, squab *Fish*: bluegill, carp, catfish, cod, dace, fish tripe, herring, king fish, mandarin fish, minnow, mullet, perch, red snapper, river bass, salmon, sea bass, sea bream, sea perch, shad, sole, sturgeon, tuna *Eggs*: chicken, duck, quail, fresh and preserved *Shellfish and other seafood*: abalone, clams, conch, crab, jellyfish, lobster, mussels, oysters, periwinkles, prawns, sea cucumbers (sea slugs), shark's fin, shrimp, squid, turtle, *wawa* fish (salamander) *Legumes*: broad beans, cowpeas, horse beans, mung beans, red beans, red kidney beans, split peas, soybeans, white beans, bean paste	More meat and poultry are consumed, though some traditional protein sources are still popular
Cereals/Grains	Wheat is the staple grain in the north, long-grain rice in the south. Fan (cereal or grain) is the primary item of the meal; ts'ai (vegetables and meat or seafood) makes it tastier. Rice is washed before cooking.	Buckwheat, corn, millet, rice, sorghum, wheat	Chinese Americans eat less fan and more ts'ai. The primary staple remains rice, but more wheat bread is eaten.
Fruits/Vegetables	Many non-Asian fruits and vegetables are popular. Potatoes, however, are not well accepted. Vegetables are usually cut into bite-size pieces before cooking. Slightly unripe fruit is often served as a dessert. Both fresh fruits and vegetables preferred; seasonal variation dictates the type of produce used. Many vegetables are pickled or preserved. Fruits are often dried or preserved.	*Fruits*: apples, bananas, custard apples, coconut, dates, dragon eyes (longan), figs, grapes, kumquats, lily seed, lime, litchi, mango, muskmelon, oranges, papaya, passion fruit, peaches, persimmons, pineapples, plums (fresh and preserved), pomegranates, pomelos, tangerines, watermelon *Vegetables*: amaranth, asparagus, bamboo shoots, banana squash, bean sprouts, bitter melon, cassava (tapioca), cauliflower, celery, cabbage (*bok choy* and *napa*), chile peppers, Chinese broccoli (*gai lan*), Chinese long beans, Chinese mustard (*gai choy*), chrysanthemum greens, cucumbers, eggplant, flat beans, fuzzy melon, garlic, ginger root, green peppers, kohlrabi, leeks, lettuce, lily blossoms, lily root, lotus root and stems, luffa, dried and fresh mushrooms (black, button, cloud ear, wood ear, enoki, straw, oyster, monkey's head), mustard root, okra, olives, onions (yellow, scallions, shallots), parsnip, peas, potato, pumpkin, seaweed (agar), snow peas, spinach, taro, tea melon, tomatoes, turnips, water chestnuts, watercress, wax beans, water convolvulus, winter melon, yams, yam beans	More temperate fruits are consumed. More raw vegetables and salads are eaten. Data on overall consumption trends are contradictory.

(*Continued*)

Table 11.1 Cultural Food Groups: Chinese (*Continued*)

Group	Comments	Common Foods	Adaptations in the United States
Additional Foods			
Seasonings	Complex, sophisticated seasoning combinations common. Various tastes appreciated, such as the moldy flavor of lily flower buds. Spice and herb preferences distinguish regional cuisines.	Anise, bird's nest, chile sauce, Chinese parsley (cilantro), cinnamon, cloves, cumin, curry powder, five-spice powder (anise, star anise, clove, cinnamon or cassia, Sichuan pepper), fennel, fish sauce, garlic, ginger, golden needles (lily flowers), green onions, hot mustard, mace, monosodium glutamate (MSG), mustard seed, nutmeg, oyster sauce, parsley, pastes (*hoisin*, sweet flour, brown bean, Sichuan hot beans, sesame seed, shrimp), pepper (black, chile, red, and Sichuan), red dates, sesame seeds (black and white), soy sauce (light and dark), star anise, tangerine skin, turmeric, vinegar	Many Chinese restaurants use MSG, but it is not usually used in the home.
Nuts/seeds	Nuts and seeds are popular snacks and may be colored or flavored.	Almonds, apricot kernels, areca nuts, cashews, chestnuts, ginkgo nuts, peanuts, walnuts; sesame seeds, watermelon seeds	
Beverages	In northern China the beverage accompanying the meal often is soup. In the south, it is tea. Alcoholic drinks, usually called wines, are rarely made from grapes. They are either beers or distilled spirits made from starches or fruit.	Beer, distilled alcoholic spirits, soup broth, tea	
Fats/oils	Traditionally lard was used if affordable. In recent years, soy, peanut, or corn oil is more common.	Bacon fat, butter, lard, corn oil, peanut oil, sesame oil, soybean oil, suet	Fat intake increases with consumption of fast foods and snacks
Sweeteners	Sugar not used in large quantities; many desserts made with bean pastes.	Honey, maltose syrup, table sugar (brown and white)	Sugar consumption has increased due to increased intake of soft drinks, candy, cakes, and pastries.

over the filling), served either fried or in soup. Spring rolls, similar to egg rolls, are made with very thin, round, wheat-flour wrappers. Dumplings can be small steamed bundles made with wontons filled with bits of shrimp, crab, and vegetables (called sui mai) or more substantial, breadlike versions, filled with spiced pork, minced beef, or sweetened bean paste, then baked, steamed, or pan-fried. Buckwheat is grown in the north and commonly made into noodles.

The Chinese eat a variety of animal protein foods. Pork, mutton, chicken, and duck are common in many regions (refer to "Regional Variations" below). Fish and seafood of all kinds are specialties. Eggs are frequently consumed. They are sometimes cooked as thin omelets in which to wrap foods or to add to mixed dishes. Century eggs, also called thousand-year-old eggs, hundred-year-old, and pine flower eggs, are duck or chicken eggs cured for three months in a lime, ash, and salt mixture. The whites become black and gelatinous; the yolks turn greenish. In Taiwan, a similar specialty called iron eggs is common. Chicken, pigeon, or quail eggs are stewed repeatedly in soy sauce, tea, or other liquids until they shrink and become flavorful and chewy. They are eaten for breakfast and snacks.[27] Other items include snakes, frogs, turtles, sea cucumbers (also known as sea slugs, shell-less echinoderms related to starfish and sea urchins), and seahorses. The Chinese also raise many kinds of insects for consumption, and arachnids such as scorpions, which are prepared fried or in soups.[28]

In China, soybeans are sometimes known as the "cow of China" as they are made into products resembling milk and cheese.[29] Soybeans are transformed into an amazing array of food products that are indispensable in Chinese cooking[29](refer to Table 11.2). Other beans are also popular, made into pastes, flour, or even thin, transparent noodles known in the United States as cellophane noodles or bean threads.

Chinese cuisine makes extensive use of vegetables. Many are those known in other regions of the world such as asparagus, broccoli, cabbage, cauliflower, eggplant, green beans, mushrooms, onions, peas, potatoes, radish, and squash. Chinese varieties may differ, however. For instance, leafy bok choy and wrinkled napa cabbage are preferred over European types; long beans, small purple eggplant, gai lan (Chinese broccoli, also called Chinese kale), gai choi (Chinese

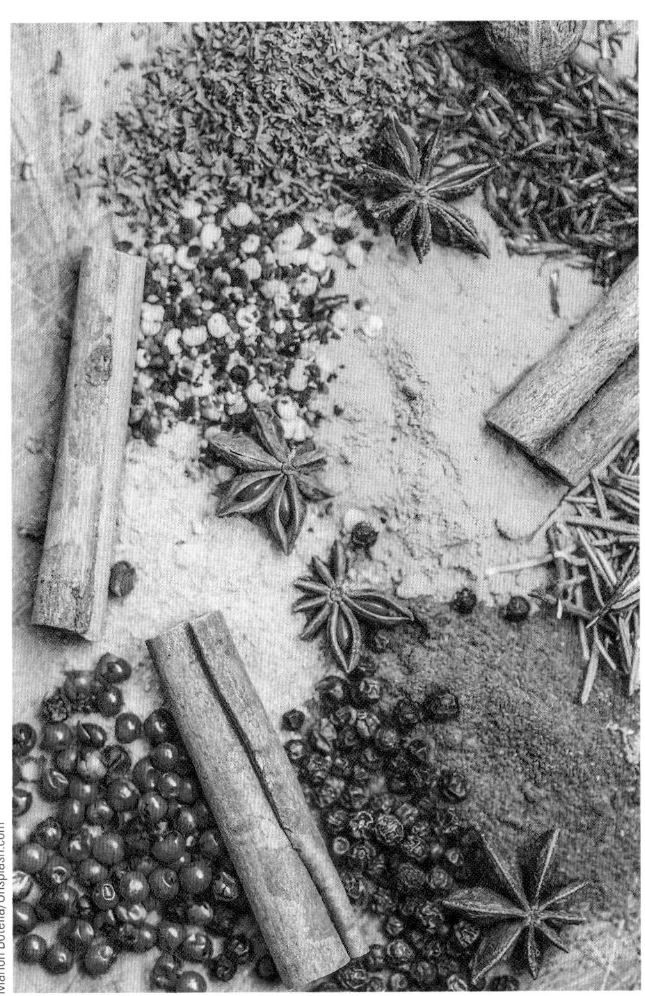

Marion Botella/Unsplash.com

▲ **Traditional herbs of China include cinnamon, anise, and turmeric, among many others.**

mustard), and the large white icicle radish are featured in many dishes. One popular squash variety is called a winter melon (when immature it is called a fuzzy melon); it is pale green and mild in flavor. Mushrooms of all types, including black mushrooms (a Japanese native called shiitake), the tiny enoki, grayish oyster mushrooms, straw mushrooms, and dried kinds such as cloud (or wood) ears flavor numerous dishes. Lily buds, snow peas (pea pods), bamboo shoots, chrysanthemum greens, water chestnuts, bitter melon, water convolvulus, and lotus root are other, more distinctively Asian, vegetables found in Chinese cuisine.

Food for Thought

Bird's nest soup may be served on special occasions in China. It is made from the cleansed nests of swifts from the South China Sea. The flavor is bland to spicy, depending on its broth, with texture as its main attraction. The dish is very expensive and is reputed to be an aphrodisiac with other health benefits. The harvesting of wild nests primarily from limestone caves has mostly been replaced by purpose-built nesting houses[30]

The Chinese eat fresh fruit infrequently, occasionally for a snack or for dessert, and it is preferred slightly unripe or even salted. Chinese dates (jujubes), persimmons, pomegranates, and tangerines are favorites. A few fruits are typically preserved in syrups, such as pungent kumquats, yellow-orange loquats, longans (dragon eyes), and litchis, a tropical fruit with creamy, jelly-like flesh.

Traditionally, people cooked with lard if they could afford it. In recent years, soy, peanut, or corn oil is more common. Until recently, sugar was not used in large quantities; many desserts were made with sweetened bean pastes.

Table 11.2 Common Chinese Soy Bean Products

Soy sauce	Cooked soybeans that are first fermented and then processed into sauce. The southern Chinese prefer light-colored soy sauce in some dishes over the darker, more opaque kind used in Japanese and some regional Chinese cooking.
Soy milk	Prepared with soaked soybeans that are first pureed, then filtered, and then boiled to produce a white, milk-like drink.
Doufu (tofu)	Made by boiling soy milk and then adding gypsum, which causes it to curdle. The excess liquid is pressed from the bean curd, producing a soft or firm, bland, custard-like product. Doufu can be purchased fresh, frozen, smoked, dried, sweetened, or in sheets to make wrapped dishes.
Fuyu (sufu)	Sometimes called Chinese cheese—bean curd is fermented in brine and 100-proof liquor. The aroma is tangy but the flavor is mild, except when chile peppers are added to the process.
Black bean sauce	Cooked fermented soybeans preserved with salt and ginger. Black beans are usually added as a flavoring in dishes.
Brown bean sauce	Similar to black bean sauce, but made with yellow soy beans.
Sweet bean sauce	Similar to soy sauce but with reduced spicing and added sugar. It is common in northern Chinese cooking.
Hoisin sauce	Thick, brownish-red sweet-and-sour sauce that combines fermented soybeans, flour, sugar, water, spices, and garlic with chiles—often used in southern Chinese cuisine.
Oyster sauce	Thick brown sauce prepared from oysters, soybeans, and brine that is also used in southern Chinese fare.
Chile bean paste	Very hot, thick paste made from brown bean sauce spiced with mashed chile peppers and vinegar. A favorite in Sichuan cuisine.

Hot soup or tea is the usual beverage accompanying a meal. The origins of wild tea lie in the eastern Himalayan corridor—Nepal, Sikkim, Bhutan, Assam, northeastern India, southeastern Tibet, northern Burma, Yunnan, Sichuan, northern Thailand, Laos, and Tonkin.[31] In addition to tea, this lush region is likely the homeland of rice, taro, bananas, citrus fruits, and more. Tea (*Camellia sinensis*), used in China for thousands of years, was introduced to western Europe in 1610 by the Dutch East India Company. There are three general types of tea: green, black (red), and oolong (black dragon). Green tea is the dried, tender leaves of the tea plant. It brews a yellow, slightly astringent drink. Black tea is toasted, fermented black-colored leaves; it makes a reddish drink. Black tea is commonly drunk in Europe and America. Oolong tea is made from partially fermented leaves and is a Taiwanese as well as a Chinese specialty. Some teas in China are flavored with fruits or flowers, such as black tea with litchis, orange blossoms, or oolong with jasmine. Other infusions of fruits or flowers are also called tea, including longan and chrysanthemum. Pearl tea, or bubble tea, made with chewy, pea-size balls of tapioca that are sucked up through large straws, was created in Taiwan and has become popular with Chinese youth worldwide.

Food for Thought

In China, a wedding tea ceremony symbolizes the union of two families. The bride and groom serve tea to their parents, in-laws, and other family. By custom, "drinking a daughter-in-law's tea" shows acceptance of the marriage.[32]

Taiwanese fare makes ample use of herbs such as basil and parsley.

A popular vodka brand is named for the warrior of Mongolia, Chinggis (Ghengis) Khan. It is made from wheat from Selenge on the Mongolian Steppes.

Dumplings shaped like animals, such as birds or frogs, are specialties in the city of Xian.

A traditional Chinese alcoholic drink is baijiu (literally "clear liquid"), a broad range of fiery grain-based liquors. Baijiu is usually made from sorghum or rice, with wheat or corn also common. The hundreds of variations of baijiu are due to centuries of differing traditions and geography.[33] Green bamboo leaf vodka, fen chiew, is another distilled drink in China. Yellow rice wine, huangjiu, comes in many types and color variations based on the fermentation process. Beer is also very popular.

Most Chinese food is cooked, and very little raw food, except fruit, is eaten. Cooked foods may be eaten cold. Common cooking methods maximize the limited fuel available and include stir-frying, steaming, deep-fat frying, simmering, and roasting. In stir frying, foods are cut into uniform, bite-size pieces and quickly cooked in a wok (a hemispherical shell of iron or steel) in which oil has been heated. The wok is placed over a gas burner or in a metal ring placed over an electric burner. Food can also be steamed in the wok. Bamboo containers, perforated on the bottom, are stacked in a wok containing boiling water and fitted with a domed cover.

The Chinese usually strive to obtain the freshest ingredients for their meals, and in most American Chinatowns it is common to find markets that sell live animals and fish. However, because of seasonal availability and geographic distances, many Chinese foods are preserved by drying or pickling.

Regional Variations China is usually divided into five culinary regions characterized by flavor or into two areas (northern and southern) based on climate and the availability of foodstuffs. In recent years, however, regional differences have diminished due to increased global influences such as social media. In a regional study of twenty types of traditional Chinese cuisines using social media, Sichuan cuisine was most favored across all regions in China.[26]

Northern This area includes the Shandong and Honan regions in Chinese cooking. The Shandong area (Beijing is sometimes included in this area, and sometimes it is considered a third division of northern cooking) is famous for Peking duck and mu shu pork, both of which are eaten wrapped in Mandarin wheat pancakes topped with hoisin, a sauce made from fermented soybeans, spices and sugar. Honan, south of Beijing, is known for its sweet-and-sour freshwater fish recipes made from whole carp caught in the Huang River. Much of the north is bordered by Mongolia, whose people eat mainly mutton.

Grilling or barbecuing is a common way of preparing meat in this area. One specialty is the Mongolian hot pot, featuring sliced meats and vegetables cooked at the table in a pot of broth simmering over a charcoal brazier. The food is eaten first, and the broth is consumed as a beverage afterward (refer to Exploring Global Cuisine—Mongolian Fare).

Northern China has a cool climate, limiting the amount and type of food produced. Traditionally, foods were often preserved, resulting in a preference for salty flavors. In general, northern Chinese staples are millet, sorghum, and soybeans. Winter vegetables such as cabbage, turnips, and onions are common. A delicacy from this area, now illegal and only sold on the black market, is braised bear paw. Hot, clear soup is the beverage that usually accompanies a meal.

Southern Southern China is divided into three culinary areas: Sichuan-Hunan, Yunnan, and Cantonese (with Fukien and Hakka regional specialties). Sichuan-Hunan (some English translations use the term *Szechuan* or *Szechwan*), which is an inland region, features fare distinguished by the use of chilies, garlic, and the Sichuan pepper fagara. Typical dishes include hot and sour soup, camphor and tea-smoked duck, and an oily walnut paste and sugar dessert that may be related to the nut halvah of the Middle East. Yunnan regional cooking is distinctive in its use of dairy products, such as yogurt, fried milk curd, and cheese. Dishes are often hot and spicy, and some of the best ham and head cheese in China are found in this area.

Cantonese cooking is probably the most familiar to Americans because the majority of Chinese restaurants in the United States serve Cantonese-style food. It is characterized by stir-fried dishes, seafood (fresh and dried or salted), delicate thickened sauces, and the use of vegetable oil instead of lard. The Cantonese are known for dim sum ("small bites," such as sui mai, pork ribs, meatballs, and other tidbits) served with tea. The staple foods of the south are rice and soybeans. As in the north, a variety of vegetables from the cabbage family are used, as well as garlic, melon, onions, peas, green beans, squashes, and a range of rootlike crops, such as taro, water chestnuts, and lotus root. Southern cooking uses mushrooms of many types to enhance the flavor of the foods and takes advantage of an abundance of fruits and nuts. Fish, both fresh and saltwater, are popular. Also important are poultry and eggs. Pork is the preferred meat. Tea is often the beverage served with meals.

Along the coast, Fujian (also referred to as Fu-chien or Fukien) provincial fare includes numerous seafood dishes, clear broths, and the use of bamboo shoots and mushrooms. Seasonings are light and ingredients are thinly sliced to enhance their flavor. Fujian cuisine is considered a main regional cooking style in China, though it is not well known outside the country. On China's central coast, chefs in the city of Shanghai specialize in new food creations and elaborate garnishes. Red cooking, also called Chinese stewing, is thought to have originated in the region around Shanghai. It is a popular braising cooking technique using light or dark soy sauce, spices, sugar, and Shaoxing cooking wine that imparts a reddish-brown color to the prepared food.

A southern regional specialty is Hakka cuisine, sometimes called the soul food of southern China. The Hakka people, their name meaning "guest families," are thought to be largely northern Han Chinese who progressively migrated south, fleeing war and poverty. They moved from the northern part of China in the twelfth century to southeast China.[34] There, they remained an insular ethnic group for several hundred years, preserving their traditional language, dress, and food. Their fare is hearty and robust, featuring dishes made with red rice wine and pungent seasonings, cooked for a lengthy time, often in clay pots. Salt-baked chicken, greens simmered with pork fat, and richly stuffed tofu are examples.

Meal Composition and Cycle

Daily Patterns The Chinese customarily eat three meals per day, plus numerous snacks. Breakfast often includes hot rice or millet porridge called congee, which in southern China may be seasoned with small amounts of meat or fish. In northern China, hot steamed bread, deep-fried crullers, dumplings, or noodles are served for breakfast. In Taiwan both southern- and northern-style breakfasts are popular. In both countries, urban lunches are usually a smaller version of dinner, including soup, rice or wheat dish, vegetables, and fish or meat. Sliced fruit may be offered at the end of the meal. The Chinese principles of yin/yang are often followed when defining meal composition. Healthy meals should be balanced, using three parts yang and two parts yin.

New Dietary Guidelines Dietary guidelines for Chinese residents were revised in 2022. These guidelines are designed for the general population of healthy individuals over the age of two in China. The guidelines are designed using the "Food Guide Pagoda," which uses five levels to recommend proportions of various food groups (refer Figure 11.4). Messages conveyed through the Pagoda are: eat a variety of foods with cereals as the base; balance eating and exercise; eat plenty of vegetables, milk, and soybeans; eat appropriate amounts of fish poultry, eggs, and lean meat; reduce salt and oil; limit sugar and alcohol; and lastly, eliminate waste and develop a new ethos of diet civilization.[35,36]

Food for Thought

Chopsticks were likely invented to retrieve food from cooking pots about 5,000 years ago. As resources became scarce around 400 BCE, Chinese chefs needed to conserve fuel, and food was cut into small pieces so it would cook more quickly; the small chunks were ideal for chopstick use. By 500 CE, chopsticks use spread into most countries that have been influenced by China, including Japan (where the chopsticks are shorter and have rounded rather than squared sides and more pointed tips) and Korea (where the chopsticks are typically made of metal, the same length as the Japanese type, but flatter). Chopsticks are found frequently in Vietnam (the Chinese type), though forks, spoons, and fingers are also commonly used. Other Southeast Asian cultures such as Thailand use chopsticks only occasionally, mostly for rice or noodles.[37]

Although the Chinese are receptive to all types of food, the composition of a meal is governed by specific rules—a balance between yin and yang foods and the proper amounts of fan and cai. *Fan* includes all foods made from grains, such as steamed rice, noodles, porridge, pancakes, or dumplings, which are served in a separate bowl to each diner. *Cai* includes cooked meats and vegetables, which are shared from bowls set in the center of the table. Fan is the primary item in a meal; cai helps people eat the grain only by making the meal tastier. A meal is not complete unless it contains fan, but it does not have to contain cai. At a banquet the opposite is true. An elaborate meal must contain cai, but the fan is usually an afterthought and may not be eaten.

Street stalls and tea houses provide snacks and small meals when away from home. Although restaurants were traditionally uncommon in rural areas, today they are found throughout the nation. The Chinese all-you-can-eat buffet, which originated in the United States, is now found in some regions. Other American restaurant ideas that have made their way to China include fast-food franchises and food courts.[13]

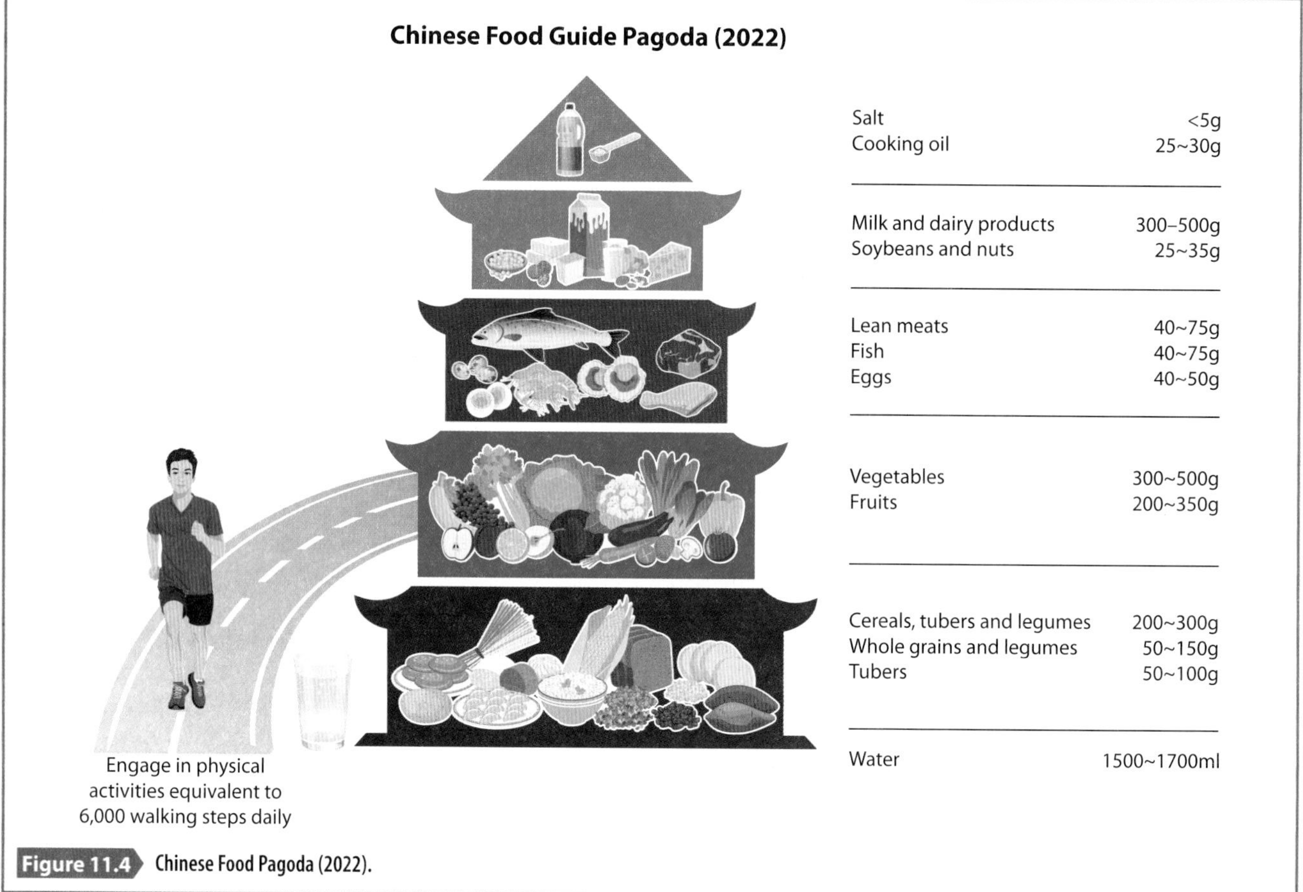

Figure 11.4 Chinese Food Pagoda (2022).

Exploring Global Cuisine

Mongolian Fare

The Mongolians once ruled an empire that stretched from China to Europe. Today, it is an independent nation reestablishing its cultural identity through shared language, customs, and cuisine.

Mongolian cuisine came from herding traditions and diets historically are based on livestock-derived foods: meat (red foods) and dairy products (white foods). This tradition continued with the addition of some grain products in the 1970s. Mongolian buuz and banš, for example, are dough envelopes filled with a mixture of onions, meat, and mutton fat similar to Chinese dumplings.[38] Meats, especially mutton, goat, beef, and blood sausages are favorites. Meat is enjoyed barbecued on a grill or over charcoal in a specially designed hot pot that sits on the table. It is also added to soups, stuffed into pancakes, and served on sesame seed buns. In the thirteenth century, an entire cooked sheep was considered a festive dish appropriate for honoring Mongol nobles.[38]

Dairy foods are numerous, prepared from cow, sheep, goat, or camel's milk. Milk is transformed into a cream (orom), creamy yogurt (tarag), yellow butter (šar tos), made from rancid cream, curd (eedem), cottage cheese (bjaslag), and different dried cheeses that can be stored throughout the winter. Fresh milk is used to prepare fermented mare's milk (ajrag) and alcohol produced from the distillation of milk (arhi), though this is often replaced by vodka in current times. Porridges, made from rice and/or foxtail millet, are cooked in a mixture of milk and yogurt, are sweet, and often sprinkled with small raisins.[34]

Flour is made from millet, buckwheat, or wheat and cooked as fried pancakes or steamed flatbreads. Typically, milky tea (süütei tsai), koumiss (a fermented milk drink), or vodka is served in a bowl and presented to guests. It is received by the guest with the right hand with the right arm supported at the elbow by the left hand. Special occasions include Lunar New Year and the Naadam festival, a three-day event featuring wrestling, archery, and horse races.

Etiquette The traditional eating utensils are chopsticks and a porcelain spoon used for soup. Teacups are always made out of porcelain, as are rice bowls. Few foods are eaten with the fingers, though that is changing somewhat in China today, where it is sometimes acceptable to pick up wrapped or stuffed items, such as dumplings by hand. All courses of a meal are traditionally served at once. Each place setting includes a bowl of rice or noodles, and each diner then takes what is desired from the communal serving plates. At the meal, all diners should take equal amounts of the cai dishes, and younger diners wait to eat until older diners have started; it is rude to reject food. It is also considered bad manners to

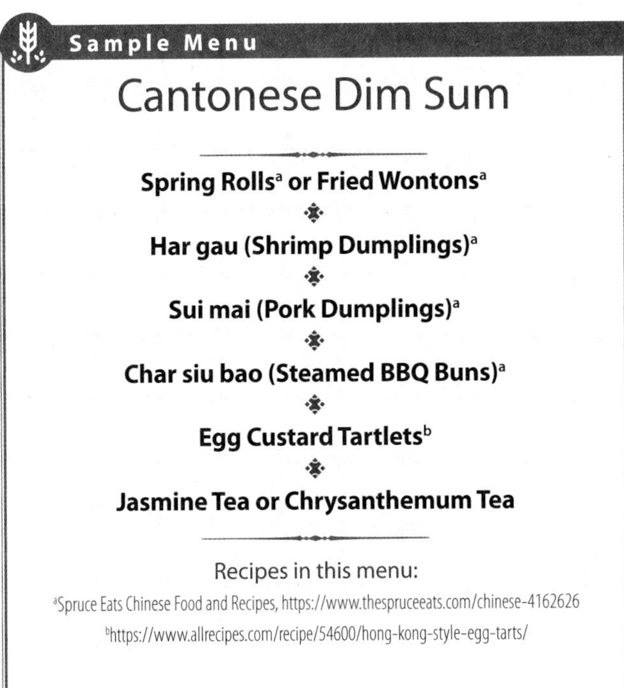
Sample Menu

Cantonese Dim Sum

Spring Rolls[a] or Fried Wontons[a]

Har gau (Shrimp Dumplings)[a]

Sui mai (Pork Dumplings)[a]

Char siu bao (Steamed BBQ Buns)[a]

Egg Custard Tartlets[b]

Jasmine Tea or Chrysanthemum Tea

Recipes in this menu:

[a]Spruce Eats Chinese Food and Recipes, https://www.thespruceeats.com/chinese-4162626

[b]https://www.allrecipes.com/recipe/54600/hong-kong-style-egg-tarts/

eat rice or noodles with the bowl resting on the table; instead, it should be raised to the mouth. It is rude to pick at your food or to lick your chopsticks. Laying your chopsticks across the top of the rice bowl or dropping them brings bad luck. It is also improper to stick chopsticks straight up in a rice bowl because in some areas this symbolizes an offering to the dead. Any bones or other debris should be placed on the small plate at each place setting, or on the table next to the rice bowl.[39]

Proper Chinese behavior at the table was first outlined over 4,000 years ago, and many practices remain unchanged.[40] Rules include not making noises while eating (except when consuming soup, when slurping facilitates cooling the soup and expresses pleasure), not grabbing food, not eating quickly, not putting food back on the communal plate after tasting it, and not picking one's teeth. Beverages, such as tea, should be served to others at the table before pouring for one's self, and the cups should not be filled to the brim. Both hands are used to offer a cup of tea, and the cup should be taken with both hands as well. Wine and other alcoholic drinks should not be consumed alone, and when the toast, "*Gambei!*" ("bottoms up") is made, everyone at the table drains his or her glass.

Though strict rules regarding dining behavior are observed in China, it is not uncommon for multiple conversations to take place at once, with frequent interruptions, at the table. It is considered polite to compliment the host throughout the meal on the deliciousness of the food and his or her good taste and wisdom.[42]

Special Occasions Traditionally, the Chinese week did not include a day of rest. Consequently, there were numerous feasts to break up the continuous workdays. Chinese festival days follow the lunar calendar and do not fall on the same day each year. Celebrations are traditionally yang occasions because heat symbolizes activity, noise, and excitement in China.[15,44,45] Yang foods, such as meats, fried dishes, and alcoholic beverages, are featured at festive banquets (refer to the "Therapeutic Uses of Food" section). Many Chinese homes are small and unsuited for entertaining groups of people, so special meals with guests are generally held at restaurants.[14]

The most important festival is New Year's, which can fall anytime from the end of January to the end of February. Traditionally the New Year was a time to settle old debts and honor ancestors, parents, and older community members. The New Year holiday season begins on the evening of the twenty-third day of the last lunar month of the year. At that time, according to cultural lore, the Kitchen God, whose picture hangs in the kitchen and who sees and hears everything in the house, flies upward to make his annual report on the family to the Jade Emperor. To ensure that his report will be good, the family smears his lips with honey or sweet rice before they burn his picture. A new picture of the Kitchen God is placed in the kitchen on New Year's Eve. Food preparation must be completed on New Year's Eve, as knives cannot

Exploring Global Cuisine

Tibetan Fare

The Tibet Autonomous Region of China has a unique fare due to the isolation provided by its locale in the Himalayan Mountains. The foundation of the diet is tsampa, a toasted flour produced from barley or buckwheat. It is traditionally mixed with the butter obtained from yak, solidified fats from yak, cow or sheep milk (called crispy oil), sugar, milk or cream, and sometimes tea to make flattened balls consumed with tea or soup. Tibetan dumplings with pleated tops and various kinds of juicy stuffing, known as momo, are popular and have spread throughout the world. The sha momo is often stuffed with yak meat, or beef outside of Tibet, and seasoned with garlic, onion, ginger soy sauce, Sichuan peppercorn, and sometimes Chinese celery.[41] Tibetans who are Buddhist do not typically eat pork, poultry, or fish. Dairy products are prevalent. Butter tea, made by churning crispy oil, milk, and salt with brewed tea, is consumed throughout the day. Sour milk, milk solids preserved from the crispy oil process, and the milk film skimmed from boiled milk and then dried are all consumed. Cabbage, radishes, onions, garlic, leeks, and potatoes are available. Wine, made from barley or buckwheat, is served on special occasions.

be used on the first day of the year because they might "cut" luck. Deep-fried dumplings, made from glutinous rice and filled with sweetmeats, and steamed turnip and rice flour puddings, are usually included in the New Year's Day meal.

During the New Year festivities, only good omens are permitted and unlucky-sounding words are not uttered. Foods that sound like lucky words, such as tangerine (good fortune), fish (surplus), chicken (good fortune), chestnuts (profit), and doufu (*fu* means "riches"), are eaten. Friends and relatives visit each other during the first ten days of the new year, and good wishes, presents, and food are exchanged. Children receive money in small red envelopes. Traditionally, the Feast of Lanterns, the fifteenth day of the first month, ends the New Year's season and is marked by the dragon dancing in the streets and exploding firecrackers to scare away evil spirits.

Ch'ing Ming, the chief spring festival, falls 106 days after the winter solstice. Families customarily go to the cemetery and tend to the graves of their relatives. Food is symbolically fed to the dead and then later eaten by the family. Sweets and alcoholic beverages are popular offerings. Duan wu, the Dragon Boat Festival, is held on the fifteenth day of the fifth month to commemorate the drowning death of a famous third-century BCE poet. A boat race and special dumplings are traditional. The Mid-Autumn Festival, or Moon Festival, occurs on the fifteenth day of the eighth lunar month, around September 22 or 23, during what is considered the brightest and biggest full moon of the year. It also coincides with fall harvest for much of the world. Traditions include family reunions and sharing moon cakes, traditional round pastries with sweet fillings, fruit, nuts, or red bean paste to commemorate the harvest moon. Several East and Southeast Asian cultures celebrate a festival around the harvest moon, with China and Korea among the largest celebrants.[45]

Food for Thought

According to the Chinese, a child is one year old at birth and becomes two years old after the New Year.

The New Year's dragon dance and firecrackers are thought to inhibit the yin element and promote the yang forces. Red, the color of yang, is used throughout the New Year's season.

In 1718, a Jesuit missionary in Quebec discovered an American species of ginseng that is nearly identical to the Chinese variety. Growing demand in China led many Americans, including Daniel Boone, to hunt the root for export.

Eating crab and persimmons together is one food taboo maintained by some older Chinese Americans because these foods represent extreme hot and extreme cold and are considered to be poisonous if mixed.

Therapeutic Uses of Food Most Chinese believe eating the proper balance of yin and yang foods is necessary to assure physical and emotional harmony and to strengthen the body against disease (refer to Chapter 1). It is felt that extra care should be taken with children's diets because they are more susceptible to imbalance. Foods fall into three categories: yin foods, yang foods, and neutral foods. Table 11.3 includes a very basic food list from the Feng Shui Institute. Foods classified as yin or yang vary from region to region. Acculturated Chinese Americans may be uncertain about some categorizations and thus identify many foods as neutral.[43]

Hot foods generally include those high in calories, cooked in oil, and irritating to the mouth and those that are red, orange, or yellow in color. Examples include most meats, eggs, chili peppers, tomatoes, eggplant, persimmons, pomegranates, onions, leeks, garlic, ginger, and alcoholic beverages. Cold foods are often low in calories, raw or boiled/steamed, soothing, and green or white in color. Many vegetables and fruits are considered cold items, as are some legumes. Pork, duck, crab, clams, shrimp, snake meat, and honey also are classified as cold in some regions. Staples, such as boiled rice and noodles, and other commonly eaten foods, such as soy sauce and red or black tea, are typically placed in a third, neutral category.[43,44,46] Some food preparations can make foods hotter or colder by the infusion or removal of heat.

Typically, hot foods are eaten in the winter by menstruating women for fatigue. Pregnancy is considered a cold condition, and birth is a dangerously cooling experience. Postpartum women often remain indoors and eat hot foods, such as chicken fried in sesame oil and pig's feet simmered in vinegar, for four to six weeks after delivery.[47] This period is known as tso yueh-tzu, "doing the month." In addition to eating warming items, raw and cooling foods are avoided, as is contact with cold air, wind, and water (bathing in hot water with ginger in it is permitted after a few days). Other conditions caused by too much yin and that respond to eating more yang foods include colds, flu, nausea, anemia, frequent urination, shortness of breath, weakness, and unexplained weight loss. It is also believed that as a person grows older, the body cools off and more hot foods should be eaten.

Conditions due to excessive yang that improve with an increase in yin food intake include constipation, diarrhea, hemorrhoids, coughing, sore throat, fever, skin problems, conjunctivitis, earaches, and hypertension. Cool foods are consumed in the summer for dry lips, and to relieve irritability.

In addition to yin and yang, some foods are believed to affect the blood or promote wound healing and are labeled pu, or bo, meaning "strengthening." This classification is separate from the concept of yin and yang but often used in conjunction with it; most strengthening foods are also categorized as hot. The yin condition of weak blood (most associated with pregnancy, postpartum, and surgery) is treated with specific hot items such as protein-rich soups made with chicken, pork liver, eggs, pig's feet, or oxtail. Other health-promoting foods identified by Chinese Americans include royal jelly (made from honey), bee pollen, lin chih (edible fungus), rattlesnake meat, dog meat, roasted beetles, barley juice, garlic,

Table 11.3 Food list from the Feng Shui Institute

Yin Food	Yang Food	Neutral Food
Almonds, apple, asparagus, bamboo, banana, barley, bean curd, bean sprouts, beer, broccoli, cabbage, celery, clams, corn, corn flour, crab, cucumber, duck, eel, fish, grapes, honey, ice creams, lemons, mushrooms, mussels, oranges, oysters, peppermint tea, pineapple, salt, shrimps, spinach, strawberries, soya beans, white sugar, tomatoes, water	Beef, black pepper, brown sugar, butter, cheese, chicken liver and fat, chilies, chocolate, coffee, eggs, smoked fish, garlic, green peppers, goose, ham, kidney beans, lamb, leeks, onions, peanut butter, roasted peanuts, potato, rabbit, turkey, walnuts, whisky, wine	Bread, carrots, cauliflower, cherries, lean chicken meat, dates, figs, milk, olives, peaches, peas, pigeon, plums, pork, raisins, brown rice, steamed white rice, sweet potato

dong gwai (angelica, a celery-like herb), fruit juice, and milk. For hypertension control, the 38 most frequently recommended foods are celery, tomato, banana, hawthorn, garlic, onion, seaweed, apple, corn, green beans, persimmon, laver, kiwi, watermelon, eggplant, carrots, mushroom, peanut, soy products, sea cucumber, buckwheat, garland chrysanthemum, spinach, honey, dairy products, vinegar, black fungus, jellyfish, green onion, shepherd's purse, soybean, potato, pear, winter melon, bitter melon, oat, pea, and tea.[48]

Ginseng is one of the better-known health-promoting Chinese foods. It is made from an herb (genus *Panax*) found in Asia and the Americas. The root is boiled until only sediment remains, then powdered for use in teas and broths. Ginseng reputedly cures cancer, rheumatism, diabetes, sexual dysfunctions, and complaints associated with aging. It is most often used today as a restorative tonic. Taro root is also thought to have therapeutic properties, such as improving eyesight, curing vaginal discharge, reducing weakness, and promoting multiple births; it will also bring good luck if eaten on the fourth day of the first lunar month.[49] Bitter orange is used to alleviate bloating and constipation. Guava, which has some hypoglycemic properties, is used for diabetes.[50] Other popular remedies include deer antlers, rhinoceros horns, and pulverized sea horse.[51,52] The concept of "like cures like" (sympathy healing) is seen in many food cures for specific illnesses.[53] Walnuts (which resemble brains) are eaten as a remedy for headaches in Hong Kong and to increase intelligence in China. Walnuts are now found to have links to an actual increase in cognition in studies that point to their antioxidant and anti-inflammatory effects.[14] The results found that walnuts are naturally high in omega-3 fatty acids, which have been linked to brain health. The nut provides anti-inflammatory benefits and prevents cells from oxidative damage. The studies found that eating as little as 1–2 ounces of walnuts per day can improve cognitive function and reduce risks for cardiovascular disease.[54,55]

Red jujubes may be consumed for strengthening blood, soups made with bones are used for treating broken bones, and male genital organs from sea otters, deer, or other animals are eaten to cure impotence. Chinese foods and herbs, such as "bird's nest" and "glucose drink" are also used in the infant weaning diet.[56,57] The weaning diet is considered the semisolid food that is added to a child's diet of formula or breast milk to increase appetite, balance the yin and yang system, restore qi, or treat diarrhea.[58–60] Based on some traditional beliefs, orange-skinned vegetables and fruits are believed to enhance the taste and flavor of soups and contribute to the yin–yang balance. Pork bone is believed to add calcium to the soup and is needed for growth. Moreover, some Chinese people believe that alligator meat will benefit the respiratory system.[61]

Some food taboos have been noted during pregnancy. Soy sauce may be avoided to prevent dark pigments on the skin, and iron supplements may not be taken because they are thought to harden the baby's bones and make birth difficult. Shellfish may also be shunned for the same reason.[62]

Contemporary Food Habits in the United States

Adaptations of Food Habits

Generally speaking, changes in the eating habits of Chinese Americans correlate with increased length of stay in the United States, and eating habit change is particularly likely in subsequent generations. Dinner often remains the most traditional Chinese meal, whereas breakfast, lunch, and snacks tend to become more Americanized.

Ingredients and Common Foods Most Americans, of Chinese descent or not, regularly consume several Chinese foods such as rice, pork, seafood, soup broth, soybean products, cooked vegetables, tea, and fruit. Though, in general, Chinese immigrants to the United States shifted toward a westernized diet. In a sample of Asian-born Chinese American college students in Florida, 59 percent said their eating habits had changed since arrival in the United States. This proportion increased with length of stay, from 38 percent among residents of less than a year to 85 percent among residents of at least three years. More American-style meals were consumed such as pizza, burgers, sandwiches, and more snack items are eaten that include fats, sweets, and dairy.[63] Meat and poultry intake increases, while some traditional protein items like pig's liver and bone marrow soup often remain popular. Greater consumption of protein foods, in addition to increased intake of fast foods, soft drinks, candy, and pastries, results in higher fat and sugar intake among more acculturated Chinese Americans.

The impact of acculturation on fruit and vegetable intake is less clear. Traditional fruits and vegetables may be replaced by more commonly available American items, such as potatoes, lettuce, apples, peaches, and watermelon.[54] Some studies have found that greater fruit and vegetable intake is associated with acculturation, education level, and income.[64,65] Among families, however, data indicate that pressure to maintain a traditional diet by older family members living at home results in a higher intake of fruits and vegetables among all members.[64,65]

Even though milk is not a familiar item in the typical Chinese diet, several studies suggest that milk, cheese, yogurt, and ice cream are accepted by Chinese Americans.[64]

One study found that dietary variety increased after immigration to the United States, and another noted that U.S.-born Chinese women have a more varied diet than Chinese American women who were foreign-born[63,66] Chinese women ate more bread, cereals, dairy foods, meats, vegetables, and other country cuisines, such as Italian and Mexican foods. In another study, acculturation was significantly associated with improved dietary variety but with lower dietary moderation.[64]

Meal Composition Skipping meals and increased snacking have been reported in Asian students and Chinese American and Chinese Canadian women.[67] Traditional foods are more likely the choice of older, less acculturated adults, and their preferences sometimes influence household meals.[67] Lunches and dinners may consist mainly of Chinese-style foods, while breakfasts are more variable. Many Chinese Americans attempt to balance hot and cold items in their diets. Other studies suggest that the use of yin and yang in the diet may diminish over time and that Chinese Americans may practice some aspects of it but without knowledge as to why certain food combinations are preferred.[68]

Food for Thought

Asian American female immigrants who have lived in the United States for a decade or longer have an 80 percent higher risk of breast cancer than more recent immigrants.[93]

Americans of Chinese descent usually celebrate the major Chinese holidays of New Year's and the Moon Festival with traditional foods. Chinese American Christians sometimes combine the spring festival of Ch'ing Ming with Easter festivities. In addition, some Chinese Americans recognize the founding of the People's Republic of China (mainland China) on October 1. The establishment of Taiwan is celebrated on October 10 with cultural performances and banquets.

Nutritional Status

Nutritional Intake The traditional Chinese diet is low in fat and dairy products and high in complex carbohydrates and sodium. As the length of stay and the number of generations living in the United States increase, the diet becomes more like the majority American diet—higher in fat, protein, sugar, and cholesterol, and lower in complex carbohydrates.[68,69] Understanding the differences between Chinese and American views on health and healthy eating can help design culturally tailored behavior change strategies. In one study on undergraduate Chinese students and what they think constitutes a healthy diet, they mentioned maintaining immunity and digestive health. The timing of eating also was important, with regular meals and more food and calories consumed in the daytime than at night. They also emphasized the consumption of fruits and vegetables.[69]

Traditionally, Chinese diets are based on vegetables, fruits, and cereals with few animal foods. However, recently, animal foods including meat, chicken, eggs, fish, and milk products are becoming popular in both urban and rural areas of China. Inadequate nutritional intake to meet Chinese dietary intake standards is still a widespread problem. Only 4.3 percent of adults receive the recommended amount of calcium of 800 mg per day. Fruit intake remains high providing a high content of vitamin C and polyphenols in citrus fruit. Boiled vegetables in the south of China are popular, while people in the north prefer stir-frying. To make vegetables more appetizing, salt and monosodium glutamate are often added. Green, black, white, or oolong tea is one of the most widely consumed beverages in China providing health benefits from the rich catechins (flavonoids) found in the leaves.[69,70]

Eating balanced meals at regular times using the circadian clock system and daily rhythms was once important to Chinese culture and frequently has been replaced by not eating at the right time, eating too much, or skipping meals altogether. This behavior has led to two types of disordered eating. Binge eating and night eating have become prevalent in younger populations of China.[70]

Dietary intake studies in China have suggested that due to rapid economic development, the diet structure has transitioned from the under-intake to the over-intake stage. There has been a movement toward the excessive intake of staple foods and meats and yet, an inadequate intake of dairy products. Some Americans of Chinese descent continue to avoid fresh dairy products because of lactose intolerance, which may be found in as many as 86 percent of Asians.[71–73] One study indicated that knowledge gaps regarding dairy products exist, and these are associated with the quantity and quality of dairy intake. The Chinese Food Guide Pagoda recommends 300–500 grams (2–3 glasses of milk) per day. Alternative calcium sources are bean curd, soy milk—if fortified with calcium—and soups or condiments made with vinegar in which bones have been partially dissolved. However, as noted previously, many Chinese Americans do consume milk, cheese, and yogurt, as well as leafy green vegetables, and calcium deficiency should not be presumed.[72,73]

Changes in dietary intake such as increased levels of meat, especially red meat or processed meat consumption, have a strong positive correlation with cancer incidence. At the same time, the incidence of being overweight in China continues to rise and has become a serious threat to personal health as well as a major public health issue.[74]

Obesity and overweight rates are growing in China. This is increasing incidences of premature mortality in Chinese populations. The prevalence estimates for overweight and obesity between 2015 and 2019 are shown on Table 11.4.[75] The overweight and obesity challenges are even higher for Chinese Americans, where approximately 42 percent are overweight or obese.[76]

Concerns that overweight and obesity rates may become problematic in this population as demographics change over time are as yet unconfirmed. Research on anthropometric measures indicates that BMI and waist circumferences underestimate obesity in Chinese Americans.[77,78] Chinese heritage was found to modify waist circumference measurements and metabolic risk factors.[79] Calculated energy requirements may differ as well. Predictive equations for basal metabolic rate (BMR) and resting energy expenditure (REE) are found to overestimate BMR and REE in adult Chinese Americans. There is a concern in some Asian nations about the increasing incidence of eating disorders in young women.[80]

In China in 2008, the Chinese Diabetes Society conducted an epidemiological survey in fourteen provinces and cities nationwide. From this survey, it has been estimated that type 2 diabetes prevalence is 9.7 percent in adults, or about 92.4 million people (43.1 million in rural areas and 49.3 in urban areas).[81] The prevalence is also correlated to the degree of economic development in a community and higher-income groups, which were two to three times higher than in low-income groups. Data on diabetes specific to Chinese Americans are sparse. Worldwide, Asian populations have shown higher prevalence rates of diabetes than European and African populations. Asian Americans are 40 percent more likely to be diagnosed with diabetes than non-Hispanic Whites.[82] The National Health and Nutrition Examination Surveys, 2011–2016 estimates that of the 14 percent of East Asians and 23.3 percent of Southeast Asian subgroups diagnosed with diabetes, 89 percent were overweight[83,84]

Data on hypertension rates among Asian Americans is lacking. The National Health and Nutrition Examination Survey estimate for Asian Americans overall is at 24.9 percent. Hypertension rates among Chinese Americans are lower than for Whites, but 19 percent of adult Chinese Americans have hypertension.[85] One study found that Chinese subjects are 30 percent more likely than Whites to have high blood pressure when adjusted for age, BMI, the prevalence of diabetes, and smoking. Asians are 20 percent more likely to suffer a stroke than Whites. Another study found that when compared to Whites, Chinese Americans who suffered from stroke had higher risk profiles, including a history of hypertension, a history of diabetes, and higher levels of blood lipids and glucose. Hypertension is considered a yang condition and is often treated by the consumption of yin foods.[85]

Table 11.4 Overweight and Obesity Prevalence Rates, 2015–2019, China

Age	Overweight	Obese
<6 years	6.8%	3.6%
6-17	11.1%	7.9%
>18	34.3%	16.4%

Food for Thought

Asian American women have the highest life expectancy (85.8 years) of any other ethnic group in the United States. Life expectancy varies among Asian subgroups: Filipino (81.5 years), Japanese (84.5 years), and Chinese women (86.1 years).[86]

A study of acculturation and diet in Chinese American women found that Chinese-language newspapers and friends were primary sources of nutrition information.[86]

Asian American adults are less likely than White adults to have heart disease and they are less likely to die from heart disease. However, cardiovascular disease rates in China increased by 60 percent between 1993 and 2003, paralleling increased overweight and obesity rates, diabetes, and hypertension.[87,88] Prevalence in the United States may also increase with these changes in first-generation immigrants, as well as with possible changes in subsequent generations.

Older cancer studies show the risk is higher in Asians than non-Hispanic Whites for stomach, liver, and intrahepatic bile duct and prostate cancer.[89,90] Liver cancer can be the result of contracting the hepatitis B virus, and Asians are 5.5 times more likely to develop chronic hepatitis B, as compared to Whites.[91] The risk of liver cancer should decrease with inoculation of the vaccine now available to prevent hepatitis B infection. The number of colorectal and breast cancer incidences in Asians has increased with the length of stay in the United States but is still less than for the non-Hispanic White population.[82,92,93] Inadequate preventive screenings and dietary changes, including lower intake of protective foods (e.g., soybean products) and higher intake of saturated fats, are thought to be factors for these increased cancer risks.[65,93–95] Infant mortality rates for Asians are lower than for non-Hispanic Whites. In Asian countries, infant deaths per 1,000 live births are 11.5 in China, 4.3 in Taiwan, 2.91 in

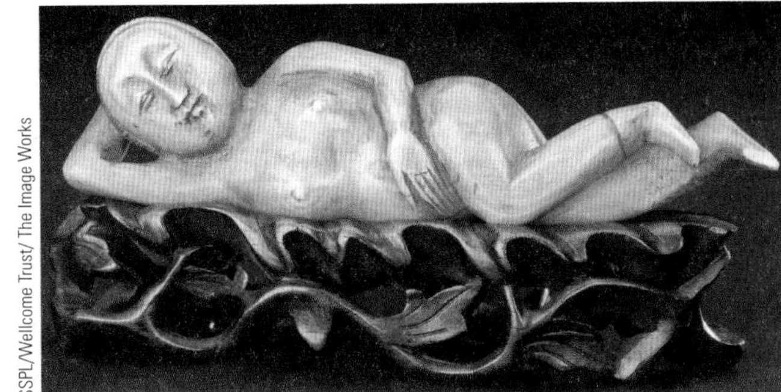

SSPL/Wellcome Trust/ The Image Works

▲ **Traditionally, Chinese women were never touched by their male health care providers. Symptoms would be discussed by pointing to an alabaster figurine, like the one shown.**

South Korea, and 22.4 in North Korea.[96–99] The infant mortality rate for Asian Americans in 2017 was 3.8 per one thousand live births.[96,97] Breastfeeding is reportedly common in China, and 65 percent of Chinese women in Australia breastfed their infants in one study. Breastfeeding rates for Asian Americans are high at 92.4 percent in 2018, however, in China, infants are breastfed for considerably longer, 83 percent were breastfeeding at 4 months, and the mean duration of breastfeeding was 10 months.[96–99]

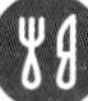

Food for Thought

In Asia, family members often stay at the hospital to provide feeding, bathing, and general care for the patient.

In Chinese culture, each ingredient has a story. Rice is thought to increase prosperity, garlic is a symbol of eternity, and bamboo shoots symbolize wealth. Citrus fruits mean abundance, luck, and wealth, and noodles, perhaps due to their shape, symbolize longevity. Legumes and seeds mean prosperity and fertility. Each bite of a meal is a wish.

Japanese

The multi-island nation of Japan is in East Asia. It is surrounded by the Pacific Ocean and lies to the east of the Eurasian continent with approximately the same latitude and range of climate as the East Coast of the United States. The capital of Japan is Tokyo, located on the island of Honshu. Today, Japan is a prosperous country of about 126 million people in a land of mountainous geography, rugged coastlines, and few mineral resources. Perhaps Japan's greatest natural resource is the sea, which provides a rich fishing ground to endow its unique cuisine.

Cultural Perspective

History of Japanese in the United States

Immigration Patterns Significant Japanese immigration to the United States occurred after 1890 during the Meiji era. The immigrants were mostly young men with four to six years of education from the rural southern provinces of Japan. Most came for economic opportunities and many eventually returned to Japan. They settled primarily in Hawaii and on the West Coast of the United States and often worked in agriculture, on the railroads, and in canneries. Like the Chinese before them, Japanese immigrants opened small businesses, such as hotels and restaurants. In contrast to the Chinese, many Japanese became farmers, ran plant nurseries, and were employed as gardeners. The Japanese prospered within their ethnic communities. Many Japanese women came to the United States as picture brides: Their marriages were arranged by professional matchmakers, and they were married by proxy in Japan. They did not usually meet their husbands until they disembarked from the ship in the United States. Among Japanese Americans, first-generation immigrants born in Japan are called Issei, second-generation Japanese Americans born in the United States are known as Nisei, and the third and fourth generations are known as Sansei and Yonsei, respectively.

The Issei were classified as aliens who were ineligible to become naturalized U.S. citizens and were often victims of discrimination. In 1913, landownership by Japanese people became illegal in California. Although the Japanese bought land in the names of their children, who were Americans by birth, the amount of land owned and leased by the Japanese was reduced by half by the 1920s. Already, in 1907, the Japanese government had informally agreed to limit the number of emigrants. Despite that agreement, the Immigration Act of 1924 authorized severe restrictions on immigration from all but European countries, effectively halting Japanese immigration.

World War II heightened the prejudice against the Japanese on the West Coast. After Japan attacked Pearl Harbor, all West Coast Japanese families, even if they were U.S. citizens, were evacuated to war relocation camps, and many remained there for the duration of the war. Most lost or sold their businesses as a result of internment. Nevertheless, many Nisei volunteered for combat duty and fought in Europe.

Current Demographics and Socioeconomic Status After the war, most Japanese Americans resettled on the West Coast, and the discriminatory laws were repealed or ruled unconstitutional. The successful postwar recovery of Japan resulted in reduced emigration to the United States, usually far below the quota allotted under current immigration laws. According to 2019 U.S. Census estimates, 1.4 million Japanese Americans live in the United States, a majority of whom reside in California or Hawaii.[100] Many West Coast cities have a section of town called "Little Tokyo" or "Japantown," and a small number of older Japanese still live in these homogeneous neighborhoods. Most Japantowns contain Japanese American–owned restaurants, markets, and other small businesses, as well as Chinese churches or Buddhist temples.

More than 95 percent of Japanese Americans live in culturally mixed urban and suburban areas. Americans of Japanese descent are unique in the high rate of citizenship, degree of assimilation, and economic mobility they have experienced.[9] Over 96 percent of all Japanese Americans have graduated from high school and 52 percent have attended college and most hold professional jobs. Only 3.9 percent of adult Japanese Americans live in poverty.[97]

Worldview

Religion Early Japanese immigrants usually joined a Buddhist temple (Pure Land sect) or a Christian church after arriving in America. The church frequently provided employment and an opportunity to learn English. Today, though this is shifting, there are more Japanese Americans who belong to Protestant faiths (33 percent) than those who follow Buddhism (25 percent).[15]

Shintoism, the indigenous religion of Japan, does not have a formal organization, but its beliefs are a fundamental part of Japanese culture. The Shinto view is that humans are inherently good. Evil is caused by pollution or filthiness—physical as well as spiritual; goodness is associated with purity. Evil can be removed through ritual purification. Shinto deities, called kami, represent any form of existence (human, animal, plant, or geologic) that evokes a sense of awe. Kami are worshiped at their shrines as a ritual expression of veneration and thankfulness. Prayers are also said for divine favors and blessings, as well as for the avoidance of misfortunes and accidents.

Family Until World War II the structure of the Japanese American family, rooted in Japanese culture, was similar to that of the Chinese due to the strong influence of Confucianism. In addition, the rigid pattern of conduct that evolved in Japan during the sixteenth century resulted in the following practices among the Issei, a term used to specify the generation born in Japan who later immigrated to another country:

1. *Koko*. Filial piety defines the relationship between parents and children, between siblings, and between individuals and their communities and rulers. (Refer to the Chinese religion section on Confucianism in the first part of this chapter for further explanation.) One outcome is that the Issei expect their children to care for them in their old age.
2. *Gaman*. Most Japanese believe it is virtuous to suppress emotions. The practice of self-control is paramount.
3. *Haji*. Individuals should not disgrace themselves, their families, or their communities. This Japanese cultural concept exerts strong social control.
4. *Enryo*. There is no equivalent word in English, but many Japanese believe it is important to be polite and to show respect, deference, self-effacement, humility, and hesitation.

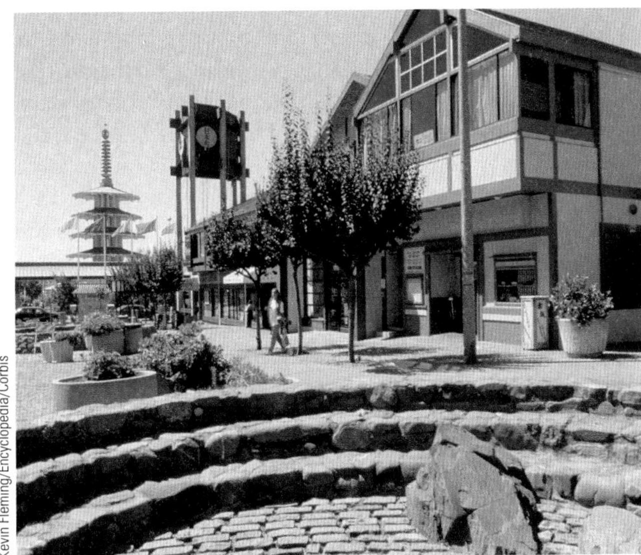

Kevin Fleming/Encyclopedia/Corbis

▲ **View of the Japantown neighborhood, San Francisco.**

Food for Thought

More than 121,000 residents of Japanese ancestry were living in Canada in 2016.

Heikegani crabs are believed to be reincarnations of warriors slain at the Battle of Dan-no-ura due to the samurai's face-like markings on their shells.

Japanese clan or village affiliation has traditionally been much weaker than in China, and Japanese immigrants arrived in the United States prepared to raise nuclear families similar to those in White America. Most Issei women worked alongside their husbands to support the family financially.

The internment of Japanese Americans during World War II, which was the result of President Roosevelt's Executive Order 9066 in February 1942 after the bombing of Pearl Harbor, brought further changes in family structure and accelerated acculturation into mainstream society after the war. The forced relocation of Japanese people in the United States also affected agriculture and what appeared on dinner plates. Once the removal began, Californians were faced with shortages of fruits and vegetables as Japanese Americans grew 95 percent of California's strawberries and one-third of the state's truck crops such as celery, peppers, snap beans, artichokes, cauliflower, cucumbers, garlic, onions, and more.[101,102]

"Relocation centers" or internment camps were situated many miles inland, often in desolate locales. The camps housed families, with the sparse possessions they could bring, in tar-papered army-style barracks. Most lived in these conditions for nearly three years or until the end of the war. Eating in common facilities, using shared restrooms, and having limited work opportunities interrupted social and cultural patterns.[103] In the camps, very low wages were paid, and the pay was the same for everyone; thus, the father could no longer be the (traditional) primary wage earner. The camps were run democratically, but positions of authority could be held only by American citizens, so the younger generation held these more prestigious jobs. The Japanese American Redress Movement was initiated as early as the 1940s and continued into the 1980s by Issei, Nisei (children born in North America whose parents were immigrants from Japan), as well as Sansei (second-generation Japanese Americans), for legislative and judicial recognition of the history and loss of internment, and collective healing.[104]

Sansei couples generally form dual-career households. Nearly 50 percent marry outside their ethnic group. The societal problems prevalent in the majority American homes, such as spousal abuse, have surfaced among Japanese Americans as well.[105] It is not known if the cultural values that have thrust Americans of Japanese descent into educational and financial success will continue in the fully assimilated fourth generation of Yonsei.

Traditional Health Beliefs and Practices Early Japanese health beliefs involved Shinto concepts of purity and pollution. Health was maintained through cleanliness and avoidance of contaminating substances such as blood, skin infections, and corpses. Botanical remedies were used, particularly purgatives, in the prevention and treatment of disease.

When Buddhism was introduced in the sixth century, the concept of harmony was applied within the context of Japanese culture to mean a person's relationship with nature, family, and society. Imbalance resulting from poor diet, insufficient sleep, lack of exercise, or conflict with family or society disrupts the proper flow of energy within the body, leading to illness. Chinese practices such as acupuncture, moxibustion, and massage were accepted as ways to restore the energy flow along the meridians of the body (refer to "Traditional Health Beliefs and Practices"). The application of yin and yang in health and diet was limited in Japan.

The more complex herbal medications of China were brought to Japan as kanpo. However, the numerous plants, animals, and minerals necessary for kanpo were not widely available on the islands, so its use was confined to the elite, urban aristocracy until recent times. Practitioners of the profession were called kanpo-i and underwent rigorous training.

Kanpo-i approached each case individually, reviewing symptoms carefully and in detail before determining the best combination of therapies and medications for the specific patient. Diagnosis was an art that recognized that symptoms may present differently in every consultation.[106] Western biomedicine was introduced to Japan in the sixteenth century with the arrival of the Portuguese. It was widely embraced; Japanese kanpo-i were required to retrain if they wished to continue working as doctors. The majority of Japanese Americans migrated to the United States when kanpo was rarely practiced, and they were often unfamiliar with its therapies.

Since 1960 Japan has been in the middle of a kanpo boom and the method is now approved for reimbursement under the Japanese health insurance policy.[107] Concerns about the side effects of biomedical therapeutics and a growing interest in holistic and herbal healing have prompted the resurgence.

Kanpo-i take a generalized approach, using natural medications with broad effects to stimulate the immune system. Some herbs also have known bacteriostatic action or anti-inflammatory properties. Small doses of the medications are taken for lengthy periods to promote gradual improvement. Physicians trained in biomedicine are also prescribing kanpo for many clients (though without the extensive education of kanpo-i); mass production of herbal medications by pharmaceutical companies began in the 1970s.

Stress-induced illness is of particular concern in Japan. Work-related fatigue and symptoms of anxiety and depression have risen dramatically in the past decade.[108] An estimated 10,000 men die annually from karoshi (literally "death from overwork," but referring to suicide). The healing industry in Japan is an estimated $30 billion-a-year business.[109] Stress-reducing therapies, called iyashi, include herbs, teas, and ten-minute massage parlors. One aquarium provides overnight accommodations in its tank rooms, where visitors can sleep to relaxing music in the company of swaying jellyfish. Spas offer specialized soaking alternatives, such as bathing in coffee, green tea, red wine, or sake, to rejuvenate and energize clients. Researchers report such activities to result in reduced levels of stress hormones as measured in saliva tests.[110] Napping on the job and at school has also gained some acceptance following studies on how short rests can improve productivity.

Traditional Food Habits

Geography and history give context to Japanese food, as it does to cuisine everywhere. The chain of volcanic islands that make up Japan was strongly influenced by Asian culture, but removed due to its location off the Asian coast. Though the foodstuffs (any substance suitable for consumption as food) eaten in Japan may have been derived from Asian sources, they were modified by Japan's relative isolation, making Japanese food preparation and presentation unique. The Japanese reverence for harmony within the body and community and with nature has resulted in a cuisine offering numerous preparation methods for a limited number of foods. Each item is to be seen, tasted, and relished. The Japanese also emphasize the appearance of the meal so that the visual appeal reflects a balance between the foods and the environment. For example, a summer meal may be served on glass dishes so that the meal looks cooler, while a September meal may include the autumn colors of red and gold.

Ingredients and Common Foods

Japan's mountainous terrain and limited arable land have contributed historically to a less-than-abundant food supply. Even today, although most have some type of garden in their homes, much of Japan's food supply is imported. Japan is the largest importer of U.S. beef, pork, and wheat products, and the second largest importer of corn.[111]

Staples and Regional Variations The basic foods of the Japanese diet are found in the cultural food groups list (Table 11.5). Several key ingredients were adopted from China, including rice, soybeans, and tea. Rice or gohan (the word for "cooked rice," and also for "meal") is the main staple eaten with almost every meal. Japan is known for its many rice paddies in rural areas. In contrast to the Chinese, the Japanese prefer short-grain rice that contains more starch and is stickier after cooking.

Rice mixed with rice vinegar, called *su*, is used in *sushi*, one of the most popular Japanese specialties in both Japan and abroad. Sushi rice is formed with fish and seafood to make decorative, bite-size mounds served with soy sauce for dipping. Types of sushi include nigiri sushi, which features rice topped with items such as sliced raw fish or squid (called sashimi), cooked octopus, crab or shrimp, omelet strips, or roe of salmon (ikura), sea urchin (uni), or flying fish (tobikko), sometimes wrapped in a strip of seaweed; maki sushi, a roll of sushi rice, often including cucumber (kappamaki), tuna, mushrooms, or other fillings, then wrapped in a sheet of seaweed and sliced into individual pieces; and

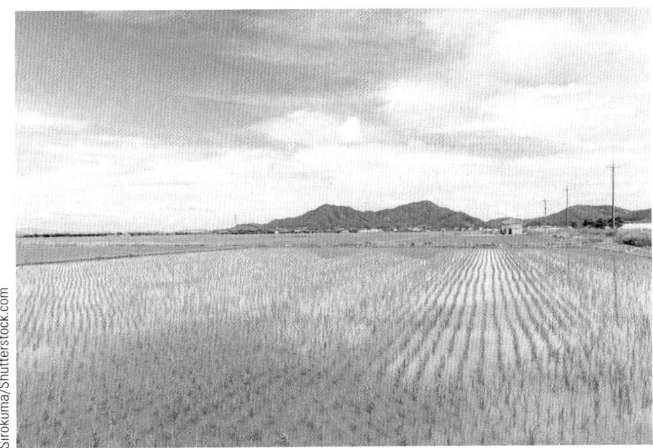
Sirokuma/Shutterstock.com

▲ Rice fields of Hirshima, Japan.

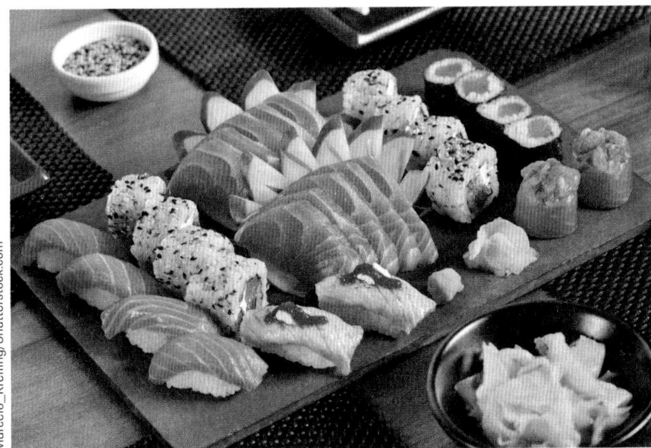
Marcelo_Krelling/Shutterstock.com

▲ Japanese sushi.

chirashi sushi, with the topping ingredients scattered over a large mound of rice and eaten with chopsticks.

Food for Thought

Sea urchin roe, called uni, is thought to enhance male sexual potency in Japan, where wholesalers pay up to $100-plus per pound for it. California imposed strict urchin harvesting laws to prevent extinction along the coast.

Rice is also made into noodles, although those made from wheat (known as udon, somen, and ramen) or buckwheat (soba) are more commonly consumed. Other noodles made from less familiar starches, such as kudzu, are also eaten.

Soybean products are an important component of Japanese cuisine. Tofu (bean curd), soy sauce (shoyu), and fermented bean paste (miso) are just a few. Miso comes in numerous varieties. Those made with the addition of rice are most popular; however, miso mixed with barley is found in western regions, and plain miso with just soybeans and salt is favored in a few central areas.[112] Red miso (akamiso) is very salty and is used most often. White miso (shiromiso) is sweeter and often used in cooked salads. Specialty misos, with added vegetables such as kombu or daikon, or seasoned with shiso, are also available. Sugar, shoyu, and vinegar are basic seasoning mixtures for foods. Teriyaki sauce ("shining broil") made from soy sauce and mirin, a sweet rice wine, is another common flavoring for foods. Shoyu and mirin can vary in strength, and the amounts used to depend on personal taste. In addition to soybeans, small, red adzuki beans are significant in Japanese cuisine, most often made into sweetened red bean paste and a popular red bean jelly dessert (similar to gelatin) called yo-kan.

Green tea is served with most meals. Tea was originally used in a devotional ceremony in Zen Buddhism. The ritual was raised to be a fine art by Japanese tea masters, and as a result, they also set the standards for behavior in Japanese society. Today, the tea ceremony and the accompanying food (kaiseki ryori) remain a cultural ideal that reflects the search for harmony with nature and within one's self. The meal features six small courses balancing the tastes of sweet,

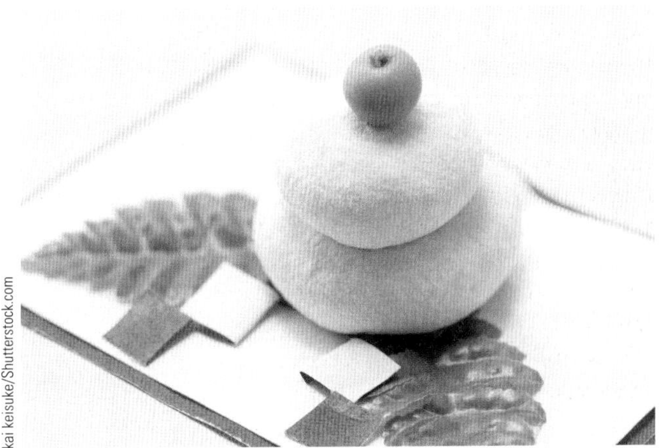
kai keisuke/Shutterstock.com

▲ Japanese sweets made from bean paste and enjoyed with tea.

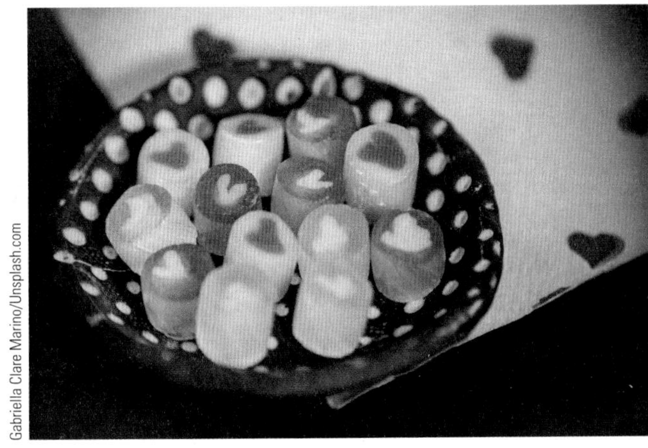
Gabriella Clare Marino/Unsplash.com

▲ Japanese sweets.

Table 11.5 Cultural Food Groups: Japanese

Group	Comments	Common Foods	Adaptations in the United States
Protein Foods			
Milk/milk products	Japanese cooking does not utilize significant amounts of dairy products. Many Japanese are lactose intolerant. Soybean products, seaweed, and small bony fish are alternative calcium sources.	Milk, butter, ice cream	First-generation Japanese Americans drink little milk and eat few dairy products. Subsequent generations eat more dairy foods.
Meat/poultry/fish/eggs/legumes	Soybean products and a wide variety of fish and shellfish (fresh, frozen, dried, smoked) are the primary protein sources in the Japanese diet. Fish and shellfish often eaten raw. Chicken is used more often than beef; price is the limiting factor in meat consumption.	*Meat*: beef, deer, lamb, pork, rabbit, veal *Poultry*: capon, chicken, duck, goose, partridge, pheasant, quail, thrush, turkey *Fish*: blowfish, bonito, bream, carp, cod, cuttlefish, eel, flounder, herring, mackerel, porgy, octopus, red snapper, salmon, sardines, shark, sillago, snipefish, squid, swordfish, trout, tuna, turbot, yellowtail, whale *Shellfish*: abalone, *ayu*, clams, crab, earshell, lobster, mussels, oysters, sea urchin roe (*uni*), scallops, shrimp, snails *Legumes*: adzuki, black beans, lima beans, red beans, soybeans	Dried fish and fish cakes are available in the United States, but some varieties of fresh fish are not. Japanese Americans eat more poultry and meat than fish.
Cereals/Grains	Short-grain rice is the primary staple of the diet and is eaten with every meal. Wheat is often eaten in the form of noodles, such as *ramen*, *somen*, and *udon*.	Wheat, rice, buckwheat, millet	Rice is still an important staple in the diet and usually eaten at dinner.
Fruits/Vegetables	Fresh fruits and vegetables are the most desirable; usually eaten only in season. Many fruits and vegetables are preserved, dried, or pickled.	*Fruits*: apples, apricots, bananas, cherries, dates, figs, grapes, grapefruits (*yuzu*), kumquats, lemons, limes, loquats, melons, oranges, peaches, pears, pear apples, persimmons, plums (fresh and pickled), pineapples, strawberries, *mikan* (tangerine) *Vegetables*: artichokes, asparagus, bamboo shoots, beans, bean sprouts, broccoli, brussels sprouts, beets, burdock root (*gobo*), cabbage (several varieties), carrots, chickweed, chrysanthemum greens, eggplant (long, slender variety), ferns, ginger, ginger sprouts and flowers (*myoga*), and pickled ginger (*beni shoga*), green onions, green peppers, gourd (*kanpyo*, dried gourd shavings), kudzu, leeks, lettuce, lotus root, *mizuna*, mushrooms (*shiitake*, *matsutake*, *nameko*), okra, onions, peas, potatoes, pumpkins, radishes, rhubarb, seaweed, snow peas, *shiso*, sorrel, spinach, squash (including *kabocha*), sweet potatoes, taro, tomatoes, turnips, watercress, yams	Fewer fruits and vegetables are eaten; freshness is less critical.
Additional Foods			
Seasonings	Sugar, *shoyu*, and vinegar are a basic seasoning mixture. *Shoyu* and *mirin* can vary in strength; amounts used will vary according to taste.	Alum, anise, bean paste (*miso*), caraway, chives, *dashi*, fish paste, garlic, ginger, mint, *mirin*, MSG, mustard, red pepper, sake, seaweed, sesame seeds, *shiso*, *shoyu*, sugar, thyme, vinegar (rice), *wasabi* (green, horseradish-like condiment)	
Nuts/seeds		Chestnut, gingko nuts, peanuts, walnuts; poppy (black and white), sesame seeds	

(*Continued*)

Table 11.5 Cultural Food Groups: Japanese (*Continued*)

Group	Comments	Common Foods	Adaptations in the United States
Beverages	Green tea is the preferred beverage with meals; coffee or black tea is drunk with Western-style foods. Sake or beer is often served with dinner.	Carbonated beverages, beer, coffee, gin, tea (black and green), sake, scotch	Japanese Americans drink less tea and more milk, coffee, and carbonated beverages.
Fats/oils	The traditional Japanese diet is low in fat and cholesterol.	Butter, cottonseed oil, olive oil, peanut oil, sesame seed oil, vegetable oil	Japanese Americans consume more fats and oils because of increased use of Western foods and cooking methods.
Sweeteners		Honey, sugar	Increased use of sugar; sweet desserts are noted.

sour, pungent, bitter, and salty. The tea used for the ceremony is not the common leaf tea usually used for meals, but rather a blend of ground, dry tea, or tea powder. Hot water is added to the tea, and the mixture is whipped together using a handmade whisk, resulting in a frothy green drink. Diners demonstrate their sophistication and sensitivity through deliberate eating of each course after expressions of appreciation for the presentation.

Food for Thought

When a family moves to a new home, they give soba noodles to the neighbors on either side and across the street as a gesture of friendship.

Kaiseki ryori meals, from 6 to 15 courses in length, can cost $100 to $300 and up per person in restaurants featuring the ceremonial menu. The meal is highly ritualized and consists of small portions, subtle flavors, and an artful presentation.

Soybean products and a wide variety of fish and shellfish (fresh, dried, or smoked) are the primary protein sources. Fresh fish and shellfish are often eaten raw. Beef, pork, and poultry are also popular but very expensive. One specialty is

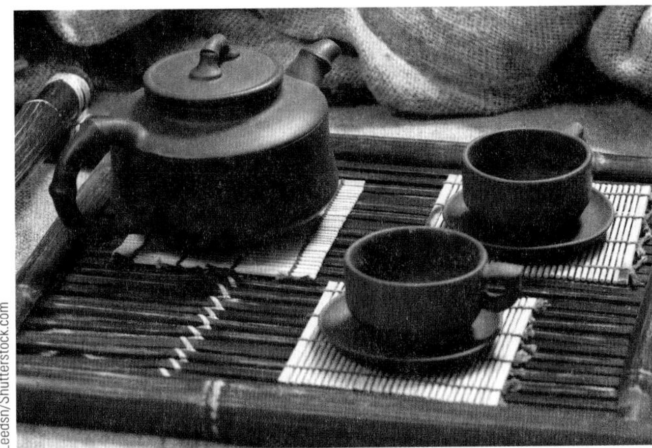

Leedsn/Shutterstock.com

▲ Drinking tea is a daily ritual for many people in Japan.

Kobe (or Tajima) beef, from a Japanese breed of cattle that are fed beer as an appetite stimulant and regularly massaged to relieve stress. It often costs more than $100 per pound. Pork is a favorite as cutlets. Chicken, which is often served as teriyaki sauce–glazed skewers, may also be very thinly sliced and served raw like sashimi.[112] Only small amounts of meat, poultry, or fish are added to the vegetables in traditional Japanese recipes. Japanese fare does not use many dairy foods.

Fresh fruits and vegetables are the most desirable and are eaten only when in season. Traditional Japanese miso soup is ever-changing based on the vegetables that are in harvest. As in China, many Asian and European varieties are consumed (see the subsection "Staples" in the Chinese part of the chapter). A few favorites include herbs and greens such as chrysanthemum greens, mizuna (potherb), and shiso (perilla, a member of the mint family—the red variety is used to color pickled foods); many tubers, including gobo (burdock root, which is shaved and leached in water to remove bitterness), sweet potatoes, a small variety of taro, and yams; and others such as daikon (a white radish similar to the Chinese radish, but longer, up to twelve inches in length), edamame (young soybean pods boiled in saltwater, then popped open for a snack, often with beer), kabocha (winter squash), shiitake mushrooms, and the winter tangerine known as mikan. Pickled vegetables are available year-round and are eaten extensively. Fresh fruit is a traditional dessert.

The Japanese use large amounts of seaweed and algae in their cooking for seasoning, as a wrapping, or in salads and soups. There are many types. Nori is a paper-thin sheet of algae that is rolled around sushi. Kombu is an essential ingredient in dashi or soup stock made from dried bonito fish and seaweed. Misoshiru is a popular soup made with dashi and miso (either red or white miso can be used). Wakame and hijiki are used primarily in soups and salads. Aonoriko is powdered green seaweed used as a seasoning agent.

Japanese dishes are classified by the way the food is prepared (refer to Table 11.6). Tempura is an example of an agemono (deep fried) dish. Adapted from a dish introduced in the sixteenth century by the Catholic Portuguese for religious fast days, it consists of shrimp and sliced vegetables—such as eggplant, carrots, sweet potato, lotus root, and green beans—lightly

Table 11.6 Selected Japanese Cooking Styles

Suimono	Clear soups, such as *dashi* or *misoshiru*
Yakimono	Broiled or grilled food (often marinated), such as *teriyaki* or *yakitori*
Nimono	Foods (usually a single item) simmered in seasoned water or broth, such as fish in sake-flavored broth, served hot or at room temperature
Mushimono	Steamed foods, such as *chawanmushi*
Agemono	Deep-fried foods, such as deep-fried tofu or *katsu*, usually served with a dipping sauce
Aemono	Fresh or cooked mixed foods tossed with thick sauces, such as salad with *miso* dressing
Sunomono	Mixed salads with vinegar dressing, such as crab and cucumber with rice vinegar and soy sauce dipping sauce
Chameshi	Rice cooked with other ingredients, such as chicken, fish, vegetables (especially mushrooms)—one specialty is rice with red adzuki beans, served for celebrations
Men rui	Noodle dishes, served hot or cold (plain or topped with fish or vegetables) with dipping sauce, or in a broth with items such as meats, seafood, tofu, and vegetables
Nabemono	Foods that are cooked at the table and one-pot dishes (usually a type of *nimono* dish), usually hearty combinations, such as *sukiyaki* and *shabu shabu*

battered and deep-fried. Katsu is another agemono dish of deep-fried breaded pork cutlets or fish filets. Sukiyaki is a simmered beef dish usually prepared at the table. The name means "broiled on the blade of the plow" and probably dates back to ancient times. The current version of sukiyaki is mislabeled, however, because it is a nimono-style (simmered), not a yakimono-style (grilled) food. *Shabu shabu*, a nabemono (one pot) dish of small pieces of beef and vegetables cooked in broth at the table, is similar to a Mongolian hot pot (refer to "Chinese Regional Specialties" above). After the meat and vegetables are cooked and eaten, the broth is ladled into bowls and consumed. Teriyaki is one type of grilled yakimono dish, as is yakitori (grilled, marinated chicken skewers). Teppanyaki is a Japanese term for stovetop grilling. The style familiar to U.S. diners was invented to take advantage of the tourist trade. Beef, chicken, shrimp, and vegetables are cooked on a hot grill in the center of a large table, then served with ponzu, a soy sauce and citrus juice mixture. Chawanmushi, a savory egg custard in which meats and vegetables are cooked, is a typical steamed mushimono (steamed) dish.[112]

Seafood, fish, fruits, and vegetables that are pickled in a mixture of miso, soy sauce, vinegar, and the residue from sake production are known as tsukemono, and they are served at nearly every meal.

Japanese foods are usually cut into small pieces if the item is not naturally easy to eat with chopsticks, and dishes are frequently modified for children, as it is believed that adult recipes are too spicy for them. Cooking style varies from region to region in Japan. Kyoto is known for its vegetarian specialties, Osaka and Tokyo are known for their seafood, and Nagasaki's cooking has been greatly influenced by the Chinese.

Meal Composition and Cycle

Daily Pattern Traditionally, the Japanese eat three meals a day, plus a snack called oyatsu. Simple meals, such as breakfast and lunch, are often ichiju—issei, meaning "soup with one side." For example, breakfast usually starts with a salty sour plum (umeboshi), followed by rice garnished with nori, soup, and pickled vegetables. A side dish such as an egg or fried fish is served with rice. A nabemono can replace the side dish, which often happens at lunchtime. The meal is typically simple and often consists only of rice topped with leftovers from the previous night. Sometimes hot tea or dashi (soup stock) is added to the rice mixture. A bowl of noodles cooked or served with meats, poultry, or fish and vegetables is popular as well. One such dish is oyakodon, which means "parent and child on rice," a mixture of boiled chicken and scrambled eggs on a bed of rice.[112]

Dinner is usually ichiju sansei, meaning "soup and three sides," including rice, soup, and tsukemono (pickles), and three dishes: a raw or vinegared fish, a simmered dish, and a grilled or fried dish.[112] Pink pickled ginger (beni shoga) garnishes many meals, and soy sauce is usually available. The pungent, green, horseradish-like condiment called wasabi may also be offered, and it is mixed in small individual bowls with soy sauce to taste. One important aspect of the Japanese diet is how protein is distributed in each meal. While protein amounts might be small, they are consumed at least three times per day. Protein distribution becomes more important to diets in the aging process.[113]

The Japanese tend not to serve meals by course. Instead, all the dishes are presented at the same time in individual portions, each food in its bowl or plate. The soup, however, is sometimes served last or near the end of the meal, and tsukemono may be placed on a communal plate for diners to add according to their personal preference. Traditionally, desserts were not common in Japan; meals usually ended with fruit.

In addition, the Japanese often eat a boxed meal called bento. A pleasing assortment of at least ten items is packaged attractively for consumption at school, picnics, or even between acts at the theater. Some restaurants specialize in bento meals.

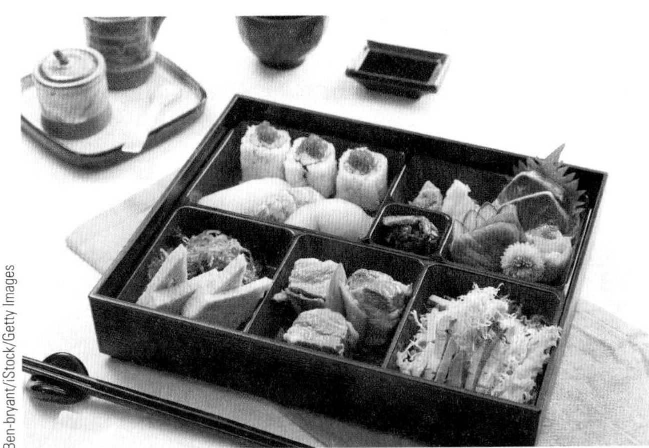
Ben-bryant/iStock/Getty Images

▲ Japanese Bento Box.

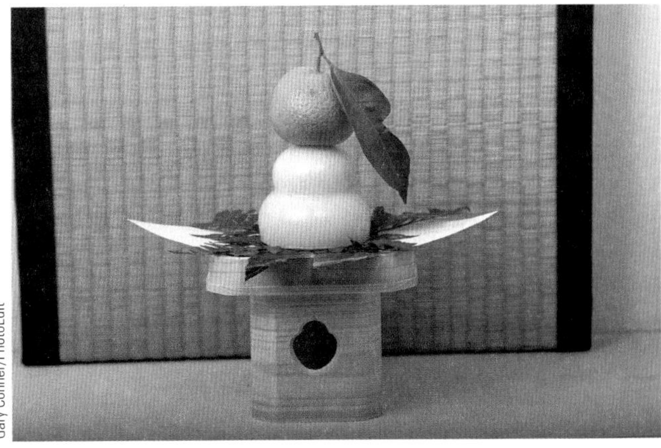
Gary Conner/PhotoEdit

▲ The *o sonae mochi* is traditional in Japanese Buddhist homes at New Year's, symbolizing prosperity and happiness in the future.

Food for Thought

Sansai ryori is a style of cooking with fresh wild herbs and vegetables such as goosefoot, mugwort, nettles, ferns, and bracken. It is considered the essence of spring.

Myoga ginger is prized in Japan for its tender shoots in the spring and its flower buds in the fall.

Kombu, a type of edible sea vegetable in the brown algae family, is eaten at celebratory occasions to symbolize happiness, as kombu in Japanese sounds similar to yorokobu, the word for rejoice. This food from the sea has been eaten and harvested in Japan for over 3,000 years.

The Japanese use 21 billion sets of disposable wood chopsticks in restaurants annually.

Snacks include several kinds of sweets, rice crackers, or fruit. Traditional Japanese confections include mochi gashi (rice cakes with sweet red bean paste), manju (dumplings), and yo-kan. Green tea is served after all meals except when Western-style food is eaten; then coffee or black tea is served. Beer or sake (rice wine, usually served warm) may be served with dinner.

Eating out is common. Numerous small restaurants specialize in certain preparations, such as sushi, yakitori, or noodle dishes. Restaurant windows often display their menu items with plastic replicas of their dishes.

Etiquette The Japanese, like the Chinese, eat with chopsticks and follow many of the same customs regarding their use (refer to the "Etiquette" subsection in the Chinese part of the chapter); the rice bowl is not held as close to the mouth, however. Soups are consumed directly from the bowl; the only dish eaten with a spoon is chawanmushi (steamed egg custard). Slurping soups and noodles are permitted and may be seen as a sign of appreciation. Tea should always be silently sipped.[42]

Traditionally the Japanese eat their meals at low tables, in a kneeling position with the heels tucked under the buttocks. In less formal situations men may sit cross-legged and women with their legs tucked to the side. Shoes are removed first. Dishes on the left are picked up with the right hand, and dishes to the right are lifted with the left hand. It is impolite to serve sake, beer, or tea to oneself. Each diner is obliged to fill his or her neighbor's glass whenever it is half-empty.

Guests are usually invited to restaurants, where the host chooses the menu in advance. The meal may include frequent toasts, particularly kampai ("bottoms up"). Games may be played at the table after the meal. Karaoke singing is common, and guests are expected to good-naturedly participate.[42]

Special Occasions In Japan, there are numerous festivals associated with the harvesting of specific crops or with local Shinto shrines or Buddhist temples, and they share many holiday traditions with the Chinese. The most important and largest celebration in Japan is the New Year celebration. Homes are cleaned thoroughly, and all debts are settled before the New Year; food is also prepared ahead so that no knives or cooking will interfere with the seven-day event. The Japanese celebrate New Year's Day on January 1. The New Year's foods consist of ten to twenty meticulously prepared dishes served in a special set of nesting boxes. Each dish symbolizes a specific value, such as happiness, prosperity, wealth, long life, wisdom, and diligence. For example, fish eggs represent fertility, mashed sweet potatoes and chestnuts protect against bad spirits, and black beans represent a willingness to keep healthy through hard work and sweat.

An important New Year's food is mochi, a rice cake made by pounding hot, steamed rice into a sticky dough. Traditionally, a Buddhist *o sonae mochi* (stacked mochi rice cakes representing older and younger generations) is set up in many homes. A large rice cake represents the foundation of the older generation and is placed on the bottom, and a smaller rice cake symbolizing the younger generation is placed atop it, followed by a tangerine indicating generations to come.

The o sonae mochi is as meaningful to the Japanese as a Christmas tree is to Americans, preserving good fortune and happiness for future generations. Another special food is ozoni, a soup cooked with mochi, vegetables, fish cakes, and chicken or eggs. A special rice wine called otoso is consumed to preserve health in the coming year. Japanese Buddhist temples usually hold an Obon festival in the second or third week of July to appreciate the living, honor the dead, and comfort the bereaved. Food and dancing are a traditional part of the holiday. Certain birthdays are considered either hazardous or auspicious in Japanese culture. When a man turns forty-two or a woman becomes thirty-three, special festivities are held to prevent misfortune. Age sixty-one marks the beginning of second childhood, and a person dons a red cap for this honor. At age seventy-seven a person puts on a long red overcoat, and at the most propitious birthday of all, age eighty-eight, the celebrant may begin wearing both the hat and the coat.

Therapeutic Uses of Food Although the use of yin and yang is not as prevalent among the Japanese as it is among the Chinese, there are many beliefs about the harmful or beneficial effects of specific foods and food combinations. Traditionally certain food pairs, such as eel and pickled plums, watermelon and crab, or cherries and milk, are thought to cause illness.

Pickled plums and hot tea, which are customarily eaten for breakfast, are believed to prevent constipation. Both pickled plums and rice porridge, called okayu, are thought to be easily digested and well tolerated during recovery from sickness.

Contemporary Food Habits in the United States

Adaptations of Food Habits

It is thought that when acculturated Japanese Americans eat a typical American diet, they may eat more rice and use more soy sauce than non-Asians. Traditional foods are still prepared for special occasions. A Westernized diet is increasingly followed even in Japan. Bread and butter are becoming staples, and consumption of meat, milk, and eggs is increasing.

Studies of Nisei and Sansei (mothers of Japanese immigrants and their daughters) show several trends in dietary acculturation.[114–116] Compared to the predominantly Japanese diet consumed by the Issei who immigrated to the United States, Nisei women in the study continued to eat rice daily but added other starches, such as bread and cereals. Traditional protein sources, including seafood, tofu, and eggs, were often replaced with more meats and dairy items. Condiments such as soy sauce and miso were consumed less often, while butter and margarine intake increased substantially. When compared to their mothers, the Sansei daughters consumed less rice and more pasta, ate less dried fish and more cheese, consumed fewer traditional preserved or pickled foods and more fresh fruits and vegetables (particularly potatoes), and used less butter and margarine. The Sansei women also ate fewer Japanese-style sweets and more salty snacks. Green tea consumption declined with the Sansei daughters, and soft drink consumption increased. Notably, meal consumption became more irregular with the Sansei, and eating out and use of takeout foods were significantly more common.

Nutritional Status

Nutritional Intake The traditional Japanese diet is high in carbohydrates (rice and potatoes) and very low in fat and cholesterol. Most cooking fats are polyunsaturated, and butter is rarely used. Japanese Americans, however, consume a more typically American diet, and this change may contribute to the increased incidence of several diseases, including gout. The westernization of meals and changing eating habits that occurred in the 1960s which has been attributed to the increased rates of gout. Compared to the Japanese diet in 1950, consumption of rice and potatoes decreased, and the intake of wheat, legumes, seeds and nuts, seaweed, vegetables, fruit, meat, seafood, eggs, milk and dairy products, oils and fats, seasoning, and spices increased.[117]

The leading cause of death for Japanese Americans is cancer and heart disease, but it is still lower than death rates for other Americans.[118] According to classic epidemiological studies, mainland Japanese Americans have a higher risk of developing colorectal cancer and heart disease than the Japanese in Hawaii, and those in Hawaii have a higher risk than the Japanese in Japan. More detailed evaluation has shown that Japanese Americans have more rapid atherosclerosis progression than Japanese men and women.[119] It has been postulated that the increase is caused by long-term lifestyle habits, including a Western-style diet and a sedentary lifestyle which is correlated to a higher intake of cholesterol and animal fat and a lower intake of dietary fiber and fish oil (omega-3 fatty acids).[120] Other cancers, such as those of the breast and prostate, have also increased in Japanese Americans as their stay in the United States lengthens, also possibly explained by lifestyle changes due to Westernized diets. However, there have been improvements in treatment and/or early detection.[121]

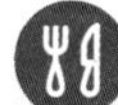

Food for Thought

Historically, rice was at times in short supply in Japan, which is perhaps why eating the round rice cakes, mochi, at New Year's represented wealth and prosperity.

Obesity rates in Japan are low compared to other countries, with of the population at 20 percent overweight and 3.5 percent obese. According to one study, U.S.-born Chinese and Japanese women had two and three times higher risk of becoming overweight/obese compared to their foreign-born counterparts.[122] Changes in diet have also been implicated in the high rates of type 2 diabetes found among Japanese American men.[123–125] Among Nisei men in one study, the rates for diabetes were twice that for similarly aged White men living in the same region of the United States and four times that for similarly aged men in Japan.[126] Data showed that

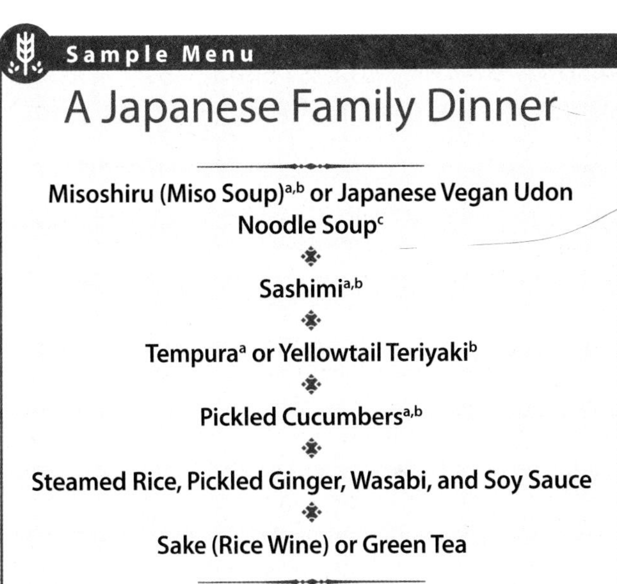

Sample Menu

A Japanese Family Dinner

Misoshiru (Miso Soup)[a,b] or Japanese Vegan Udon Noodle Soup[c]

Sashimi[a,b]

Tempura[a] or Yellowtail Teriyaki[b]

Pickled Cucumbers[a,b]

Steamed Rice, Pickled Ginger, Wasabi, and Soy Sauce

Sake (Rice Wine) or Green Tea

Recipes in this menu:

[a]Fukushima, S. 2001. *Japanese home cooking*. Boston: Periplus.

[b]*Yasuko-san's Home Cooking* at http://www.nsknet.or.jp/~tomi-yasu/index_e.html

[c]The Spruce Eats at https://www.thespruceeats.com/japanese-udon-noodle-soup-3377950

the Japanese American men were consuming carbohydrate, protein, and fat proportions similar to the overall American diet, but with fewer total calories. (A third of Japanese Americans are overweight and obesity is higher in U.S.-born Japanese Americans than in foreign-born Japanese Americans, though total rates are low.)[127] However, insulin resistance and metabolic syndrome were greater in Japanese American men when compared to Japanese subjects, and increased intra-abdominal fat deposits were found.[128,129]

Among women, intra-abdominal fat increased with menopause. Intra-abdominal fat deposition was found predictive of type 2 diabetes in Japanese Americans independent of total adiposity, family history, and other risk factors.[130–132] A genetic predisposition for diabetes combined with increased fat consumption, especially animal fats, may account for the disproportionately high rates.

Food for Thought

Even though anyone can have the enzyme issue that causes alcohol intolerance, people of East Asian descent are more likely to have inherited the gene. This inherited condition causes immediate skin flushing (reddening) and may even result in heart palpitations when alcohol is consumed.[133]

Earlier studies suggest older Japanese Americans may have a low intake of calcium because of the limited consumption of dairy products.[139] The Japanese have a high incidence of lactose intolerance. Although seaweed, tofu, and small bony fish contain calcium, they may not be eaten in adequate amounts to provide sufficient intake. The prevalence of osteoporosis may be higher than among Whites (refer to Cultural Controversy—Dairy Foods, BMD, and Osteoporosis).[138] Calorie consumption and meat intake have also been found to decline with age in Japanese Americans. Recent studies have suggested that muscle strength is associated with healthy bone status. Physical activity and movement help prevent sarcopenia (muscle loss) in older adults which reinforces the notion of using them or losing them. This is an important message for older Japanese adults who may be at risk for osteoporosis.[134,140,141] Protein is also important to prevent sarcopenia. Older adults may benefit from proportionally more protein in their diets, evenly distributed across the day for muscle health. Consumption of protein foods throughout the day every 3–4 hours has been the focus of several research studies.[113]

The traditional Japanese diet tends to be high in salt from soy sauce, dashi, miso, monosodium glutamate (MSG), dried preserved fish, and pickled vegetables. Rates of conditions sometimes linked to high-sodium diets, such as hypertension, stroke, and stomach cancer, are extremely high in Japan but have been dropping as the Japanese adopt Western fare.[135]

Infant mortality rates for Japanese Americans are lower than those for the general population.[96] However, a study comparing pregnancy outcomes in Japanese Americans noted that U.S.-born mothers are significantly more likely to have low-birth-weight infants than foreign-born mothers.[136,137]

Food for Thought

Korea is called *Choson* which, though disputed, some interpret to mean "Land of Morning Calm."

Japanese Americans often believe that the health care provider is a knowledgeable authority figure who will meet their needs without assistance. Most Americans of Japanese descent expect to be directed in their health care with specific suggestions for improvement. Criticism of a client's health habits can lead to embarrassment and loss of effective communication. Concrete, structured approaches based on information gathered through an unhurried, in-depth interview that determines the degree of acculturation and personal preferences are most effective.

Koreans

The mountainous peninsula that forms Korea is suspended geographically and culturally between China and Japan. Korea has historically been caught in the middle of both

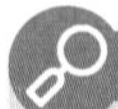

Cultural Controversy

Dairy Foods, BMD, and Osteoporosis

Osteoporosis, which means "porous bone," affects 10 million women and 2 million men in the United States. Another 16 million have low bone mineral density (BMD), which may put them at risk of developing the disease. Osteoporosis is characterized by reduced height, a stooped spinal deformity, and over 1.5 million bone fractures annually, most often of the spine, the hip, and the wrist. The causes of osteoporosis are not completely understood. Contributing factors include ethnicity, family history, low calcium intake, insufficient weight-bearing exercise, smoking, high alcohol consumption, and low levels of estrogen in women and testosterone in men.[138]

White women have long been considered at the highest risk for osteoporosis. In particular, thin White women have been thought most vulnerable because higher body mass is related to better BMD. Asian women have a lower incidence of hip fracture than White women, but the prevalence of vertebral fractures among Asians seems to be as high as that in White individuals. Protective factors that lower the risk for fracture in Asians may be diminishing, however. Hip fracture rates are rising dramatically in Japan, Hong Kong, and among the Chinese in Singapore.[139]

Dietary recommendations regarding osteoporosis have traditionally emphasized a high intake of calcium-rich foods. Dairy foods are considered good sources because in addition to calcium they also contain vitamin D, which enhances the absorption of the mineral. Although many Asians do not eat dairy foods, it has been thought that they obtained adequate calcium from eating small fish with bones (e.g., sardines), mineral-rich fish sauces, and ample dark green leafy vegetables. Some scientists also suggest that soybean intake may be protective, slowing bone mineral loss after menopause.[140] Yet, if the prevalence of low BMD and osteoporosis among Asians is higher than previously calculated, and if fractures are increasing, do non-dairy foods provide adequate calcium intake? Or, if the intake of traditional calcium-rich foods declines with acculturation in the United States (and Westernization worldwide), are dairy foods needed to provide the calcium no longer being consumed?[141,142]

More research on the bioavailability of calcium in different foods and the role of diet in the development of BMD, osteoporosis, and fractures is needed to determine whether dairy food recommendations are sensible for all Americans or simply ethnocentric.

Perspectives on Aging Well

Reaching Your Triple Digit Birthday—Diet Secrets of Centenarians

What is the secret to reaching 100? Well, it's usually a combination of genetics, lifestyle choices (especially diet), and just plain luck. While an individual can't control the genes they were born with, how they live their lives and the choices that they make can have a huge influence.

The connection between mind, body, and spirit is crucial. For the Japanese, eating a healthy diet is a key part of the equation. One of the largest groups of centenarians lives in Okinawa, Japan. Many studies have been conducted with this group, that looked at the role of their diets in relation to cardiovascular health and disease. The Okinawan diets are loaded with antioxidants—heavy on grains, vegetables, and daily consumption of fish. In particular, cold-water varieties such as tuna, mackerel, and salmon were the most common. These types of fish contain high concentrations of Omega-3 fatty acids, which have been linked to reducing the risk of heart disease and breast cancer. Once again fish gets a gold star for being a superfood![143–145]

Vegetables, -in particular the yellow-green varieties (spinach, kale, broccoli, squash, sweet potatoes, carrots), and fruit like melon, also contain high amounts of antioxidants. On average, the Okinawan centenarians consume at least seven ½ cup servings of vegetables daily, and an equal number of grains (mostly whole grains). They also eat small amounts of food throughout the course of the day. In short, the average Okinawan's diet is far richer in complex carbohydrates and plant-based foods, and lower in fat, than the average American's.[145]

For those wanting to reach a triple-digit birthday, consider the other traits of centenarians. These include daily exercise, a positive outlook on life, and the love of learning new things (many centenarians have cell phones and iPads, and know how to Google). They surround themselves with friends and celebrate aging. And last but not least, centenarians have one more thing in common. Most live in environments that exhibit clean air, good water, low stress, and unspoiled nature. Ponce de Leon's fountain of youth may be in our own backyard![145]

Chinese and Japanese expansionism yet has maintained a homogeneous population with an independent, distinctive character. Little land is arable, and the climate fluctuates between cold, snowy winters and hot, monsoonal summers that limit agriculture significantly. The peninsula is currently divided into two nations. The Democratic People's Republic of Korea (North Korea), with the capital city of Pyongyang, has a communist government. The Republic of Korea (South Korea), with the capital city of Seoul, is a democracy. Both nations desire the reunification of Korea through political and military domination of the other.[146]

Food for Thought

The status of Koreans in the United States during World War II was unique. Many remained technically Japanese citizens (due to Japan's annexation of Korea after years of war from 1910 to 1945) and as such were declared enemy aliens (although none were interred).[146] References say some wore "I am Korean" buttons to distinguish themselves from Japanese residents during World War II.[147]

There were approximately 198,000 Canadians of Korean ancestry in the 2016 Census.

Cultural Perspective

History of Koreans in the United States

Immigration Patterns Early Korean immigration to the United States was severely restricted by the isolationist policies of Korea. A small number of Koreans arrived before 1900, most of whom were Protestants seeking to escape discrimination and further their education in America.

Food for Thought

The economic success of South Korea has lured thousands of second-generation Korean Americans to immigrate there, where they have taken positions in marketing, public relations, and the entertainment industry.

Between 1903 and 1905 about 7,500 Korean people, mostly young men in their twenties, immigrated to work in Hawaiian sugarcane fields. Most were from the lower economic classes, had been city-dwelling Koreans already uprooted from their more conservative communities in the countryside, and had had contact with Christian missionaries before departure. They overwhelmingly affiliated themselves with Christian institutions after arriving in Hawaii.[148] By 1924, about 2,000 "picture brides" from Korea arrived to join the earlier immigrants. This abruptly ended with the Immigration Act of 1924, which banned all Asian immigrants. The next wave of immigration occurred after the War Bride Act of 1946 facilitated the immigration of Korean wives of American servicemen and children that were adopted into American families. Between 1950 and 1964, approximately 6,000 Korean students, businessmen, and politicians entered the United States. The 1965 Immigration and Naturalization Act made family reunification possible and increased the annual number of immigrants from Korea arriving in the United States (reaching 30,000 in 1976).[149]

Current Demographics The Korean immigrant population has increased dramatically in recent years. According to 2019 Census estimates,[150] over 1.9 million Koreans are living in the United States, over half of whom have arrived since 1980. More than 54 percent of Koreans in America were born in Korea, and 36 percent of those have become citizens.[150] Large numbers of immigrants to the United States relocated first from North Korea to South Korea, seeking greater freedom. Koreans coming to America often hope to find economic opportunity and to avoid any North Korean–South Korean conflict that may arise in the future. Large numbers of Koreans have settled in California, particularly Los Angeles and the New York metropolitan area.

Socioeconomic Status Korean families in America working together toward the success of a small business and the purchase of a home are common. Contributing factors include high achievement in education and professionalism; quick mastery of English; over 58 percent of individuals have college degrees; and large numbers work in management and professional positions.

Worldview

Religion In 2014, South Korea had no majority religious group. Researchers found a plurality of people had no religious affiliation (46 percent) and the remaining were Christians (29 percent) and Buddhists (23 percent).[151] Smaller numbers adhere to shamanism (belief in natural and ancestral spirits) and Ch'ŏndogyo or religion of the heavenly way, formerly known as Tonghak or "Eastern learning" (a mixture of Confucianism, Taoism, Buddhism, shamanism, and Roman Catholicism), an indigenous Korean religion.[152] In North Korea, all religious beliefs other than national political ideology and self-reliance are suppressed.

Today, 71 percent of Korean Americans identify themselves as Christian (61 percent Protestant and 10 percent Catholic), and there are 4,454 Korean Christian churches in the United States. Six percent of Korean Americans identify themselves as Buddhists.[152]

Family Hundreds of years of Confucianism in Korea have significantly influenced family structure regardless of current religious affiliation. Family is highly valued, and loyalty to one's immediate and extended family is more important than individual wants or needs. Generational ties are more important than those of marriage, and parents are especially close to their children. Korean Americans often invite family members in Korea to join them in the United States, and extended families are not uncommon.

In Korea, the father is always the head of the family; if a father is unable to fulfill that role, the eldest son (even if still a child) takes on that responsibility. Birth sequence orders life's events within the family and older sons are traditionally awarded privileges, such as advanced education, that younger children and daughters are denied. Though changing since Korea opened more to the outside world in the nineteenth century, the role of women traditionally is to take care of the house and care for children.[153] Parenting tends to be authoritative, and any child over the age of five years exhibiting inappropriate behavior brings disrespect to the entire family. Older family members are esteemed and cared for in Korea. The most important passages in a person's life are the completion of a baby's first 100 days, marriage, and 61st birthday.[154] People over the age of 60 are given much respect and encouraged to relax and enjoy life.

Many changes occur in the Korean family after immigration to the United States. For example, the marriage bond often becomes more important than obligations to parents. Few older Koreans maintain traditional arrangements of living with an eldest son's family. Some live with unmarried children or with married daughters or live alone.[15] The dominance of men within the family has declined with increased participation of women in the workplace, yet most married women assume total responsibility for their home and their

New American Perspectives

Korean

Michael Han, Foodservice Management

I am a Korean American born in South Korea, and my parents moved to the United States in 1979 when I was eight months old. Members of my father's family came over first and then we followed.

We pretty much ate Korean meals at home. Most meals consisted of short-grain (sticky) rice, and kimchi, with a soup/stew. The soup contains meat (including Spam) and vegetables. My father really likes meat, so we probably had more than other Korean families, and really unusual is that he added butter as well. Now he adds olive oil instead because his cholesterol is too high. Once in a while, we would have Korean barbecue, but that was for special occasions or as a treat. Dessert was mostly fruit.

When I was young, I wanted to eat more American food. For a while, my mom would make pancakes for breakfast on the weekend, and when she stopped, I was really upset. Now I eat American food for breakfast and lunch but not dinner, and I usually have rice once a day. My aunt has taken over making kimchi for the family, but I don't live that close to her, so I only get it once in a while. When I do have it—I eat it all the time, so my supply lasts only a week.

In general, it would be hard to get Koreans in the United States to modify the amount and type of rice they eat, and I don't think they would ever give up pickled, spicy vegetables like kimchi.

job and often are not paid for their work if employed in a family-owned business.

Traditional Health Beliefs and Practices Family spirituality has a great influence on health and emotional well-being, especially for the older Korean population. Traditional Korean concepts related health to happiness, to the ability to live life fully, to function without impairment, and to not be a burden on one's children.[15] A good appetite is a significant indicator of health. Family togetherness, interdependence, and coping are important themes for well-being and lifestyle choices.[155]

The Korean system of health and illness is closely related to Chinese precepts (refer to the section "Traditional Health Beliefs and Practices" in the Chinese part of the chapter). The proper balance of eum (yin) and yang must occur to maintain health, influenced by the relationships of the five evolutive elements (fire, water, wood, metal, and earth) and ki (vital energy). Too much or too little of these forces results in illness. For example, cold, damp, heat, or wind can enter a body through the pores and then interfere with ki and weaken yang. Symptoms of the imbalance include indigestion, arthritis, and asthma. Other disruptive causes such as physical exhaustion, eating too much or too little food, and spiritual intervention (by ancestors or supernatural deities) may also result in disease.[156]

Both digestion and circulation are prominent in the maintenance of health, because energy is absorbed into the body through the stomach when food is mixed with air or one of the forces, and the blood distributes this vital energy. Good-quality food is restorative, but too much food can block ki, resulting in cold hands and feet, cold sweats, or even fainting.[15] A few Koreans attribute diabetes to eating too much rich food, such as meat, sugar, or honey, and getting too little exercise. Blood conditions that interfere with the distribution of vital energy include a lack of blood; a drying or hardening of the blood (typical in old age, causing indigestion, neuralgia, and body aches); and bad blood, caused by a sudden fright, which can result in chronic pain.

Korean-specific folk illnesses often include somatic complaints that are an expression of psychological distress.[157] Excessive emotions such as joy, sadness, depression, worry, anger, fright, and fear are believed to result in certain physical conditions. Hwabyung, attributed most often to anger, victimization, or stress, is associated with poor appetite, indigestion, stomach pain, chest pain, shortness of breath, weight gain, and high blood pressure among other symptoms. A study of middle-aged Korean women found that nearly 5 percent suffered from hwabyung, with rates higher in women of lower socioeconomic status, those who lived in rural areas, those who were separated or divorced, and those who smoked or drank alcohol.[158] Han, which causes a painful lump in the throat, occurs when a person suffers disappointments and regrets, such as guilt over the neglect of one's children, parents, or spouse. Shinggyongshaeyak, resulting from stress (especially from oversensitivity and lack of happy interactions with family and friends), can cause insomnia, weight loss, and nervous collapse. Traditional cures include the use of a shaman or spiritual mediator (mansin or mudang) to determine whether the cause of an illness is due to disharmony with one's ancestors or natural and supernatural forces.[158] Sacred therapeutic rituals to rectify such spiritual disruptions are conducted with the patient, the family, and sometimes the community.

Hanyak is the traditional approach to natural cures in Korea. It is typically practiced by a hanui. When a client visits a hanui, he or she obtains a medical history, observes how the patient looks, listens to the quality of the voice, and takes the patient's pulse. More than twenty-four pulse conditions are defined, from floating to sunken, and smooth, vacant, or accelerated.[158] Hanyak medications are classified according to their plant, animal, or mineral source, and mixed in ways to balance um (yin), yang, and ki. Other physical therapies to restore harmony and vital energy, such as acupuncture, moxibustion, cupping, and sweating (refer to Chapter 2), may also be applied. In the United States, the hanui may use some biomedical procedures in conjunction with traditional practices. It has been reported that some hanui take blood pressure and body temperatures. Some even offer the convenience of taking hanyak prescriptions in pill form so that bitter-tasting broths or teas are avoided.[159–161]

Many professional Korean health practices have been popularized and may be used as home remedies. In the United States, where access to traditional healers may be limited in some regions, the mother or grandmother in the home often takes responsibility for administering these cures.[159] Some Koreans believe that a person's fate is determined by the forces of um and yang at the moment of birth. Christian Koreans may believe strongly in faith healing and fate as determined by God. However, it does not appear to influence their desire for health care or practicing health-promoting lifestyles.[160]

Traditional Food Habits

Ingredients and Common Foods Korean cuisine is a distinctly hearty Asian fare that is highly seasoned and instantaneously recognizable as Korean by its flavors and colors. Sweet, sour, bitter, hot, and salty tastes are combined in all meals, and foods are often seasoned before and after cooking. Five colors—white, red, black, green, and yellow—are also important considerations in the preparation and presentation of dishes. Food is important to Korean cultural identity and even the most Westernized urban dwellers still emphasize grains, especially rice, and fresh vegetables.[154]

Staples Korean cooking is based on grains flavored with spicy vegetables and meat, poultry, or fish side dishes. Korean staples are listed in Table 11.7. Steam-cooked rice is the foundation of the Korean diet and its cooking is an important skill; the rice must be neither underdone nor overcooked and mushy. Though short-grain varieties are usually preferred, both a regular and glutinous (sticky) type, the latter most often in sweets, is also traditional. Long-grain rice is available but not common. Millet and barley are used, most often as extenders for rice.

Noodles are also an important staple and are made from wheat, buckwheat, mung beans, and from the starch of sweet potatoes and the kudzu plant (a pervasive vine).[162] The buckwheat variety is often used in cold dishes. Fritters, dumplings, and pancakes flavored with scallions, chili pepper, and sometimes fish or meat placed directly in the batter before cooking are other popular grain dishes.[163]

A traditional Korean meal is not complete without kimchi, a mixture of various pickled vegetables such as cabbage, radish, green onion, and cucumber. Some types of kimchi are spicy (using red chili pepper powder), while others are not. Garlic is always added, however. Ambient bacteria in the environment results in fermentation, which gives kimchi its pungent flavor and beneficial bioactive compounds.[164] Non-fermented vegetables are also served at every meal. Chinese cabbage (both bok choy and napa), European cabbage, and a long white radish (similar but not identical to the Japanese daikon radish) are eaten most often. Eggplant, cucumbers, perilla (a mint-family green also called shiso), chrysanthemum greens, bean sprouts, sweet potatoes, and winter melon are also very popular. Vegetables are added to soups and braised dishes and are often served individually as hot or cold side dishes.[164] Seaweed is eaten as a vegetable, including kelp and laver (called kim). Kim is brushed with sesame oil, salted, and toasted to make a condiment. The seaweed called wakame in Japan, miyeok in Korea, is an edible brown sea vegetable usually sold dried that has high nutritional value and is used in Korean soups.[165] Fruits are eaten mostly fresh. Crisp, juicy Asian pears (known as apple pears in the United States) are very popular; apples, cherries, jujubes (red dates), plums, melons, grapes, tangerines, and persimmons are also common.

Food for Thought

The preparation of kimchi every autumn can be a special family event for Koreans. In the past, a family's wealth was demonstrated by the ingredients in their kimchi, with rare vegetables and fruits used by the most affluent. Koreans consume over 2 tons annually.

South Korea is the largest consumer of Spam® outside the United States.

It is believed that a Portuguese Catholic priest introduced chili peppers into Korea in the sixteenth century. They were quickly adopted and have become ubiquitous in the cuisine.

Fish and shellfish are eaten throughout Korea. Fresh fish dishes are preferred near the coast or in river regions, but dried or salted fish is more common in the inland areas. Saewujeot, a Korean fermented fish sauce, is made from tiny shrimplike crustaceans. Saewujeot flavors many dishes. Beef and beef variety cuts cubed, thinly sliced, or eaten as small marinated ribs, are often barbecued or grilled at the table over a small charcoal brazier or gas grill.[166] Bulgogi, grilled strips of marinated beef flavored with garlic, onions, soy sauce, and sesame oil, is a favorite of many Koreans. Another Korean specialty is the fire pot (sinsullo), similar to the Mongolian hot pot, featuring beef or liver, cooked egg strips, sliced vegetables (e.g., mushrooms, carrots, bamboo shoots, onions), and nuts that are cooked in a seasoned broth heated over charcoal. After the morsels of food have been eaten, the broth is served as a soup. Chicken and poultry are not especially popular in Korea, though that is also shifting. Soybean products, however, are common, including soy sauce and soy paste. Bean curd, made from soybeans (tobu) or mung beans (cheong-po), is a favorite. Mung beans, adzuki beans, and other legumes are steamed and added to many savory and sweet dishes. Nuts, such as pine nuts, chestnuts, and peanuts, and toasted, crushed sesame seeds are frequent additions as ingredients or garnish.[167]

Table 11.7 Cultural Food Groups: Koreans

Group	Comments	Common Foods	Adaptations in the United States
Protein Foods			
Milk/milk products	Milk and milk products are generally not consumed or used in cooking.		Milk, yogurt, and cheese product consumption increases.
Meat/poultry/fish/eggs/legumes	Beef and beef variety cuts are especially popular. Barbecuing is a popular method for cooking meat. Fish and shellfish, either fresh, dried, or salted, are eaten throughout Korea. Soybean products are added to many dishes.	*Meat*: beef, variety meats (heart, kidney, liver), oxtail, pork *Fish and shellfish*: abalone, clams, codfish, crab, cuttlefish, jellyfish, lobster, mackerel, mullet, octopus, oysters, perch, scallops, sea cucumber, shad, shrimp, squid, whiting *Poultry and small birds*: chicken, pheasant *Eggs*: hen *Legumes*: adzuki, lima beans, mung beans, red beans, soybeans	Beef, pork, and poultry consumption rises. Fish is eaten frequently. Many still consume tofu several times a week. Younger Korean Americans may consume more pork products.
Cereals/Grains	Rice is the most important component of the Korean diet. Noodles made from wheat, mung bean, or buckwheat flours are an important staple.	Barley, buckwheat, millet, rice (short-grain glutinous), wheat	Rice consumption declines, but it is still eaten every day. Breads, cereals, and pasta popular with well-acculturated Korean Americans.
Fruits/Vegetables	A wide variety of fruits are consumed. Vegetables are often pickled and are eaten at every meal.	*Fruits*: apples, Asian pears, cherries, dates (jujubes, red date), grapes, melons, oranges, pears, persimmons, plums, pumpkin, tangerines *Vegetables*: bamboo shoots, bean sprouts, beets, cabbage (Chinese, European), celery, chives, chrysanthemum leaves, cucumber, eggplant, fern, green beans, green onion, green pepper, leaf lettuce, leeks, lotus root, mushrooms, onion, peas, perilla (*shiso*), potato, seaweed (*kim*), spinach, sweet potato, turnips, water chestnut, watercress, white radish	Increased intake of fruits and vegetables is noted. The majority eat *kimchi* daily.
Additional Foods			
Seasonings	Sweet, sour, bitter, hot, and salty tastes are combined in all meals. Dishes are often seasoned during and after cooking.	Chile peppers (*gochujang*—fermented chile paste), Chinese parsley (cilantro), chrysanthemum greens, cinnamon, garlic, ginger root, green onions, MSG, hot mustard, red pepper sauce, pine nuts, rice wine, *saewujeot* (fermented fish sauce), sesame seed oil, sesame seeds, soy sauce, sugar, vinegar, sea salt	
Nuts/seeds		Chestnuts, gingko nuts, hazelnuts, peanuts, pine nuts, pistachios, sesame seeds, walnuts	
Beverages	Herbal teas are popular, as well as rice tea. They are commonly served after the meal. Soup or barley water is used as a beverage with the meal.	Barley water, beer, coffee, fruit drinks, green tea, honey water, jasmine tea, magnolia flower drink, rice tea, rice water, rice wine, *soju* (sweet potato vodka), spiced teas (ginseng, cinnamon, ginger), wines made from other ingredients	Hot barley water is still the preferred beverage and is served after the meal. Increased consumption of soft drinks.
Fats/oils	Animal fat is rarely used.	Sesame oil, vegetable oils	
Sweeteners	Sweets are made for snacks and special occasions.	Honey, sugar	Cookies and other sweets popular with Korean American youth.

Seasonings are the soul of Korean cooking. Garlic, ginger root, black pepper, chili peppers, scallions, and toasted sesame in the form of oil or crushed seeds flavor nearly all dishes. Ginseng is added to some soups such as samgyetang (ginseng chicken soup). Prepared condiments, such as soy sauce, toenjang (fermented soybean paste), fish sauce (saewujeot), and hot mustard are also frequently added to foods. Gochujang, a fermented jamlike chili paste, is usually prepared by families in the spring and then traditionally stored for use throughout the year in black pottery crocks. Marinades and dipping sauces are common.[167]

Soup or thin barley water can be used as a beverage. Herbal teas are very popular; ginseng tea flavored with cinnamon is a favorite. Ginger, cinnamon, or citron can also be used separately to make a spice tea. A common drink is rice tea, made by pouring warm water over toasted, ground rice or by simmering water in the pot in which rice was cooked. On special occasions, wine might be served. Wines are made from rice and other grains; some include various flower blossoms or ginseng as flavorings. Beer is also well-liked. Milk and other dairy products are generally not consumed or used in cooking.

Meal Composition and Cycle

Daily Patterns Three small meals, with frequent snacking throughout the day, are typical in Korea. Breakfast was traditionally the main meal in Korea, but today is more likely to be something light, eaten on the run. Soup is almost always served at breakfast, along with rice (usually as gruel). Eggs, meat or fish, or vegetables may top the meal. Kimchi and dipping sauces are the usual accompaniments.

Lunch is typically noodles served with a broth of beef, chicken, or fish and garnished with shellfish, meat, or vegetables. Supper is more similar to breakfast, but with steamed rice. In many modern homes, it has become the main meal of the day. Snacks are widely available from street vendors, including grilled and steamed tidbits of all types. Sweets, such as rice cookies and cakes, or dried fruit (especially persimmons) are also popular snacks.

Rice is considered the main dish of each meal. Everything else is served as an accompaniment to the rice and is called panch'an. For dinner, at least one meat or fish dish is included, if affordable, and two or three vegetables are usually served. Kimchi is always offered. Soup is very popular and is served at most meals. Individual bowls of rice and soup are served to each diner, and panch'an dishes are served on trays in the center of the table for communal eating. Wine may be served before the meal with appetizers such as batter-fried vegetables, seasoned tobu, pickled seafood, meatballs, or steamed dumplings. Dessert is seldom eaten, although fresh fruit sometimes concludes the meal. Hot barley water or rice tea is served with the meal.

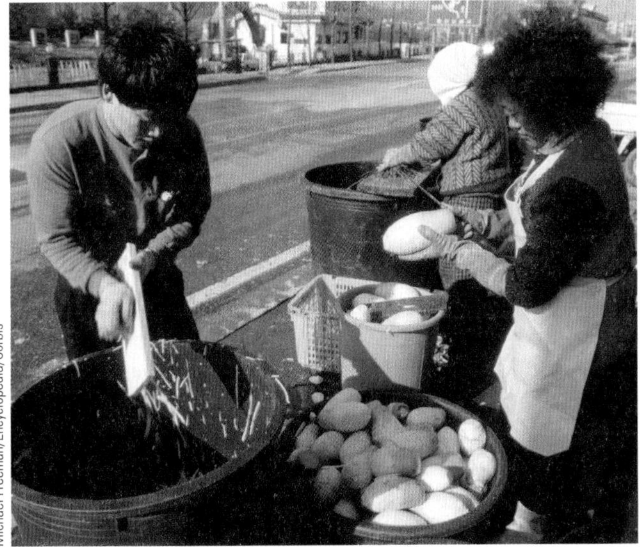

Michael Freeman/Encyclopedia/Corbis

▲ **Korean street vendors shredding daikon for the preparation of the spicy vegetable pickle kimchi.**

Drinking is a social ritual practiced mostly by men. Distilled beverages like soju, a sweet potato vodka, are consumed with snacks like spicy squid or chili peppers stuffed with beef.

A special category of food, called anju, is considered an alternative to a full meal. Analogous to tapas in Spain (refer to Chapter 6), they are small dishes especially suited to eating while socializing and drinking.[164] Examples include scallion-flavored pancakes usually accompanied by Korean rice wine, mukhuli, Japanese-style sashimi, quail eggs, bits of pork, raw crab in chili paste, or dumplings. These items are often served as appetizers in Korean American restaurants.

 **Food for Thought**

At Korean weddings, sweetened dates rolled in sesame seeds are tossed at the bride by her in-laws to ensure health, prosperity, and numerous children.

Boyak, a restorative herbal medicine in Korea, is often given as a gift, particularly to one's parents, to promote long life.

Etiquette Chopsticks and soup spoons are usually the only eating utensils used in Korea. In the past, seating was around a low, rectangular table on the floor (today most tables are set with chairs). Traditionally, older diners are served first, and children are served last at the meal. It is considered polite to fill the soy sauce dish of the people one is sitting beside. Food is always passed with the right hand, and a communal beverage may be passed for all to share.

Special Occasions Korean cooking was historically divided into everyday fare and cuisine for royalty. The traditions of palace cooking and food presentation, including the use of numerous ingredients in elaborate dishes, are seen today in meals for special occasions. At a meal celebrating a birthday or holiday, or one shared with guests, more dishes are served and both wine and dessert are offered. For special occasions, Koreans offer a thick drink of persimmons or dates, nuts, and spices, or a beverage made with molasses and magnolia served with small, edible flowers floating on top.

Both Koreans and Korean Americans celebrate several holidays throughout the year. The first is New Year's, called Sol, a three-day event at which traditional dress is worn and the older people in the family are honored. Festivities include feasts, games, and flying kites. On the first full moon, in a tradition reflecting ancient religious rites, torches are lighted, and firecrackers are set off to frighten evil spirits away. Shampoo Day (Yadu Nal) on June 15 is when families bathe in streams to ward off fevers. Thanksgiving (Chusok) is a fall harvest festival; duk, steamed rice cakes filled with chestnuts, dates, red beans, or other items, are associated with the holiday.

A special ceremony is observed on a child's first birthday when the child is dressed in traditional clothing and

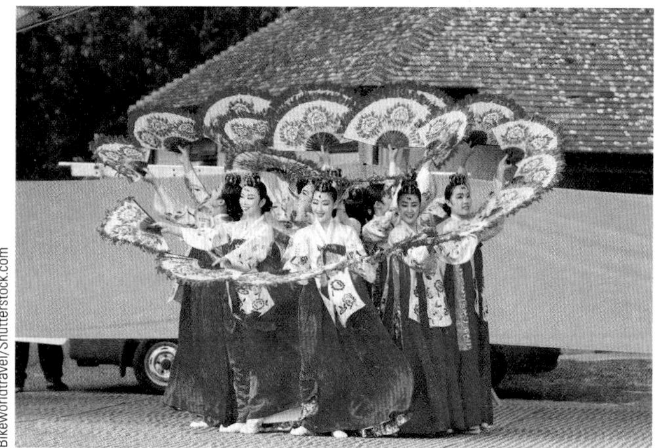
Bikeworldtravel/Shutterstock.com

▲ Korean Americans celebrate Sol, or the New Year, on the first full moon.

placed among stacks of rice cakes, cookies, and fruit. Family and friends offer the child objects symbolizing various professions, such as a pen for writing or a coin for finance, and the first one accepted is thought to predict his or her future career.[154]

Therapeutic Uses of Food Many Koreans follow the yin and yang food classification system, or eum yang in Korean. Little has been reported about specific foods, although Koreans are believed to adhere to categorizations similar to other Asians: cold foods include mung beans, winter melon, cucumber, and most other vegetables and fruits; meats (e.g., beef, mutton, goat), chili peppers, garlic, and ginger are considered hot (yang) foods.

Preparation of healthy, tasty food is an important way that Korean women show affection for family and friends.[153,155] Good appetite is considered a sign of good health. Foods that are believed to be health-promoting include bean-paste soup, beef turnip soup, rice with grains and beans, broiled seaweed, kimchi, and ginseng tea. Ginseng products are often used to promote health and stamina and alleviate tiredness. One very popular tonic, called boyak, combines ginseng and deer horn or bear gallbladder.[157]

More than one-half of Korean American respondents in one survey reported using ginseng, with older women more likely to use such products than men or younger women.[168] Other home remedies commonly used include ginger tea, yoojacha (hot citrus beverage), bean sprout soup, and lemon with honey in hot water. Restorative herbal medicines, vitamin supplements, meat soups, bone marrow soup, and samgyetang (game-hen soup) also were mentioned by subjects as useful when feeling weak.

A study of pregnant Korean American women suggests that certain foods, such as seaweed soup, beef, and rice, are thought to build strength during pregnancy.[169] Food taboos during pregnancy often involve the concept of "like causes like." For instance, eating blemished fruit may result in a baby with skin problems. Although most food avoidance was attributed to personal preference and availability, many of the women acknowledged familiarity with the traditional beliefs. Korean women traditionally consumed seaweed soup, miyuk kook, three times a day for seven weeks after the birth of a child to restore their strength.

Traditional Korean medicine (acupuncture, moxibustion, cupping, and herbal medicine) is often widely used before the introduction of conventional medicine. Consequently, there is a dual health care system made up of traditional and conventional medicine based on a patient's choice. Traditional Korean medicine has been covered by Korea's mandatory National Health Insurance since 1987.[170]

Contemporary Food Habits in the United States

Adaptations of Food Habits

Ingredients and Common Foods Korean Americans keep many traditional Korean food habits after immigrating to the United States. Many eat rice and kimchi daily.[171,172] Beef, pork, and fish continue to be consumed and sesame oil/seeds and vegetable oils are used more often than butter or mayonnaise. Condiments such as soy sauce, soybean paste, gochujang (a fermented chili paste), and garlic, remain popular and tofu (tobu in Korea) is eaten often.

An older national study of mostly first-generation Korean Americans found regular consumption continued of some traditional dishes and ingredients, such as rice, kimchi, garlic, scallions, Korean soup, sesame oil, Korean stew, soybean paste, and gochugang, the savory, sweet and spicy gochugang. Frequently consumed American foods included oranges, low-fat milk, bagels, tomatoes, and bread. Regularly eaten foods common to both cultures included onions, coffee, apples, eggs, beef, carrots, lettuce, fish, and tea. The researchers found that most respondents had access to Korean items, but as participation in American social life increased, acceptance of American foods increased. Persons who had someone familiar with Korean fare to cook for them were more likely to continue eating traditional dishes than those who cooked for themselves.[173]

Another study reported that well-acculturated Korean American mothers were less likely to prepare Korean dishes at home and were more likely to dine out.[174] Research on Korean, Korean American, and American adolescents found that Korean American teens adopted a diet in-between that of traditional Korean and American food patterns, eating less rice and kimchi, and more cookies, other sweets, and soft drinks.[175] Despite these earlier findings, Korean food remains close to the cultural identity of Korean Americans and is increasingly popular in American mainstream culture.[176]

It should be noted that many changes in the traditional diet have been observed in Korea. As the Korea National Health and Nutrition Examination Survey (2016–2018) states, ultra-processed food intake has increased causing an increase in high-calorie, high-sugar, and high-fat foods. These foods are low in fiber, protein, minerals, and vitamins. Ultra-processed foods account for one-fourth of daily energy intake.[177]

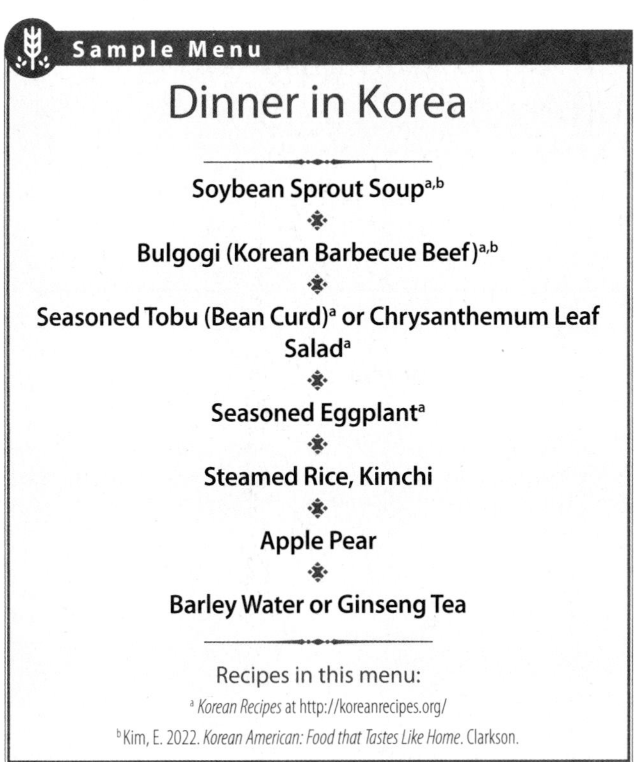

Sample Menu

Dinner in Korea

Soybean Sprout Soup[a,b]

Bulgogi (Korean Barbecue Beef)[a,b]

Seasoned Tobu (Bean Curd)[a] **or Chrysanthemum Leaf Salad**[a]

Seasoned Eggplant[a]

Steamed Rice, Kimchi

Apple Pear

Barley Water or Ginseng Tea

Recipes in this menu:

[a] *Korean Recipes* at http://koreanrecipes.org/

[b] Kim, E. 2022. *Korean American: Food that Tastes Like Home*. Clarkson.

Korean American Cuisine Koreans have blended their traditional flavoring and cooking techniques into American foods. One of the better-known dishes is the Korean taco, a Mexican corn tortilla with Korean-style fillings, such as bulgogi (grilled beef) and kimchi. This style of taco started in a food truck in Los Angeles and rapidly spread across the country, especially in metropolitan areas. Other examples of Korean fusion dishes are kimchi quesadillas, short rib sliders, and Korean fried chicken.

Meal Composition and Cycle Little has been reported regarding Korean American meal composition and cycle. It is assumed that because Korean meal and snacking patterns are similar to those in the United States, three meals a day remain common. Survey data suggest that hot barley water served after meals is still the preferred beverage of Korean Americans. Acculturation and/or length of stay has been found to increase the frequency of eating out for Korean Americans.[174]

Korean Americans observe traditional Korean holidays (refer to "Special Occasions" in this section) as well as other events, such as Buddha's birthday (April 8), Korean Memorial Day (June 6), South Korean Constitution Day (July 17), and Korean National Foundation Day (October 3). Fathers are honored on June 15. In addition, Christian Americans of Korean descent celebrate the major religious holidays.

Nutritional Status

Nutritional Intake Few health studies focusing on Korean Americans have been published. Most research on Asian Americans combines heterogeneous Asian and sometimes Pacific Islander populations. One study found that Korean Americans maintained a relatively traditional diet and that even with the addition of some American foods, 60 percent of calories came from carbohydrates and only 16 percent from fat.[152] Higher intakes of vitamins A and C, beta-carotene, niacin, and fiber are associated with a more traditional diet. High sodium intake is also common when Korean foods are preferred. Korean Americans who adopt more American foods are reported to consume more calories and have higher intakes of total fat, saturated fat, cholesterol, B1, vitamin E, folate, iron, and zinc. Calcium, which is often deficient in the Korean diet, is increased with the use of dairy products. A survey of Korean Americans conducted in a midwestern city found that those with the least-healthy eating habits were younger, not married, less educated, and more acculturated to mainstream American culture.[176–178]

Traditional Korean diets are composed of a variety of fermented foods which provide healthy bacteria to the gut. The westernized diet, on the other hand, has few varieties of microorganisms to add to the gut microbiome.[178,179] The traditional Korean diet has high levels of digestible and non-digestible carbohydrates and low levels of animal protein compared to the westernized diet. Obese and overweight individuals are more prone to develop microbial dysbiosis and metabolic disturbances. Traditional Korean foods may help treat these conditions.

Self-reported health behaviors and medical disorders indicate that 22 percent of Korean Americans smoke cigarettes, less than 10 percent drink moderately or heavily, 40 percent are physically inactive, and 30 percent are overweight or obese. Their reported medical disorders were: 4.4 percent heart disease and 17 percent hypertension, 4 percent type 2 diabetes, 11 percent ulcers, cancer was less than 2 percent, and hepatitis B was 6 percent.[162,180–183]

Age-adjusted mortality rates for Korean Americans are lower than for the general population, although infant mortality rates are somewhat higher than those for Whites.[184] The more common cause of death among Koreans is stomach cancer; higher incidences of stomach, liver, and esophageal cancers have been found among Korean Americans as compared to White Americans.[185,186] However, the self-reported incidence of digestive diseases decreased with increased length of residence in the United States but increased with more servings of rice or rice dishes.[187] The rate of hepatitis B (responsible for most liver cancer) is very high in Korean Americans.

Other research also reported high blood pressure rates in Korean Americans but were not consistent in being higher or lower than the U.S. average. In Korea, hypertension affects 42 percent of the population.[188] No correlation with diet (including alcohol, spicy food, or salt intake) was noted.[180] Korean Americans diagnosed with high blood pressure are less likely to take hypertension medications or to follow their physician's advice on losing weight or lowering sodium intake. Incidence of death from heart disease also is very low.[162,180–182]

In 2017, Korea was estimated to have the second lowest obesity rate at 5.3 percent of the population. Information on obesity in Korean Americans is limited and there are gaps in the data.[179] More recently, a literature review determined that first-generation, foreign-born Koreans had significantly higher five-year increases in BMI, which was not associated with the length of U.S. residence that is normally seen in other foreign-born Americans.[178,179]

Korean Bug Business

South Korea has one of the most advanced edible bug industries in Asia. The industry grew by 84 percent in 2016. The Ministry of Food and Drug Safety has approved 10 edible insects: grasshoppers, silkworm pupae, silkworm larvae, mealworm larvae, two-spotted crickets, Kolbe beetle larvae, Japanese rhinoceros beetle larvae, darkling beetles, and Western honeybee larvae. Most of these insects are rich in protein and unsaturated fatty acids, making them highly sought after as a food of high nutritional value.[189]

Food for Thought

As with other Asians who use moxibustion or cupping, health care providers need to determine the cause of burns and bruises on clients before assuming abuse has occurred.

Health and Longevity Takeaway

Koretaka Ueda is approaching his 100th birthday. His youthful enthusiasm and energy for life are contagious. Every day, Koretaka, who grew up in Hiroshima, Japan goes to the library, tends his rice fields, and walks 3000 steps, rain or shine. Clearly, there were no signs of muscle loss (sarcopenia) in this gentleman. "Health is like a battle against yourself—the tendency is to become more dependent and weaker as you age, but in fact, it is just the opposite. If you can walk upstairs, then do it. Appreciate your health- *arigato u gozai mash ta*," he advises.

Any amount and type of physical activity may slow aging deep within our cells. Understanding how cells age is complex. Biological and chronological ages rarely match. A cell could be relatively young in terms of how long it has existed but function slowly or erratically, as if elderly.

In addition, regular exercise and physical activity can reduce the risk of developing some diseases and disabilities that develop as people grow older. In some cases, exercise is an effective treatment for many chronic conditions. For example, studies show that people with arthritis, heart disease, or diabetes benefit from regular exercise. Exercise also helps people with high blood pressure, balance problems, or difficulty walking.

Comfort Food

Tomie Kurisu—Hiroshima, Japan

Food rituals can reflect what is most admired in a culture. Tea ceremonies in Japan are marked by four basic principles : harmony (wa), respect (kei), purity (sei), and tranquility (jaku).

What is a favorite comfort food that you consider traditional from your home culture?

TK: I have so many comfort foods, but if I were to pick one, it would be the tea ceremony where we drink green tea called matcha together with Japanese sweets to balance the bitter taste of the tea. I love this ceremony because it is an artistic (I am an artist), a spiritual process aimed at bringing harmony and peace to guests.

Did you eat this food together with community? Where was it eaten?

TK: In my home, we serve tea with delicate sweets in the shape of flowers. It is enjoyed in the company of guests and provides a time to slow down and connect with people. To honor friendships and talk for hours while sipping tea.

Additional RECIPE TO TRY

Perpetual Miso Soup

Makes about 6 servings

Experiment by adding different seasonal vegetables

½ cup dried seaweed (wakame is recommended)

½ cup shiro miso (white fermented soybean paste)

6 cups Dashi (a stalk make from fish and kelp)*

½ pound tofu, drained and cut into ½ inch cubes

½ cup thinly sliced scallion greens—green onions

2 cups of cooked garden vegetables in season

To make the soup:

Combine wakame with warm water and cover by 1 inch. Let stand 15 minutes, or until reconstituted. Drain. Stir together miso and 1.2 cup Dashi in a bowl until smooth. Heat remaining dashi in a pan over high heat until hot and gently stir in tofu, cooked vegetables, and reconstituted wakame. Simmer for 1 minute and remove from heat. Immediately stir in the miso mixture and scallion greens and serve.

Nutritional information (per serving):

calories 62; fat 5 g (1.0 saturated fat); sodium 161 mg; total carbohydrate 5 g; protein 7 g

*If you don't have Dashi, chicken broth may be substituted, or for vegan Dashi substitute shiitake mushrooms and dried seaweed. Soak them for about 30 minutes, then boil the mixture for 10 minutes.

Discussion Starters

Examining the Diet of Asian Americans

In small groups of three or four, compare and contrast the diet and culture of Chinese Americans, Japanese Americans, and Korean Americans, with each group focusing on a different aspect of the diet and culture of these groups:

Group A: The food habits and the typical eating etiquette and meal composition of these three immigrant groups

Group B: Issues involved in counseling these immigrant groups on diet and health

Group C: Attitudes within each immigrant group toward diet, health, and medical treatment, notably attitudes toward traditional home culture medical treatment and U.S. biomedicine

Group D: Amount of obesity, diabetes, hypertension, and other diseases within each immigrant group

Within your group, try to come to a consensus on what findings to report to the rest of the class. Before breaking up, assign a number to each group member: A1, A2, A3, A4; B1, B2, and so forth. Form new groups with all the 1's in a group; all the 2's in another group; all the 3's another group; and so on. In your new group, report the findings of your previous group, and, as a group, discuss the relationship between traditional attitudes toward diet and health and changes in diet and health due to immigration to the United States.

Review Questions

1. List the countries for each region of Asia: East Asia, Southeast Asia, and South Asia.
2. Visit a Chinese restaurant or just look at the menu. Can you tell which region of China the recipes represent? How? Why do so many Chinese restaurants in the United States cook Cantonese style (Guangdong)?
3. What are the basic tenets of Confucianism, Taoism, and Buddhism? How might these religions influence Asian food culture?
4. Describe what is meant by Traditional Chinese Medicines, Kanpo, and Hanyak. How might these be integrated into the Chinese, Japanese, and Korean meanings of a balanced diet and life?
5. What are the staples of the Asian diet? Describe some common foods derived from soybeans. What are different types of tea from Asia—describe how they differ, including their tastes.
6. How did the Chinese influence the cuisine and worldview of the Koreans and the Japanese? Provide two examples of their influence, one each in Korea and Japan.

Reflection

1. Fermented foods and their effects on gut health is an up-and-coming area of nutrition research. Some think of the gastrointestinal tract as the "second brain" and it is so linked to other areas of the body and health. Think of your diet and consider ways you could add a daily dose of microbes to your diet by consuming fermented food. What would you consume?
2. Sarcopenia is a prevalent medical condition in older adults. For many, it is the beginning of the deterioration of health. How can sarcopenia be prevented? What is the role that protein plays in the prevention of sarcopenia and how does this pertain to your own diet?

References

1. Carnes, T., & Yang, F. 2015. *Asian American religions*. Oxford University Press. Retrieved from https://doi.org/10.1093/acrefore/9780199340378.013.502
2. Wright, D.C. 2020. *The history of China*. ABC-CLIO.
3. Mark, Joshua J. 2012. Ancient China. *World History Encyclopedia*. World History Encyclopedia.
4. Shelke, K. 2016. *Pasta and noodles: A global history*. Reaktion Books.
5. World Population Review. 2022. Retrieved from https://worldpopulationreview.com/countries/china-population; and World Bank.
6. The World Bank. 2022. Population, total—China. Retrieved from https://data.worldbank.org/indicator/SP.POP.TOTL?locations=CN
7. Lee, H.R. 2015. The untold story of Chinese restaurants in America. *Scholars Strategy Network, 20*.
8. Editors at IBISWorld. 2022 Chinese Restaurants in the US Market 2005–2028. Retrieved from https://www.ibisworld.com/industry-statistics/market-size/restaurants-united-states/ (accessed on January 3, 2023).
9. U.S. Census Bureau. n.d. Selected population profile in the U.S. *2020 American Community Survey 1-5-Year Estimates*. Retrieved from https://data.census.gov/cedsci/table?q=asian%20us%20total&y=2020 (accessed March 22, 2022).
10. U.S. Census Bureau. 2019. *Asian alone or in combination with one or more other races, and with one or more Asian categories for selected groups*. Retrieved from https://www.census.gov/data/tables/2019/demo/race/ppl-ac19.html.
11. Budiman, A. 2021. Chinese in the U.S. Fact Sheet. Pew Research Center. Retrieved from https://www.pewresearch.org/social-trends/fact-sheet/asian-americans-chinese-in-the-u-s/.
12. Pew Research Center. 2017. Top 10 U.S. metropolitan areas by Chinese population. Retrieved from https://www.pewresearch.org/social-trends/chart/top-u-s-metro-areas-chinese-population/.
13. Pew Research Center. April 9, 2021. *Key facts about Asian origin groups in the U.S.* Retrieved from https://www.pewresearch.org/fact-tank/2021/04/29/key-facts-about-asian-origin-groups-in-the-u-s/ (accessed March 22, 2022).
14. Wang, L.L.C. 2014. Chinese Americans. In R.V. Dassanowsky & J. Lehman (Eds.), *Gale encyclopedia of multicultural America*. Farmington Hills, MI: Gale Group.
15. Pew Research Center. 2012. Asian Americans: A Mosaic of Faiths. Pew Research Center.
16. Foy, G. 2014. Buddhism in China. *Asia Society*.
17. Britannica. n.d. Central Asia and China. Retrieved from https://www.britannica.com/topic/Buddhism/Central-Asia-and-China

18. Yu, P. L. 2020. How Taiwanese death rituals have adapted for families living in the US. *The Conversation*.
19. Xu, H.Y., Zhang, Y.Q., Liu, Z.M., Chen, T., Lv, C.Y., Tang, S.H., . . . & Huang, L.Q. 2015. ETCM: an encyclopedia of traditional Chinese medicine. *Nucleic Acids Research*, 47(D1), D976–D982.
20. Britannica, T. Editors of Encyclopedia. July 28, 2021. *Traditional Chinese medicine. Encyclopedia Britannica*. Retrieved from https://www.britannica.com/science/traditional-Chinese-medicine
21. Tang, J.L., Liu, B.Y., & Ma, K.W. 2008. Traditional Chinese medicine. *The Lancet*, 372(9654), 1938–1940.
22. Lu, M. & Busemeyer, J.R. 2014. Do traditional Chinese theories of Yi Jing ("Yin-Yang") and Chinese medicine go beyond western concepts of mind and matter. *Mind and Matter*, 12(1), 37–59.
23. Luo, Y., Wang, C.Z., Hesse-Fong, J., Lin, J.G., & Yuan, C.S. 2015. Application of Chinese medicine in acute and critical medical conditions. *The American Journal of Chinese Medicine*, 47(06), 1223–1235.
24. Holman, C.T. 2017. *Treating emotional trauma with Chinese medicine: Integrated diagnostic and treatment strategies*. Singing Dragon.
25. Wu, A.P., Burke, A., & LeBaron, S. 2007. Use of traditional medicine by immigrant Chinese patients. *Family Medicine-Kansas City*, 39(3), 195.
26. Zhang, C., Yue, Z., Zhou, Q., Ma, S., & Zhang, Z.K. 2019. Using social media to explore regional cuisine preferences in China. *Online Information Review*, 43(7), 1098–1114.
27. Hiufu Wong, Maggie. 2015. 40 of the best Taiwanese foods and drinks. CNN. Retrieved from edition.cnn.com (accessed on March 15, 2022).
28. Feng, Y., Chen, X.M., Zhao, M., He, Z., Sun, L., Wang, C.Y., & Ding, W.F. 2018. Edible insects in China: Utilization and prospects. *Insect Science*, 25(2), 184–198.
29. Fu, J.C. 2018. The Tyranny of the Bottle: Vitasoy and the Cultural Politics of Packaging. *Worldwide Waste: Journal of Interdisciplinary Studies*, 1(1).
30. Babji, A.S., Nurfatin, M.H., Etty Syarmila, I.K., & Masitah, M. 2015. Secrets of edible bird nest.
31. Van Driem, G.L. 2019. The tale of tea: *A comprehensive history of tea from prehistoric times to the present day*. In The Tale of Tea. Brill.
32. Lo, A. 2021. Things you should know about the Chinese tea ceremony. Brides. Retrieved from https://www.brides.com
33. Sandhaus, D. 2015. *Drunk in China: Baijiu and the World's Oldest Drinking Culture*. University of Nebraska Press.
34. Furstenau, N.M. 2021. *Green chili and other impostors*. University of Iowa Press.
35. Yang, Y.X., Wang, X.L., Leong, P.M., Zhang, H.M., Yang, X.G., Kong, L.Z., . . . & Su, Y.X. 2018. New Chinese dietary guidelines: Healthy eating patterns and food-based dietary recommendations. *Asia Pacific Journal of Clinical Nutrition*, 27(4), 908–913. Retrieved from https://search.informit.org/doi/10.3316/ielapa.762435308484087
36. Food and Agriculture Organization of the United Nations. 2016. Food-based dietary guidelines—China. Retrieved from https://www.fao.org/nutrition/education/food-based-dietary-guidelines/regions/countries/china/en/ (accessed March 23, 2022).
37. Bramen, L. 2009. The history of chopsticks. Smithsonian. Retrieved from https://www.smithsonianmag.com/arts-culture/the-history-of-chopsticks-64935342/#:~:text=According%20to%20the%20California%20Academy,retrieve%20food%20from%20cooking%20pots
38. Ruhlmann, S. 2016. Are buuz and banš traditional Mongolian foods? Strategy of appropriation and identity adjustment in contemporary Mongolia. *In Eating Traditional Food* (pp. 100–117). Routledge.
39. De Mente, B.L. 2016. *Etiquette guide to China: Know the rules that make the difference!* Tuttle Publishing.
40. Li, Y. January 2016. The comparison of Chinese and western table manners. In *2nd International Conference on Education Technology, Management and Humanities Science*, pp. 1–4.
41. DiStefano, J. 2015. butter tea, yak jerky, and momos galore: An introduction to Tibetan cuisine. Serious Eats. https://www.seriouseats.com/tibetan-cuisine-introduction-dishes-to-know
42. De Mente, B.L. 2016. *Etiquette Guide to China: Know the rules that make the difference!* Tuttle Publishing.
43. Feng Shui Institute. Retrieved from https://feng-shui-institute.org/Feng_Shui/yinyang_food.html (accessed March 23, 2022).
44. Newman, J.M. 1998. Chinese ingredients: Both usual and unusual. In J.M. Powers (Ed.), *Cathay to Canada: Chinese cuisine in transition*. Willowdale, Canada: Ontario Historical Society.
45. Murray, L. September 25, 2015. *Shine on, Harvest Moon Festival. Encyclopedia Britannica*. Retrieved from https://www.britannica.com/story/shine-on-harvest-moon-festival
46. Geck, M.S., Cabras, S., Casu, L., García, A.J.R., & Leonti, M. 2017. The taste of heat: How humoral qualities act as a cultural filter for chemosensory properties guiding herbal medicine. *Journal of Ethnopharmacology*, 198, 499–515.
47. Ding, G., Niu, L., Vinturache, A., Zhang, J., Lu, M., Gao, Y.U., . . . & Shanghai Birth Cohort Study. 2020. "Doing the month" and postpartum depression among Chinese women: a Shanghai prospective cohort study. *Women and Birth*, 33(2), e151–e158.
48. Zou, P. 2016. Traditional Chinese medicine, food therapy, and hypertension control: a narrative review of Chinese literature. *The American Journal of Chinese Medicine*, 44(08), 1579–1594.
49. Zhang, Y. 2021. Diet according to traditional Chinese medicine for health and longevity. In *Nutrition, Food and Diet in Ageing and Longevity*. Springer, Cham, pp. 331–356.
50. Cheng, J.T. & Yang, R.S. 1983. Hypoglycemic effect of guava juice in mice and human subjects. *American Journal of Clinical Nutrition*, 11, 74–76.
51. Li, C. 2020. Deer antlers: traditional Chinese medicine use and recent pharmaceuticals. *Animal Production Science*, 60(10), 1233–1237.
52. Wu, F., Li, H., Jin, L., Li, X., Ma, Y., You, J., . . . & Xu, Y. 2013. Deer antler base as a traditional Chinese medicine: a review of its traditional uses, chemistry and pharmacology. *Journal of Ethnopharmacology*, 145(2), 403–415.
53. Ma, G. 2015. Food, eating behavior, and culture in Chinese society. *Journal of Ethnic Foods*, 2(4), 195–199.
54. Chauhan, A. & Chauhan, V. 2020. Beneficial effects of walnuts on cognition and brain health. *Nutrients*, 12(2), 550.
55. Rajaram, S., Valls-Pedret, C., Cofán, M., Sabaté, J., Serra-Mir, M., Pérez-Heras, A., . . . & Ros, E. 2017. The Walnuts and Healthy Aging Study (WAHA): Protocol for a nutritional intervention trial with walnuts on brain aging. *Frontiers in Aging Neuroscience, 8*.
56. Sit, C., David, L., & Yeung, L. 2001. The growth and feeding patterns of 9 to 12 month old Chinese Canadian infants. *Nutrition Research*, 21, 505–516.
57. Lee, A. & Brann, L. 2015. Influence of cultural beliefs on infant feeding, postpartum and childcare practices among Chinese-American mothers in New York City. *Journal of Community Health*, 40(3), 476–483.
58. Liu, S., Sucher, K., & McProud, L. 2005, August. Use of Chinese herbs for Chinese infant feeding in the San Francisco Bay Area. *Journal of the American Dietetic Association*, 105(8, Suppl.).
59. Li, C. 2020. Deer antlers: Traditional Chinese medicine use and recent pharmaceuticals. *Animal Production Science*, 60(10), 1233–1237.
60. Wu, F., Li, H., Jin, L., Li, X., Ma, Y., You, J., . . . & Xu, Y. 2013. Deer antler base as a traditional Chinese medicine: A review of its traditional uses, chemistry and pharmacology. *Journal of Ethnopharmacology*, 145(2), 403–415.
61. Yun, W. 1996. *A growing kid*. Hong Kong, China: Sun Ya.
62. Campbell, T. & Chang, B. 1981. Health care of the Chinese in America. In G. Henderson & M. Primeaux (Eds.), *Transcultural health care*. Menlo Park, CA: Addison-Wesley.
63. Tseng, M., Wright, D.J., & Fang, C.Y. 2015. Acculturation and dietary change among Chinese immigrant women in the United States. *Journal of Immigrant and Minority Health*, 17(2), 400–407.

64. Kirshner, L., Yi, S.S., Wylie-Rosett, J., Matthan, N.R., & Beasley, J.M. 2020. Acculturation and diet among Chinese American immigrants in New York City. *Current Developments in Nutrition*, 4(1), nzz124.
65. Rosenmöller, D.L., Gasevic, D., Seidell, J., & Lear, S.A. 2011. Determinants of changes in dietary patterns among Chinese immigrants: A cross-sectional analysis. *International Journal of Behavioral Nutrition and Physical Activity*, 8(1), 1–8.
66. Beasley, J.M., Yi, S.S., Ahn, J., Kwon, S.C., & Wylie-Rosett, J. 2015. Dietary patterns in Chinese Americans are associated with cardiovascular disease risk factors, the Chinese American Cardiovascular Health Assessment (CHA CHA). *Journal of Immigrant and Minority Health*, 21(5), 1061–1069.
67. Serafica, R.C. 2014. Dietary acculturation in Asian Americans. *Journal of Cultural Diversity*, 21(4), 145.
68. Liu, A., Berhane, Z., & Tseng, M. 2010. Improved dietary variety and adequacy but lower dietary moderation with acculturation in Chinese women in the United States. *Journal of the American Dietetic Association*, 110(3), 457–462.
69. Banna, J.C., Gilliland, B., Keefe, M., & Zheng, D. 2016. Cross-cultural comparison of perspectives on healthy eating among Chinese and American undergraduate students. *BMC Public Health*, 16(1), 1015. Retrieved from https://doi.org/10.1186/s12889-016-3680-y
70. Sun, S., Li, H., Liu, G., & Zhang, J. 2020. A critical review of the association between nutrition and health in modern Chinese diet. *Journal of Food and Nutrition Research*, 8(7), 337–346. doi: 10.12691/JFNR-8-7-5.
71. Zhao, A., Szeto, I.M.-Y., Wang, Y., Li, C., Pan, M., Li, T., Wang, P., & Zhang, Y. 2017. Knowledge, attitude, and practice (KAP) of dairy products in Chinese Urban population and the effects on dairy intake quality. *Nutrients*, 9, 668. Retrieved from https://doi.org/10.3390/nu9070668
72. Wang, Y.G., Yan, Y.S., Xu, J.J., Du, R.F., Flatz, S.D., Kuhnau, W., & Flatz, G. 1984. Prevalence of primary adult lactose malabsorption in three populations of northern China. *Human Genetics*, 67, 103–106.
73. Yang, Y.X., He, M., Cui, H.M., Bian, L.H., Jianyu, L., Cheng, W.F., Xu, H.F., & Feng, W. 1999. Study on the incidence of lactose intolerance of children in China. *Journal of Hygiene Research*, 28, 44–46.
74. Chinese Nutrition Association. 2016. *Dietary Guidelines for Chinese Residents 2016*. People's Medical Publishing House: Beijing, China, p. 3.
75. Pan, X., Wang, L., & Pan, A. 2021. Epidemiology and determinants of obesity in China. *The Lancet Diabetes & Endocrinology*, 9(6), 373–392. Retrieved from https://doi.org/10.1016/S2213-8587(21)00045-0 (accessed March 24, 2022).
76. Xu, Y., Wang, L., He, J., Bi, Y., Li, M., Wang, T., . . . & 2010 China Noncommunicable Disease Surveillance Group. (2013). Prevalence and control of diabetes in Chinese adults. *JAMA*, 310(9), 948–959.
77. Chooi, Y., Ding, C., & Magkos, F. 2015. The epidemiology of obesity. *Metabolism, 92*, 6–10. Retrieved from https://doi.org/10.1016/j.metabol.2018.09.005
78. Wang, L.L.C. 2014. Chinese Americans. In R.V. Dassanowsky & J. Lehman (Eds.), *Gale encyclopedia of multicultural America*. Farmington Hills, MI: Gale Group.
79. Lear, S.A., Chen, M.M., Frohlich, J.J., & Birmingham, C.L. 2002. The relationship between waist circumference and metabolic risk factors: Cohorts of European and Chinese descent. *Metabolism*, 51, 1427–1432.
80. Hoek, H. 2016. Review of the worldwide epidemiology of eating disorders, *Current Opinion in Psychiatry*, 29(6), 336–339. doi: 10.1097/YCO.0000000000000282
81. Weng, J., Ji, L., Jia, W., Lu, J., Zhou, Z., Zou, D., Zhu, D., Chen, L., Chen, L., Guo, L., Guo, X., Ji, Q., Li, Q., Li, X., Liu, J., Ran, X., Shan, Z., Shi, L., Song, G., Yang, L., . . . & Chinese Diabetes Society 2016. Standards of care for type 2 diabetes in China. *Diabetes/Metabolism Research and Reviews*, 32(5), 442–458. Retrieved from https://doi.org/10.1002/dmrr.2827 (accessed March 24, 2022).
82. U.S. Department of Health and Human Services, Office of Minority Health. Diabetes and Asian Americans. 2017. Retrieved from https://minorityhealth.hhs.gov/omh/browse.aspx?lvl=4&lvlid=48 (accessed March 24, 2022).
83. Cheng, Y., Kanaya, A., Araneta, M., et al. 2015. Prevalence of diabetes by race and ethnicity in the United States, 2011–2016. *JAMA*, 322(24), 2389–2398. Retrieved from https://jamanetwork.com/journals/jama/article-abstract/2757817 (accessed March 24, 2022).
84. National Diabetes Statistics Report. 2020. Estimates of diabetes and its burden in the U.S. Retrieved from https://www.cdc.gov/diabetes/pdfs/data/statistics/national-diabetes-statistics-report.pdf (accessed March 24, 2022).
85. Jung, M., Lee, S., Thomas, S., & Juon, H. 2015. Hypertension prevalence, treatment, and related behaviors among Asian Americans: An examination by method of measurement and disaggregated subgroups. *Journal of Racial and Ethnic Health Disparities*, 6(3), 584–593.
86. Baluran, D.A. & Patterson, E.J. 2021. Examining ethnic variation in life expectancy among Asians in the United States, 2012–2016. *Demography*, 58(5), 1631–1654.
87. Newman, J.M. 2000. Chinese meals. In H.L. Meiselman (Ed.), *Dimensions of the meal: The science, culture, business, and art of eating*. Gaithersburg, MD: Aspen.
88. Ma, G., Li, Y., Wu, Y., Zhai, F., Cui, Z., Hu, X., . . . & Wang, Y. 2005. The prevalence of body overweight and obesity and its changes among Chinese people during 1992 to 2002. *China Journal of Preventive Medicine*, 39, 311–315.
89. Wang, Y., Mi, J., Shan, X.Y., Wang, Q.J., & Ge, K.Y. 2007. Is China facing an obesity epidemic and the consequences? The trends in obesity and chronic disease in China. *International Journal of Obesity*, 31, 177–188.
90. National Cancer Institute. 2013. *Seer cancer statistics review, 1975–2010*, Tables 2.15 through 24.15. Retrieved from http://seer.cancer.gov/csr/2010sections.html (accessed March 12, 2015).
91. Gomez, S.L., Clarke, C.A., Shema, S.J., Chang, E.T., Keegan, T.H.M., & Glaser, S.L. 2010. Disparities in breast cancer survival among Asian women by ethnicity and immigrant status: A population-based study. *American Journal of Public Health*, 100(5), 861–869.
92. Centers for Disease Control and Prevention. 2012. *Healthy people 2010 database*, Table 14-03a. Retrieved from http://wonder.cdc.gov/scripts/data2010 (accessed March 12, 2015).
93. Miller, B.A., Chu, K.C., Hankey, B.F., & Ries, L.A.G. 2008. Cancer incidence and mortality patterns among specific Asian and Pacific Islander populations in the US. *Cancer Causes Control*, 19(3), 227–256.
94. Jenkins, C.N.H. & Kagawa-Singer, M. 1994. *Cancer*. In N.W.S. Zane, D.T. Takeuchi, & K.N.J. Young (Eds.), *Confronting critical health issues of Asian and Pacific Islander Americans*. Thousand Oaks, CA: Sage.
95. Wong, S.T., Gildengorin, G., Nguyen, T., & Mock, J. 2005. Disparities in colorectal cancer screening rates among Asian Americans and non-Latino whites. *Cancer*, 104, 2940–2947.
96. The World Factbook. Country comparisons—infant mortality rate. Retrieved from https://www.cia.gov/the-world-factbook/field/infant-mortality-rate/country-comparison
97. U.S. Department of Health and Human Services, Office of Minority Health 2017 Infant Mortality and Asian Americans. Retrieved from https://www.minorityhealth.hhs.gov/omh/browse.aspx?lvl=4&lvlid=53
98. Centers for Disease Control. 2018. Breast feeding report card. Retrieved from https://www.cdc.gov/breastfeeding/data/nis_data/analysis.html.
99. Li, Q., Tian, J., Xu, F., & Binns, C. 2020. Breastfeeding in China: A review of changes in the past decade. *International Journal of Environmental Research and Public Health*, 17(21), 8234. doi: 10.3390/ijerph17218234.

100. U.S. Census Bureau. 2019. Japanese alone or in any combination. Retrieved from https://data.census.gov/cedsci/table?t=022%20-%20Japanese%20alone%3A041%20-%20Japanese%20alone%20or%20in%20any%20combination (accessed March 24, 2022).
101. Burton, J.F., Farrell, M.M., Lord, F.B., & Lord, R.W. 2010. A brief history of Japanese American relocation during World War II. Confinement and Ethnicity: An Overview of World War II Japanese American Relocation Sites.
102. Tokunaga, Y. 2015. Japanese internment as an agricultural labor crisis. *Southern California Quarterly*, 101(1), 79–113. Retrieved from https://doi.org/10.1525/scq.2019.101.1.79
103. Educator Resources Series. 2022. Japanese-American incarceration during World War II. The National Archives and Records Administration. Retrieved from https://www.archives.gov/education/lessons/japanese-relocation#background
104. Asaka, M. 2019. The Movement for Japanese American Redress. *In Oxford Research Encyclopedia of American History*.
105. Hoeffe, E.M., Rastogi, S., Kim, M.O., & Shahid, H. 2012. *The Asian population: 2010*. U.S. Census Bureau. Retrieved from http://www.census.gov/prod/cen2010/briefs/c2010br-11.pdf (accessed March 12, 2015).
106. Hashizume, S. & Takano, J. 1983. Nursing care of Japanese American patients. In M.S. Orque, B. Bloch, & L.S.A. Monrroy (Eds.), *Ethnic nursing care: A multicultural approach*. St. Louis: Mosby.
107. Lock, M. 1990. Rationalization of Japanese herbal medication: The hegemony of orchestrated pluralism. *Human Organization*, 49, 41–47.
108. World Health Organization. 2001. *Legal status of traditional medicine and complementary/alternative medicine: A worldwide review*, pp. 155–159. Retrieved from http://apps.who.int/medicinedocs/pdf/h2943e/h2943e.pdf (accessed April 18, 2015).
109. Pollack, R. & Kuo, I. 2004. *Advances in the treatment of anxiety disorders—Transcultural issues*. Retrieved from http://www.medscape.com/viewarticle/47156
110. Faiola, A. 2006, June 6. Sleeping with the fish for inner peace. *San Jose Mercury News*, p. 9A.
111. Marie, Kimberly. 2018. United States agricultural exports to Japan remain promising. International Agricultural Trade Report. USDA Foreign Agricultural Service.
112. Hosking, R. 2015. *A dictionary of Japanese food: Ingredients & culture*. Tuttle Publishing.
113. Paddon-Jones, D., Campbell, W., Jacques, P., Kritchevsky, S., Moore, L., Rodriguez, N., & van Loon, L. 2015. Protein and healthy aging. *The American Journal of Clinical Nutrition*, 101(6), 1339S–1345S. Retrieved from https://doi.org/10.3945/ajcn.114.084061 (accessed March 25, 2023).
114. Tani, Y., Fujiwara, T., Doi, S., & Isumi, A. 2015. Home cooking and child obesity in Japan: Results from the A-CHILD study. *Nutrients*, 11(12), 2859.
115. Serafica, R.C. 2014. Dietary acculturation in Asian Americans. *Journal of Cultural Diversity*, 21(4), 145.
116. Kudo, Y., Falciglia, G.A., & Couch, S.C. 2000. Evolution of meal patterns and food choices of Japanese American females born in the United States. *European Journal of Clinical Nutrition*, 54, 665–670.
117. Takashi, K. 2021. Modification of dietary habits for prevention of gout in Japanese people: Gout and the Japanese diet. *American Journal of Health Research*, 9(5), 117–127. Retrieved from http://ajohealthres.org/article/656/10.11648.j.ajhr.20210905.12 (accessed on March 24, 2022).
118. Toru, O., Hiroshi, A., Kazuhiro, S., Kazuhiro, S., Kiyohiko, Hatake., & Isseu, K. 2020. Cardio-oncology in Japan: The rapidly rising sun. *JACC: CardioOncology*. Retrieved from https://www.jacc.org/doi/full/10.1016/j.jaccao.2020.10.014 (accessed on March 24, 2022).
119. Wenkam, N.S. & Wolff, R.J. 1970. A half century of changing food habits among Japanese in Hawaii. *Journal of the American Dietetic Association*, 57, 29–32.
120. Watanabe, H., Yamane, K., Fujikawa, R., Okubo, M., Egusa, G., & Kohno, N. 2003. Westernization of lifestyle markedly increases carotid intima-media wall thickness (IMT) in Japanese people. *Atherosclerosis*, 166, 67–72.
121. Kimura, R. & Egawa, S. 2018. Epidemiology of prostate cancer in Asian countries. *International Journal of Urology*, 25(6), 524–532. Retrieved from https://onlinelibrary.wiley.com/doi/full/10.1111/iju.13593 (accessed March 24, 2022).
122. Singh, G. & DiBari, J. 2015 Marked disparities in pre-pregnancy obesity and overweight prevalence among US Women by race/ethnicity, nativity/immigrant status, and sociodemographic characteristics, 2012–2014. *Journal of Obesity*. Retrieved from https://www.hindawi.com/journals/jobe/2019/2419263/ (accessed on March 24, 2022).
123. Sekikawa, A., Curb J.D., Ueshima H., El-Saed A., Kadowaki T., Abbott R.D., . . . & ERA JUMP 77 (Electron-Beam Tomography, Risk Factor Assessment Among Japanese and U.S. Men in the Post-World War II Birth Cohort) Study Group. 2008. Marine-derived n-3 fatty acids and atherosclerosis in Japanese, Japanese-American, and white men—A cross-sectional study. *Journal of the American College of Cardiology*, 52, 417–424.
124. Fujimoto, W.Y., Bergstrom, R.W., Newell-Morris, L., & Leonetti, D.L. 1989. Nature and nurture in the etiology of type 2 diabetes mellitus in Japanese Americans. *Diabetes/Metabolism Reviews*, 5, 607–625.
125. Nakanishi, S., Okubo, M., Yoneda, M., Jitsuiki, K., Yamane, K., & Kohno, N. 2004. A comparison between Japanese Americans living in Hawaii and Los Angeles and native Japanese: The impact of lifestyle Westernization on diabetes mellitus. *Biomedicine & Pharmacotherapy*, 58, 571–577.
126. Pierce, B.L., Austin, M.A., Crane, P.K., Retzlaff, B.M., Fish, B., Hutter, C.M., . . . & Fujimoto, W.Y. 2007. Measuring dietary acculturation in Japanese Americans with the use of confirmatory factor analysis of food-frequency data. *American Journal of Clinical Nutrition*, 86, 496–503.
127. Tsunehara, C.H., Leonetti, D.L., & Fujimoto, W.Y. 1990. Diet of second generation Japanese American men with and without noninsulin-dependent diabetes. *American Journal of Clinical Nutrition*, 52, 731–738.
128. U.S. Department of Health and Human Services. n.d. *Obesity and Asian Americans*. Retrieved from http://minorityhealth.hhs.gov/omh/browse.aspx?lvl54&lvlid555; and Centers for Disease Control and Prevention. 2008. *Health characteristics of the Asian adult population: United States, 2004–2006*, Table 2. Retrieved from http://www.cdc.gov/nchs/data/ad/ad394.pdf (accessed March 12, 2015).
129. Bergstrom, R.W., Newell-Morris, L.L., Leonetti, D.L., Shuman, W.P., Wahl, P.W., & Fujimoto, W.Y. 1990. Association of elevated fasting C-peptide level and increased intra-abdominal fat distribution with development of NIDDM in Japanese American men. *Diabetes*, 39, 104–111.
130. Yoneda, M., Yamane, K., Jitsuiki, K., Nakanishi, S., Kamei, N., Watanabe, H., & Kohno, N. 2008. Prevalence of metabolic syndrome compared between native Japanese and Japanese Americans. *Diabetes Research and Clinical Practice*, 79(3), 518–522.
131. Pribila, B.A., Hertzler, S.R., Martin, B.R., Weaver, C.M., & Savaiano, D.A. 2000. Improved lactose digestion and intolerance among African-American adolescent girls fed a dairy-rich diet. *Journal of the American Dietetic Association*, 100, 524–528.
132. Lee, C.G., Fujimoto, W.Y., Brunzell, J.D., Kahn, S.E., McNeely, M.J., Leonetti, D.L., & Boyko, E.J. 2010. Intra-abdominal fat accumulation is greatest at younger ages in Japanese American adults. *Diabetes Research and Clinical Practice*, 89, 58–64.
133. Editors at Cleveland Clinic. 2022. Alcohol intolerance. Retrieved from https://my.clevelandclinic.org/health/diseases/17659-alcohol-intolerance

134. Tachiki, T., Kouda, K., Dongmei, N., et al. 2015. Muscle strength is associated with bone health independently of muscle mass in postmenopausal women: the Japanese population-based osteoporosis study. *The Journal of Bone and Mineral Metabolism*, 37, 53–59. Retrieved from https://doi.org/10.1007/s00774-017-0895-7 (accessed March 25, 2022).
135. Morimoto, Y., Maskarinec, G., Conroy, S.M., Lim, U., Shepherd, J., & Novotny, R. 2012. Asian ethnicity is associated with a higher trunk/peripheral fat ratio in women and adolescent girls. *Journal of Epidemiology*, 22(2), 130–135.
136. Ikeda, N., Inoue, M., Iso, H., Ikeda, S., Satoh, T., Noda, M., . . . & Shibuya, K. 2012. Adult mortality attributable to preventable risk factors for non-communicable diseases and injuries in Japan: a comparative risk assessment. *PLOS Medicine*, 9(1), e1001160. doi: 10.1371/journal.pmed.1001160. Epub January 24, 2012.
137. Alexander, G.R., Mor, J.M., Kogan, M.D., Leland, N.L., & Kieffer, E. 1996. Pregnancy outcomes of US born and foreign-born Japanese Americans. *American Journal of Public Health*, 86, 820–824.
138. Pouresmaeili, F., Kamalidehghan, B., Kamarehei, M., & Goh, Y.M. 2018. A comprehensive overview on osteoporosis and its risk factors. *Therapeutics and Clinical Risk Management*, 14, 2029.
139. Thambiah, S.C. & Yeap, S.S. 2020. Osteoporosis in South-East Asian countries. *The Clinical Biochemist Reviews*, 41(1), 29.
140. Liu, J., Curtis, E.M., Cooper, C., & Harvey, N.C. 2015. State of the art in osteoporosis risk assessment and treatment. *Journal of Endocrinological Investigation*, 42(10), 1149–1164.
141. Polzonetti, V., Pucciarelli, S., Vincenzetti, S., & Polidori, P. 2020. Dietary intake of vitamin d from dairy products reduces the risk of osteoporosis. *Nutrients*, 12(6), 1743.
142. Flammini, L., Martuzzi, F., Vivo, V., Ghirri, A., Salomi, E., Bignetti, E., & Barocelli, E. 2016. Hake fish bone as a calcium source for efficient bone mineralization. *International Journal of Food Sciences and Nutrition*, 67(3), 265–273.
143. Willcox, C., Willcox, B., Shimajiri, S., Sayuri, K., & Makoto, S. 2007. Aging gracefully: A retrospective analysis of functional status in Okinawan centenarians. *The American Journal of Geriatric Psychiatry*, 15(3), 252–256. Retrieved from https://doi.org/10.1097/JGP.0b013e31803190cc
144. Pietri, P. & Stefanadis, C. 2021. Cardiovascular aging and longevity: JACC state-of-the-art review. *Journal of the American College of Cardiology*, 77(2), 189–204. Retrieved from https://www.sciencedirect.com/science/article/pii/S0735109720378682 (accessed March 25, 2022).
145. Buettner, D. & Skemp, S. 2016. Blue zones: Lessons from the world's longest lived. *Journal of Lifestyle Medicine*,*10*(5), 318–321. Retrieved from https://journals.sagepub.com/doi/10.1177/1559827616637066 (accessed March 25, 2022).
146. Blakemore, E. 2020. How Japan Took Control of Korea. History. Retrieved from https://www.history.com/news/japan-colonization-korea
147. Ho, J. 2021. Anti-Asian racism, Black Lives Matter, and COVID-19. *Japan Forum*, 33(1), 148–159.
148. Yoo, D. 2010. *Contentious spirits: Religion in Korean American history, 1903–1945*. Stanford University Press.
149. Chin, S. 2015. History of Korean immigration to American, from 1903 to present. Retrieved from https://sites.bu.edu/koreandiaspora/issues/history-of-korean-immigration-to-america-from-1903-to-present/ (accessed March 20, 2022).
150. U.S. Census Bureau. 2019. Korea, including South Korea and North Korea. Retrieved from https://data.census.gov/cedsci/table?t=771%20-%20Korea,%20including%20South%20Korea%20and%20North%20Korea (accessed March 24, 2022).
151. Connor, P. 2014. Facts about South Korea's growing Christian population. *Pew Research Center*, 12.
152. Britannica, T. Editors of Encyclopaedia. May 1, 2020. *Chŏndogyo*. *Encyclopedia Britannica*. Retrieved from https://www.britannica.com/topic/Chondogyo
153. *Women's role in contemporary Korea*. 2022. Asia Society Center for Global Education. Retrieved from https://asiasociety.org/education/womens-role-contemporary-korea (accessed March 20, 2022).
154. Im, H.B., Lew, Y.I., Hahn, H-b., Lee, C., & Yu, W-i. March 24, 2022. South Korea. *Encyclopedia Britannica*.
155. Kim, S.S., Kim-Godwin, Y.S., & Koenig, H.G. 2016. Family spirituality and family health among Korean-American elderly couples. *Journal of Religion and Health*, 55, 729–746. Retrieved from https://www.britannica.com/place/South-Korea.
156. Purnell, L. & Fenkl, E. 2015. *Handbook for culturally competent care*. Springer International Publishing.
157. Chin, S.Y. 1992. This, that, and the other: Managing illness in a first-generation Korean American family. *Western Journal of Medicine*, 157, 305–309.
158. Park, Y.J., Kim, H.S., Schwartz-Barcott, D., & Kim, J.W. 2002. The conceptual structure of hwa-byung in middle-aged Korean women. *Health Care for Women International*, 23, 389–397.
159. Pang, K.Y.C. 1989. The practice of traditional Korean medicine in Washington, DC. *Social Science and Medicine*, 28, 875–884.
160. Kim, M., Han, H.R., Kim, K.B., & Duong, D.N. 2002. The use of traditional and Western medicine among Korean American elderly. *Journal of Community Health*, 27(2), 109–120.
161. Purnell, L. & Fenkl, A. 2020. *Textbook for transcultural health care: A population approach*, 5th ed. Springer International Publishing.
162. Heiniger, L.E., Sherman, K.A., Shaw, L.K., & Costa, D. 2015. Fatalism and health promoting behaviors in Chinese and Korean immigrants and Caucasians. *Journal of Immigrant and Minority Health*, 17(1), 165–171.
163. Korean Food Foundation. 2015. *The Korean kitchen: 75 healthy, delicious and easy recipes*. Hollym International Corp.
164. Oh, S.H., Park, K.W., Daily III, J.W., & Lee, Y.E. 2014. Preserving the legacy of healthy Korean food. *Journal of Medicinal Food*, 17(1), 1–5.
165. Albuquerque, C.R., Maihara, V.A., De Lima, C.B., & Silva, P.S.C. 2015. Seaweeds as source of the essential elements. *Brazilian Journal of Radiation Sciences*, 7(2A).
166. Kim, B. & Ram, C. 2018. *Korean BBQ: Master your grill in seven sauces (a cookbook)*. Ten Speed Press.
167. Kim, K. and Wharton, R. 2018. Korean home cooking: classic and modern recipes. Abrams.
168. Kwak, J. 1998. *Dok Suni: Recipes from my mother's Korean kitchen*. New York: St. Martin's Press.
169. Yom, M.S., Gordon, B.H.J., & Sucher, K.P. 1995. Korean dietary habits and health beliefs in the San Francisco Bay Area. *Journal of the American Dietetic Association*, 95(Suppl.), A–98.
170. Choi, J., Kang, S., You, C., & Kwon, Y. 2015. The determinants of choosing traditional Korean medicine or conventional medicine: Findings from the Korea health panel. *Evidence-Based Complementary and Alternative Medicine*, Vol. 2015. Retrieved from https://www.hindawi.com/journals/ecam/2015/147408/ (accessed March 24, 2022).
171. Park, K. 2018. *The Korean American dream: Immigrants and small business in New York City*. Ithaca, NY: Cornell University Press. Retrieved from https://doi.org/10.7591/9781501724558
172. Ahn, Roy. 2009. Home run: My journey back to Korean food. *Gastronomica*, 9(4), 12–15. Retrieved from https://doi.org/10.1525/gfc.2009.9.4.12
173. Kim, K.K., Yu, E.S., Chen, E.H., Cross, N., Kim, J., & Brintnall, R.A. 2000. National health status of Korean Americans: Implications for cancer risk. *Oncology Nursing Forum*, 27, 1573–1583.
174. Kim, J. & Chan, M.M. 2004. Acculturation and dietary habits of Korean Americans. *British Journal of Nutrition*, 91, 469–478.
175. Park, S.Y., Paik, N.Y., Skinner, J.D., Ok, S.W., & Spindler, A.A. 2003. Mothers' acculturation and eating behaviors of Korean American families in California. *Journal of Nutrition Education*, 35, 142–147.

176. Kim, S.H., Kim, M.S., Lee, M.S., Park, Y.S., Lee, H.J., Kang, S.A., . . . & Kwon, D.Y. 2016. Korean diet: Characteristics and historical background. *Journal of Ethnic Foods*, 3(1), 26–31.
177. Shim, J.S., Shim, S.Y., Cha, H.J., Kim, J., & Kim, H.C. 2022. Association between ultra-processed food consumption and dietary intake and diet quality in Korean adults. *Journal of the Academy of Nutrition and Dietetics*, 122(3), 583–594.
178. Shin, J., Jung, S., Kim, S., Kang, M., Kim, M., Joung, H., Hwang, G., & Shin, D. 2015. Differential effects of typical Korean versus American-style diets on gut microbial composition and metabolic profile in healthy overweight Koreans: A randomized crossover trial. *Nutrients*, 11(10), 2450. Retrieved from https://doi.org/10.3390/nu11102450 (accessed on March 25, 2025).
179. Nam, G.E. & Park, H.S. 2018. Perspective on diagnostic criteria for obesity and abdominal obesity in Korean adults. *Journal of Obesity & Metabolic Syndrome*, 27(3), 134–142. Retrieved from https://doi.org/10.7570/jomes.2018.27.3.134 (accessed March 25, 2022).
180. Yang, E.J., Chung, H.K., Kim, W.Y., Bianchi, L., & Song, W.O. 2007. Chronic diseases and dietary changes in relation to Korean Americans' length of residence in the United States. *Journal of the American Dietetic Association*, 107(6), 942–950.
181. Kim, M.T., Kim, K.B., Juon, H.S., & Hill, M.N. 2000. Prevalence and factors associated with high blood pressure in Korean Americans. *Ethnicity & Disease*, 10(3), 364–374.
182. Kim, M.J., Ahn, Y.H., Chon, C., Bowen, P., & Khan, S. 2005. Health disparities in lifestyle choices among hypertensive Korean Americans, non-Hispanic Whites, and Blacks. *Biological Research for Nursing*, 7(1), 67–74.
183. Shin, C.N. & Lach, H. 2011, December 15. Nutritional issues of Korean Americans. *Clinical Nursing Research*, 20, 162–180.
184. Lauderdale, D.S. & Kestenbaum, B. 2002. Mortality rates of elderly Asian American populations based on Medicare and Social Security data. *Demography*, 39, 529–540.
185. Baker, L.C., Afendulis, C.C., Chandra, A., McConville, S., Phibbs, C.S., & Fuentes-Afflick, E. 2007. Differences in neonatal mortality among whites and Asian American subgroups: Evidence from California. *Archives of Pediatrics and Adolescent Medicine*, 161(1), 69–76.
186. Kim, K.E. 2003. Gastric cancer in Korean Americans. *Korean and Korean American Studies Bulletin*, 13, 84–90.
187. McCracken, M., Olsen, M., Chen, M.S. Jr., Jemal, A., Thun, M., Cok-kinides, V., . . . & Ward, E. 2007. November–December. Cancer incidence, mortality, and associated risk factors among Asian Americans of Chinese, Filipino, Vietnamese, Korean, and Japanese ethnicities. *CA: A Cancer Journal for Clinicians*, 57(6), 380.
188. Yang, E.J., Chung, H.K., Kim, W.Y., Bianchi, L., & Song, W.O. 2007, June. Chronic diseases and dietary changes in relation to Korean Americans' length of residence in the United States. *Journal of the American Dietetic Association*, 107(6), 942–950.
189. Kim, T.K., Yong, H.I., Kim, Y.B., Kim, H.W., & Choi, Y.S. 2015. Edible insects as a protein source: A review of public perception, processing technology, and research trends. *Food Science of Animal Resources*, 39(4), 521–540. Retrieved from https://doi.org/10.5851/kosfa.2019.e53 (accessed on March 25, 2021).

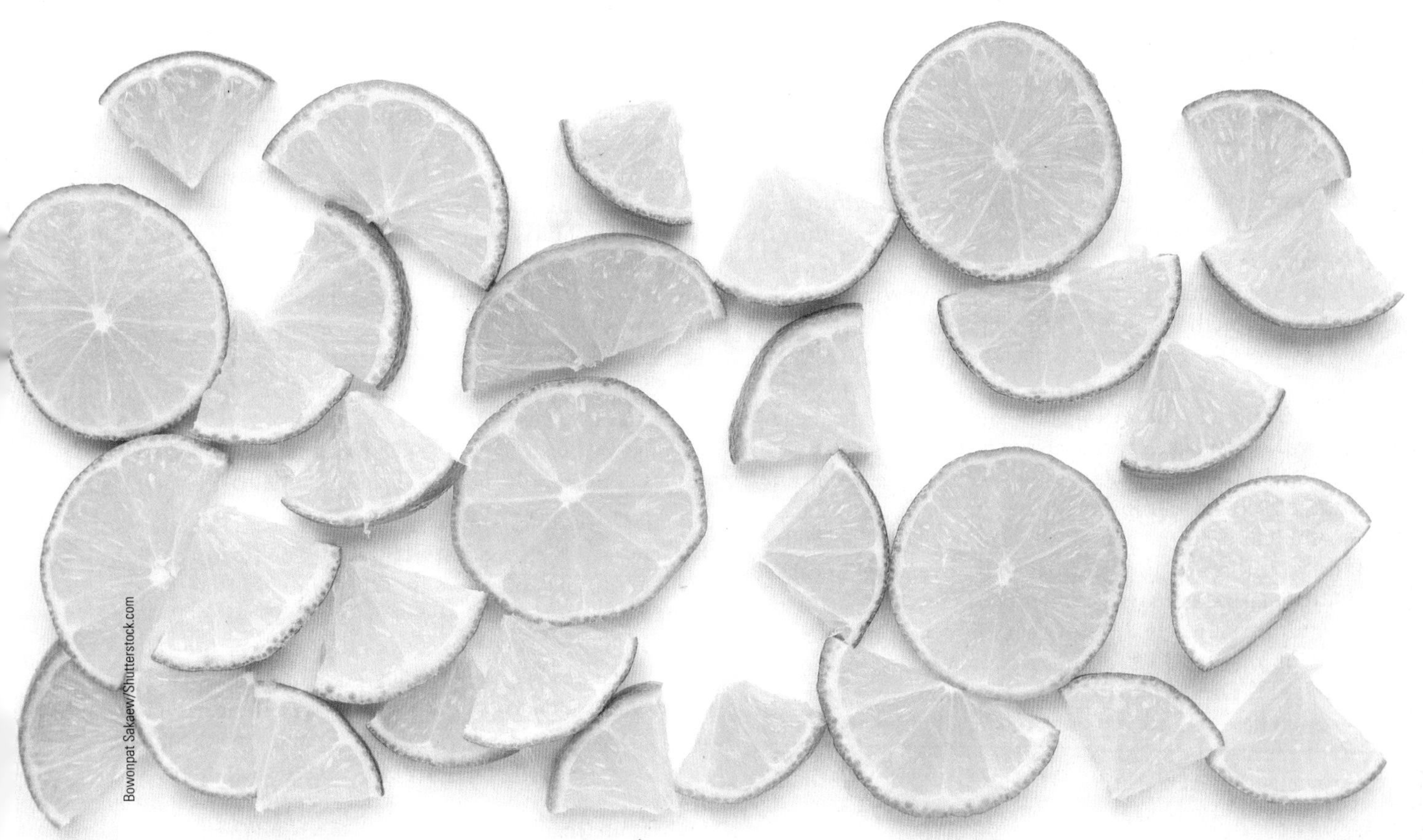

Southeast Asians and Residents of Oceania

Chapter 12

Learning Objectives

12.1 Explain how the agriculture and geography of the mainland and island regions in Southeast Asia and Oceania affect food production and regional patterns of intake.

12.2 Identify the immigration patterns, historical socioeconomic influences, and current locations of Southeast Asians and residents of Oceania in America today.

12.3 Differentiate the religions, family structures, and traditional health beliefs and practices of the people of Southeast Asia and residents of Oceania before and after immigration to the United States.

12.4 Compare the differences and similarities among staple foods and preparation techniques within Southeast Asia and Oceania regions.

12.5 Compare key foods for each of the food groups within Southeast Asia and Oceania and see how these foods have been adapted by immigrants in the United States.

12.6 Differentiate the traditional meal composition and cycles and compare these to the meal composition and cycles of Southeast Asians and residents of Oceania living in the United States today.

12.7 Describe regional specialties and dishes in the diets of the different Southeast Asian cultures and the Oceania nations.

12.8 Identify health concerns associated with the nutritional intake of these groups.

Southeast Asians and the residents of Oceania, those living in 14 Pacific Island countries including New Zealand and Australia, enjoy similar tropical environs and may share some common ancestors. However, their cultures have diverged markedly over the centuries. The countries of Southeast Asia have developed under hundreds of years of Chinese influence and sometimes domination. Throughout history, migrants from China settled heavily in the region, and Southeast Asian countries, for the practical purposes of trade, often went along with the Chinese-imposed worldview of the emperor invoking heaven's will.[1] Spanish expansionism in the Philippines and French occupation in Vietnam were also significant. In contrast, Asian and European contact in the Pacific Islands was limited until the eighteenth century, and subsequent foreign influence almost completely overwhelmed the traditional indigenous societies. This section discusses the cultures and cuisines of the Southeast Asians who have immigrated in substantial numbers to the United States—Filipino, Vietnamese, Cambodian, and Laotian communities—as well as those Oceania groups with significant American populations—Native Hawaiians, Samoans, Guamanians, and Tongans.

Southeast Asians

Cultural Perspective

History of Southeast Asians in the United States

Immigration Patterns Most Filipinos immigrate to the United States for educational and economic opportunities. In contrast, the majority of mainland Southeast Asians who have come to the United States have arrived since the 1970s as refugees from the political conflicts of the region (refer Figure 12.1).

Food for Thought

The only Filipinos allowed to apply for U.S. citizenship before 1946 were those who had enlisted in the U.S. Navy, Naval Auxiliary, or Marine Corps during World War II; had served at least three years; and had an honorable discharge.

The Philippines Substantial immigration from the Philippines to the United States started in 1898 after the country became a U.S. territory. Approximately 113,000 young Filipinos traveled to the Hawaiian Islands between 1909 and 1930 to work in the sugarcane fields. Many of these immigrants later moved to the U.S. mainland. These early immigrants were considered U.S. nationals and carried U.S. passports, yet they were not allowed to become citizens or own land. Most were from the island of Ilocos. Because they were not permitted to bring their wives or families, social and political clubs replaced the family as the primary social structure.

In 1924, the immigration of Filipinos slowed as a result of Asian exclusion laws (refer to Chapter 11 for more information). After World War II, it became legal for Filipinos to become U.S. citizens, and the number of immigrants increased. Significant numbers of Filipinos arrived in the United States after 1965 when the U.S. immigration laws were changed, and by 1980 more than 350,000 had emigrated to mostly urban areas. Two-thirds of the Filipinos who arrived after World War II qualified for entrance as professional or technical workers. Yet, discrimination against Asians often forced Filipinos into low-paying jobs. "Little Manilas" formed in many California cities, and similar homogeneous neighborhoods were found in Chicago, New York City, and Washington, DC, where some Filipinos opened small service businesses to meet the needs of their community.

Vietnam Vietnamese immigration to the United States is characterized by three distinct waves. The first occurred when South Vietnam fell to the North in 1975, and 60,000 Vietnamese left the country with the assistance of the United States. Another 70,000 managed to flee on their own. Most of these refugees had been employed by the United States or were members of the upper classes. They immigrated as intact family groups and were able to bring their property with them. From 1975–1977, another wave of Vietnamese left for political or economic reasons, often escaping by sea. Many left their families and what little money they had to find freedom. The third phase of immigration started in 1978, when increasing numbers of ethnic Chinese living in Vietnam fled the country, again by boat. This wave of immigration was accelerated by the Chinese invasion of northern Vietnam in 1979. This second group of people who came by sea left with no financial resources, and many lost family members escaping in unseaworthy vessels that were easy prey for pirates. After being rescued, they often lived for several months, even years, in refugee camps in various Southeast Asian countries before coming to the United States. In addition, the United States and Vietnam developed the Orderly Departure Program (ODP) in 1979 to bring imprisoned former South Vietnamese soldiers and the approximately 8,000 Amerasians, children of U.S. fathers and Vietnamese mothers, to the United States.

Cambodia and Laos Cambodian and Laotian immigration to the United States did not begin until the United States granted asylum to the residents of the refugee camps along the border with Thailand from 1976–1979. International concern about the large numbers of refugees and the conditions in the camps prompted accelerated admittance of Southeast Asian immigrants worldwide. Many of the refugees were members of tribal populations who lived in the isolated mountainous regions of Southeast Asia, including the Hmong and Mien (ethnic Chinese populations who migrated south to escape persecution in the eighteenth century).

Current Demographics and Socioeconomic Status

Filipino The Filipino American population has more than doubled since 1980. According to 2019 Census estimates, over 4 million Filipinos live in the United States.[2] Almost half reside in California, with more than

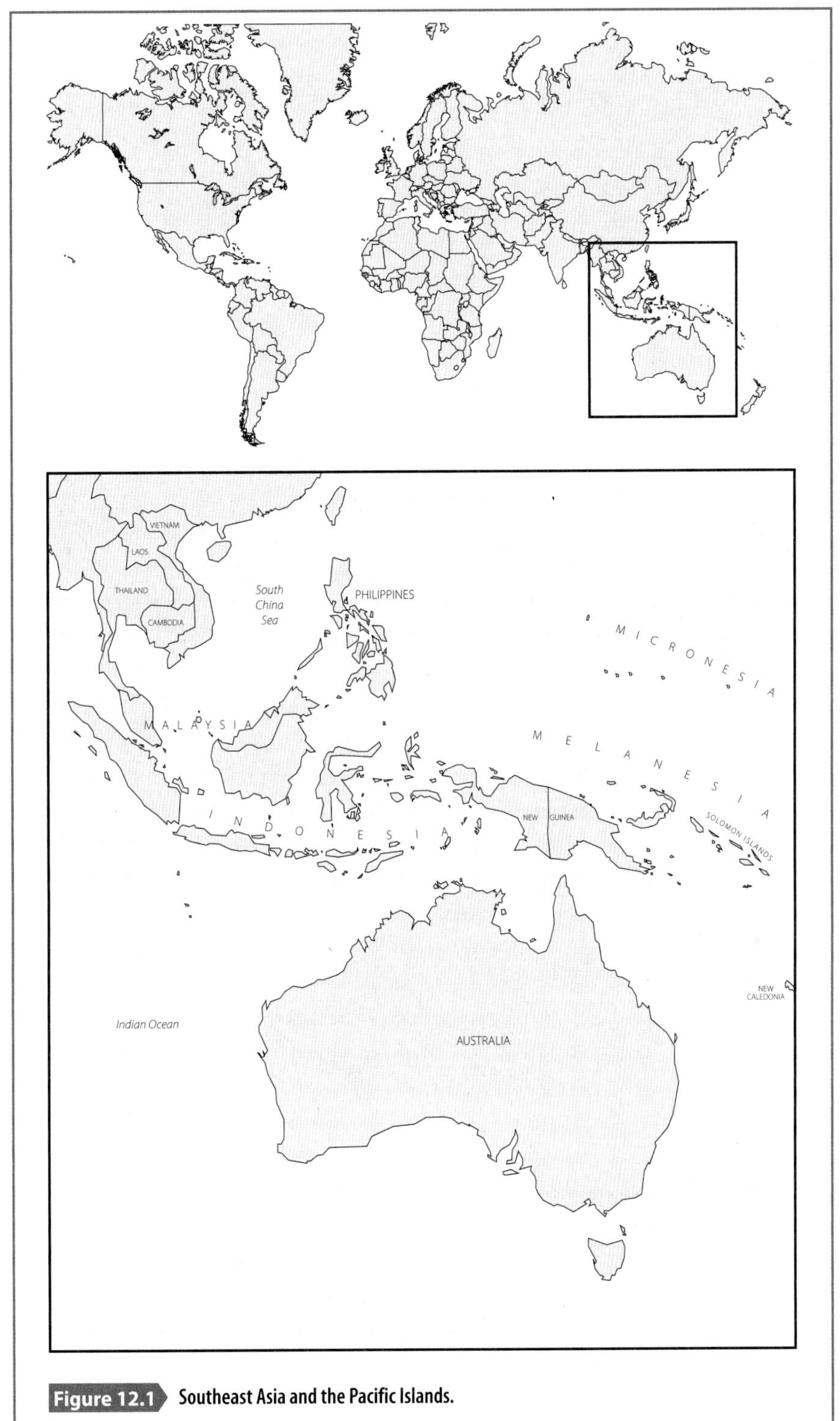

Figure 12.1 Southeast Asia and the Pacific Islands.

200,000 Filipinos also residing in Hawaii, 150,000 in Chicago, 250,000 in New York, 120,000 in Seattle, and 150,000 in Las Vegas. It should be noted that Filipino Americans are a very heterogeneous group who come from different cultural groups within the Philippines and often speak a variety of native languages.

Over 50 percent of Filipino Americans are foreign-born and citizenship rates are higher than in other Asian groups. Educational attainment is also high. Nearly 38 percent of Filipino Americans hold college degrees.[2] Family poverty rates are approximately half that of the general U.S. population both due to higher earnings and, sometimes, to pooled income of several adults living in each household.[3]

Vietnamese More than 1.3 million Vietnamese have entered the United States since 1975, and the total Vietnamese

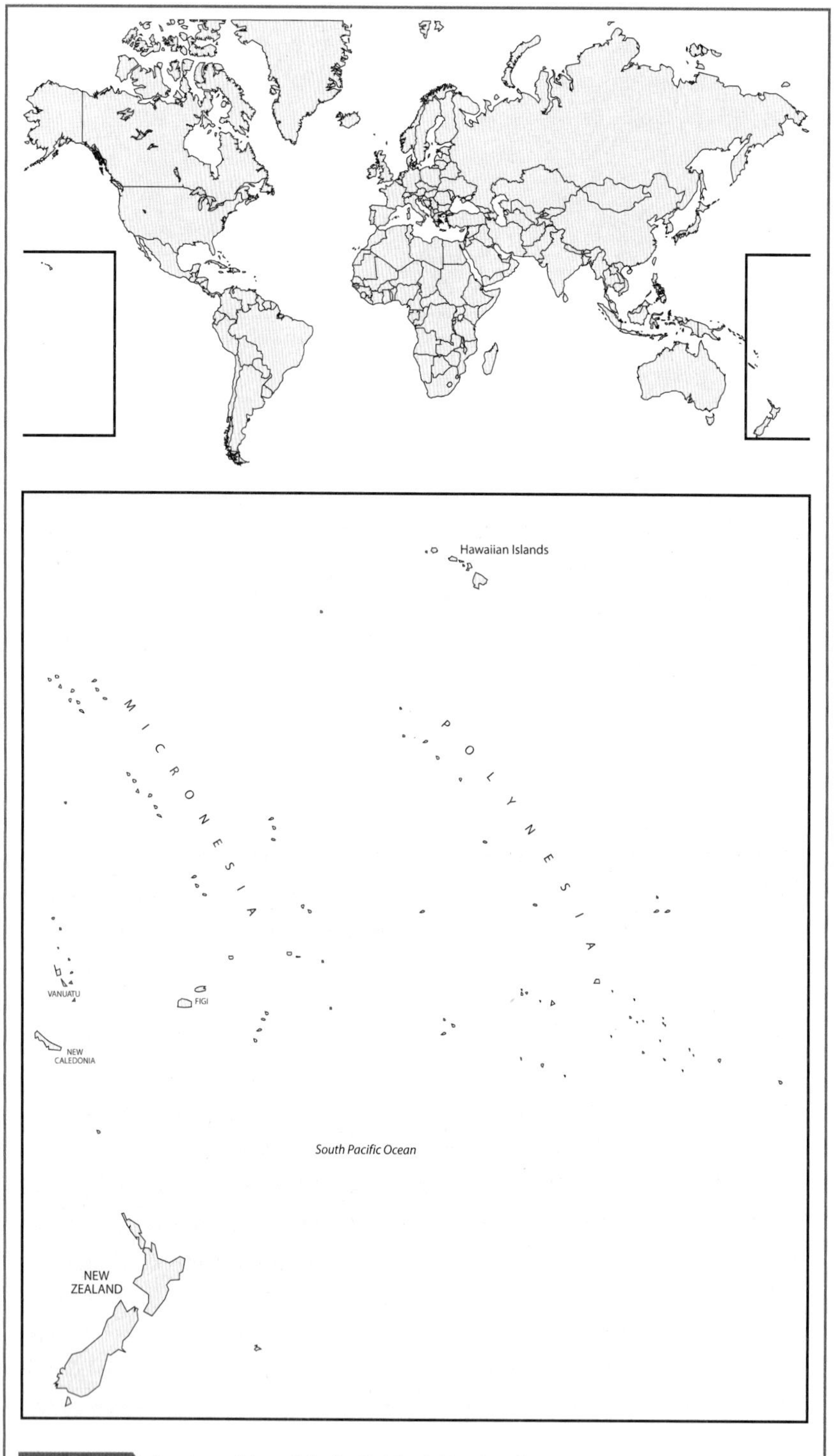

Figure 12.1 Southeast Asia and the Pacific Islands (Continued).

population, including those born in America, was estimated at over 2.1 million in 2019 by the U.S. Census. Some were initially sponsored by American agencies or organizations, which provided food, clothing, and shelter in cities throughout the United States until the Vietnamese could become self-supporting. Many Vietnamese Americans have since relocated to the western and Gulf states, perhaps because the climate is similar to that of Vietnam.[4]

Food for Thought

There were over 901,218 Canadians of Filipino heritage in the 2016 Canadian Census.[6]

In 1972, the karaoke machine was invented in the Philippines by Roberto del Rosario, who outsourced production to Japan. Karaoke remains popular today among Filipino Americans perhaps due to its early introduction in the Philippines.[5]

Vietnamese Americans live primarily in urban areas. Many are young and live in large households with grandparents and other relatives. The first wave of Vietnamese immigrants was well-educated, could speak English, and had held white-collar jobs in Vietnam. Many of them had to accept blue-collar jobs initially and had difficulties supporting their extended families. The second and third waves of Vietnamese Americans were less prepared for life in the United States because they often had no English language skills, were illiterate, had less job training, and did not have support from an extended family.

Language acquisition has been important in the Vietnamese community, and many immigrants have decided to assimilate as quickly as possible. However, over 80 percent do not speak English at home. Education is highly valued, and a child's academic achievement is considered a reflection on the whole family. Vietnamese have high rates of employment, and more than 50 percent have professional or service-related employment. Those who obtain college degrees often prefer technical professions, such as engineering. Median family income is slightly higher than the U.S. average, and the poverty rate for Vietnamese in the U.S. is at the national average of 12 percent.[4]

Food for Thought

In 2016, the Canadian Census reported over 1,063,330 residents of Southeast Asian heritage, 240,615,000 of whom were Vietnamese.[7]

The two major Hmong dialect and cultural groups are the Green Hmong and the White Hmong. The colors refer to women's traditional dress. In the past there was little intermarriage between the two dialect groups, but in recent decades it has become more common.[8,13]

The U.S. Census reported that in 2019, 327,000 Thais were living in the United States, with most having settled in Los Angeles, New York, and Texas.

Cambodian The 2019 U.S. Census identified approximately 339,000 Americans of Cambodian descent. Nearly half of Cambodian Americans reside in California, with the greatest populations found in Long Beach and Stockton. Another large Cambodian community has developed in Lowell, Massachusetts. Texas, Pennsylvania, Virginia, New York, Minnesota, and Illinois also have significant numbers of immigrants.

Adjustment to America has been slower for some Cambodians, many of whom came from rural regions where they worked as farmers. They have a high unemployment rate, and those who work have found employment in professional and service jobs, manufacturing, transportation, and manual labor. Median family income is slightly above the national average, but 13 percent of Cambodians live below the poverty level. Low levels of education have limited economic success for many Cambodian Americans—55 percent of adult men and women have a high school education and 16 percent have a college degree.[9]

Laotian Over 254,000 Laotians live in the United States, according to 2019 U.S. Census figures. Most Laotians have settled in Sacramento and California cities with larger populations in the San Francisco Bay Area. Outside of California, Seattle, Dallas, Fort Worth, and Minneapolis–Saint Paul also have a significant number of Laotians.[9]

Approximately 56 percent of adults have a high school degree, 27 percent have some college, and 14 percent have a Bachelor's degree or higher. Many Laotians hold jobs in transportation and as machine operators, fabricators, and laborers, and it is estimated that only 13 percent live in poverty.[10]

More than 46 percent of American Hmong over 25 years old have a high school degree, 31 percent have some college, and over 17 percent have a college degree. Median family income is above the national average. The poverty rate is at 17 percent, higher than the national average (13 percent) in the United States for the same period.[8]

Worldview

Religion Many Southeast Asians hold beliefs dating back to the ancient religions prevalent before the introduction of Hinduism, Buddhism, Catholicism, and Islam. Most believe in spirits and ghosts, especially of ancestors, who can act as guardians against misfortune or cause harm and suffering. Ideas about spirit intervention have often been incorporated into Eastern and Western religious practices or survive as significant superstitions. Overall, in the United States, Asian Americans are Christian (42 percent), unaffiliated (26 percent), Buddhist (14 percent), Hindu (10 percent), Muslim (4 percent), Sikh (1 percent), and other (2 percent).[11]

Filipino The majority of Americans of Filipino descent are Roman Catholics (65 percent), while others are Protestant (21 percent), Buddhist (1 percent), and those religiously unaffiliated (8 percent)[11]. Religion significantly affects the worldview of Filipinos, especially elders. Many hold that those who lead a good life on earth will be rewarded with life after death. Human misfortunes come from violating the will of God. One should accept one's fate because supernatural forces control the world. Time and providence will ultimately solve all problems.

Vietnamese Forty-three percent of Vietnamese Americans are Buddhists, and 30 percent are Roman Catholic. Small numbers of Protestants (6 percent) also are found and 20 percent are unaffiliated.[11] Buddhism in Vietnam is primarily Mahayana (which recognizes a large body of scripture written up to 400 years after the original canon). This makes it unique among the nations of Southeast Asia (which mostly follow Theravada Buddhism and adhere to the original scriptures alone). Mahayana is a blend of Chan (Zen) and Pure Land, with some Tien-Tai influence as well, and is considered one of the three main branches of Buddhism. Buddhism first reached Vietnam between the first and third century BCE from India and China and bases its philosophies on the teachings of Siddartha Gautama (commonly referred to as the Buddha). Mahayana Buddhists believe that you become awakened when you understand the true nature of reality.

Followers seek to understand this reality and actualize it through compassion. They consider themselves as part of a greater force in the universe (refer to Chapter 4 for more information about Buddhism).

Cambodian The predominant religion in Cambodia is Theravada Buddhism, in which a person attains enlightenment as a result of their efforts, reveres the historical Buddha, and does not pay homage to numerous buddhas and bodhisattvas of the Mahayana Buddhist tradition. Making merit through good deeds, participation in religious rituals, and the support of monks and temples is critical to one's progress through reincarnation. Although some Cambodian Americans have converted to Christian faiths, most practice Buddhism, often in temples established in apartments or homes.

Laotian Almost all Laotians are also Theravada Buddhists. Making merit for Laotians includes the expectation that every man will devote some time in his life to living as a practicing monk, either before marriage or in his old age. In the United States, men find it difficult to fulfill their obligation to the faith. Women may become nuns for periods in their lives as well, especially if widowed. Most Laotians in the United States worship at Buddhist temples alongside Cambodians or Thais who share their religious practices.

About half the Hmong population in the United States is now Christian as a result of French and American missionary work in Laos and conversions after arrival. Many Hmong, fleeing war in Laos, came as refugees between 1975 and 2000. During resettlement, young Hmong were separated from the older community members left in Thai refugee camps and lost their knowledge of traditional spiritual rituals.[12] Baptists, Presbyterians, Mormons, Jehovah's Witnesses, and members of the Church of Christ have actively recruited the Hmong. The other half of Hmong Americans practice animism, shamanism, and ancestor worship (Ua Dab). They believe that the world is divided into two spheres—that which is visible, containing humans, nature, and material objects, and that which is invisible, containing spirits. The shaman acts as an intermediary between the two; some spirits, such as those of ancestors, are available to those who aren't shamans. Women are generally responsible for making contact with these more accessible spirits.

Food for Thought

Hmong ancestors are fed at every festive occasion with a little pork and rice placed in the center of the feast table.

In Thailand, miniature temples or traditional houses are built and posted on pedestals next to a home to shelter the family from spirits. Spirit house traditions are found in several Southeast Asian countries.

It has been suggested that many Hmong became Protestants because they believed it was necessary to gain entry to the United States or in deference to their church sponsors. Some try to combine ancestor worship with their new faiths so as not to offend the spirits.[13] Small numbers of other Hmong belong to a modern Hmong religion called *Chao Fa* ("Lord of the Sky"), started by a prophet in the 1960s who encouraged the Hmong to break with both Laotian and Western ways.

Family Southeast Asians share high esteem for the family, respect for elders, and interdependence among family members. Behavior that would bring shame to the family's honor is avoided, as is a direct expression of conflict. Social acceptance and smooth interpersonal relationships are emphasized.

Filipino The Filipino family is highly structured. At the center is the extended family, containing all paternal and maternal relatives. Kinship is extended to friends, neighbors, and fellow workers through the system of compadrazgo. Lifelong relationships are initiated through shared Roman Catholic rituals, particularly the selection of godparents and the baptism of new babies. Community obligations created through this system include shared food, labor, and financial resources.

The first Filipino immigrants were often unmarried men hoping to make their fortune and return to the Philippines. Some who came between 1903–1935 were seeking higher education. Others who came during this time were recruited to work in Hawaii as plantation workers.[14] They developed surrogate family systems of fellow workers who lived together, with the eldest man serving as patriarch. More recent immigrants have come as whole families and have been able to maintain much of their social organization.

Filipino children are adored by their families and are typically indulged until the age of six. At that time, socialization through negative feedback can begin. Children are taught to be obedient and respectful, to contain their emotions and avoid all conflict, and to be quiet and shy. Politeness is emphasized.[14,15] People must avoid shaming themselves or their families; discord is minimized by the use of euphemisms and by sending go-betweens in sensitive situations. The prestige of a family may be measured by how well children adhere to traditional values. Though Filipino parents often support their children in advanced education and professional careers, women may be discouraged from attending schools where they would be beyond family supervision.[15]

Food for Thought

When Cambodians wed, a Buddhist monk cuts a lock of hair from both the bride and groom to mix symbolically in a bowl.

A Cambodian proverb says, "Travel on a river by following its bends, live in a country by following its customs."[16]

Some Filipino proverbs are: "All food is tasty in famine;" "A fly on the water buffalo's back is taller than the water buffalo;" and "Don't empty the water jar until the rain falls."[14]

Vietnamese The extended Vietnamese family has been modified in the United States to adapt to American norms. Close relatives are encouraged to move into homes next door or in the same neighborhood.

Families are in transition. The father is traditionally the undisputed head of the household, but patriarchy is diminishing as women attain higher levels of education and professional achievement. American-style dating has become common. Although most Vietnamese marry within their ethnic group, women are more likely than men to wed non-Vietnamese mates. Divorce is uncommon.[17]

The level of intergenerational conflict is reportedly high.[17] Children are often the first to learn English and acculturate more easily than their parents, sometimes causing value conflicts and loss of respect for elders. The role of older family members is also changing. Old age is valued in Southeast Asia, but in the United States older relatives are often physically isolated from their peers and even from younger family members. They may also be linguistically isolated within the larger community.

Cambodian Large extended families are common in Cambodia, where children are considered treasures. Cambodians are notable in that their traditional kinship system was bilateral, emphasizing both the paternal and maternal lines. The family was primarily a matriarchy until the 1930s when French influence strengthened the authority of the father. Today, men are responsible for providing for their families, while women make all decisions regarding the family budget.

It has been difficult for Cambodian Americans to retain their traditional family structure in the United States. A large percentage of Cambodian homes are headed by single women, possibly due to the large numbers of men killed during conflicts in Cambodia. Furthermore, Cambodian American women often are formally educated, and their financial contributions are needed to help support the whole family. Differences between immigrants who have lived most of their lives in Cambodia and the children of these immigrants raised in the United States (with no memory of Cambodia) can be enormous in terms of language, acculturation, and values.[16]

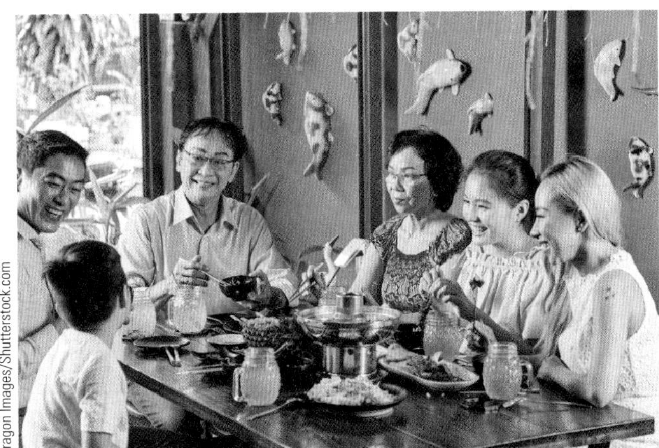
Dragon Images/Shutterstock.com

▲ **The traditional Vietnamese extended family home is less common in the United States, but relatives often live near each other.**

Laotian Most families are agriculturally based in Laos. Extended members live together and work together in the fields to support the whole family. In Laos, men represent the family in village affairs, and women run the home. Great significance is given to the site of the family's house; it is believed that as long as the site exists, the family will exist.

Extended families are still important to Laotian Americans and relatives aid each other with social and economic support. Family structures of mother-father-and-children living in one home have become the norm, although extended members tend to live nearby each other. Women have attained nearly equal status with men in the United States, and it is not unusual for Laotian men to share responsibility for household chores.[18]

Hmong Hmong-American families are among the youngest and largest in the United States: in 2010, half the Hmong population of the United States was younger than 20[13]. The typical Hmong family size is about six members; the Asian American average is 3, and the White American average is 2.6.[19] These large families are usually nuclear, reflecting the number of children rather than relatives. Extended family members are often located nearby, and families frequently congregate with other families from the same traditional clan from Laos, sometimes pooling resources.[13] In households of foreign-born Hmong in the United States, 45 percent live in multigenerational households; among all Hmong in the United States, both foreign and U.S.-born, 36 percent live in multigenerational households.[20]

Men remain the heads of households in the United States. Women are traditionally held in high regard in their roles as mothers, yet it has been noted that fathers are assuming a much larger role in child care in the United States.[21,22] Children are the heart of the home, and much of family life revolves around them. At age five, however, children are expected to behave like adults. As in some other Southeast Asian groups, a generation gap has developed between recently arrived immigrants and their Westernized children.

Traditional Health Beliefs and Practices Southeast Asian health concepts typically combine facets of multiple belief systems. Indigenous ideas about the origins of illness center on the supernatural world, particularly the intervention of malevolent spirits or the ghosts of angry ancestors. Chinese medical practices involving yin and yang, the five evolutive elements (refer to Chapter 11) of fire, water, wood, metal, and earth, and/or *ki* (vital energy) are considerations in some areas of mainland Southeast Asia, while the hot–cold theory is more prevalent in the Philippines (refer to Chapter 9).

Religious precepts regarding rewards for making merit, or performing good deeds, and punishment for violating God's will are also involved in health maintenance. In the most general terms, keeping healthy requires personal harmony with the supernatural world, nature, society, and family fulfilled through one's obligations to one's ancestors, one's religion, and one's kin and community. Illness is usually defined by its cause, not its symptoms.

Most Filipinos adhere to the concept of bahala na, meaning that life is controlled by the will of God and by supernatural forces. If a person behaves properly, shows consideration of others and sensitivity in relationships, fulfills debts and obligations, shows gratitude, and avoids shame, they are rewarded with health in this life and eternal life after death.[10] Many Filipinos believe that illness is a punishment for transgressions against God. Religious medals are worn for protection from evil.[14,23,24]

Spanish control of the islands administered through Mexico led to the adoption of some aspects of humoral medicine in the Philippines, including not only the hot–cold theory but also the condition commonly known as wind or air (mal aire in Mexico; refer to the section titled "Traditional Health Beliefs and Practices" in Chapter 9).

Supernatural illnesses in the Philippines are most often due to the unhappy ghosts of one's ancestors, although witchcraft, or the powers of animal spirits, may also be involved. *Usog* or *tuyaw* occurs when a person transmits illness through the power of the evil eye or the use of hands, fingers, words, or even physical proximity. Undesirable traits or conditions can be transferred magically through contact with a person or object.[25] Some Filipino Americans who believe in supernatural causes of disease do not think that these forces apply in the United States, because ghosts and spirits cannot cross the ocean, nor can they survive in the noisy cities where many Filipinos now live.

Food for Thought

Hmong marriages are traditionally formalized at a two-day feast featuring a roasted pig.

In the Philippines, health is maintained through the balance of natural and supernatural elements. A person is thought to be predisposed to certain illnesses, and the timing of external events contributes to the development of disease. There are seven common Filipino cultural terms related to health and illness in Filipino culture. These include:

Namamana – Inheritance

Lihi – Conception or maternal cravings

Pasma – Hot and cold syndrome

Sumpa and Gaba – Curse

Namalingo – Mystical and supernatural causes

Kaloob ng Diyos – God's will[25]

Additionally, unbalanced conditions, such as working too much, overeating, excessive drinking, inadequate diet or sleep, unhygienic conditions, infections, accidents, emotional stress (especially fright or anxiety), or loss of self-esteem, may increase a person's vulnerability, as do factors such as the season and the weather.

Three practices are used to produce balance: heating, protection, and flushing. It is widely believed that a warm body is needed to prevent illness. Heating means that a person balances hot and cold—whether through exposure to the elements or through eating the right proportions of foods classified as hot or cold—so that warmth is maintained and overheating is avoided. For example, cold or cooling foods, such as orange juice, are not consumed first thing in the morning. Bathing, often twice per day, is also used to maintain warmth in the body. Any imbalance, whether too hot or too cold, is believed to cause illness by reducing blood flow, causing loss of appetite, and lowering the body's ability to fight off sickness. For example, a nursing mother who becomes overheated by too much sun or from exposure to a hot kitchen may find that her milk has become rancid, producing colic or diarrhea in the baby.[26] Specifics on the application of hot and cold classifications and treatment vary tremendously from person to person.

Protection safeguards the body from natural and supernatural forces. For instance, a layer of fat is needed to protect the body from external cooling. Wind is of special concern. It may cause disease directly through drafts or be absorbed through the pores or any wounds. Wind that is too cold or too hot is thought to affect the blood, causing increased or decreased circulation, resulting in a general malaise and increased susceptibility to illness. A postpartum woman might avoid bathing for 9–40 days after the birth of the baby to prevent wind from entering her vagina; a newborn's umbilicus is bound to keep wind from entering that opening; and coconut oil may be rubbed into the skin to block the pores. Whooping cough and mental illnesses are two of the more serious conditions that can be caused by wind.[27]

Activities of daily living, such as household chores, are often considered physical activities by Filipino women. There are barriers and belief systems around rigorous physical activity for health and disease management. It is important to be able to view health interventions from culturally relevant perspectives to make them meaningful.[28] Flushing is used to cleanse the body of impurities or evil forces through perspiration, flatulence, vomiting, or menstrual blood. Vinegar mixed with water, salt, and chili peppers is one example of a flushing treatment, taken to stimulate sweating.

Several types of traditional healers are common in the Philippines: midwives, masseurs, curers (who diagnose through evaluation of the pulse), arbularyos (herbalists), and shamans, who cure supernaturally caused illnesses through the use of folk remedies. In urban regions, where belief in ghosts and spirits is not as prevalent, faith healers are gaining in popularity. Faith healers do not diagnose illness but cure it through prayer, anointing with oil, and the laying on of hands, which transmits sacred healing energy to the patient. The role of the community in providing social support and balance is an important factor in helping individuals maintain a healthy balance of physical and emotional health.[29,30]

Vietnamese Americans have high regard for the American medical establishment. Medical doctors are held in the highest esteem. However, traditional Vietnamese views on health are more related to personal destiny. How one behaved in past lives and the number of good deeds performed by one's ancestors determine one's experiences in this life. Current behavior, such as pleasing good spirits and avoiding evil spirits, can also impact health.[17] Similar to the Filipinos, pregnant Vietnamese women may avoid funerals or ugly objects or leaving their homes at the times malevolent spirits are active (noon and 5:00 p.m.). The use of divination, through fortune-telling, astrology, or physiognomy (the shape of the body, especially the head, as it correlates to the mind), is popular for predicting how a person might expect his or her life to proceed and what interventions might be needed to prevent certain negative experiences.[17,31]

Traditionally, the Vietnamese believe that the human body is sustained by three separate souls: one that encompasses the life force, one that represents intelligence, and one that embodies emotions. In addition, nine vital spirits assist the souls. Soul loss can be an important and life-threatening reason for illness. Typically, strong feelings, especially fright, can cause the soul to leave the body.

The Chinese medical system is commonly used by ethnic Chinese Vietnamese and by some other Vietnamese as well. Maintaining a balance of yin and yang, especially through diet and the treatment of disease, is a primary consideration in health. Like the Filipinos, wind (or air) is sometimes seen as a cause of illness. Some Hmong are also concerned with hot, cold, and wind as well. Hmong women are reportedly thought to be in a cold condition immediately following birth (having lost hot blood) and must avoid cold drinks, cold drafts and wind, and sexual intercourse to reestablish balance. In one recent study looking at traditional, complementary, and alternative medicine in Southeast Asian countries, the most common self-help practices in the past 12 months included praying for your health (30.1 percent), meditation (13.9 percent), and relaxation techniques (9.9 percent).[31]

Cambodians, Laotians, and Hmong are also concerned with spiritual intervention in health. Laotians identify 32 spirits that oversee the 32 organs of the body.[18] The Hmong recognize the world of the invisible, where the spirit of every animal, tree, and rock resides, amid the souls of the living, ancestor spirits, caretaker spirits, and evil spirits. Ancestor spirits require special consideration because if they become angry, they may leave their progenies or fail to protect them from evil. The Laotians have elaborate rituals called baci, mostly performed on all special occasions by older men who are or have been monks, that bind the spirits to their possessor. Among the Hmong, the loss of one's soul, usually due to strong emotional distress, is the single most important cause of illness. It generally results in malaise and weight loss, leading to more serious disease. Related to soul loss is the condition called ceeb, or fright illness. Ceeb typically occurs in children (although it can happen to adults as well) if they are in an accident, chased by a dog, startled by a noise, or plunged into cold water. The soul becomes disconnected; the blood cools down and slows, resulting in a chilling effect that begins in the extremities and can progress to the vital organs.[32–34]

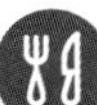

Food for Thought

In parts of Southeast Asia, the opium poppy is traditionally grown in home herb gardens for use as a pain killer.[35] Opium was known to ancient Greek and Roman physicians as well, and used as a pain killer, to induce sleep, and to help other ailments. The poppy plant, *Papaver somniferum*, produces opium, a powerful narcotic whose derivates include morphine, codeine, heroin, and oxycodone.

Traditional Cambodian healers, known as krou Khmer, may be found in many Cambodian American communities. Some techniques used by these healers are massages, herbal medicines, and "coining" with a copper coin dipped in a balm applied to acupuncture points of the body.[16]

Unique to Southeast Asians in the United States is the unexplained condition known as sudden unexpected nocturnal death syndrome (SUNDS) when a seemingly healthy person dies in his or her sleep. It is especially prevalent among Cambodians, Laotians, and Hmong, although it may occur in other immigrants from the mainland as well. Although biomedical hypotheses have been proposed to account for the fatal syndrome, such as heart irregularities or sleep apnea, none has been proven. It is now believed the phenomenon known as sleep paralysis is involved. Some researchers believe that death is caused within the cultural context of the nightmare experience. Specifically, the nightmare spirit, dab tsog, enters the room at night and the dreamer "wakes" to the sensation of the spirit sitting on his or her chest; they are unable to move and are terrified. Although many immigrants report having experienced nightmares in Southeast Asia, the attack by the spirit does not usually result in death. Cultural disruptions are believed to have intensified the episodes. Guilt and depression create increased vulnerability to fatal nightmare experiences. Posttraumatic stress disorder, panic attacks, exposure to chemical warfare agents, or blood electrolyte imbalances may be other risk factors.[36–38]

Food for Thought

Laotians often wear strings tied around the wrist at occasions such as weddings, for a newborn and mother, at a death, or for illness, to bind the 32 kwan (parts of the soul) and keep them from wandering and creating an imbalance that may lead to illness and bad luck.

Traditional healers are typically specialized practitioners among mainland Southeast Asians. They may provide services for broken bones, skin infections, or objects stuck in the throat. Hmong herbalists (kws tshuaj) treat natural disorders, such as menstrual problems, impotence, infertility, stomach disorders, and diarrhea, with teas and poultices.[24] Hmong shamans treat patients for spiritual disorders at great personal risk due to interaction with the spirit world. They heal conditions such as mental illness, hypertension, diabetes, breathing difficulties, and fainting. In many cases, they often deal with lost souls. Magic healers are not spiritually chosen for their profession but may interface with the spirit world to treat injuries and stones (such as those found in kidneys, or those placed in bodies by evil spirits). Monks may lead religious rituals. Among most Southeast Asians, minor illnesses may be treated by anyone with healing experience, typically a grandmother or mother in the home. The family takes responsibility for the illness of an individual and will usually exhaust all remedies available within the house before seeking outside help.[39]

Botanical remedies are very popular with many mainland Southeast Asians living in the United States. Cambodians, Laotians, and Hmong sometimes maintain herb gardens for easy access to therapeutic ingredients. Some immigrants frequent Chinese herbalists or will buy imported products from Asia.[40] Kws tshuaj (herbal medicine experts) sell tshuaj ntsuab (fresh herbs), tshuaj qhuav (dried roots or bark), as well as other organic substances (e.g., rhinoceros bones/skin/dried blood, dried bear, sea cucumber and snake gall bladders, etc.). Herbs and other substances are prepared as teas, broths, steam inhalants, or balms.[40,41] Physical therapies may include massage; cupping (a heated cup or a cup with a small amount of burning paper is placed over a certain spot on the body until the fire goes out, leaving a round red spot on the skin); moxibustion (burning a small bundle of herbs on the skin or using a lit cigarette); and coining (rubbing a coin or spoon dipped in tiger balm or eucalyptus ointment across the skin with pressure), scratching, or pinching affected areas. In most cases, the therapy is used to release any bad wind or excess heat and to restore balance to the body. Health care providers must consider the potential use of complementary and alternative medicine and its importance in these cultures. It is also important to understand specific herbal remedies and how they may react with conventional medicines.

Food for Thought

Mien rituals involving ancestor spirits require a genealogical record of the family going back ten generations. Mien (Yao) people often live in parts of Laos and Thailand; they do not have a country of their own.

Religious rituals are also used to intervene on behalf of an ill person. Hmong soul callers perform the "Mandate of Life" ceremony to return a lost soul to its host body, and the Mien people appeal to ancestor spirits to protect family members and assist in healing. These rituals sometimes include animal offerings. A butchered animal, typically a chicken, pig, or occasionally a cow, is purchased from a packinghouse before the ceremony; then it is cooked and consumed after the rite as part of a feast. Its soul is offered in exchange for the victim's missing soul.[40,41] In Vietnam, small shrines are sometimes constructed to appease ancestor spirits or the souls of premature infants who have died and still wander the earth. Offerings may also be made to the Goddess Quang Am for good health. Among Catholic Vietnamese and Filipinos, appeals are made to the Virgin Mary; group prayer has assumed significance for many Protestant Southeast Asians.

It has been noted that Christian Hmong often avoid the use of shamans, soul callers, and other traditional practitioners, depending on the clergy and the power of prayer to promote physical and spiritual healing. Herbs, however, may still be used at home.[41]

Traditional Food Habits

The cuisines of Southeast Asia have many ingredients in common, but food preparation methods and meal patterns reflect the outside cultures that have influenced each nation. For example, the Vietnamese often serve cream-filled French pastries for dessert, whereas Filipinos frequently have Spanish-style custard flan. As in China and Japan, the staple foods are rice (primarily long grain), soybean products, and tea. A meal is not considered complete unless rice is included. Instead of soy sauce, however, Southeast Asians often season their food with strongly flavored fermented fish sauces and fish pastes.

Ingredients and Common Foods

Staples

Filipino Filipino fare reflects the predominantly Malayan ancestry of Filipino people, with overlays of Chinese, Japanese, East Indian, Indonesian, and Islamic culture. This tapestry of multicultural influences, along with indigenous tribal influence, creates a unique cuisine. The distinction of Filipino food from other Southeast Asian nations is the major influence of Spanish and American colonization.[42–44] There are three principal flavors in Filipino cooking: sweet, salty, and sour. Combined, they make a bold and heady cuisine. Garlic, brought with chilies and tomatoes by the Spanish in the 1500s, is a main ingredient in most recipes. One popular Filipino preparation, adobo, combines marinated chicken, pork, and sometimes fish or shellfish, that is fried with garlic in lard and then braised in vinegar, garlic, chili peppers, bay leaf, and peppercorn with whatever vegetables are on hand, such as plantains, potatoes, greens, or bamboo shoots.[45] Filipinos traditionally used a clay pot for cooking but now use a large wok called a kawali, especially for frying. They tend to cook food longer than the Chinese do, to allow it to absorb more flavor and fat. The common foods of the Philippines are listed in Table 12.1. Researchers found that outside influences on Filipino food include the following:

Chinese—soybeans, curds, certain pork and beef cuts, various types of noodle soup (pansit mami, bihon, sotanghon), steamed buns with fillings (siopao), dumplings (siomai), crullers, and cooking with oil in a wok.

Spanish—stuffed capons, beef rolls, stews of meats, sausages, and vegetables (cocido, puchero), leche flan, soft meringue rolled with custard filling (brazo de Mercedes), and nutty meringue/buttercream layer cake (sans rival).

American—frozen and pressure-cooked foods, food that is portable and quick

Others—pizza, sukiyaki, Mongolian barbecue, roast beef.[44]

Table 12.1 Cultural Food Groups: Filipino

Group	Comments	Common Foods	Adaptations in the United States
Protein Foods			
Milk/milk products	Filipinos make one of the few native cheeses in Asia, from *carabao* (water buffalo) milk. U.S. influence has resulted in the availability of many Western dairy products. Many Filipinos may be lactose intolerant. In desserts, coconut milk is frequently used in place of cow's milk.	Evaporated milk (cow, goat), white cheese (*carabao*) Consumption	Consumption of milk and other dairy products has increased.
Meat/poultry/fish/eggs/legumes	Protein intake is often dependent on income.	*Meat:* beef, *carabao*, goat, pork, monkey, variety meats (liver, kidney, stomach, tripe), rabbits *Poultry and small birds:* chicken, duck, pigeon, sparrow *Fish and shellfish:* anchovies, bonita, carp, catfish, crab, crawfish, cuttlefish, *dilis*, mackerel, milkfish, mussels, prawns, rock oyster, salt cod, salmon, sardines, sea bass, sea urchins, shrimp, sole, squid, swordfish, tilapia, tuna *Eggs:* chicken, fish *Legumes:* black beans, black-eyed peas, chickpeas, lentils, lima beans, mung beans, red beans, soybeans, white kidney beans, winged beans	Consumption of fish has decreased; intake of meat, poultry, and eggs has increased.
Cereals/Grains	Rice is the main staple and is usually eaten at every meal.	Corn, oatmeal, rice (long- and short-grain, flour, noodles), wheat flour (bread and noodles)	Rice is not usually eaten at breakfast but is eaten at least once per day.
Fruits/Vegetables	Vegetables are often consumed in mixed stews, stir-fries, and soups. Braised vegetables may be consumed as entrée or side dish. Pickled fruits and vegetables are very popular.	*Fruits:* apples, avocados, banana blossoms, bananas (100 varieties), breadfruit, *calamansi* (lime), citrus fruit, coconut, durian, grapes, guava, jackfruit, Java plum, litchi, mangoes, melons, papaya, pears, persimmons (*chicos*), pineapples, plums, pomegranates, pomelo, rambutan, rhubarb, star fruit, strawberries, sugar cane, tamarind, watermelon *Vegetables:* amaranth, bamboo shoots, bean sprouts, beets, bitter melon, burdock root, cabbage, carrots, cashew nut leaves, cassava, cauliflower, celery, Chinese celery, drumstick plant (sili leaves), eggplant, endive, garlic, green beans, green papaya, green peppers, hearts of palm, hyacinth bean, *kamis*, leaf fern, leeks, lettuce, long green beans, mushrooms, nettles, okra, onions, parsley, pigeon peas, potatoes, pumpkins, purslane, radish, safflower, snow peas, spinach, sponge gourd, squash blossoms, winter and summer squashes, sugar palm shoot, swamp cabbage, sweet potatoes, taro leaves and roots, tomatoes, turnips, water chestnuts, watercress, yams	More green vegetables are consumed. More raw vegetables and salads are eaten.

(Continued)

Table 12.1 Cultural Food Groups: Filipino (*Continued*)

Group	Comments	Common Foods	Adaptations in the United States
Additional Foods			
Seasonings	Food is spicy, but the variety of spices used is limited. Regional cooking is differentiated in part by seasoning preferences.	*Atchuete* (annatto), *bagoong*, *baggongalamang*, chile peppers, garlic, lemon grass, *patis*, seaweed, soy sauce, turmeric, vinegar	
Nuts/seeds		Betel nuts, cashews, *kaong* (palm seeds), peanuts, pili nuts	
Beverages		Soy milk, cocoa, coconut juice, coffee with milk, tea	Chocolate milk is substituted for soy milk. Soft drinks are popular.
Fats/oils	Traditional diet is considerably higher in fat than are other Asian cultures.	Coconut oil, lard, vegetable oil	
Sweeteners		Brown and white sugar, coconut, honey	

Rice is the foundation of the diet, and the long-grain variety accompanies the meal. It is typically steamed or fried (the preferred method of serving leftover rice). Garlic fried rice is a favorite, topped with bits of meat, sausages, and a fried egg. Vinegar, additional garlic, and a spicy vegetable/fruit pickle called atchara are added to taste. A common bread, pan de sal, is made from rice flour. Noodles are also used extensively. Pancit is a popular dish made with rice, wheat, or mung bean noodles mixed with cooked chicken, ham, shrimp, or pork in a soy and garlic-flavored sauce. Short-grain, glutinous rice is used for sweet desserts such as puto, a fluffy cake made from rice, sugar, and sometimes coconut milk.

The amount of meat, poultry, or fish a family eats depends on economic status, as it does in most cultures. Pork, chicken, and fish are popular, added as available to mixed dishes such as sinigang, a soup of fish or meat cooked in water with sour fruits, tomatoes, and vegetables; puchero, a beef, chicken, sweet potato, tomato, and garbanzo bean stew with an eggplant sauce; gulay, fried fish with vegetables; and lumpia, the Filipino version of egg rolls, stuffed with pork, chili peppers, and vegetables like hearts of palm. Other traditional dishes popular for special occasions include chicken relleno, a whole chicken stuffed with boiled eggs, pork, sausage, and spices; paella, a Spanish recipe for saffron-flavored rice typically topped with chicken, sausage, pork, seafood, tomatoes, and peas; and lechon, a whole roasted pig.

Filipinos use all parts of the animal in their cooking; in addition to the pork meat, for example, the pig variety cuts might show up in various soups or mixed stews, such as dinuguan, consisting of diced pork, chicken, or entrails cooked in pig's blood and seasoned with vinegar and hot green chili peppers or sausage such as garlicky longaniza. The skin is commonly fried to make sitsaron (similar to the Mexican chicharrónes or U.S. cracklings), which are eaten as snacks or pulverized to top noodle dishes.

Due to the U.S. influence in the Philippines, many Western dairy products are available, but fresh cow's milk is used infrequently. Evaporated milk is a common ingredient in leche flan, a custard, and in halo-halo, a parfait-like dessert consisting of shaved ice, coconut milk, mung beans, purple yam pudding (ube), boiled palm seeds (kaong), corn kernels, pineapple jelly, and other ingredients. Halo-halo can be bought premixed with just the shaved ice needed for completion. Rural Filipinos use carabao (water buffalo) milk to make one of the few native kinds of cheese in Asia, kesong puti. Carabao milk is also popular in desserts, such as ice cream, flan, and pastille candies.

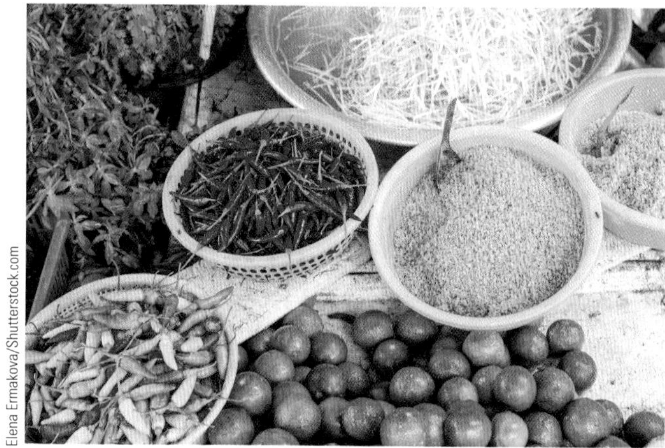
Elena Ermakova/Shutterstock.com

▲ **Traditional Foods of Southeast Asia and Oceania.**

A common seasoning, used instead of salt and found throughout Southeast Asia, is fermented fish paste or sauce. In the Philippines, the powerful paste is called bagoong and tastes somewhat like anchovies, although it can be made from a variety of fish. A similar paste made of shrimp is known as bagoong-alamang. Patis is a translucent amber fish sauce. To obtain the popular sour–cool taste, palm vinegar, or a paste made from either the cucumber-like vegetable called kamis or the pulp of the tamarind pod, may be used. Kinilaw, a Filipino specialty, uses sour ingredients to marinate and pickle raw foods, including fruits and vegetables, but also meats, organs, and seafood. Bagoong, patis, lime (calamansi) wedges, and vinegar flavored with chilies are frequently placed on the table so that each diner may add saltiness or sourness to taste.

A principal food in many Pacific Islands is the coconut, and it is widely used in Filipino cooking. In addition, copra (dried coconut kernels used for oil extraction) is an important export crop. It takes approximately one year for a coconut to mature, but if picked at six months, the soft, jellylike coconut meat can be eaten with a spoon and is a popular delicacy. The coconut plant provides several food products, including beverages, cooking liquids, and even a vegetable. The sweet, clear liquid found in young coconuts is the juice or water. It is consumed fresh but is not used in cooking. Coconut cream, which is used for cooking along with coconut milk, is the first liquid extracted from grated, mature coconut meat. After the cream is removed, coconut milk is made by adding water to the meat and then squeezing the mixture. Coconut milk is used primarily in special dishes. Coconut palm blossom sap can be fermented to produce a strong alcoholic drink called tuba, which, when distilled, is known as lambanog. Hearts of palm, sometimes called palmetto cabbage, is the firm, greenish inner core of the tree; it is used as a vegetable. Bananas, durian (a large, strong-smelling, sweet fruit with a creamy texture), jackfruit, mango, papaya, and pineapples are also popular.

Food for Thought

In Filipino culture, sticky, glutinous rice cakes symbolize the cohesiveness of the family.

Among the more unusual Filipino specialties is balut, eaten occasionally as a snack. These partially developed duck eggs are soft-boiled and sold warm by street vendors. Salt and a little vinegar are added to the embryonic birds before they are popped whole into the mouth.

Durian odor, which has been likened to rotting onions mixed with gasoline, is so strong that some apartment buildings in Asia ban the fruit. The taste is said to be custard-like and garlicy, with a creamy cheesecake texture.

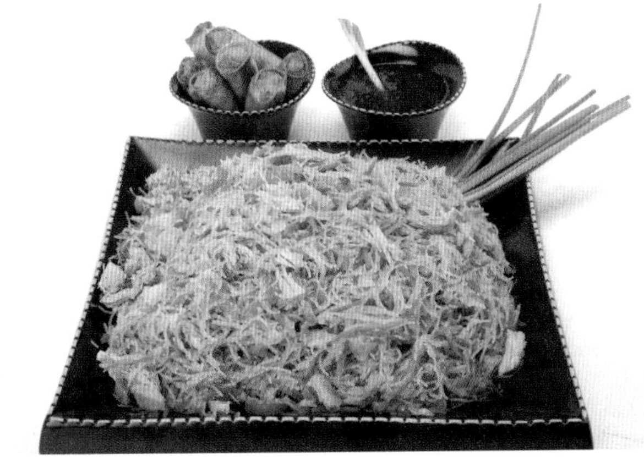

▲ Two traditional Filipino dishes—lumpia (similar to an egg roll) and pancit (noodles cooked with meat or shrimp in a soy- and garlicflavored sauce).

Michael Cocita/Shutterstock.com

Regional cooking styles are divided into four regions in the Philippines: Luzon (the largest group of islands, also home to the nation's capital, Manila), Bicolandia, the Viscayan Islands, and Mindanao. Luzon is made up of various ethnic groups, and the cuisine has been strongly influenced by the Spanish. Ocean fish, such as prawns, milkfish (bangus), and halibut, as well as the ample use of anchovy sauce and shrimp paste, are preferred in the northern areas. Foods are typically boiled or steamed. Saluyot ("okra leaves"—not related to okra), a spinach-like green with a slippery texture when cooked, and drumstick plant leaves, called sili, are especially popular in the north.

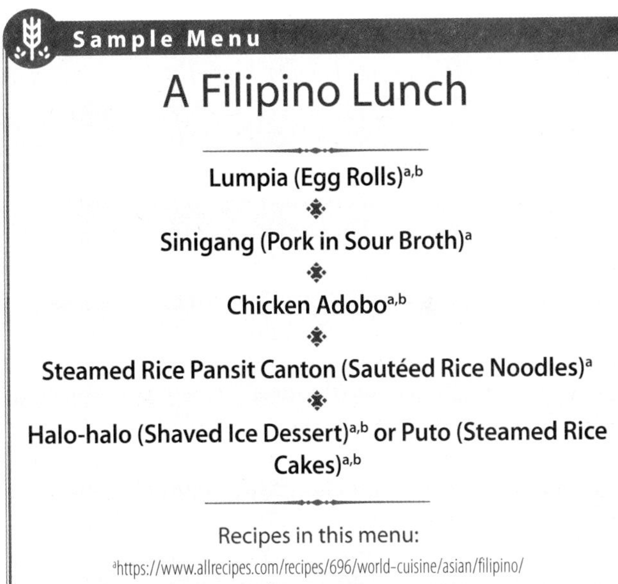

Sample Menu

A Filipino Lunch

Lumpia (Egg Rolls)[a,b]

Sinigang (Pork in Sour Broth)[a]

Chicken Adobo[a,b]

Steamed Rice Pansit Canton (Sautéed Rice Noodles)[a]

Halo-halo (Shaved Ice Dessert)[a,b] or Puto (Steamed Rice Cakes)[a,b]

Recipes in this menu:

[a]https://www.allrecipes.com/recipes/696/world-cuisine/asian/filipino/

[b]*Filipino Recipes* at http://www.filipinofoodrecipes.net/

Food for Thought

Adobo describes not only a dish but a cooking technique in Filipino cuisine. To qualify as adobo, meat (usually chicken or pork) is braised in vinegar, bay leaves, garlic, salt, and black pepper. A "new" innovation of adding soy sauce, and other special preferences, can be a topic of heated debate.[45]

Rice is grown in the central region of Luzon, known for its freshwater fish and richly sauced dishes flavored with onions and garlic. One delicacy is rellenong manok, a deboned chicken stuffed with sausage, vegetables, and ground pork mixed with raisins and spices, topped with a tangy red sauce. Stir-frying is the most common cooking technique. Coconut products and tropical fruits predominate. Sweetened rice dishes such as suman, a snack made from rice (cassava or plantains can be used) steamed in banana leaves or corn husks, are a specialty.

Bicolandia is an ethnically homogeneous region that came in contact with both Malaysian and Polynesian cooking. Foods are spicy and hot with chili peppers, balanced by copious use of coconut milk and cream. Taro leaves cooked in coconut milk with ginger and chilies are one example of the unique blend of foods found in this area. Viscayan Islands fare also reflects its heritage—abundant use of seafood (including a distinctive fermented shrimp paste called guinamos) and seaweed, as well as many dessert specialties, such as candies and pastries, developed due to the sugarcane plantations in the area. The Mindanao region was heavily influenced by the Indonesians and Malaysians. The many ethnic groups living there are predominantly Muslim, so little pork is consumed (refer to Chapter 4). Sauces made from peanuts and chilies are popular, as are curries and other spicy dishes, such as piarun (fish spiced with chilies) and tiola sapi (boiled beef curry).

Vietnamese, Cambodian, and Laotian Ingredients are similar in all the mainland Southeast Asian countries, but recipes, flavor preferences, and meal patterns vary. Indigenous fish and seafood, tropical fruits and vegetables, and glutinous rice were the foundation of the native diets. The Chinese introduced long-grain rice, soy products, stir-frying, hot pots, fried pastries, and chopsticks to areas they ruled. French regional occupation popularized such items as French bread, meat pâtés, asparagus, potatoes, pastries, and strong coffee. Indian and Malaysian influence is seen in the curries and coconut milk–flavored dishes of eastern and southern Southeast Asia. The common foods of mainland Southeast Asians are listed in Table 12.2.

Rice, both long and short grain, is the staple of the diet. Rice products, such as noodles, paper, and flour, are used extensively. In Vietnam, rice paper is used as egg roll or wonton wrappers. In the dish cha gio, the moistened paper is wrapped around a variety of meats, fish, vegetables, and herbs and then deep-fried. Often the rice paper is filled with meat, fresh herbs, and vegetables at the table. Dried rice noodles (sticks) are called pho, which is also the name of the popular noodle-based soup in Vietnam. In Laos, the sticky, glutinous short-grain rice is more prevalent than long-grain types (traditionally formed into small balls to use as scoops for other foods), and the very thin Chinese-style rice noodles are common. Wheat is used to make French bread, noodles, and some pastries.

Fried noodles topped with meats and vegetables are a favorite. Fish and shellfish are the predominant protein food on the mainland. Even landlocked Laos depends on freshwater varieties. Fish, shrimp, and squid are often preserved through salting and drying. Poultry is widely available, and pork or goat is eaten in wealthier areas. Beef is used occasionally. Religious prohibitions often influence which meats are consumed. Like other Asians, the people of mainland Southeast Asia do not use appreciable amounts of dairy products. However, soy milk is a common beverage. Soy products, particularly a chewier version of tofu (soybean curd) called tempeh, are common.

Mainland Southeast Asians frequently consume vegetables, cooked in stir-fries and stews or uncooked in salads and pickles. Especially noteworthy are the many shredded vegetables and unripe fruits, such as cabbage, papaya, carrots, cucumber, radishes, jicama, and bean sprouts topped with fish, poultry, meat, or peanuts and spicy hot dressing. One example is goi go, a Vietnamese specialty featuring cabbage and chicken. Greens and leaves are often used to wrap foods, such as collard greens for Cambodian steamed fish and la lot (betel leaves) used for Vietnamese spring rolls stuffed with minced beef. Further, fresh herbs and spices, including basil, coriander leaves, chili peppers, galangal (similar to young ginger root), garlic, ginger, makrut lime leaves, lemongrass,

Table 12.2 Cultural Food Groups: Mainland Southeast Asian

Group	Comments	Common Foods	Adaptations in the United States
Protein Foods			
Milk/milk products	Most Southeast Asians do not drink milk and may be lactose intolerant. Sweetened condensed milk is used in coffee; whipping cream is used in pastries.	Sweetened condensed milk, whipping cream	It is expected that younger Southeast Asians will increase their use of dairy products. Ice cream is popular; milk and cheese are often disliked.
Meat/poultry/fish/eggs/legumes	The traditional Southeast Asian diet is low in protein. Fish, poultry, and pork are common; most parts of the animal are used (brains, heart, lungs, spleen).	*Meat:* beef, lamb, pork, goat, venison; variety meats of all types *Poultry and small birds:* chicken, duck, quail, pigeon, sparrow, doves *Eggs:* chicken, duck (both embryonic and unfertilized), fish *Fish and shellfish:* almost all varieties of freshwater and saltwater seafood, fresh and dried *Legumes:* chickpeas, lentils, mung beans (black and red), soybeans and soybean products (tempeh, tofu, soy milk), winged beans	Meat, lamb, and eggs are eaten more; fish, shellfish, and duck are eaten less because of price.

(Continued)

Table 12.2 Cultural Food Groups: Mainland Southeast Asian (*Continued*)

Group	Comments	Common Foods	Adaptations in the United States
Cereals/Grains	Rice is the staple grain and is usually eaten with every meal. French bread is commonly eaten.	Rice (long- and short-grain, sticks, noodles), wheat (French bread, cakes, pastries)	Intake of baked goods increases.
Fruits/Vegetables	Hearty garnishes of fresh vegetables are commonly added to dishes. The Vietnamese eat a considerable amount of fruit and vegetables, fresh and cooked. Fruit is often eaten for dessert or as a snack.	*Fruits:* apples, bananas, cantaloupe, coconut, custard apple, dates, durian, figs, grapefruit, guava, jackfruit, jujube, lemon, lime, litchi, longans, mandarin orange, mango, orange, papaya, peach, pear, persimmon, pineapple, plum, pomegranates, pomelo, raisins, rambutan, roselle, sapodilla, star fruit, soursop, strawberries, tamarind, watermelon *Vegetables:* amaranth, arrowroot, artichokes, asparagus, bamboo shoots, banana leaves and flowers, betel leaves, beans (yard long and string), bitter melon, breadfruit, broccoli (Chinese and domestic), cabbage (domestic, Chinese, savoy, napa), calabash, carrot, cassava (tapioca), cauliflower, celery (domestic and Chinese), chayote squash, Chinese chard, Chinese radish (*daikon*), chrysanthemum, corn, cucumber, eggplant (domestic and Thai), leeks, lotus root, luffa, matrimony vine, mushrooms (many varieties), mustard (Chinese greens), okra (domestic, lady finger), peas, peppers, potato, pumpkin (flowers, leaves), spinach, squash, sweet potatoes (tubers, leaves), taro (root, stalk, leaf, shoots), tomatoes, turnips, water lily greens, water chestnuts, water convolvulus, was gourd, yams	Use of fruits and vegetables is dependent on availability and price. It is expected that use of fruits and vegetables will decline. Fresh vegetables and herbs are sometimes grown in backyard gardens.
Additional Foods			
Seasonings	Fermented fish sauce, as well as soy sauce, is often used. Fresh herbs are very popular garnishes in Vietnamese dishes; typical Cambodian fare is delicately seasoned; Thai dishes are frequently very hot and spicy, with several types of curry and chile peppers especially popular.	Allspice, alum, basil, black pepper, borax, cayenne pepper, chile pepper, chives, cinnamon, coconut milk, fresh coriander, curry powder, fennel, galanga, garlic, ginger, makrut lime leaves, lemon grass, lemon juice, lily flowers, lotus seed, mint, MSG, *nuoc mam* (and other fermented fish sauces and pastes), paprika, saffron, star anise, tamarind juice, vinegar	
Nuts/seeds		Almonds, betel nuts, cashews, chestnuts, macadamia nuts, peanuts, pili nuts, walnuts; locust seeds, lotus seeds, pumpkin seeds, sesame seeds, watermelon seeds	Peanut butter is often disliked.
Beverages	Beverages are usually drunk after the meal or with snacks or desserts.	Coffee, tea, sweetened soybean milk, a wide variety of fruit and bean drinks, hot water, hot soup, beer	Carbonated drinks have increased in use.
Fats/oils		Bacon, butter, lard, margarine, peanut oil, vegetable oil	The Vietnamese have increased their use of butter and margarine.
Sweeteners	Sweets are luxury foods.	Cane sugar, candy	The use of sweetened products has risen in the United States.

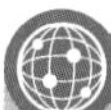

Exploring Global Cuisine

The Cooking of the Diverse Cultures in Oceania: Malaysia, Singapore, and Indonesia

Malaysia, which includes a western section contiguous with Thailand and an eastern section on the island of Borneo, extends south into the gap between Southeast Asia, the Philippines, and Australia (refer to Figure 12.1). At its tip is the independent city-nation of Singapore. Indonesia, comprised of over 10,000 islands (mostly uninhabited), arches eastward from Malaysia and includes Bali, Kalimantan (the Indonesian portion of Borneo), Java, New Guinea, and Sumatra. The region lies along the equator and contains a majority of the world's tropical rainforests. The fertile land is conducive to the cultivation of the herbs and spices brought by Asian, Middle Eastern, and European traders, including chili peppers, cinnamon, cloves, cumin, ginger, nutmeg, and pepper. Parts of Indonesia are still known as the Spice Islands.

The cuisines of Malaysia, Singapore, and Indonesia have been greatly influenced by the diversity of their populations: native Malays, Chinese, Asian Indians, Pakistanis, Europeans, Thais, Eurasians, Melaka Portuguese (Malaysian Portuguese), and Peranakan. Further, the numerous religious practices of the region—Islam, Hinduism, Buddhism, Christianity, and Judaism—have played a role in the fare. Today, Malaysia and Indonesia are predominantly Muslim nations (except Bali, which is mostly Hindu), while Singapore is primarily Christian.

Rice, both long-grain and sticky-glutinous, is the foundation of the diet. It is often steamed, but it is also popularly fried, prepared as sticky rice balls, and especially as noodles. Noodles are typically stir-fried, added to soups, or topped with mixed vegetables, fish, or meat. They are eaten at nearly all meals, and often for snacks. One Indonesian favorite is nasi goring—Chinese fried rice topped with a European-introduced fried egg. Steamed rice in Malaysia is often served with both an Indian-influenced meat or fish and a Chinese stir-fried vegetable. Fish is very common (often fried) and eaten by all groups except some vegetarian Buddhists (who prefer tofu- or tempeh-based dishes). Beef and poultry are popular but costly in much of Malaysia and Indonesia, while pork is uncommon in the majority of Muslim areas. The exception is Singapore, a wealthier nation, which includes abundant meat and egg dishes in its fare. Temperate vegetables introduced from the Middle East and Europe, such as tomatoes, eggplants, and potatoes, are usually added to soups and rice dishes instead of being served separately. Salads are popular, however, an example of which is Indonesian gado gado, a mixture of cooked vegetables (including cabbage, green beans, and carrots) dressed with peanut sauce.
Tropical fruits are eaten at nearly every meal—fresh, preserved, in baked goods and puddings, and deep-fried as fritters.

Coconut flavors many foods, and seasonings are used liberally, including chilies, fresh coriander, ginger, lemongrass, pandanus leaf, pepper, and turmeric. Lemons, limes, unripe mangoes, tamarind, or vinegar are usually added for a sour taste. The most distinctive cooking in the region is Nyonya fare, found especially in Singapore, which combines Chinese preparations (often pork-based) with Malaysian seasonings, particularly coconut, turmeric, and lemongrass.

All courses are served at once in Malaysian, Singaporean, and Indonesian meals, and the dishes are categorized by preparation technique, not ingredients. For example, sambals are fried dishes seasoned with chilies (or the name for just a chili dipping sauce); satays are delicate, grilled kebabs (of Middle Eastern origin) served with dipping sauces; croquettes (from the Dutch influence) are fried rice, meat, vegetable; or fruit fritters; and sayur are soupy dishes with ample sauce for dipping rice balls. In most areas, forks and spoons are used (knives are rarely used). One tradition is universal in the region: street vendors. Meals and snacks are usually available around the clock at food stalls and small eateries, and al fresco dining is a daily event. Singapore has one of the most renowned street food scenes in the world. Many of these eateries have earned Michelin stars, a hallmark of culinary excellence.

and mint, are often added to foods as they are served, providing distinctive flavors and color to many dishes. Both Laotian laap, a spicy ground meat or fish dish (traditionally prepared uncooked), and Vietnamese grilled lemon grass beef, bo nuong xa, are served with a substantial garnish of basil, mint, and coriander leaves. Due to the strong influence of the French, the Vietnamese also frequently eat asparagus, green beans (haricots), and potatoes; though the French had less impact on the cuisine of surrounding nations, subsequent Vietnamese rule has popularized these vegetables in other regions as well.

Tropical fruits are available, although in some areas bananas and plantains are the only fruit widely consumed. Banana leaves are used to wrap rice, vegetables, and meats for steaming in both Cambodia and Laos. Pineapple, papaya, limes, mangoes, and mangosteens are common, as are soursop, star fruit, guavas, custard apples, durian, jackfruit, and tamarind (a pod with very tart pulp). Oranges, lemons, melons, and sugarcane are also popular.

Food for Thought

In Vietnam, com, meaning cooked rice, is the same word used for "food."

Mahayana Vietnamese Buddhists who are not strict vegetarians often practice a vegetarianism diet 6 days per month: the 8th, 14th, 15th, 23rd, and the last two days of the lunar month.

"Without fish sauce or salt, life is nothing," according to a Vietnamese saying.

In Vietnam, foods are customarily seasoned with a salty sauce made from fermented fish called nuoc mam. It can be transformed into a hot sauce, nuoc cham, with the addition of chilies, vinegar, sugar, garlic, and citrus fruit juice. In Cambodia, the fermented fish sauce is called tuk-trey; a stronger fish paste is also used, known as prahoc. The Laotian version of fish sauce is nam pa; pa dek is the fermented fish paste.

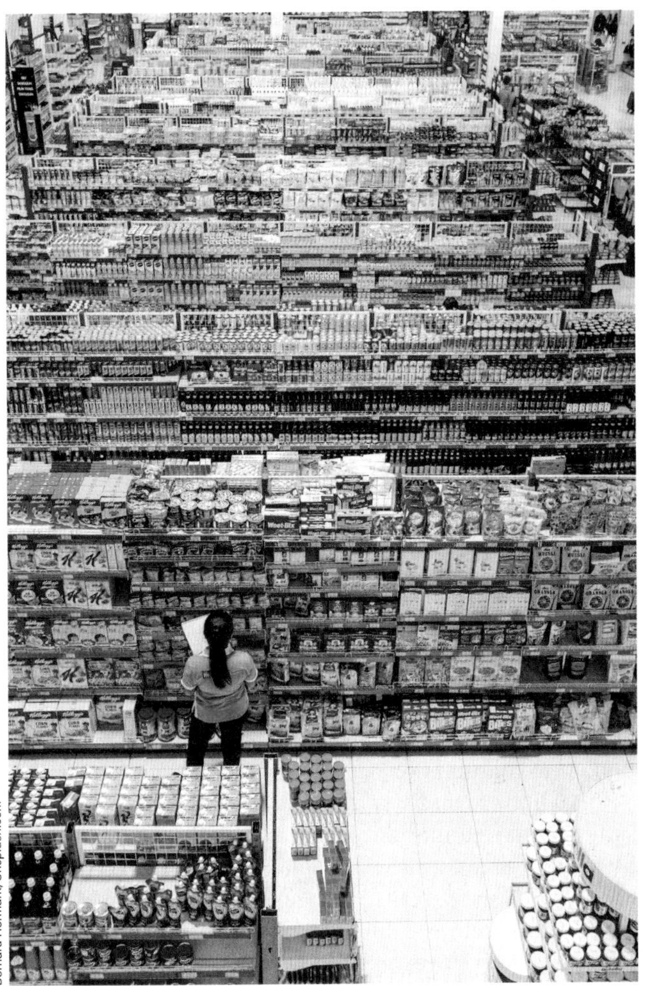
Bernard Hermant/Unsplash.com

▲ The rise in processed food trends in Asia can be readily seen in grocery stores.

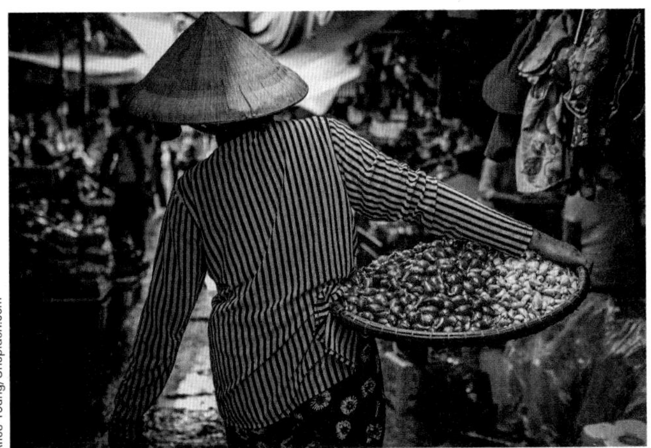
Alice Young/Unsplash.com

▲ Shoppers choose from a wide selection of tropical fruits and vegetables in a Southeast Asian traditional street market.

Tea is the preferred beverage throughout mainland Southeast Asia. In Vietnam, it is served before and after meals but not during the meal. Tea is often blended with flowers such as rose petals, jasmine blossoms, chrysanthemums, and lotus blossoms (which are especially popular). Coffee is popular in French-influenced areas, usually served with large amounts of sweetened condensed milk added to it. Broth is traditionally consumed at meals, and in less afluent, rural regions, such as where the Hmong live, it is the only beverage besides water that is commonly available. In wealthier areas, men may drink beer, and women and children consume soft drinks during meals. Soybean drinks and fruit drinks are common; rice wine or whiskey is served on special occasions.

Food for Thought

Banh mi, a soft wheat bread sandwich filled with tasty Vietnamese-spiced meats, first came to Vietnam through soldiers during the French colonization with the name "baguette," though banh mi usually has a fluffier texture than classic French baguettes, and crispier crust due to Vietnamese cooking techniques used.[46]

Hot pots, stir-fried foods, and chao (rice gruel similar to congee) are especially popular. Soups are a specialty, particularly pho bo ha noi, a delicate broth to which rice noodles, sliced beef, bean sprouts, herbs, and other seasonings are added immediately before serving. Mein go is a chicken noodle soup served similarly. Other favorites include stuffed tofu, bun cha (grilled pork over noodles), and snails (stir-fried, simmered in beer, or minced with garlic). The central region is known for sophisticated gastronomy. Presentation is emphasized and seasonal cooking reigns. Specialties include a sauce similar to nuoc mam made from shrimp called mam tom, shrimp pâté grilled on sugar cane, spicy pork sausages, sweet soups, vermicelli soups, and both sweet and salty rice cakes. The climate of the South is tropical. Cooking is simpler and seasoning is stronger; curries and spicy Indonesian-style peanut sauces are favorites. Coconut milk and caramel flavor many dishes. Clay pot cooking is common. One specialty is tidbits of grilled meats, fresh vegetables, and fruits such as guava, mango, green papaya, pineapple, or starfruit wrapped in a lettuce leaf, according to personal preference, that can be dipped in salty or spicy sauces. Sweets are more popular in the south than in other areas.

Khmer cooking in Cambodia features northern Indian, Malaysian, and Chinese elements. Although French cooking is much admired, it has never been integrated into the Khmer

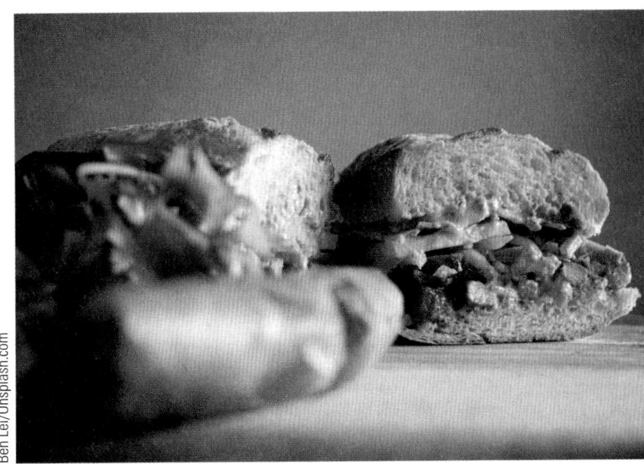
Ben Lei/Unsplash.com

▲ Vietnamese banh mi sandwich.

kitchen.[47] Aromatic seasonings are preferred, particularly the paste known as kroeung, made fresh for each dish from pulverized herbs and spices such as galangal, garlic, makrut lime leaves, lemongrass, shallots, and turmeric. A touch of spice is achieved with chili peppers, though it is usually moderated by the use of coconut milk. Sweet ingredients, such as ripe fruit or sugar, are often included as a contrast to the sour flavor provided by vinegar, lime juice, or tamarind. Salty fish sauce or soy sauce is always added, as are bitter herbs for balance. Amok, fish in coconut milk steamed in a banana or collard leaf, is a national favorite as is num banh choc, a rice noodle and fish soup. In some areas, dishes featuring wild foods such as land crabs, snakes, and locusts are found.

Laotians prefer sticky rice over long-grain types. Added vegetables and fish make up the basic diet, with eggs, poultry, and beef included as affordable. In rural areas, game such as deer, squirrels, ducks, quail, lizards, frogs, snakes, and grasshoppers are common. Meats are frequently stewed or grilled, though a salty beef jerky prepared with nam pa, a fish sauce, is a specialty. Coconut cream or milk, nam pa and pa dek (thick fish paste), lime juice, fresh coriander leaves, garlic, lemongrass, and mint are typical seasonings. Hot chili peppers add heat to most foods, though the extent of their use varies regionally. Spicy salads consisting of fresh vegetables or shredded immature papaya topped with lime juice, palm sugar, and chili pepper dressing are popular. Chinese and French influence via Vietnam is seen in some areas where French bread, croissants, spring rolls, and a soup similar to pho are popular foods.

Hmong fare traditionally differs from Laotian cooking and shares some similarities with Vietnamese cuisine. Long-grain rice is favored and stir-frying, steaming, and roasting are common preparation methods. Although rice and vegetables are the foundation of the diet, families sometimes raise chickens, ducks, pigeons, and pigs. These foods are supplemented with wild game and fish, crabs, and snails. Seasonings, however, are similar to Laotian, though the Hmong use soy sauce in addition to fish sauces. Hmong who were forced from the mountains to the lowlands during Southeast Asian conflicts have added many Laotian foods to their meals.

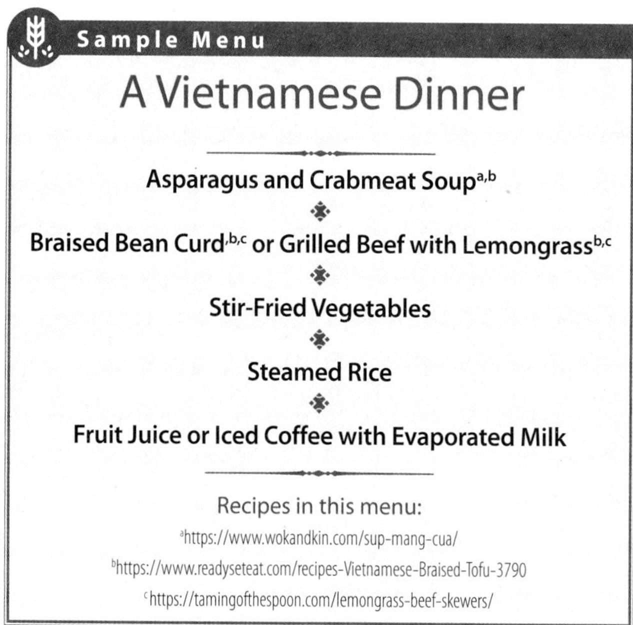
Sample Menu

A Vietnamese Dinner

Asparagus and Crabmeat Soup[a,b]

Braised Bean Curd[b,c] or Grilled Beef with Lemongrass[b,c]

Stir-Fried Vegetables

Steamed Rice

Fruit Juice or Iced Coffee with Evaporated Milk

Recipes in this menu:

[a] https://www.wokandkin.com/sup-mang-cua/

[b] https://www.readyseteat.com/recipes-Vietnamese-Braised-Tofu-3790

[c] https://tamingofthespoon.com/lemongrass-beef-skewers/

Meal Composition and Cycle

Daily Pattern

Filipino The traditional meal pattern in the Philippines is three meals a day. Breakfast is often garlic fried rice with eggs or broiled fish, sausage, or meat, plus coffee or hot chocolate; bread may be substituted for rice. Especially popular are sweet, cheesy rolls called ensaymada. Lunch and dinner are often large meals, characteristically including soup, rice, a crispy or chewy dish (such as fried fish), a salty dish (meat or poultry cooked in fish sauce or soy sauce), a sour dish (flavored predominantly with vinegar or tamarind), a noodle dish, and often, an adobo dish. Fresh fruit or dessert concludes the meal. The diets of Filipino Americans have changed substantially, with twice as many calories from protein and three times as many from fat. Dairy consumption, meat consumption, fat, and sugar have also increased.[48]

In addition to meals, two snacks, called meriendas, are consumed in the mid-morning and late afternoon. Meriendas may be small or may consist of substantial amounts of food, such as fritters, pastries, fruits, ensaymadas (spiral-shaped pastry made with sweet yeast dough), lumpia (fried spring rolls), or almost anything else except rice, which is served only at meals.

Vietnamese and Other Mainland Southeast Asians Mainland Southeast Asians eat two or three meals a day with the number of meals and the amount of food consumed often based on income. Snacking is uncommon. Southeast Asians do not usually associate particular foods with breakfast, lunch, or dinner. For example, soups are especially popular and are often consumed with every meal.

In Vietnam, the traditional diet is usually low-fat and plant-focused. Breakfast is large and may consist of soup with rice noodles topped with meat or poultry; a boiled egg with meat and pickled vegetables on French bread; chao with bits of leftover meat and vegetables; steamed rice cakes or Chinese-style crullers; or sticky rice or boiled sweet potatoes with sugar, coconut, and chopped roasted peanuts. A strong cup of coffee may accompany the meal. Lunch and dinner typically include rice, fish or meat, a vegetable dish, and a broth with vegetables or meat. Fresh vegetables and pickled garnishes are served with the meal. All items are served at once, and individual diners place whatever foods they wish over their portion of rice and flavor it as desired with nuoc mam and other condiments. French bread with meat or shrimp pâté may be substituted for a lunch or dinner meal. In the late afternoon, tea or coffee may be enjoyed with a sweet custard, pastry, candy, or a piece of fruit. Rice is consumed at almost every meal. Pho is a rice noodle soup made with beef or chicken broth has become quite popular in the United States.

Cambodians also often eat family style. Soups are often served for breakfast and accompany the main course at nearly every other meal. Steamed or fried rice or rice noodles are the centerpieces of lunch and dinner, accompanied by grilled or steamed freshwater fish and seafood, and less frequently poultry, pork, or beef. Fresh salads are common. Fruit is often eaten as a dessert, though very sweet rice or corn dishes are also popular. Tea and coffee with condensed milk are usually consumed with the meal, and fruit juices, soft drinks, and beer may be available. In Laos glutinous (sticky) rice, fish, poultry or meat, soup, and a cooked vegetable dish or fresh salads make up most meals. Chili pepper paste is the standard condiment. Tea, coffee with condensed milk, and rice wine or rice whiskey round out the menu.

Food for Thought

Turo-Turo are fast food stands or small restaurants in the Philippines specializing in rice bowls topped with foods according to the customer's preference. Other hot items are also available.

Most Filipinos today eat with utensils, but the traditional way of eating is kamayan, or "with hands." As it is in other Asian nations, the tactile experience of hand-eating is a literal connection to land and nourishment. A Filipino kamayan is also a family-style meal, usually served over banana leaves. During colonization, eating with your hands was considered lowly and improper by the colonizers.[49]

Etiquette Filipinos often dine at tables equipped with lazy Susan turntables so that dishes are accessible to everyone. Traditionally, no one starts eating until the eldest at the table begins. Many Filipinos use a Western style of dining with forks, knives, and spoons. Others employ just forks and spoons. The spoon is used to hold the food down while the fork is used to pull bits away. The food is then pushed onto the spoon with the fork and eaten. Chopsticks may be used for Chinese dishes. Small mounds of rice are rolled between the index finger, middle finger, and thumb to form a ball that is dipped into a sauce, then pressed into a bit of meat or poultry, and popped whole into the mouth. It is considered rude to take the last bits of food from the central platter.[50]

In Vietnam, it is polite to wait for the eldest person to be served and then, after everyone else is served, to ask him or her if it is okay to eat. It is a breach of good manners to refuse any offer of food, yet when served, only small amounts of any single dish should be taken. If sufficient amounts remain, seconds will be offered.[52] Throughout mainland Southeast Asia, an empty plate or cup indicates that the diner is still hungry or thirsty. Leaving a small amount of food or beverage signals satiety.

Traditional dining in Vietnam is done on a low table with the family gathered around, sitting cross-legged on mats. Both hands customarily rest on the table while dining, and conversation is limited. In contrast, dinner is a time for socializing in Laos. The food is served on a low rattan tray, and women gather on one side, the men on the other side. Each diner eats from the dishes as desired.

A variety of utensils are used to eat in Southeast Asia mainland nations. Chopsticks are used for most dishes in most of Vietnam, though spoons and fingers are considered appropriate for certain foods and in some regions. Rural Laotians often eat with their fingers, using balls of sticky rice to scoop up fish, meats, vegetables, and sauce; however, spoons are used as needed. In urban areas forks are now common. Hmong typically employ forks and spoons, and Cambodians use spoons, chopsticks, or fingers dependent on the food.

Special Occasions

Filipino In the predominantly Catholic Philippines, religious festivals and saints' days are numerous (refer to Chapter 4). On all special occasions, it is customary to serve plenty of food buffet-style with a roasted pig (lechon) as the centerpiece. The Filipinos claim to have the longest Christmas season in the world, from the first Sunday of Advent in late November or early December to January 6. The midnight Mass celebrated on Christmas Eve is usually followed by the traditional medianoche—a midnight supper of fiesta foods such as roast ham, sweet potatoes, and banana flower salad—or nilaga—a dish made of boiled meat, onions, and vegetables whose name means "good life"—and hot chocolate. Other specialties eaten during the Christmas season are puto bumbong, a rice flour delicacy cooked in a whistling bamboo kettle, and bibingka, a glutinous rice cake cooked in a clay pan topped with salted egg slices, kesong puti cheese, and a bit of coconut.

A midnight Mass is also held on New Year's Eve, but many Filipinos attend parties to celebrate the holiday instead. Again, a midnight supper consisting of celebratory foods is traditional. There is also a superstition that eating seven grapes in succession as the clock strikes midnight will bring good luck in the coming year. For birthdays, the pancit is eaten to ensure a long life.

There are numerous Filipino practices and customs associated with Easter, beginning with observances on Ash Wednesday. Late on Easter Eve, young children are awakened to partake of special meat dishes, such as adobo and dinuguan, in the belief that if they do not do so, they will become deaf. In May, fiestas honoring the Virgin Mary often include family feasts.

Vietnamese and Other Mainland Southeast Asians Of all Vietnamese holidays, Tet, the New Year's celebration, is the most important. Tet is observed at the end of the lunar year (end of January or beginning of February) just after the rice harvest.

In Vietnam, the first Tet ritual is an observance at the family gravesites. Offerings of cake, chicken, tea, rice, and alcohol, as well as money, are made at the graves, and then the family picnics on the offerings.

The second ritual, held on the 23rd day of the 12th lunar month, is to celebrate the departure of the Spirit of the Hearth, Ong Tao. He is represented by three stones on which the cooking pots are placed and is honored by a small altar. Like the Chinese Kitchen God, Ong Tao returns to the celestial realm each year and reports on the family's behavior. After the family makes an offering to symbolize his departure, they share a feast including glutinous rice cakes and a very sweet soybean soup. One week later the family celebrates Ong Tao's return to their hearth. The following day is the first day of Tet. Guests (especially those with favorable names, such as Tho, meaning "longevity") are entertained with tea, rice alcohol, red-dyed watermelon seeds, candied fruits, and vegetables.

Food for Thought

Hospitality is very important to Filipinos, and food gifts to express love or appreciation are common.

Special dishes prepared for the week-long celebration include banh chung, sticky rice cakes filled with meat and beans and boiled in banana leaves, squid soup, stir-fried young seasonal vegetables, pork with lotus root, and sometimes a special shark fin soup.

Many Vietnamese, including those in the United States, celebrate the Buddhist holiday called Trung Nguyen, or Wandering Souls Day. It occurs in the middle of the seventh lunar month and is celebrated with a large banquet prepared in honor of the lost souls of ancestors. Traditionally, the Vietnamese did not commemorate birthdays but rather honored their ancestors on the anniversary of their death with a special celebration and meal. Everyone's birthday is celebrated at the beginning of a new year on New Year's Day. In the United States, it is now more common for Vietnamese people to celebrate birthdays.

The largest holiday of the year in Cambodia is also the New Year's Day celebration, Chaul Chnam, which begins on April 13th and lasts for three days. Prayers and special foods like fried coconut and fried bananas rolled in coconut are offered to the New Year Angel, who descends with either blessings or ill will. The Water Festival, held in November after the seasonal rains have ended, features colorful floats in local rivers.

Most Laotian holidays are religious in origin and are celebrated at local temples. Pha Vet, which occurs in the fourth lunar month, commemorates the life of Buddha. Boon Bang Fay, held in the sixth lunar month, also honors the Buddha with a fireworks display. Among the Hmong and other Laotians, the New Year's celebration is a major event. It begins with the first crow of a rooster on the first day of the new moon in the twelfth lunar month, usually in December. The highlight of the festivities is the world renewal ritual, which involves an elder who chants while holding a live chicken. He circles a tree three times clockwise to remove the accumulated evil of the previous year and then circles the tree three more times counterclockwise to invoke good fortune in the upcoming year. The bad luck collects in the blood of the chicken, which is traditionally taken to a remote location and slaughtered. Customarily considered a good time to meet future wives and husbands, New Year's was the one time each year when Hmong from different clans celebrated together.

Therapeutic Uses of Food

Filipino When the Spanish came to the Philippines, they introduced the hot–cold theory of health and diet (refer to Chapter 9). Foods are classified as being hot or cold based on their innate qualities or their effect on the body, not on their spiciness or temperature. Although the classification of certain foods varies regionally, avocados, alcoholic beverages, coconuts, nuts, legumes, spices, chili peppers, and fatty meats are generally considered hot items; tropical fruits, vegetables, milk and dairy foods, eggs, fish, and lean or inexpensive meats are regarded as cold. A balance is attempted at meals between hot and cold elements. The many ingredients chosen in Filipino dishes are thought to ensure this balance.

Some illnesses are characterized as hot or cold and are treated with foods of the opposite category. Diarrhea and fevers are hot; colds and chills are cold. Other food beliefs are based on sympathetic qualities ("like causes like"). Sometimes the meaning behind therapeutic food use is more obscure; horseradish leaves and broth seasoned with ginger are believed to promote milk production in nursing mothers, and fish heads and onions are considered brain food by some Filipinos. Honey, as well as certain herbs such as thyme, marjoram, and chamomile, is used to treat diabetes. Licorice root is considered a general tonic, especially beneficial during times of stress. Some older Filipinos have adopted the Asian Indian practice of chewing areca nuts (also called betel nuts), which is believed to prevent tooth decay, although it leaves permanent stains.[51]

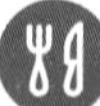

Food for Thought

A feast is held by the Hmong following the birth of a child. Included are two chickens representing the parents, a boiled egg signifying the child, and a small lit candle symbolic of the ancestor spirits whose blessing and protection are sought.

Feu is a Laotian beef noodle soup similar to Vietnamese phở.

The Department of Health in the Philippines has approved several herbal remedies as safe and effective, including ampalaya (bitter melon, prepared as a side dish or as a juice) for diabetes, bawang (garlic) to lower blood cholesterol levels and reduce blood pressure, ulasaming bato (pepperomia, which is eaten as a salad or brewed into tea) for arthritis and gout, and sambong (an indigenous herb) as a diuretic.[51]

Kratom (*Mitragyna speciosa*) is a medicinal plant that is smoked, chewed, or brewed and can be bought in local coffee shops in some regions of Southeast Asia. It has been used traditionally to fight fatigue and used as a drink in social settings. It has also been used for common ailments such as fever, cough, hypertension, diabetes, pain, and anxiety. In urban areas adulterated kratom cocktails are being consumed by younger people as a euphoric recreational drug.[52]

Vietnamese and Other Mainland Southeast Asians Many Vietnamese follow the Chinese yin–yang theory of health and diet (refer to the section titled "Therapeutic Uses of Food" in Chapter 11). Yin is known as âm and yang is called duong. As in the hot–cold system, classification is based on intrinsic characteristics rather than temperature or spiciness. Examples of duong (hot) foods are red meat, unripe fruit, ginger, garlic, coffee, and alcoholic beverages. Âm (cold) items include noodles, bananas, oranges, gelatin, and ice cream.[53] Some foods, such as rice, pork, eggs, chicken broth, teas, and sweets, are classified as neutral. Not only must a balance be maintained within a meal, but extremes are also avoided during certain conditions, such as pregnancy. As with Filipinos and other Asians, illnesses are defined as âm and duong and are sometimes caused by eating too many âm or too many duong foods. During pregnancy, which is duong, hot foods are avoided, and equilibrium is restored by eating foods of the opposite type; during the postpartum period, which is âm, cold foods are avoided. Yin and yang concepts are less prevalent among Cambodians and Laotians, although some hot and cold beliefs exist regarding specific foods and certain conditions.

The Chinese medical system details other influential elements in health, including the five flavors of sour, bitter, sweet, pungent, and salty; these tastes are harmonized in many Vietnamese dishes. Vietnamese believe that ingestion of specific organ meats will benefit the like internal organs. For example, consumption of liver will produce a stronger liver. Some Vietnamese believe that eating gelatinous tiger bones (produced by prolonged cooking) will make them strong. Concurrently, some foods may be injurious because they resemble certain disorders. Pregnant women may refuse to eat ginger because the multilobed root is thought to cause polydactyly (too many digits) in babies.[53]

Food taboos and perinatal food avoidance are commonly practiced across Southeast Asia. Cambodians may drink water with bitter melon for fevers. Vietnamese women may consume large amounts of salty foods during pregnancy,[54] and mothers may avoid feeding chicken or duck to their babies to prevent them from becoming deaf or mute.[54] Hmong women eat a diet of rice, chicken broth, black pepper, and herbs for a month after giving birth, and some clans have specific taboos against eating certain foods, such as heart.[55,56]

Contemporary Food Habits in the United States

Adaptations of Food Habits

Filipino Most Filipino Americans can obtain traditional foodstuffs without much difficulty, although some of the familiar tropical fresh fruits and vegetables are not available. Research shows that most Filipinos still eat rice every day but not with every meal, and their diets tend to contain a greater variety of foods, especially more milk, green vegetables, meat, and sweets than they did in the Philippines.[57–60] Meriendas are not eaten as often as in the Philippines.

Filipinos born in the United States frequently consume a typical American diet. Breakfast consists of cereal, toast, eggs or meat, juice, and coffee; sandwiches, salads, and sodas are common at lunch; and dinner is usually a meat or fish dish served with rice or potatoes, followed by dessert. Traditional Filipino items may appear at some meals, such as eating longaniza sausage at breakfast or eating halo-halo (a layered treat, sometimes topped with vanilla ice cream) for dessert.[61]

Vietnamese and Other Mainland Southeast Asians A study conducted in Washington, DC, found that 30 percent of the Vietnamese households surveyed had changed their eating habits since coming to the United States.[62,63] Although most continued to eat rice at least once a day, they ate more bread or instant noodles at lunch and more cereal at breakfast. Respondents also reported consuming more meat and poultry and less fish and shellfish than in Vietnam, mainly because of cost. Pork and pork products were still preferred to beef. They also reported consuming fewer bananas but more oranges, fruit juices, and soft drinks. Research indicates that Vietnamese Americans have higher BMI (body mass index) and abdominal obesity than their counterparts in the Philippines. These factors increase the risks of chronic disease.[61]

A recent study indicates that Asian American youth in general consume milk, fruit, meat, unenriched white rice, vegetables, and high-fat and high-sugar items in diets characterized by both Asian and American foods.[64] A sample of Hmong adults in central California revealed their struggle in making healthier food choices with both American and Hmong food while trying to preserve their culture and identity. Rice was cited as a staple consumed at every meal. Foods such as desserts were not part of Hmong food traditionally and fruit was considered nontraditional or consumed as an appetizer for special occasions. Understanding of food patterns and health was found to be strong, and most felt traditional foods were healthier. Participants felt younger Hmong generations did eat traditional food, though the practice of passing on traditional food preparation, recipes, and cultural traditions was becoming less common due to the acculturation of the Western culture.[65]

Food for Thought

Some young Hmong women avoid eating gizzards because they are believed to toughen the placenta and make birth difficult.

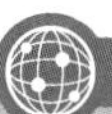

Exploring Global Cuisine

Thai Fare

There are approximately 12 times more Filipino Americans and six times more Vietnamese Americans than there are Thai Americans in the United States. Yet Thai cooking is more familiar to the general population than either Filipino or Vietnamese fare. The popularity of Thai cuisine and the proliferation of Thai restaurants in the United States began in the 1980s due in part to a planned push by the Thai government to standardize training in Thai cuisine and send chefs around the world. Then, too, Americans began going to Thailand during the 1950s and 1960s in the military or as Peace Corps volunteers and Fulbright fellows, and Thai students that came to U.S. universities early on stayed and opened restaurants. These groups began creating cookbooks and introducing and popularizing the cuisine in the United States.[66] In 2008, Thai restaurants were 16 percent of the total U.S. market share in the restaurant industry. They introduced distinctive cuisine in many parts of the United States, even where few Thai Americans live.[67]

The country of Thailand is located on the southern end of the archipelago that is Southeast Asia. The hot, monsoonal climate is ideal for rice cultivation. Long-grain rice is the foundation of the diet, though short-grain sticky rice is used for snacks and desserts and is preferred in the regional Issan cuisine of the northeast (similar to Cambodian fare, also known for its culinary use of insects).[68] Noodles made of rice, wheat, or mung beans are also common. Both tropical and temperate fruits and vegetables are prominent in the cuisine. Seafood from the lengthy coast, especially shrimp, is popular. Dried herring-like fish (which are sometimes smoked as well) are often flaked into rice for added flavor. Beef, chicken, and pork are common. Duck is a favorite. Favorite dishes include som tum, also known as Thai papaya salad, made with fresh, crisp green papaya slices mixed with local tomatoes, chilies, garlic, and fish sauce; larb, a typical Isaan dish, made with minced meat mixed with ground toasted rice, shallots, spring onions, mint leaves, and seasoned with chili, lime juice, and fish sauce.[69]

Thai food differs from that of its Southeast Asian neighbors because of its flavors. It can be one of the hottest cuisines in the world, with lavish use of chili peppers. Several varieties of basil, fresh coriander leaves and root, galangal, garlic, ginger root, makrut lime leaves, lemon grass, mint, and tamarind are typical seasonings. In addition, curried dishes are eaten daily. There are three types: yellow curries, which are smooth, mild, Indian-like sauces that include spices such as cardamom and turmeric; red curries, which are often hotter sauces that typically include ample red chilies and coconut milk; and green curries, which are prepared with fresh green chilies cilantro, makrut lime leaf and peel, and basil. Fermented fish products, such as nam pla (similar to the Vietnamese sauce called nuoc mam) and kapi (a paste made from fish or shrimp), are added to most dishes. Nam prik, a sauce that combines nam pla or kapi with other ingredients like garlic, peppers, shallots, lime juice, tamarind, palm sugar, and peanuts, complements dishes such as yam (fresh vegetables rolled up into a leafy package and dipped into the nam prik), salads (nam prik is the dressing), noodle dishes, dumplings, fried or grilled foods, and highly spiced raw pork called nam. Noodle dishes are usually eaten for breakfast and lunch. Phad Thai—stir-fried noodles cooked with bits of meat, seafood, and vegetables bound with eggs, then topped with peanuts and nam prik—is an example. Sweets such as coconut custards, sweet sticky rice with mango, and fruit jellies are preferred snacks.

Some types of Thai cooking began as a court cuisine, and this heritage is most obvious in dishes that use the freshest ingredients, have no bones, pits, or stones, and in which all flavors are perfectly balanced, including spiciness. Some dishes in this category include *sangkaya fak ton*, steamed pumpkin stuffed with coconut custard, mieng kum or a wild betel leaf-wrapped appetizer, and gaeng ranjuan—beef soup with fermented shrimp paste.[70,71] Royal cuisine or not, Thai dinner often includes appetizers, such as deep-fried chicken wings stuffed with ground pork and shrimp or pastries shaped like delicate flowers. The main meal traditionally features steamed rice, soup, a curried dish, a fried dish, and a salad of raw vegetables and grilled poultry, beef, or seafood. Mee krob, a volcanic-looking mound of stir-fried noodles and meats or seafood cooked with sugar until caramelized, is a favorite addition. Various nam prik accompany the dishes. All dishes are served at the same time. Fingers and spoons are the usual implements, and forks are available for pushing food into the spoon. The meal usually concludes with elaborately carved fruits.

Food purchasing and preparation as well as meal patterns continue to change. Southeast Asian American women report that men frequently help with shopping or cooking. Vietnamese, Cambodian, and Laotian adolescents often are involved in food purchases, and surveys indicate as many as 60 percent of girls and 35 percent of boys have total responsibility for fixing dinner each evening. Southeast Asian women living in the United States are more likely to have a job or to attend adult education classes than in their homeland, relinquishing some household responsibilities to other family members. Further, many families report a significant decline in eating meals together.[72]

Nutritional Status

Nutritional Intake

Filipino Life expectancy rates for Filipino Americans are higher than for the general U.S. population at 78.8 years in 2019. Life expectancy in the Philippines was 71.3 years in 2019.[73] The traditional Filipino diet is higher in total fat, saturated fat, and cholesterol than most Asian diets, and urban Filipinos living in the United States tend to have an even higher intake of these dietary components.[74] Median body mass indexes (BMIs) in men and women are close to those of Whites in the United States, while rates of overweight and obesity are higher than in most other Asian groups. The percent of obese Asian men age 20 and over was 14.2 percent, and slightly higher for Asian women at 16 percent in 2018.[75,76] Filipino Americans have high rates of hypertension and serum cholesterol levels, equal to those of White Americans. Twenty-seven percent of Filipinos have reported being told that they had hypertension. Heart disease is the leading cause of death in mortality statistics for Filipinos, and strokes are the second. Filipinos develop type 2 diabetes (9 percent) more often than most other Asians. Filipina women are at an increased risk for developing gestational diabetes during pregnancy. Filipina women in the United States have been found to have larger waist circumferences and a higher percentage of visceral adipose tissue than White women despite lower overweight and obesity rates, suggesting more research is needed on metabolic syndrome (which is also higher in Filipinas) in non-obese populations.[76–78]

Many are lactose intolerant and calcium intake may therefore be limited. Dried fish, fish sauce, and fish paste may provide calcium, but amounts vary depending on the source and quality of the product. Some Filipinos may be at risk for calcium deficiency, particularly newer immigrant women during pregnancy and postpartum.[11]

Infant mortality rates are slightly below those for the general population.[79] When compared to other Asian groups, Filipino neonates are also at increased risk for death from infection and post neonatal infants from respiratory distress syndrome.[80] Breastfeeding rates in Southeast Asia and the Pacific have declined over the last 15 years. It has been estimated that the exclusive breastfeeding rate has decreased from 31 percent to 29 percent overall in Cambodia (refer to Figure 12.2). Breastfeeding can prevent up to 50 percent of child deaths due to diarrhea, can improve cognition and reduce monetary costs for families and governments in Southeast Asia. For these reasons, breastfeeding promotion has become a national priority.[80]

In addition, Filipino rates for hyperuricemia (resulting in gouty arthritis) and glucose-6-phosphate dehydrogenase deficiency (causing anemia unrelated to iron intake) are also higher than for White Americans. It should also be noted that alpha thalassemia (hemoglobin H disease) is also prevalent and results in hypochromic microcytic anemia, especially during an infection or when oxidant drugs are taken.

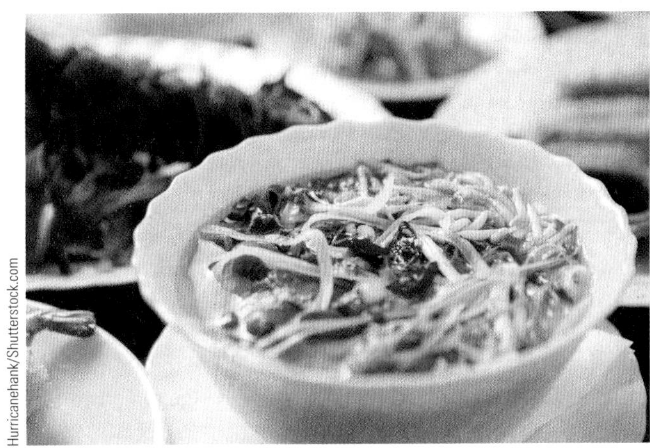

Hurricanehank/Shutterstock.com

▲ Vietnamese soup called pho has become very popular in the United States.

Vietnamese and Other Mainland Southeast Asians Food intake data suggest that the calcium intake of mainland Southeast Asians is low, although this observation does not account for fish sauces and other traditional foods that may contain sufficient calcium.[77] An analysis of broth made with acidified bones reported that one tablespoon provided nearly as much calcium as one-half cup of milk.[78] Vietnamese have been reported to have high rates of lactose intolerance.

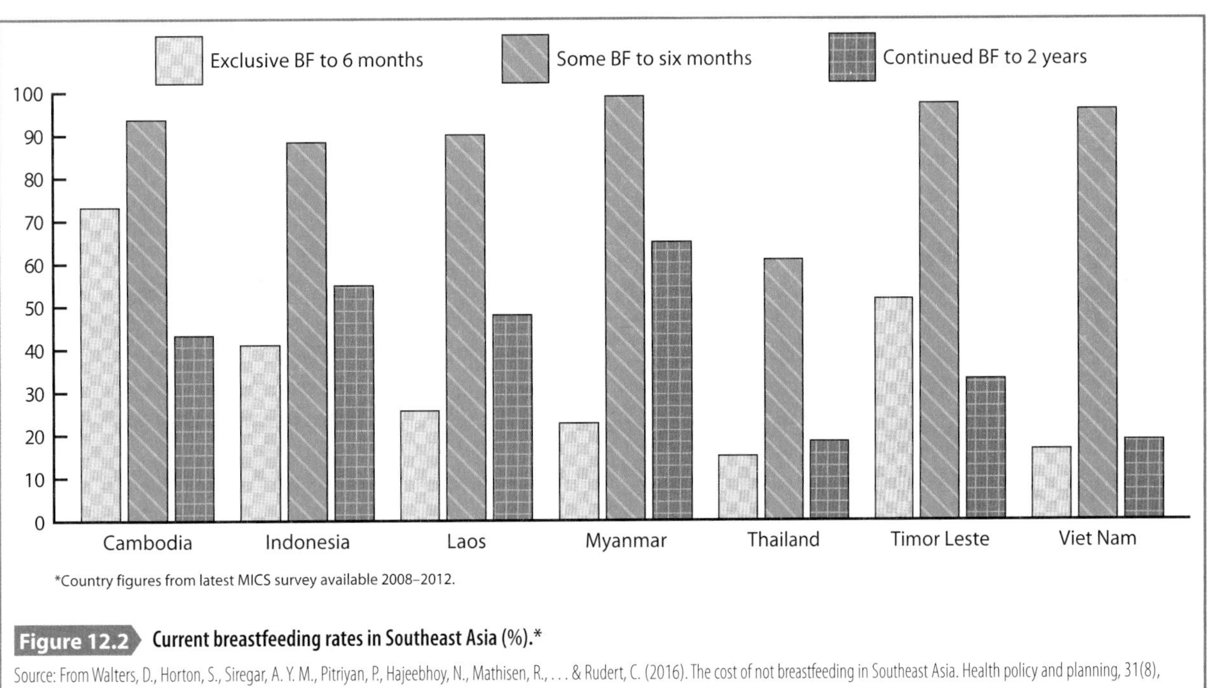

Figure 12.2 **Current breastfeeding rates in Southeast Asia (%).***

Source: From Walters, D., Horton, S., Siregar, A. Y. M., Pitriyan, P., Hajeebhoy, N., Mathisen, R., . . . & Rudert, C. (2016). The cost of not breastfeeding in Southeast Asia. Health policy and planning, 31(8), 1107–1116.

 **Food for Thought**

Certain Filipino dishes are very high in purines (a naturally found substance in some foods that produce uric acid crystals upon digestion that can build up in joints), a concern for patients with gout; dinu-guan, a savory stew, often includes pork liver, kidney, heart, and small intestine which are high in purines.

Very little health and nutrition research has investigated the children and grandchildren of Southeast Asian immigrants from specific countries, but other studies have shown that diet and health risk factors are correlated to the adoption of American culture and lifestyle. As previously mentioned, Asian American women have the highest life expectancy (86.7 years) of any other ethnic group in the United States. The following health conditions are more common for these ethnic groups: cancer, heart disease, stroke, unintentional injuries (accidents), and type 2 diabetes (at a lower BMI).[81] Asian Americans also have a high prevalence of the following conditions and risk factors: chronic obstructive pulmonary disease, hepatitis B, HIV/AIDS, smoking, tuberculosis, and liver disease.[81–83] Thalassemia, a genetic form of anemia, is more common in Southeast Asians and is not due to an iron deficiency. In a study of California Asian groups, Cambodian and Laotian women had adverse maternal risk profiles and higher death rates than Whites for neonates, postnatal infants, and infants. Prenatal screening is important for the diagnosis and treatment of thalassemia.[84]

 **Food for Thought**

Mien people from southern China or southeast Asia now in California, are at high risk for trichinosis infection due to the use of raw pork in dishes such as laap.

Southeast Asians typically calculate age on a lunar calendar, often starting with being one year old at birth. Reported age may differ as much as two years from Western chronological age, which can distort the use of standardized growth curves. Some Vietnamese parents may claim, however, that their children are younger than they are to enroll them in lower school grades.

Numerous studies have noted that the now older refugees from mainland Southeast Asia are at special risk for mental health problems, due to the horrors of war, difficulties in escape, lengthy camp confinement, and the extreme cultural differences between their homeland and the United States and some instances of racial prejudice and discrimination.[85,86] Post-traumatic stress disorder is common. One study of the Hmong suggests, however, that levels of depression, anxiety, hostility, and other symptoms of adjustment problems may gradually resolve with a length of stay. Adherence to traditional health beliefs varies, often according to whether new religious faiths have been adopted; Christian churches may strongly discourage ancestor and spirit worship. Some studies suggest that the majority of immigrants continue certain practices, such as the use of botanical home remedies and coining (refer to the section "Traditional Health Beliefs and Practices"), for many years after arrival although the costs and inconvenience of some traditional cures, including difficulties in obtaining animals and herbs, the disintegration of clan ties, and the scarcity of shamans present barriers in some communities. Southeast Asians frequently develop a medical pluralism, accepting those theories and therapeutics most congruent with their acculturation experiences.[87,88]

Because the postpartum period is defined as yin (cold), women avoid exposure to cold and wind (refer to the section "Traditional Health Beliefs and Practices"). Clients may

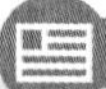 **New American Perspectives**

Han Le, Student

I was born in Vietnam but came to the United States when I was about a year old. My parents left Vietnam in 1976. My grandparents got us and about 35 other people out on a boat. We first went to a refugee camp in Malaysia, and after a few months, we were able to settle in Southern California.

At home, we ate a traditional diet, and I still do. Rice and noodles are staple foods. Breakfast is a French baguette with pâté and ham (there is a lot of pork in the diet). Lunch is soup or a bowl of rice with one entrée, usually a leftover from dinner. There are always three things for dinner: (1) always soup, (2) a stewed meat entrée, and (3) vegetable stir-fry. Fruit is usually served as dessert. Snacks are commonly fruit or sticky rice. Western foods that I eat now are dairy products such as milk, cheese, and yogurt; cereal for breakfast; and more sweets for dessert. I lost all my baby teeth due to cavities because I was given so much candy. In Vietnam, only children from wealthy families got candy, so it was a real treat here.

When we first came over, our neighbors gave my parents cereal to try, and they liked it. At that time my parents hardly spoke or read English, and there were very few Vietnamese markets. Because the cereal box had pictures of cats and dogs on it, when they went to the grocery store they bought a box of something with pictures of cats or dogs on it, but it turned out to be pet food. They ate the whole box, but they did put sugar on it because it wasn't sweet enough. This was not an uncommon problem when the Vietnamese first immigrated to the United States. A friend was enrolled in WIC (Women, Infants, and Children) while she was pregnant and had vouchers to buy WIC food at the market. She recognized the word *cheese* and she bought cream cheese and ate one package every day during her pregnancy.

When counseling Vietnamese, it is important to remember that our meal is not complete unless it contains rice or noodles. Therefore, you should not recommend eliminating these elements of the diet but rather just decrease their amount.

refuse to get out of bed soon after giving birth and refuse to take a shower or wash their hair. Âm foods, such as cold beverages and vegetables, may be refused even if prepared in a culturally sensitive manner. Women may consume alcoholic beverages because they are duong, and alcohol is also thought to cleanse the reproductive system and promote milk production. Hmong women also consider the postpartum period a cold condition.[88]

An in-depth interview is critical to determine the patient's country of origin (a patient may be offended if grouped with all other Southeast Asians), length of time in the United States, and any immediate health problems. The degree of acculturation and personal food preferences should also be noted.[88]

Oceania

Oceania encompasses some 10,000 islands and their inhabitants. Polynesia, Micronesia, and Melanesia are the three areas that make up the Pacific region. Polynesia includes the major islands and island groups of Hawaii, American Samoa, Western Samoa, Tonga, Easter Island, Tahiti, and the Society Islands. The 2,000 small islands of Micronesia include Guam, Kiribati, Nauru, the Marshall and Northern Mariana Islands, Palau, and the Federated States of Micronesia. Although the boundaries of Melanesia are not exact, it includes the nations of Fiji, Papua New Guinea, Vanuatu, the Solomon Islands, and the French dependency on New Caledonia.

Although the area is geographically similar, consisting of mostly small, tropical coral or volcanic islands, Oceania is racially and culturally diverse. European, American, and Japanese influences have been extensive. Today there are greater numbers of some Oceania communities living in the United States than in their native homelands.

Cultural Perspective

History of Oceania Immigrants in the United States

Immigration Patterns The migration of population groups has been very fluid among Polynesia, Micronesia, and Melanesia. As conditions on one island grew too crowded, colonization of surrounding islands occurred. That trend continues, with economic opportunity as the primary motivation for residents of Oceania to immigrate to the United States and other nations.

Hawaiians When British explorer James Cook first arrived in Hawaii, approximately 300,000 Native Hawaiians were living on the islands. European diseases introduced by the explorers and missionaries decimated the population, and by 1910 only a little more than 38,500 persons of Hawaiian ancestry remained. A high rate of intermarriage has resulted in a population with few Hawaiians of full native heritage. A large number of Hawaiians have migrated to the mainland United States, but the census figures do not reflect such interstate relocations.

Samoans In 1951, the Pago Pago naval base that employed many Samoans moved to Hawaii, and many Samoans followed. Increasing population pressures and a deteriorating economy encouraged further immigration. Once in Hawaii, Samoans sometimes move to the mainland United States in search of broader job availability and wider educational opportunities for their children. A chain of immigration between Hawaii and the West Coast has been created, with Samoans established on the mainland helping extended family members settle nearby.

Guamanians Following the attainment of citizenship in 1950, many Guamanians enlisted in the U.S. armed forces seeking better employment. Some moved to Hawaii and the West Coast of the U.S. mainland. By the early 1970s, approximately 12,000 Guamanians had immigrated, mostly Chamorros (native Micronesians). Major populations have settled in San Diego, Los Angeles, San Francisco, the Seattle area, and Hawaii.[89]

Tongans The immigration of Tongans to the United States did not begin until population pressures in the 1960s decreased economic opportunities in Tonga. Under the strict hereditary social structure, only the eldest son in a family may inherit the land, leaving younger men with little economic mobility. Unlike most other residents of Oceania, Tongans usually immigrate directly to the U.S. mainland rather than settling first in Hawaii.

New Zealand and Australia Oceania is dominated by the larger land masses of Australia, New Zealand, and New Guinea. These islands have mountain ranges, deserts, and semi-arid land. New Guinea has highland rainforests and a tropical climate similar to other Pacific islands. The first wave of immigration from Australia and New Zealand came in the 1850s for the California gold rush.[90,91] Assimilation has not been difficult for the majority of this group due to their native language being English.

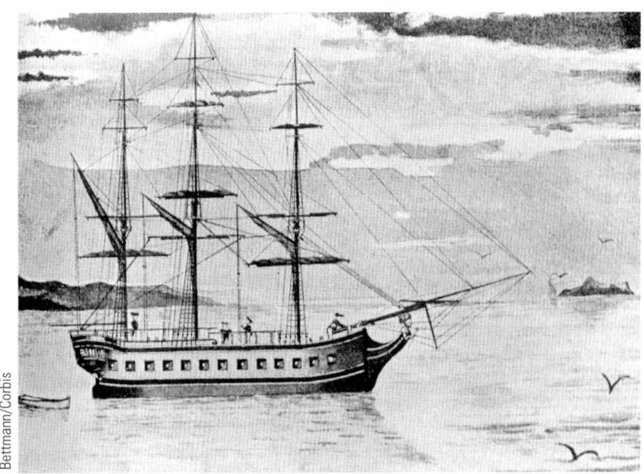
Bettmann/Corbis

▲ A rendering of the Resolution, the ship used by James Cook to explore Polynesia. Many Pacific Islander cultural traditions disappeared after European discovery of the islands in the eighteenth century.

Current Demographics and Socioeconomic Status

Hawaiians More than 1.4 million U.S. citizens self-identified as Native Hawaiians and Pacific Islanders (NHPI) in the 2021 U.S. Census estimate (note: NHPIs are referred to in this text as residents of Oceania). Over half a million are Native Hawaiians, and Samoans are the next largest group with under 200,000. More than half of NHPI people live in Hawaii and California. Scant socioeconomic data are available, but reports indicate that some Hawaiians occupy the lowest economic strata in the state of Hawaii, along with other Pacific Islander immigrants, living mostly in rural and semi-rural regions. Hawaiian heritage is less of a handicap on the mainland, where Hawaiians have a cultural advantage over other Pacific Islanders (through extensive exposure to U.S. society) and often enter the middle class. Overall, median family income is higher than the national average, and poverty rates are lower (9 percent) than the total U.S. figure. Over 92 percent have a high school degree and 33 percent have a college degree.[92]

Samoans Probably more Samoans are living outside Samoa than in American and Western Samoa combined. Over 213,439 Samoans total (alone and in combination with another ethnicity) are U.S. residents. The largest groups are found in Honolulu, Los Angeles, the San Francisco Bay Area, and Salt Lake City.[93]

Though nearly one-third of Samoans in the United States work in office and sales jobs, and 18 percent hold management and professional positions, another 30 percent of Samoans in the United States are employed in unskilled or semiskilled labor such as assembly line jobs, construction, janitorial or maintenance jobs, or as security guards. Median family income is lower than the national average.[94]

Guamanians The 2020 U.S. Census statistics indicate over 182,000 Guamanians are residing in the United States. Many are Chamorros, indigenous people of Guam, although the self-identification figures are unclear on the exact percentage. The Chamorros often become part of Pacific Islander communities (with Samoan and Tongan immigrants). Large populations of Guamanians are found in Hawaii, California, Washington State, and Washington, DC.[95]

Over one-quarter of Guamanians work in professional or management positions, and nearly one-third are employed in office and sales jobs. Their median family income is above the U.S. average. Nearly 50 percent of Guamanian adults have attended college, though graduation rates are well below the national average. Additionally, 22 percent of adults have not graduated from high school.[95]

Tongans Over 61,000 Tongans live in the United States according to U.S. 2020 Census figures.[97] Many are Mormons and are aided in their immigration by their church, and most move to communities of other immigrants from Oceania in San Francisco, Los Angeles, Dallas, Fort Worth, and Salt Lake City.[95]

Regarding educational attainment in the U.S. Tongan community, 81 percent of adults have graduated from high school. Median family income is higher than the national average.

New Zealand and Australia The number of U.S residents reporting Australian and New Zealand ancestry is about 128,018 according to the. the 2019 U.S. Census statistics. Of these, 12.5 percent completed high school, 31 percent attained a Bachelor's degree, and 30 percent attained a graduate degree. Twenty-one percent are in professional jobs and 33 percent are in education.[95]

Worldview

Religion Residents of Oceania follow a wide variety of religions, often according to which missionary groups were active in their homeland. Hawaiians practice mostly Protestantism, Buddhism, or Shintoism. Samoans are largely Methodist, Catholic, Mormon, and Anglican. Chomorros (people of Guam) are primarily Catholic, and Tongans in the United States are mostly Mormon. Religion is often prominent in daily life, and ministers usually are held in high esteem. In Samoa, nightly readings from the Bible are common in most homes, and prayers are offered at every meal.[96–98] People in New Zealand are 51 percent Christian (predominantly Anglican, Roman Catholic, and Presbyterian, but also other Christian denominations, including 1.6 percent Māori Christian). Other are Hindu (1.5 percent), Buddhist (1.3 percent), and nonreligious (31.1 percent).[99] Although many indigenous Māori are Christian today, traditional spirituality included a respect for the land, knowledge that Earth Mother gives birth to all things, and living in unity with nature.[100] In Australia, 52.1 percent of people are Christian (usually Catholic or Anglican), 29.6 percent are nonreligious, 2.6 percent follow Islam, 2.4 percent are Buddhist, 1.9 percent are Hindu, and just over 10 percent are not affiliated or "other."[101] Aboriginal peoples in Australia have practiced spirituality in which the spirit ancestors in the Creation made all the plants, animals, and people, and then gave the country meaning by shaping it and establishing the law. All beings strive to live in agreement with that legacy, and in celebration and reverence for past events called the Dreaming.[102]

Family Although most native religions were abandoned, many concepts central to Oceania culture remained within the structure of families. For example, on many islands, social rank and power were established by birth order within the extended kinship system or clan, and even within families, younger siblings deferred to their older brothers and sisters. Older family members were respected. The senior patriarch in the group, whether in the village or a family, managed all group matters. In Hawaii, people were segregated by gender under the *kapu* system, each with specific roles and responsibilities. Extended families were the foundation of society, and children were raised usually by grandparents, aunts and uncles, and even remote kin rather than by just the parents. Household composition was flexible, and all members were obligated to support the extended family, resulting in the substantial redistribution of resources. Generosity and sharing were highly valued. Any social transgressions committed by the individual were the responsibility of the whole family. In Samoa, if the violation was severe, the family could be disinherited from their land and stripped of any social title.[103]

Food for Thought

Over 45,000 Fijians live in the United States. Most are of Asian-Indian descent and were originally indentured laborers in Fiji. Though overall educational attainment can be low, median family income approaches the national average, and poverty rates are significantly lower than the norm.[104]

Certain fish in Hawaii were reserved for royalty and, traditionally, women rarely consumed fish, although they were permitted to eat shellfish.

In Samoa, a serious offense by an individual can be ameliorated by an ifoga (literally "a lowering"). The extended family positions themselves in front of the victim's home and remains there until invited in and forgiven. They formally apologize through the presentation of gifts and cash.

Some of these same practices are continued by Oceania people today. Unlike many immigrant groups, they typically maintain extended families in the United States. Responsibility for child rearing is shared among family members (children may move freely between homes), and household chores are assigned according to age and gender. The oldest man (or occasionally the oldest woman) in the home assumes control, collecting everyone's paycheck (or weekly contribution) and providing for the household needs. The good of the whole family is considered before the benefit of the individual, and most are guided by their desire to avoid disgracing their family. In Guam, this interdependence is known as inafa'maolek and extends not only to family and community but to national affiliation as well.[98,103]

The stresses of acculturation in the United States usually occur due to moving from a society in which there is little anonymity (with individual behavior reflecting on the whole family or village) to a society in which people from Oceania are often marginalized or even invisible if misidentified as Asians or Filipinos. Most maintain close contact with their homeland and fulfill their obligation to the family by sending financial support. Trips back to the islands for political and social events are common.

Traditional Health Beliefs and Practices Religion and medicine were closely linked in Oceania culture, and the loss of many traditional health beliefs and practices occurred with the adoption of nonnative faiths. Although folk healers specializing in herbs, massage, or religious and/or spiritual intervention work in Pacific Islander communities both in Hawaii and on the U.S. mainland, their current use is not well documented. Traditional practitioners are identified with a broad range of Eastern and Western religious affiliations and offer a wide spectrum of services. Their clientele is also extremely diverse, often crossing ethnic or religious lines to seek effective care.[105,106]

Many Native Hawaiians believe lokahi, harmony between individuals, nature, and the gods, is essential to good health. Hawaiian healers typically practice massage (ho'olomilomi—used for conditions such as childbirth, asthma, congestion, bronchitis, inflammation, and rheumatism), herbal medicine (la'au lapa'au), and/or conflict resolution (ho'ononpono, meaning "make things right"—used to remove emotional obstacles to healing). Meditation, deep breathing, and Chinese Traditional Medicine may also be employed. Healing is initiated at the end of each session with spiritual blessings.[107]

It is reported that more than 300 Hawaiian botanicals and animal- or mineral-based cures were available traditionally, with over 58 remedies for respiratory problems alone.[108,109] Today, only 30 plants are estimated to be used regularly. Examples include aloe vera for burns, hypertension, diabetes, and cancer; plantain leaves to reduce blood sugar levels in diabetes; polokai (black nightshade) for asthma, coughs, and colds; and wild ginger for gastrointestinal problems, ulcers, and asthma. Native Hawaiians also practice home remedies. For example, drinking seawater followed by freshwater is believed to be a general tonic.[110]

Samoans believe that health is maintained through a good diet, cleanliness, and harmony in interpersonal relationships. An individual is at high risk of illness if they do not fulfill family obligations or support village life. The concept of balance is essential: disruptions in interpersonal relationships, working too hard, sleeping too little, or eating the wrong foods can cause dislocation of the to'ala (the center of one's being, located just beneath the navel) to another part of the body, where it induces pain, poor appetite, or other symptoms. Treatment typically requires the restoration of balance. A family may get together to openly air disputes so that harmony can be re-established, or massage by an elder may be used to gently coax the to'ala back into position. A traditional Samoan healer may be consulted to cure certain folk

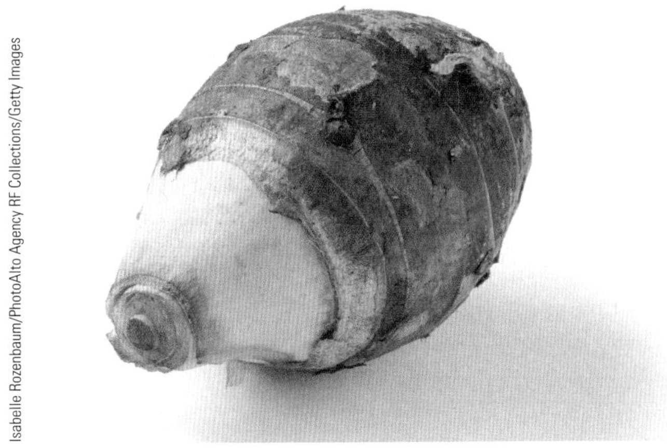

Isabelle Rozenbaum/PhotoAlto Agency RF Collections/Getty Images

▲ **Taro root, a staple of the Native Hawaiians and Pacific Islanders, is served boiled or pounded into a paste called poi. The leaves are also consumed.**

illnesses, particularly those due to supernatural causes, such as spirit possession by malevolent ghosts or the actions of ancestor spirits angered by a person's conduct.[111-113]

Traditional medicine in New Zealand and Australia emphasizes close interaction between the physical and the non-physical. The blending of traditional indigenous healing techniques with modern techniques has been well accepted. Many natural medicines are available at health shops, along with pharmaceutical medicines from pharmacies. New Zealand has had a national health care system in place for years providing free medicine and treatment to its residents. The average life expectancy is higher than average (73 years) in Australia at 83 years and 82 years in New Zealand.[114,115]

Traditional Food Habits

Though beautiful pottery, likely for food cooking and storage, is evident, the cooking in early Oceania developed without the use of metal pots, pans, and utensils. The indigenous cuisine was probably based on breadfruit, taro, cassava, yams, and perhaps pigs and poultry. Fruits were also widely available, although those often associated with the Pacific region, such as coconuts and bananas, were not introduced from Indonesia until approximately 1000 C.E. Other items, including sugar cane and pineapple, were brought by European plantation owners.

The ancestors of contemporary Aboriginal people first arrived in Australia over 50,000 years ago and they were sustained as hunter-gathering groups by strict protocols for foraging, and maintaining food harvesting limits. In general, there was seasonal bounty which they keenly understood needed to be nurtured. Indigenous food culture included wild freshwater and marine fisheries. Women gathered plant foods, shellfish, seaweed, ground insects, and small burrowing animals. Men of the community fished and hunted more mobile animals such as wallabies, kangaroos, and emus. Protein sources included insects, crustaceans, shellfish, fish, eels, reptiles, birds, and mammals. Fruit, seeds, nuts, sporocarps (seed-like growths on ferns), foliage, stems, galls, gums, leaf exudates, roots, tubers, and fungi were sought. Though some of the food gathered was eaten while on the move, the bulk was taken back to the main camp at the end of the day for cooking and eating by the rest of the group. Older people controlled the food distribution, determined by age, gender, and kinship obligations. Relative to what early European settlers ate, the Aboriginal foods were bountiful.[106]

In New Zealand, the Māori body of knowledge (mātauranga) interacts with the ecosystem for sustainable food for the community. Though food sovereignty has been encroached upon after European settlement, historically, collecting, harvesting, processing, cooking, and sharing traditional foods nourish both physical and spiritual well-being. For the Māori, food practices preserve the environment and regenerate the community.[115]

Ingredients and Common Foods

Staples Starchy vegetables are the mainstay of the traditional Pacific Islander diet (Table 12.3). These include the root taro, which is a little denser and more glutinous than the white potato; breadfruit, with a fluffy, breadlike interior; cassava; and yams. These foods were often cooked and then pounded into a paste. In Hawaii, taro root paste eaten fresh, or partially fermented, is called poi (a word that originally referred to the pounding method). When food was scarce, the Native Hawaiians survived on the purplish-colored poi, sometimes with a little seaweed or fish added to it. Although taro root is also a staple in Samoa, it is usually boiled but not pounded. Arrowroot is used to thicken puddings and other dishes. The Europeans introduced wheat, and bread is eaten in some areas; for instance, Portuguese sweet bread is known as Hawaiian bread in Hawaii. Asian settlers popularized both short- and long-grain rice, as well as noodles.[116]

More than 40 varieties of seaweed are consumed. Cooked greens, including the leaves of the taro root, yam, ti plant, and sweet potatoes, are very popular. One specialty is to wrap foods in ti or taro leaves, then steam the packets for several hours. The musky flavor of the leaves permeates the entire dish, called laulau in Hawaii.[117] Another specialty known as lu'au (taro root) is made by cooking taro root leaves with water, salt, onions, stock, and chicken or octopus, with coconut milk.

Fish and seafood are abundant in the Pacific Islands, and in some regions, they were eaten at every meal. Mullet is one of the most popular fishes, but many others, including mahimahi ("dolphin fish," not related to the mammal), salmon, shark, tuna, and sardines are also consumed. A tremendous variety of shellfish is available, such as clams, crabs, lobster, scallops, shrimp, crawfish, and sea urchins, as well as many local species. Eel, octopus, squid, and sea cucumbers are also eaten. Although some fish and seafood were stewed or roasted, some were also eaten uncooked, marinated in lemon or lime juice, which turns the fish opaque much the same as cooking it. A popular Hawaiian specialty is lomi-lomi, made with marinated chunks of salmon, tomatoes, and onions served with or without poi as an appetizer. A similar Samoan dish, called oka, is also made with chunks of raw fish marinated in a mixture of lemon juice and coconut cream.

Food for Thought

Traditionally, Samoan men obtained striking *pe'a* tattoos from midtorso to knees as a marker of maturity. While missionaries to the region disapproved, the practice was never fully abandoned.

Fish hooks are symbolic of good luck in Hawaii.

Pork is the most commonly eaten meat, especially for ceremonial occasions. Traditionally it was cooked in a pit called an imu in Hawaii, ahima'a in Tahiti, and an umu in Tonga. A fire was built over the stones lining the pit, and when the coals were hot, layers of banana leaves or palm fronds were added. The pig and other foods, such as breadfruit and yams, were placed on the leaves, then covered with more leaves and sealed with dirt. In some cases, water was poured over

Table 12.3 Cultural Food Groups: Residents of Oceania

Group	Comments	Common Foods	Adaptations in the United States
Protein Foods			
Milk/milk products	Milk and other dairy products are uncommon. Many Pacific Islanders are lactose intolerant.		Increased intake of milk has occurred.
Meat/poultry/fish/eggs/legumes	Pork is the most commonly eaten meat. Soybean products are used by Asian residents. Winged beans are a popular legume on some islands.	*Meat:* beef, pork *Poultry and small birds:* chicken, duck, squab, turkey *Eggs:* chicken, duck *Fish and shellfish:* ahi, clams, crabs, crawfish, eel, lobster, *mahimahi,* mullet, octopus, salmon, sardines, scallops, sea cucumber, sea urchin, shark, shrimp, swordfish, tuna, turtle, whale *Legumes:* beans (long, navy, soy, sword, winged), cowpeas, lentils, pigeon peas	Dietary changes often occur before immigration. Dietary changes often occur before immigration. Many are dependent on imported foods such as canned meats and fish.
Cereals/Grains	Europeans introduced wheat bread, and Asians brought rice and noodles.	Rice, wheat	Increased intake of bread and rice is noted.
Fruits/Vegetables	Starchy vegetables are the mainstay of the diet. They were often cooked and pounded into a paste. More than 40 varieties of seaweed are eaten. Cooked greens are popular. Fruits are an important ingredient. Immature coconuts are considered a delicacy. Arrowroot is used to thicken puddings and other dishes.	*Fruits:* acerola cherry, apples, apricot, avocado, banana, breadfruit, citrus fruits, coconut, guava, jackfruit, kumquat, litchis, loquat, mango, melons, papaya, passion fruit, peach, pear, pineapple, plum, prune, soursop, strawberry, tamarind *Vegetables:* arrowroot, bitter melon, burdock root, cabbage, carrot, cassava, cauliflower, *daikon,* eggplant, ferns, green beans, green pepper, horseradish, jute, kohlrabi, leeks, lettuce, lotus root, mustard greens, green onions, parsley, peas, seaweed, spinach, squashes, sweet potato, taro, *ti* plant, tomato, water chestnuts, yams	The traditional starchy vegetables have decreased in use and may only be consumed at special occasions.
Additional Foods			
Seasonings	Food is not highly seasoned but often flavored with lime or lemon juice and coconut milk or cream.	Curry powder, garlic, ginger, mint, paprika, pepper, salt, scallions or green onions, seaweed, soy sauce, tamarind	
Nuts/seeds	Nuts are a core ingredient.	Candlenuts (*kukui*), litchi, macadamia nuts, peanuts	
Beverages	Coconuts provide juice for drinking and sap for fermentation.	Cocoa, coconut drinks, coffee, fruit juice, *kava* (alcoholic beverage made from pepper plant), tea	Increased consumption of sweetened fruit beverages and soft drinks has occurred.
Fats/oils	Coconut oil and lard are the preferred fats.	Butter, coconut oil or cream, lard, vegetable oil and shortening, sesame oil	Use of vegetable oils and mayonnaise has increased.
Sweeteners		Sugar	

the rocks just before the pit was closed, steaming the foods instead of baking them. The pit was left sealed for hours until the food was completely cooked.

Chicken is widely available, as are eggs. Limited grazing land kept beef from becoming a frequently eaten item. Milk and other dairy products are also uncommon. Soybean products are used by Asian residents, and winged beans are a popular legume on some islands.

Fruits and nuts are important ingredients in Pacific Islander cuisine. Bananas, candlenuts (kukui nuts), citrus fruits, coconuts, pineapples, guavas, litchis, jackfruit, mangoes, melons, papayas, passion fruit, and *vi* (ambarella) are a few of the widely available varieties. Fruits are eaten fresh or added to dishes such as Samoan papaya and coconut cream soup (supo 'esi) and deep-fried dumplings filled with pineapple or bananas (pani keki). Coconuts provide juice for drinking, sap for fermentation, and milk or cream used in numerous stewed dishes (coconut milk can also be made into foods resembling cheese and buttermilk). Immature coconuts are considered a delicacy throughout the Pacific. Haupia, a traditional gelatin-like Hawaiian dessert, is made from coconut milk sweetened with sugar.

Traditional Pacific Islander fare was not highly seasoned. The flavors of lime or lemon juice, coconut milk or cream, and salt predominate, with the occasional use of ginger, garlic, tamarind, and scallions or onions. Coconut oil and lard are the preferred fats, providing a distinctive taste to many dishes. Foreign spices, such as Asian Indian curry blends, and sauces, such as soy sauce, have been incorporated into some dishes.

In contemporary Australia, Vegemite®, a thick brown and savory paste made from brewer's yeast and flavored with vegetable extract and spices, is often spread on toast or crackers. The salty concoction, somewhat similar to British Marmite, is beloved in Australia. Many people in the country eat about 84 pounds of chicken a year, and about 73 pounds of beef, while lamb and mutton consumption has fallen to about 31 pounds and pork consumption to about 55 pounds. Overall, Australian meat consumption is about three times the world average. Only one in 10 Australian adults eats sufficient vegetables unless it's potatoes (about 137 pounds).[118]

In New Zealand, several favorite foods stem from Māori traditions such as indigenous shellfish tuaua, and steam-cooked meat, potatoes, and root vegetables wrapped in leaves and placed in a basket laid on heated stones within a deep pit (hangi). Other popular dishes include lamb, sausage sizzles, and whitebait fritters, made by cooking fish with eggs and flour to produce a crispy omelet, as well as kumara (sweet potatoes) baked at times in a traditional hangi earth oven, and also made into croquettes and chips as a snack. Mince pies, a pastry filled with meat and gravy, is a portable food, and kiwifruit on its own or as a garnish for pavlova dessert is popular.

Meal Composition and Cycle

Daily Patterns Traditional meals included poi (boiled taro root), breadfruit, or green bananas; fish or pork; and greens or seaweed. In Samoa, Guam, and Tonga, most dishes are cooked in coconut milk or cream. Although the evening supper was generally the largest meal, little distinction was made between the foods served at the two or three daily meals. When food was pit-cooked, amounts suitable for two or three days at a time were prepared. Fresh fruit was eaten as snacks. Beverages made from coconut juice or sap were common. Asians introduced various teas, including those made from lemongrass and orange leaves. In Samoa, a drink made from ground cacao beans mixed with water called koko samoa is traditional. Kava, a bland, mildly intoxicating beverage, remains a popular drink in many regions. It is made from the chewed or ground root of the native pepper plant, mixed with water in a stone bowl. It reputedly tastes a little like dirt or licorice.

Traditional meals in New Zealand and Australia resemble European patterns, however, meats may be consumed at higher consumption rates. Breakfasts are made up of toast and cereals. Lunch and dinner include beef, lamb, and seafood are often covered with sauce and served in the form of meat pies called pasties or as a barbecue grilled steak or chop.[119,120]

Etiquette Most people from Oceania consider hospitality an honor, and outsiders are usually exempt from traditional manners. In Samoa, for example, it is considered rude to eat in front of someone without sharing. When eating a meal, respect should be shown for the food because it represents the host's generosity; this includes not talking during the meal. Most hosts will not eat until a guest is satisfied. As in many societies, it is impolite to refuse food, although a guest is not obligated to eat every morsel served. At some Samoan celebrations, for example, a large box of food may be placed on the table for each guest. The diner samples items from the box until full then brings the remaining food home to share with his or her extended family.

Special Occasions Throughout Oceania, special events were commemorated with feasting, often including pit-roasted foods. In Hawaii weddings, childbirth, completion of a canoe or house, or a prolific harvest or abundant catch was celebrated with a luau, featuring a whole pig, poultry, fish, and vegetables cooked in an imu (earth oven). In Samoa, the feast is sometimes preceded by a kava ceremony, in which the beverage, often used for relaxation, is distributed ritualistically to guests who are expected to drain the cup in one gulp. Traditionally kava was offered as a gesture of hospitality and for special occasions. In Tonga, where umu-cooked food accompanies celebrations such as the commemoration of a royal birthday, special coconut frond stretchers are woven for transporting the massive amounts of food prepared for the occasion.

Food for Thought

Hawaii is a leader in aquaculture. As early as 1778, Captain Cook reported 360 fish farms on the island of Kauai, producing an estimated 2 million pounds of fish annually.

The enzyme papain, extracted from papayas, is used in some meat tenderizers. In Hawaii, papaya juice is applied to jellyfish stings to reduce the pain.

Red salt, made from salt mixed with iron-rich earth, is a Hawaiian specialty, traditionally reserved for important feasts.

When drinking kava, it is considered polite to drip a few drops onto the ground and say "manuia" as a blessing before quaffing.

Holidays celebrated in Oceania are usually those associated with religious affiliation. In addition, Hawaiians also honor Prince Kuhio on March 26th and the Kamehameha Dynasty on June 11th. Samoans feast nearly every Sunday, and almost all denominations celebrate White Sunday on the third Sunday of October, venerating children. After a special service featuring religious recitations by children, a festive meal is served, and children are waited on by the adults in their extended family. Guamanians celebrate their Liberation Day on July 21st with parades, fireworks, and feasting. King Tuafa'ahau Tuopu IV's birthday is a national holiday in Tonga. New Zealand and Australia celebrate mostly Christian holidays. The holiday seasons, however, are reversed in the southern hemisphere, meaning Christmas, December 25th, could be spent at the beach.[119,120]

Food holds particular importance within most Pacific Island cultures. Sharing food is a way of demonstrating generosity and support for family and the village. It is also a way of expressing prosperity or social standing. Many events are celebrated with feasting, and food is eaten to excess as

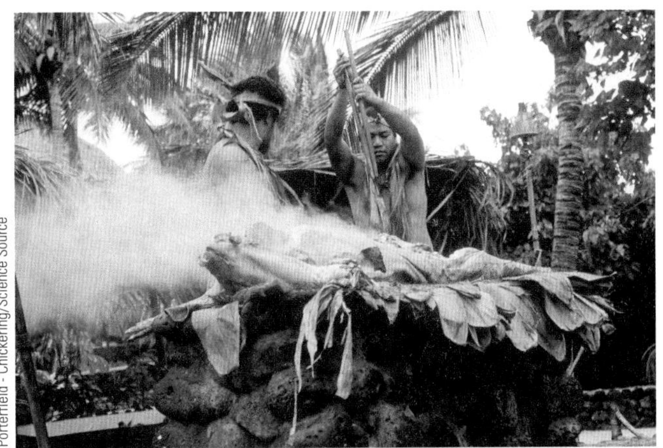
Porterfield - Chickering/Science Source

▲ Pork was traditionally the most commonly eaten meat in Hawaii, particularly for ceremonial occasions. The pig and other foods were cooked in a stone-lined pit over coals.

part of the ceremony in some regions. Traditionally, gender roles were defined by food interactions. Boys and girls were often raised similarly until the age of eight or nine, at which time they were separated for training in food procurement (farming and fishing) or food preparation (cooking and food storage). Throughout Oceania, gifts of food are given often. Because the gifts are given without expectation of reciprocity, it is a serious affront to reject any item presented.

Therapeutic Uses of Foods Numerous botanicals are used by Native Hawaiians as cures. Most notable is the pepper plant (*Piper methusticum*—related to the betel vine), which is used to make kava or awa. It is sometimes used medicinally as an analgesic or narcotic. In diluted form, it is used as a sedative and given to teething infants. Noni (Indian mulberry) is consumed as a juice for anorexia, renal problems, urinary tract infections, hypertension, diabetes, and musculoskeletal pain, to boost the immune system, and to prevent cancer. Noni fruit juice is considered a functional food supplement and is native to Hawaii. The drink's anti-inflammatory properties may contribute to preventing diseases of inflammation. Turmeric is consumed as a blood cleanser,[121] and breadfruit is made into tea to treat high blood sugar and elevated blood pressure. Poi, a starchy Polynesian food made from pounded taro root, is a major dietary staple of the Pacific Islands and may have beneficial health effects as a probiotic.[122]

Mustards are a popular exported commodity in Australia and New Zealand. These products are high in polyunsaturated fats and other phytochemicals. They have been used for medicinal purposes in traditional medicinal systems. Leaves of several varieties of the plant have more vitamin A than spinach and more vitamin C than oranges.[123] A relatively new species of superfood grown in Australia is finger lime. The fruit extracts have been used to reduce inflammation.[124]

Sample Menu

A Native Hawaiian Dinner

Lomi-Lomi (Marinated Salmon)[a,b]

Chicken Lu'au (Chicken with Spinach Leaves)[b]

Poi (Fermented Taro Root)[c] with raw onions

Haupia (Coconut Dessert)[d,c]

Fruit Juice or Coffee

Recipes in this menu:

[a]https://www.allrecipes.com/recipe/84860/lomi-lomi/

[b]https://www.food.com/recipe/easy-chicken-luau-420038

[c]*Polynesian Cultural Center* at https://www.polynesia.com/recipes/side-dishes/hawaiian-poi

[d]https://www.seriouseats.com/haupia-hawaiian-coconut-pudding-recipe

Contemporary Food Habits in the United States

Adaptations of Food Habits

Ingredients and Common Foods In Hawaii, today's population often eats fare that combines elements of Eastern and Western foods, typified by the plate lunch: rice heaped with one or two types of meat, poultry, or fish (such as teriyaki beef, spaghetti and meat sauce, fried mahi-mahi, pit-cooked pork, curry, or Spam) covered with gravy, served with a scoop of macaroni or potato salad, and eaten with chopsticks. Soy sauce is the most common condiment. Japanese sweet black-bean pastry, Portuguese sweet bread, Chinese noodles or crispy duck, and Korean kimchi are common. These dishes, emerging from Hawaii's past, as well as typical American dishes, are widely consumed. Snacking is prevalent and may include noodles topped with meat (saimin), steamed pork rolls (manapua), or a large ball of glutinous rice with a bit of pickled daikon or teriyaki tuna tucked in the middle (musubi). Crack seed is especially popular, consisting of dried, salted, and sugared fruits (e.g., guava, sliced ginger, lemon peel, mango, plum) that provide a sweet-and-sour flavor experience. Some are also seasoned with spices, such as anise. The seed kernels (in whole preserved fruit) are traditionally cracked open with the teeth, adding extra flavor and giving a descriptive name to the treats. The flavor is salty-sour-sweet with just a touch of bitterness. The custom of eating preserved fruit was brought into Hawaii by plantation workers from Zhongshan in southern China, who began arriving in Hawaii—then a kingdom—as contract laborers in the mid-nineteenth century.[125,126]

The dietary changes made by other groups in Oceania often begin before immigration to the mainland United States. Most are highly reliant on imported foods in their homelands, particularly processed items such as canned meats and fish, cooking oil, mayonnaise, cookies, breakfast cereals, and soft drinks. Providers of processed foods were primarily countries with economic links to the region, such as France, Australia, New Zealand, and the United States.[127] Many times, imported processed food is high in fat or sugar, or both, causing health concerns. Six out of the 10 countries with the world's highest diabetes prevalence are in the Pacific Islands, according to the International Diabetes Federation. The costs of local foods drive purchases of imports—for example, a package of instant noodles costs 26–70 U.S. cents, while locally grown cassava or sweet potato tubers cost 21 times that amount in Honiara, the capital of the Solomon Islands.[128] Access to native foods in Samoa, such as taro and coconut, appears limited.[129,130] Nutrient-rich native foods, such as fish, yams, papayas, and mangoes, were rarely consumed by Guamanian children in another older study.[131] Traditional starches, such as taro root and cassava, are often reserved for special-occasion feasts.[132]

Little has been reported on Oceania immigrant food habits in the United States. An older study comparing the intakes of Western Samoans (living in a less affluent, less Westernized culture) to those of American Samoans (living in a more affluent, more Westernized culture) found that the Western Samoans ate a diet higher in total fat due to a reliance on coconut cream compared to a diet higher in protein, cholesterol, and salt due to higher consumption of processed foods eaten by American Samoans.[133]

Older studies on Samoans who have moved to Hawaii show diets with a greater variety of foods; traditional foods contribute only minimally to daily intake, and items such as rice, bread, sugar, beef, canned fish, milk, soft drinks, and sweetened fruit beverages make up most of the diet.[134] Available health statistics indicate that a diet substantially higher in fat and simple carbohydrates and lower in fruits, vegetables, and fiber has been adopted by many immigrants.

Meal Composition and Cycle Three meals each day are common for most people in Oceania. Breakfast is most often cereal with coffee. More traditional meals may be eaten for lunch and dinner; a few Hawaiians still eat poi once or twice a day. Fruit appears more often as part of the meal rather than as a snack. It is believed that Sunday feasting among Samoans is still prevalent.

Nutritional Status

Nutritional Intake Fishing contributes to food security not only for consumption but also for income generation. Dietary patterns have, however, been shifting from reliance on traditional low-fat diets that were based on fish, leafy greens, and complex carbohydrates to more modern diets higher in sugar and fat. Packaged cereals, noodles, rice, and sugar-sweetened beverages have taken place of locally produced plants and animals. Diseases related to overconsumption coupled with malnutrition and vitamin and mineral deficiencies in children have become major health concerns.[135]

An older study of children in Guam found that three-quarters consumed fruits and vegetables less than once daily, and Native Hawaiian and Pacific Islander adults consume approximately one fruit or vegetable daily on average. Rice, meat, powdered fruit drinks, milk, and fortified cereals were the primary sources of vitamins and minerals in the diets of Guamanian children in other research. Low intakes of calcium, vitamin E, and folate were identified.[136,137]

Food for Thought

Areca nuts are used throughout Oceania, and in Hawaii, they are considered a stimulant. Guamanians are especially fond of chewing them. The practice is traditionally passed from grandparent to grandchild and is common at social occasions. Chomorrans (indigenous people of Guam) chew them after meals.

Those who live in the Pacific Islands have high rates of smoking, alcohol consumption, and obesity. In 2016, 24 percent of the adult population was overweight, and 51 percent of the adult population was considered obese. This is almost three times more than the obesity rate of the Asian American population. Samoans were 5.6 times more likely to be obese as compared to the overall Asian American population.[138] Obesity may be caused by overeating (within the context of family and church activities) combined with inadequate physical exercise. In addition, traditionally, being overweight was an aesthetic preference in many of the Oceania cultures. Heredity may also be a factor and/or it may be due to the change in the types and amount of foods consumed plus lower levels of physical activity. Additionally, researchers have found that when Pacific Islanders are compared to Whites with the same percentage of body fat, the Pacific Islanders have higher BMIs, suggesting greater nonfat density. Body mass index cutoffs for overweight and obesity that are standardized for Whites may need to be modified.[138]

Many who live in the Pacific Islands value a larger body size. One older study in Hawaii found that they believe Whites and Europeans should be slim, but that Hawaiians should have larger body sizes. Though Samoans living in westernized New Zealand identified a slim body as ideal. However, many who had a higher-than-normal BMI did not consider themselves to be obese and were positive about their body size and health. Research in Micronesia reported that many mothers of overweight children associate thinness with illness.[139,140]

The risk for type 2 diabetes is also high for the Pacific Islander population. In 2018, they were 2.5 times more likely to be diagnosed with diabetes compared to the non-Hispanic White population. In 2018, American Samoans had the highest diabetes rates among Pacific Islander subpopulations (22 percent). This is almost three times higher than the non-Hispanic White population. It is postulated that Samoans may be especially susceptible to kidney damage associated with hypertension because end-stage renal failure is a common cause of death in American Samoan diabetes patients.[141] Leading causes of death among the Pacific Island population are cancer, heart disease, unintentional injuries (accidents), stroke, and diabetes. The leading cause of death for Native Hawaiians and Pacific Islanders was cancer, heart disease, and COVID-19 in 2020. They are 30 percent more likely to be diagnosed with cancer, as compared to non-Hispanic

Whites. American Samoan women are twice as likely to be diagnosed with, and to die from, cervical cancer, as compared to non-Hispanic Whites. American Samoan men are eight times more likely to develop liver cancer, and Native Hawaiian men are 2.4 times more likely to be diagnosed with the same disease, as compared to non-Hispanic Whites. In Hawaii, Native Hawaiian men have the highest mortality rate for all types of cancer, as compared to other ethnic groups in Hawaii, and Native Hawaiian women have the highest incidence rate for all types of cancer, as compared to other ethnic groups in the state. In the U.S. territory of Guam, the incidence rate was higher for all cancer types in the Micronesian population, as compared to other ethnic groups in Guam from 2008–2012.[142]

Nutrition risk factors of New Zealand and Australia tell a different story. The New Zealand Ministry of Health reported that in 2020–2021, approximately 1 in 3 adults were classified as obese (34.3 percent). This increase from 2019 was primarily seen in women. For specific ethnic groups, the rates were higher, with 71.3 percent of Pacific Islander, 50 percent of Maori, 32 percent of European/Other, and 18 percent of Asian adults ranked as obese.[143] In 2018, an estimated 36 percent of Australians are overweight, and 31 percent were obese. Men were more likely to be overweight and obese than women. The highest overweight prevalence was found in the lowest socioeconomic areas.[144] The leading causes of death in both countries are cancer and cardiovascular disease.

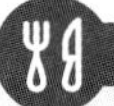

Food for Thought

Research on Asian, mixed ethnicity, and White adolescent girls in Hawaii found that all groups could benefit from an increased intake of fruits, vegetables, and calcium-rich foods.[145]

Many residents of Oceania are lactose intolerant; it is estimated that 50 percent of Samoan adults do not tolerate milk.[146]

In Guam, an extremely high prevalence of both amyotrophic lateral sclerosis (called letigo) and Parkinsonism dementia (known as bodig) has been reported. Incidence has decreased significantly, however, suggesting environmental causes may be to blame.[147]

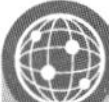

Exploring Global Cuisine

Australian and New Zealand's Oceania Fare

Despite being part of Oceania—which includes Micronesia, Fiji, Kirbati, Marshall Islands, Nauru, Palau, Papua New Guinea, Samoa, Solomon Islands, Tonga, Tuvalu, and Vanuatu—the food culture of Australia and New Zealand has only a few similarities today with earlier people of the region. The large island continent of Australia and the two-island nation of New Zealand are thought to have been initially populated by people from Southeast Asia. Centuries later, Polynesians traveled to New Zealand, intermingling with the existing native peoples to become the Māori. Despite a shared heritage, the cooking of Southeast Asia and the Pacific Islands and the fare of Australia and New Zealand are quite different. British colonization of the countries in the eighteenth and nineteenth centuries overwhelmed the original inhabitants and their culinary traditions.

Meat is the mainstay of the Australian and New Zealand diets. Beef is most popular in Australia, especially steak served with fried eggs or stuffed with oysters (carpetbagger steak). Lamb is favored in New Zealand (and also well-liked in Australia), typically roasted and served with mint sauce or barbecued. Other meats and poultry are uncommon in both nations, though some wild game, particularly venison, boar, duck, and pheasant, is found in New Zealand. Fish and seafood, however, are eaten often, including shrimp, oysters, scallops, spiny lobster, and crawfish (called yabbies in Australia). Most meats and fish are simply prepared, by roasting, pan-frying, braising or poaching, and grilling. Traditionally, the seasoning was very limited, but today, an international array of herbs and spices are used. For example, in New Zealand, Asian Indian lamb curries and Greek gyros are popular. Minced and ground meats appear in numerous dishes. In Australia, shepherd's pie (ground lamb topped with mashed potatoes) and hamburgers topped with fried eggs and beet slices are common. Battered, fried sausages are a favorite snack in New Zealand. In both nations, individual steak, sausage, bacon and egg, or fish pies (consumed with tomato sauce or ketchup) are popular.

Numerous fruits and vegetables are grown in a mild climate. Potatoes, beets, peas, carrots, and corn are typical accompaniments to meals, though more exotic produce, such as eggplants, feijoas, kiwifruit (Chinese gooseberries), pineapple, and tamarillos are also available. Bread rounds out the meal. Sweets are eaten daily. Scones are common, as are biscuits (cookies) such as lamingtons (chocolate coconut) and ANZAC biscuits (oatmeal cookies provided to the Australian and New Zealand Army Corps during the world wars). Puddings and custards are especially popular. Both countries claim pavlova, a meringue and fruit dish topped with whipped cream, as a national dessert. Three meals each day are the norm. In Australia, an afternoon break for tea or beer is customary, and in New Zealand, many people break for morning and afternoon tea. Australia is noteworthy for its beers and hearty wines, beverages that New Zealand is also successfully producing. In tandem with these foodways, efforts are being made toward the recognition of the food sovereignty of the indigenous peoples of New Zealand. This is especially interesting as traditional foods incorporate ecological knowledge to create sustainable food systems.[148]

The Aboriginal foods of Australia, often called bush tucker, include bandicoot, seeds, nuts, duck, emu, goose, turkey, kangaroo, wombat, emu, duck, fish, shrimp, carpet snakes, lizards, crab, crocodile, various fish, witchetty grubs, and wild plants such as yams, onions, wattle seeds, and quandong (a peach-like fruit), cashews, and berries.[149] Most foods were prepared simply over a fire, in the ashes, or boiled. Research shows that where traditional foods remain an integral part of the Aboriginal diet, there is no evidence of diabetes or cardiovascular disease. Once non-traditional foods were integrated into the contemporary diets of Aboriginal Australians, lifestyle-related chronic disease rates rose.[149] Foods introduced by Polynesians formed the foundation of the Māori diet in New Zealand, such as kumara (sweet potatoes), taro, and ti plants. Native greens and fruits were also available. Fish, seafood, birds, and sea mammals provided protein (there were no indigenous land mammals in the islands). The Polynesian influence is also seen in the use of the hangi, a pit-roasting method similar to imu used for ceremonial occasions. Māori food presence in the dominant New Zealand culture is growing. Since 2008, Maori cookbooks have been published and have appeared in mainstream bookshops.[150]

One study reported that weight-loss interventions based on traditional Hawaiian foods were well accepted by Native Hawaiians, particularly those who emphasized cultural values and provided group support. However, most participants found it difficult to adhere to the diet long-term, citing difficulties in obtaining fresh produce and the pressures of an obesogenic environment.[151] A study in Micronesia found significant cultural conflict in homes where mothers attempted to restrict the food intake of their overweight children. Food is associated with love, and grandparents who perceive grandchildren as too thin often accuse mothers of inadequate care.

An in-depth interview should be used to determine if a client has any traditional health beliefs or practices regarding a specific condition and if religious affiliation is a factor. Due to the paucity of research, coworkers or a client's family members may provide significant information regarding particular Oceania groups.

Health and Longevity Takeaway

"Longevity spinach," popular in Southeast Asia, is not actually spinach, but a light green, semi-succulent vining plant scientifically called *Gynura procumbens*. It often looks like thick ground cover and is known for its highly-nutritious superfood qualities. It is rich in vitamin K, polyphenols, flavonoids, and other nutrients. It can be eaten raw in salads or smoothies or sauteed or steamed like regular spinach. Longevity spinach grows well in warmer climates and prefers partial shade. It also grows well in pots on the patio. This is a great addition to salads to boost their already powerful anti-aging properties.

Food for Thought

Samoan women are traditionally treated to a rich coconut drink called vaisalo after childbirth.

Comfort Food—Vietnam

Sarah Duong's story

In many immigrant families, comfort food at home can be something not widely eaten in the majority United States culture. Sarah Duong was born in the United States, but her parents were born in Vietnam. This opened a flavor world to her outside mainstream culture in Kansas City.

What is a favorite comfort food that you consider traditional from your home culture?

SD: My comfort food is steamed buns. These are similar to a sandwich in pouch form that has meat inside. It's my favorite because they are a quick source of meat and protein and are easy and simple to make. The texture is fluffy and I love them served warm. Making steamed buns with my parents in Kansas City, all of us in the kitchen together, is a favorite memory of mine. Cooking gave us a chance to talk, laugh, and enjoy quality time with each other. Everyone had their role in the baking process. We usually made an abundance of steamed buns because we would freeze them. It takes about an hour to make from scratch.

Did you eat this food together with community? Where was it eaten?

SD: Normally, steamed buns are eaten for breakfast as a meal at the kitchen table in my family but I also enjoy them for a snack because they are easy to grab when I'm on the run. When I go back home there is not a large Vietnamese community, so it is usually my mom, dad, and I who eat steamed buns together.

Here is Sarah's recipe:

Steamed Buns

Serves 4 (12 buns)

Dough Mixture:

4 cups of self-rising flour
1 cup of milk
3/4 cup of white sugar

Pork mixture:

10 dried mushrooms
3/4 pound ground pork
1/2 cup white onion, chopped
2 green onions, finely chopped
1/8 cup frozen green peas
1/8 cup carrot, diced
1 Chinese sausage (such as lap cheong)
1 teaspoon granulated white sugar
1/4 tsp. ground black pepper
1 tsp. sesame oil
2 Tbsp. oyster sauce
3 chicken eggs hard-boiled and cut into quarters
12 cupcake liners

Mix the flour, milk, and sugar for the dough in a large bowl. Next, hydrate the dried mushrooms in a bowl of hot water until they are soft. Then, mix the pork, mushrooms, chopped white and green onion, peas, carrots, sausage, 1 tsp. sugar, pepper, oil, and oyster sauce in a bowl. Divide the mixture into 12 equal-sized balls and make a hole in the middle to fit one ¼-sized piece of egg inside. Wrap each ball around the egg so that it is all-encompassing and to where you cannot see the egg anymore. Using a steamer, cook the balls for 4 minutes and then take them out of the steamer and set them to the side. Divide the dough into 12 equal balls and then flatten the balls. Put the pork ball into the middle of the flat dough. Wrap the dough around the ball and pinch the top. Then, place the dough balls into the cupcake liners, put the balls into the steamer for 10 minutes, and serve.

Nutritional Information (per serving):

calories 844; protein 44 g; carbohydrates 153 g; dietary fiber 5 g; sugar 55 g; fat 11 g; saturated fat 3.6 g; cholesterol 209 mg; sodium 219 mg

(Continued)

Comfort Food—Vietnam (*Continued*)

Sarah Duong's story

Additional RECIPE TO TRY

Vietnamese Iced Coffee

Makes 1 Serving

2 Tbsp. dark-roast ground coffee with chicory
2 Tbsp. light or low-fat sweetened condensed milk
Options: a dash of cinnamon, cocoa

Steep coffee grounds in a French press with 1 cup boiling water for 4 minutes. Pour through a coffee filter into a mug or heat-proof glass. Stir in condensed milk until blended. Add in optional spices. Add ice, stir, and serve.

Nutrition Information (per serving):
calories 163; protein 4 g; carbohydrates 30 g; fat 3 g; saturated fat 2 g; cholesterol 10 mg

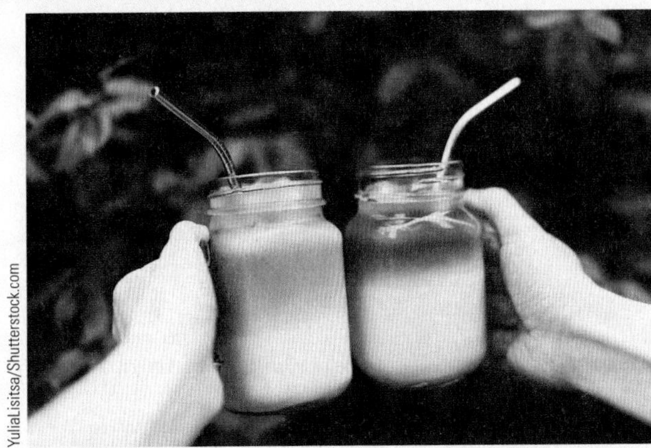

YuliaLisitsa/Shutterstock.com

▲ **Vietnamese iced coffee. Coffee beverages in Southeast Asia may accompany meals or snacks.**

Discussion Starters

Working with Differences in Diet and Culture

In small groups of three or four, compare and contrast the diet and culture of Filipino, Vietnamese, Cambodian, and Laotian Americans, with each group focusing on a different aspect of the diet and culture of these groups:

Group A: The food habits and the typical eating etiquette and meal composition of these four immigrant groups

Group B: Issues involved in counseling these immigrant groups on diet and health

Group C: Attitudes within each immigrant group toward diet, health, and medical treatment, notably attitudes toward traditional home culture medical treatment and U.S. biomedicine

Group D: Amount of obesity, diabetes, hypertension, and other diseases within each immigrant group

Within your group, try to come to a consensus on what findings to report to the rest of the class. Before breaking up, assign a number to each group member: A1, A2, A3, A4; B1, B2, and so forth. Form new groups with all the 1's in a group, all the 2's in another group, all the 3's another group, and so on. In your new group, report the findings of your previous group, and, as a group, discuss the relationship between traditional attitudes toward diet and health and changes in diet and health due to immigration to the United States.

Review Questions

1. Choose one typical Filipino dish and describe it. Explain how it conforms to the principles of Filipino cooking. Select one or two ingredients and discuss whether they are due to an influence from another culture and why that might have happened.
2. Describe the traditional health and dietary beliefs for the prevention and treatment of disease in one Southeast Asian immigrant group. How does the concept of "balance" for the maintenance of health fit within Southeast Asian health beliefs?
3. Pick one type of traditional healer used in Southeast Asian countries. Describe this type of healer's practice and research whether they currently practice in the United States.
4. List the indigenous foods of the Pacific Islands. Pick two from your list, describe how they might be prepared today, and discuss whether they are considered to have any special dietary or health properties.
5. Processed meat products, such as Spam, are common in the Filipino, Native Hawaiian, and Pacific Islander diets. What is Spam, where does it come from, and how did it become prevalent in the Oceania diet? Include a recipe using Spam.

Reflection

1. The acculturation process of coming to the United States often hurts the nutrition and health of immigrants. For example, there is a misperception that bottle-feeding infants may be healthier and more convenient, when in fact breastmilk is better for infant health. Considering the low breastfeeding rates in most Southeast Asian cultures, what types of education/social media campaigns, etc., may be beneficial in encouraging women to breastfeed their babies?

References

1. Stuart-Fox, M. 2004. Southeast Asia and China: The role of history and culture in shaping future relations. *Contemporary Southeast Asia*, 26(1), 116–139. http://www.jstor.org/stable/25798674
2. Pew Research Center. April 29, 2021. Filipinos in the U.S. Fact Sheet. Retrieved from https://www.pewresearch.org/social-trends/fact-sheet/asian-americans-filipinos-in-the-u-s/
3. Budiman, A. April 29, 2021. Filipinos in the U.S. Fact Sheet. Pew Research Center. Retrieved from https://www.pewresearch.org/social-trends/fact-sheet/asian-americans-filipinos-in-the-u-s/
4. Budiman, A. April 29, 2021. Vietnamese in the U.S. Fact Sheet. Pew Research Center. Retrieved from https://www.pewresearch.org/social-trends/fact-sheet/asian-americans-vietnamese-in-the-u-s-fact-sheet/
5. Melindy, B. 2014. Filipino Americans. In R.V. Dassanowsky & J. Lehman (Eds.), *Gale encyclopedia of multicultural America*, 3rd ed. Farmington Hills, MI: Gale Group. Vol. 2.
6. Republic of the Philippines Embassy of the Philippines Ottawa, Canada. May, 2016. Filipiinos in Canada. Retrieved from https://ottawape.dfa.gov.ph/index.php/2016-04-12-08-34-55/filipino-diaspora.
7. Wikipedia. 2016. South Asian Canadians. Retrieved from https://en.wikipedia.org/wiki/South_Asian_Canadians
8. Budiman, A. April 29, 2021. Hmong in the U.S. Fact Sheet. Pew Research Center. Retrieved from https://www.pewresearch.org/social-trends/fact-sheet/asian-americans-hmong-in-the-u-s/
9. Budiman, A. April 29, 2021. Cambodian in the U.S. Fact Sheet. Pew Research Center Retrieved from https://www.pewresearch.org/social-trends/fact-sheet/asian-americans-cambodians-in-the-u-s/
10. Budiman, A. April 29, 2021. Laotians in the U.S. Fact Sheet. Pew Research Center Retrieved from https://www.pewresearch.org/social-trends/fact-sheet/asian-americans-laotians-in-the-u-s/
11. Liu, J. 2012. Asian Americans: A mosaic of faiths. Pew Research Center. Retrieved from https://www.pewresearch.org/religion/2012/07/19/asian-americans-a-mosaic-of-faiths-overview/
12. Borja, M.M. 2014. To follow the new rule or way": Hmong refugee resettlement and the practice of American religious pluralism (Doctoral dissertation, Columbia University).
13. Bankston, C.L. 2014. Hmong Americans. In T. Riggs (Ed.), *Gale Encyclopedia of Multicultural America/* 3rd ed., Vol. 2. pp. 331–344. Retrieved from https://link.gale.com/apps/doc/CX3273300087/GVRL?u=multi_america&sid=bookmark-GVRL&xid=a797a7d4
14. Melendy, H.B. 2014. Filipino Americans. In T. Riggs (Ed.), *Gale Encyclopedia of Multicultural America*. 3rd ed., Vol. 2, pp. 119–135. Retrieved from https://link.gale.com/apps/doc/CX3273300072/GVRL?u=multi_america&sid=bookmark-GVRL&xid=e4910a6c
15. Tuazon, N. 2021. People of Filipino Heritage. In: Purnell, L., Fenkl, E. (eds) Textbook for transcultural health care: A population approach. Springer, Cham. Retrieved from https://doi.org/10.1007/978-3-030-51399-3_14.
16. Bankston, C.L., III. 2014. Cambodian Americans. In T. Riggs (Ed.), *Gale Encyclopedia of Multicultural America*, 3rd ed., Vol. 1, pp. 381–393. Retrieved from https://link.gale.com/apps/doc/CX3273300040/GVRL?u=multi_america&sid=bookmark-GVRL&xid=cdeb834b.
17. Bankston, C.L., III. 2014. Vietnamese Americans. In T. Riggs (Ed.), *Gale Encyclopedia of Multicultural America*, 3rd ed., Vol. 4, pp. 499–512. Retrieved from https://link.gale.com/apps/doc/CX3273300187/GVRL?u=multi_america&sid=bookmark-GVRL&xid=59cf1766.
18. Bankston, C.L. 2014. Laotian Americans. In T. Riggs (Ed.), *Gale Encyclopedia of Multicultural America*, 3rd ed., Vol. 3, pp. 53–64. Retrieved from https://link.gale.com/apps/doc/CX3273300111/GVRL?u=multi_america&sid=bookmark-GVRL&xid=00e90476
19. Pfeifer, M.E. & Thao, B.K. (Eds.). 2013. State of the Hmong American community. Washington, DC: Hmong National Development.
20. Budiman, A. 2021. Hmong in the U.S. Fact Sheet. Pew Research Center. Retrieved from https://www.pewresearch.org/social-trends/fact-sheet/asian-americans-hmong-in-the-u-s/
21. Vang, C.Y., Nibbs, F., & Vang, M. (Eds.). 2016. *Claiming place: On the agency of Hmong women*. University of Minnesota Press.
22. Mouavangsou, K. 2018. Because I am a daughter: A Hmong woman's educational journey. *Journal of Southeast Asian American Education and Advancement*, 13(1), 4.
23. Maneze, D., Ramjan, L., DiGiacomo, M., Everett, B., Davidson, P.M., & Salamonson, Y. 2018. Negotiating health and chronic illness in Filipino-Australians: a qualitative study with implications for health promotion. *Ethnicty & Health*, 23(6), 611–628. doi: 10.1080/13557858.2017.1294656.
24. Bhimla, A., Yap, L., Lee, M., Seals, B., Aczon, H., & Ma, G.X. 2017. Addressing the Health Needs of High-Risk Filipino Americans in the Greater Philadelphia region. *Journal of Community Health*, 42(2), 269–277. Retrieved from https://doi.org/10.1007/s10900-016-0252-0.
25. Abad, P.J., Tan, M.L., Baluyot, M.M., Villa, A.Q., Talapian, G.L., Reyes, M.E., Suarez, R.C., Sur, A.L., Aldemita, V.D., Padilla, C.D., & Laurino, M.Y. 2014. Cultural beliefs on disease causation in the Philippines: challenge and implications in genetic counseling. *Journal of Community Genetics*, 5(4), 399–407. Retrieved from https://doi.org/10.1007/s12687-014-0193-1.
26. Berdon, J.S., Ragosta, E.L., Inocian, R.B., Manalag, C.A., & Lozano, E.B. 2016. Unveiling Cebuano traditional healing practices. *Asia Pacific Journal of Multidisciplinary Research*, 4(1), 51–59.
27. Lopez, M.L. (2006). *A handbook of Philippine folklore*. UP Press.
28. Ceria-Ulep, C.D., Serafica, R.C., & Tse, A. 2011. Filipino older adults' beliefs about exercise activity. *Nursing Forum*, 46(4), 240–250. Retrieved from https://doi.org/10.1111/j.1744-6198.2011.00238.x
29. Lagarde, J., Laurino, M.Y., San Juan, M.D., Cauyan, J., Tumulak, M., & Ventura, E.R. 2019. Risk perception and screening behavior of Filipino women at risk for breast cancer: implications for cancer genetic counseling. *Journal of Community Genetics*, 10(2), 281–289. Retrieved from https://doi.org/10.1007/s12687-018-0391-3
30. Purnel, L.D. & Fenkl, E.A. 2020. *Textbook for transultural health care: A Population approach*, 5th ed. Springer.
31. Peltzer, K., Pengpid, S., Puckpinyo, A., Yi, S., & Anh, Le Vu. 2016. The utilization of traditional, complementary and alternative medicine for non-communicable diseases and mental disorders in health care patients in Cambodia, Thailand *BMC Complementary and Alternative Medicine*, 92. DOI: 10.1186/s12906-016-1078-0.
32. Peltzer, K. & Pengpid, S. 2015. Utilization and practice of traditional/complementary/alternative medicine (T/CAM) in Southeast Asian Nations (ASEAN) Member States. *Studies on Ethno-Medicine*, 9(2), 209–218, DOI: 10.1080/09735070.2015.11905437.
33. Kpobi, L. & Swartz, L. 2018. Implications of healing power and positioning for collaboration between formal mental health services and traditional/alternative medicine: the case of Ghana. *Global Health Action* 11:1.
34. Peltzer, K., Thang Nguyen Huu, Nguyen Bach Ngoc, Supa Pengpid. 2017. The use of herbal remedies and supplementary products among chronic disease patients in Vietnam. *Studies on Ethno-Medicine*, 11(2), 137–145. Retrieved from https://www.tandfonline.com/doi/abs/10.1080/09735070.2017.1305230
35. Nuttall, P. & Flores, F.C. 1997. Hmong healing practices used for common childhood illnesses. *Pediatric Nursing*, 23, 247–214.
36. Hinton, D.E., Pich, V., Chhean, D., & Pollack, M.H. 2005. The ghost pushes you down: Sleep paralysis-type panic attacks in a Khmer refugee population. *Transcultural Psychiatry*, 42, 46–47.
37. Pols, H., Thompson, M.C., & Warner, J.H. 2017. Translating the body: medical education in Southeast Asia.
38. Rehman, S.U., Choe, K., & Yoo, H.H. 2016. Review on a traditional herbal medicine, Eurycoma longifolia Jack (Tongkat Ali):

its traditional uses, chemistry, evidence-based pharmacology and toxicology. *Molecules*, 21(3), 331.

39. Ng, A.W., Poon, S.L., Huang, M.N., Lim, J.Q., Boot, A., Yu, W., . . . & Rozen, S.G. 2017. Aristolochic acids and their derivatives are widely implicated in liver cancers in Taiwan and throughout Asia. *Science Translational Medicine*, 9(412).
40. Lee, G.Y. & Lett, D. 2010. Hmong religious practice in Australia.
41. Her-Xiong, Y. & Schroepfer, T. 2018. Walking in two worlds: Hmong end of life beliefs & rituals. *Journal of Social Work in End-of-Life & Palliative Care*, 14(4), 291–314.
42. Tuazon, N. 2021. People of Filipino heritage. In: Purnell, L. & Fenkl, E. (eds), *Textbook for transcultural health care: A population approach*. Springer, Cham. Retrieved from https://doi.org/10.1007/978-3-030-51399-3_14
43. Zibart, E. 2010. *The ethnic food lover's companion: A sourcebook for understanding the cuisines of the World*. Menasha Ridge Press.
44. Florendo, J. 2019. Colonizing the Filipino palate. *Unpublished Paper. Presented at the 12th DLSU Arts Congress, Manila, Philippines.* Retrieved from https://www. dlsu. edu. ph/wp-content/uploads/pdf/conferences/arts-congress-proceedings/2019/FAC-03. pdf (accessed October 27, 2020).
45. Lazor, D. 2019. An Introduction to Filipino cuisine. Serious Eats. Retrieved from https://www.seriouseats.com/what-is-filipino-food-cuisine.
46. Owen, J. 2005. New rodent discovered at Asian food market. *National Geographic News*, May 16. Retrieved from http://news.nationalgeographic.com/news/2005/05/0516_050516_new_rodent.html
47. O'Neill, M. 2001, July 23. Letter from Cambodia: Home for dinner. *The New Yorker*, pp. 55–63.
48. Vargas, P. & Jurado, L.F. 2015. Dietary acculturation among Filipino Americans. *International Journal of Environmental Research and Public Health*, 13(1). Retrieved from https://doi.org/10.3390/ijerph13010016
49. Noche, C. 2017. What eating with my hands means to me (and 6 other Filipinos). Food52. Retrieved from https://food52.com/blog/19423-what-eating-with-my-hands-means-to-me-and-6-other-filipinos
50. Foster, D. 2000. *The global etiquette guide to Asia*. New York: Wiley.
51. Philippine Herbal Medicine. 2006. Retrieved from http://herbal-medicine.philsite.net/index.htm.
52. Singh, D., Narayanan, S., Vicknasingam, B., Corazza, O., Santacroce, R., & Roman-Urrestarazu, A. 2017. Changing trends in the use of kratom (*Mitragyna speciosa) in* Southeast Asia. *Human Psychopharmacology: Clinical and Experimental*, 32:e2582. Retrieved from https://doi.org/10.1002/hup.2582
53. Avieli, N. 2011. Making sense of Vietnamese cuisine. *Education About Asia*, 16(3), 42–45.
54. Köhler, R., Sae-tan, S., Lambert, C., & Biesalski, H.K. 2018. Plant-based food taboos in pregnancy and the postpartum period in Southeast Asia—A systematic review of literature. *Nutrition & Food Science*, 48, 949–961. Retrieved from https://doi.org/10.1108/nfs-02-2018-0059
55. Smith, T.J., Tan, X., Arnold, C.D., Sitthideth, D., Kounnavong, S., & Hess, S.Y. 2022. Traditional prenatal and postpartum food restrictions among women in northern Lao PDR. *Maternal & Child Nutrition*, 18(1), e13273.
56. Barennes, H., Sengkhamyong, K., René, J.P., & Phimmasane, M. 2015. Beriberi (thiamine deficiency) and high infant mortality in Northern Laos. *PLoS Neglected Tropical Diseases*, 9, e0003581.
57. Vargas, P. & Jurado, L.F. 2016. Dietary acculturation among Filipino americans. *International Journal of Environmental Research and Public Health*, 13(1), 16.
58. Dela Cruz, F.A. n.d. *Food intake and dietary acculturative changes of first generation Filipino Americans*. Western Institute of Nursing, 2010, Meeting Abstract.
59. Dela Cruz, F.A., Lao, B.T., & Heinlein, C. 2013. Level of acculturation, food intake, dietary changes, and health status of first-generation Filipino Americans in Southern California. *Journal of the American Association of Nurse Practitioners*, 25(11), 619–630.
60. Angosta, A.D. & Kirsten E. Speck. 2014. Assessment of heart disease knowledge and risk factors among first-generation Filipino Americans residing in southern Nevada: A cross-sectional study. *Clinical Nursing Studies*, 2(2), 123.
61. Vargas, P.P. 2015. Acculturation, dietary pattern and health indicators among Filipino American immigrants in New Jersey (doctoral dissertation). The William Paterson University of New Jersey.
62. Tran, T.V., Vatcher, R., Lee, H.N., Phan, P.T. & Nguyen, T.N. 2013. Household income and vegetable consumption among white, Chinese, Korean and Vietnamese Americans. *International Journal of Social Science Studies*, 1(2), 31–43.
63. Vargas, P. & Jurado, L.F. 2016. Dietary acculturation among Filipino americans. *International Journal of Environmental Research and Public Health*, 13(1), 16.
64. Diep, C.S., Foster, M.J., McKyer, E.L.J., Goodson, P., Guidry, J.J., & Liew, J. 2015. What are Asian-American youth consuming? A systematic literature review. *Journal of Immigrant and Minority Health*, 17(2), 591–604.
65. Yang, J. 2020. *The Culture of Food: An Exploratory Study of Food Choices in the Hmong People with Diabetes*. Doctoral dissertation, University of California, Davis.
66. Padoongpatt, M. 2017. *Flavors of empire: Food and the making of Thai America*, Vol. 45. University of California Press.
67. 2008 Restaurant Industry Pocket FactBook. National Restaurant Association. (2008). Washington, DC.
68. Gampell, J. 2006. Letter from Ubon: In northeast Thailand, a cuisine based on bugs. *The New York Times*, June 22. Retrieved from http://travel2.nytimes.com/2006/06/22/travel/22webletter.html
69. Sanguankiattichai, N. 2019. Michelin Guide Magazine. Retrieved from https://guide.michelin.com/th/en/article/features/10-must-try-isaan-dishes-and-where-to-find-them-in-bangkok
70. Nualkhair, C. 2019. Michelin Guide Magazine. Retrieved from https://guide.michelin.com/th/en/article/features/a-guide-to-royal-thai-cuisine
71. Steinberg, R. 1970. *Pacific and Southeast Asian cooking*. New York: Time-Life Books.
72. Rigg, J. 2015. *Challenging Southeast Asian Development. The shadows of success*. Routledge Pub. London.
73. NCHS Data Brief, Number 427. December 2021. Retrieved from https://www.cdc.gov/nchs/products/databriefs/db427.htm (accessed April 19, 2022.
74. Capua, John E. Spring 2013. Dietary acculturation among Filipino immigrants. Thesis.
75. dela Cruz, F.A., Lao, B.T., & Heinlein, C. 2013. Level of acculturation, food intake, dietary changes, and health status of first-generation Filipino Americans in Southern California. *Journal of the American Association of Nurse Practitioners*, 25(11), 619–630.
76. CDC Health of Asian or Pacific Islander Population. Table 26. Retrieved from https://www.cdc.gov/nchs/faststats/asian-health.htm (accessed April 18, 2022).
77. Djibo, D.A., Araneta, M.R.G., Kritz-Silverstein, D., Barrett-Connor, E., & Wooten, W. 2015. Body adiposity index as a risk factor for the metabolic syndrome in postmenopausal Caucasian, African American, and Filipina women. *Diabetes & Metabolic Syndrome: Clinical Research & Reviews*, 9(2), 108–113.
78. Hedderson, M.M., Darbinian, J.A., & Ferrara, A. 2010. Disparities in the risk of gestational diabetes by race-ethnicity and country of birth. *Paediatric and Perinatal Epidemiology*, 24(5), 441–448.
79. Palaniappan, L.P., Wong, E., Shin, J.J., Fortmann, S.P., & Lauderdale, D.S. 2009. Asian Americans have a greater prevalence of metabolic syndrome despite lower body mass index. *Circulation*, 119, e363 [Abstract].

80. Walters, D., Horton, S., Yudistira, A., Siregar, M., Pitriyan, P., Hajeebhoy, N., Mathisen, R., Thi, L., Phan, H., Rudert, C. 2016. The cost of not breastfeeding in Southeast Asia. *Health Policy and Planning,* 31(8), 1107–1116. Retrieved from https://doi.org/10.1093/heapol/czw044
81. Fu, H. & VanLandingham, M.J. 2012. Disentangling the effects of migration, selection and acculturation on weight and body fat distribution: Results from a natural experiment involving Vietnamese Americans, returnees, and never-leavers. *Journal of Immigrant and Minority Health,* 14(5), 786–796.
82. Sangalang, C.C., Becerra, D., Mitchell, F.M. et al. 2019. Trauma, Post-migration stress, and mental health: A comparative analysis of refugees and immigrants in the United States. *Journal of Immigrant Minority Health,* 21, 909–919. Retrieved from https://doi.org/10.1007/s10903-018-0826-2.
83. Tu, J.V., Chu, A., Rezai, M.R., Guo, H., Maclagan, L.C., Austin, P.C., Booth, G.L., Manuel, D.G., Chiu, M., Ko, D.T., Lee, D.S., Shah, B.R., Donovan, L.R., Sohail, Q.Z., and Alter, D.A. 2015. Incidence of major cardiovascular events in immigrants to Ontario, Canada. *AHA/ASA Journals,* 132(16), 549–1559.
84. Li, C-K. 2017. New trend in the epidemiology of thalassaemia. *Best Practice & Research Clinical Obstetrics & Gynaecology, 39,* 16–26.
85. Wyatt, L.C., Ung, T., Park, R., Kwon, S.C., & Trinh-Shevrin, C. 2015. Risk factors of suicide and depression among Asian American, Native Hawaiian, and Pacific Islander youth: A systematic literature review. *Journal of Health Care for the Poor and Underserved,* 26(20), 191.
86. Sue, S. 1999. Merging past, present and future in cross-cultural psychology. 1st ed., p. 536.
87. Lee, S.Y., Martins, S.S., & Lee, H.B. 2015. Mental disorders and mental health service use across Asian American subethnic groups in the United States. *Community Mental Health Journal,* 51(2), 153–160.
88. Sangalang, C.C., Jager, J., & Harachi, T.W. 2017. Effects of maternal traumatic distress on family functioning and child mental health: An examination of Southeast Asian refugee families in the US. *Social Science & Medicine,* 184, 178–186.
89. Swain, L. 2014. Pacific Islander Americans. *Gale Encyclopedia of Multicultural America,* Vol. 3, 3rd ed.
90. Cuthbertson, K. 2014. Australian Americans. *Gale Encyclopedia of Multicultural America,* Vol. 1, 3rd ed.
91. Knight, J. 2014. New Zealander Americans. *Gale Encyclopedia of Multicultural America,* Vol. 3, 3rd ed.
92. U.S. Census Bureau. July 1, 2021. Quick Facts Hawaii (accessed April 7, 2022).
93. U.S. Census Bureau. April 30, 2020. Asian and pacific Islander Population in the United States. Retrieved from https://www.census.gov/library/visualizations/2020/demo/aian-population.html.
94. HRSA Fact Sheet 9-30-2020. FY 2020 American Samoa. US department of health and Human Service. Retrieved from file:///C:/Users/seann/Downloads/HDW_FactSheet.pdf (accessed April 19, 2022).
95. U.S. Census Bureau. 2019. American Community Survey. Retrieved from https://data.census.gov/cedsci/table?t=931%20-%20Australia%20and%20New%20Zealand%20Subregion&tid=ACSSPP1Y2019.S0201 (accessed April 18, 2022).
96. Winters, E. & Swartz, M. 2014. Hawaiians. In T. Riggs (Ed.), *Gale Encyclopedia of Multicultural America,* 3rd ed., Vol. 2, pp. 317–329. Retrieved from https://link.gale.com/apps/doc/CX3273300086/GVRL?u=multi_america&sid=bookmark-GVRL&xid=0a55b5ac
97. Swain, L. 2014. Pacific Islander Americans. In T. Riggs (Ed.), *Gale Encyclopedia of Multicultural America,* 3rd ed., Vol. 3, pp. 401–410. Retrieved from https://link.gale.com/apps/doc/CX3273300137/GVRL?u=multi_america&sid=bookmark-GVRL&xid=3699b4fe
98. Spear, J.E. 2014. Guamanian Americans. In T. Riggs (Ed.), *Gale Encyclopedia of Multicultural America,* 3rd ed., Vol. 2, pp. 263–273. Retrieved from https://link.gale.com/apps/doc/CX3273300082/GVRL?u=multi_america&sid=bookmark-GVRL&xid=1d693ffd
99. Sinclair, K. and Dalziel, R. New Zealand: People. Britannica. Retrieved from https://www.britannica.com/place/New-Zealand/People.
100. Lockhart, C., Houkamau, C.A., Sibley, C.G., & Osborne, D. 2019. To be at one with the land: Māori spirituality predicts greater environmental regard. *Religions,* 10(7), 427. Retrieved from https://doi.org/10.3390/rel10070427
101. Hughes, C. 2018. Distribution of religious affiliation in Australia in 2016. Statista. Retrieved from https://www.statista.com/statistics/959996/distribution-of-religious-affiliation-australia/
102. Jones, D.S. & Clarke, P.A. 2018. Aboriginal culture and food-landscape relationships in Australia: Indigenous knowledge for country and landscape. *Routledge Handbook of Landscape and Food,* pp. 41–60.
103. Winters, E. & Swartz, M. 2014. Hawaiians. In T. Riggs (Ed.), *Gale Encyclopedia of Multicultural America,* 3rd ed., Vol. 2, pp. 317–329. Retrieved from https://link.gale.com/apps/doc/CX3273300086/GVRL?u=multi_america&sid=bookmark-GVRL&xid=0a55b5ac
104. Pew Research Center. 2018. Statistical portrait of the Foreign Born. Retrieved from https://www.pewresearch.org/hispanic/wp-content/uploads/sites/5/2020/08/Pew-Research-Center_Current-Data_Statistical-Portrait-of-the-Foreign-Born-2018.pdf
105. Hughes, C. 2018. Distribution of religious affiliation in Australia in 2016. Statista. Retrieved from https://www.statista.com/statistics/959996/distribution-of-religious-affiliation-australia/
106. Jones, D.S. & Clarke, P.A. 2018. Aboriginal culture and food-landscape relationships in Australia: Indigenous knowledge for country and landscape. *Routledge Handbook of Landscape and Food,* pp. 41–60.
107. Kaholokula, J.K.A., Ing, C.T., Look, M.A., Delafield, R., & Sinclair, K.I. 2018. Culturally responsive approaches to health promotion for Native Hawaiians and Pacific Islanders. *Annals of Human Biology,* 45(3), 249–263.
108. Matsuno, R.K., Pagano, I.S., Maskarinec, G., Issell, B.F., & Gotay, C.C. 2012. Complementary and alternative medicine use and breast cancer prognosis: a pooled analysis of four population-based studies of breast cancer survivors. *Journal of Women's Health,* 21(12), 1252–1258.
109. Young, B. 2016. Early Physicians of Hawaii and Reflections on the Emergence of Hawaiian Doctors.
110. Cnnruc, H.K. Hawaiian health practitioners in contemporary society.
111. Yamada, A.M., Vaivao, D.E.S., & Subica, A.M. 2019. Addressing mental health challenges of Samoan Americans in Southern California: Perspectives of Samoan community providers. *Asian American Journal of Psychology,* 10(3), 227.
112. Howard, A. 1986. Samoan coping behavior. In P.T. Baker, J.M. Hanna, & T.S. Baker (Eds.), *The changing Samoans: Behavior and health in transition.* New York: Oxford University Press.
113. Kinloch, P. 1985. *Talking health but doing sickness: Studies in Samoan health.* Wellington, New Zealand: Victoria University Press.
114. Braithwaite, J. 2009. Overview of the Health care System in Australia & New Zealand. *Health Management,* 9(1).
115. Huambachano, M.A. 2019. Indigenous food sovereignty: Reclaiming food as sacred medicine in Aotearoa New Zealand and Peru. *New Zealand Journal of Ecology,* 43(3), 1–6. Retrieved from https://www.jstor.org/stable/26841826.
116. Wong, K.A. & Kataoka-Yahiro, M.R. 2017. Nutrition and diet as it relates to health and well-being of Native Hawaiian Kūpuna (elders): a systematic literature review. *Journal of Transcultural Nursing,* 28(4), 408–422.
117. Titcomb, M. 2021. Native use of fish in Hawaii. In *Native Use of Fish in Hawaii.* University of Hawaii Press.
118. Symons, M. 2014. Australia's cuisine culture: a history of our food. Australian Geographic. Retrieved from https://www.australiangeographic.com.au/topics/history-culture/2014/06/australias-cuisine-culture-a-history-of-food/
119. Cuthbertson, K. 2014. Australian Americans. Gale Encyclopedia of Multicultural America, 3rd ed., Vol. 1. Retrieved from Australian Americans - Document - Gale eBooks (accessed April 18, 2022).

120. Knight, J. 2014. New Zealander Americans. Gale Encyclopedia of Multicultural America, 3rd. ed., Vol 1. Retrieved from Australian Americans - Document - Gale eBooks (accessed April 18, 2022).
121. Lee, D., Yu, J.S., Huang, P., Qader, M., Manavalan, A., Wu, X., . . . & Kim, K.H. 2020. Identification of anti-inflammatory compounds from Hawaiian noni (Morinda citrifolia L.) fruit Juice. *Molecules*, 25(21), 4968.
122. Brown, A.C., Ibrahim, S.A., & Song, D. 2016. Poi history, uses, and role in health. In *Fruits, vegetables, and herbs*, Academic Press, pp. 331–342.
123. Williams, P.M. 1996. Te Rongoa Maori: Maori Medicine. In *Birkenhead: Reed Books*. Auckland, New Zealand: Penguin Books, p. 79
124. Cornara, L., Xiao, J., Smeriglio, A., Trombetta, D., & Burlando, B. 2020. Emerging exotic fruits: New functional foods in the European market. *EFood*, 1(2), 126–139.
125. Liu, R. 2019. The enduring appeal of Hawaii's Preserved fruits. *New York Times Style Magazine*. Retrieved from https://www.nytimes.com/2019/09/11/t-magazine/crack-seed.html.
126. Winters, E. & Swartz, M. 2014. Hawaiians. In T. Riggs (Ed.), *Gale Encyclopedia of Multicultural America*, 3rd ed., Vol. 2, pp. 317–329. Retrieved from https://link.gale.com/apps/doc/CX3273300086/GVRL?u=multi_america&sid=bookmark-GVRL&xid=0a55b5ac
127. Snowdon, W., Raj, A., Reeve, E., Guerrero, R. L., Fesaitu, J., Cateine, K., & Guignet, C. 2013. Processed foods available in the Pacific Islands. *Globalization and Health*, 9(1), 1–7.
128. United Nations Office for the Coordination of Humanitarian Affairs. 2014. Trade and transfat in the Pacific. Retrieved from https://www.thenewhumanitarian.org/analysis/2014/11/17/trade-and-transfat-pacific
129. Farrell, P., Thow, A.M., Schuster, S., Vizintin, P., & Negin, J. 2019. Access to a nutritious diet in Samoa: local insights. *Ecology of Food and Nutrition*, 58(3), 189–206.
130. Hardin, J. 2021. Life before vegetables: Nutrition, cash, and subjunctive health in Samoa. *Cultural Anthropology*, 36(3), 428–457.
131. Hanna, J.M., Pelletier, D.L., & Brown, V.J. 1986. The diet and nutrition of contemporary Samoans. In P.T. Baker, J.M. Hanna, & T.S. Baker (Eds.), *The changing Samoans: Behavior and health in transition*. New York: Oxford University Press.
132. Pobocik, R.S. & Richer, J.J. 2002. Estimated intake and food sources of vitamin A, folate, vitamin C, vitamin E, calcium, iron, and zinc for Gaumanian children aged 9 to 12. *Pacific Health Dialog*, 9, 193–202.
133. Fitzpatrick-Nietschmann, J. 1983. Pacific Islanders—migration and health. *Western Journal of Medicine*, 139, 848–853.
134. Shovic, A.C. 1994. Development of a Samoan nutrition exchange list using culturally accepted foods. *Journal of the American Dietetic Association*, 94, 541–543.
135. Charlton, K.E., Russell, J., Gorman, E., Hanich, Q., Delisle, A., Campbell, B., & Bell, J. 2016. Fish, food security and health in Pacific Island countries and territories: a systematic literature review. *BMC Public Health*, 16(1), 1–26.
136. Asian & Pacific Islander American Health Forum. 2012. Asian American, Native Hawaiian, & Pacific Islander maternal health disparities—San Francisco, CA. Retrieved from http://www.apiahf.org/si...sue%20Brief%20final.pdf
137. LeonGuerrero, R.T. & Workman, R.L. 2002. Physical activity and nutritional status of adolescents on Guam. *Pacific Health Dialog*, 9, 177–185.
138. CDC. 2020. Summary Health Statistics: National Health Interview Survey: 2016. Table A-15a.
139. Lameko, V. 2020. Obesity in Samoa: culture, history and dietary practices.
140. Brewis, A.A., McGarvey, S.T., Jones, J., & Swinburn, B.A. 1998. Perceptions of body size in Pacific Islanders. *International Journal of Obesity and Related Metabolic Disorders*, 22, 185–189.
141. CDC. 2021. Summary health statistics: National Health Interview Survey: 2018. Table A-4a. Retrieved from http://www.cdc.gov/nchs/nhis/shs/tables.htm
142. CDC. 2017. Selected Health Conditions Among Native Hawaiian and Pacific Islander Adults: United States, 2014.
143. Ministry of Health. 2020/21. Obesity statistics. Retrieved from https://www.health.govt.nz/nz-health-statistics/health-statistics-and-data-sets/obesity-statistics (accessed April 19, 2022).
144. Australian Institute of Health and Welfare. July 23, 2020. Overweight and Obesity. Retrieved from https://www.aihw.gov.au/reports/australias-health/overweight-and-obesity (accessed on April 19, 2022).
145. Daida, Y., Novotny, R., Grove, J.S., Acharya, S., & Vogt, T.M. 2006. Ethnicity and nutrition of adolescent girls in Hawaii. *Journal of the American Dietetic Association*, 106, 221–226.
146. Stride, P. 2016. Polynesian bones. *Journal of Advances in Medicine and Medical Research*, 16, 1–9.
147. Steele, J.C. 2005. Parkinsonism-dementia complex of Guam. *Movement Disorders*, 12, S99–S107.
148. Huambachano, M.A. 2019. Indigenous food sovereignty. *New Zealand Journal of Ecology*, 43(3), 1–6.
149. Ferguson, M., Brown, C., Georga, C., Miles, E., Wilson, A., & Brimblecombe, J. 2017. Traditional food availability and consumption in remote Aboriginal communities in the Northern Territory, Australia. *Australian and New Zealand Journal of Public Health*, 41(3), 294–298.
150. Morris, C. 2013. Kai or Kiwi? Māori and 'Kiwi'cookbooks, and the struggle for the field of New Zealand cuisine. *Journal of Sociology*, 49(2–3), 210–223.
151. Boyd, J.K. & Braun, K.L. 2007. Supports for and barriers to healthy living for Native Hawaiian young adults enrolled in community colleges. *Preventing Chronic Disease*, 4(4), 1–12. Retrieved from http://www.cdc.gov/pcd/issues/2007/oct/07_0012.htm

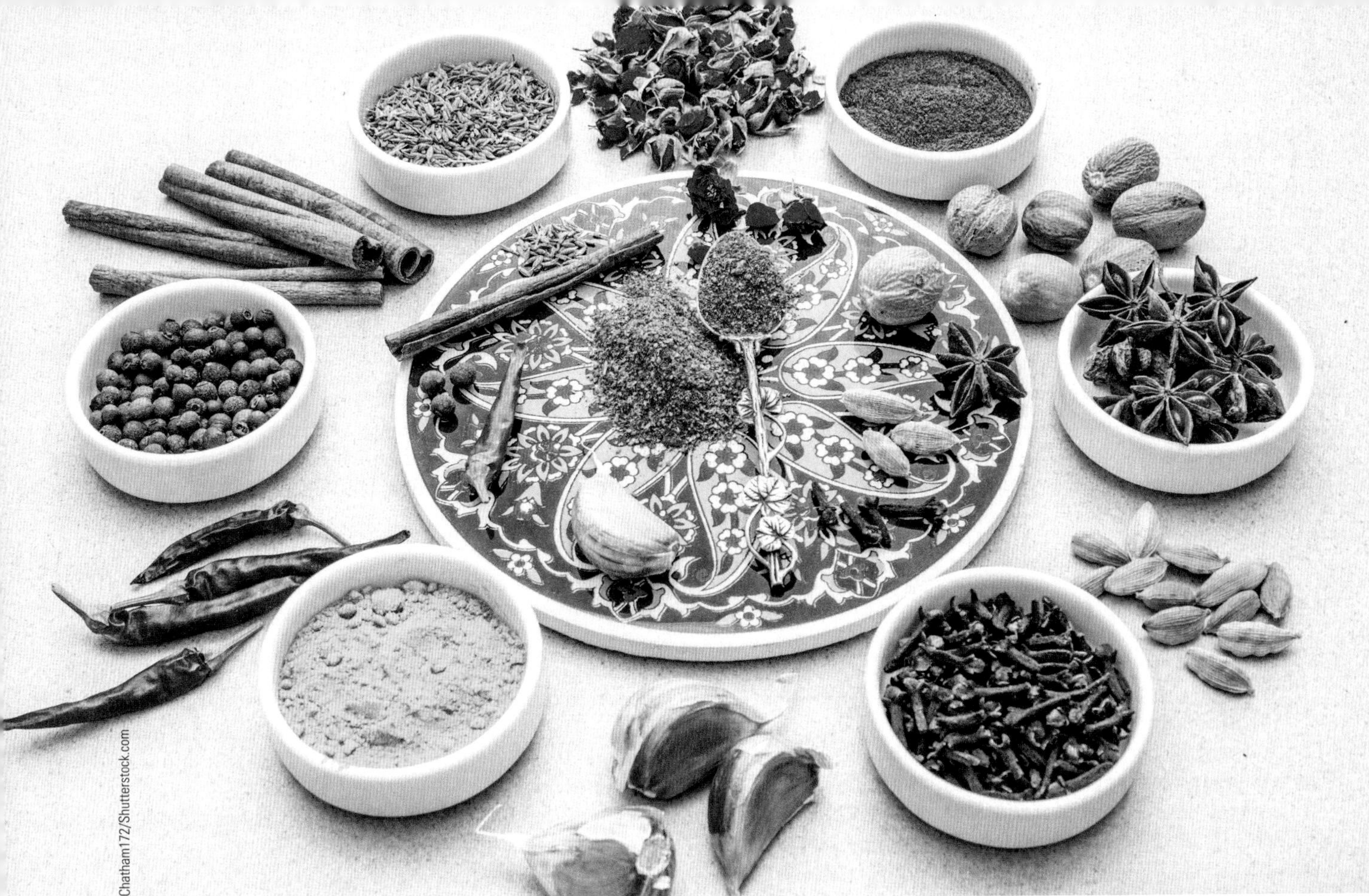
Chatham172/Shutterstock.com

People of the Balkans and the Middle East

Chapter 13

Learning Objectives

13.1 List the countries that are in the Balkan region and those that are in the Middle East.

13.2 Identify the immigration patterns, historical socioeconomic influences, and current locations of the people of the Balkans and the Middle East who are in the United States today.

13.3 Differentiate the religions, family structures, and traditional health beliefs and practices of the people of the Balkans and the Middle East before and after immigration to the United States.

13.4 Describe the differences between the staples and regional variations in ingredients—both for the nations of the Balkans and the Middle East.

13.5 Identify key foods for each of the food groups for the nations and regions of the Middle East and the Balkans and how these foods have been adapted by immigrants in the United States.

13.6 Describe the impact of religion on the foods of the Middle East and list each celebration that has specific dishes associated with it.

13.7 Identify health concerns associated with the nutritional intake of these groups.

The southeast European nations of the Balkan Peninsula and the countries of the Middle East are near central Europe, Africa, and Asia. The region has traditionally been a cultural crossroads of ideas, values, and material goods and is often considered the cradle of Western civilization. Many immigrants from the Balkans and the Middle East have come to the United States in search of education, economic opportunity, and political stability. They frequently retain a strong ethnic identity, exhibited in their religious faith and their maintenance of traditional food culture. This chapter examines the cuisine of the Balkans and the Middle East, its role in the U.S. diet, and the changes that have occurred in the United States.

The Balkans and the Middle East

Cultural Perspective

The Balkan nations include Greece, Albania, Bosnia-Herzegovina, Montenegro, Serbia (including the two autonomous provinces Kosovo and Vojvodina), the Republic of Macedonia, Croatia, Slovenia, Bulgaria, and Romania. Countries in the Middle East include Bahrain, Egypt, Iran, Iraq, Israel, Jordan, Kuwait, Lebanon, Oman, Saudi Arabia, Syria, Turkey, United Arab Emirates, and Yemen (Figure 13.1). In addition, several notable groups do not have a homeland in the region, including the Palestinians (an Arab ethnic group), the Kurds (an Indo-European ethnic group), and the Chaldeans and Assyrians (Semitic ethnic groups).

Geographically, much of the Balkans is considered temperate in climate and is suited to agriculture. In Greece, however, and in most of the Middle East, aridity limits cultivation. Even in the desert regions, distinct areas of arable land exist along the seacoasts and in some plains and valleys, such as the Fertile Crescent (a plain in Iraq fed by the Euphrates and Tigris Rivers) and the Nile River valley of Egypt.

Food for Thought

An Arab is commonly defined as a person who speaks Arabic—the term does not refer to a particular religious belief though many Arabs are Muslim. Arabs are Semitic, meaning speakers of a family of languages that include Hebrew, Arabic, Aramaic, and certain ancient languages. Arab people inhabit much of the Middle East and North Africa. Iranians, also called Persians, speak Farsi. The Turks, whose nation is geographically divided between Europe and Asia, speak modern Turkish, a language that is traced to the Altay region in the Eurasian steppes and is now written with the Latin alphabet.

Greece dominated or greatly influenced its Balkan and Middle Eastern neighbors in ancient times, and, in turn, it was conquered and ruled by the Turkish Ottoman Empire for four centuries in the modern era. These hundreds of years of Greek and Turkish hegemony facilitated the spread of products, especially foods, throughout the region and stretched cultural influence to both the southern states of the former Soviet Union (refer to Chapter 7) and North Africa. Despite such commonalities, however, populations within the nations of the Balkans and the Middle East are very diverse in religious affiliation. Judaism, Christianity (particularly Eastern Orthodox), and Islam all have substantial numbers of followers in the region. Faith is fundamental to daily life in both the Balkans and the Middle East.

History of People of the Balkans and the Middle East in the United States

Immigration Patterns

Balkans Immigration from Greece has occurred primarily in two waves. The first lasted from the late 1800s to the 1920s when the restrictive Immigration Act of 1924 was imposed; the second wave started after World War II and has not yet ended. The early Greek immigrants were mostly young men from rural agricultural areas who came to America primarily for economic opportunities. Many came to make their fortune and go back to their homeland—approximately 30 percent of early Greek immigrants returned to Greece. A bitter civil war from 1946 to 1949 and a military coup in 1967 resulted in numerous Greek refugees who sought asylum in the United States. While most settled in New York, Detroit, Chicago, and other cities of the Midwest, a large community developed in Tarpon Springs, Florida, with many members employed in sponge diving. Some Greeks were attracted to mining and railroad work in the West.

Food for Thought

Until 1992, the nations of Serbia, Croatia, Slovenia, Bosnia-Herzegovina, Montenegro, and Macedonia were the states of a single country known as Yugoslavia.

During the 1850s and 1860s, numerous Croatian immigrants from the area of Dalmatia arrived in the United States. Most migrated to the southern and western regions where they had a substantial impact on the oyster fisheries of Mississippi and the fig, apple, grape, and plum horticulture of northern California. The many Serbians, also known as Serbs, who immigrated to the United States in this period were often unskilled laborers who obtained industrial jobs in the Northeast. Croatian and Serbian immigration increased following World War II, including professionals, such as engineers and physicians, seeking better job opportunities.

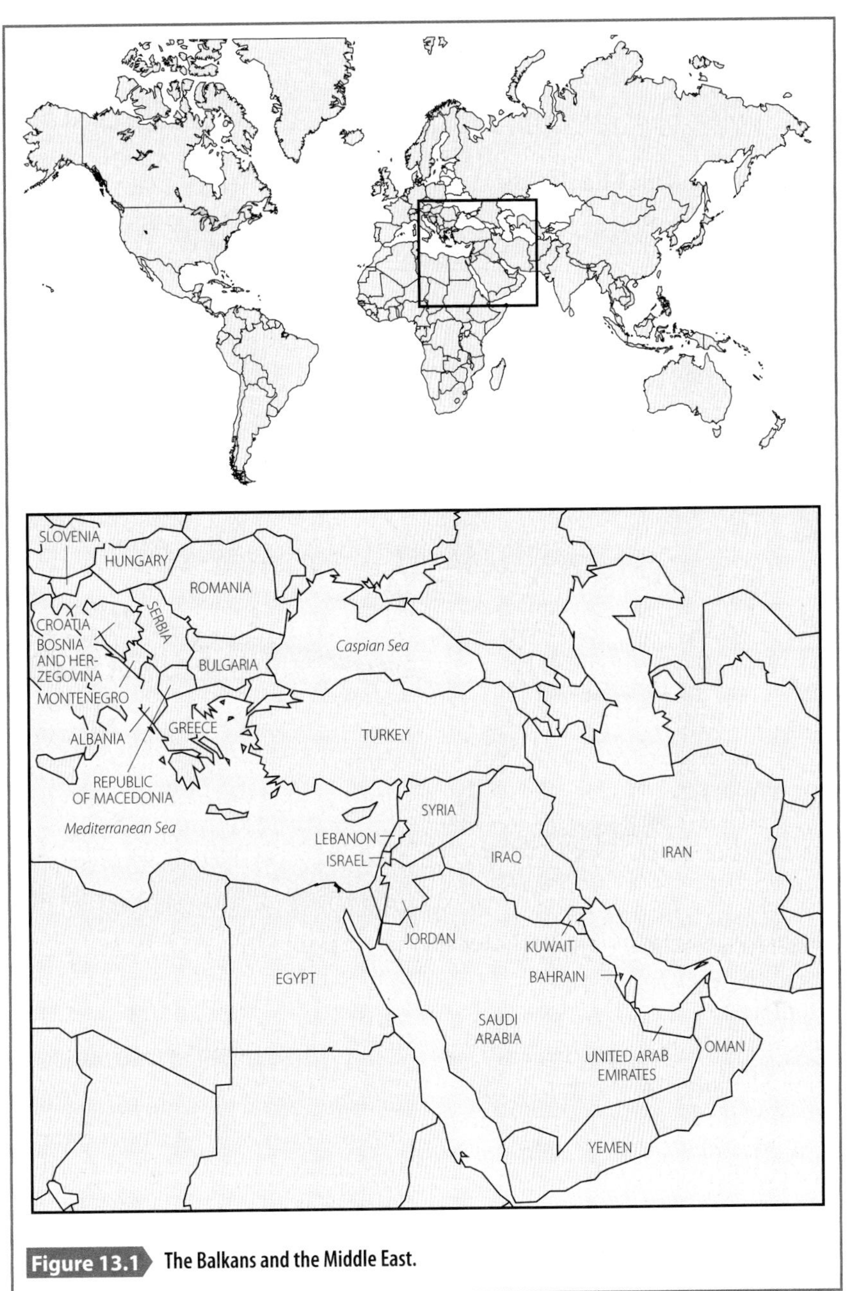

Figure 13.1 The Balkans and the Middle East.

Food for Thought

Though large numbers of Kurds have been displaced due to conflicts in the Middle East, most refugees—over 500,000—have gone to Europe. Much smaller numbers have come to the United States, particularly Nashville, Salt Lake City, and San Diego.

Around the turn of the twentieth century, an elite group of Arab artists, writers, and poets settled in New York City. They called their literary circle the Pen League; the best-known member was Kahlil Gibran, author of *The Prophet*.

The largest number of Slovenian immigrants arrived between 1880 and World War I, though exact figures are not available because many were listed as Austrians. Most were farmers seeking economic opportunity. They settled initially in the rural Midwest, forming self-sustaining ethnic communities with Slovenian churches, schools, businesses, and social organizations.

Middle East Statistics on immigration from the Middle East are inexact. Until 1900, all immigrants from the area were called "Egyptians." Later arrivals were typically termed "Syrians" or "Turks from Asia." More specific nationalities have been recognized since the 1930s, yet it has only been in recent years that Palestinian has been defined as an immigration category, and it is standard practice to combine Chaldeans with Assyrians.

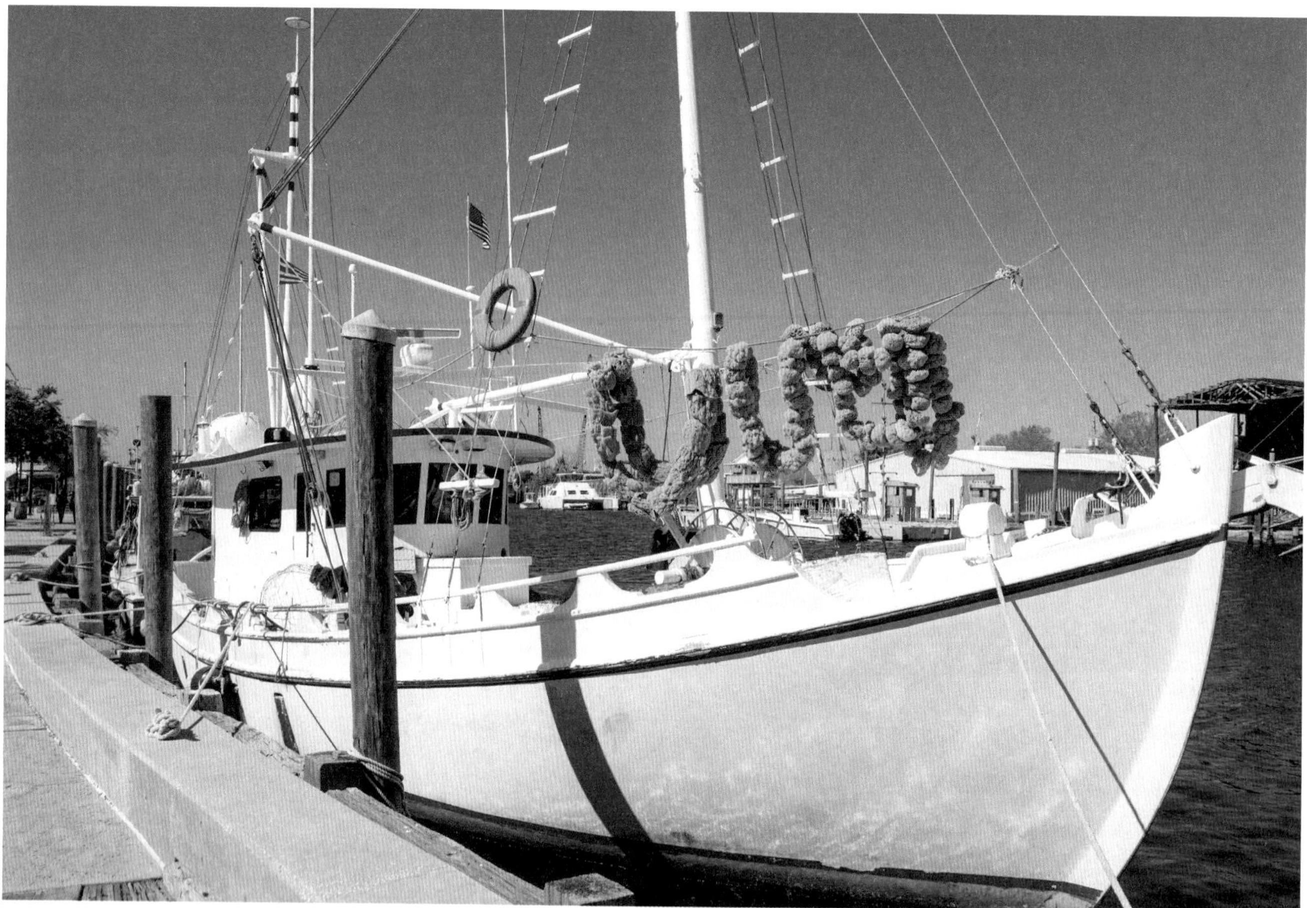
iStock.com/Benedek

▲ A large Greek community developed in Tarpon Springs, Florida, with members employed in sponge diving.

Early Arab immigrants arrived at the turn of the twentieth century seeking economic opportunity. Most were Christians from the area that is today Lebanon and Syria, although small numbers of Turkish Muslims also came during this period. Most settled in New England and the Midwest and were employed in the textile, shoe, and wire factories.

The major influx of Middle Easterners began in the years following World War II. A high percentage of immigrants from Jordan, Egypt, Lebanon, Iraq, and Syria were Christian Palestinians who initially fled Israel when it was declared a state. After first settling in refugee camps, many later immigrated to the United States when Israel won the 1967 war against neighboring Arab countries. Political unrest and the Islamic revolution in Iran led to a large exodus of Persians beginning in 1976. Many were members of the wealthy Iranian elite; fewer were Jewish and Christian, including Chaldeans and Assyrians. In addition, many Turks and Arabs who came to the United States for their college education elected to stay in the country to establish their careers. A similar situation is reported for Israelis, who immigrated in small but steady numbers to America for advanced education and professional, managerial, or technical jobs.

Current Demographics and Socioeconomic Status

Balkans Nearly 1.2 million people claimed Greek ancestry in the 2019 U.S. Census estimates. New York City has the largest concentration of Greek Americans, followed by California, Illinois, Massachusetts, and Florida. In recent years, Greek Americans have moved progressively south and west in the United States. Early Greek immigrants preferred to live in urban areas. The Greeks sought economic independence by opening small businesses, especially in candy production and restaurants. Greek Americans can be found in all occupations, particularly managerial, professional, technical, and service jobs.[1]

Over 400,000 Croatian Americans and 184,000 Americans of Serbian descent lived in the United States in 2019.[1] Most originally settled in the mining regions of Pennsylvania, Ohio, and other midwestern states; mining also attracted sizable populations to Colorado, Nevada, Arizona, and California. More than 179,000 Slovenian Americans were identified in the 2019 U.S. Census data.[1] Although many Slovenian immigrants also became involved in mining, others moved to industrial urban areas in search of jobs. Forty percent live in Ohio, with Cleveland having the largest Slovenian community in the nation. Other states with notable Slovenian populations include Pennsylvania, Minnesota, Wisconsin, California, Colorado, Michigan, Florida, and New York. Many Croatians, Serbians, and Slovenians who first arrived in the United States were unskilled laborers in agriculture or industry. Education was valued and second-generation immigrants obtained the training needed to secure white-collar employment. Over time, most Americans of Croatian, Serbian, and Slovenian descent have assimilated into the U.S. mainstream, working in all sectors of the economy. Incomes are usually at or over the U.S. average.[2–4]

Beginning in the early 1990s, nearly 200,000 Bosnian refugees seeking refuge from ethnic cleansing in that region were resettled in the United States. Many left their homeland suddenly, with little time to pack or prepare for life in a new country. Nearly all are Muslim, and most were not comfortable in the small number of Bosnian Serbian or Bosnian Croatian communities already scattered throughout the United States. A majority have chosen to live in homogeneous Bosnian Muslim neighborhoods in New York, St. Louis, Chicago, Salt Lake City, St. Petersburg, Florida, and Waynesboro, Pennsylvania. Significant populations are found in California as well. Though approximately half of the Bosnian refugees arrived unskilled in any profession, today 68 percent of their young adults are attending institutions of higher education.[5]

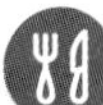

Food for Thought

The 2016 Canadian census lists over 271,405 residents of Greek ancestry, 133,965 Croatians, and much smaller populations of Serbians and Slovenians.

Middle Easterners Demographic figures for Middle Easterners are more problematic. Some older immigrants may deny their Arab ancestry due to a history of discrimination in the West, and more recent arrivals may refuse cooperation with government-sponsored surveys due to negative experiences in their homelands and fear of mistreatment following the September 11, 2001 attacks on the United States. Immigration figures suggest, however, that Arabs are one of the fastest-growing ethnic groups in the nation, increasing from approximately 200,000 in 1970 to over 2 million in 2019.

In 2019, the Census estimated 481,000 self-declared Americans from Lebanon, 179,000 from Syria, 279,000 from Egypt, 118,000 from Morocco, 93,000 from Jordan, and 176,000 from Iraq.[1] A movement toward pan-Arab Americanism is seen in the number of U.S.-born Arabs who are selecting "Arab" or "Arabic" as their background instead of national affiliation.[6,7] Two-thirds of Arabs have settled in California, New York, and Michigan. The largest concentration of Arabs (including those from areas other than the Middle East) is in the Detroit metropolitan area.[6,7] Most Arabs choose urban areas of residence, and ethnic neighborhoods have developed in cities with substantial Arab populations. These communities help preserve Arab culture within what is often viewed as an alien American society.

Early Arab immigrants found it easy to assimilate into American society, in part because a majority of them were Christian. Many survived as peddlers and then later opened family businesses, usually dry goods or grocery stores. A tradition of entrepreneurship among Arabs continues today, and nearly one in five owns his or her own business. Even families that started with unskilled employment or small businesses have made substantial economic progress through schooling. Nearly every Arab American group in the 2021 Census reported that 50 percent had a college degree or higher, and median family income was above the U.S. average.[1]

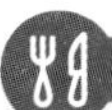

Food for Thought

McDonald's and Walmart sell halal foods like halal Chicken McNuggets™ at certain U.S. locations.

Persia was the conventional European name for Iran, used until the early twentieth century; many Iranian immigrants prefer the designation Persian American.

Over 468,000 Americans of Iranian heritage were living in the United States according to 2019 Census figures. Nearly half reside in Southern California, and another large population is found in New York City.[1] Many who immigrated following the 1979 Iranian revolution were among the well-educated elite who spoke English fluently and were skilled in a profession, such as engineering, medicine, pharmacy, dentistry, and law. Others arrived in the United States with substantial savings from their livelihood in Iran. This group has been economically successful in the United States. It is also reported that many Iranian immigrants are self-employed.[8] Data on foreign-born Iranians show that over half hold college degrees, and median household income far exceeds that of the average U.S. family. Turkish Americans numbered 212,000 in the census estimates of 2019. Immigration before 1965 was severely limited by quotas, yet included a disproportionate number of engineers and physicians. Since that time, the number of Turkish immigrants has increased, with most seeking educational and occupational opportunities.[9] Homogeneous neighborhoods, supported by Turkish American organizations, have been established in many cities, including New York City, Boston, Chicago, Detroit, Los Angeles, San Francisco, and Rochester, New York. Smaller populations are found in New England, the Midwest, and parts of the South, including Maryland, Virginia, Texas, and Georgia. Census statistics on foreign-born Turkish Americans indicate higher rates of high school and college graduation than the U.S. norm, and median household income above the U.S. family average. Turkish Americans are found in most employment sectors and are solidly middle-class in socioeconomic status.[9]

Most Israelis today come to the United States for educational and professional opportunities; many are of European heritage and are typically middle- or upper-income. According to the 2019 U.S. Census, there were 144,000 Israeli Americans. Some arrivals are also seeking security and escape from the political unrest in their home region. Most possess the job skills that ensure an easy transition in the United States, and over half hold professional, managerial, or technical positions. They are prominent in the fields of medicine, technology, architecture, entertainment, and education. Approximately one-third are self-employed in the garment industry, electronic industry, or small businesses catering to the Israeli community, including restaurants, nightclubs, and retail shops.[10] Their average earnings are believed to be higher than the U.S. norm.

Worldview

Religion In the Balkans and the Middle East, religion is often a defining factor in life. Although affiliation varies, strong devotion is common. Many congregations remain insular in the United States, serving the needs of a specific ethnic group, and there is little interest in proselytizing to outsiders.

Balkans The ethnicity of Greek immigrants was affirmed mostly by religion; it was said that a person was not Greek by birth but through an active affiliation with the Greek Eastern Orthodox Church. The first Greek Orthodox Church in America was founded in New Orleans in 1864. Most Greek Americans today still belong to the church, which continues to be the center of Greek community life. The word *orthodox* comes from the Greek for "correct" (*orthos*) and "worship" (*doxa*). A fundamental belief of the Greek Orthodox faith is that an individual attains complete identification with God through participation in the numerous religious services and activities sponsored by the church. Although the Greek Orthodox Church is conservative and traditionally resistant to change, some accommodations have been made in the United States; for instance, the service typically is conducted both in Greek and English, and modern organ music accompanies the liturgy (refer to Chapter 4 for more information about Greek Orthodoxy).

Most people from Serbia also belong to the Eastern Orthodox faith as members of the Serbian Orthodox Autonomous Church. A majority of people from Croatia and Slovenia are devout Roman Catholics, worshiping primarily in multiethnic congregations. A small number of Slovenians are Protestants known as Windish. Windish churches have helped maintain Slovenian ethnic identity through services conducted in a Slovenian dialect. Small populations of Croatian Muslims are found in Cleveland and Chicago.

Early Bosnian Croat immigrants were mostly members of the Catholic Church, and Bosnian Serb immigrants followed the Eastern Orthodox religion. An estimated 68 Serbian Orthodox churches exist in the United States, serving both the worship and social needs of each community. The majority of recent Bosnian refugees are Sunni Muslims. In St. Louis, Missouri, for instance, an estimated 70,000 Bosnians, many of them Muslim, call the city home. The majority of this group arrived in the 1990s, fleeing civil war at home.[11] Regardless of faith, many Bosnians are more secular than observant, attending services on major holidays only, or not at all. Intermarriage between Bosnians of different religious beliefs is not uncommon.[6]

Middle Easterners Early Arab immigrants were primarily Christians belonging to the Eastern Orthodox (particularly the Egyptian Coptic Church) or the Latin rite Maronite, Melkite, or Chaldean churches. Although Christian Arabs are still a majority in America, more recent immigrants follow Islam, and the number of Arab Muslims in the United States is growing rapidly. Of all Muslims living in the United States, 14 percent are from the Middle East or North Africa.[12] Overall, there are 3.45 million followers of Islam in the United States and most (55 percent) belong to the Sunni sect. The others are Shiite (16 percent) and the rest identify with neither group.[13] Many Arab Muslims in the United States have made several adaptations to accommodate their religious practices to American society. Most significantly, the Friday Sabbath prayer has been moved to Sunday, and many Muslims cannot fulfill their obligation to pray five times daily due to work or school limitations (refer to Chapter 4 for more information about Islam).

Although 40 percent of Iranians in the United States are members of the Muslim Shiite community, 20 percent identify with Christianity, Judaism, Zoroastrianism, and Baha'ism (which preaches gender equality, world brotherhood, and pacifism) in equal portions; the remaining 40 percent do not identify with a particular religion.[14] Most Turkish Americans are Sunni Muslims and many worship at Arab or Pakistani mosques.

Presumably, most Israeli Americans are followers of Judaism. However, unlike other Middle Eastern groups, Israelis who immigrate may be among the least religious in Israel. Many, upon arrival, choose to join Reform congregations or are unaffiliated with a synagogue.

Family

Balkans The traditional Greek home is strongly patriarchal. The head of the household is the unquestioned authority, with responsibility for supporting the immediate family and elder parents. In addition, he is accountable for the family's reputation within the community. The Greek term for this pride and obligation to family is philot imo, meaning "love of honor." Each family member is expected to behave in ways that maintain family dignity and status.

Obligation to family and community has lessened somewhat in the Greek American community. Extended families have become less common due to assimilation pressures and secondary migration to other areas of the country. Children are doted on, and parents often put their welfare first. Yet obedience and respect for elders are expected, and intergenerational conflict is less common among Greek Americans than in many other immigrant groups.

Greek women had traditionally focused on family, home, and church. Even after coming to the United States, many Greek American women continued in this role. Today, they balance their duty to family and community with personal interests in education or pursuing a career. Education is valued by Greek men and women.

Croatian and Serbian families are also traditionally patriarchal. Extended families are the norm, often including friends as well as relatives. Among Croatians, communal living may involve taking in boarders. Both Croatians and Serbians have become well-acculturated in the United States. The tradition of older generations caring for children has allowed many Croatian and Serbian women to take advantage of educational and career opportunities, and the authority of the father has lessened. Slovenian Americans are also assimilated. The extended family structure typical in Slovenia is rarely found among Slovenians in the United States, who prefer nuclear families. American women of Slovenian descent are active in the home, church, and Slovenian schools and are increasingly involved in politics.

Food for Thought

The tall white hats worn by professional chefs are thought to have originated when the Byzantine Empire invaded Greece and Greek chefs fled to nearby monasteries for protection, adopting the monks' large stovepipe hats to fit in.[15] Another story involves creating the pleats in the hat to resemble the royal crown in Assyrian culture. And yet another story claims a chef for Henry III lost a hair in the king's soup so he was beheaded and all chefs thereafter were required to wear hats. The contemporary chef's hat was adopted around 1900.[16]

Of the 90,000 Jews living in Iran in 1987, 55,000 have since left, including 35,000 who have immigrated to the United States.[14]

Bosnians traditionally maintained extended family homes, but conflict in the region and migration to urban areas has resulted in more nuclear families living apart from relatives.[17] In the United States, the extended family structure is important to newer arrivals but difficult for some refugees who had no family members already established in the country. While strong family bonds support new immigrants, Bosnian women (who are not employed outside the home) and older family members are often dependent on extended family and may become isolated within the larger community. As is true of other immigrant populations, Bosnian immigrants in the United States are attracted to established communities of other Bosnians partly because many are separated from immediate family and it often takes years to reunite.[18] Traditionally, Bosnian husbands and wives both work but responsibility for the home remains with the wife. Bosnian children assimilate quickly to American culture, and some parents are frustrated by their inability to instill Bosnian cultural values and maintain the Bosnian language within the home.

Food for Thought

Bosnian pita, a phyllo pastry often filled with meat, cheese, and potatoes, or spinach and cheese, is distinctive. In other parts of the former Yugoslavia, pitas that are meat-filled are called burek. A pita meat pie is often the final course of a meal or is served as a light supper on its own.

Almost all Bosnian family names end with the suffix *ic*, which essentially means "child of," much like the use of the suffix "son" in names such as Johnson. Women's first names tend to end in the letter *a* or *ica*, pronounced EET-sa.[18]

Middle Easterners Traditionally, Arab cultures center on a strong patriarchal family whose honor must be maintained. The family demands conformity and subordination of individual will and interest, but in return, the members of the family are protected and can identify with the family's status. Families often live with extended members in a single home or, for well-to-do Arabs, in a family compound. An exception is Egyptians, who traditionally live in nuclear family groups.[19]

The teachings of the Qur'an state that men and women are considered equal but with different roles and responsibilities. Children are valued in Arab families, and sacrifice for the good of the children is common. Men are obligated to provide economic security for children, while women are expected to socialize them, including the preservation of religious and cultural values. It is the role of women to provide love and comfort in the home as well. The relationship between mothers and daughters is very intimate. There is also a strong bond between mothers and sons, especially the firstborn son.[20,21]

Courtship as a prelude to marriage in Arab culture often involves input from the bride and groom's nuclear and extended families. An engagement may be viewed as a time to get to know the potential partner before deciding whether or not to marry.[21] Only after an engagement announcement is made are young men and women allowed to date, and then only when chaperoned. A family's honor is related to the modesty and chastity of the women in the home: A woman is chaste before her wedding and faithful after. Actual or alleged violations of moral codes by a young woman are considered evidence that her mother has failed in her responsibilities; inappropriate sexual conduct also disgraces her relatives. Interethnic marriages are strongly discouraged by both Muslims and Christians, especially for women. For many, it is preferable to marry someone of a different ethnic group and the same religious affiliation than to marry outside the religion. Most Iranians and Turks establish homes similar to those of Arabs, headed by the father or eldest sons, and centered on an extended family network for support. Immigration to the United States often results in difficulties in maintaining an extended family household for many Middle Easterners. Family ties remain strong among Arabs, Iranians, and Turks; however, nuclear families are the norm for most immigrants. It is still common for grandparents to live with their children and grandchildren, yet in some more acculturated families (such as in many Lebanese homes) daughters are no longer solely responsible for the care of older family members, but a duty they now share with their brothers.[22–24]

The role of women of Middle Eastern heritage in the United States is changing for those who are engaged in American society, and the customarily strict separation of private and public spheres has blurred with increased numbers of women seeking college degrees and professional careers.[7,24] For example, dating is becoming more accepted as segregation of the sexes cannot be maintained in most schools, nor in the U.S. workplace. More traditional Middle Eastern women are sometimes isolated in their home life. Some Iranian women, for instance, feel that their limited authority has decreased since arriving in the United States, that they spend more time on household chores, and that they are less involved in family decisions and mosque activities. More acculturated Arab women may also experience serious setbacks in acceptance of their Americanized conduct every time a large influx of new and conservatively minded Middle Eastern women settles in their area.[7]

Many second-and third-generation Middle Easterners in the United States think that their parents are old-fashioned. The adoption of American practices, such as personal autonomy and self-determination, contradicts the Middle Eastern emphasis on doing what is best for the good of the family, increasing intergenerational conflict between parents and children. Acculturation also may result in the reduction of a father's authority in some Middle Eastern homes, though filial respect is usually retained. Pressures for children to adhere to family expectations—from participation in arranged marriages to denial of college attendance—can be substantial, however, and not all children reject the values of their parents. Although some Arab groups, such as Egyptians and Syrians, are especially well acculturated, and some subgroups within each population are fully integrated within the U.S. society, resistance to American culture can be strong among a small number of Middle Eastern immigrants. The attempt to retain ethnic identity takes many forms, and it cannot be assumed that assimilation is automatic, especially for new immigrants who may to return to their homeland when conflicts subside or are fearful of discrimination in the United States. For example, some Arab immigrants seek to insulate their families from the influences of American society by isolating them within homogeneous enclaves. Other communities open their doors for increased interaction; for example, after the September 11, 2001, Al Qaeda attacks, some Turkish American communities coordinated interfaith dialogs and conferences. This was done to foster an understanding of their faith and culture, and allow other Americans to get to know them better.[9]

A majority of Israelis live in nuclear families. After arrival in the United States, the nuclear family structure continues with support from Jewish organizations and a network of Israeli American groups. Israeli American women are typically well-educated and over half are employed outside the home, often in professional positions. Israeli immigrants are often concerned that their cultural values will be lost if their children become acculturated, and a great concern is the preservation of their identity within the U.S. culture.[10] Many Israeli parents, like American Jewish parents, strive to preserve ethnic identity by enrolling their children in religious training and Jewish summer camps, and by sending them to Israel to learn about their heritage.

Traditional Health Beliefs and Practices

Balkans In many parts of the Balkans, physical fitness is thought essential to good health and is also considered necessary in the development of good character. Team sports, water activities, gymnastics, skiing, hiking, and bicycling are common forms of exercise. Among some Greeks, eating a good diet, relaxing, adequate sleep, and keeping a positive mental attitude are equally important to maintaining health.[2,3,25,26]

Traditionally, most health care was provided by grandmothers or mothers at home. Many people kept an herbal pharmacy available for the preparation of therapeutic teas. In Greece, castor oil is taken to clean the bowels, quinine is used to relieve pain, chamomile tea is sipped to get rid of cramps, and a sore throat is treated with honey and lemon. Examples of Bosnian cures also include chamomile, as well as elder, rose hips, and mint.[18] Greek cupping (refer to Chapter 2 for more information) is similar to the Asian method, except that the skin is cut with a razor first to allow the blood out. to treat colds and chest ailments. More severe conditions and serious injuries are treated by neighborhood experts, for instance, the midwives and bone-setters used in Croatia. Some people in the Balkans believe that the evil eye of one who envies a person can cause accidents or illness. Greeks may use ritual prayer, the sign of the cross, or wear blue amulets with an eye in the center or garlic as a precaution against a jealous gaze. When receiving a compliment (a form of envy), it is also customary to spit two or three times to keep harm away. The peoples of the Balkans give special magical healing power to stones with holes. Alternative medicine is very well-known and mystical. There is also a belief in the healing power of sacred or healing water.[27]

Food for Thought

The Sufis, members of an ascetic and mystical Islamic sect, define health as an existential state of abstinence, patience, and self-examination, resulting in harmony with the universe.

Zamzam water from the Mecca Valley is collected by Muslims who complete the hajj (pilgrimage to Mecca) to be shared with family and friends at home—it is thought to have curative powers.

Middle Easterners Traditional humoral medicine is important in the health practices of Iranians. Though traditional humoral theories identify four bodily humors, in practice

Iranians are concerned primarily with hot and cold. Each person is born with a physiological temperament dependent on the ratio of humors, which varies by gender, age, and race—women, for instance, are considered colder than men, and younger persons are hotter than older people—and can be influenced by diet, climate, geographic location and certain conditions, such as childbirth.[28] Sickness can be caused by consuming too many hot items or too many cold foods (refer to the "Therapeutic Uses of Food" section), but individual conditions and symptoms are not classified as being hot or cold. Iranians are also concerned with the amount of blood they have, which in turn is associated with numerous ailments, including thinness (due to lack of proper nourishment), weakness, irritability, lethargy, and headaches. Kam Kuhn—blood deficiency due to excessive bleeding from injuries, menstruation, or a poor diet that prevents the making of blood—is the source of these symptoms.

Iranians use the term narahati for undifferentiated feelings of physical and emotional discomfort. Most often it is expressed privately and in a nonverbal form through sullenness, anorexia, and, among women, bouts of crying. Expressions of anger are considered the public expressions of the condition and are usually discouraged because anger is a lack of control that can upset the social order and cause others to become narahat. Sorrow or grief is another public expression, but in contrast to anger, sadness is considered the poetic manifestation of fully experiencing the tragedy of the human condition. Naharati qalb (heart distress) is a folk condition typified by fluttering of the heart due to the strong expression of anger or sadness.[29]

A long-standing tradition of home health care exists among Middle Easterners. Folk remedies are common, such as rubbing *ko'hl* (a dark powder made mainly from the chemical element antimony and used mostly as a cosmetic) on the umbilical cord of an infant to help it dry. Herbal therapies are especially prevalent, and it is believed that approximately 200 plant species are used in Arab traditional medicine today.[30] Examples include yarrow for diabetes and *khella* (a member of the parsley family) for kidney disorders. One recent study looked at the use of self-medication with antibiotics (SMA) in the Middle East and found that the prevalence of SMA ranged from 19% to 82%. Most of these were penicillin left over from pharmacies without prescriptions or friends/relatives and were taken for upper-respiratory track problems.[31] Palestinians use most traditional remedies as both food and medicine; for instance, caraway is used for digestive disorders and to increase milk flow in nursing mothers; mallow is used as a laxative; and olive oil to treat urinary tract infections, prostate conditions, and cancer.[32,33] Other cures include snakeroot as a diuretic, lavender for kidney stones, and rue as an analgesic and sedative. A popular herbal "wonder drug" for cancer that has spread through the Middle East is *Ephedra foeminea* (Alanda). This is concerning as the drug could interfere with the cytotoxic effects of chemotherapy. In Iran, foxglove blossoms are used especially for nervous conditions, and some digestive problems, to strengthen the blood, relieve fear, and for pains of unknown etiology; arugula seeds are taken to clean dirty blood and for fever, constipation, and nausea; and mint tea with coriander seeds is used to promote sleep.[30,34,35] In Turkey, nettle, oleander, and thyme are used therapeutically for cancer. Other commonly used herbal remedies include St. John's wort, rosemary, sage, and hawthorne. In one recent study of individuals with type 2 diabetes in Saudi Arabia (which has the second highest rate of diabetes in the Middle East), 68 percent were frequent consumers of herbal remedies, especially cinnamon, ginger, and fenugreek, which were used to treat the disease.[36]

Cupping (refer to Chapter 2) is used by some Middle Easterners to cure chronic leg pain, paralysis, headaches, and obesity. Another therapy that is sometimes applied is called *wasm* or cauterization.[37,38] A heated iron rod is used to place symbolic burn marks on the patient, for example, below the anus to treat diarrhea and under the ear lobe to cure a toothache. The burns are then treated with special herbal poultices. This practice has decreased over the years due to several adverse events and problems such as severe burns, wound infections, and worsening of the disease due to delayed treatment. Although superstition is discouraged in Islam, many Arabs retain some beliefs in magic and supernatural causes of illness. As in the Balkans, the evil eye is feared by some Arabs, who may place blue beads on infants to protect them, or wear amulets. In Iran, some believe the evil eye is the cause of cheshm-i-bad, the occurrence of a sudden or unexplained illness.[30,34] Some Arabs attribute mental illness to possession by the devil or by jinn (spirits who can be good or evil).

Iranians often put their health into the hands of God. Taqdir, meaning "God's will," is thought to determine all aspects of life and, ultimately, death. Throughout the Middle East, illness is sometimes seen as a punishment from God. However, biomedical practice is well established in the Middle East, and for the most part, Western therapies are considered strong and effective.[14]

Traditional Food Habits

The origins of many Balkan and Middle Eastern dishes may never be known because the geographic, political, and economic history of the region has resulted in similar food cultures. Many ingredients in the Balkans and the Middle East, including wheat, olives, and dates, are indigenous. Sheep were first domesticated in the region over 10,000 years ago. Other foods, such as rice, chickpeas, and lemons, gained widespread acceptance after introduction. Yet most countries in the area claim one dish or another prepared by all ethnic groups to be their own invention.

Culinary commonalities extend beyond the arbitrary designation of the Balkan and Middle Eastern nations. As previously mentioned, North Africa is sometimes considered part of the Middle East and shares numerous dishes of the region. In addition, the southern nations of the former Soviet Union, the southern regions of central Europe, and parts of South Asia exhibit influences as well.

The most significant differences in Balkan and Middle Eastern foods are due to various religious dietary restrictions and proximity to other global cuisines. For example, the Christian populations of Croatia, Serbia, and Slovenia frequently consume pork, a favorite of neighboring central Europeans. Yet, Christian Greeks, who have no pork prohibitions, eat it only occasionally, preferring lamb and goat, similar to adjacent Middle Easterners. Alcoholic beverages are banned for Muslims and are avoided in most Middle Eastern nations, though widely consumed in Turkey, perhaps due to historical associations with nearby Russia (beet soup is also popular). But despite these distinctions, foods are far more similar than different.

Ingredients and Common Foods

Staples The common ingredients used in Balkan and Middle Eastern cooking are listed in Table 13.1. Wheat, thought to have been cultivated first in this region, is consumed at every meal as bread. Leavened loaves are typical in Greece and the other Balkan nations, and leavened as well as unleavened flatbreads are more common in Middle Eastern countries. However, both loaves and flatbreads are found throughout the region. Pita or pida, a thin, round Arabic bread with a hollow center (sometimes known as pocket bread in the United States), is a common type, as is lavash, a larger, crisp flatbread (also called cracker bread).

 **Food for Thought**

The olive tree, which grows in the coastal areas of the eastern Mediterranean, southeastern Europe, northern Iran, western Asia, and northern Africa, is one of the oldest cultivated trees on the planet, with evidence dating back more than 7,000 years. Olive trees are important in the context of religion—olives are mentioned several times in the Bible, both in the New and Old Testaments. It is also praised as a blessed tree and fruit in the Holy Qur'an.[39]

Besides bread, wheat dough is also used to make pies and turnovers prepared in a variety of sizes and shapes. Bread dough, shortcrust, or paper-thin pastry sheets called filo or phyllo are all used. Savory pies may contain meat, cheese, eggs, or vegetables. Desserts are usually filled with nuts or dried fruits. An example of a fried meat or cheese-filled pastry that can be served hot or cold is called a sanbusak. Traditionally half-moon-shaped, sanbusak is popular in Syria, Lebanon, and Egypt. A similar turnover is called burek in Slovenia and boereg in Bulgaria and Romania. Fatayer is another specialty served as a snack, featuring bread dough topped with cheese, meat, or spinach and baked like a pizza. Tiropitas are Greek flaky turnovers stuffed with cheese. In Serbia, a cheese and egg pie called gibanica is popular. A dessert called baklava or paklava made with filo dough can be purchased at every bakery and café throughout the Balkans and Middle East. The sheets of dough are layered with a walnut, almond, or pistachio filling and then soaked in a syrup

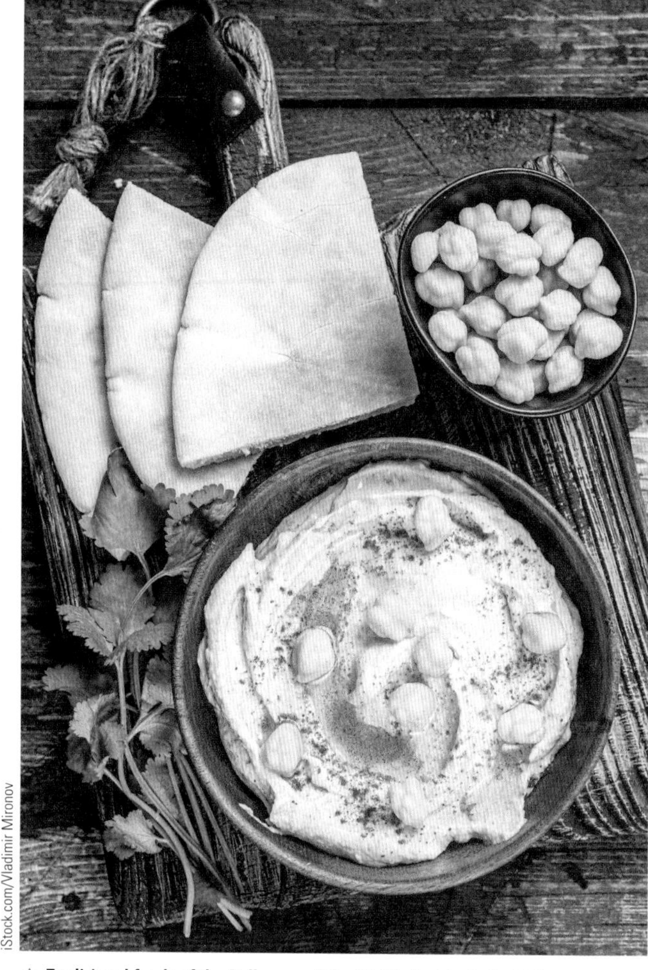

iStock.com/Vladimir Mironov

▲ Traditional foods of the Balkans and the Middle East include chickpea hummus, pita bread, and parsley.

flavored with honey, brandy, rose water, or orange blossom water. It is often cut into diamond shapes.

Raw kernels of cracked whole wheat are used in several Balkan and Middle Eastern dishes. When the kernels are first steamed and then dried and crushed to different degrees of fineness, the cracked wheat is called burghul or bulgur. Un-ripened, roasted and crushed wheat kernels are known in Arabic markets as freekeh. All varieties of wheat kernels are typically cooked as side dishes or made into tabouli, a popular salad containing onions, parsley, mint, and various fresh vegetables. Another Arab specialty is kish'ka, made by blending bulgur with yogurt, drying the mixture in the sun, then grinding it into a powder that can later be reconstituted with water to make a filling for pita or thinned enough for soup. In Serbia, wheat kernels are cooked with sugar, dried fruits, and ground nuts to make koljivo.

Dumplings filled with meat are called cmoki in Slovenia and are stuffed with fruit for dessert. In Turkey, cheese or meat dumplings are known as manti. A few pasta dishes are found in the Balkans, such as the Greek pasta with baked lamb or goat and tomatoes called yiouvetsi and macaroni baked with cheese, ground meat, tomato sauce, and bechamel

Table 13.1 Cultural Food Groups: Balkans and Middle East

Group	Comments	Common Foods	Adaptations in the United States
Protein Foods			
Milk/milk products	Most dairy products are consumed in fermented form (yogurt, cheese). Whole milk is used in desserts, especially puddings. Sour cream and whipped cream are common in northern Balkan nations. High incidence of lactose intolerance is reported.	Cheese (goat's, sheep's, cow's, and camel's), milk (goat's, sheep's, camel's, and cow's), yogurt; buttermilk, cream	More cow's milk and less sheep's, camel's, and goat's milk are drunk. Ice cream is popular. Feta is the most common Middle Eastern cheese available in the United States.
Meat/poultry/fish/eggs/legumes	Lamb is the most popular meat. Pork is eaten only by Christians, not by Muslims or Jews. Jews do not eat shellfish. In Egypt, fish is generally not eaten with dairy products. Legumes are commonly consumed.	*Meat:* beef, kid, lamb, pork, rabbit, veal, many variety cuts *Poultry:* chicken, duck, pigeon, turkey *Fish and shellfish:* anchovies, bass, bream, clams, cod, crab, crawfish, eels, flounder, frog legs, halibut, lobster, mackerel, mullet, mussels, oysters, redfish, salmon, sardines, shrimp *Eggs:* poultry, fish *Legumes:* black beans, chickpeas (garbanzo beans), fava (broad) beans, lentils, navy beans, red beans; peanuts	Lamb is still very popular. More beef and fewer legumes are eaten.
Cereals/Grains	Some form of wheat or rice usually accompanies the meal in the Balkans and Middle East.	Bread (wheat, barley, corn, millet), barley, buckwheat, corn, farina, millet, oatmeal, pasta, rice (long-grain and basmati), wheat (bulgur, couscous)	Bread and grains are eaten at most meals. Pita bread is commonly available.
Fruits/Vegetables	Fruits are eaten for dessert or as snacks. Fresh fruit and vegetables are preferred, but if they are not available, fruits are served as jams and compotes and vegetables as pickles. Eggplant is very popular. Vegetables are consumed often; sometimes stuffed with rice or a meat mixture.	*Fruits:* apples, apricots, avocado, barberries, bergamots, cherries, currants, dates, figs, grapes, lemons, limes, melons (most varieties), oranges, peaches, pears, plums, pomegranates, quinces, raisins, strawberries, tangerines *Vegetables:* artichokes, asparagus, beets, broccoli, brussels sprouts, cabbage, carrots, cauliflower, celeriac, celery, corn, cucumbers, eggplant, grape leaves, green beans, green peppers, greens, Jerusalem artichokes, leeks, lettuce, mushrooms, okra, olives, onions, peas, pimientos, potatoes, spinach, squashes, tomatoes, turnips, zucchini	Fewer fruits and vegetables are consumed. Olives are still popular.
Additional Foods			
Seasonings	Numerous spices and herbs are used. Lemons are often used for flavoring.	*Ajowan,* allspice, anise, basil, bay leaf, caraway seed, cardamom, cayenne, chervil, chives, chocolate, cinnamon, cloves, coriander, cumin, dill, fennel, fenugreek seeds, garlic, ginger, gum arabic and mastic, lavender, linden blossoms, mace, *mahleb,* marjoram, mint, mustard, nasturtium flowers, nutmeg, orange blossoms or water, oregano, paprika, parsley, pepper (red and black), rose petals and water, rosemary, saffron, sage, savory, sorrel, *sumac,* tamarind, tarragon, thyme, turmeric, *verjuice,* verbena, vinegar	
Nuts/seeds	Ground nuts are often used to thicken soups and stews.	Almonds, cashews, hazelnuts, peanuts, pine nuts, pistachios, walnuts; poppy, pumpkin, sunflower, sesame seeds	

(Continued)

Table 13.1 Cultural Food Groups: Balkans and Middle East (*Continued*)

Group	Comments	Common Foods	Adaptations in the United States
Beverages	Coffee and tea are often flavored with cardamom or mint, respectively. Aperitifs are often anise flavored. Alcoholic beverages are prohibited for Muslims, but consumed in most of the Balkans, Turkey, and Israel.	Coffee, date palm juice, fruit juices, tea and herbal infusions, yogurt drinks; beer, wine, brandy	
Fats/oils	Olive oil is generally used in dishes that are to be eaten cold. For most deep-frying, corn or nut oil is used; olive oil is preferred for deep-frying fish. Clarified butter (*samana*) is also popular. Sheep's tail fat is a delicacy.	Butter, olive oil, sesame oil, various nut and vegetable oils, rendered lamb fat	Olive oil is still popular.
Sweeteners	Coffee and tea are heavily sweetened. Dessert syrups are flavored with honey, rose water, or orange-flower water.	Honey, sugar	

sauce called pastitsio. A dish similar to Italian pasta with beans is prepared. In the Middle East, vermicelli is often added to rice, and noodles are found in a few dishes, such as Syrian chicken with macaroni.

In addition to wheat, rice is also a staple item in Middle Eastern cuisine and is found in some Balkan regions. The long-grain variety is used to make pilaf, called plov in Uzbekistan, a dish that commonly accompanies meat or poultry. The rice is first sautéed in butter or oil in which chopped onions have been browned. It is then steamed in chicken or beef broth. Saffron or turmeric may be added to give the dish a deep yellow color.

Polo is the Iranian version of pilaf, but a final step in its preparation produces rice with a crunchy brown crust known as the tah dig. A more fragrant variety of rice, basmati, is used in Iran for khoresh, rice topped with stewed meat, poultry, or legumes. Rice is frequently added to soups and stuffings for poultry and vegetables in both the Balkans and the Middle East.

A large variety of legumes are another important ingredient in both Balkan and Middle Eastern cooking. Cooked, pureed chickpeas are the base for hummus, often served as an appetizer or as a dip. Ground chickpeas or fava beans are sometimes formed into small balls and then fried and served as a main course (ta'amia) or in pita bread with raw vegetables (falafel). A common breakfast food is foul, which is slowly simmered fava or black beans topped with chopped tomato, garlic, lemon juice, olive oil, and cilantro (fresh coriander leaves). Lentils are especially popular in the soups of some areas.

Food for Thought

In the Balkans and the Middle East, burek is a filled filo-like pastry often sold at street food stalls.

Many vegetables are used, although eggplant is the most popular in the Middle East, Greece, and southern Balkan regions. A traditional cooking method dating to the Middle Ages in the Middle East (yakhni in Arabic; yiachni in Greek) is a meat or vegetable preparation stewed simply with onions, tomato, garlic, and herbs in a small amount of water. Vegetable salads of freshly sliced tomatoes or cucumbers are common as are cold, cooked vegetable salads. Vegetables are frequently stuffed with a meat or rice mixture. Moussaka or musaka is a Balkan specialty made with minced lamb, eggplant, onions, and tomato sauce baked in a dish lined with eggplant slices. The Turks prefer imam bayildi (meaning "the priest fainted"), eggplant filled with tomatoes, onions, and garlic, stewed in olive oil which is served cold.[40] Grape or cabbage leaves are stuffed to make the specialties known as dolma or sarma. Potatoes, particularly enjoyed in the northern Balkan nations, are also found in some Middle Eastern stews and side dishes. Vegetables are frequently enjoyed raw, mixed in a salad, or preserved as pickles. Sauerkraut is eaten in Croatia, Serbia, and Slovenia.

The olive tree contributes in many ways, particularly to Greek and Middle Eastern cooking. Olives prepared in a Middle Eastern marinade of aromatics sometimes have a much stronger flavor than European or American olives; they often accompany the meal or are served as an appetizer (refer to Table 13.2). The olive is also a source of oil, which is frequently used in food preparation, although butter, clarified butter (samana), and most vegetable oils, as well as rendered lamb fat and margarine, are found in the Balkans and the Middle East. Olive oil is generally used in dishes that are to be eaten cold. For most deep-frying, corn or nut oil is used, but olive oil is preferred for deep-frying fish.

Fruits are preferred fresh, eaten for dessert or as snacks. Apricots, cherries, figs, dates, grapes, melons, pomegranates, and quince are favorites. Pears, plums, and pumpkins are well-liked in the more temperate climates of the northern

Table 13.2 Glossary of Selected Olives

Olives originated in the Middle East and spread throughout the Mediterranean. They are picked unripe (green, with dry, firm flesh and a bitter taste) or when fully ripened (black, oilier, soft textured, and milder in flavor). Raw olives are inedible and must be cured in salt (also called dry-cured) or in a brine, oil, wine, or lye solution before they can be consumed. Both the stage at which they are harvested and the type of curing process affect the flavor of the final product.

Aleppo (Middle East)	Small, dry-cured black olive (with wrinkled, chewy texture) named after a Syrian city
Amphissa (Greek)	Dark purple olives with nutty flavor
Gaeta (Italy)	Medium black olives, dry-cured (with wrinkled texture) or brine-cured (with smooth purplish flesh)
Kalamata (Greece/Middle East)	Large, deep-purple with crunchy texture—salt-cured, packed in vinegar (sometimes with preserved lemon in Morocco)
Kura (Middle East)	Large green olive with hard flesh cracked to allow penetration of brine, bitter flavored, also called Middle Eastern cracked green
Manzanilla (Spain)	Small to large green olive usually pitted and stuffed with other ingredients (e.g., pimento, garlic, almonds)
Middle Eastern Green	Small, brine-cured olives packed with olive oil, herbs, and often chili peppers
Moroccan Dry-Cured	Medium black, dry-cured with wrinkled flesh and bitter flavor, used mostly in cooking
Nabali (Middle East)	Dark green olive with soft texture, brine-cured, and often packed with lemon, garlic, and vinegar—grown in Israel (including the Palestinian territories) and Jordan; also called *mushhan, baladi*, or Roman olives
Naphlion (Greece)	Dark green, brine-cured, packed in olive oil
Niçoise (France)	Small, sour, salt-cured purplish black olives
Picholine (France)	Small, mild, salt-cured light green olives
Sicilian (Italy)	Very large, green olive, brine-cured, somewhat sour
Thassos (Greece)	Small, dry-cured black olives (with wrinkled texture), intense tart flavor

Balkan nations. A distinctive characteristic of Middle Eastern fare is the addition of fruits to savory dishes; apricot sauce tops meatballs in Egypt and chicken in Syria. Fruits are also often served dried or as jams and compotes. Slatko is a Balkan specialty featuring fruits simmered in thick syrup. Fruit juices (especially lemon) and syrups flavor many foods.

Fresh milk is not widely consumed in the Balkans or Middle East, though it is used in puddings and custards. Dairy products are usually fermented into yogurt or processed into cheese. Yogurt is eaten as a side dish and served plain (unsweetened) or mixed with cucumbers or other vegetables. It is diluted to make a refreshing drink. Cheese is usually made from goat, sheep, or (in the Middle East) camel's milk. The most widely used cheese is feta, a salty, white, moist cheese that crumbles easily. Myzithra, a soft pot cheese, is a by-product of the feta process. Labneh or labni is a fresh cheese made by draining the whey from salted yogurt overnight. Haloumi is a springy, semisoft cheese that is sometimes flavored with mint. It holds its shape when cooked, and pieces can be grilled quickly on both sides for a hot treat. Kaseri is a firm, white, aged cheese, mild in flavor and similar to Italian provolone. Kashkaval is a hard, tangy ewe's milk cheese, sometimes called the cheddar of the Balkans.

Almost all meats and seafood are eaten in the Balkans and the Middle East, except pork in Muslim countries and pork and shellfish among observant Jews in Israel. Lamb is the most widely used meat, though pork is very popular in the northern Balkan areas. Grilling, frying, grinding, and stewing are the common ways of preparing meat in the region. A popular dish is kabobs, marinated pieces of meat threaded onto skewers and then grilled over a fire. Vegetables, such as onions or tomatoes, are sometimes added to the skewers. Souvlaki or shawarma is very thin slices of lamb (or chicken) layered onto a rotisserie with slices of fat (resulting in a single roast), grilled, then carved and served. In Greece, thin slices of souvlaki are folded into pita bread with tomatoes, cucumber, and yogurt to make the sandwich-like treat gyros. Meatballs, called kofta, are favorites, eaten as snacks or served with stewed vegetables. A whole roasted lamb or sheep is a festive dish prepared for parties, festivals, and family gatherings.

Food for Thought

Eggplant "caviar," which is a cooked salad, and baba ganoush, a smoked eggplant puree, are very popular appetizer dishes served throughout the Middle East.

The term yogurt is believed to be from the Turkish word yoğurmak, which means to thicken, coagulate, or curdle. In Syria and Lebanon, the fermented milk product is called laban; in Egypt, laban zabadi; and in Iran, mast.

Camel's milk, unlike other commonly consumed animal milks, is high in vitamin C.

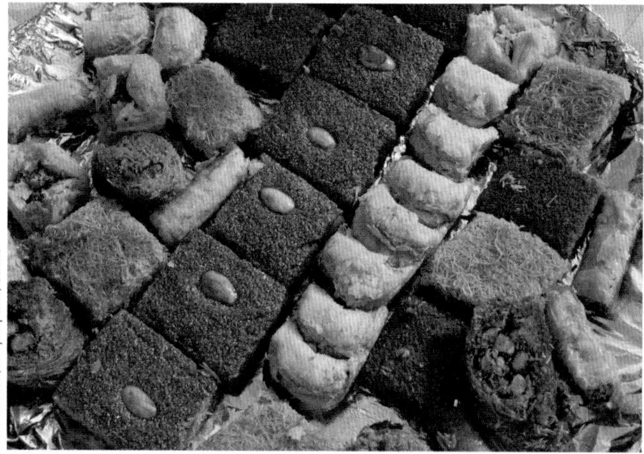
Dave Bartruff/Encyclopedia/Corbis

▲ Assorted Egyptian pastries made with filo dough, couscous, and nuts.

Numerous spices and herbs are used in the Balkans and Middle Eastern seasoning as a result of a once-thriving spice trade with India, Africa, and Asia. Common spices and herbs are dill, garlic, mint, cardamom, cinnamon, oregano, parsley, and pepper. Sumac, ground red berries from a nontoxic variety of the plant, is sprinkled over salads to give a slightly astringent flavor; it is mixed with thyme to make the Arabic seasoning mix called za'atar. Other typical Middle Eastern spices include mahleb, made from the ground pits of a cherry-like fruit, and ajowan, small, black carom seeds with a thyme-like flavor. The juice of unripe lemons, verjuice, is used to provide a sour taste to dishes. Ground nuts are often used to thicken soups and stews. Sesame seeds are crushed to make a thick sauce, tahini, which is used as an ingredient in Arabic cooking and in a sweet dessert paste known as halvah.

Fruit juice is popular as a beverage throughout the Balkans and the Middle East, and sometimes fruit syrups or flower extracts are mixed with ice (or in the past, snow) to make the refreshing beverage known as sharbat in Arabic or şerbet in Turkish (the origin of the English word "sherbet"). Coffee is a favorite (refer to "Is Coffee Beneficial for Health?" later in this chapter) across the entire region, consumed throughout the day at home and in cafés. It is frequently flavored with cardamom and copious amounts of sugar. Traditionally, the drink is made in a long-handled metal briki, producing a strong, very thick, and often sweet brew served in small cylindrical cups. It is called "Turkish coffee" in Turkey and "Serbian coffee" in Serbia. Tea is equally popular in many nations and is served sweetened and flavored with mint, or fruit such as dates or raisins.

The Balkan countries are well known for their wines and distilled spirits. Cviček is a rosé served throughout Slovenia, and a high-proof brandy made from plums called sljivovica is available in both Serbia and Slovenia. Best known in the United States are the Greek specialties retsina (white wine with a resinous flavor), ouzo and arak (anise-flavored aperitifs), and metaxia (orange-flavored brandy). Although observant Muslims do not drink alcohol, several Middle Eastern nations (e.g., Iraq, Israel, and Turkey) produce wines and spirits. Raki, a Turkish version of arak, is traditionally consumed with appetizers.

Regional Variations

Balkans All Balkan nations combine both European and Middle Eastern elements in their cooking. The noteworthy division is between the more European-influenced fare of Bosnia-Herzegovina, Croatia, Romania (refer to Exploring Global Cuisine: Romanian Fare), Serbia, Slovenia, and the other northern nations and the foods of the southern countries, including Albania (refer to Exploring Global Cuisine: Albanian Fare) and Greece, with a decidedly more Middle Eastern flavor (Greek cooking is considered in the discussion of Turkish fare in the following section).

The use of pork and veal, the selection of fruits and vegetables, and the popularity of fresh dairy products are all characteristics of central European cooking in the northern Balkans. German-style sausages, pork roasts, and hams are frequently consumed. Veal is popular for stew and is sometimes seasoned with paprika. One popular dish found in most of the Balkan countries is ćevapi (or ćevapčići), grilled elongated kebobs of spicy minced meat that are often eaten on somun (a thick pita bread) or lepinja (a small, flat roll). In Bosnia, they are usually made with beef, or a beef and lamb mixture served with chopped onions, cottage cheese, and an extra-rich sour cream called kajmak. Large, thin meat patties made from lamb and beef, known as pljeskavica, are considered the national dish of Serbia but are also a favorite with Bosnians and Croatians. Middle Eastern–style grilled meats are also found in some areas, especially in Bosnia-Herzegovina.

Potatoes, cabbage, and cucumbers are typical vegetables, and many families gather wild mushrooms. Ajyar, made with roasted red bell peppers and eggplant, seasoned with garlic and vinegar, is popular throughout the Balkans. It comes in many versions, from sweet to hot (flavored with chili peppers), and is served as a condiment with grilled meats, as a salad on a mezze plate (typically with a selection of sliced sausages or smoked meats, cheeses, hard-boiled eggs, and sliced tomatoes) or spread on bread. Vegetables are sometimes stuffed with meat and rice mixtures similar to those in the Middle East, but with a Balkan flavor due to the use of bell peppers, onions, potatoes, or cabbage leaves. In Bosnia-Herzegovina, Serbia, and elsewhere, these stuffed items are called sarma or dolma and may be served in the tureen in which they have been heated.[41] Cooler-weather fruits such as apples, berries, peaches, pears, and plums are common. They are found in desserts, such as sweet dumplings and strudels, and preserved as compotes. Fruit juices are favorites and an important industry in the region.

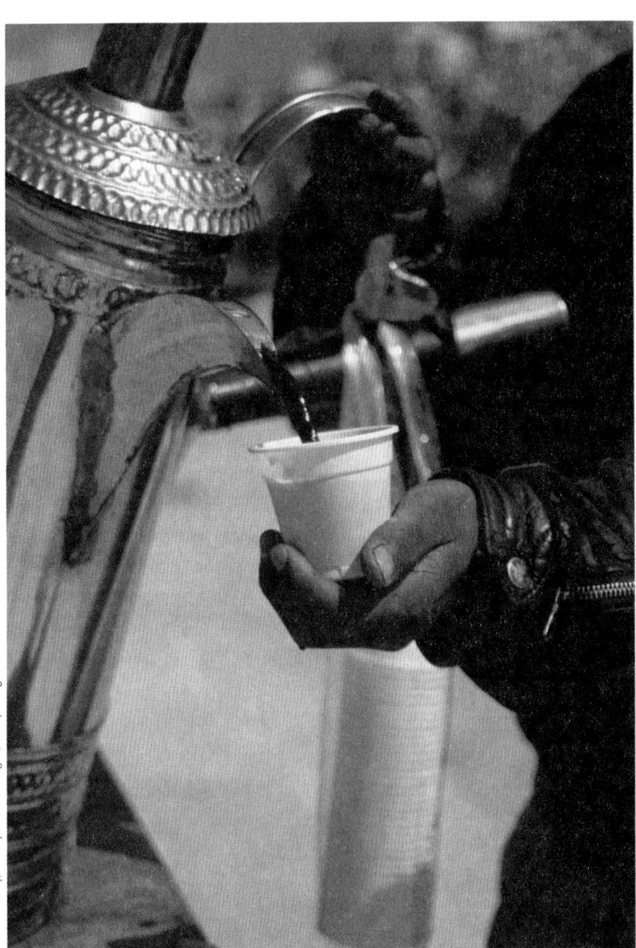

Mark Daffey/Lonely Planet Images/Getty Images

▲ **Middle Eastern coffee is preferred strong, thick, and sweet and is sometimes flavored with cardamom.**

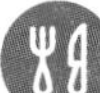 **Food for Thought**

In the Middle East, coffee is often consumed highly sweetened; at funerals or special occassions bitter kahwah saadah, or "black coffee," can be offered.

The Arabs were the first to mix gum arabic with sugar to produce chewing gum.

The Greeks prefer to chew on the licorice-flavored resin *mastic* (source of the verb masticate).

Buttermilk is frequently consumed and fresh cheeses are well-liked, often combined with herbs for mezze or mixed with eggs and honey or sugar for cheese-filled dessert pastries. Cream enriches soups, stews, casseroles, and sauces. Sour cream or whipped cream tops many dishes. A specialty dairy product found throughout the region is thick, crème fraiche-like smetana (in Slovenia), vrhnje (in Croatia), or pavlaka (in Bosnia-Herzegovina). In Croatia, it is added to cottage cheese and seasoned with onions, garlic, radish or horseradish, and paprika, then eaten with cornbread.

The definitive northern Balkan treat is a sweet yeast bread rolled with a rich walnut, butter, cream, and egg filling. It is widely known as potica and in some areas as povitica or kolachki. Some versions are more savory, flavored with tarragon—others are sweeter, with dried fruits. Variations include cream cheese, poppy seed, and pumpkin fillings. Whipped cream tops many sweet versions.

Middle Eastern There are two schools of thought about the number of regional cooking areas in the Middle East. One identifies three culinary areas: Greek/Turkish, Iranian, and Arabic, and the other defines five divisions: Greek/Turkish, Arabic, Iranian, Israeli, and North African (refer to Exploring Global Cuisine: Moroccan Cooking). Certainly, every region has some unique recipes and cooking methods, but the similarity in fare throughout the region is striking.

The cooking of Greece and Turkey has evolved through an extensive exchange of ingredients and preparation techniques. Both cuisines feature more meat (especially grilled), fish and seafood, cheese, butter, and olive oil than in the fare of neighboring Middle Eastern countries. Both the Greeks and Turks prefer using flatware to fingers when eating. Similar distinguishing dishes include filo dough layered with spinach and feta filling (spanakopita in Greece, ispanakli borek in Turkey); fish roe (caviar) dip made with olive oil and bread (taramasalata in Greece and tarama in Turkey); salads with fresh greens, tomato, cucumbers, olives, and lemon juice–olive oil vinaigrette (the Greek version adds feta cheese; the Turkish recipe includes more vegetables, such as green peppers); the lemony, egg-enriched sauce used to thicken soups and top meat and vegetable dishes (avgolemono in Greece, tebiye in Turkey); yogurt cake; and anise-flavored alcoholic beverages. Yet many differences exist. Greeks prefer small pastries, such as the specialty butter cookie, kourabiedes, for snacking and dessert, while the Turkish sweet tooth is more often satisfied with fruit compotes, rich custards, and candy, including lokum, also known as Turkish delight. More significantly, consumption due to religious affiliation varies. Feasting and fasting rules for the Eastern Orthodox of Greece and the Muslims of Turkey differ tremendously (refer to Chapter 4).

Arab fare, based originally on the cooking of nomadic communities and later influenced by the foods of surrounding nations, features more grains, legumes, and vegetables than the Greek, Turkish, Israeli, or Iranian diet. In Syria and Lebanon, the national dish is kibbeh, a mixture of fine cracked wheat, grated onion, and ground lamb pounded into a paste. This mixture can be eaten raw or grilled, and with a great deal of dexterity, it can be made into a hollow shell, then filled with a meat mixture, and deep-fried. In Jordan, a specialty is mansaf—flatbread layered with yogurt is placed on a communal platter and then topped with a mound of rice pilaf and shredded lamb or chicken. A broth mixed with whey or yogurt is poured over the top,

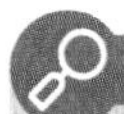

Cultural Controversy

Is Coffee Beneficial for Health?

Despite the importance of wheat in the diet of Western nations, it can be argued that the most important Middle Eastern product consumed worldwide is coffee. Coffee is indigenous to Ethiopia, but it was the Arabs who first brewed and popularized the beverage after it was introduced to the region sometime around the tenth century. Today, coffee is one of the most commonly consumed beverages in the world, with over 2.5 billion cups are consumed annually. Coffee is currently grown in over 50 countries and is second only to petroleum in global trade activity and value. The International Coffee Organization reports that world consumption of coffee in 2020/21 was 167 million bags, up 2 percent from the previous year, and it is becoming increasingly common in tea-drinking nations such as Japan, China, and India.[42,43]

It is said that a Sufi sheikh was the first to note the ability of coffee to promote wakefulness, and it became widely used by worshippers to increase stamina and produce a mystical euphoria.[44] The Sufis called it qahwah (thought to be the origin of the term coffee), a word originally used for wine. By the early 1500s, it had become a secular beverage consumed in Middle Eastern social settings, especially coffee houses, where men could drink and discuss the matters of the day. The coffeehouses attracted philosophers and poets, and in Istanbul, they were known in jest as schools of knowledge. Some Islamic leaders became concerned that coffee was a stimulant or even an intoxicant that encouraged radical thinking and was therefore haram or non-permissible. This led to the closure of coffeehouses in some areas, but efforts to enforce a permanent ban among Muslims failed due to coffee's broad popularity, and a later understanding of the beverage as an aid, perhaps, to sharpen the mind.

During this period, coffee was successfully grown in the Arabian Peninsula nations, and the product was improved by dark-roasting the beans. The beverage spread with the expansion of the Turkish Ottoman Empire, especially in southern Europe, where the social tradition of coffeehouses was well accepted. The Middle East became the first major exporter of beans through the Yemenese port of Mocha. However, some sixteenth-century Catholics believed that coffee was the beverage of Satan, due to its association with infidels. The popular legend is that plans to prohibit coffee were foiled when Pope Clement VIII asked to taste the brew and immediately claimed it was so good that Christians should make it their own.[45]

Historical controversies aside, the most significant issue regarding coffee in modern times is its health impact. Coffee contains numerous active ingredients, most notably caffeine and chlorogenic acid. Caffeine is an alkaloid that is classified with cocaine and amphetamines as a central nervous system stimulant. Chlorogenic acid is a phenolic compound that works as an antioxidant. Over the years, coffee has developed a bad reputation, related to studies on the development of ulcers, heart disease, cancer, and birth defects. Beginning in the 1980s, many health-conscious people began to cut consumption or switch to decaffeinated coffee.[46,47]

Recent research, however, is leading to the redemption of the beverage. Coffee has been exonerated as a causative agent in many gastrointestinal disorders, in most cardiovascular conditions, and in almost all cancers.[46,47] Specifically, several recent studies have linked coffee consumption to decreased risk of colorectal cancer.[48,49] Instead, research suggests that moderate consumption of three to five cups each day may actually offer health benefits, reducing the risk of metabolic syndrome, coronary heart disease,[50,51] type 2 diabetes, several cancers, rheumatoid arthritis, and possibly Alzheimer's disease.[50–52] Studies on the effect of coffee on hypertension are contradictory. Green coffee even may be more beneficial as an anti-inflammatory.[52] Researchers caution that coffee is not for everyone and that people with hypertension, children, elders, and pregnant women are most susceptible to adverse effects.

then the dish is garnished with nuts. The national dish of Egypt is ful medames, cooked fava beans seasoned with oil, lemon, and garlic, sprinkled with parsley, and served with baladi, a whole-wheat type of pita bread. Many soups and stews include legumes, and some salads include grains, such as tabouli. Pieces of pita bread are added to many dishes as well. Tharid is a casserole of layered flatbread with meat stew found in many Arab nations. Fatout is a popular preparation in Yemen, combining toasted bread with honey, scrambled eggs, or any other food; fattoush is a Lebanese favorite with greens, tomatoes, radishes, cucumbers, onions, and pieces of pita bread. Another feature of Arab cooking is the use of a variety of meat. Lamb, goat, and beef are costly; thus, all parts of the animal are used, with brains, chitterlings, heads, and feet considered delicacies. Pacha is an Iraqi soup of sheep heads, stomach, and trotters served with ample bread and pickled vegetables.

Iran is the most eastern of Middle Eastern nations. It spans a region between the warm Persian Gulf and the cold Caspian Sea, encompassing several agricultural climates suited to a wide variety of fruits and vegetables. Its dominance of the Middle East, parts of the Balkans, and areas of India during the Persian Empire dispersed indigenous products such as spinach, pomegranates, and saffron throughout the region.

Later trade routes between China and Syria (the Silk Road) and between India and Africa crossed through Iran, introducing rice, tea, eggplants, citrus fruits, tamarind, and garam masala (a spice blend from India commonly made from cinnamon, pepper, cardamom, mustard seeds, coriander, cloves, mace, and nutmeg and used in sauces, lentil dishes, and soups) from these eastern cuisines. Though the cooking of Iran, usually called Persian cuisine, is very similar to other Middle Eastern foods, it is famous for its sophisticated rice dishes and its use of fruits for flavoring. The national dish is chelo kebab, which is thinly sliced pieces of marinated, charcoal-grilled lamb served over rice seasoned with butter, egg yolks, saffron, and sumac. Soups and sauces are given a

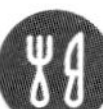 Food for Thought

Syrian food is often spicier than that of other Arab nations. They are known for their small baked lamb pies seasoned with cayenne called sfeehas. Sfeehas are also popular in Lebanon and other areas of the Middle East.

Tharid, made with pieces of bread in a hearty vegetable or meat stew, was reputedly Mohammed's favorite dish.

The Iranians call all bread *nan* and bake many varieties, such as nan-e lavash and nan-e barbari, in a clay bread oven known as a tanoor. *Naan* flatbreads, found in Indian cuisine, were likely developed about 2,500 years ago after yeast being used for brewing in Egypt came into India.[53] Naan are baked in tandoor ovens.

Israelis born in Israel are nicknamed sabra after the cactus of the same name because the fruit is tough and prickly on the outside but sweet inside. A U.S. native plant known as the prickly pear cactus was first exported to the Middle East in the nineteenth century.

sweet and sour taste by combining different ripe and unripe fruits, such as oranges, barberries, cherries, dates, grapes, plums, pomegranates, quinces, and raisins with astringent seasonings, including lemon juice, vinegar, tamarind, and sumac.

Israel probably has the most varied foods and food culture because its cuisine blends indigenous Middle Eastern cooking with that of the many Jewish immigrant groups who have settled in the area since nationhood. Hummus and pita bread may appear at the same meal as German schnitzel, Hungarian-style goulash, or Italian pasta.[53–56] American immigrants introduced bagels; Russians brought kasha and borscht. Chocolate mousse cake, Linzer torte, and coconut macaroons are as popular as baklava. Furthermore, observant Israeli citizens adhere to the kosher laws of the Jewish religion (refer to Chapter 4 for more information on Jewish dietary practices).

Meal Composition and Cycle

Daily Patterns

Balkans People in Balkan countries usually eat three meals a day. The main meal is at midday, and in the hotter climates, a short nap follows. Dinner is lighter and is served in the cooler evening hours. Snacking is prevalent.

In the northern regions, a light breakfast of bread with preserves or honey and tea or coffee is most common. Lunch usually includes soup, a casserole of meats and vegetables, or a fish dish, bread and cheese, and a fruit compote or pastry for dessert. Dinner is often leftovers or another soup or stew; sweet dumplings may also be served. Wine is the typical beverage for both lunch and dinner, though buttermilk, fruit juices, and soft drinks are consumed in some areas. In urban regions, street vendors ply pastries and ice cream throughout the day. Late evening visits to cafés or coffee houses often include small kebabs, meatballs, vegetable salads and pickles, and other tidbits to accompany coffee, wine, or plum brandy.

In Greece and the southern Balkan nations, the traditional breakfast typically consists of bread with cheese, olives, or jam plus coffee or tea. The main meal, eaten in the early afternoon, usually begins with mezze or appetizers, such as hummus, baba ganoush, tiropitas, and dolmas, often consumed with a small glass of ouzo: the actual selection of included items varies by the inclination of the homemaker and affordability. Next, a meat stew, meatballs, kebabs, vegetables stuffed with chopped meat, or a bean dish is served with a salad of raw seasonal vegetables, yogurt or cheese, and fruit for dessert. Roasted or baked whole meats are served on weekends, accompanied by cooked vegetables, salad, and dessert. Late afternoon and early evening are times when neighbors and friends may drop by for some sweets and a cup of coffee or a glass of ouzo. A light supper is served in the late evening. Throughout the day, mezze are widely available from street vendors and cafés for snacking.

Middle East In most Arabic countries, coffee or tea is often served first for breakfast around 7:00 or 8:00 a.m., followed by a light meal that might include bread, cheeses, beans, eggs, olives, jam and bread, and plain yogurt. Lunch is the main meal of the day, eaten in the early afternoon. It is customarily bread, rice, or bulgur, and a vegetable or legume casserole, a meat or poultry stew, or, where available, a fish or seafood dish. Fresh or cooked vegetable salad or onions and olives are common side dishes. Additional items, depending on region and affordability, may include a selection of mezze (such as hummus, tabouli, vegetables in yogurt, and bowls of nuts), a soup, and cheeses. Dessert is usually included, typically a piece of fresh fruit, a pastry, or a custard or pudding. Diluted yogurt drinks (ayran and doogh), which provide a daily dose of probiotics or water, are served while eating, followed by sweetened tea or coffee. Dinner in the early evening is light, consisting of foods similar to those eaten at breakfast, soup, or leftovers from lunch. All the dishes in a meal are customarily served at once in Egypt, Iraq, and Yemen, and in courses in Jordan, Lebanon, and Syria.[55]

Turkish meals vary slightly from the Middle Eastern pattern. Breakfast (often served a little later than in Arabic nations) varies regionally, but is often substantial, with leavened bread or simit (a chewy or crunchy ring-shaped roll resembling a bagel in shape, but richer in flavor—also found in Greece where they are called koulouri), cheese, butter, tomatoes, olives, and jam served with sweetened tea. Eggs, soups, or sausages are common additions in some areas. Lunch, eaten around noon, and dinner, served between 6:00 and 8:00 p.m., are also plentiful meals, especially dinner, which is the main meal of the day. It begins with a selection of mezze (mezeler in Turkish) served with raki. Items may include lamb meatballs, dolma, stuffed mussels, fried squids, baba ganouj, hummus, and vegetable salads. These appetizers

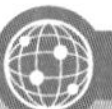

Exploring Global Cuisine

Romanian Fare

Romania is a nation poised between the West and the East. Some describe Romanian food as "pastoral" with Turkish and Hungarian overtones. However, there are also many Italian and central European influences. Beef, veal, mutton, lamb, pork, chicken, goose, and duck are popular. Freshwater fish such as pike and catfish are harvested from the Danube and other rivers. Cabbage, red and green peppers, leeks, tomatoes, onions, radishes, and lettuce are common vegetables. Temperate fruits, particularly grapes, plums, and berries, are eaten. Other common foods include walnuts, filberts, olives, sour cream, and sheep and goat cheeses. The national bread is mamaliga, which is like Italian polenta. It is sliced and spread with butter or topped with cheese, meats, or fruit for dessert. Another specialty is pastrama (from the Turkish meaning "to keep"), which is lamb, beef, pork, or goose cured (spicing varies, from garlic and black pepper to allspice, nutmeg, and hot red pepper) and then smoked. Ground meats are also popular, made into patties, stuffed into cabbage leaves, or as sausages. One-dish meals such as stews and soups are eaten with whole-grain bread; one example is ciorba, a soup made with vegetables (e.g., peppers, onions, sauerkraut, tomatoes) and meat (usually ground) or fish and then flavored with sour ingredients (e.g., sauerkraut juice, pickle juice, or vinegar). Cake is a traditional dessert, but custards (including one similar to Italian zabaglione) and soufflés are also eaten. Romanian beverages include wine (red, white, sweet, dry) and tuica, a plum and wheat brandy. Most Romanians belong to the Eastern Orthodox Church and adhere to the numerous feasting and fasting days of the church calendar.

are followed by a course featuring vegetables such as eggplant, tomatoes, or leeks stewed in olive oil. Kebabs, casseroles, or stews are the centerpiece of the meal, served with pilaf and bread. Fresh fruit such as melon, baklava, or rice pudding follows, and the sweets are consumed with coffee. In some regions, tripe soup with vinegar and garlic may be eaten after dinner and served with alcoholic beverages. Turkish meals are typically served in courses.

In Iran, breakfast is usually a selection of flatbreads served with feta or other cheeses, sweetened whipped cream, and jam. In some regions, offal soup or halim (a savory wheat porridge with meats and vegetables) is preferred.[60] Lunch and dinner are similar, usually with rice, a meat or poultry dish (roasted, or as kebabs or ground meat), often a vegetable salad, flatbreads, some feta cheese or yogurt, and a selection of chopped herbs (such as mint, basil, and dill). A meat or vegetable stew is frequently substituted for the meat or poultry course, served over the rice. Fruit, especially melon or grapes, is a typical dessert, and tea or a yogurt drink accompanies the meal. Traditionally, the dishes are all served at one time and eaten communally.

Weekday breakfasts in Israel are customarily light: coffee with some pita and olive oil and za'atar, European-style bread with jam or other spread, or a selection of cheeses, yogurt, and chopped vegetables and fruit. Sabbath breakfasts, however, are somewhat heartier. European Jews may choose coffeecakes or pancakes, and Middle Eastern Jews may select bureks, kataif (a sweet, stuffed pancake), or sabikh (an Iraqi dish of pita bread topped with fried eggplant, hard-boiled egg, tahini, and a mango pickle). The traditional Israeli breakfast buffet

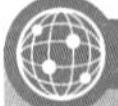

Exploring Global Cuisine

Albanian Fare

Albania was little known to most Americans until the 1998 civil war in the Serbian province of Kosovo focused attention on the plight of the Kosovar Albanians. Albanians, living in a country bordered by Greece, Macedonia, Serbia, and Montenegro, have often been involved in regional discord and shifting national boundaries.[57] Years of foreign rule have left their mark on Albanian cuisine: pastitsio (macaroni, ground lamb, cheese, and tomatoes topped with béchamel sauce) and feta from Greece, versions of imam bayaldi (stuffed eggplant) and halvah (a sesame/sugar sweet) from Turkey, omelets and tomato sauces from Italy, boereg (stuffed pastries) from Armenia, and borscht from Russia. Dolmas, kofta, shish kebabs, moussaka, and baklava are also popular.

In the least wealthy rural regions of Albania, farmers and shepherds are often limited to a diet of cornmeal bread, cheese, and yogurt, with added lamb or mutton when affordable. In wealthier areas, three meals a day are typical with a mid-afternoon snack of thick Turkish-style coffee or tea consumed with pastries, nuts, or fresh fruit, called sille. A complete lunch or dinner begins with mezze (appetizers), such as salads, pickles, fish and seafood, omelets, spit-roasted lamb or entrails, and a baked variety of meats. Examples include liptao, a feta cheese salad garnished with bell pepper, deli meats, sardines, and hard-boiled egg; and soup-like tarator, yogurt flavored with garlic and olive oil and mixed with vegetables, such as cucumber. These are usually consumed with a glass of the distilled Turkish specialty, raki, or a beverage made from fermented cabbage called orme. The meal follows with soups, meat, or cheese-stuffed vegetables or casseroles; pilaf-like dishes or pies filled with vegetables, cheese, and/or ground meats called byrek; and an assortment of vegetable side dishes and pickles. Dessert may include pastries but is typically a fruit compote. Few legumes are consumed, but nuts (especially walnuts) are added to numerous sweet and savory dishes.

One of the most distinctive characteristics of Albanian fare is that there is little cross-over between vegetable and fruit dishes. Vegetables may be side dishes, or pickled; fruits are eaten fresh, as preserves, or in desserts. Pies are never have a vegetable-sweetened filling, for example.[57,58]

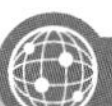

Exploring Global Cuisine

Moroccan Cooking

Morocco, although located in northwestern Africa, the majority of its population identifies as Middle Eastern. It is one of five nations that make up the Maghreb, a region of North Africa differentiated from the Middle East by its substantial populations of nomadic Berbers, also including the countries of Algeria, Tunisia, Mauritania, and Libya. Although there are very few immigrants to the United States from the Maghreb, many Moroccan restaurants have opened offering the flavors of North Africa.

The cooking of Morocco is predominantly Berber in origin, strongly influenced by the spice trade from Asia, neighboring Arabic fare, and, to a much lesser degree, through interchange with sub-Saharan Africa and the southern European countries of the Mediterranean. It is noteworthy for its exquisite seasonings. Spices, such as allspice, anise, cardamom, cayenne, cumin, cinnamon, cloves, mace, malagueta pepper (refer to Chapter 8), nutmeg, turmeric, and saffron, are combined with herbs, including basil, fresh coriander, lavender, marjoram, mint, verbena, and za'atar. One mixture, ras el hanout, includes between ten and 25 ingredients, depending on the chef and its intended purpose; medicinal herbs such as belladonna or reputed aphrodisiacs (such as the pulverized beetle known as "Spanish fly") may also be added.[58] Garlic, onions, lemons (some preserved through brining), almonds, and sweet peppers also flavor many dishes, and some are heated with the chili pepper and garlic paste condiment called harissa (from Tunisia, where foods are preferred very spicy). Rose water and orange blossom water are also commonly used. Foods are also flavored by the preferred cooking fats of the region, zebeda (a sour fresh butter) and smen (a preserved clarified butter often seasoned with herbs; it is traditionally stored for months underground until cheese-like).

Couscous is a staple eaten throughout the Maghreb, where it is known by many names. It is made from grains of semolina wheat (other grains prepared the same way, such as barley and millet, are also called couscous) mixed with water and processed into very small pellets and dried. To prepare couscous, these granules are mixed with water and rolled between the palms of your hands to form tiny beads. It is traditionally cooked in a specialized steamer known as a couscousière. The word couscous is also used to describe the finished dish: the steamed grain topped with a mixture of lamb with chickpeas and vegetables, fish with fennel, dates with cinnamon (for dessert), or other popular versions.[58,59] Moroccan stews, tagines, are slow-cooked in ceramic pots and feature any combination of meats, poultry, fish, organ meats, vegetables, and fruits. Mechoui is spit-roasted lamb or kid. The meat is first rubbed with cumin and garlic and then cooked until it can be pulled off with the fingers. Bastilla or b'stila (from the Spanish word for pastry or pie, pastel) is the quintessential Moroccan dish: sheets of warqa (a dough similar to filo, though thinner) enclose layers of ground almonds mixed with sugar and cinnamon alternating with pigeon or chicken meat. The layers are bound with a lemony egg sauce, and the pie is baked until golden. The crispy crust is often sprinkled with sugar and cinnamon before serving. Cooked or marinated vegetable salads usually start a meal, and fresh fruit and nuts add the finishing touch. While some foods are eaten with a fork or a spoon, many require a piece of bread and agile fingers. Eating is done with the right hand only, using the thumb and first two fingers.

associated with kibbutz life is offered at some restaurants, featuring a more typically Middle Eastern selection of flatbreads, cheeses, vegetables, and olives, often with added eggs, baked goods, and other selections. The midday meal is the largest in most homes, beginning with hummus or tahini served with pita bread, then a salad—often cucumbers, tomatoes, and onions—followed by items appropriate to a meat or dairy meal (refer to Chapter 4 for more information on the laws of Kashrut). The evening meal, typically eaten around 8:00 or 9:00 p.m., is usually light with cheeses, yogurt, salads, and eggs. Some families serve all the dishes of the meal at once, while others serve them in courses, often depending on heritage. Street stands offer falafel, kebabs, shawarma, and other snacks, and fast-food restaurants, especially those serving hamburgers or pizza, are popular with many Israelis. Fruit juices, soft drinks, and beer are common meal beverages.

Etiquette Throughout the Balkans and the Middle East, hospitality is a duty and a family's status is measured by how guests are treated. Guests, even uninvited ones, are made to feel welcome and are automatically offered food and drink. In the Balkans, it is likely to be fruit compotes and candies to eat and buttermilk, coffee, or plum brandy to drink. In Greece, ouzo or arak are offered as beverages. In the Middle East, it may be a few dates and water or an extensive choice of mezze served with coffee, tea, or raki. Even if food is initially refused, it will be offered again, and a guest must accept it because refusal is considered an insult. Invited guests bring a gift, often candy or other sweets, which the host must open immediately and serve. Hospitality is even offered to clients in the office setting, and failure to make guests or clients comfortable may create extreme embarrassment for all parties.[22]

In the Middle East, etiquette varies by region. Usually, food is shared from a central, communal plate and served by the host. The host will also offer second helpings as soon as the guest's plate is cleared. Many meals are eaten while sitting on the floor or cushions. A dignitary or head of the family is often served the best portion first. In Saudi Arabia and other nations of the Arabian peninsula, the honored seat at the table is in the middle of the table, whereas in Egypt, it is at the head of the table. In some areas, such as some parts of Yemen, it is customary for women to eat separately from men.[61] Guests are traditionally entertained in a separate room before the meal, at which thyme scented water is provided so they may wash their hands. A dining table might be a large, round metal tray, resting on a low stool or platform, and the diners sit around it on cushions. Western-style dining is found occasionally, especially in Middle Eastern restaurants. In Iran, food is traditionally served on a rug. The meal is set out in several serving bowls placed on the table or rug and then shared by the diners. After the meal, the guests leave the table, wash their hands, and then have coffee or tea.

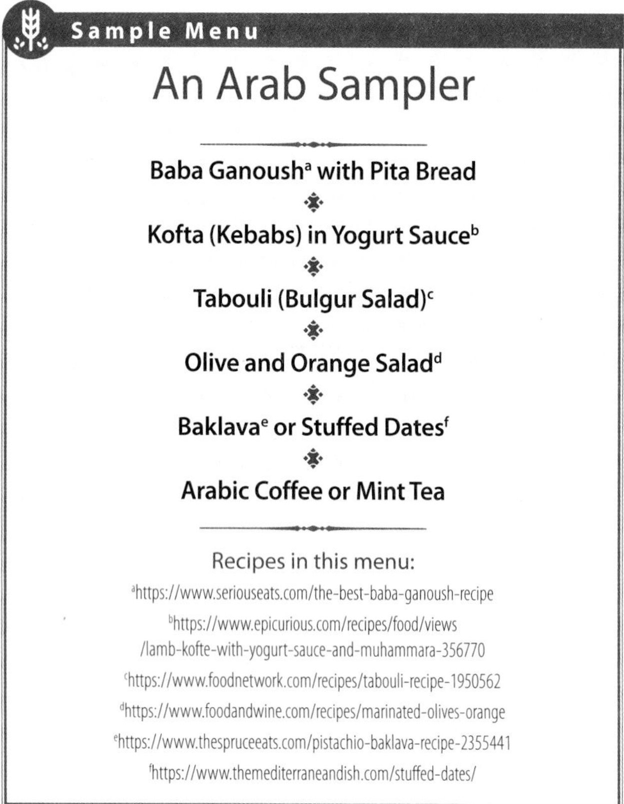

Sample Menu

An Arab Sampler

Baba Ganoush[a] with Pita Bread

Kofta (Kebabs) in Yogurt Sauce[b]

Tabouli (Bulgur Salad)[c]

Olive and Orange Salad[d]

Baklava[e] or Stuffed Dates[f]

Arabic Coffee or Mint Tea

Recipes in this menu:

[a]https://www.seriouseats.com/the-best-baba-ganoush-recipe

[b]https://www.epicurious.com/recipes/food/views/lamb-kofte-with-yogurt-sauce-and-muhammara-356770

[c]https://www.foodnetwork.com/recipes/tabouli-recipe-1950562

[d]https://www.foodandwine.com/recipes/marinated-olives-orange

[e]https://www.thespruceeats.com/pistachio-baklava-recipe-2355441

[f]https://www.themediterraneandish.com/stuffed-dates/

Food for Thought

"Spoon sweets" (seasonal fruits, vegetables, nuts, or rose petals preserved in a heavy, sweet syrup) are a Greek specialty specifically reserved for guests, offered by the spoonful on arrival as a sweet welcome.

Several rules of etiquette apply to eating in the Middle East. One should always wash one's hands before eating. In Muslim regions, the guests thank Allah before and after the meal. Some Middle Easterners may say "Sahain!" ("good appetite!") to start the meal, and "Daimah" (may there always be plenty) to end it.[62] Three fingers of the right hand are used if forks or spoons are not offered. The left hand should not be used in any food-related manner (including passing food), and traditionally women should not touch any food that is to be eaten by a Muslim man who is not her immediate family member. Rice should be taken from the communal bowl and rolled into a small ball with the fingers before dipping it into stews or sauces. Licking the fingers after eating is expected, and appreciation is shown in some areas by making eating noises. It is rude to fill one's own cup, and it is expected that a diner will refresh his or her neighbor's cup as soon as it is half empty. It is also considered polite to continue eating until everyone else is finished because if one person stops the others feel compelled to stop, too. One should leave a little food on one's plate to indicate satisfaction with the abundance of the meal. Most conversation takes place before and after the meal, and limited discussion of pleasant and joyful things takes place while dining. It is important to compliment the host and hostess on their hospitality.

Special Occasions In Balkan and Middle Eastern countries, food plays an important role in the celebration of religious occasions and in the observance of certain events such as weddings and births. In the Eastern Orthodox Church, there are numerous feast and fast days (refer to Chapter 4). The most important religious holiday for the Greeks is Easter. Immediately after midnight Mass on Holy Saturday, the family shares the first post-Lenten meal. It traditionally begins with red-dyed Easter eggs and continues with mayeritsa, a soup made of the lamb's internal organs, sometimes flavored with avgolemono, a tart egg yolk and lemon sauce. The Easter Sunday meal usually consists of roast lamb, rice pilaf, accompanying vegetables, cheese, yogurt, and a special Easter bread called lambropsomo that is decorated with whole-dyed eggs. Dessert usually includes sweet pastries made with filo dough and koulourakia, a traditional Greek sweet bread cookie, sometimes shaped into a hairpin twist or wreath or coiled in the shape of a snake (a creature that the pagan Greeks worshiped for its healing powers). Easter is preceded by the pre-Lenten holiday of Apokreas, which is similar to Carnival or Mardi Gras and features costumed events and parties with ample merrymaking, food, and music. In addition to religious holidays, Greek Americans typically celebrate Greek Independence Day on March 25th. It is commemorated with parades in traditional dress, folk dancing, songs, and poetry readings.

The Easter meal in Croatia is typically lamb or ham and pogaca, an Easter bread with painted eggs on top that is similar to the Greek lambropsomo. Christmas Eve features a meal of cod, and a stuffed cabbage and sauerkraut dish is customary on Christmas. Among Serbians, the most auspicious day of the year is Krsna Slava, Patron Saint's Day. This holiday dates back to the worship of protective spirits in pagan times; today, each family honors its self-chosen patron saint with a sumptuous feast and dancing that may last for two to three days. The family customarily announces the annual open house with a small advertisement in the local newspaper. Krsni kolac is a ritual bread prepared for the occasion, decorated with the religious Serbian emblem "Samo sloga Srbina spašava" ("Only unity will save the Serbs") as well as grapes, wheat, birds, flowers, barrels of wine, or other representations made in the dough. Slovenians celebrate St. Nick's Feast. Gifts are distributed to children by St. Nick, dressed as a bishop, who admonishes the youngsters to be good. The grape harvest and winemaking are traditionally commemorated with numerous festivals and St. Martin's Feast.

There are also feasts and fasts connected with Islamic religious observances. Traditional festive foods vary from country to country and may also vary seasonally since the Muslim calendar is lunar, and holidays fall at different times each

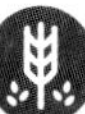
Sample Menu

A Greek Mezze

Olives and Cheeses (such as Kaseri or Myzithra)

Taramosalata (Caviar Dip)[a] or Hummus (Chickpea Dip)

Tzatziki (Cucumber Yogurt Dip)[b]

Pita Bread

Spanakopita (Spinach and Cheese Triangles)[c]

Dolmas (Stuffed Grape Leaves)[d] with Avgolemono[e]

Ouzo or Wine

Recipes in this menu:

[a]https://cooking.nytimes.com/recipes/1019414-taramasalata

[b]https://www.allrecipes.com/recipe/145409/greek-tzatziki/

[c]https://www.allrecipes.com/recipe/18417/spanakopita-greek-spinach-pie/

[d]https://www.foodnetwork.com/recipes/tyler-florence/dolmades-stuffed-grape-leaves-recipe-1940988

[e]https://www.foodandwine.com/recipes/avgolemono-chicken-soup-rice

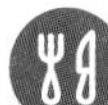
Food for Thought

In Yemen, qat (the herb with amphetamine-like properties called khat in Ethiopia—refer to Chapter 8) is frequently chewed in social and business settings.

In Greek Orthodox tradition, the egg represents life, and red is the color of the blood Christ shed. The breaking of the red-dyed egg symbolizes the resurrection.

For New Year's Day, the Greeks prepare a sweet spicy bread called vasilopita with a coin baked into it—the person who gets the piece with the money has good luck in the upcoming year (the Serbs have the same tradition for Christmas Day).

Kahk is a sweet Egyptian biscuit or cookie made with ample butter and nuts that is served on all special occasions.

Some non-Christian Arab Americans celebrate the birth of Jesus on Christmas; Jesus is considered a prophet in Islam.

year. Iftar is the meal that breaks the fast during Ramadan, the month in which Muslims fast from sunrise to sunset; it is common to dine with relatives and neighbors. The meal usually starts with a beverage, preferably water, followed by an odd number of dates and coffee or tea. A large meal, served after prayers, includes moist and hearty dishes. Regular items eaten during Ramadan include soups, fruit juices, cheeses, and fresh or dried fruit. Traditional sweets include kataif, which refers to a pancake or a shredded wheat dough dessert, and, in Turkey and Iran, rose-flavored rice puddings. In some Muslim homes, the post-fast meal is considered a feast with elaborate dishes that emphasize the Muslim virtues of hospitality and community, while in other homes a more moderate meal is thought to be in keeping with the purposes of the fast.[62] The dawn meal is usually light, and salty foods are avoided because water is not allowed during the fast.

The holiday Eid al-Fitr follows the end of Ramadan and is described as a cross between the feasting of Thanksgiving and the festivity of Christmas. Typically, family, friends, and neighbors gather to celebrate; in areas with large Muslim populations, Eid al-Fitr may be held at the local fairgrounds with games, rides, and many food vendors. The other major holiday observed by Arab Muslims is Eid al-Adha, the Feast of Sacrifice held in conjunction with the annual pilgrimage to Mecca (refer to Chapter 4).

In Turkey, Eid al-Fitr is known as Seker Bayram, meaning "sugar festival." It is traditional to exchange small gifts with friends, and for four days children are given sweet treats, such as lokums or chocolates. On the tenth day of the first lunar month of the Islamic calendar, Turks celebrate the martyrdom of Mohammed's grandson and the day Noah was able to leave the ark. They prepare asure, or Noah's pudding, made from the ingredients remaining after the receding of the flood waters: fresh and dried fruits, nuts, and legumes. Kurban Bayram is a day of remembrance for when the prophet Abraham nearly sacrificed his son Ishmael. Families customarily sacrifice a sheep or a goat and distribute it to family, friends, and community charities. Another special occasion in Turkey is National Sovereignty and Children's Day on April 23rd. It commemorates the establishment of the Grand National Assembly in 1923 and specifically honors all children. The following day has become Turkish American Day in the United States, featuring parades in traditional dress and other festivities.

In Iran, the most significant holiday of the year is Muharram, which commemorates the martyrdom of the grandson of Mohammed in the seventh century. It is a time of communal mourning and penitence for Shiites and often features sholeh zard, a sweet rice pudding flavored with saffron. Another celebration marking the spring equinox is Nau Roz, which features a meal, called haft-sinn, including a ceremonial table setting where the Qur'an, a mirror (to reflect life), sweets, bread, cheese, and seven items starting with the letter *s* in Farsi representing rebirth, good fortune, love, happiness, health, and other wishes for the new year are displayed. Foods and other goods starting with *s* may include serke (vinegar), seeb (apple), sanjed (dried fruit or olives), sumagh (sumac), samanu (a sweet sprouted wheat kernel pudding), seer (garlic), sonbul (hyacinth), sabzi (sprouted seeds), or sekeh (coins). Readings from the Qur'an are followed with a traditional meal of herbed rice (sabzu polo) and an herbed omelet (kukuye sabzi) served with fish. The number seven probably

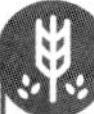

Sample Menu

A Persian Lunch

Olives and Pistachios

Khoresh-e Fesenjan (Chicken Stew with Walnuts and Pomegranate over Rice)[a]

Salad-e Shirazi (Cucumber, Tomato, and Onion Salad)[a]

Feta Cheese and Lavash

Fresh Fruit or Sholeh Zard (Saffron Pudding)[a]

Black or Cardamom-flavored Tea

Recipes in this menu:

[a]*Iranian/Persian Recipes* at http://www.iranchamber.com/recipes/recipes.php

relates to the seven days of the week or the seven planets of the ancient solar system. On the thirteenth day of Nau Roz, it is customary to have a picnic.

Food for Thought

In Greece and the Middle East, sugared almonds (Jordan almonds) are served at weddings and are thought to ensure sweetness in married life.

La Tavla de Dulce, a fancy platter of treats such as rose jam and candied orange peel, was a traditional way of showing Jewish Sephardic hospitality—warm, gracious, and very sweet—to guests.[63]

The traditional holidays of the Jewish calendar are observed in Israel (refer to Chapter 4 for Jewish food practices). The Shabbat, or Sabbath, occurs from sunset Friday to sunset on Saturday evening. Traditionally, the Friday night meal is served on a table set with white linen and includes the symbolic Kiddush cup of wine that is shared by all diners. In Ashkenazi homes, a representative menu could include gefilte fish, a leavened, braided loaf of egg-rich bread called challah, a roast chicken, a noodle pudding called kugel, and fruit or cake and tea for dessert. In Sephardic households, a more Middle Eastern meal would be typical, such as pilaf, roast lamb, cooked eggplant or stuffed dolma, pita bread, and honey-soaked filo pastries with coffee for dessert. Jews from other regions have favorite Sabbath menus as well. For example, an Ethiopian family might serve chicken doro wat (stew) and caraway-flavored dabo bread. Because all work, including cooking, is prohibited on the Sabbath, the more observant prepare food during the day on Friday or leave it cooking overnight so that it can be consumed on Saturday. Stews that can simmer overnight on the stovetop are popular dishes for the midday meal following morning services, such as cholent, also known as hamin in Israel. Every family has its own version, though most include beans and potatoes. The Lebanese and Syrians use white beans, the Brazilians use black beans, and the Moroccans add rice. Most Ashkenazi recipes use beef brisket, and some Sephardic versions include sausages. In most homes, whole eggs cooked in their shells are buried in the stew. Other religious holidays offer a similar variety of food traditions based on the nationality of origin. Israelis also observe the secular Yom Ha-Atzma'ut, Independence Day, on the fifth day of Iyar (a spring month in the Jewish lunar calendar). Celebrants view parades, hold barbecues, and watch fireworks. Street vendors sell falafel, ears of corn, and numerous sweets, including candied fruits and nuts, sesame seed candy, and European cakes and tortes with whipped cream.

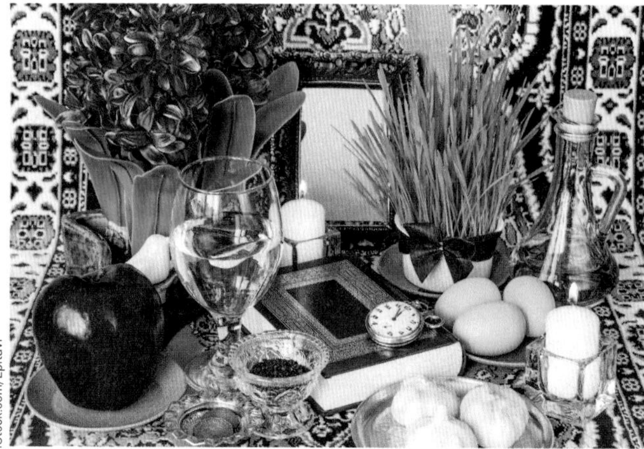

iStock.com/Epitavi

▲ A traditional Haft-Sin table is an ancient Persian tradition displayed at Nowruz, the Iranian new year. It is comprised of an arrangement of seven items that all begin with the letter "S" in the Farsi language.

Therapeutic Uses of Food Fresh foods are considered best, and canned or frozen foods are often avoided by Middle Easterners to preserve health. The amount of food eaten is of special concern in the diet. Ample meals are needed to prevent illness, and poor appetite is regarded as a disease in itself or as a generalized complaint signifying that one's life is not as it should be. Food deprivation is believed to cause illness.[64]

Some Middle Easterners also believe that illness can be triggered by hot cold shifts in food, especially in people with weak or susceptible constitutions. For instance, in Iran, it is believed that eating too many hot foods may result in headaches, sweating, itching, and rashes. Excessive amounts of cold foods can cause dizziness, nausea, and vomiting.[29,34] Foods and drinks of the opposite category can ameliorate these conditions. For example, citrus fruits or a sour lemonade called ablimu are used for headaches and acne. Nausea is treated with tea or a sweet similar to rock candy. Classifications can vary, but examples of hot foods include lamb, eggs, onions, garlic, carrots, bell peppers, apples, dates, quinces, chickpeas, wheat, almonds, walnuts, pistachios, honey, and tea. Cold foods can include beef, cucumbers, tomatoes, eggplant, grape leaves, grapes, lemons, sour cherries, apricots, mulberries, pomegranates, rice, yogurt, coffee, and beer. The temperature (not spiciness) can cause a shift in the body from hot to cold and vice versa, and it is believed the digestive system must have time to adjust to one extreme before a food of the opposite temperature can be introduced. In addition, though illness may be related to hot-cold imbalances, Iranians do not consider certain conditions as being hot or cold. Thus, a symptom such as coughing requires specific treatment unrelated to classification: consuming cold turnips is considered beneficial, whereas cold pickles are deemed harmful.[65]

Some Middle Easterners also believe certain combinations of incompatible foods are damaging to health. For example, Egyptians do not consume fish at the same time as dairy products. Other Middle Easterners avoid eating sour foods with milk and legumes with cheese. Iranians believe consumption of melon with yogurt causes wind in the stomach and gastrointestinal disorders.

Herbal medicine is frequently used in the Middle East among pregnant women. Peppermint, ginger, thyme, chamomile, sate, aniseed, fenugreek, and green tea are often used for treating gastrointestinal disorders, nausea, and vomiting. Green tea is used as a laxative and a relaxing agent. It is thought that herbal medicines are more effective and have fewer side effects than modern medicine during pregnancy. Many special foods are associated with childbirth. Eggs cooked in garlic and chicken soup are frequently consumed by Lebanese women after childbirth. When a woman gives birth to a girl in Iran, coldness is neutralized with a diet high in hot foods to ensure a child of the opposite sex in the next pregnancy. Saffron custard garnished with nuts is thought to help Iranian women regain strength postpartum, while Palestinian women consume oats, coriander, or fennel.[66]

Food is often thought of as medicine in the Middle East, especially in Arabic nations.[67] Turnips are considered good for the kidneys and urinary tract, whereas cauliflower is beneficial for the respiratory system. Red onion bulbs and their leaves (which are added to salads) are consumed to help with diabetes and cancer. They are also eaten to ease liver disease, which is treated with asparagus and artichokes. Many foods have a multiplicity of therapeutic uses. Some Palestinians, for example, consider garlic to be good for colic, nausea, kidney infections, intestinal worms, ulcers, genitourinary infections, prostate conditions, tumors, and as an aphrodisiac.[67]

Contemporary Food Habits in the United States

Adaptations of Food Habits

There is scant information on the adaptation of Balkan or Middle Eastern diets in the United States. It is assumed that, as in other immigrant groups, increasing length of stay is correlated with Americanization of the diet, with traditional dishes prepared and eaten only for the main meal or special occasions. It is less likely that religious dietary practices, such as adherence to halal or kosher law, change significantly after arrival in the United States.

Ingredients and Common Foods Greek Americans still use olive oil extensively, although they use less of it than their immigrant relatives.[68] Salads still accompany the meal, and fruit is often served for dessert. Vegetables are prepared traditionally. Lamb is still very popular; for special occasions, roasted leg of lamb is substituted for the whole animal. Consumption of beef and pork has increased, whereas consumption of legumes has decreased. Cereal and grain consumption among Greek Americans remains high, and bread, rice, or cereal products are usually included in every meal. Greek Americans consume more milk than their immigrant parents, and ice cream is very popular.

One earlier study of first-generation Egyptians found that traditional wheat bread remained commonly consumed, though intake of legumes, especially fava beans, was somewhat lower than when the immigrants had lived in Egypt. Snacking and eating out had become much more prevalent, and soft drinks were more popular.[69]

Food for Thought

The demand for properly slaughtered (halal) meat among Muslims in the United States has led to exponential growth in Arab halal markets.

Greek weddings in the United States offer a blend of Greek and American foods, e.g., the wedding cake is served along with baklava.

Meal Composition and Cycle Greek Americans maintain traditional meal patterns, but the main meal of the day is now dinner.[70] Many prefer an American-type breakfast and lunch, but dinner is often more traditional. However, they have

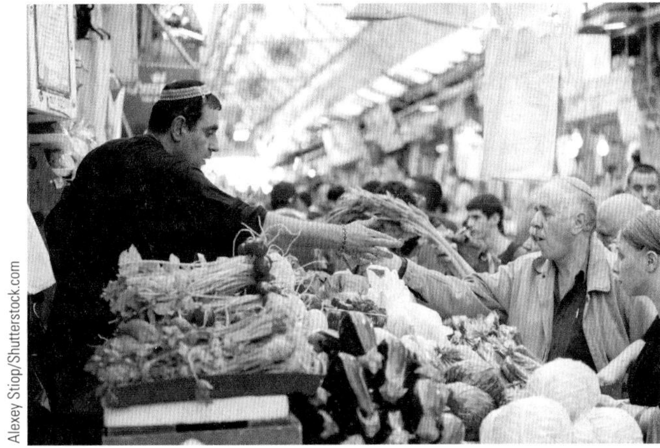

Alexey Stiop/Shutterstock.com

▲ A Middle Eastern market.

adapted Greek recipes to make them less time-consuming to prepare and to include fewer fats and spices. It is assumed that the meal pattern for most Americans of Croatian, Serbian, and Slovenian heritage is much acculturated.

After immigration to Canada and the United States, Arab Americans may have a substantial midday meal, but like the Greeks, the main meal of the day has become dinner.[70]

Nutritional Status

Nutritional Intake Very little has been reported on the nutritional composition of the Balkan American or Middle Eastern American diet. However, research on the diets of nations bordering the Mediterranean (particularly Greece) often reports that the traditional diet there, one that is low in saturated fats and high in monounsaturated fats and omega-3 fatty acids (due to a low intake of meats combined with high consumption of olive oil, fruits, and vegetables), lowers the risk of cardiovascular disease and cancer. The prevalence of at least one daily carbonated soft drink consumption is still less than 10 percent. Studies on the impact of the Mediterranean diet[71] on the development of metabolic syndrome conditions (including obesity, hypertension, and type 2 diabetes) have been contradictory, but support improvement in risk factors associated with the heart.[72–74] There are many varieties of the Mediterranean diet, which makes classification of its food components challenging, and often study results give mixed results. What is known is that the number of people consuming this traditional diet is declining with the Westernization of the region. Since the 1960s, the Greeks have been consuming significantly less olive oil and more alcohol. Overweight and obesity rates in Greece are nearly 50 percent for women and almost 67 percent for men.[75] In Lebanon, over 70 percent of adult men and 58 percent of adult women are overweight. A recent study in Lebanon found younger adults were eating fewer fruits, vegetables, and legumes, while consuming more meat and sugar and drinking more soft drinks and alcoholic beverages, than older adults.[75] Similar trends are seen in Saudi Arabia where, in 2019, over 62 percent of men and 56 percent of women are overweight.[75] Dietary guidelines were introduced in 2012 which were aimed at reducing trans fat and sodium, increasing exercise, and promoting more vegetable and fruit consumption.

Sparse data on Bosnian immigrants have shown that compared to general American population studies, Bosnian Americans have greater coronary heart disease risk.[76] Providers report a need for diet and exercise counseling due to diets high in sugar, fat, and meat, and low in salads, fruits, and grains. Some refugees have stated they have little time for exercise beyond work-related physical activity.

Research suggests that Arab men living in the Arabian Peninsula region may be as susceptible to the clustering of risk factors in metabolic syndrome as some other ethnic groups, such as Asian Indians (refer to Chapter 14 for more information). A high prevalence of undiagnosed type 2 diabetes and hypertension, high rates of insulin resistance, low levels of high-density lipoprotein (HDL) cholesterol, and a tendency toward abdominal obesity were found. Coronary heart disease, diabetes, hypertension, and cancer are the primary health concerns in Arab countries.[77] Studies of men and women in Turkey, where cardiovascular disease is the most common cause of death, have also reported strikingly low serum levels of HDL cholesterol unrelated to diet, obesity, or lifestyle.[78,79] Obesity and diabetes incidence are rapidly increasing as a result of urbanization, low physical activity, and unhealthy eating. Turkey has prioritized WHO risk factor reduction targets over the next 20 years to reduce the cost of cardiovascular disease, which has been estimated in the billions.[78,79] Worldwide, one of the greatest relative increases in type 2 diabetes is expected to occur in the eastern Mediterranean region.

Data on cancer incidence in Arab/Chaldean adults indicate that, when compared to the non-Arab White population, the men have disproportionately high rates of leukemia, multiple myeloma, and liver, kidney, and urinary bladder cancers, while women have greater proportions of leukemia and thyroid and brain cancers. However, the leading causes of cancer-related deaths in Arab Americans are lung, colorectal, and breast cancers.[80,81]

The effects of Ramadan fasting have been explored among Muslims. Although hunger increases in some fasters, one study showed that there were no significant changes in body weight.[82–84] Although there is a keen interest in modified fasting as a mechanism for weight management and diabetes control, results have been mixed. Ramadan fasting may be a healthy nonpharmacological means for improving the cardiovascular and overall health of individuals. A majority of pregnant women go through Ramadan, and one study suggested that with certain precautions, such as excluding women with medical risk factors (including diabetes and history of preterm deliveries or renal stones), increased prenatal visits, avoiding strenuous exercise, staying cool, and consumption of extra fluids before dawn, fasting was safe for many of the women.

The Middle East has a tradition of high breastfeeding initiation rates. This high rate was attributed to a strong social network of support for the practice. In Turkey, mothers sometimes nurse their sons longer than daughters because breast milk is believed to increase strength. Exclusive breastfeeding is less likely to be practiced by working mothers.[85] Though rates of celiac disease in the Middle East are estimated to be below those in northern Europeans (refer to Chapter 6), it is considered the primary cause of chronic diarrhea in Iran and may contribute to iron deficiency, malnutrition, rickets, and short stature in children. Thalassemia syndromes may also be prevalent in Middle Easterners. Women from the Middle East also have high rates of vitamin D deficiency.[86]

Comfort Food

Sima's Iranian Family Comfort

In the Middle East, an Iranian family may associate dishes with a particular family member, a significant person or moment lived, and those foods become comfort foods for a cultural and/or personal connection. These foods, much like they do in other parts of the world, help shape identity. For Sima, they bring back both particular people and a lived experience.

What is a favorite comfort food that you consider traditional from your home culture?

S: Growing up in Iran, tahchin was a family favorite of mine. The smell of this baked chicken and rice casserole, combined with saffron filled my house with warm sweet smells. There is nothing like the unique smell of saffron baking into the rice. My mom told me the secret to a great tahchin recipe is keeping it moist and not letting it dry out. It's the yogurt and oil that keeps it moist. I would smell it as it baked in our kitchen, while I would do my homework.

Did you eat this food together with the community? Where was it eaten?

S: When my father got home from work, I would help set a tablecloth on the rug, and set the dishes, forks, and spoons out. The tahcheen would go in the middle, with other side dishes, like Persian cucumber dip, salad, and raw greens like parsley, surrounding it. We would all sit around the meal, eating, laughing, telling jokes, and discussing our day. Now that I am an adult with my own family, I try to have this wonderful food at least once a month.

Here is Sima's recipe:

Tahchin (Crispy Saffron Chicken and Rice Casserole)

Makes about 10 servings

½ cup olive oil, plus oil to drizzle the rice
2 medium yellow onions (½ onion grated and 1½ onions, thinly sliced to sauté)
¼ tsp. ground turmeric
2 cups basmati rice, rinsed
4 cups water
1 Tbsp. plus 2 tsp. kosher salt, plus more to season onions
1 medium egg
1½ cups thick Greek low-fat plain yogurt
1 tsp. saffron threads, crushed and dissolved in ¼ cup hot water
1 Tbsp. ground cumin
2 Tbsp. freshly squeezed lemon juice
1½ pounds boneless, skinless chicken thighs (cooked and shredded)
2 Tbsp. room temperature ghee or unsalted butter (optional)

Preheat oven to 400°F. Spread 3 Tbsp. of the olive oil over the bottom of a 9 x 13 x 2 inch glass baking dish. Place it in the oven to warm up. Sautee the sliced onions until translucent, add turmeric, and a little salt if desired, and set aside. Place the rice in a fine-mesh strainer and rinse until it is no longer cloudy. In a 3-quart pot, combine the rice, 4 cups of water, and 1 Tbsp. of salt, bringing it to a boil. Cook at a gentle boil, reducing the heat to medium-high until the rice grains soften but are not mushy and most of the water is absorbed (about 10-15 minutes). Pour the rice into a strainer and run it under cold water to cool it down. Drizzle it with olive oil. In a large mixing bowl, beat the egg using a fork or a whisk, add 1½ cups of yogurt, 2 Tbsp. of oil, the saffron water, 1 Tbsp. of cumin, 1 tsp. of salt, and 2 Tbsp. of lemon juice, and mix well until it achieves a cohesive consistency (about 1 minute). Add the cooked rice to the yogurt mixture and gently mix through. It will be bright yellow. Remove the baking dish from the oven and add half of the rice-yogurt mixture to the bottom and sides of the dish. Pat it down firmly. Then layer the chicken and sauteed onions over the rice and top with the remaining rice yogurt mixture. Use a spoon or your hands to compact the rice. Cover with tin foil and poke small holes in the middle of the foil to allow steam to release. Cook for 75–90 minutes. The sides should become golden brown. Let cool for 5 minutes. Add ghee or butter so that it melts into the dish. Holding the serving platter tightly over the dish, grab onto the handles on both sides of the baking dish and invert it onto the platter. The crispy bottom should be facing up and the dish should be intact.

Nutritional information (per serving):

calories 360; fat 16 g (saturated fat 4 g); sodium 800 mg; carbohydrate 32 g; fiber 1 g; protein 23 g

And additional RECIPE TO TRY (Bulgarian)

Banitsa

Serves 12 people

4 large eggs
2 cups yogurt (Bulgarian, if possible), plus more for serving
12 oz feta cheese
½ tsp. baking soda
1 pound phyllo sheet
¾ cup unsalted butter

Preheat the oven to 375°F. Grease a 12-inch baking pan with butter or cooking oil spray. In a large bowl, beat together the eggs and yogurt until smooth. Crumble in the feta cheese, add the baking soda, and whisk together. Unroll the thawed phyllo sheets and cover with a towel. Place one of the sheets on a clean working surface and spread it with butter. Add the cheese-yogurt mix in a thin line across the long side nearest you. Tightly roll up the phyllo sheet to the other long side. Place seam side down at the edge of the baking dish. Repeat with the remaining phyllo sheets, continuing to wrap them around the edge of the pan, coiling in towards the center. Brush the top with butter. Bake in the preheated oven till the top is golden brown or about 45 minutes to 1 hour. After baking, cover with a towel to let cool for about 15 minutes and serve with remaining yogurt.

Nutritional information (per serving):

calories 348; fat 21 g (saturated fat 12 g); sodium 660 mg; carbohydrate 26 g; fiber 1.5 g; protein 11 g

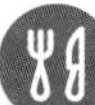

Food for Thought

The most common ailments that traditional healers in Saudi Arabia treat are abdominal pain, flatulence, low back pain, sadness, depression, and headache. In an earlier study, about 42 percent of the 1,408 people studied consulted traditional healers sometimes, and 23.9 percent had done so in the last 12 months.[87]

Traditional healers in Saudi Arabia have a shared worldview of their society which includes beliefs in magic, evil eye, and possession. They typically perform religious-based practices, such as reading the Holy Qur'an, as a source of healing.[88]

Health and Longevity Takeaway

A good night's sleep is essential for a good memory, but daytime naps can have the same effect on boosting memory and decreasing stress. Mid-day napping is common in Middle Eastern countries and may be one of the secrets to their longevity. One of the latest trends is a "coffee nap" or "Nappuccino." Try drinking a caffeinated drink like coffee, followed by a 20-minute nap. Since it takes caffeine about 20–30 minutes to take effect, the nap and caffeine provide an extra energy boost.

Discussion Starters

Diet and Culture of Balkan and Middle Eastern Americans

In small groups of three to four, compare and contrast the diet and culture of Balkan Americans and Middle Eastern Americans, with each group focusing on a different aspect of the diet and culture of these groups:

Group A: The food habits and the typical eating etiquette and meal composition of these two immigrant groups

Group B: Issues involved in counseling these immigrant groups on diet and health

Group C: Attitudes within each immigrant group toward diet, health, and medical treatment, notably attitudes toward traditional home culture medical treatment and U.S. biomedicine

Group D: Amount of obesity, diabetes, hypertension, and other diseases within each immigrant group

Given the scarcity of data in some cases, you may have to draw hypotheses about the diet, food habits, and so on of these groups from what we know about diet, food habits, and the like of nonimmigrants.

Within your group, try to come to a consensus on what findings to report to the rest of the class. Before breaking up, assign a number to each group member: A1, A2, A3, A4; B1, B2, and so forth. Form new groups with all the 1's in a group, all the 2's in another group, all the 3's another group, and so on. In your new group, report the findings of your previous group, and as a group, discuss the relationship between traditional attitudes toward diet and health and changes in diet and health due to immigration to the United States.

Review Questions

1. What food flavors and food ingredients are associated with the Balkan and Middle Eastern countries? Why might they be similar? Describe two recipes, one from the Balkans and one from the Middle East, that contain filo (phyllo) dough.
2. What is meant by the "evil eye"? How might you protect yourself from it?
3. What countries make up the Balkans and the Middle East? Pick either the Balkans or the Middle East and map the religions found in that region. Pick one religion, describe a recipe eaten for a holiday of that religion, and explain how the recipe reflects the ingredients of the region.
4. What are common health problems associated with people from the Balkans or the Middle East? Select one group and a health disorder, and describe that group's cultural beliefs regarding the cause and appropriate treatment of that disorder.
5. In several countries from these two regions, food and illness may be classified as "hot" or "cold." What does this mean? Provide examples

Reflection

In most countries, herbal medicines are commonly used first, before seeking care in westernized healthcare systems. This is especially true in Middle Eastern countries where a majority of the population has been found to use this form of medicine for primary care. Health care practitioners do not typically ask about herb uses. How can practitioners be culturally sensitive toward longstanding belief systems and bridge the gap between herbal usage and pharmaceutical medicine for their patients?

References

1. U.S. Census Bureau. 2019. People reporting ancestry. American Community Survey. Retrieved from https://data.census.gov/cedsci/table?q=B04006&t=Ancestry&tid=ACSDT1Y2019.B04006&hidePreview=false (accessed April 20, 2022).
2. Ifkovic, E. 2014. Croatian Americans. In R.V. Dassanowsky & J. Lehman (Eds.), *Gale encyclopedia of multicultural America*. Farmington Hills, MI: Gale Group.

3. Stevanovic, B. 2014. Serbian Americans. In R.V. Dassanowsky & J. Lehman (Eds.), *Gale encyclopedia of multicultural America*. Farmington Hills, MI: Gale Group.
4. Gobetz, E. 2014. Slovenian Americans. In R.V. Dassanowsky & J. Lehman (Eds.), *Gale encyclopedia of multicultural America*. Farmington Hills, MI: Gale Group.
5. Miller, O. 2014. Bosnian Americans. *Gale encyclopedia of multicultural America*. Vol. 1, 3rd ed. Farmington Hills, MI: Gale Group.
6. Arab American Institute. Retrieved from http://www.aaiusa.org/pages/demographics/ (accessed April 20, 2015).
7. Abraham, N. 2014. Arab Americans. In R.V. Dassanowsky & J. Lehman (Eds.), Gale encyclopedia of multicultural America. Vol. 1, 3rd ed. Farmington Hills, MI: Gale Group.
8. Riggs, T. 2014 Iranian Americans. *Gale encyclopedia of multicultural America*. Vol. 2, 3rd ed., pp. 433–443. Retrieved from https://link.gale.com/apps/doc/CX3273300095/GVRL?u=multi_america&sid=bookmark-GVRL&xid=25ae5e45
9. Altschiller, D. 2014. Turkish Americans. In R.V. Dassanowsky & J. Lehman (Eds.), *Gale encyclopedia of multicultural America*. Vol. 4, 3rd ed. Farmington Hills, MI: Gale Group.
10. Rudolph, L.C. 2014. Israeli Americans. In R.V. Dassanowsky & J. Lehman (Eds.), *Gale encyclopedia of multicultural America*. Vol. 2, 3rd ed. Farmington Hills, MI: Gale Group.
11. Zurcher, A. 2016. America's 'invisible' Muslims. BBC. Retrieved from https://www.bbc.com/news/magazine-37663226 (accessed April 21, 2022).
12. Pew Research Center. 2017. U.S. Muslims concerned about their place in society, but continue to believe in the American dream. Retrieved from https://www.pewresearch.org/religion/2017/07/26/demographic-portrait-of-muslim-americans/.
13. Lipka, M. 2017. Muslims and Islam: key findings in the U.S. and around the world. Retrieved from https://www.pewresearch.org/fact-tank/2017/08/09/muslims-and-islam-key-findings-in-the-u-s-and-around-the-world/
14. Iranian Americans. 2014. In T. Riggs (Ed.), *Gale encyclopedia of multicultural America*. 3rd ed., Vol. 2, pp. 433–443. Retrieved from https://link.gale.com/apps/doc/CX3273300095/GVRL?u=multi_america&sid=bookmark-GVRL&xid=25ae5e45.
15. Vos, H. 2016. In "This history and significance of the chef's toque." Auguste Escoffier School of Culinary Arts. Retrieved from https://www.escoffier.edu/blog/world-food-drink/a-history-of-the-chefs-hat/
16. Guignier, B. The chef's hat through the ages. *Alimentarium Magazine*. Retrieved from https://www.alimentarium.org/en/magazine/history/chef%E2%80%99s-hat-through-ages.
17. Alić, A. 2020. Structural and functional changes in Bosnian family-disappearance of the "Sofra". *European Journal of Social Sciences*, 3(2), 68–84.
18. Miller, O. 2014. Bosnian Americans. In T. Riggs (Ed.), *Gale encyclopedia of multicultural America*. Vol. 1, 3rd ed., pp. 331–341. Retrieved from https://link.gale.com/apps/doc/CX3273300036/GVRL?u=multi_america&sid=bookmark-GVRL&xid=2de475de.
19. Mikhail, M. 2014. Egyptian Americans. In T. Riggs (Ed.), *Gale encyclopedia of multicultural America*. Vol. 2, 3rd ed., pp. 61–71. Retrieved from https://link.gale.com/apps/doc/CX3273300067/GVRL?u=multi_america&sid=bookmark-GVRL&xid=d9d7623b
20. Beitin, B.K., & Aprahamian, M. 2014. Family values and traditions. In *Biopsychosocial perspectives on Arab Americans*. Springer, Boston, MA: Springer, pp. 67–88.
21. Ajami, J., Rasmi, S., Abudabbeh, N., Amer, M., & Awad, G. 2015. Traditions and practices throughout the family life cycle. *Handbook of Arab American psychology*, p. 103.
22. Rahimieh, N. 2015. *Iranian culture: Representation and identity*. Routledge.
23. Wehbe-Alamah, H.B. 2014. Folk care beliefs and practices of traditional Lebanese and Syrian Muslims in the Midwestern United States. *Leininger's culture care diversity and universality*, pp. 137–181.
24. Ahmed, L. 2021. *Women and gender in Islam: Historical roots of a modern debate*. New Haven, CT: Yale University Press. Retrieved from https://doi.org/10.12987/9780300258172.
25. Karageorgou, D., Magriplis, E., Mitsopoulou, A.V., Dimakopoulos, I., Bakogianni, I., Micha, R., . . . & Roma, E. (2019). Dietary patterns and lifestyle characteristics in adults: Results from the Hellenic National Nutrition and Health Survey (HNNHS). *Public Health*, 171, 76–88.
26. Boshnjaku, A., & Krasniqi, E. Life expectancy's relationship with behavioral factors and polypharmacy in Western Balkan countries.
27. Nestor, V. 2017. Traditional rituals and beliefs in the peoples of the Balkans. *ANGLISTICUM. Journal of the Association-Institute for English Language and American Studies*, 3(12), 107–112.
28. Abu-Rabia, A. 2015. *Indigenous medicine among the Bedouin in the Middle East*. Berghahn Books.
29. Purnell, L.D., & Fenkl, E.A. 2019. Transcultural diversity and health care. In *Handbook for culturally competent care*. Springer, Cham, pp. 1–6.
30. Abu-Rabia, A. 2005. Herbs as food and medicine source in Palestine. *Asian Pacific Journal of Cancer Prevention*, 6, 404–407.
31. Alhomoud, F., Aljamea, Z., Almahasnah, R., Alkhalifah, K., Basalelah, L., & Alhomoud, F.K. 2017. Self-medication and self-prescription with antibiotics in the Middle East—do they really happen? A systematic review of the prevalence, possible reasons, and outcomes. *International Journal of Infectious Diseases*, 57, 3–12.
32. Ben-Arye, E., Mahajna, J., Aly, R., Ali-Shtayeh, M. S., Bentur, Y., Lev, E., . . . & Samuels, N. 2016. Exploring an herbal "wonder cure" for cancer: a multidisciplinary approach. *Journal of Cancer Research and Clinical Oncology*, 142(7), 1499–1508
33. Jaradat, N.A., Al-Ramahi, R., Zaid, A.N., Ayesh, O.I., & Eid, A.M. 2016. Ethnopharmacological survey of herbal remedies used for treatment of various types of cancer and their methods of preparations in the West Bank-Palestine. *BMC Complementary and Alternative Medicine*, 16(1), 1–12.
34. Saad, B., Azaizeh, H., & Said, O. 2005. Tradition and perspectives of Arab herbal medicine: A review. *eCAM*, 2, 475–479.
35. Ogur, R., Korkmaz, A., & Bakir, B. 2006. Herbal treatment usage frequency, types and preferences in Turkey. *Middle East Journal of Family Medicine*, 4, 38–44.
36. Alqathama, A., Alluhiabi, G., Baghdadi, H., Aljahani, L., Khan, O., Jabal, S., . . . & Alhomoud, F. 2020. Herbal medicine from the perspective of type II diabetic patients and physicians: what is the relationship? *BMC Complementary Medicine and Therapies*, 20(1), 1–9.
37. Arishy, A., Alnamazi, N., Mashraqi, M., Alomaish, A., Moafa, A., Alfaifi, K., . . . & Ghazwani, S. 2022. Knowledge and attitude of parents towards traditional cauterization and its practice on their children in Jazan region, Saudi Arabia. *Medical Science*, 26(122).
38. Aboushanab, T., & AlSanad, S. 2019. An ethnomedical perspective of Arabic traditional cauterization; Al-Kaiy. *Advanced Journal of Social Science*, 4(1), 18–23.
39. Hashmi, M. A., Khan, A., Hanif, M., Farooq, U., & Perveen, S. 2015. Traditional uses, phytochemistry, and pharmacology of olea europaea (Olive). *Evidence-based complementary and alternative medicine: eCAM*, 541591. Retrieved from https://doi.org/10.1155/2015/541591
40. Nickles, H.G. 1969. *Middle Eastern cooking*. New York: Time-Life Books.
41. Rolek, B. 2021. Serbian stuffed cabbage (sarma). *The Spruce Eats*. Retrieved from https://www.thespruceeats.com/serbian-stuffed-cabbage-recipe-sarma-1136569.
42. International Coffee Organization. March, 2022. Retrieved from https://ico.org/ (accessed April 25, 2022).
43. Davidson, A. 1999. *The Oxford companion to food*. New York: Oxford University Press.
44. Coffee Culture and History in the Middle East. Middle Eastern Coffee Culture and History. Retrieved from www.kopiluwakdirect.com (accessed April 25, 2022).
45. Packard, D.P.K & McWilliams, M. 1993. May/June. Cultural foods heritage of Middle Eastern immigrants. *Nutrition Today*, 6–12.
46. Gökcen, B.B., & Şanlier, N. 2019. Coffee consumption and disease correlations. *Critical reviews in food science and nutrition*, 59(2), 336–348.
47. Schmit, S.L., Rennert, H.S., Rennert, G., & Gruber, S.B. 2016. Coffee consumption and the risk of colorectal cancer. *Cancer Epidemiology and Prevention Biomarkers*, 25(4), 634–639.

48. Barrea, L., Pugliese, G., Frias-Toral, E., El Ghoch, M., Castellucci, B., Chapela, S.P., de los Angeles Carignano, M., et al. 2021. Coffee consumption, health benefits and side effects: a narrative review and update for dietitians and nutritionists. *Critical Reviews in Food Science and Nutrition*, pp. 1–24.
49. Bosso, H., Barbalho, S.M., de Alvares Goulart, R., & Otoboni, A.M. M.B. 2023. Green coffee: economic relevance and a systematic review of the effects on human health. Critical Reviews in Food Science and Nutrition, 63(3), 394–410.
50. Rodríguez-Artalejo, F., & López-García, E. 2017. Coffee consumption and cardiovascular disease: A condensed review of epidemiological evidence and mechanisms. *Journal of Agricultural and Food Chemistry*, 66(21), 5257–5263.
51. Ghavami, H.S., Khoshtinat, M., Sadeghi-Farah, S., Kalimani, A.B., Ferrie, S., & Faraji, H. 2021. The relationship of coffee consumption and CVD risk factors in elderly patients with T2DM. *BMC Cardiovascular Disorders*, *21*(1), 1–7.
52. Wierzejska, R. 2017. Can coffee consumption lower the risk of Alzheimer's disease and Parkinson's disease? A literature review. *Archives of Medical Science: AMS*, 13(3), 507.
53. Dash, M. 2014. Food story: how naan and kulcha became India's much-loved breads. *The Indian Express*. Retrieved from https://indianexpress.com/article/lifestyle/food-wine/food-story-how-naan-and-kulcha-became-indias-much-loved-breads/
54. Raviv, Y. 2015. *Falafel nation: Cuisine and the making of national identity in Israel*. University of Nebraska Press.
55. Zibart, E. 2001. *The ethnic food lover's companion: Understanding the cuisines of the world*. Birmingham, AL: Menasha Ridge Press.
56. Avieli, N. 2018. *Food and power: A culinary ethnography of Israel*. Vol. 67. University of California Press.
57. Jurgens, J. 2014. Albanian Americans. In T. Riggs (Ed.), *Gale encyclopedia of multicultural America*. Vol. 1, 3rd ed., pp. 61–73. Retrieved from https://link.gale.com/apps/doc/CX3273300015/GVRL?u=multi_america&sid=bookmark-GVRL&xid=b936a85c
58. Duruz, J. 2016. Ras el Hanout and Preserved Lemons: Memories, Markets and the Scent of Borrowed Traditions. In *Cooking Cultures: Convergent Histories of Food and Feeling*, p. 201.
59. Hutcherson, A. 2021. A guide to couscous: the history, different types and how to cook with it. *The Washington Post*. Retrieved from https://www.washingtonpost.com/food/2021/05/14/couscous-moroccan-pearl-israeli/
60. Batmanglii, N.K. 2000. *New food of life: Ancient Persian and modern Iranian cooking and ceremonies*. Washington, DC: Mage.
61. Foster, D. 2002. *The global etiquette guide to Africa sand the Middle East*. New York: Wiley.
62. Dresser, N. 2011. *Multicultural manners: Essential rules of etiquette for the 21st century*. New York: John Wiley & Sons.
63. Lohman, S. 2022. Hamin: a Sephardic sabbath stew. American Jewish Historical Society, a Smithsonian Affiliate. Retrieved from https://ajhs.org/blog/hamin-sephardic-sabbath-stew
64. Seidal, K. 2001. Serving the guest, Sufi cookbook and art gallery. Retrieved from Serving the Guest: A Sufi Cookbook and Art Gallery (www.superluminal.com) (accessed April 26, 2022).
65. Egherman, T. May 3, 2016. The hot and cold secrets of the Persian kitchen. Global voices-Middle East. Retrieved from The Hot and Cold Secrets of the Persian Kitchen. Global Voices (accessed April 26, 2022).
66. John, L.J., & Shantakumari, N. 2015. Herbal medicines use during pregnancy: a review from the Middle East. *Oman Medical Journal*, 30(4), 229.
67. Attum, B., Hafiz, S., Malik, A., & Shamoon, Z. 2021. Cultural competence in the care of Muslim patients and their families. In StatPearls [Internet]. Treasure Island, FL: StatPearls Publishing.
68. Papadimitriou, A., Foscolou, A., Itsiopoulos, C., Thodis, A., Kouris-Blazos, A., Brazionis, L., . . . & Sidossis, L.S. 2022. Adherence to the Mediterranean diet and successful aging in Greeks living in Greece and abroad: the epidemiological Mediterranean Islands Study (MEDIS). *Nutrition and Health*.
69. Maamoun, M., Sucher, K.P., & Hollenbeck, C. 2006. *Food habits and acculturation among first generation Egyptians living in the San Francisco Bay Area (SFBA)*. Unpublished master's thesis, San Jose State University.
70. Theodoratus, R. *The acceptance of Greek foods in America*. Ann Arbor, 1001, 48105-2722. Retrieved from: https://aadl.org/files/cooks/repast/2005_Spring.pdf
71. D'Innocenzo, S., Biagi, C., & Lanari, M. 2019. Obesity and the Mediterranean diet: a review of evidence of the role and sustainability of the Mediterranean diet. *Nutrients*, 11(6), 1306.
72. Martínez-González, M.A., Salas-Salvadó, J., Estruch, R., Corella, D., Fitó, M., Ros, E., & Predimed Investigators. 2015. Benefits of the Mediterranean diet: insights from the PREDIMED study. *Progress in Cardiovascular Diseases*, 58(1), 50–60.
73. Mentella, M.C., Scaldaferri, F., Ricci, C., Gasbarrini, A., & Miggiano, G.A. D. 2019. Cancer and Mediterranean diet: a review. *Nutrients*, 11(9), 2059.
74. Martínez-González, M.A., Gea, A., & Ruiz-Canela, M. 2019. The Mediterranean diet and cardiovascular health: A critical review. *Circulation Research*, 124(5), 779–798.
75. World Obesity. 2019. Global Obesity Observatory. Adults. Retrieved from https://data.worldobesity.org/country/greece-80/#data_prevalence (accessed April 25, 2022).
76. Bourdillon, M.T., Akhter, A.S., Vrtikapa, D., *et al.* 2018. Cardiovascular health in St. Louis Bosnian-Americans. *Journal of Immigrant Minority Health,* 20, 1147–1157. Retrieved from https://doi.org/10.1007/s10903-017-0641-1.
77. Al-Rethaiaa, S.S., Fahm, A.E., & Al-Shwaiyat, N.M. 2010. Obesity and eating habits among college students in Saudi Arabia: A cross sectional study. *Nutrition Journal*, 9(39).
78. Tokgozoglu, L., Kayikcioglu, M., & Ekinci, B. 2021. The landscape of preventive cardiology in Turkey: Challenges and successes. *American Journal of Preventive Cardiology*, 6, 100184.
79. Balbay, Y., Gagnon-Arpin, I., Malhan, S., Öksüz, M.E., Sutherland, G., Dobrescu, A., . . . & Habib, M. 2019. The impact of addressing modifiable risk factors to reduce the burden of cardiovascular disease in Turkey. *Turk Kardiyol Dern Ars*, 47(6), 487–497.
80. Abuelezam, N.N., & El-Sayed, A.M. 2021. The health of Arab Americans in the United States: An update. *Handbook of healthcare in the Arab world*, pp. 739–764.
81. Jadalla, A.A., Hattar, M., & Schubert, C.C. 2015. Acculturation as a predictor of health promoting and lifestyle practices of Arab Americans: A Descriptive study. *Journal of Cultural Diversity*, 22(1).
82. Mazidi, M., Rezaie, P., Chaudhri, O., Karimi, E., & Nematy, M. 2015. The effect of Ramadan fasting on cardiometabolic risk factors and anthropometrics parameters: a systematic review. *Pakistan Journal of Medical Sciences*, 31(5), 1250.
83. Meo, S.A., & Hassan, A. 2015. Physiological changes during fasting in Ramadan. *Journal of Pakistan Medical Association*, 65(5 Suppl 1), S6–14.
84. Lessan, N., & Ali, T. 2019. Energy metabolism and intermittent fasting: the Ramadan perspective. *Nutrients*, 11(5), 1192.
85. Alzaheb, R.A. 2017. Factors influencing exclusive breastfeeding in Tabuk, Saudi Arabia. *Clinical Medicine Insights: Pediatrics*, 11, 1179556517698136.
86. Lips, P., Cashman, K.D., Lamberg-Allardt, C., Bischoff-Ferrari, H.A., Obermayer-Pietsch, B., Bianchi, M.L., . . . & Bouillon, R. 2019. Current vitamin D status in European and Middle East countries and strategies to prevent vitamin D deficiency: a position statement of the European Calcified Tissue Society. *European Journal of Endocrinology*, 180(4), P23–P54.
87. Al-Rowais, N., Al-Faris, E., Mohammad, A. G., Al-Rukban, M., & Abdulghani, H.M. 2010. Traditional healers in Riyadh region: reasons and health problems for seeking their advice. A household survey. *Journal of Alternative and Complementary Medicine*, 16(2), 199–204. Retrieved from https://doi.org/10.1089/acm.2009.0283
88. Alosaimi, F.D., Alshehri, Y., Alfraih, I. *et al.* 2015. Psychosocial correlates of using faith healing services in Riyadh, Saudi Arabia: a comparative cross-sectional study. *International Journal of Mental Health Systems,* 9, 8. Retrieved from https://doi.org/10.1186/1752-4458-9-8.

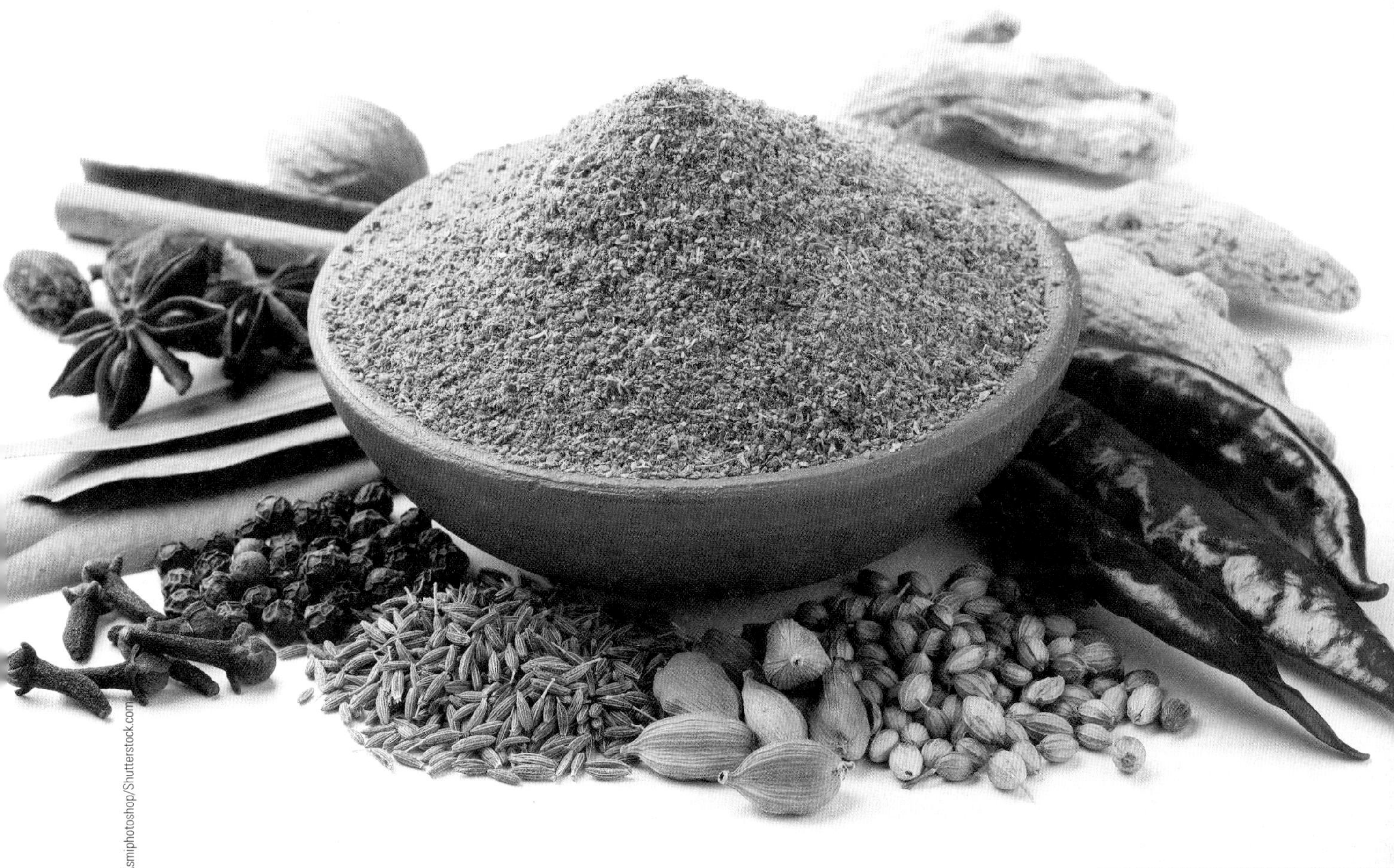
Asmiphotoshop/Shutterstock.com

Chapter 14

South Asians

Learning Objectives

14.1 Differentiate the regions of South Asia and discuss how these relate to food production and intake.

14.2 Identify the immigration patterns, historical socioeconomic influences, and current locations of Asian Indians and Pakistanis in the United States today.

14.3 Compare the typical religions, family structures, and traditional health beliefs and practices of Indians and Pakistanis—before and after immigration.

14.4 Describe the differences between the staples and regional variation in ingredients between the regions of India and the regions of Pakistan.

14.5 Identify key foods and foodways for each of the food groups for Asian Indians and Pakistanis and how these foods have been adapted by immigrants in the United States.

14.6 Describe vegetarianism's historical context and current-day impact on these cultures.

14.7 Describe the impact religion has on foods, foodways, hospitality, and medicine for these cultures.

14.8 Identify health concerns associated with the nutritional intake of these groups.

South Asia is the geographic region comprising the nations of India, Pakistan, Bangladesh, Sri Lanka, Nepal, and Bhutan (refer to Figure 14.1). Immigrants from South Asia, mostly those from India and Pakistan, comprise one of the fastest-growing populations in the United States. The South Asian subcontinent contains the fertile Indus and Ganges River basins and parts of the Himalayan mountain range; it varies in climate from extensive desert regions to jungle forests to the world's largest mountain glaciers.

India is a culturally complex country with more than 1.38 billion people—over four times that of the United States. The sophisticated civilization began roughly 8,000 years ago in the Indus Valley of northern India and is the source of some of the most influential religions, art, architecture, and foods in the world.[1,2] The total population of the early Indus civilization is thought to have been upward of 5 million, and its territory stretched over 900 miles along the Indus River. The two best-known excavated cities of the Indus civilization, also called the Harrapan civilization, are Harappa and Mohenjo-Daro. The first discovery of Harappa was in 1829 CE, making it a late-comer, after Egypt and Mesopotamia, for study by archeologists.

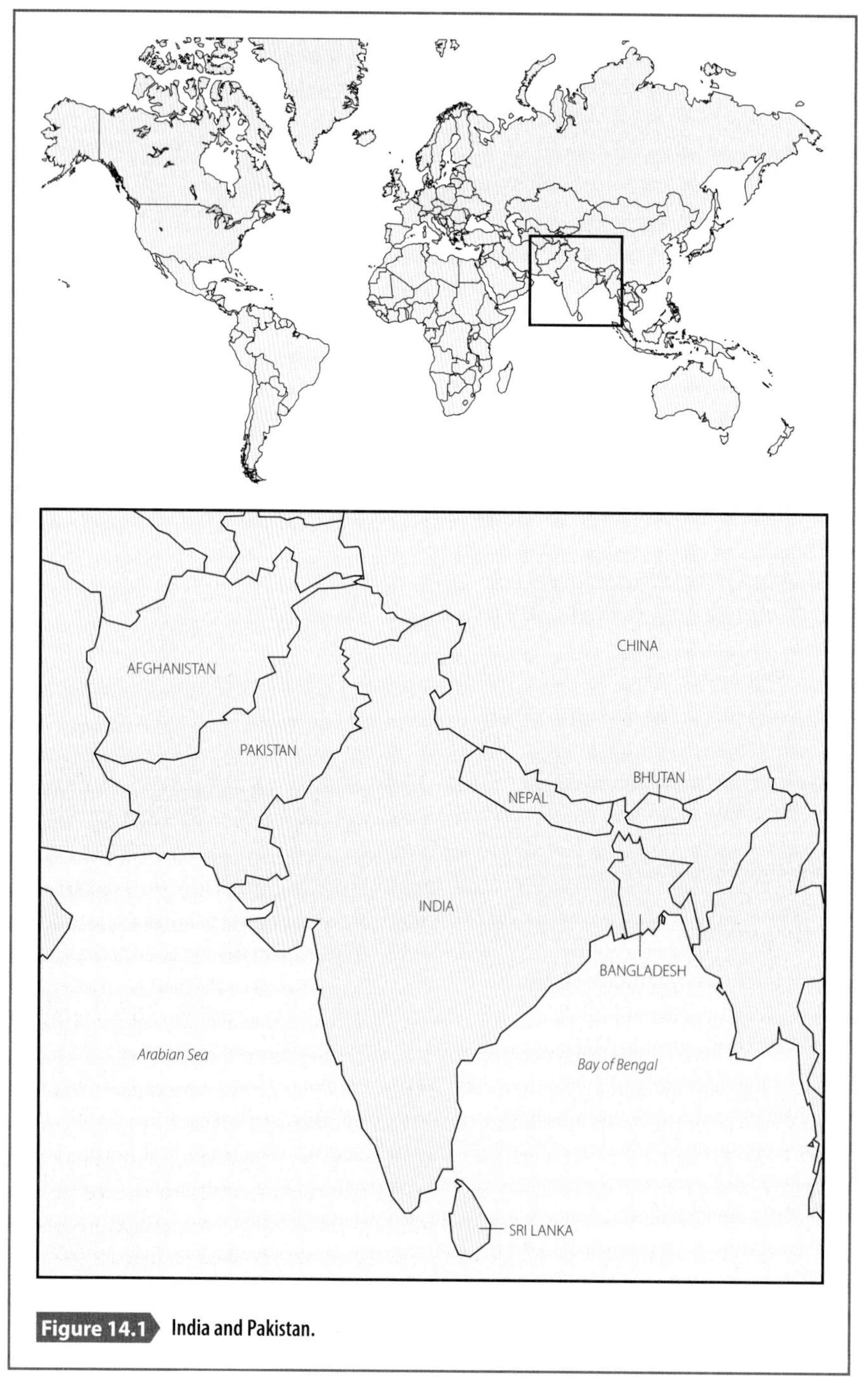

Figure 14.1 India and Pakistan.

The people of India are as diverse as its geography and climate. People entered India from different parts of the world at different periods and virtually every racial and religious group is represented on the subcontinent. As a result, India has a varied population and diversified ethnic composition with wide-ranging customs. One result of this history is that there are currently 22 separate languages recognized by the Indian government, though only Hindi or English are used for official purposes. In addition, more than 270 languages with 10,000 speakers or more are spoken in India, and there are hundreds of dialects.[3]

Food for Thought

Fewer than 238,000 Sri Lankans, Nepalese, and Bhutanese combined have immigrated to the United States. The 2019 Census reported that 261,000 Bangladeshis are estimated to live in the nation (over half of them in New York City), most of whom have arrived since 1990.[4]

The Islamic Republic of Pakistan, located to the northwest of India, encompasses some of the most rugged terrains in the world. The Himalayas stretch across the north, including the second-highest peak in the world, K2. The Hindu Kush mountain range defines the northwestern region. From these mountains spills the Indus River, supplying the plains of the south before emptying into the Arabian Sea.

One day before Indian independence from Britain on August 15, 1947, Pakistan was partitioned from India by the British as a result of calls for a Muslim homeland. It was a bitter split. Wars and numerous conflicts between the countries have been fought since independence, and tensions continue over the province of Kashmir, with both countries stationing armies along the border. Pakistan is divided into four provinces, each with its own cultural groups and languages: Punjab (spilt from the state of the same name in India), Sindh, Baluchistan, and the North-West Frontier Province (NWFP).

Although India and Pakistan share a past, Asian Indians and Pakistanis each bring distinctive contributions when they immigrate to the United States, particularly in their traditional foods and food habits. This chapter examines the customary diets of India and Pakistan and the changes that occur when immigrants from these countries move to America.

South Asians

Cultural Perspective

History of Asian Indians and Pakistanis in the United States

The majority of people from Pakistan and India arriving in the United States are not escaping political or economic pressures in their homelands. In addition, since 1965, when the Immigration and Nationality Act was implemented, the majority of South Asian immigrants have been from the upper socioeconomic classes. They were somewhat acculturated at the time of arrival, often fluent in English, and acquainted with many American customs.

Immigration Patterns

Asian Indians The first immigrants to the United States from India were members of the Sikh religion, who arrived on the West Coast in the early twentieth century. Many were employed by the railroads, and others established large farms. They faced overt discrimination and persecution. Anti–Asian Indian feelings brought about the expulsion of Asian Indians from Washington logging communities and, in 1907, sparked violent riots in California. Although such extreme bigotry lessened over time, the Asian Indian immigrant population remained small until after World War II.

Food for Thought

The term Indian can refer to South Asian or Indian Americans from Asia. Native people of the Americas are often called by their tribal affiliation or by the terms Native American, First Nations, or Indigenous people.

In the early 1900s, it was not unusual for single Sikh men living in the United States to marry Mexican American women and start families due to the Immigration Act of 1917. The Act, which banned Asians and other non-White people from entering the United States, kept Sikh men from going to India to marry (if they left the United States, they may not have been allowed to return). California's anti-miscegenation laws were also a cause of this unique subculture's existence.

In the 2016 Canadian census, 1,963,330 individuals identified themselves as South Asian.[5]

The change in immigration laws (the Immigration and Nationality Act of 1965 abolished National Origins Formula which kept non-Western and non-Northern European groups from immigrating) encouraged Asian Indians, especially well-educated urban professionals, to come to the United States starting in the 1960s. Economic and social adjustment was a priority for this group, although many Asian Indian traditions continue within the privacy of the home. These immigrants formed a self-reliant community and discouraged comparison or identification with other ethnic groups.

Pakistanis Though Muslims from northern India certainly came to the United States before the founding of Pakistan, immigration from the nation technically began in 1947. However, before 1965, only 2,500 Pakistanis moved to the United States. Beginning in 1965, when immigration quotas were lifted, the number of immigrants from Pakistan have increased significantly.

Current Demographics and Socioeconomic Status

Asian Indians According to U.S. Census estimates for 2019, over 4.6 million Asian Indians live in the United States. Over 90 percent of Indian Americans are foreign-born, and most of them have arrived since 1970.[6] Asian Indians have settled throughout the United States, but especially in the metropolitan areas of California, New York, and New Jersey, as well as in Illinois, Maryland, Massachusetts, Michigan, Ohio, Pennsylvania, and Texas. There are also several Asian Indian settlements in the agricultural regions of California.[4]

Some Asian Indians coming to the United States in recent years are from regions where Indian immigration in the past has been substantial, such as East Africa, Fiji, and Guyana. These immigrants often form separate enclaves.

The relative affluence of Americans of Asian Indian heritage is due mostly to a well-educated population: nearly 54 percent held a college or graduate degree in 2019. Many were employed in professional or white-collar occupations in India, such as college professors, engineers, physicians, and scientists, and most continue their careers in the United States. Nearly 69 percent of Indian Americans hold management or professional jobs. Newer immigrants have found success in small-business and franchise ownership involving many members of their extended family. Motel and hotel ownership is especially common for some immigrants, and it is estimated that over 50 percent of these businesses nationwide are run by Indian Americans. Median family income is well above the national norm, and family poverty rates are below average at 6 percent.[6]

Many Asian Indians come to the United States to complete their college or postgraduate education. They are often unmarried or have left their spouses and children in India. Sometimes families join the student in America after they have become financially established.

Pakistanis As of 2019, Census figures suggest the number of Pakistani Americans is less than 554,000, more than 50 percent of whom are foreign-born immigrants, and nearly all of whom have arrived since 1980.[4] A majority have come from large cities and the largest population settled in the New York City metropolitan area and Chicago.[6]

The immigrants who first arrived after 1965 were typically well-educated professionals seeking employment in professions such as law, medicine, computer technology, and teaching. Many students obtaining advanced degrees also chose to stay in the United States. Over 57 percent of Pakistani Americans hold a college degree. However, Pakistanis are often grouped with Asian Indians and Arabs in data collection, so little is known specifically regarding their socioeconomic status. It is believed that most Pakistani Americans are solidly middle-class or upper-middle-class. Homeownership is valued and may be higher than average compared to other recent immigrant groups. Family income for Pakistani Americans is similar to the U.S. median. However, 15 percent of Pakistani families were living in poverty as of 2019.[6,7]

Worldview

India is a country of diverse cultures. The notion of a singular worldview in a country of over 1.4 billion people seems far-fetched, especially when you consider the population's various religious backgrounds—Hindus, Muslims, Sikhs, Christians, and Jains—and a variety of languages and regions (former princely states) with pronounced cultural differences. Yet, even in early times, travelers from Europe, China, and Arab nations have seen commonality among India's peoples, an underlying unity in apparent diversity.

Through thousands of years, India has been in constant transformation: encounters with other civilizations and cultural forces such as Islam in medieval times, European colonialism, and more recently, West-centric globalization. The custom of the culture is hierarchical with large differences in power and prestige between, for example, the chief executive and the office assistant. The people from India also tend to stand out in humane orientation—that is, the degree to which people are caring, altruistic, generous, and kind. Overall, India and South Asia, in general, are oriented toward collectivism, or the degree to which people feel solidarity with small groups such as their family or circle of friends. This feeling of loyalty to family and, further, to caste in India, can sometimes make collaboration with outside groups, or large organizations, challenging.[8]

The Caste System in India The traditional Indian caste system, which influences the social structure of many Asian Indian groups, is the Hindu method of ordering an individual's role in society. A more encompassing term is jati, which is the organization of all aspects of Hindu life, including actions, places, things, and symbols, not just people. Caste categories are hereditary. There are four main castes associated with certain professions (although members are not necessarily employed in these jobs): the Brahmins (priests), Kshatriyas (soldiers), Vaisyas (merchants or farmers), and the Sudras (serfs). These castes are divided into more than 1,000 subcastes, usually according to occupation. Existing outside the caste system are Dalits (officially, Scheduled Caste), individuals historically and pejoratively called "untouchables," who often only had access to "menial" work such as garbage disposal and sewage cleaning. Although changing (laws discriminating against untouchables were repealed in 1949), faced with exclusion and discrimination for centuries, many Scheduled Caste people end up with little or no access to education.[9] The group continues to occupy the lowest stratum in Indian society, a concern for many. However, there are signs of change. Researchers found that people belonging to lower castes generally do not feel there is widespread caste discrimination in India today. For instance,

13 percent of the lowest classes say there is a lot of discrimination against them, and 87 percent say there is not. Christians are more likely than other religious groups in India to say there is a lot of discrimination against lower caste groups (three in ten). A strong majority (82 percent) of people in the lower castes say they have not *personally* felt caste discrimination in the past 12 months. Members of the Scheduled Castes are slightly more likely than members of other castes to say they have personally faced caste-based discrimination (17 percent) in the last 12 months. Caste-based discrimination is more commonly reported in some parts of India, however, and appears to be highest in the northeast (there, 38 percent of respondents say they experienced discrimination because of their caste in the last 12 months).[10]

The caste system has existed in some form in India for at least 3,000 years. Many people interact socially within their caste, and marriages are primarily between members of the same caste. Americans of Asian Indian descent, too, often continue to identify with their caste. As with all cultural practices, it is important to remember that even within a group there is a great diversity of individual beliefs and customs.

Food for Thought

The term *yoga* comes from a Sanskrit word that means yoke or union. Traditionally, yoga is a method that joins the individual self with the divine, and develops the mind-body connection in an individual. It is one of the longest-surviving philosophical systems in the world, perhaps beginning 5,000 years ago. Yoga also aids people of all age groups to improve strength and flexibility and rejuvenate the body. In the United States, estimates say that 11 million Americans or more practice yoga at least occasionally.

A reverence for all life, called ahimsa, is fundamental to Asian Indian ideology. It is reflected in the religions native to India, as well as in the vegetarian diet that many Indians follow.

Religion

Asian Indians The influence of religion on Indian culture is ubiquitous. Every aspect of life and death is affected not only by individual religious affiliation but also by the Hindu ideology that pervades Indian society. Religious pluralism has long been a core value in India, which has a large majority of Hindu people, with smaller communities of Muslims, Christians, Sikhs, Buddhists, Jains, and other groups (refer to Chapter 4 for more information about the major Indian religions).

Hinduism Nearly 80 percent of Indians are Hindus.[11] Hinduism is an ancient faith, believed to have developed in India between 2000 and 1500 BCE from the Aryan hymns and prayers known as the Vedas mixed with elements from traditional Dravidian religion. It is unique in that it is not a single religion, but a compilation of many traditions and philosophies. Hindus recognize one God, Brahman, the eternal origin, who is the cause and foundation of all existence. Many manifestations (avatars), divinities, and mythological stories exist to represent different ways to approach and access this truth. Followers believe there are multiple paths to reaching God, and for most Hindus, God is in everyone and everything.

Many Hindu temples now exist in the United States in regions where Asian Indians have settled, with services and religious ceremonies conducted by Brahmin priests (who are sometimes employed part-time in other occupations). However, temple attendance may be limited to significant religious events and daily prayer is often offered at home in a sacred space set aside for the family. These small private altars emphasize that God's presence is everywhere, and symbolically present in the home.

Islam Today the Islamic religion in India is second only to Hinduism in the number of followers. Followers of Islam account for 14.2 percent of the population.[11] Islam was brought to India by traders from Persia, and it expanded with the Muslim invasions of the northern regions beginning in about 700 CE. The Islamic Moghul Empire then dominated the country for nearly 800 years. The five pillars of Islam are the profession of faith (shahada), prayer (salat), alms (zakat), fasting (sawm), and pilgrimage (hajj). The influence of Islam is seen today mostly in northern India.

Buddhism Buddhism arose in northeastern India between the fourth and sixth centuries BCE. Intense religious activity and social change marked the era. In many instances, the ferment was due to those who wanted changes in Hinduism. Many new communities developed at the time Buddhism did, such as the Jains who stressed the need to free the soul from matter, and many shared the same vocabulary as Hinduism—nirvana (transcendent freedom), atman (self or soul), yoga (union), karma (causality), buddha (an enlightened one), samsara (eternal recurrence or becoming), and dharma (rule or law), and most involved the practice of yoga.[12] Buddhism is often described as a philosophy of life. It's growth was led by a charismatic, ascetic founder, known as Gautama Buddha who broke away from his Hindu family beliefs. The basic teachings of the Buddha are based on three universal truths: nothing is lost in the universe, everything changes, and the law of cause and effect. Followers study the cause of suffering and the path to its end. After about the second and third century CE, Buddhism expanded beyond the Indian subcontinent into Central Asia and China. After the Muslim invasions and the sacking of the Indian monasteries in the twelfth and thirteenth centuries CE, there was little interest in a resurgence in India, however. Today, Buddhism is followed by less than 1 percent of people in India. After 1950, however, there has been a resurgence of Buddhism caused, in part, by Tibetan refugees and by Scheduled Caste (Dalit) conversions.

Jainism This branch of Hinduism developed at about the same time Buddhism emerged. The Jains believe that all living beings have souls and practice non-violence which extends from speech, to thoughts, and everyday life. Some wear masks to prevent breathing in insects and sweep a path in front of them to prevent stepping on any creatures. Orthodox Jains are strict vegetarians. Approximately 5 million Indians are Jains; in the United States, there are approximately 80,000 Jains.[13] Many groups have established their own temples for worship.

Sikhism The Sikh religion was founded by Guru Nanak in the sixteenth century. Sikhs recognize that all humans are equal, including men and women, reject idolatry, and have no clergy system or ritual. They refer to the divine as Waheguru or the Wondrous Enlightener. Sikh beliefs include five articles of faith worn by male initiates on the body: kesh, uncut hair covered in a turban; kara, a steel bracelet symbolizing strength and integrity; kirpan, a ceremonial sword to emphasize martial strength; kanga, a small wooden comb to keep hair in place, symbolizing cleanliness and order; and kachhera, cotton shorts for chastity and readiness for battle. In the United States, many Sikhs continue these traditions, though some men forgo uncut hair to better fit into American society.[14] In the early twenty-first century, there were nearly 25 million Sikhs worldwide, the majority of them in the Indian state of Punjab.[15] About 500,000 Sikhs live in the United States.[16]

Christians It is estimated that Christians make up 2.4 percent of the Indian population.[17] One form of Christianity emerged from the influence of St. Thomas, who is said to have landed on the coast of Kerala in 52 CE and converted local Hindu and Jewish populations, and possibly from Nestorian missionaries in the sixth century CE, and again from the work of Christian missionaries during the Western colonial period, particularly after the 1800s. After the arrival of the Portuguese in 1498, old conflicts of Christendom began on the Indian subcontinent, and the Roman Catholic Church became dominant among Christians in the Kerala region for a time.[18] Syrian Christians do not observe Hindu dietary laws, but they do participate in the caste system. Many own lands and often operate their farms with labor from low-caste Hindu communities. Syrian Christians often have strong positions in the plantation industry, growing cardamom, tea, coffee, and rubber, and they are successful entrepreneurs, owning factories and small businesses; others hold professional jobs in teaching, science, and medicine.[18] Another Christian community developed at the former Portuguese colony of Goa, farther north along the southwest coast. Approximately half of the citizens are Catholic, known as Goan Christians, and the city is dedicated to St. Catherine.

Zoroastrianism More than 1,200 years ago the Parsis (or Parsees, meaning Persians) fled from religious persecution in Persia to northern India. The religion they brought, Zoroastrianism, named for the Iranian prophet Zoroaster (or Zarathustra), is an ancient faith that venerates Ahura Mazda, the wise god. The sacred fires of Zoroastrianism are tended in temples protected from the sun and from the eyes of unbelievers.[19] The Parsis have adapted many of their practices to blend into Indian society but have maintained their faith through the private schooling of their children.

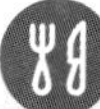

Food for Thought

The Taj Mahal, one of India's most widely recognized buildings, was built by the Mughal emperor Shah Jahan (1628–1658) to honor his wife Mumtaz Mahal who died in childbirth. It is admired for its harmonious proportions, the way its white marble reflects hues according to the intensity of the sun or moonlight, and the blend of Indian, Persian, and Islamic styles. The Taj Mahal was designated a UNESCO World Heritage site in 1983.[20]

In India, marriage is traditionally considered the beginning of a relationship from which love develops over time.

Judaism Four small Jewish communities were established in India when Jews fled persecution in Greece, Palestine (under Roman domination), Iraq, and Germany. The largest populations are found in Mumbai, Kolkata, and Kochi, where the oldest synagogue in India was built along India's Malabar Coast. After it was destroyed in the sixteenth century by the Portuguese, the newer Paradesi Synagogue was built in 1568 under the protection of the Raja of Kochi. The community became a prosperous trading community in Kerala and controlled a major portion of the world's spice trade for a time.

Animism The oldest religions in India are those practiced by the small tribal populations that live in isolated regions of the Himalayas. They worship spirits associated with natural phenomena, which, as a religious practice, is known as animism. In the past, they have practiced such varied social customs as polyandry (having more than one husband) and headhunting.

Family

Asian Indians The husband is the head of the household in the traditional Indian family. Traditionally, the wife does not work outside the home and is expected to perform all duties related to housekeeping and child care. She obtains help in these responsibilities from the extended family or, if affordable, from household paid help. If the wife does hold a job, she can depend on the help of relatives. Children are expected to show respect for their elders; parents may strongly prefer what career a child should pursue. Dating is uncommon in India, and many marriages are arranged by families based on similarities in caste, education, religion, and upbringing between prospective husbands and wives.

Traditionally, the ethic of joint family over that of the nuclear family as a unit of care is prevalent. Older people in the family are treated with respect, and younger people are encouraged to maintain family integrity, which is valued more highly than developing individual capacities. Young Asian Indians usually do not seek a radical shift between generations, in contrast to the West.[8] In the United States, most Indian Americans live in nuclear families, and strains in the traditional structure often occur. Asian Indian women are more likely to work in America than in their homeland, yet they lack the support system of an extended family. Older family members may also find themselves cut off from their traditional role of advisers and may not have opportunities for involvement in certain religious activities that would fill their lives in India. Some Asian Indians find it difficult to adjust to these changes. Children who grow up in the United States usually insist on making their own career choices. Dating has become more acceptable, but some parents strongly discourage relationships with persons of other ethnic or religious backgrounds.[7] Though fewer parents choose their child's spouse, many Asian Indian children still defer to their parents' opinions; young potential grooms in the United States sometimes ask their families in India to find suitable wives for them.

Older members of the family are well respected in Indian culture, and it is considered auspicious to have a senior at any social function. Older women are considered experts in family matters. Traditionally, the oldest sons are expected to care for their parents, who, in turn, often help out with caring for children in the family. Some Indian Americans continue the practice of having aging parents in the home, and others (with parents who still live in India) host their mothers or fathers for months at a time.

The family is seen as the way to preserve Indian values and beliefs while living in the United States. Many consider themselves bicultural—Indians at home but Americans at work.[21] Most Asian Indians have found successful adjustment in the United States through educational and economic achievement in American public life while maintaining an emphasis on Asian Indian culture within the privacy of their home life.

Pakistanis The traditional Pakistani home is strongly patriarchal. The husband is often the only wage earner in the family, and the wife is expected to stay inside the house to raise the children.[22,23] She will go outside the home to do essential chores such as shopping, but other activities usually require that she be accompanied by her husband. Faith is the centerpiece of family life for Muslims, and modesty for women is prized.

Women are not allowed to have contact with unrelated men after puberty, and inappropriate touching could disgrace the entire family and make a young girl unsuitable for marriage. In the United States, most households include the immediate members, though close relatives such as grandparents or aunts and uncles may live in the home for extended periods. Some women prefer a traditional role. They may remain at home throughout the day and may never acquire English language skills. Others straddle a middle ground, working during the day, interacting with non-Pakistanis, and returning at night to don traditional garb and perform customary religious and family chores.

Pakistani Americans vary in assimilation to western life. While many first-generation Pakistani American women continue holding traditional roles in the family, second-generation Pakistani American women may be more likely to launch professional careers. Like many South Asians, Pakistani Americans value education and careers in the sciences, medicine, and pharmacy are valued. Young women are encouraged to enter these careers. Dating is discouraged for girls and marriage is expected to be within their ethnicity and with parental approval. Increasingly, however, young Pakistani Americans make their own marriage decisions, and "love" marriages are more acceptable, though young women generally have less freedom to date or socialize than their male counterparts.[23]

Traditional Health Beliefs and Practices

Asian Indians Traditional medicine in India has a long and distinguished history. Several systems have developed over several thousand years, the most important of which is Ayurvedic medicine, which established the humoral concepts of the body that were later adopted in Greece and eventually evolved into biomedicine as it is practiced today.

Ayurvedic medicine, which is based on the idea of balance in bodily systems and uses diet, herbal treatments, and yogic techniques to achieve it, developed into its current form between 500 BCE and 500 CE. Ayurveda is based on Sanskrit texts and the writings of practitioners. Ayur means "longevity" and veda means "science or knowledge." Many times, this is translated as the science of life. Ayurvedic physicians, called vaidyas, are trained at government-supported schools that grant degrees based on an established curriculum. Their diagnosis focuses on who the person is that has the illness: their tastes, their work habits, their character, and their life history. Evaluation of the pulse, the face, the eyes, and the nails provides further data. A person's constitution, including temperament and preferences in food, is of great and effective use in diagnosis and treatment.

Food for Thought

Deepak Chopra, an Indian-born physician, popularized Ayurvedic medicine in the United States through his best-selling books and videos.

Ayurvedic therapy uses diet, herbal remedies, and meditation to reestablish equilibrium between the sick person and the universe, including the social, natural, and spiritual worlds. Diet is considered the most significant component.

Food for Thought

Meditation is a practice that encourages a heightened state of awareness by focusing attention. As practitioners gradually incorporate meditation teachings into everyday life, they may approach spiritual enlightenment. It is practiced by Hindus and Buddhists, and by some Christians and Muslims as well. Many meditation practices are associated with yoga.

Homeopathy is well-accepted throughout India and Pakistan.

Pakistani hakims sometimes use exotic preparations, such as those made from opium poppies, in their treatment programs.

Foods are classified as hot or cold depending on their effect on the body and must be balanced for each condition (refer to the "Therapeutic Uses of Food" section later in this chapter). Of nearly 10,000 plants used for medicinal purposes in India, 1200 to 1500 are officially in the Ayurvedic pharmacopeia. Because the mind, body, and soul are all considered to be interconnected parts of the whole system, meditation is used to address the imbalance in the spirit of a person.

Ayurvedic medicine has declined somewhat in popularity in India as Westernized medicine has become more established. It is frequently perceived as a paraprofessional practice, despite accreditation programs for Ayurvedic doctors. Folk beliefs about health and illness are found in some regions. In India, folk medicine is a humoral system that identifies four humors—yellow bile, black bile, phlegm, and blood—and four qualities—heat, cold, moisture, and dryness. Health is sustained through the balance of these humors and qualities. Illness is treated by complementary remedies; for example, disease due to too much cold is cured with a hot therapy. Diet is an important therapeutic tool, and advanced conditions are often treated first with a fast, or limitation of intake, to allow the digestive system to rest. There is limited research on the effects of Asian Indian fasting behavior on glycemic control. Intermittent fasting is a well-documented lifestyle modification that can provide benefits as a mode of type 2 diabetes and weight management.[24] Siddha medicine, another humoral system, developed within Tamil culture and is found mostly in southern India. Older practices, such as the use of shamans, bonesetters, and snakebite healers, are found in some rural regions.

Home remedies such as herbal infusions and poultices are prevalent in India, often derived from Ayurvedic prescriptions or other traditional practices, but administered by home diagnosis. Many are known to have pharmacological activity, and several are contraindicated in certain medical conditions or toxic in some preparations. Examples include aloe vera for obesity, liver problems, and both high and low blood sugar levels. Licorice root is used for indigestion and stomach aches, urinary tract problems, constipation, colds, and coughs. Black nightshade is considered helpful for heart disease and liver problems. Nannari sharbat is a traditional herbal beverage used to treat dehydration. Diabetes is treated with numerous cures, including pellitory, neem, gudmar, and puncture vine.[25] Recent surveys of more remote areas of the country have identified numerous previously unknown plants used by local inhabitants, many with demonstrated therapeutic properties.[26–28] Often medications available only through prescription in the United States can be purchased over the counter in India. Widespread use of antibiotics and mixing of therapeutics have been reported.

Pakistanis Little has been reported on the traditional health beliefs and practices of Pakistanis, though it has been noted that complementary care may be sought concurrently with biomedicine.[29–31] Pakistan has a very sophisticated use of herbal and biodiverse medicines due to the rich flora and diversity of plants grown in their climatic and topographical regions. Out of 6,000 flowering plant species, 2,000 are considered to have medicinal properties.[32,33] Therapeutic herbs or botanicals are used to maintain balance in the body and to cure a variety of ailments, such as common colds, coughs, cancer, leprosy, and reproductive disorders. Respondents who used such services reported that they believed hakims, physicians using traditional remedies in India and Muslim countries, were reliable and inexpensive; those who did not visit hakims questioned their effectiveness and safety. Ayurvedic medicine is also available. Prophetic healing, prayer, and home remedies such as honey are often used to treat minor conditions or to seek protection from malignant influences.[34,35]

Traditional Food Habits

Foods in India vary from north to south, east to west, and region to region, depending on the settlement story of the region, land and rainfall, religion, and caste group. Traditional grains include rice, wheat, millet, amaranth, buckwheat, and barley, and entire palates revolve around these. From the rice-based idli (savory rice cake) and dosas (thin rice-flour crepes) of the south, the variety of wheat bread and sauces of the northwest, to the fish and rice dishes in the northeast, plus much more, the cooking of India is intriguing, diverse, and wonderous. The cooking methods of Pakistan are considered similar to northern Indian fare, though with Persian and Afghani influences that include a greater emphasis on meat dishes and a preference for onions, ginger, and garlic.

Ingredients and Common Foods

Staples

India Few foods are eaten throughout all of India. Grains and legumes predominate in frequently vegetarian cooking, with added vegetables and fruits. Dairy items often supplement the diet. The types of ingredients and preparation methods vary by locality and, often, according to religious practices.

Rice is the grain most commonly consumed, and the average Indian eats half a pound of it each day. This amount, however, varies considerably by region; rice is most popular in the southern and eastern areas of the nation. Wherever it is consumed, long-grained rice is preferred for many dishes, though hundreds of varieties of rice give cooks a choice for pairing with seasonal foods as textures, aromas, and subtle flavors vary. Wheat, used primarily in bread, is another staple. Legumes are consumed daily by nearly all Asian Indians. Dal (or dhal) is the term for dried beans, peas, and lentils, which come hulled, skinned, whole, and split (in some literature the English word pulse is used instead). Dal is also the name for the dish made when they are boiled and seasoned. They are also commonly added to rice or soups, prepared as seasoned purees, or ground into flour to make distinctive bread (refer to Table 14.1).

Dairy foods are significant in most regions. Fermented milk products such as yogurt are found throughout most of the country, as is the cooking fat ghee, which is pure, clarified butter. Other common cooking fats used include coconut oil, sesame oil, soybean oil, and mustard oil. Seasonings are distinctive. Masalas are mixtures of spices and herbs that can be either fresh and "wet" or dried and powdered. Coriander, cumin, fenugreek, turmeric, black and cayenne pepper, cloves, cardamom, cinnamon, and chili peppers are often included in a blend, garam masala, that varies by family. A much-simplified version of this is often sold as "curry powder" in Western countries. These same spices, used in various ways (whole in hot oil, roasted, and dried) and added to foods at various times (when heating the cooking fat, at the end of cooking as a tempering method, and so forth), have a role in ancient Indian food preparations for medicinal purposes as well as for flavor. In addition to flavor, spice properties can be antibacterial, antispasmodic, antioxidant, and antiseptic, and they have been used to balance blood sugar and gastrointestinal distress for millennia.[36] Other typical spices and herbs include ajwain (carom or lovage seeds), amchoor (unripe mango powder), asafetida (a pungent powdered resin), coconut, fresh coriander, garlic, mint, saffron, tamarind (the sour pulp of a bean pod), fenugreek, and more. Beyond these generalities, the staples of the Indian diet are best classified by region.

The greatest division in diet is seen between northern and southern India. Northern cuisine is characterized by the use of wheat, tea, a large number of eggs, garlic, dried or pickled fruits and vegetables, and use of dry masalas that are fragrant rather than piquant. These foods are typical of a cooler climate, where wheat grows better than rice and where fruits, vegetables, herbs, and spices are available only seasonally. Boiling, stewing, and frying are the most common forms of cooking. In the south, steaming is the preferred method of food preparation. Rice, coffee, fresh and fermented pickles, chutney, pachadi (which can be a yogurt or other "pounded" side dish), "wet," spicy-hot masalas, fresh fruits, vegetables, herbs, and spices are fundamental to the cuisine. Again, these foods reflect the regional agricultural conditions and approaches to traditional health where food is considered medicine.

Many Asian Indians are vegetarians, and most use some milk products but avoid eggs (refer to Exploring Global Cuisine: Vegetarianism in India). Pork is eaten in some communities in the west, especially where the Portuguese introduced Christianity, lamb, goat, and beef are eaten in many areas of the north, and fish and poultry are eaten in several coastal regions. The cultural food groups list is found in Table 14.2.

Table 14.1 Selected South Asian Dals

English	Hindi	Common Preparations
Black lentils (black gram)	*Urad dal*	Black skins with creamy insides—boiled, added to rice or vegetables, seasoned with mustard oil (Bengal); often ground for flatbreads (e.g., pappadams) or fermented and combined with rice flour to make flatbreads (e.g., idli, dosas).
Black-eyed peas	*Lobia*	Boiled, seasoned with onions, ginger, garlic (in the north), ginger, asafetida, mustard oil (in the west), or coconut (in the south).
Chickpeas (Bengal gram)	*Channa dal*	Most commonly used dal in India—boiled, added to curries, chutneys, rice (pulao); pureed (sambar); roasted whole for snacks; ground into flour (besan) and added to curries, used for deep-fried fritters; made into thick, sweet puddings for dessert.
Green peas	*Mutter dal*	Boiled, added to curries, rice (pulao) or pureed.
Hyacinth beans	*Valor*	Boiled, often seasoned with coconut, ginger, and jaggery; sprouted in soups, salads.
Lima beans	*Pavta*	Boiled, mixed with vegetables (especially potatoes, eggplant), added to curries; made into fritters or patties.
Madras beans (horse gram)	*Kulith*	Assertive earthy flavor—boiled, added to curries; powdered for soup.
Mung beans (green gram)	*Moong dal*	Brownish green—boiled with spices, added to rice (khichri), made into dumplings; sprouted for salads.
Red lentils	*Masur dal*	Salmon colored—boiled, often mashed and added to meat for kebabs or curries (most common in the north).
Yellow lentils (yellow split peas)	*Toor (Arhar) dal*	Pale yellow—boiled, often pureed with seasonings, or added to rice (khichri); mashed with other dals or rice to make pancakes (adai).

Table 14.2 Cultural Food Groups: South Asian

Group	Comments	Common Foods	Adaptations in the United States
Protein Foods			
Milk/milk products	In general, milk is considered a beverage for children in India; consumed by some adults in Pakistan. Fermented dairy products are popular.	Fresh cow's, buffalo's, ass's milk; evaporated milk; cream used in Pakistan; fermented milk products (yogurt, *lassi*); fresh curds very popular; fresh cheese (paneer); milk-based desserts, such as kheer, khir, *kulfi*, *barfi*, and Pakistani puddings.	Much cheese is consumed by Asian Indians; ice cream is popular with Asian Indians and Pakistanis.
Meat/poultry/ fish/eggs/ legumes	A sophisticated vegetarian cuisine exists in India; legumes are a primary protein source; meat and poultry are very popular in Pakistan. Hulled, split legumes, grains, and seeds, such as lentils, are known as dals. Legumes are typically prepared whole or pureed, or used as flour to prepare baked, steamed, or fried breads and pastries. Beef avoided by Hindus; pork prohibited for Muslims.	*Meats:* beef, goat, mutton, pork *Poultry:* chicken, duck *Fish and seafood:* Bombay duck, carp, clams, crab, herring, lobster, mackerel, mullet, pomfret, sardines, shrimp, sole, turtle *Eggs:* chicken *Legumes:* beans (kidney, mung, etc.), chickpeas, lentils (many varieties and colors), peas (black-eyed, green)	Consumption of legumes decreases; meat intake increases. Meat may be added to traditional Indian vegetarian dishes. Fast foods are popular.
Cereals/Grains	More than 1,000 varieties of Indian rice are cultivated. Basmati is preferred in Pakistan. Wheat used mostly in northern India and Pakistan; rice in southern India. Most breads (*roti*) are unleavened.	Rice (steamed, boiled, fried, puffed), wheat, buckwheat, corn, millet, sorghum	Use of American-style breads occurs in place of ***roti***; breakfast cereals are popular
Fruits/Vegetables	More than 100 types of fruit and 200 types of vegetables are commonly used in India. Fruits and vegetables may be used in fresh or preserved pickles, called *rayta* (northern India/Pakistan), *pachadi* (southern), or chutney. Fruits often costly in Pakistan.	*Fruit:* apples, apricots, avocados, bananas (several types), coconut, dates, figs, grapes, guava, jackfruit, limes, litchis, loquats, mangoes, melon, nongus, oranges, papaya, peaches, pears, persimmons (*chicos*), pineapple, plums, pomegranate, pomelos, raisins, starfruit, strawberries, sugarcane, tangerines, watermelon *Vegetables:* agathi flowers, amaranth, artichokes, bamboo shoots, banana flower, beets (leaves and root), bitter melon, Brussels sprouts, cabbage, carrots, cauliflower, collard greens (*haak*), corn, cucumbers, drumstick plant, eggplant, lettuce, lotus root, manioc (tapioca), mushrooms, mustard greens, okra, onions, pandanus, parsnips, plantain flowers, potatoes, pumpkin, radishes (four types, leaves and roots), rhubarb, sago palm, scallions, spinach, squash, sweet potatoes (leaves and roots), tomatoes, turnips, yams, water chestnuts, water convolvulus, water lilies	Decreased variety of fruits and vegetables is available; decreased vegetable intake results for Asian Indians. More fruit juice is consumed by Asian Indians. Salad is well accepted by Asian Indians. Use of canned and frozen produce increases.

(Continued)

Table 14.2 Cultural Food Groups: South Asian (*Continued*)

Group	Comments	Common Foods	Adaptations in the United States
Additional Foods			
Seasonings	Aromatic (northern) and hot (southern) combinations of fresh or dried spices and herbs accentuate or complement food flavors. Pakistani fare similar to northern Indian but with ample use of ginger, garlic, and onions.	*Ajwain, amchoor*, asafetida, bay leaf, cardamom (two types), chiles, cinnamon, cloves, coconut, fresh coriander, coriander seeds, cumin, dill, fennel, fenugreek, garlic, kewra, lemon, limes, mace, mint, mustard, nutmeg, pepper (black and red), poppy seeds, rose water, saffron, tamarind, turmeric	Spice use depends on availability.
Nuts/seeds	Nuts and seeds of all types are popular; used to thicken korma sauces in India and garnish desserts in Pakistan.	Almonds, betel nuts and leaves, cashews, peanuts, pistachios, sunflower seeds, walnuts	*Paan* tray may be limited to betel nuts and spices.
Beverages	Tea is common in northern India/Pakistan, coffee in southern India. Coffeehouses are favored meeting places.	Coffee, tea, water flavored with fruit syrups, sugarcane, spices, or herbs; alcoholic beverages such as fermented fruit syrups, rice wines, beer	Increased consumption of soft drinks and coffee is noted for Asian Indians. Alcoholic beverages are widely accepted by Asian Indians (women may abstain); consumed by very few Pakistanis.
Fats/oils		Coconut oil, ghee (clarified butter), mustard oil, peanut oil, sesame seed oil, sunflower oil	Purchased ghee is often made from vegetable oil instead of butter.
Sweeteners		Sugarcane, *jaggery* (unrefined palm sugar), molasses	Candy and sweets are enjoyed by Asian Indians but not overconsumed; cookies may replace flatbreads as snacks for Pakistanis.

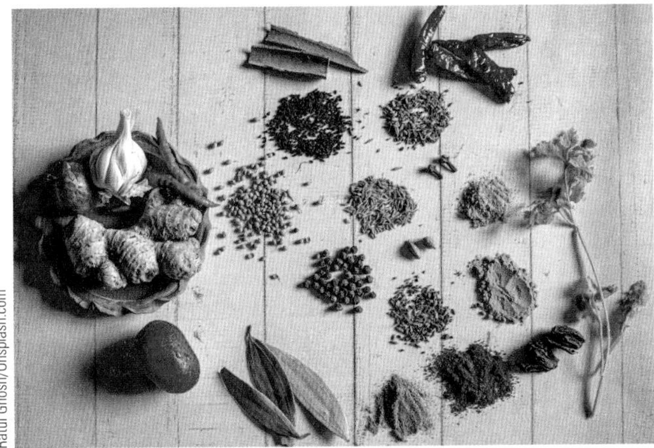

Ratul Ghosh/Unsplash.com

▲ **Traditional foods of India are often flavored with the expert use of herbs and spices such as black pepper, cardamom, cloves, fresh coriander (cilantro), cinnamon, coriander seeds, cumin, chilies, garlic, ginger root, mint, bay, mustard seeds, nutmeg, and turmeric, among other varieties.**

Pakistan Pakistani fare is distinctive for its ample use of garlic, ginger, and onions in many savory and even some sweet dishes. Wheat is the staple of Pakistan, and flatbreads, similar to those in northern India, accompany every meal. Dalia, the Pakistani version of Middle Eastern bulgur, is cooked with water or milk to make porridge. Other commonly consumed grains include rice, usually the floral and nutty-flavored basmati rice cooked as pulao (and similar to Turkish pilau) and khichri (mildly spiced mixture of rice and lentils). Corn is popular in some areas, typically ground into meal and made into bread flavored with mustard greens and served with butter. Barley, sorghum, and millet are available but consumed less frequently. Legumes, especially chickpeas and lentils, are served daily, usually as one of several side dishes. One favorite is chole, chickpeas or whole dried peas cooked with ginger, garlic, onions, tomatoes, chili peppers, cumin, and turmeric. Besan (chickpea flour) is used for breads and batters for fried foods.

Dairy foods from cows and water buffaloes are another staple in the diet. Whole-milk yogurt (dahi) is used to prepare raitas (yogurt and vegetable side dishes) that are often eaten with every meal. Lassi (the diluted yogurt beverage found in India), paneer (Indian-style pot cheese much like ricotta from Italy), fresh milk, cream, and ice cream are other common dairy foods, consumed regularly or added to other dishes.

Lamb, mutton, goat, beef, and chicken are Pakistani favorites. Pork is rarely eaten due to the Muslim majority, and nearly all meats are processed according to Islamic halal guidelines (refer to Chapter 4). Meat or poultry is served at lunch and dinner if affordable. Beef stew, called nihari,

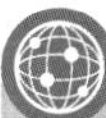

Exploring Global Cuisine

Vegetarianism in India

The ancient Indian diet featured a variety of meats, such as beef, buffalo, horses, sheep, goats, and pork, in addition to wild game including deer, alligator, and tortoise. The vegetarian ethic entered India slowly, probably beginning with the Aryans. Later, prohibitions were extended to the milk cow and the draft bull, as well as the village pig (a useful scavenger) and the village cock. Over time, a more general concern for animal life developed, and the principals of ahimsa (respect for all living things and avoidance of violence present in the Hindu, Buddhist, and Jainism tradition) developed. The Vedas, the oldest and sacred texts of Hinduism, say that all creatures manifest the same life force and merit equal compassion; by 1500 to 500 BCE vegetarianism was encouraged. Indian culture, however, is highly diverse with correspondingly diverse food habits, and any generalization is risky. It is suggested, however, that only in India, with its enormous variety of available fruits, vegetables, and grains, could such a broad acceptance of a vegetarian diet prevail.[37]

There has been a surge in vegetarianism in the last 10 years worldwide, partly due to concerns for the environment, health concerns, and animal rights. The U.S. sales of plant-based foods have increased 31% from 2017 to 2020.[38] Yet the definition of vegetarianism in India is elusive. It is usually considered a symbol of piety in the Brahmin castes and may be a necessity among low-income families. Abstinence from meat and poultry is most common; however, nearly all Indian vegetarians consume milk products, and some eat eggs. Except in the state of Gujarat (where the influence of Jainism has been especially strong), a large percentage of people living in coastal regions eat fish, sometimes justifying it as the fruit of the sea. Other Indians practice vegetarianism only on days of religious observance or as they age and become more devout. Overall, it is believed that about 30 percent of Indians are strict vegetarians, abstaining from all meat, poultry, fish, and eggs but consuming milk, yogurt, and other dairy products.

is an example of pot roasting (dum), a popular preparation technique. Braising (korma or qorma) is also common, as is the Indian charcoal tandoori style of cooking. Bhuna is a method of slowly frying wet seasonings (such as onions, ginger, and garlic), then adding dry spices to make a thick paste, then vegetables, and finally bits of meat to make a curried dish. Biryani rice is another specialty, a highly seasoned pilau (including saffron) with added meat. Yogurt or amchoor is used to marinate both meats and poultry. Minced and ground meat dishes are especially popular, and meats are sometimes extended with ground legumes. Kabobs can be grilled or pan-fried patties; kofta are fried meatballs (sometimes dipped in besan batter first) served with a curry sauce. Ghee is the preferred cooking fat, although some Pakistanis must use less costly vegetable oils.

Food for Thought

The word *curry* is believed to be the English adaptation of a southern Indian term for "sauce," kari. Curry powder is not a single spice but a complex blend of seasonings that vary according to the cook and the dish.

The word curry is rarely used in India. Each dish, made uniquely, has its own name. Reducing the entire subcontinent's cuisine to one word is seen as an erasure of the diversity of Indian food traditions.[39]

In India, each family may have their own recipe for garam masala, a mix of ground fresh spices sprinkled over a dish for an enhancing burst of flavor.

In 2018, the Supreme Court in New Delhi, ruled it cannot direct the entire country to be vegetarian and did not hear a petition to ban all meat exports.[40]

Both tropical and temperate vegetables and fruits are available, though not consumed in large amounts. Apples, apricots, cabbage, carrots, cauliflower, cucumbers, dates, grapes, guavas, mangos, onions, oranges, papayas, peas, plums, pomegranates, potatoes, pumpkin, spinach, tamarind, and watermelon are common. Vegetables are typically added to raitas, chutneys, curried dishes, and stews. Desserts are popular, especially ice cream and puddings made from rice, besan (chickpea flour), carrots, bread, or vermicelli noodles. Cardamom, cloves, ginger, poppy seeds, aniseed, saffron, almonds, or pistachios flavor many sweets. One unique pudding dating from the Moghul period includes both ginger and garlic. Fried fritters are consumed, as are ladoos, balls made from sweetened besan and garnished with nuts. A dairy dessert specialty is ras malai, common to West Bengal in India, Bangladesh, and Pakistan, which may be best described as a rich cheese-based creamy treat. Special-occasion desserts may be garnished with silver leaf. Tea is consumed throughout the day. It is usually heavily sweetened and boiled with milk, and at times flavored with cinnamon or cardamom. Other popular beverages include lassi, sharbat (fruit juice), and sugarcane juice. Carbonated drinks are less common, and alcohol is prohibited for Muslims.

Regional Variations

Northern India The influences of the Moghul period are still found in the cooking of northern India, where Muslim influence was most prominent. The royal court fare of that time featured lavish meat and rice dishes flavored with expensive aromatic seasonings, nuts, dried fruits such as raisins, and yogurt or cream. Ample use of ghee and sugar was also characteristic. Many similarities between the foods of this region, Pakistan and modern-day Iran, are still evident due to this shared history.

Basmati rice is commonly served as a pilaf in northern India, and biriyani with seasoned chicken, lamb, or beef is popular. Meatballs (kofta) made with ground meats or with meat and dal mixtures are a specialty, as are skewered pieces of broiled or grilled meats (kabobs). Northern specialties include korma—a curried lamb dish with a nut and yogurt-thickened sauce—and masala chicken. Peanut and sesame oils are used in many preparations. The dishes of the north, particularly in Kashmir (which borders Pakistan and has a significant Muslim population), are often seasoned with saffron.[41]

Many varieties of bread—that are fried, baked, stuffed, fermented, delicate, thin, fat, laminated, unleavened, leavened, plain, or seasoned—are eaten daily throughout the country. Examples include whole-wheat flatbreads, such as chapatis, which are cooked on a griddle without oil until they puff up, and deep-fried puris. Paratha, a griddle-fried roti, is used as a wrapping for spiced vegetable fillings. A rich, leavened bread of the region, called sheermal, is flavored with saffron. The grains used for bread include wheat, rice, pearl millet, sorghum, finger millet, mung bean, and chickpea flour. Fresh cheese similar to ricotta sometimes made from buffalo milk, called paneer, is added to many dishes, or it is skewered and grilled in some recipes. Milk desserts are favored, such as carrot pudding (gajar halwa) and rice pudding with cardamom (kheer).

In northern and northwestern India a special cylindrical clay oven heated with charcoal and called a tandoor is used. Tandoori cooking is identified particularly with lamb and chicken dishes (the meat is often marinated in a spicy yogurt sauce before cooking), although the leavened bread known as naan is also typically baked in a tandoor. This method of cooking is associated with the state of Punjab, and though few homes have tandoor ovens, it has been popularized throughout the nation (and with many visitors) by specialty restaurants.

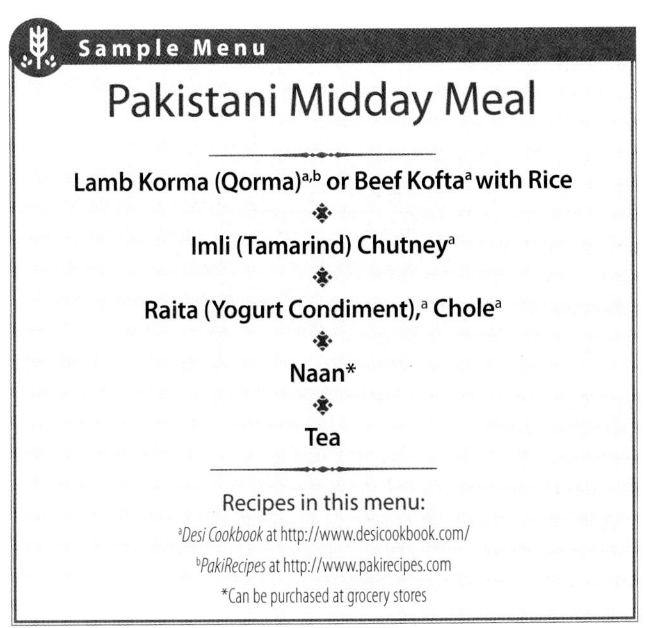

Sample Menu

Pakistani Midday Meal

Lamb Korma (Qorma)[a,b] or Beef Kofta[a] with Rice

Imli (Tamarind) Chutney[a]

Raita (Yogurt Condiment),[a] Chole[a]

Naan*

Tea

Recipes in this menu:

[a]*Desi Cookbook* at http://www.desicookbook.com/

[b]*PakiRecipes* at http://www.pakirecipes.com

*Can be purchased at grocery stores

Food for Thought

Green tea is often made in a samovar in the Indian state of Kashmir, a method that may have been introduced to the region from Russia via central Asia.

Samosas—triangular, deep-fried turnovers with spicy potato, vegetable, cheese, or meat stuffings and served with chutney—are thought to be variations of Middle Eastern sanbusak.

A comfort food in many parts of India is khichri, a combination of vegetables sautéed with rice and dal in an ample amount of ghee. In some regions of India, khichri is usually served with kadhi, a sauce made with yogurt and besan.

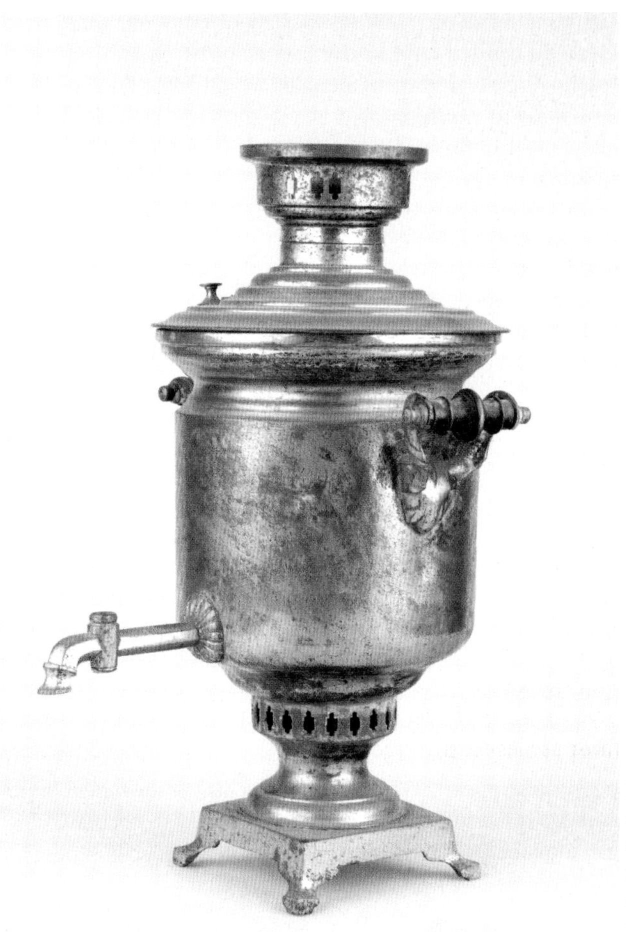

Algimantas Barzdzius/Shutterstock.com

▲ **Traditional Indian samovar for making tea.**

The northwestern region is characterized by a large percentage of Hindus and Jains and high numbers of vegetarians. In the state of Punjab, where the national capital Delhi is situated, many cooler-weather vegetables associated more with temperate climates than tropical ones, such as cabbage, carrots, cauliflower, potatoes, tomatoes, and turnips, are used. Onions and garlic are common seasonings. Dairy products, including milk and buttermilk in addition to yogurt and paneer, are consumed more often in this area than in any other Indian region.[42] In the state of Rajasthan, barley, millet, and, later, corn were the primary grains grown in the region and are featured in many breads. Today, wheat is becoming much more prominent. Aromatic spices such as cumin and cardamom are found in many dishes, and red chilies add zing. A little farther south is the state of Gujarat, which specializes in vegetarian dishes flavored with green chilies and ginger.[42] Sweet-and-sour dishes are also featured, usually achieved by pairing sugar with a sour fruit indigenous to the region called kokum (related to mangosteen and tamarind). The combination is found in savory dishes as well as in desserts, and especially in the drink kokum sharbat.

Coastal India The coastal region offers several seafood specialties and fish prepared in a variety of ways, including fried, steamed, boiled, and stuffed with herbs. For example, in the northeastern state of Bengal (which includes the city of Kolkata—formerly known as Calcutta), prawns are a specialty even in the more inland areas. Freshwater fish, mostly those from numerous rivers and estuaries, are consumed by most Bengalis every day. A favorite cooking method along the coast is bhapa, packets of fish (or vegetables) wrapped in banana leaves, steamed, and seasoned with mustard seed and spices, such as cumin, asafetida, and nigella (a small black seed with subtle bitterness called kalonji in Hindi). A dessert version steams sweetened yogurt. The inland dishes of Bengal are noteworthy for their use of poppy seeds. Mumbai (formerly known as Bombay), located on the west coast in the state of Maharashtra, boasts a dried, salted fish—which is thin, bony, and has a strong aroma when dried—known as Bombay duck, also common to the Bay of Bengal and Kolkata. Other coastal foods eaten by the people of Maharashtra include numerous fish dishes as well as shrimp, crab, and lobster. In inland areas, Marathi people are known for adding peanuts to their dishes, and for bhakris, a crispy, traditional flatbread made from rice flour (sorghum flour is used in some rural areas) and cooked on an ungreased griddle. The tiny state of Goa, which is south of Mumbai, is home to many Christians. Fish is eaten daily, but pork is also popular. The most famous dish of the region is vindaloo, a hot-and-sour pork dish seasoned with coconut, vinegar, tomatoes, and ample chili peppers. The dish, combining the Portuguese *carne vinha d'alhos* (meat marinated in wine vinegar and garlic) with Indian ingredients, developed after the arrival of Portuguese traders along the Malabar Coast in 1498.

Southern India The menus of the south feature numerous steamed and fried rice dishes. Coarse red rice with a smoky flavor called rosematta is favored in some parts of southeastern India, including the state of Tamil Nadu, and may be mixed with other grains.[43] Crispy puffed rice with tamarind chutney is a snack called bhelpuri. Other grains, such as semolina wheat, are also popular cooked as a cereal known as uppama, which may include vegetables. Dals, particularly chickpeas and lentils, accompany nearly every meal in the form of a spiced lentil-based stew known as sambar or as a thin, crisply fried roti called pappadams. Fermented black lentil flour mixed with rice flour is used at breakfast for steamed cakes called idli and for fried rice-flour crepes called dosas, often served with spicy potatoes. A mixture of different dals (and sometimes rice) is cooked, seasoned with chili peppers, and mashed into a thick, unfermented puree that is fried for the savory pancakes known as adai, traditionally served with jaggery or coconut chutney. Fresh milk curds are also served for breakfast.

Spiced vegetable dishes, such as aviyal, include such southern ingredients as bananas, banana flowers, bittermelons, coconut, drumstick plant, green mango, and jackfruit seeds, in addition to potatoes, cauliflower, and eggplant. Pandanus leaves (fragrant screw pine) add antioxidants and are used to season some dishes. Coconut milk is often used in curries and sauces, and coconut oil is commonly used for frying.[43] Refreshing yogurt-based pachadi and spicy, pickled fruits or vegetables or chutney, accompany the main course. In the state of Kerala (in the southwest), fewer people are vegetarians than in some other regions of the nation, fish or seafood is eaten often, as is chicken. Black pepper is a favorite seasoning, often combined with coconut, green chilies, and curry leaves (a herb reminiscent of lemongrass), anise, and asafetida combined. A large Muslim population prepares traditional biryanis and cooks lamb with garlic, anise, and ground chili peppers. In the large state of Andhra Pradesh, dishes are typically seasoned with tamarind (which is also used for beverages), gongura (the leaves of roselle, a type of hibiscus also used in African cooking), and red chili peppers. Andhran fare is reputedly the hottest in all of India. Throughout the South, deep-fried salty foods and sweets are favored snacks, such as the syrup-soaked, orange-colored pretzels called jalebis.

Pakistan Pakistani fare consists of many regional variations. In Punjab, the royal cooking style of the Moghul period still influences a preference for elaborate, rich dishes. Tandoori fare is popular, and the karahi—a deep, cast-iron pot shaped something like a wok—is used to deep-fry foods. Fish is a common food in Sindh, which has a lengthy coastline, and is prepared as fritters, kabobs, steamed, or in sauces. Spit-roasted meats are a specialty in Baluchistan. Called sajji, the whole lamb or chicken is skewered on a small pole, then the

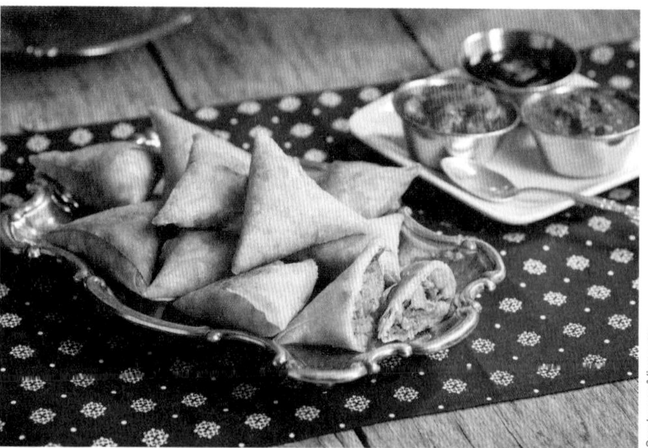
iStock.com/Viennetta

▲ **Samosas, spicy deep-fried turnovers.**

poles are inserted into the dirt around a large fire. The poles are rotated by hand as the meat cooks, assuring even roasting. The North-West Frontier Province, which is populated by distinct communities, has a simple cuisine that emphasizes rice, dal, and lamb. More locally, in the valley of Hunza, a distinctive fare developed due, in part, to the limitations of its high altitude. Wheat predominates, traditionally baked as a flatbread in hot ashes. Maltash, a strongly flavored aged butter, is prized, and kurutz, a salty dry cheese, flavors soups. Wild thyme and turmeric are common seasonings. Apricots and apricot kernels are eaten as snacks, while oil extracted from the kernels is used in cooking.[44]

Food for Thought

A French colony on the east coast of India at Puducherry (formerly, Pondicherry) introduced baguettes, croissants, pâté, and French-style desserts into the regional fare.

The English words pepper, sugar, and orange are all derived from Asian Indian terms for those foods.

Balti cooking, from the Kashmir region (claimed by both Pakistan and India), uses a wok-like karahi pan to stir-fry aromatic dishes seasoned with fresh coriander, mint, and fenugreek served with flatbreads instead of rice.

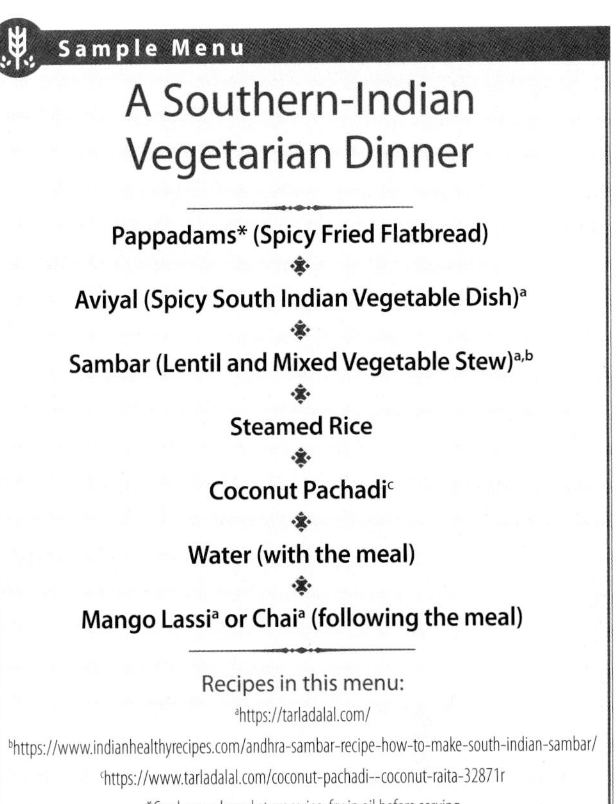

Sample Menu

A Southern-Indian Vegetarian Dinner

Pappadams* (Spicy Fried Flatbread)

Aviyal (Spicy South Indian Vegetable Dish)[a]

Sambar (Lentil and Mixed Vegetable Stew)[a,b]

Steamed Rice

Coconut Pachadi[c]

Water (with the meal)

Mango Lassi[a] or Chai[a] (following the meal)

Recipes in this menu:

[a]https://tarladalal.com/

[b]https://www.indianhealthyrecipes.com/andhra-sambar-recipe-how-to-make-south-indian-sambar/

[c]https://www.tarladalal.com/coconut-pachadi--coconut-raita-32871r

*Can be purchased at groceries; fry in oil before serving

Religious Variations In addition to region, religious affiliation may greatly influence food habits, especially in India. Religious groups have varying dietary practices, yet their cooking is Indian in flavor.

The relationship between food and spirituality is very complex in Hinduism. Eating is an integral part of each person's spiritual journey and defines one's role within society (refer to the sections "Special Occasions" and "Role of Food in Indian Society and Etiquette"). For example, each caste traditionally was associated with different food habits. Brahmans were generally vegetarians. Kshatriyas consumed meat, and vaishyas consumed meat depending on their locale and whether it was available—farmers often had more access than merchants. Sudras ate meat, but typically only when it was provided for them as leftovers, or was affordable.

Food for Thought

The chai you find in coffeehouses today has a history dating back thousands of years. Tea was first chewed or drank as a soup by the forest inhabitants of the eastern Himalayas. Later, perhaps 5,000 to 9,000 years ago, masala chai (spiced tea) may have begun in an ancient royal court as a healing Ayurvedic beverage made of milk and aromatic spices. Black tea became part of the beverage more recently.[45]

Muslims avoid all pork and pork products but are not vegetarians. Orthodox Jains may eat only foods that avoid injury to any life and are therefore strict vegetarians. In addition, there are 22 prohibited foods (e.g., fruit with small seeds or tender new greens) and 32 other items that may have the potential for life to exist, including root vegetables, because insects might be killed when the tubers are harvested, and honey, because bees might be killed when it is gathered from the hive. They also refuse to eat any foods made with eggs and many avoid blood-colored foods such as tomatoes and watermelon. Water must be boiled (and re-boiled after six hours)—if boiled water is unavailable, distilled water may be permitted.[37,42] Sikh cuisine is noted for its use of wheat, corn, and sugar and complete abstinence from alcohol and beef (pork is permitted). Sikhs are also prohibited from consuming halal meat. Some Sikhs are vegetarians and may avoid eggs. Many Sikh dishes are prepared in pure ghee, which gives them a richness not found in some other religious fare. The Syrian Christians are renowned for their beef (tenderized by mincing or marinating), duck, and wild boar dishes. Goan Christians are unique in Indian cooking for their use of pork. They make Western-style sausages and have such specialties as a vinegar-basted hog's head stuffed with vegetables and herbs. Most Jews in India keep kosher. The Parsis blend Indian and Persian elements in their cuisine, exemplified by dishes such as dhansak, an entrée combining lamb, tripe, lentils, and vegetables. Eggs, such as ekuri—spicy scrambled eggs—are especially popular.

Due to a large Muslim majority, dietary variations due to religious practice are limited in Pakistan. The small number of Hindu, Christian, Sikh, and Zoroastrian Pakistanis are assumed to adapt their food habits in ways appropriate to their faith (refer to Chapter 4).

Meal Composition and Cycle

Daily Patterns

Asian Indians Though not consistent across regions and classes, meal patterns in India vary less than the foods served. Two full meals with substantial snacks are typical. Early risers enjoy a rich coffee or tea boiled with milk and sugar.

Breakfast, usually eaten between 9:00 and 11:00 a.m., consists of rice or roti (usually whole-wheat flatbread), a pickled fruit or vegetable, and a sambar or other dal dish, which may be left over from the previous evening. At 4:00 or 5:00 p.m., similar foods or snack items are eaten with coffee or tea. The main meal of the day follows between 7:00 and 9:00 p.m.[46] Texture, color, and balance of seasoning are all important factors in an Indian meal. A menu customarily includes at least one rice dish; a seasoned vegetable, legume, or meat dish; a vegetable legume side dish; a baked or fried roti; a fruit or vegetable pickle; and a yogurt raita or pachadi. Sometimes a dessert is served, usually fruit.

Water is the most common drink consumed with meals, though milk and buttermilk are also prevalent. Sugarcane juice, fruit juice, and sodas are popular in urban areas. Alcoholic beverages are not widely consumed, though rice beer, home-brewed rum made from molasses, toddy (a brandy-like drink made from palm sap), and melon wine are a few traditional beverages still popular in some rural regions. Many Westernized Asian Indians, particularly men, drink beer or Scotch whisky.

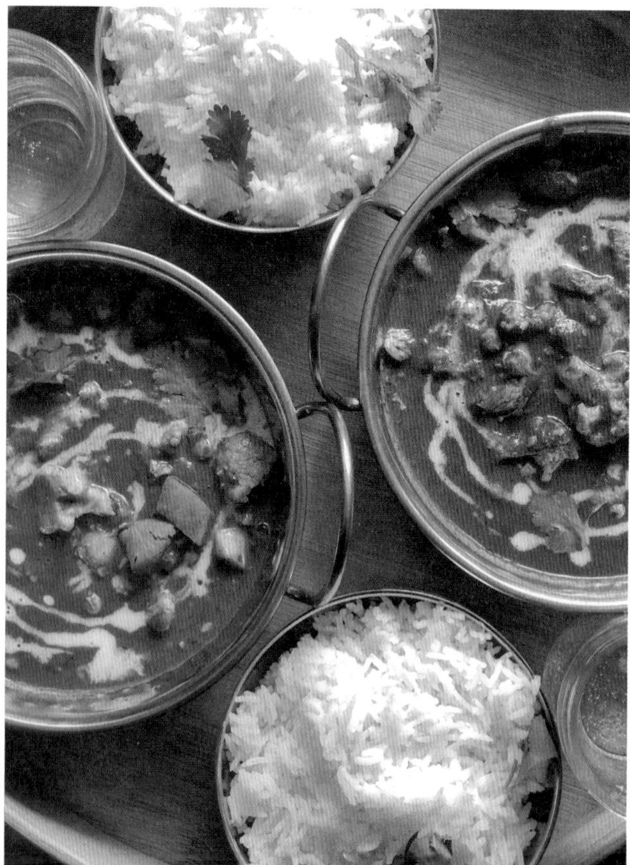

Andy Hay/Unsplash.com

▲ Traditional lunch with basmati, a long-grain aromatic variety of rice.

Courses are not presented sequentially in an Indian meal. Often, they are placed on the table all at once, although diners are expected to understand the order foods should be eaten in. Typically, rice and dal are eaten first, then vegetable dishes, then the heavier protein, with cooling raita to complete the meal. Chutneys or pickles are often eaten between these courses to clear the palate. Traditionally, an individual serving of rice or bread is served surrounded by a selection of other foods, such as vegetables, dals, fish, raita or pachadi, and pickled fruits or vegetables. Diners may combine tastes and textures according to personal preference. Although not all diners partake, traditionally, the meal concludes with passing the paan tray. Paan is a combination of betel (areca) nuts and spices, such as anise seed, cardamom, and fennel, wrapped in large, heart-shaped betel leaves secured with a clove. It is chewed to freshen the breath and aid digestion.

Snacking is very popular in India. In cities and small towns, snacks are sold in numerous small shops and by street vendors. In villages, they are prepared at home. A clear distinction is made between meals and snacks. Many Indian languages have specific words to define each form of eating. In southern India, and elsewhere throughout the subcontinent, the word tiffin is used to distinguish a snack from a meal. A meal is not a meal unless the traditional staple prepared in the traditional manner, such as boiled rice in southern India (or roti in northern India), is served. This means that no matter how substantial the snack—and some include more food than a meal—it is still called tiffin.

Spicy snacks served with chutney often consist of batter-fried vegetables, pancakes with or without a filling, or fried seasoned dough made from wheat or lentils. Savory salad-like mixtures of diced fruit and vegetables (sometimes with added meat or shrimp) and flavored with amchoor or tamarind, called chaat, are popular. Snacks sweetened with sugarcane, molasses, or jaggery are usually milk-based, as are the saffron-spiced kheer (also called payasam), the Indian ice cream called kulfi, and the candy barfi, although nuts, coconut, sesame seeds, or lentils are also used. Bengalis are noted for their sweetshops, which prepare numerous specialties, such as sandesh chomchom, rasogolla, pantua (delicate sweets based on chhana, a ricotta-like simple cheese), and patishapta (rice-flour crepes filled with coconut and jaggery).[47] A snack may also include a cooling beverage, such as the sweetened, yogurt drink called lassi or the sweet-sour lime drink, nimbu pani, sometimes sprinkled with spices. This drink, considered the world's first lemonade, was quickly popular once citrus fruits were exported out of Asia into Europe.

Restaurants are becoming increasingly popular in India serving Indian regional cuisines, and Western fast-food franchises are found in many cities. Chinese and Thai establishments are also common, particularly in urban areas.

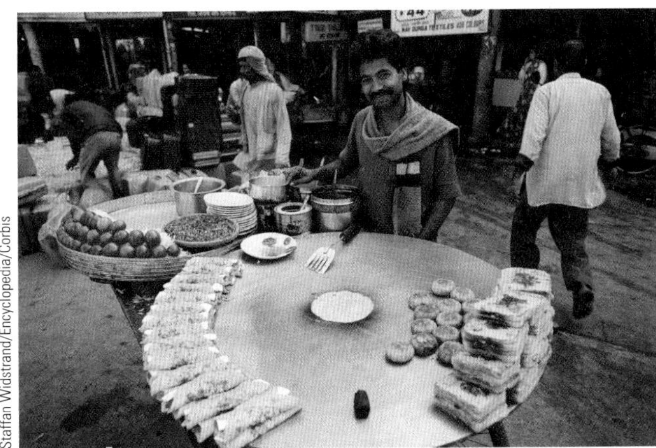

Staffan Widstrand/Encyclopedia/Corbis

▲ Fast food street vendor sells his food in Karachi, Pakistan.

Pakistanis Breakfast, if consumed, is a light meal in Pakistan, consisting of fried flatbreads such as puris, a sweetened porridge, or a legume dish. Traditionally, however, only two meals a day are eaten. Lunch and dinner are large meals and, if affordable, include a meat, poultry, or fish dish, as well as side dishes such as chole (chickpeas with onion, ginger, and tomato), raitas, and other fresh vegetable or fruit salad-like mixtures, chutneys, and pickles selected for a balance of flavors and textures. Flatbreads and tea are served with the meal.

Dessert often follows, and paan may be chewed afterward. Khat, a plant with mild amphetamine-like properties, is often added to the betel-leaf roll (refer to Chapter 8). Snacking is common and hearty, including fried items such as meat, poultry, or fish fritters and patties, stuffed pastries and flatbreads, kabobs, sandwiches, spicy salad-like mixtures, roast beef or chicken, and, in urban areas, Western fast food.

Food for Thought

Traditionally, six tastes (sweet, sour, salty, bitter, pungent, and astringent) were balanced in an Indian diet. These were ideally eaten specifically to each individual's needs for health balance.

McDonald's restaurants in India do not serve beef hamburgers but offer instead selections such as paneer wraps and spicy potato burgers—all items made with egg-free mayonnaise.[48]

The decorative dot, called bindi, that Hindu, Sikh, Buddhist, and Jain women apply to their foreheads can represent joy or prosperity and is placed at the point of the inner third eye. Today, it is often an easy-to-apply self-adhesive sticker and comes in many colors and styles as a fashion trend.

Traditionally, meals were served on large trays and eaten with the hands while sitting on the floor. Many Pakistanis today consume their meals at tables using flatware and cutlery.[49]

Special Occasions

Asian Indians Another aspect of Indian culture affecting daily diet is the concept of feasting and fasting. As with other Indian food habits, feasting and fasting activities are complex and vary greatly from person to person and group to group. No occasion passes in India without some special food observance: regional holidays, community celebrations, and personal events such as births, weddings, funerals, and illness. A devout Hindu may feast or fast nearly every day of the year (refer to Chapter 4).

Feasting Feasts, in addition to commemorating an occasion, serve as a method of food distribution throughout the community. They are generally observed by presenting prasada (a Sanskrit word meaning "favor" or "grace") in the form of food and sweets of many kinds, to an appropriate holy figure during puja (worship). This act is thought to consecrate the food, which is then distributed to all members of the community. The food insecure throughout India often depend on feast days for sustenance.

Some foods are associated with certain concepts. Rice and bananas both symbolize fertility, for example. Betel leaves represent auspiciousness; ghee, purity; salt, hospitality and pleasantness; mango, hospitality, and auspiciousness; and betel nuts and coconuts, hospitality, sacredness, and auspiciousness.

Most festivals are Hindu in origin, and although many are observed nationwide, each is celebrated differently according to the region. Holi is a spectacular holiday in the north, featuring reenactments of Krishna's life, fireworks, and colored powders tossed everywhere. Celebrants snack at festival bazaar booths. Dussehra is a ten-day holiday observed in both the north and the south. Special dishes are prepared each day, culminating in an enormous feast on the last evening after a torchlight parade in some regions of ornamented elephants. Diwali, the festival of lights, is celebrated everywhere with gifts of sweets. Another holiday, Janmashtami, commemorates the birth of Krishna. As a boy, Krishna and his friends would steal butter or curds (yogurt) hung high in earthen containers. This story is recreated during the celebration as young boys attempt to break elevated clay pots full of curds.

Non-Hindu harvest festivals also feature feasts. They are dedicated to wheat in the North and rice in the South. At the four-day rice festival, Pongal (literally meaning "to boil" or "overflow" in Tamil), a mixture of boiled sweet rice (also called Pongal) is served. The ten-day festival of Onam in Kerala culminates with a feast served by the local women, including 30–40 dishes ranging from fiery curries to foods sweetened with a combination of molasses, milk, and sugar.

Asian Indian Muslims may dine with friends on Eid al-Fitr at the end of Ramadan and Eid al-Adha (refer to Chapter 13). Christians celebrate Christmas and Easter in India, often with great community support. Park Street in Kolkata, for example, is lighted festively for Christmas and thousands visit the sight.

Fasting Fasting is also associated with special occasions in India. It accompanies both religious and personal events. An orthodox Hindu may fast more days a week than not. However, the term *fast* includes many different food restrictions in India, from avoidance of a single food item to complete abstinence from all food. A person might adopt a completely vegetarian diet for the day or eat foods believed to be spiritually purer, such as those cooked in milk (refer to the section "Role of Food in Indian Society and Etiquette" in this chapter).

Muslims in India also fast, notably during the month of Ramadan. No food or drink is consumed between sunrise and sunset (refer to Chapter 4 for more information). Sikhs may fast on the days of the full moon along with ritual bathing and giving away of charity.[50]

Pakistanis Most Pakistanis follow the Islamic calendar, fasting for the month of Ramadan and celebrating the feast days of Eid al-Fitr and Eid al-Adha (refer to Chapter 4). Several secular holidays are also observed, including Pakistan Day (March 23), Independence Day (August 14), and the birthday of the national founder, Mohammad Ali Jinnah (December 25). Special occasions are marked by dishes that use costly ingredients, such as silver leaf and nuts, and feature numerous sweets.

Role of Food in Indian Society and Etiquette The importance of food in Indian culture goes far beyond mere sustenance. Sanskrit texts describe its importance as central in the cycle of life. The Second Anuvaka, Taittiriya Upanishad says:

> All beings that exist on earth are born of food; then they live by food, then again to the food they go at the end. So verily, food is the oldest of all creatures.

Many Hindu dietary customs are meant to lead to purity of mind and spirit. Pollution is the opposite of purity, and polluted foods should be avoided or ameliorated.

The Hindu classification system of jati is used to evaluate the relative spiritual purity of all foods. Purity is determined by the ingredients, how they are prepared, who prepared them, and how they are served. Some foods, such as milk, are inherently pure. Raw foods that are naturally protected by a husk or a peel are less susceptible to pollution. Pakka (meaning "cooked") foods are those that are fried or fat-basted during preparation, preferably in ghee. Pakka foods are relatively unrestricted due to their high degree of purity, often include fried bread and many sweets, and are considered appropriate for serving at temples and community feasts. Kaccha (meaning "undercooked") foods are those that are boiled in water, baked, or roasted. Kaccha foods are thought to be more susceptible to pollution and must, therefore, be treated carefully during serving and consumption.

Some foods, such as alcohol and meat, are innately polluted and by their very nature impure. All leftovers, unless completely untouched by the consumer or by other foods that have been eaten, are considered polluted, which points to ancient food safety techniques passed through generations.

The traditional role of women in food preparation is extremely important throughout Indian culture. Feeding the family is often an Indian woman's primary household duty. She is responsible for overseeing the procurement, storage, preparation, and serving of all meals. Because arranged marriages are common, training in kitchen management is often considered essential for a Hindu woman in obtaining good marriage offers. It is generally believed that a woman cannot be completely substituted for in the kitchen, for she imparts a special sweetness to food. If the wife is unable to perform food-related duties, a daughter or daughter-in-law may substitute, and in multi-family homes, the mother-in-law assumes control of the kitchen. If servants help in meal preparation, it is still important for the woman of the house to serve the food directly from the chula (stove) to the table. However, the roles of women in India are changing. In 2020, women accounted for 20 percent of the labor force in India, a misleadingly low figure because the Indian women who are in farming, manufacturing, in construction, and home-based business activities do not factor into the GDP. According to an Oxfam study, women's ability to undertake paid work is determined by a combination of economic considerations and social norms.[51]

Food for Thought

Food served in brass dishes is thought to be less vulnerable to "pollution" than food in clay dishes. Traditionally, clay dishes and bowls were designed to be used once and thrown back to the earth where they were absorbed (recycled).

Traditionally, only foods cooked and served by a member of an equal or superior caste could be consumed by any Hindu, and only members of the same caste ate together. Today, more modern Hindus adhere to alimentary rules only during holy services and holidays, if at all. Most Westernized Indians eat in restaurants and use convenience products in cooking, ignoring how and by whom the food was prepared.[42]

Food for Thought

Many Brahmins were historically employed as cooks because everyone could eat food prepared by this caste.

Cow's milk is thought to increase intelligence; buffalo's milk is believed to strengthen the body.

Garlic is found in many Ayurvedic remedies, and an old Indian proverb says: "Garlic is as good as ten mothers."

Curcumin, a chemical found in turmeric, has anti-inflammatory and immunomodulatory properties and has been reported to be beneficial in arthritis, asthma, cardiovascular disease, diabetes, Alzheimer's disease, and some cancers.[52]

The consumption of foods considered to be polluted also varies among Hindus. Historically, laborers and warriors were allowed to eat meat to help keep up their strength. Some Brahmin subcastes, though primarily vegetarian, permit the consumption of impure foods that are plentiful in their region, such as fish in the coastal areas and lamb in the north. Other sects are so rigid that even inadvertent intake of polluted food results in spiritual disaster. Members of the International Society for Krishna Consciousness (refer to Chapter 4) believe when there is no other food, meat eating is acceptable to keep from starving, but otherwise as all species have a soul, it is sinful.

Hospitality is highly valued in Hindu homes, where serving a guest is considered equivalent to serving God.[42] Traditionally, the head of the household was responsible for assuring that any guests, pregnant women, or older adults were well fed before he could sit down to eat. The order of serving today is more likely to be guests, oldest men, remaining male diners, children, and then women. In some situations, men and women may be separated while eating. However, more Westernized Asian Indians are often relaxed about these customs, and in some homes, each diner goes their own way at meals.[42]

Food is traditionally served in small individual bowls from serving trays called thalis. The thalis may be silver or brass, with matching bowls. Sometimes, thalis are simply banana leaves and the bowls earthenware, which is becoming in vogue again today with chefs emphasizing traditional meal styles and recyclability. Only the right hand is used in dining, which may be done with spoons, forks, and knives, or with just the fingers. While it varies by region, usually only the fingertips are used to delicately scoop of food with bits of bread or dexterously roll bread around items that are then eaten.[53] Food being served to others should never be directly touched with the hand, nor should a diner refill his or her glass, waiting instead for neighboring diners to do so, and carefully tending to their neighbor's drinks whenever their glass is half empty. If alcohol is served, a guest is expected to make a toast to the health of the host (after the host toasts the guests).

Therapeutic Uses of Food

Asian Indians Ayurvedic medicine is based on the premise that each human is a microcosm of the universe. As such, the body experiences the three inevitable laws of nature (also called universal tendencies) of creation (sattwa), maintenance (rajus), and dissolution (tamas). The fundamental elements of fire, water, and wind also have their counterparts in the humors of the body—bile (pitta), phlegm (kapha), and wind (vata). Pitta regulates metabolic activities and resulting heat. Kapha provides structure and support through bone and flesh, and vata represents the movement of muscle and semen. Health is maintained through a careful balance of humors and substances in the body according to each person's internal constitution and external experiences.[54–56]

When pitta is in balance, digestion is comfortable and a person is content; balanced kapha produces physical and emotional stability, strength, and stamina; vitality and creativity are the results of balanced vata.[57] Good digestion is critical because food is transformed into the body's humors and substances when it is cooked by the digestive agnis ("fires"), producing food juices and wastes. Indigestible food is harmful because it is believed to accumulate in the intestines and decompose, sending toxins into the bloodstream; excessive waste or too little waste is an imbalance that causes illness.

Foods are classified according to which humor they enhance or inhibit. For example, pomegranate[58] increases vata and reduces pitta and kapha. Molasses does the opposite: it increases pitta and kapha and reduces vata. Some foods are also grouped according to their universal tendencies. Mung beans, for instance, are considered sattvic (pure and balanced), chili peppers are rajasic (stimulating), and meats are tamasic (foods that can dull the mind). Furthermore, the hot–cold classification system is used for foods, depending on how they affect the body. The specific identification of an item as hot or cold varies regionally; for example, lentils and peas are considered hot in western India, but cold in northern India. Generally, wheat, spices, and seasonings (except mustard and sesame seeds), chicken, and oils are classified as hot; rice, leafy vegetables, fruits (except mango, papaya, and jackfruit), dairy products, honey, sugar, pickles, and condiments are considered cold. The hot or cold nature of a food can be altered through the method of preparation. The use of hot spices or roasting may make a cold food hot; conversely, soaking a hot food in water or blending it with yogurt can change it into a cold food. Many foods are considered incompatible in Ayurvedic medicine, such as honey with ghee, rice with vinegar, and honeydew melon with yogurt, because of conflicting properties which overwhelm the agnis and diminish digestion.[55]

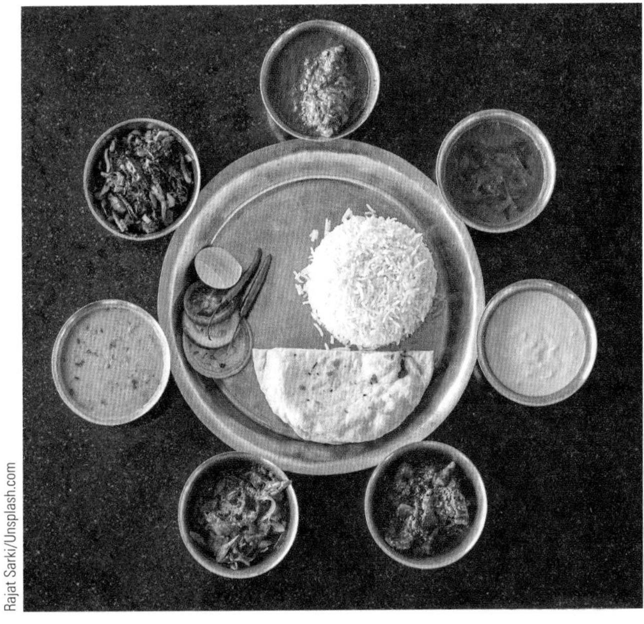
Rajat Sarki/Unsplash.com

▲ **Traditional Indian thali, featuring a selection of rice, roti (flat bread), dal (lentils), flavorful fish, vegetables, chutney, and yogurt-based pachadi or raita.**

Although a balance of foods according to humoral effect, universal tendencies, and hot-cold is believed essential to health, the exact proportions of each change with age, gender, physical condition, and the weather. Traditionally, six seasons are recognized, each with certain dietary recommendations. During winter, when digestion is thought to be strongest, roasted or sour and salty dishes are preferred as well as sweets; in summer and during the monsoons, when digestion is thought to be weak, salty, sour, and fatty foods are avoided. The way foods are eaten is as important as which foods are consumed. To maximize digestion of foods, a person should eat in a quiet atmosphere, sip warm water throughout the meal, and sit for a short while after dining.[55]

Pregnancy is considered to be a normal and healthy condition; however, certain food taboos are sometimes followed. Women especially avoid extremes in foods that are too hot or too cold. Lime juice with honey is a general tonic, believed to prevent excessive bleeding at birth, while cow's milk (particularly with almonds and saffron) and rice porridge are thought to ensure the proper development of the fetus. Fenugreek seeds in buttermilk are given for nausea, and butter or ghee is believed to make the body supple and ease the delivery of the baby.

Food taboos for infants and young children may also be practiced. A survey of Indian mothers found that many believed spicy foods and mangoes were too hot and caused diarrhea, bananas caused colds, and fried foods were considered difficult to digest and the source of coughs.

Numerous dietary remedies are listed for minor illnesses. Barley water is consumed for a fever; vomiting is treated with milk. Coconut water, buttermilk, anise seed oil, and pomegranate flowers are all considered helpful for diarrhea. A powder called ashta choornam (a mixture of asafetida, salt, ginger, pepper, cumin, and ajwain) is added to honey for indigestion. Ginger tea or garlic soup is used to treat colds. Gooseberries and hibiscus flower tea are considered general tonics.[37] Bittermelon and fenugreek seeds—used to treat diabetes—have been found to work clinically as hypoglycemic agents.[59]

Pakistanis Limited data suggest that a hot-cold system of classification is used by some Pakistanis. Items considered hot and therefore avoided during summer include beef and potatoes. Cold foods avoided during winter include chicken, fish, and fruit. Folk remedies are very common in Pakistan, for everything from colds and flu to asthma and jaundice.[60] Eggs, curds (yogurt), ginger, honey, and poppy seeds are just a few of the foods used therapeutically. For infant care, Pakistanis may believe that colostrum is like stale milk and until the breast milk comes in the baby is given cow's milk and a mixture of food called ghutti (honey, butter mixed with sugar, and other liquids). In addition, some believe that certain foods should be restricted during children's illness. Breast milk should not be given if the child has diarrhea, and the child has a fever, milk and rice are withheld.[61]

Contemporary Food Habits in the United States

Adaptations of Food Habits

Asian Indians Americans of Asian Indian descent have usually been exposed to American or European lifestyles in India and may be familiar with a Westernized diet before immigration to the United States. Yet even the most acculturated Indian Americans continue some traditional food habits. Most accept American foods when eating out, but many prefer Asian Indian foods when at home.

Food for Thought

Asian Indians who are practicing Muslims rarely eat pork in the United States. They may drive long distances to purchase halal or kosher meats to fulfill traditional Muslim dietary laws.

Ingredients and Common Foods Numerous changes can occur with immigration including diet. For example, when coming to the United States, often higher levels of fat intake and fewer fruits and vegetables are eaten which impacts health.[62,63] Two earlier studies of Asian Indian college students in Pennsylvania suggested that acculturation takes place in two phases.[64,65] Typically, the first lasts for two to three years, often while the immigrant is a student. Interaction with mainstream American society may be limited during this period. The recent immigrant prefers to associate with members of the same caste, regional, or linguistic group; experience with American foods often includes only fast foods. Young Asian Indian students are often unable to cook and may rely heavily on purchased meals. Many Asian Indian immigrants will eat hamburgers because of their availability and low cost. Sometime during the next ten years, Asian Indians who stay in the United States longer than four years enter the second phase of acculturation. They are usually employed by American businesses and are raising families. They keep their social interactions with Americans separate from those with other Indian Americans. They might serve meat and alcohol to American guests, for example, and vegetarian dishes to Indian guests.[64,65]

Early research on Asian Indian immigrants reported some vegetarians become meat eaters when living in America. In one early study, one-third of those who were vegetarians in India became nonvegetarians in the United States.[66] The "meatification" of human diets in South Asia is on the rise, as it is for immigrants to the United States.[67,68] A study of software engineers living in northern California found that acculturation resulted in increased acculturation and consumption of meat.[69]

As yet, the reasons vegetarians become nonvegetarians have not been stated conclusively. It has been suggested that vegetarianism may lose its social and cultural significance in the United States. Availability of choice is also a potential reason why vegetarian options in restaurants in the United States have been increasing. Data regarding the influence of factors such as gender, income, region of origin in India, and length of stay in America have been contradictory. Variables that affect acculturation include gender (men tend to change their food habits more readily than women because women are the traditional food preparers in Indian society), age (children raised in the United States prefer American foods), marital status (single unmarried men are the most acculturated, married men in the United States with their families in India next, and married men with families in the United States are least acculturated), caste (depending on whether caste members used meat or alcohol in India), and region (Asian Indians from rural areas are often stricter vegetarians than those from the cities).

Meal Composition and Cycle

Asian Indian eating patterns may become more irregular in the United States, possibly because of the pressures of a faster-paced lifestyle. Breakfast is the meal most commonly omitted; snacking occurs between one and three times per day and may be more common in women than in men. Many Americans of Asian Indian descent eat American foods for breakfast and lunch. Traditional Indian evening meals are preferred if native foods and spices are available. Yet dinners at home may also be influenced by U.S. food habits in that more meat, poultry, or fish may be eaten, and American breads may be served in place of roti.

Research on Asian Americans illustrates many of these changes. Dinner is now the main meal of the day, and breakfast is a little larger than is traditional, usually consisting of toast or cereal and milk, with tea. Lunch, unless brought from home, was typically pizza, a salad, or a sandwich. Rice remains the core of the evening meal, and 60 percent of households reported serving it daily. Fish consumption, closely associated with cultural identity for some, actually increases in American homes compared to those in India. Fish is served with rice and dal, seasoned with cumin, fennel, fenugreek, nigella seed, and mustard seed. The portion size of fish has doubled to about eight ounces, and this meal is eaten at approximately half of all dinners. Rice with other items, for example, roast chicken, is consumed at other main meals. Dishes are usually prepared in an Indian style by sautéing, stewing, or braising.[68]

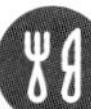

Food for Thought

Chaat houses, specializing in the small, usually cold dishes of mixed grains, fruits, vegetables, legumes, and meats topped with a tangy dressing, are trendy gathering spots for Asian Indian Americans. In India, chaat houses are popular eateries as well.

Iron intake may be low among some Indian American vegetarians; however, substantial amounts of iron are obtained through the use of traditional iron cookware.[70]

Pakistanis Many Pakistani Americans are believed to consume at least one traditional meal each day, usually, dinner, when the family can gather and discuss the day's events.[7] American-style convenience foods are popular for breakfast and lunch; cereals, pizza, hamburgers, sandwiches, fried fish, and cookies replace the flatbreads, stews, and curries typically consumed for these meals. Current research on Pakistani immigrants has suggested major changes in meal patterns with frequent dining out and eating fast foods. Western desserts and snacks were also more frequently consumed. Consumption of potatoes, dairy, oil, animal protein, and fish increased and beans, lentils, fruits, and vegetables decreased.[71]

Nutritional Status

Nutritional Intake Recent research on Asian Indians is noteworthy for the dramatic health changes that have occurred among urban Indians in India and immigrants to Western nations, suggesting the adverse effects of dietary differences and a sedentary lifestyle. Dietary acculturation studies have reported an alteration in vegetarian practices among immigrants. These include a change in consumption of ghee, yogurt, Indian bread, rice dishes, and tea from frequent to low moderate upon migration. There is also an increase in fruit juice, cheese, American bread, dry cereal, soft drinks, and coffee. There also has been a shift in the use of hydrogenated vegetable oils as compared to olive oil and increased consumption of fried/fast/processed foods. This has been referred to as "contaminated vegetarianism".[55,72,73] In comparison, there is little data on Pakistani and other South Asian immigrants, especially those in the United States.

Asian Indians Data on the nutritional status of Indian Americans suggest that in general, many meet recommended intakes for grains and vegetables but do not meet those for fruits, dairy products, or meats, poultry, and fish.[7,74] Intake of dietary fat for Indian Americans approximates that of the U.S. population but is often higher than fat intake in India. In one study looking at first-generation Asian Indian adolescents in the United States, intake of saturated fat exceeded recommended daily recommendations and potassium, magnesium, calcium, vitamin D, and fiber intakes were insufficient in nearly all study participants. Sodium intake also exceeded recommendations. Energy, carbohydrate, and protein intakes seem to increase with the length of stay in the United States.[74]

Obesity rates among Asian Indian Americans are lower than among African Americans and Whites in the United States, and the average body mass index (BMI) is less than that found in Blacks, Mexican Americans, and Whites. However, BMI tends to increase with urbanization and migration, and Asian Indians have a higher percentage of body fat in relation to BMI than other groups. Asian Indians have increased amounts of visceral fat (fat stored within the abdominal cavity and around several vital organs), even in non-obese persons. Percent of visceral fat is correlated with an increased risk of serious health problems and cannot often be seen—someone can be thin on the outside and fat on the inside. Since a higher percentage of body fat, fat patterning, and abdominal adiposity are associated with increased rates of insulin resistance and dyslipidemia, this suggests that some Asian Indians who are not overweight by national standards are, nonetheless, metabolically obese.[75] In 2002, the World Health Organization (WHO) recommended establishing new BMI standards for Asian populations: ideal weight (18.5 to < 23.0 kg/m^2), a moderate-risk public health action point (23.0 kg/m^2), and a high-risk public health action point (27.5 kg/m^2). In 2009, India's health ministry enacted even lower BMI ranges for overweight (23.0 to < 25.0) and obesity (≥ 25.0).[76,77]

Studies reveal that twenty percent of Asian Indian men are overweight and 4.7 percent are obese. Seventeen percent of Asian Indian women are overweight and 6 percent of women are obese. High rates of insulin resistance and dyslipidemia, especially high triglyceride levels and low high-density lipoprotein (HDL) cholesterol levels, are associated with increased risk for type 2 diabetes and cardiovascular disease in Asian Indians.[78] Data show that Asian Indians develop diabetes and cardiovascular disease at an earlier age and have higher prevalence rates than Whites and most other ethnic groups.[73,79–81] These high rates have been referred to as the "Asian Indian Phenotype" which predisposes Indians to hyperinsulinemia, insulin resistance, dyslipidemia with hypertriglyceridemia, and low high-density lipoprotein cholesterol levels. The overall prevalence of diabetes in Indian Americans has been estimated to average 13 percent in adults, compared to 9.3 percent for the general U.S. population, and is higher than rates for other Asian Americans, Black Americans, Latinx Americans, White Americans, and many Native American groups. Rates of cardiovascular disease for Indian Americans are higher than for Whites, and data show that it has an earlier onset and higher mortality rates when compared to deaths from all other causes.[82] Cardiovascular risk was found to increase in Asian Indian immigrants with a length of stay in one study. Hypertension rates in Indian Americans are variable—slightly below the prevalence in Whites in some studies and above the average in others.[80,81] Researchers are studying numerous other factors related to these issues in an attempt to fully understand the role of genetic predisposition and environmental influence (such as diet, inactivity, and stress) in the condition.

It should be noted that the traditional Asian Indian vegetarian diet has many health-promoting features. The traditional diet is low in fat and high in fiber and uses many anti-inflammatory, antimicrobial, and chemopreventative properties. Research outcomes that have studied South Asians' dietary intake and its effect on health have been inconsistent, partly due to vegetarian contamination as previously discussed. One recent study of over 1000 Asian Indians living in the United States showed a lower prevalence of type 2 diabetes for those who adopted a healthy lifestyle, vegetarian, and/or plant-based dietary practices.[83] The most prevalent cancers in Asian Indians are of the lung, breast, and prostate. Colorectal cancers, leukemias, and liver cancers are also common.[84]

Despite high socioeconomic status, few births to teen mothers, and good prenatal care, overweight Asian Indian women in one study were more likely to have adverse birth outcomes than Black, White, and Asian Americans.[85] These included high levels of low birth weight, special needs, and fetal mortality. Other research comparing perinatal outcomes among Asians and Pacific Islanders reported Asian Indian/Pakistani women had the highest risk for preterm delivery, gestational diabetes, and low birth weight at term.[86] A variety of factors may be involved in producing high-risk factors such as vitamin D deficiency, obesity, stress, etc. Studies in Canada and Britain have found that South Asian women were more likely than Whites to become insulin resistant during late pregnancy, and nearly half of all Asian Indian women who developed gestational diabetes had metabolic syndrome following birth.[87–89] Scientists are uncertain as to why this paradox of poor birth outcomes in a population with few environmental risk factors exists.

Early initiation of breastfeeding is important in promoting newborn health. Breastfeeding prevents newborn infections, averts newborn death due to sepsis, pneumonia, diarrhea, and hypothermia, and facilitates sustained breastfeeding. It is common practice in India to avoid breastfeeding colostrum to newborns due to various concerns such as causing indigestion or diarrhea or that it is bad for the infant's health.[90] Foods such as ghee and fenugreek are believed to increase milk production. Prelacteal feeds were prepared for the infants during this period, including honey (which is thought by some Asian Indians to help rid the infant of meconium) and water with sugar, glucose, or jaggery and seasonings such as asafetida, cumin, and aniseed.[91]

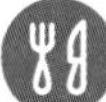

Food for Thought

Even though India has been a dairying culture for millennia, Asian Indians may have difficulty digesting fresh milk. Some feel the traditional fermentation of milk into yogurt, the making of butter by churning yogurt, and the use of clarified butter (where the milk solids are strained away), and the culturing of milk into cheese which reduces the lactose levels, led to a population that did not need to develop the ability to digest lactose after weaning age, unlike the dairying cultures of Europe.[92]

Conditions that may be of concern in some Asian Indians and Pakistanis include beta-thalassemia, which is a commonly inherited disorder, and a high prevalence of glucose-6 phosphate dehydrogenase deficiency in some tribal groups from the North-West Frontier Province of Pakistan.

Pakistanis Little has been reported on the consumption patterns of Pakistani Americans. Malnutrition has been noted in some regions of Pakistan where droughts limit the food supply, and some studies estimate stunting occurs in 40–50 percent of all Pakistani children. Growth retardation has been linked to growth hormone and vitamin D deficiency. Rural children have been found at potential risk for underconsumption of micronutrients even when ample food is available. Vitamin D deficiency has also been linked to low bone mineral density and a risk for early osteoporotic fractures in both men and women.

In contrast, overconsumption is more of a concern for Pakistanis living in urban areas and Westernized nations. Children living in Pakistani cities were found to have a high intake of calories, sugar, total fats, and cholesterol.[93–95] Overweight and obesity rates are similar to that of India, with 25 percent of men overweight and 12 percent obese. Women are higher with 30 percent being overweight and 22 being percent obese. Adults living in wealthier neighborhoods of Karachi reported higher rates of type 2 diabetes and cardiovascular disease when compared to those living in impoverished Karachi households. Of particular concern is a fat distribution pattern that favors abdominal fat, even at recommended weight levels.[78]

Health and Longevity Takeaway

Could the traditional Asian Indian fast be one of the secrets to healthy aging? There have been numerous animal and human clinical trials that have shown that intermittent fasting can lead to improvements in health conditions such as obesity, diabetes, cardiovascular disease, cancers, and neurological disorders. The evidence has been less clear for lifespan effects, but new research on prolonged fasting cycles has been linked to promoting stem cell-based regeneration. The ketogenesis effect (increased ketones in the bloodstream) from fasting may enhance the body's defenses against oxidative and metabolic stress and can initiate the removal or repair of damaged molecules.[96]

Practitioner Perspectives

Asian Indian

Gita Patel, MS, RD, CDE, LD

I am from India and have been a practitioner in the United States for close to 30 years, and many of my clients are South Asians. I would describe the typical South Asian meal as containing a lot of variety on the plate—grains (rice and bread), beans (lentils), salad ingredients in the raytas, along with vegetables. The meal also contains several condiments, such as pappadams and pickled mangos—all these ingredients help balance the meal, which is important because many South Asians from India are vegetarians. For South Asians living in the United States, the typical fast foods that have crept into the diet tend to be those that can be vegetarian, such as pizza. Inexpensive convenience foods are bagels, pasta, and ramen noodles. Many South Asians will go out to eat in Mexican and most Asian restaurants.

Preparation of South Asian food is labor intensive, and back home there are often servants to help in the kitchen. Here, especially for younger South Asian men who are not married, the ingredients may be hard to find, and they will have to prepare their own food. So, it is not uncommon that they will go out to eat and, even though they are vegetarian, will sometimes even eat hamburgers.

South Asians have a very high rate of type 2 diabetes and heart disease, so my advice to many of my clients is to eat smaller portions of rice and bread, increase their intake of vegetables and lentils, and be aware of the sodium content in food, especially pickles. I always ask about desserts and sweets in their diet since they are common in the diet. I never tell my clients to eliminate bread and rice from their diet because I know they won't do it. Instead, I tell them how much they can eat. Same with fruit, but I tell them to eat whole fruit and not consume it as juice.

Comfort Food—Northeast India

A First-Generation Story

Chandra is the first generation in her family to grow up in the United States. Since she was born overseas but came to the United States when she was very young, she is sometimes told she is part of the .5 generation. Both her parents are from India and moved the family to America when Chandra was just 18 months old. Chandra grew up with many of her parent's Indian traditions especially when it came to food.

What is a favorite comfort food that you consider traditional from your home culture?

C: My favorite comfort food growing up was keema. It's a very homey dish in northeastern India made of minced lamb, though other ground meat can be substituted. My family usually had it with rice, thought it is equally good with bread such as roti (wheat flat bread) or luchi (fried puffy bread).

(Continued)

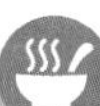

Comfort Food—Northeast India (*Continued*)

A First-generation story

The aroma that rose from the pan as my mom cooked was warm, spicy, and irresistible. I loved it when mom would substitute tiny cubes of potatoes for the traditional peas. Mom would always tell me the health reasons certain ingredients were added to the food as she cooked—the tomato (or sometimes yogurt) was to help balance acidity, turmeric was for the heart, ginger for digestion—and I now that I'm older, I really appreciate how ingrained food and medicine were in my family home culture.

Is this food eaten together with community? Where was it eaten?

C: I grew up in the Midwest and most people I knew had never heard of the food from my family's homeland. Since keema is a simple dish that is normally eaten at home and not in large community celebrations, I did not share this "home food" with my friends. I helped my mom make keema a lot and learned to make it myself when I was young. My memories of comfort are tied to memories of cooking beside my mom in her kitchen in Kansas. I always tried hard to not have to chop the onions, but otherwise cooking with mom is a cherished memory.

Here is Chandra's family recipe for keema:

Serves 4

2 Tbsp. vegetable oil
1 bay leaf
4 whole cloves
4 whole cardamom pods
½ stick cinnamon
1 dried red chili
1 medium onion, finely chopped
½ tsp. sugar
1 pound lean minced meat (lamb, turkey, or beef)
1 inch of fresh ginger root, finely chopped or mashed, or 1 teaspoon dried ginger powder
¼–½ tsp. cayenne or to taste
1 tsp. salt
½ medium tomato, cut into 2 pieces, or ¼ cup plain yogurt
¾ cup frozen green peas, or 1 medium potato, peeled and cut into small ½-inch cubes
¼–½ tsp. garam masala (optional)

Heat the oil in a medium-sized, heavy pan. When hot, add bay, cloves, cardamom, cinnamon, and dried chili, and let sizzle for five seconds. Add chopped onions and fry until the edges start to turn brown. Push onions to the side and add sugar to the oil. Let the sugar heat through and begin to caramelize, stirring a little, before mixing it into the rest of the onions. Add the minced meat and fry until browned. If needed, drain excess fat. If using potatoes, add them now. Add ginger, cayenne, and salt. Add the tomato pieces. Continue to fry, stirring frequently to avoid sticking, about 10 minutes. Add enough water to come just to the top of the meat. If using peas, add them now. Reduce heat and simmer uncovered for 15 minutes. Keema should be moist, with a little "sauce," not completely dry. If desired, add garam masala. Serve with rice or Indian bread.

Nutritional Information (per serving):
calories 308; protein 34 g; carbohydrates 6.8 g; dietary fiber 2 g; sugars 2.5 g; fat 15 g; saturated fat 4 g; cholesterol 102 mg; sodium 672 mg

Discussion Starters

Comparing Native Diet and Culture to That of Immigrants in the United States

In small groups of three to four, compare and contrast the diet and culture of Asian Indian and Pakistani immigrants to the United States with the diet and culture of immigrants to the United States from the Balkans and the Middle East (refer to Discussion Starter from Chapter 13) and from Vietnam, Cambodia, and Laos (refer to Discussion Starter from Chapter 12). Again, each group of students is to focus on a different aspect of the diet and culture of these groups:

Group A: The food habits and the typical eating etiquette and meal composition of these three immigrant groups

Group B: Issues involved in counseling these immigrant groups on diet and health

Group C: Attitudes within each immigrant group toward diet, health, and medical treatment, notably attitudes toward traditional home culture medical treatment and U.S. biomedicine

Group D: Amount of obesity, diabetes, hypertension, and other diseases within each immigrant group

Within your group, decide on what findings to report to the rest of the class. Before breaking up, assign a number to each group member: A1, A2, A3, A4; B1, B2, and so on. Form new groups with all the 1's in a group; all the 2's in another group; all the 3's another group; and so on. In your new group, report the findings of your previous group, and as a group, discuss how traditional attitudes toward diet and health in these immigrant groups relate to the changes in diet and health due to immigration to the United States.

Review Questions

1. List the countries that comprise South Asia. List and briefly describe at least four religions practiced in this region. What are the similarities and differences regarding religion between Pakistan and India?
2. Describe the vegetarian diet of Hindus. Which animal foods are allowed and which are not consumed? What are the staples of the diet? How would the Hindu diet differ from that of the Sikhs and Muslims? What would make a food pure or polluted? Are there regional differences in staples used in India and Pakistan? Describe at least three types of bread consumed in India.
3. What are masalas, and when are they used in South Asian cooking? Describe regional variations in South Asian cuisine. What is curry?
4. Briefly explain Ayurvedic medicine. How does food fit into the Ayurvedic system?
5. What is metabolic syndrome? How does it affect Asian Indians, and how may their diet contribute to its development?

Reflection

Taking into consideration Ayurveda, how important is it when making dietary and lifestyle change recommendations, to consider an individual's set of physical, physiological, and psychological attributes? For example, taste preference, sweet, sour, or salty tastes, genetics, or family history for physiological predispositions or emotions and mood.

References

1. Pandey Mukherjee, J. 2016. Indus era 8,000 years old, not 5,500; ended because of weaker monsoon. *The Times of India*. Retrieved from https://timesofindia.indiatimes.com/india/indus-era-8000-years-old-not-5500-ended-because-of-weaker-monsoon/articleshow/52485332.cms
2. Mark, J.J. 2020. Indus Valley Civilization. *World History Encyclopedia*. Retrieved from https://www.worldhistory.org/Indus_Valley_Civilization/
3. Press Trust of India. 2018. More than 19500 mother tongues spoken in India: Census. *Indian Express*. Retrieved from https://indianexpress.com/article/india/more-than-19500-mother-tongues-spoken-in-india-census-5241056/
4. U.S. Census Bureau. 2019. American Community Survey 1 Year Estimates. B05006. Selected Population Profile in the U.S. Retrieved from https://data.census.gov/cedsci/table?q=B05006%3A%20PLACE%20OF%20BIRTH%20FOR%20THE%20FOREIGN-BORN%20POPULATION%20IN%20THE%20UNITED%20STATES&hidePreview=true&tid=ACSDT1Y2019.B05006&vintage=2018
5. Census in Brief. 2017 Ethnic and cultural origins of Canadians: Portrait of a rich heritage. Retrieved from https://www12.statcan.gc.ca/census-recensement/2016/as-sa/98-200-x/2016016/98-200-x2016016-eng.Cfm (accessed April 27, 2022).
6. Pew Research Center. April 29, 2021. Indians in the U.S. Fact Sheet. Retrieved from https://www.pewresearch.org/social-trends/fact-sheet/asian-americans-indians-in-the-u-s/ (accessed April 28, 2022).
7. Pavri, T. 2014. Asian Indian Americans. In R.V. Dassanowsky & J. Lehman (Eds.), *Gale Encyclopedia of Multicultural America*. 3rd ed., Vol. 3. Farmington Hills, MI: Gale Group.
8. Kakar, S. & Kakar, K. 2009. *The Indians: Portrait of a people*. Penguin Books India.
9. CJP Editors. 2018. Caste discrimination and related laws in India. Citizens for Justice and Peace (CJP). Retrieved from https://cjp.org.in/caste-discrimination-and-related-laws-in-india/
10. Sahgal, N., Evans, J., Salazar, A.M., Starr, K.J., & Corichi, M. 2021. Attitudes about caste. Pew Research Center.
11. Kramer, S. 2021. Key findings about the religious composition of India. Pew Research Center. Retrieved from https://www.pewresearch.org/fact-tank/2021/09/21/key-findings-about-the-religious-composition-of-india/
12. Snellgrove, D.L., Kitagawa, J.M., Reynolds, F.E., Nakamura, H., Tucci, G., & Lopez, D.S. 2021. Buddhism. *Encyclopedia Britannica*. Retrieved from https://www.britannica.com/topic/Buddhism
13. Pariona, A. 2020. Countries with the largest Jain populations. WorldAtlas. Retrieved from https://www.worldatlas.com/articles/countries-with-the-largest-jain-populations.html
14. Stabin, T. 2014. Sikh Americans. In T. Riggs (Ed.), *Gale Encyclopedia of Multicultural America*. 3rd ed., Vol. 4, pp. 179–192.
15. McLeod, W.H. 2020. *Sikhism. Encyclopedia Britannica*. Retrieved from https://www.britannica.com/topic/Sikhism
16. Sikh Coalition, New York, NY. 2022. "About Us." Retrieved from https://www.sikhcoalition.org/about-us/
17. Salazar, A.M. 2021. 8 key findings about Christians in India. Pew Research Center. Retrieved from https://www.pewresearch.org/fact-tank/2021/07/12/8-key-findings-about-christians-in-india/
18. Syrian Christians in India. Worldmark Encyclopedia of Cultures and Daily Life. Retrieved from https://www.encyclopedia.com/humanities/encyclopedias-almanacs-transcripts-and-maps/syrian-christians-india (accessed April 25, 2022).
19. Britannica, T. Editors of Encyclopaedia. 2019. Parsi. *Encyclopedia Britannica*. Retrieved from https://www.britannica.com/topic/Parsi
20. Britannica, T. Editors of Encyclopaedia. 2021. Taj Mahal. *Encyclopedia Britannica*. Retrieved from https://www.britannica.com/topic/Taj-Mahal
21. Inman, A.G., Howard, E.E., Beaumont R.L., & Walker, J.A. 2007. Cultural transmission: Influence of contextual factors in Asian Indian immigrant parents' experiences. *Journal of Counseling Psychology*, 54(1), 93–100.
22. Habiba, U., Ali, R., & Ashfaq, A. 2016. From patriarchy to neopatriarchy: Experiences of women from Pakistan. *International Journal of Humanities and Social Science*, 6(3), 212–221.
23. Pavri, T. 2014. Pakistani Americans. In T. Riggs (Ed.), *Gale Encyclopedia of Multicultural America*. 3rd ed., Vol. 3. pp. 425–436. Retrieved from https://link.gale.com/apps/doc/CX3273300139/GVRL?u=multi_america&sid=bookmark-GVRL&xid=348124bc
24. Kalra, S., Bajaj, S., Gupta, Y., Agarwal, P., Singh, S. K., Julka, S., . . . & Agrawal, N. 2015. Fasts, feasts and festivals in diabetes-1: Glycemic management during Hindu fasts. *Indian Journal of Endocrinology and Metabolism*, 19(2), 198.
25. Sarkar, P., Dh, L.K., Dhumal, C., Panigrahi, S.S., & Choudhary, R. 2015. Traditional and ayurvedic foods of Indian origin. *Journal of Ethnic Foods*, 2(3), 97–109.
26. Chhetri, D.R., Parajuli, P., & Subba, G.C. 2005. Antidiabetic plants used by Sikkim and Darjeeling Himalayan tribes, India. *Journal of Ethnopharmacology*, 99, 199–202.
27. Katewa, S.S., Chaudhary, B.L., & Jain, A. 2004. Folk medicines from tribal areas of Rajasthan, India. *Journal of Ethnopharmacology*, 92, 41–46.
28. Mahishi, P., Srinivasa, B.H., & Shivanna, M.B. 2005. Medicinal plant wealth of local communities in some villages in Shimoga District of Karnataka, India. *Journal of Ethnopharmacology*, 98, 307–312.
29. https://geriatrics.stanford.edu/ethnomed/pakistani/fund/pakistani_americans.html
30. https://libraryguides.umassmed.edu/diversity_guide/pakistani

31. D'Avanzo, C. 2008. *Mosby's pocket guide to cultural health assessment*. Elsevier Health Sciences.
32. Hussain, F., Shah, S.M., & Sher, H. 2007. Traditional resource evaluation of some plants of Mastuj, District Chitral. *Pakistan Journal of Botany*, 39(2), 339–354.
33. Nisar, M.F., Ismail, S., Arshad, M., Majeed, A., & Arfan, M. 2011. Ethnomedicinal Flora of District Mandi Bahauddin, Pakistan. *Middle East Journal of Scientific Research*, 9, 233–238.
34. Shaikh, B.T. & Hatcher, J. 2005. Complementary and alternative medicine in Pakistan: prospects and limitations. *Evidence-Based Complementary and Alternative Medicine*, 2(2), 139–142.
35. Hussain, W., Badshah, L., Ullah, M., Ali, M., Ali, A., & Hussain, F. 2018. Quantitative study of medicinal plants used by the communities residing in Koh-e-Safaid Range, northern Pakistani-Afghan borders. *Journal of Ethnobiology and Ethnomedicine*, 14(1), 1–18.
36. Kumar, V. 2020. RETRACTED ARTICLE: Seven spices of India—from kitchen to clinic. *Journal of Ethnic Food*, 7, 23. Retrieved from https://doi.org/10.1186/s42779-020-00058-0
37. Achaya, K.T. 1994. *Indian food: A historical companion*. Delhi: Oxford University Press.
38. Taylor Sen, C. 2020. How Indian Vegetarianism Disrupted the Way the World Eats. Retrieved from: https://arrow.tudublin.ie/cgi/viewcontent.cgi?article=1215&context=dgs
39. Borges, A., 2017. This cartoon perfectly nails how foreigners stereotype all Indian food as 'curry.' BussFeed India. Retrieved from https://www.buzzfeed.com/andreborges/people-really-love-this-guys-cartoon-about-people-who-think
40. Rautray, S. 2018. Cannot direct entire country to turn vegetarian, says Supreme Court. *The Economic Times*. Retrieved from https://economictimes.indiatimes.com/news/politics-and-nation/cannot-direct-entire-country-to-turn-vegetarian-says-supreme-court/articleshow/66189978.cms?from=mdr
41. Government of India-Indian Culture. n.d. Food and Culture. Retrieved from Food and Culture | Indian Culture (accessed April 28, 2022).
42. Sen, C.T. 2004. *Food culture in India*. Westport, CT: Greenwood Press.
43. Zibart, E. 2001. *The ethnic food lover's companion: Understanding the cuisines of the world*. Birmingham, AL: Menasha Ridge Press.
44. Flowerday, J. 2006. *Cooking in Hunza*. Saudi Aramco World, May/June. Retrieved from http://www.saudiaramcoworld.com/issue/200603/cooking.in.hunza.htm
45. Goodwin, L. 2020. The history of masala chai. *The Spruce Eats*. Retrieved from https://www.thespruceeats.com/the-history-of-masala-chai-tea-765836
46. Rau, S.R. 1969. *The cooking of India*. New York: Time-Life Books.
47. Furstenau, N.M. 2021. *Green chili & other impostors*. University of Iowa Press.
48. The Travel. May 6, 2020. What does McDonald's In India Serve? Check out these delicious menu items. Retrieved from What Does McDonald's In India Serve? Check Out These Delicious Menu Items (thetravel.com) (accessed April 28, 2022).
49. Etiquette scholar. n.d. Pakistan Dining Etiquette. Retrieved from Pakistan Dining Etiquette (www.etiquettescholar.com) (accessed April 27, 2022).
50. News 18. July 27, 2018. Guru Purnima - and its history, significance and rituals. Retrieved from Guru Purnima – and Its History, Significance and Rituals (news18.com) (accessed April 28, 2022).
51. The Hindu. January 21, 2019. Inequality has 'female face' in India, women's unpaid work worth 3.1% of GDP: Oxfam. Retrieved from https://www.thehindu.com/news/national/inequality-has-female-face-in-india-womens-unpaid-work-worth-31-of-gdp-oxfam/article26048261.ece (accessed April 20, 2022).
52. Waite, S. & Linja, S. 2017. *The Alzheimer's prevention food guide*. Rockridge Press.
53. Laura. March 2, 2022. Indian Dining Etiquette. Retrieved from https://www.asiahighlights.com/india/dining-etiquette (accessed May 2, 2022).
54. Sarkar, P., Dh, L.K., Dhumal, C., Panigrahi, S.S., & Choudhary, R. 2015. Traditional and ayurvedic foods of Indian origin. *Journal of Ethnic Foods*, 2(3), 97–109.
55. Payyappallimana, U. & Venkatasubramanian, P. 2016. Exploring Ayurvedic knowledge on food and health for providing innovative solutions to contemporary healthcare. *Frontiers in Public Health*, 4, 57.
56. Niemi, M. & Ståhle, G. 2016. The use of ayurvedic medicine in the context of health promotion–a mixed methods case study of an ayurvedic centre in Sweden. *BMC Complementary and Alternative Medicine*, 16(1), 1–14.
57. Ray, M., Ghosh, K., Singh, S., & Mondal, K.C. 2016. Folk to functional: an explorative overview of rice-based fermented foods and beverages in India. *Journal of Ethnic Foods*, 3(1), 5–18.
58. Ganguly, S. 2017. Medicinal utility of pomegranate fruit in regular human diet: A brief review. *International Journal of Forestry and Horticulture*, 3(1), 7–18.
59. Chevallier, A. 2016. *Encyclopedia of Herbal Medicine: 550 Herbs and Remedies for Common Ailments*. Penguin.
60. Ramzan, S., Soelberg, J., Jäger, A.K., & Cantarero-Arévalo, L. 2017. Traditional medicine among people of Pakistani descent in the capital region of Copenhagen. *Journal of Ethnopharmacology*, 196, 267–280.
61. Samina, R., Adeela, R., & Nurazzura, M.D. 2017. The perceptions and the practices of folk medicines among youths in Pakistan. *Pertanika Journal of Social Sciences & Humanities*, 25(2).
62. Serafica, R.C. 2014. Dietary acculturation in Asian Americans. *Journal of Cultural Diversity*, 21(4), 145–151.
63. Venkatesh, S. & Weatherspoon, L.J. 2018. Reliability and validity of an Asian Indian dietary acculturation measure (AIDAM). *Health Education & Behavior: The Official Publication of the Society for Public Health Education*, 45(6), 908–917. Retrieved from https://doi.org/10.1177/1090198118775479
64. Mahadevan, M. & Blair, D. 2009. Changes in food habits of south Indian Hindu Brahmin immigrants in State College, PA. *Ecology of Food and Nutrition*, 48(5), 404–432.
65. Gupta, S.P. 1976. Changes in food habits of Asian Indians in the United States: A case study. *Sociology and Social Research*, 60, 87–99.
66. Karim, N., Bloch, D.S., Falciglia, G., & Murthy, L. 1986. Modifications of food consumption patterns reported by people from India, living in Cincinnati, Ohio. *Ecology of Food and Nutrition*, 19, 11–18.
67. Jakobsen, J. & Hansen, A. 2020. Geographies of meatification: An emerging Asian meat complex. *Globalizations*, 17(1), 93–109.
68. Venkatesh, S. & Weatherspoon, L.J. 2018. Food behaviors and dietary acculturation of Asian Indians in the US. *Journal of Nutrition Education and Behavior*, 50(6), 529–535.
69. Maheshwary, S. & Ashwini, W. 2010. Acculturation, food habits and physical activity in South Asian software engineers living in the United States, MS project, San Jose State University.
70. Kollipara, U.K. & Brittin, H.C. 1996. Increased iron content of some Indian foods due to cookware. *Journal of the American Dietetic Association*, 96, 508–510.
71. Parackal, S. 2017. Dietary transition in the south Asian diaspora: implications for diabetes prevention strategies. *Current Diabetes Reviews*, 13(5), 482-487.
72. Lesser, I.A., Gasevic, D., & Lear, S.A. 2014. The association between acculturation and dietary patterns of South Asian immigrants. PloS one, 9(2), e88495.
73. Enas, E.A., Mohan, V., Deepa, M., Farooq, S., Pazhoor, S., & Chennikkara, H. 2007. The metabolic syndrome and dyslipidemia among Asian Indians: A population with high rates of diabetes and premature coronary artery disease. *Journal of the Cardiometabolic Syndrome*, 2, 267–275.

74. Martyn-Nemeth, P., Quinn, L., Menon, U., Shrestha, S., Patel, C., & Shah, G. 2017. Dietary profiles of first-generation South Asian Indian adolescents in the United States. *Journal of Immigrant and Minority Health*, 19(2), 309–317.
75. Frysh, P. August 26, 2021. What is visceral fat? WebMD. Retrieved from https://www.webmd.com/diet/what-is-visceral-fat (accessed on April 29, 2022).
76. Expert Consultation WHO. 2004; Appropriate body-mass index for Asian populations and its implications for policy and intervention strategies. *Lancet*, 363(9403), 157–163.
77. Misra, A., Chowbey, P., Makkar, B.M., Vikram, N.K., Wasir, J.S., Chadha, D., . . . Concensus Group. 2009. Consensus statement for diagnosis of obesity, abdominal obesity and the metabolic syndrome for Asian Indians and recommendations for physical activity, medical and surgical management. *Journal of the Association Physicians India*, 57, 163–170.
78. World Obesity n.d. Global obesity observatory. Retrieved from https://data.worldobesity.org/country/pakistan-167/ (accessed April 28, 2022).
79. Centers for Disease Control and Prevention. 2014. *National diabetes statistics report: Estimates of diabetes and its burden in the United States*, 2014. Atlanta, GA: U.S. Department of Health and Human Services.
80. Unnikrishnan, R., Gupta, P.K., & Mohan, V. 2018. Diabetes in South Asians: phenotype, clinical presentation, and natural history. *Current Diabetes Reports*, 18(6), 1–7.
81. Ayyappa, K.A., Shatwan, I., Bodhini, D., Bramwell, L.R., Ramya, K., Sudha, V., . . . & Vimaleswaran, K.S. 2017. High fat diet modifies the association of lipoprotein lipase gene polymorphism with high density lipoprotein cholesterol in an Asian Indian population. *Nutrition & Metabolism*, 14(1), 1–9.
82. Vimaleswaran, K.S., Bodhini, D., Lakshmipriya, N., Ramya, K., Anjana, R.M., Sudha, V., . . . & Radha, V. 2016. Interaction between FTO gene variants and lifestyle factors on metabolic traits in an Asian Indian population. *Nutrition & Metabolism*, 13(1), 1–10.
83. Misra, R., Balagopal, P., Raj, S., & Patel, T.G. 2018. Vegetarian diet and cardiometabolic risk among Asian Indians in the United States. *Journal of Diabetes Research, 2018*.
84. Thompson, C.A., Gomez, S.L., Hastings, K.G., Kapphahn, K., Yu, P., Shariff-Marco, S., . . . & Palaniappan, L.P. 2016. The burden of cancer in Asian Americans: a report of national mortality trends by Asian ethnicity. *Cancer Epidemiology and Prevention Biomarkers*, 25(10), 1371–1382.
85. Kutchi, I., Chellammal, P., & Akila, A. 2020. Maternal obesity and pregnancy outcome: in perspective of new Asian Indian guidelines. *The Journal of Obstetrics and Gynecology of India*, 70(2), 138–144.
86. Puthussery, S. 2016. Perinatal outcomes among migrant mothers in the United Kingdom: Is it a matter of biology, behaviour, policy, social determinants or access to health care? *Best Practice & Research Clinical Obstetrics & Gynaecology*, 32, 39–49.
87. Kousta, E., Efstathiadou, Z., Lawrence, N.J., Jeffs, J.A., Godsland, I.F., Barrett, S.C., . . . Johnston, D.G. 2006. The impact of ethnicity on glucose regulation and the metabolic syndrome following gestational diabetes. *Diabetologia*, 49, 36–40.
88. Retnakaran, R., Hanley, A.J., Connelly, P.W., Sermer, M., & Zinman, B. 2006. Ethnicity modifies the effect of obesity on insulin resistance in pregnancy: A comparison of Asian, South Asian, and Caucasian women. *Journal of Clinical Endocrinology and Metabolism*, 91, 93–97.
89. Hedderson, M.M., Darbinian, J.A., & Ferrara A. 2010. Disparities in the risk of gestational diabetes by race-ethnicity and country of birth. *Paediatric and Perinatal Epidemiology*, 2(5), 441–448.
90. Sharma, I.K. & Byrne, A. 2016. Early initiation of breastfeeding: a systematic literature review of factors and barriers in South Asia. *International Breastfeeding Journal*, 11(1), 1–12.
91. Varma, S., Wagle, A., & Sucher, K. 2010. *Dietary behaviors and practices of pregnant and lactating South Asian women living in the United States*. San Jose State University, San Jose, CA. Master's project.
92. Wiley, A.S. 2014. Cultures of milk. In *Cultures of Milk*. Harvard University Press.
93. Osei-Kwasi, H.A., Nicolaou, M., Powell, K., Terragni, L., Maes, L., Stronks, K., . . . & Holdsworth, M. 2016. Systematic mapping review of the factors influencing dietary behaviour in ethnic minority groups living in Europe: a DEDIPAC study. *International Journal of Behavioral Nutrition and Physical Activity*, 13(1), 1–17.
94. LeCroy, M.N. & Stevens, J. 2017. Dietary intake and habits of South Asian immigrants living in Western countries. *Nutrition REVIEWS*, 75(6), 391–404.
95. LeCroy, M.N., Bryant, M., Albrecht, S.S., Siega-Riz, A.M., Ward, D.S., Cai, J., & Stevens, J. 2021. Obesogenic home food availability, diet, and BMI in Pakistani and White toddlers. *Maternal & Child Nutrition*, 17(3), e13138.
96. Longo, V.D., Di Tano, M., Mattson, M.P., & Guidi, N. 2021. Intermittent and periodic fasting, longevity and disease. *Nature Aging*, 1(1), 47–59.

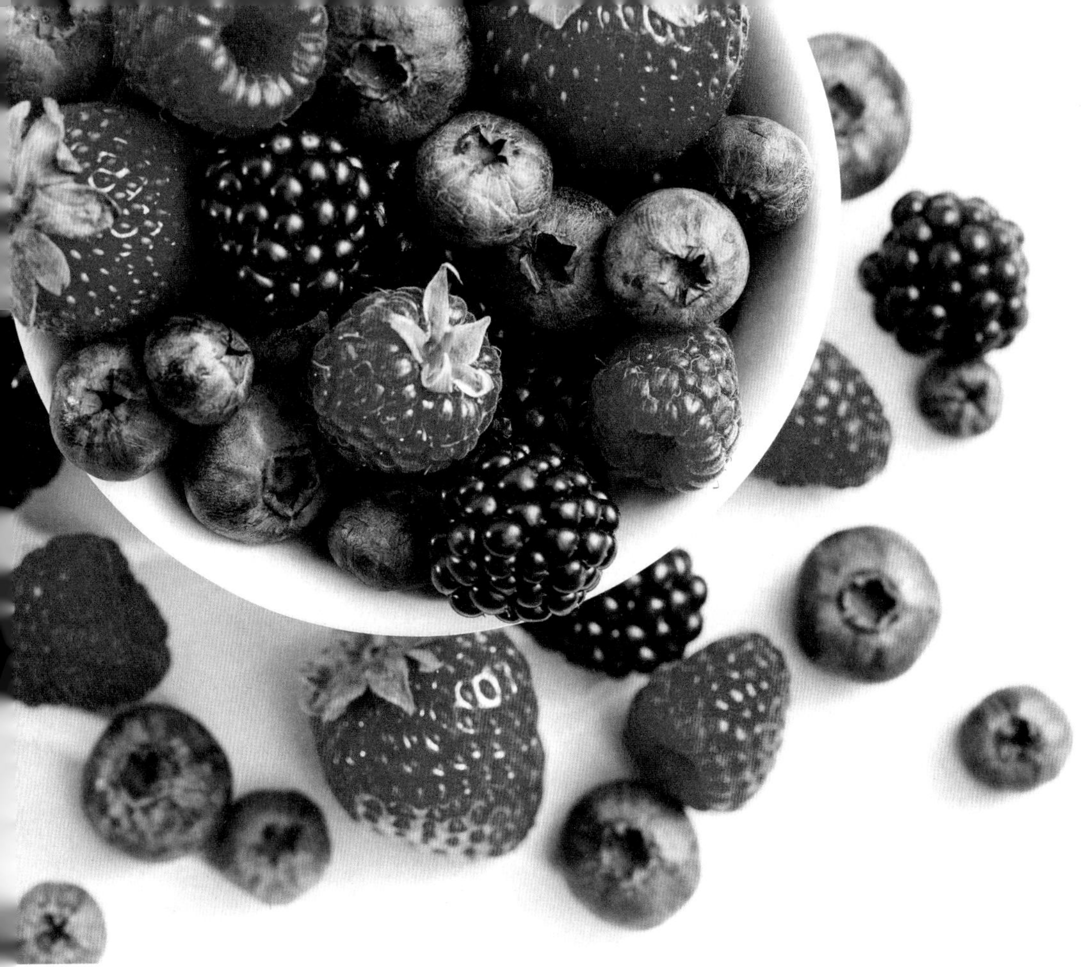

Romariolen/Shutterstock.com

Chapter 15

Regional Americans

Learning Objectives

15.1 List the regions of the United States and the states that form each regional grouping.

15.2 Identify the settlement patterns of each of the regions and states.

15.3 Compare the indigenous ingredients to the foods introduced by the settlers and relate these to regional dishes.

15.4 Discuss the regional variation in staple ingredients within each of the regions.

15.5 Identify key agricultural products produced by each state.

15.6 Describe regional specialties and dishes for each region.

In Boston, they eat beans. In Philadelphia, they eat cheesesteaks. In Kansas City, they eat barbecue. And in Seattle, they drink café lattes. A person from Montana is no more likely to eat grits (ground hominy) than a person from Mississippi is likely to eat Rocky Mountain oysters (deep-fried beef testicles). Just as certain fare is associated with ethnicity and religious affiliation, local food preferences are central to American regional identity. This chapter profiles the Northeast, South, Midwest, and West regions and examines traditional fare, noting significant culinary variations and trends in U.S. regional food habits.

American Regional Food Habits

What Is Regional Fare?

Regional fare has traditionally been homestyle food prepared with local ingredients, dependent on agricultural conditions and seasonal availability. Most families made do with what they could grow, gather, or barter. Local foods are the most significant of several factors that influence the development of a particular regional cuisine. The spicy cooking of the Southwest with its emphasis on corn, beans, and chilies could not have been created in the upper Great Lakes area, which produces wheat, fish, and dairy foods. Before the advent of food preservation and refrigerated shipping, local items were not only freshest and tastiest but also most economical because they were grown nearby. Strong associations with place and food suggest the importance placed on the superior quality of local items. Even today, with a global assortment available, there is a certain cachet to Maine lobsters, Vermont maple syrup, Georgia peaches, Florida oranges, Idaho potatoes, and Washington apples (refer to Figure 15.1).

Ethnic and religious practices also affect the development of regional fare, particularly specialty foods. Jewish bagels in New York, German doughnuts called fastnachts in Pennsylvania, Cajun French–style sausages in Louisiana, West African–influenced hoppin' John in South Carolina, southern Italian–flavored pizza in Chicago, Cornish pasties in Michigan, and Mexican-inspired chili con carne in Texas are just a few examples. Most regional cuisine is a blend of several ethnic elements, such as the Native American-British dishes of New England, the African–French–Spanish–British–Native American mélange that is southern fare, and the northern Italian–Mexican–Asian mix found in California cuisine.

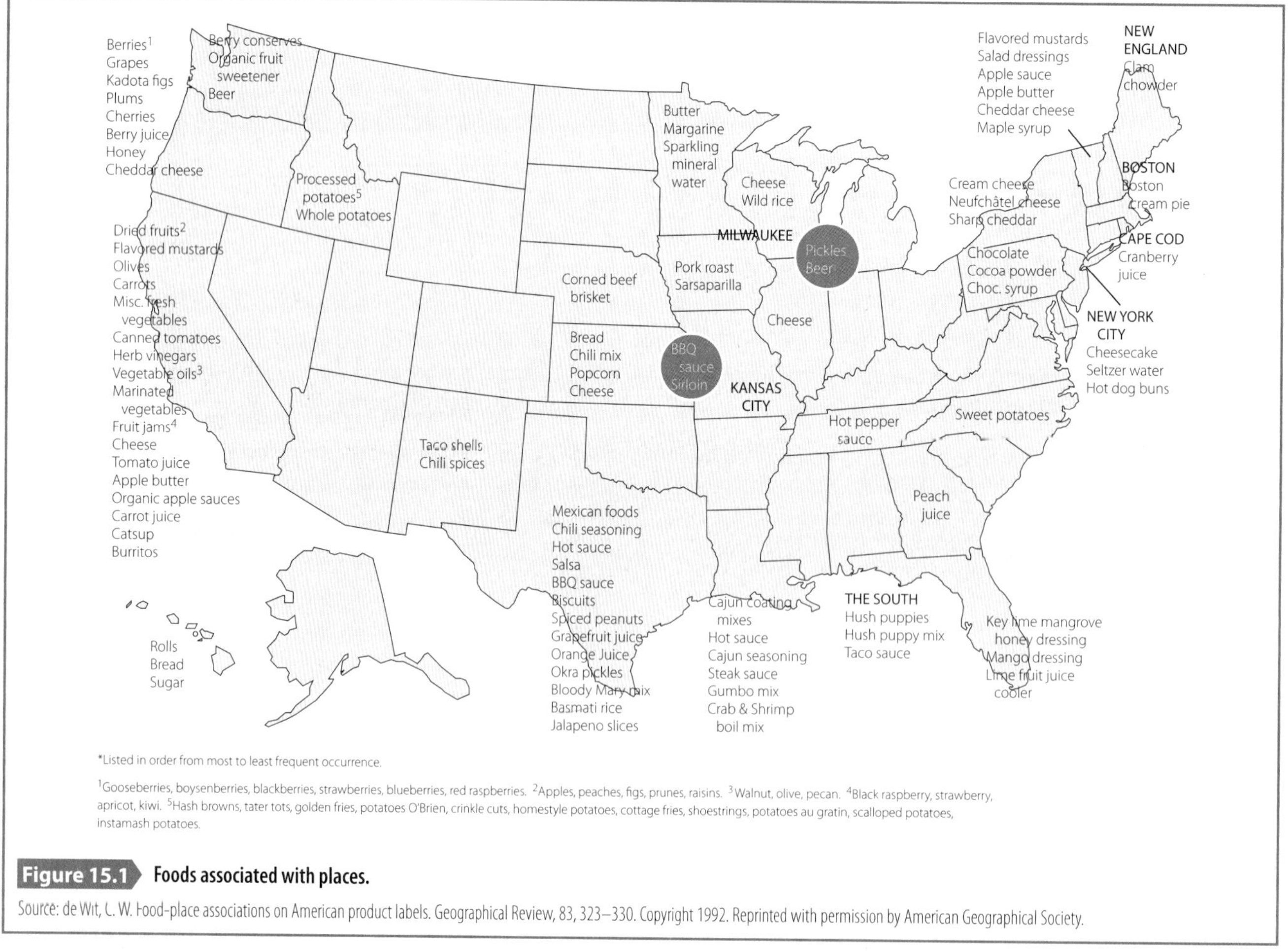

*Listed in order from most to least frequent occurrence.

[1]Gooseberries, boysenberries, blackberries, strawberries, blueberries, red raspberries. [2]Apples, peaches, figs, prunes, raisins. [3]Walnut, olive, pecan. [4]Black raspberry, strawberry, apricot, kiwi. [5]Hash browns, tater tots, golden fries, potatoes O'Brien, crinkle cuts, homestyle potatoes, cottage fries, shoestrings, potatoes au gratin, scalloped potatoes, instamash potatoes.

Figure 15.1 Foods associated with places.

Source: de Wit, C. W. Food-place associations on American product labels. Geographical Review, 83, 323–330. Copyright 1992. Reprinted with permission by American Geographical Society.

Religious food habits are a factor in areas where large numbers of a specific faith have congregated. For instance, the majority of Mormons live in Utah, and Mormons typically do not drink alcohol, tea, coffee, or other stimulating beverages. Alcohol purchases in Utah are more strictly controlled with more restrictions as to what and where they can be sold. Sweets are allowed, however, and are well integrated into family activities.

A third factor in regional foods is local history, which is often associated with certain dishes. A good example is the Kentucky stew called burgoo. Legend has it that the mixture of poultry and red meat with vegetables dates back to the Civil War when French chef Gustave Jaubert, serving in the Confederate cavalry at Lexington, created the stew from native blackbirds, game, and greens. Others say it originates from the bulgur porridge sailors ate in the 1700s. Or, that it is a spin-off of Brunswick stew, to which Native Americans, Virginians, and Georgians have some claim. There is no single recipe for the dish, but today it typically includes chicken, pork, beef, or lamb; and cabbage, potatoes, tomatoes, lima beans, corn, and okra. It is seasoned with cayenne. Burgoo is traditionally served at picnics, political rallies, and sporting events, including Derby Day.

Current trends can influence regional fare as well. Some dishes sweep through one region but never gain national acceptance, such as caviar pie (layered hard-boiled eggs, scallions, caviar, and sour cream) in the Southeast, or loco moco (a bowl with rice topped with a ground beef patty, then an egg over easy, and gravy) in Hawaii. Other trends start regionally and then catch on countrywide, such as the salsas of the Southwest.

Economics contributes to the popularity of certain foods. One study found that some of the best markets for beer in the country are in areas with the least household income. Wine appears more popular with upper-income populations in the United States,[1,2] although more recently brewpubs have risen in popularity with this group as well. The number of brewpubs in the United States increased substantially from 2006 to 2020.[3,4]

People living in the United States spend 6.4 percent of their household income on food. In 2020, the average annual household food expenditure was $7,316. Households with incomes in the lowest quintile spent an average of $4,099 on food which is 27 percent of their income. Whereas households with incomes in the highest quintile spent an average of $12,245 on food, which is 7 percent of their income.[5] Due to lower spending power, lower-income households purchase cheaper, less healthful foods (often higher in fat and sugar) compared to higher-income households.[6,7]

The blending of physical, cultural, historic, current, and economic conditions in a region produces a characteristic flavor imparted to the foods from the environment, what researchers call a "taste of place," from the French *goût de terroir*.[8,9] Elementally, the taste of place is the identification of certain ingredients or dishes within an area. At a deeper level, it is the emotional connection between people and a local heritage, an appreciation for the regional characteristics that create flavors unlike those found anywhere else in the nation, or the world.[10]

Regional Divisions

The United States has been divided in numerous ways. Sometimes regions are delineated by terrain, as in the Great Plains, or marked by major rivers or mountain ranges, as in the Mississippi River Valley or the Appalachians. Sometimes areas are defined by similarities in climate, as in the Sun Belt; by economic affiliation, as in the Steel Belt and Silicon Valley; or by the characteristics of the population, as in the Bible Belt and in the old term Indian Lands. Historical divisions, such as the Mason-Dixon Line, or political divisions, including state boundaries, can also be used. Geographers suggest that traditional regions contain elements of all these variables, characterized as a synergistic relationship between a people and the land that develops over time and is specific to the locality. Such regional identity is dynamic, more of a process than a delineation, and subject to changes in population, economy, ecology, and other factors.[11,12] However, geographic considerations are used to set arbitrary regional divisions independent of cultural relationships.

The U.S. Census Bureau and the U.S. Department of Commerce list four regions with nine subdivisions for data collection purposes: Northeast, Midwest, South, and West. Although these categories group together states with distinctively different cuisines, such as Florida and Texas, or Alaska and Hawaii, most demographic and food consumption data are presented in this four-region format (refer to Figure 15.2).[13] It is useful for detecting broad trends, as long as results are not overgeneralized to smaller populations that may observe alternate regional boundaries.

The Northeast

Regional Profile

The states of the U.S. Northeast include those of New England (Connecticut, Maine, Massachusetts, New Hampshire, Rhode Island, and Vermont) and those of the Mid-Atlantic region (New Jersey, New York, and Pennsylvania). The New England area features a rugged, irregular Atlantic coastline with many protected bays. Rolling hills and valleys that gradually become densely forested mountains extend west. The region is noted for its spectacular autumn weather and colorful fall foliage, followed by harsh winters. The Mid-Atlantic states are farther south and more temperate in climate. Sandy beaches and estuaries line the long coast. The ridges, river valleys, and fertile plateaus of the Adirondack, Appalachian, Blue, Catskill, and other mountain ranges crisscross much of the three states. Freshwater lakes dot the region and provide the northern boundary along Lake Ontario and Lake Erie.

Despite differences in climate and geography, the entire Northeast shares a common early history of sophisticated

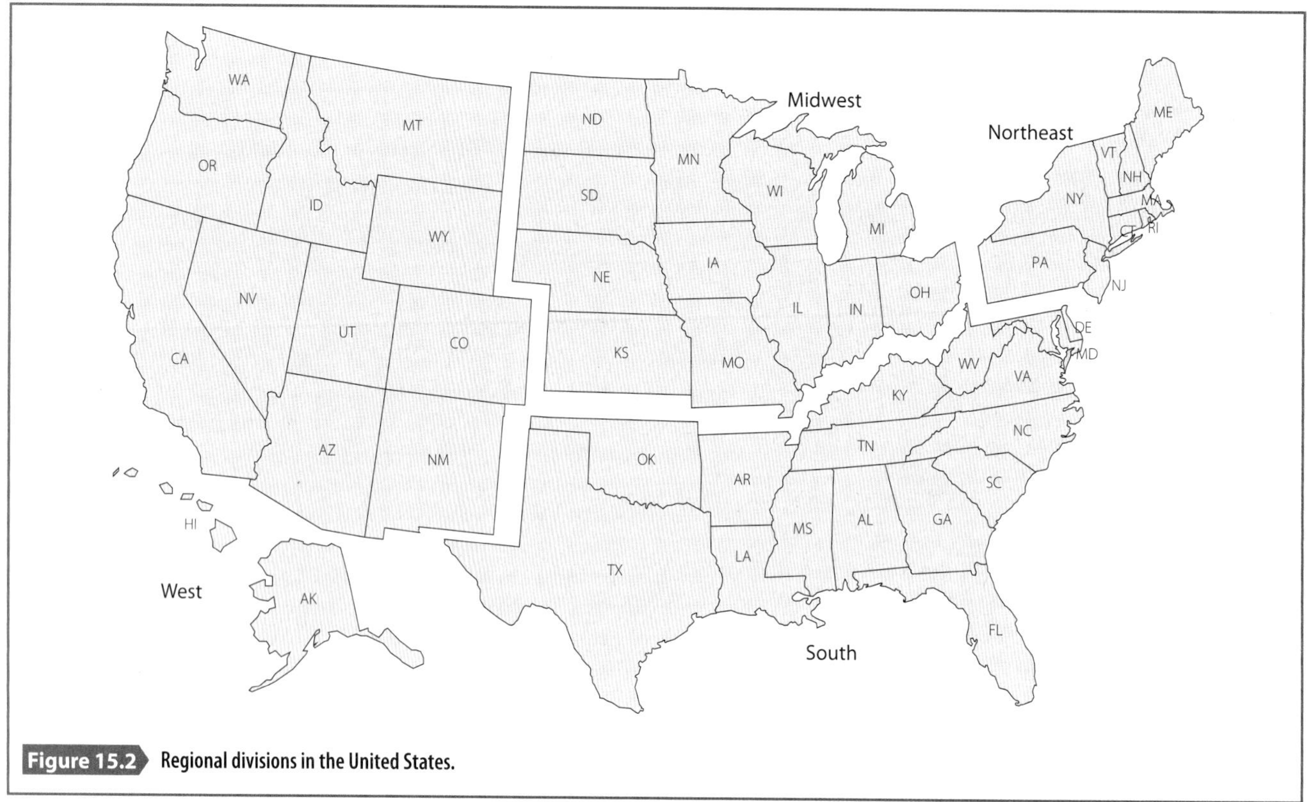

Figure 15.2 Regional divisions in the United States.

Native American societies supplanted by European settlements. The colonial immigrants from England, Germany, the Netherlands, and France were followed by newcomers from Ireland, Italy, Portugal, Poland, and other central and eastern European countries, particularly in the Mid-Atlantic states. African Americans from the South and more recent immigrants from the Caribbean, Central America, Africa, and Asia have added to the diversity of some parts of the Northeast (refer to each chapter on ethnic food habits for more immigration details and Table 15.1).

Seventeen percent of the total U.S. population is found in the Northeast.[13] Over nine million of those individuals (16 percent) were born in another country. Thirty-one percent of those living in the Northeast region are Asian and 44 percent are Latinx. Disproportionately large populations of Black and Latinx Americans reside in New York and New Jersey. Yet, the rest of the Northeast is still predominantly White, including large percentages of Italians, Ukrainians, Portuguese, French Canadians, Russians, Lithuanians, Slovaks, and Poles. Nearly half of all American Jews also live in the Northeast, primarily in New York, New Jersey, and Massachusetts.[13]

As noted in Table 15.1, the Northeast had a total population of 57.6 million in 2020. The median age was 40 years. The median household income was $72,698, compared to $64,994 nationally. The poverty level is lower than the national rate at 11.6 percent. The largest number of immigrants to the northeast come from Latin America (44 percent), and Asia (31 percent). The predominant races are White (61 percent), Hispanic (15 percent), Black (11 percent), and Asian (7 percent).

Table 15.1 Northeast Region Profile 2020

	Northeast Region	United States
Population	57,609,148	326,569,308
Median age	40 years	38 years
Median household Income	$72,698	$64,994
Poverty	11.6%	12.8%
Education:		
High School	89.7%	88.5%
> Bachelor's degree	37.7%	32.9%
Place of Birth:		
Europe	17%	11%
Asia	31%	31%
Africa	6%	5%
Oceana	0%	1%
Latin America	44%	50%
North American	2%	2%
Race & Ethnicity:		
White	61%	60%
Black	11%	12%
Native	0%	1%
Asian	7%	6%
Islander	0%	0%
Other	1%	0%
Two Races	2%	3%
Hispanic	15%	18%

U.S. Census Bureau (2020). *American Community Survey 5-year estimates*. Retrieved from Census *Reporter Profile page for Northeast Region* http://censusreporter.org/profiles/02000US1-northeast-region/

Traditional Fare

The cooking of the Northeast features the abundance of the Atlantic, the plenty of native and introduced produce, and the freshwater wealth of the many rivers and lakes (refer to Table 15.2). In New England, seafood—such as clams, lobster, scallops, and fish, especially cod—has been prominent. Indigenous game, including wild turkey and venison, supplemented the poultry, pork, and beef brought by early immigrants. The foundation of the diet was traditionally corn, and many dishes of the region reflect its importance. Beans have also made a substantial contribution. Root vegetables such as potatoes, onions, beets, turnips, rutabagas, and carrots were quickly added to the vegetable selection. Wild berries, including blueberries, cranberries, gooseberries, and cloudberries (which look like bleached blackberries), grapes, and beach plums were the main fruits consumed until the apple orchards planted by immigrants became productive. Maple sugar sweetened many foods in New England. Even when molasses and cane sugar became widely available, maple syrup was preferred for many dishes.

The warmer weather and fertile lands of the Mid-Atlantic states have provided even more native foods than New England. The coastal waters offer clams, oysters, mussels, scallops, and crabs, while the estuaries shelter ducks, geese, and turtles. Passenger pigeons once darkened the skies with their massive numbers, and bison roamed the area around Lake Erie. Freshwater fish such as catfish, eels, pickerel, salmon, shad, smelt, trout, and whitefish were plentiful; at one time, shad, a flavorful relative of the herring, was the most numerous of all freshwater fish in the United States. Both the flesh and roe were commonly eaten.

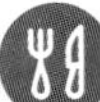

Food for Thought

Fudge was originally a maple sugar candy popular in New England in the 1800s. When cocoa powder became widely available after the invention of the cocoa press in 1828, eating chocolate was developed. The press could inexpensively pulverize the cacao beans into a fine powder which was then mixed with liquids and other ingredients and poured into molds for confections.[14]

Shad migrate from the ocean up freshwater rivers to spawn in early summer. Shadberries (also known as juneberries) are a popular treat that ripen at the same time the fish arrive each year.

Salmon served with fresh peas is a Fourth of July tradition for many New Englanders.

Introduced foods also flourished in the region. Cabbage, potatoes, yams, carrots, peas, apples, pears, cherries, peaches, and strawberries were easily grown. Tomatoes thrived in the hot summers. Although New Jersey is now one of the most

Table 15.2 Northeastern Specialties

Group	Foods	Preparations
Protein Foods		
Milk/milk products	Cream; cheddar and cream cheese	Cream soups, sauces, puddings; ice cream
Meats/poultry/fish/eggs	Native game, particularly venison and turkey Preserved meats, such as corned beef, pastrami, salt pork, ham, bacon, sausages Seafood prevalent, especially clams, lobster, oysters, scallops Salt and freshwater fish, such as salt cod and shad Numerous beans (e.g., cranberry, kidney, lima)	New England boiled dinner; scrapple; red-flannel hash Fish stews, soups; clam chowder; clam bakes; oyster or lobster loafs Cod cakes; shad bakes; *gefilte* fish Baked beans; succotash
Cereals/Grains	Corn, wheat, rye	Cornmeal porridges, puddings, and breads Dumplings Baked goods—savory and sweet pies, cakes, doughnuts, waffles, pretzels, bagels
Fruits/Vegetables	Apples, blueberries, cranberries, grapes Cabbage, fiddlehead fern fronds, potatoes	Applesauce, apple butter; fruit puddings, pies Coleslaw; sauerkraut; ferns on toast; potatoes—mashed, fried, creamed, baked, scalloped, hashed, as croquettes, salad
Additional Foods		
Seasonings	Salt, pepper, onions, saffron	
Nuts/seeds	Black walnuts, butternuts	
Beverages	Apple cider, hard cider, applejack; ale, beer; rum, whiskey; wine	New York State white, red, sparkling wines; sherry, port
Fats/oils	Lard, butter	
Sweeteners	Maple sugar; molasses	Maple sugar candies, maple syrup pie; chocolates

industrialized states in the nation, it is still known as the Garden State due to the success of these early agricultural efforts. Wheat, which was difficult to grow in New England, did well in the Mid-Atlantic. At one time, New York provided all the wheat consumed in the Northeast and much of the South.

New England

The cuisine of New England has been shaped predominantly by Native American preparation techniques combined with British homestyle cooking. Roasting, boiling, and stewing are preferred. Dishes are often made with cream, and strong seasonings are avoided. People of the region take pride in simple fare.

The immigrants of the early seventeenth century were mostly tradespeople, inexperienced in farming and husbandry. History abounds with tales of how the first settlers were dependent on the skills and generosity of local Native Americans in preventing starvation (refer to Chapter 5). Corn dishes were especially significant. Cornmeal porridge cooked into a mush-like consistency was a Native American food called samp by the early colonists. It was often prepared with another cornerstone of the Indian diet, beans. New Englanders used cornmeal to adapt the traditional wheat-based English dish known as hasty pudding. The settlers would pour cornmeal porridge into a loaf pan to firm up overnight, then slice it and serve it topped with cream. This new dish, often flavored with maple syrup or molasses, was named Indian pudding.

Steamed, baked, and boiled puddings were eaten daily in New England homes. They were known as grunts (steamed dough and berries), slumps (baked puddings), and flummeries (a British molded oatmeal or custard pudding). As in England, a pudding could be savory or sweet and was generally served at the beginning of the meal. Breads were also a mainstay. Many were dense and baked without any leavening (reliable leavenings such as baking powder and baking soda were not available until the mid-1900s). Homegrown yeast from potatoes, hops, or the dregs of beer barrels were used in some recipes. Cornbread cooked in a skillet over the fire was most common. Rye, which grows well in cooler climates, was often combined with Native American cornmeal to make a popular bread called ryaninjun (from "rye 'n' Indian"). Stewed pumpkin was sometimes added for a moister loaf. Boston brown bread is a traditional recipe of the region—a steamed loaf made with whole-wheat and rye flours (sometimes with cornmeal as well) and flavored with molasses.

Pork, cod, or beef flavored most main dishes. Long winters required that most meats and fish be preserved, and few recipes called for fresh cuts. Salt pork, bacon, smoked pork, dried salt cod, corned beef, and dried beef were common, usually braised or stewed with vegetables. The New England boiled dinner was typical. This one-pot meal is still popular throughout the region and usually includes corned beef brisket simmered for hours with potatoes, onions, carrots, turnips, and, traditionally, beets. Cabbage is added toward the end of the cooking time. Seasoning is mild, often just a little black pepper. Leftovers are often chopped up the next day and heated in a skillet with a little cream and sometimes some bacon and more onions to make another New England specialty known as a red-flannel hash, so called because the cooked beets would bleed into the other ingredients during frying. A dried salt cod and potato version of the New England boiled dinner is prepared in Massachusetts, called Cape Cod turkey. Plymouth succotash is another example. Although this Native American dish (refer to Chapter 5) is often associated with southern fare today, it was popular in the Northeast during colonial times. It combined corned beef, turkey or chicken, beans, corn, potatoes, and turnips. Other variations featured just vegetables or combinations of meats, poultry, and fish.

Food for Thought

The oldest continually operating cheese factory in the United States was founded in 1822 in Healdville, Vermont.

The Maine bean pot is based on the Native American method of placing the ingredients in a pot that is then buried in a pit over embers, a so-called bean hole.

During the colonial period, dried salt cod was exchanged for fruit in the Mediterranean and for molasses in the Caribbean (the molasses was then used to make rum). Cod traders in Massachusetts became wealthy and were nicknamed the "codfish aristocracy."

Other popular dishes included dried beef rehydrated in boiling water and served with cream sauce over bread or potatoes (precursor to what is called chipped beef today) and fried salt pork topped with cream gravy. New England states without access to the coast were more dependent on meat, poultry, and dairy products. Today, New Hampshire is acknowledged for the quality of its butter, and Vermont is famous for its cheeses, such as cheddar and the similar, but milder, Colby.

Beans were eaten regularly in early New England. Best known are baked beans flavored with molasses or maple syrup and salt pork, a recipe adapted from the Native American dish. Traditionally, the Puritans prepared a large pot of beans on Saturday morning, simmered them over the fire all day, and then ate them with Boston brown bread for dinner to start the Sabbath (observed from sundown to sundown). Leftovers were kept warm on the hearth for Sunday breakfast and lunch, often codfish cakes.[15] Boston is still known as Beantown due to its long association with baked beans. In Maine, a version of baked beans called bean pot is made with indigenous yellow-eye, cranberry, or kidney beans.

Pies made with suet pastry were served at many meals. Savory kinds included an American version of the British steak and kidney pie, chicken pot pie (later topped with biscuits instead of pie crust), a ground pork and onion pie seasoned with allspice called tourtière introduced by French Canadians in the region (served traditionally at Christmas or on New Year's Day), clam pie, lobster and oyster pie, and salt-cod pie covered with mashed potatoes. Sweet pies were also popular, especially apple pies, made with fresh apple slices, dried rings, or even applesauce. Mincemeat, a traditional English treat combining savory and sweet ingredients, was featured at many meals because the filling of meat, dried fruits, nuts, and rum or other alcoholic preservatives aged well, becoming tastier over time. Today, fried pies (fried applesauce turnovers flavored with cinnamon) and apple pie topped with sliced cheddar cheese are Vermont favorites, while in New Hampshire, apple pie is sometimes drenched in maple syrup. Blueberry pie is a specialty in Maine.

No discussion of New England fare is complete without further detailing fish and shellfish use in coastal areas. In Massachusetts, for example, cod helped sustain the earliest populations, and Cape Cod, the peninsula that curls out into the Atlantic, was so named in 1602 for an abundance of the fish. The Puritans used it in boiled and baked dishes, soups, stews, hash, and, most notably, codfish cakes. These cakes, which are also called codfish balls, are still a sign of regional affiliation for some residents of the Boston area. In Connecticut, shad was enjoyed by the Native Americans of the region but disdained by the earliest Europeans in the area due to its multitude of tiny, difficult-to-remove bones. By the mid-eighteenth century, Connecticut residents had changed their opinion of shad, especially the roe, which they fried quickly in butter. Traditionally, Native Americans would plank the fish and slowly cook it at the edge of hot coals, a method still practiced today at shad bakes where the fillets are placed on an oak board with strips of bacon, then grilled or smoked.

Lobster is a specialty, especially in Maine. The Native Americans of the area consumed the meat, used the discarded shells for fertilizer, and formed the claws into pipes. British settlers mostly added lobster meat to mixed fish dishes, and later colonialists added it to salads, sauces, soups, and fried croquettes. Commercial trapping began in the late 1800s with the advent of shipping by train and the development of the canning industry. The lobster supply diminished rapidly, increasing its prestige and popularity—today trapping regulations are strict. In addition to steamed or grilled lobster tail, a specialty in Maine and other coastal areas is lobster rolls, which take two forms (both served on toasted, fluffy white bread buns): plain meat drenched in butter, or meat mixed with mayonnaise, celery, onions, and lemon juice.[15]

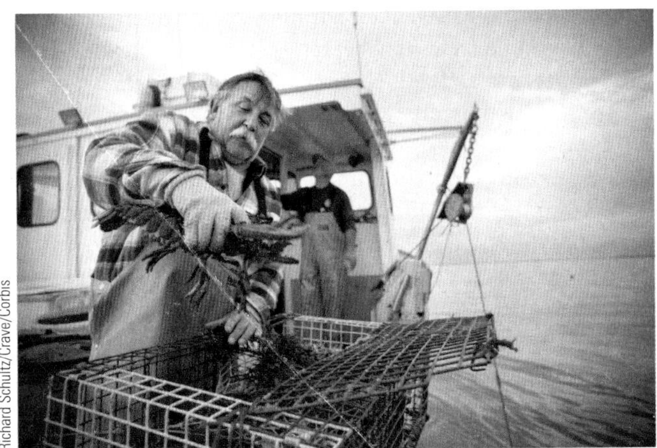

Richard Schultz/Crave/Corbis

▲ **Lobster is a specialty of Maine, though it is also trapped in other New England coastal states.**

Clams, oysters, and scallops are also New England favorites. The clambake, in which clams, corn, and other items such as onions, potatoes, or lobster are steamed in a pit on the beach, shares some similarities with Native American seafood feasts. Clams are also featured in the cream-based soup known as clam chowder. One version, the cream-based Boston clam chowder, is known nationally. It is typically garnished with Boston crackers or oyster crackers, the slightly sweet, small, dry biscuits invented by Massachusetts sea captains for use on long journeys aboard ship. In Rhode Island tomato-based red clam chowder, a soup inaccurately attributed to Manhattan, is popular. Clams called steamers are just that—steamed and served with broth and melted butter (a bucket of steamers is often the first course of a lobster dinner). Oysters were typically prepared with cream and breadcrumbs in a dish called scalloped oysters or served in oyster stew. In Rhode Island, they were especially popular among the nineteenth-century elite, who served them in pies (raw oysters in a cream sauce topped with biscuit dough), as patties, creamed, curried, and, for New Year's Eve, pickled, with eggnog to wash them down. Today, they are commonly broiled with bacon or breaded and deep-fried. Bay, sea, and Digby scallops are prepared similarly to oysters. In Maine, two less common shellfish specialties are found. The first is mussels (the state provides nearly two-thirds of those shellfish consumed nationally), and the second is sea urchin roe (uni), served at local restaurants and sushi bars, or exported to Japan.[16]

There are two fruits particularly associated with the New England area. The first is cranberries, known as sassamanesh by some eastern Native Americans and as ibimi or bitter berry by Pequots and Leni-Lenape people, who ate them fresh with maple syrup, or dried and added to pemmican. Dutch and German settlers introduced the term Kranbeere, meaning "crane berry," because the flower resembles the head of a crane. Cranberries grow exceptionally well in the sandy peat bogs of eastern Massachusetts, where they were first cultivated in the early 1800s. They are used primarily in juices and sauces, though in recent years, dried cranberries have become popular as snacks or added to baked goods. The second fruit is wild or low-bush blueberries, which are used mostly in baked goods. Maine grows nearly 100 percent of this variety in the United States.

New England desserts are mostly fruit based. In addition to the puddings and pies already discussed, pandowdies

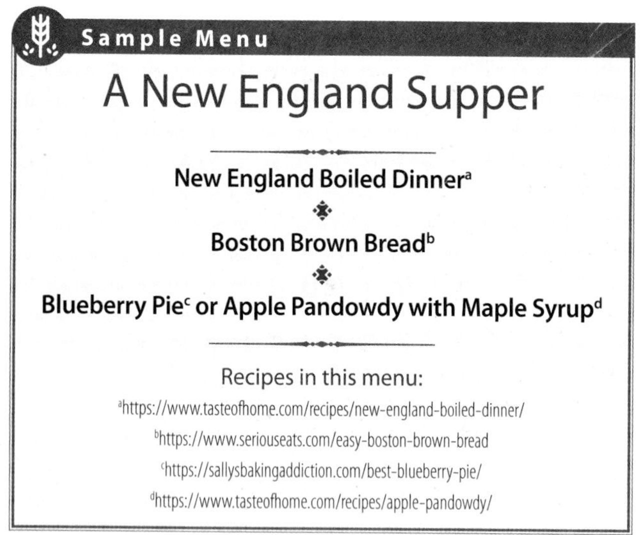

Sample Menu

A New England Supper

New England Boiled Dinner[a]

Boston Brown Bread[b]

Blueberry Pie[c] **or Apple Pandowdy with Maple Syrup**[d]

Recipes in this menu:

[a]https://www.tasteofhome.com/recipes/new-england-boiled-dinner/

[b]https://www.seriouseats.com/easy-boston-brown-bread

[c]https://sallysbakingaddiction.com/best-blueberry-pie/

[d]https://www.tasteofhome.com/recipes/apple-pandowdy/

(baked fruit layered with bread), shortbreads (fruit preserves, biscuits, and cream), and roly-polies (fruit rolled up in biscuit dough, then baked) were other favorites. Pound cakes and fruitcakes were enjoyed but were difficult to make before commercial leavening and reliable ovens were available.

No sweet is as associated with New England, particularly Vermont, as is maple syrup. The sweet sap of the sugar maple tree had long been used by Native Americans of the Northeast to cook beans and meats and to flavor other items (refer to Chapter 5). Syrup was an everyday sweetener in colonial kitchens throughout the region until cane sugar became more affordable. Maple syrup production peaked in the 1880s, and the sweet has since become costly. Vermont specialties include sugar-on-snow (hot syrup poured over fresh snow to make a chewy taffy eaten with pickles or doughnuts), maple syrup pie (with a filling of cream, eggs, and syrup), and maple sugar candies.

Food for Thought

One New England dessert popular throughout the nation is chocolate chip cookies, which were created by Ruth Wakefield in 1930 at the Toll House Inn in Whitman, Massachusetts.

Boston cream pie, a favorite in New England, is not a pie but a custard-filled white cake covered with chocolate icing. It probably derives from a popular colonial dessert called "pudding cake" that included cake, custard, and usually fruit or jam.

Tea and apple cider were consumed daily in colonial times. Hard cider, an alcoholic beverage caused by the fermentation of sugars in apple cider, was also favored. Many New Englanders would start their day with a pint of beer or ale made from barley, corn, pumpkins, persimmons, or spruce bark. Rum, as well as whiskey made from rye, was available. Wine from dandelions or gooseberries was a specialty, and an American version of the English drink called syllabub, containing apple cider, sherry or wine, and whipped cream, was served on special occasions. Today, apple cider remains a regional specialty, particularly in New Hampshire.

Mid-Atlantic

Many of the influences on New England fare are seen in the foods of the Mid-Atlantic states as well. Native American fare was combined with immigrant preferences to produce a new regional cuisine. Unlike New England, where most of the colonists were from England, many settlers in New Jersey, New York, and Pennsylvania came from the Netherlands and Germany. They provided a distinctively different flavor to foods, including greater use of pork (especially sausages) and dairy products, more baked goods, and stronger seasonings. Later immigrants from southern and eastern Europe contributed many specialties. Further, the warmer climate and fertile farmlands offered a greater variety of ingredients to the cooks of New York, New Jersey, and Pennsylvania.

The Dutch in the mid-1600s brought wheat to the New York area, which at the time was known as New Netherland. They also grew barley, buckwheat, and rye. Although these were preferred grains, the Dutch used what they called "turkey wheat" (corn) to make a boiled milk and cornmeal porridge known as suppawn that was eaten daily at breakfast. This same porridge was topped with meats and vegetables for lunch, then baked to make the hearty dish called hutspot, an American adaptation of a stew common in the Netherlands.

Dairy cattle provided ample milk, butter, and cheese. The Dutch were among the first settlers wealthy enough to import sugar, brandy, chocolate, and numerous spices, including pepper, cloves, cinnamon, and saffron. Many Dutch specialties of the region have made their way into American cooking, including pickled cabbage; Kool sla (from the Dutch word for "cabbage"), now known as coleslaw; and headcheese, a ball-shaped sausage made from the head and feet of the hog. Doughnuts, crullers, pancakes, and waffles were also introduced by the Dutch.

During the same period, German immigrants arrived in the United States. Some sought religious freedom (mostly Mennonites, with smaller numbers of Amish, Schwenkfelders, and other sects) who made their home in the tolerant colony of Pennsylvania (refer to Chapter 7). They became known as the Pennsylvania Dutch, a corruption of the German word Deutsch, which means "German." Although some German religious communities remained isolated (and are even to this day), many German immigrants gradually became integrated into the broader populations of Pennsylvania and surrounding states. Likewise, many German foods of the region have become an indistinguishable part of U.S. cuisine.

Pork was the foundation of the German diet, and immigrants brought ham, pork chops, pork schnitzel (pounded into thin slices), bacon, salt pork, pickled pig's knuckles, souse (jellied pig's feet loaf), maw (stomach stuffed with meat and vegetables), and a German version of headcheese. Every part of the hog was used, and leftovers would be stretched with lima beans to make a Pennsylvania version of baked beans with ham (*bohne mit schinken un'grumberra*) or dried green beans and potatoes. The best-known leftover dish is scrapple, still popular throughout the state. Scrapple is a combination of ground pork or sausage, cornmeal porridge, and spices formed into a loaf, sliced into thick slabs when firm, and fried in butter. It is typically served with fried eggs, applesauce, and maple syrup. In addition, smoked and fresh sausages were consumed daily. Chicken stews and soups, made substantial with homemade noodles or dumplings, were also popular with the Pennsylvania Dutch. Beef was used in the braised roast known as sauerbraten and in the smoked, cured dried beef called Bündnerfleisch.

Asparagus, green peas, sugar peas (called Mennonite pod peas), and rhubarb are a few of the vegetables favored by the Pennsylvania Dutch. Potatoes are eaten mashed, fried, creamed, baked, scalloped, hashed, as croquettes, as dumplings, in stews and soups, and as potato salad. Cabbage is also ubiquitous, mostly as sauerkraut and slaw. Apples are particularly popular—fresh, as applesauce, in pastries, as cider, and in preserves such as the thick, sweet spread known as apple butter. Many fruits and vegetables are pickled or preserved. Examples include spiced pears, pickled watermelon rind, sweet pickles, and corn relish. Dark rye bread, cornbread, yeast rolls, potato rolls, cinnamon rolls and sticky buns, streuselkuchen (coffeecakes with a sugar crumb topping), fastnachts (doughnuts), and buckwheat pancakes are just a few of the baked goods found in the region. The Pennsylvania Dutch are also known for numerous desserts, especially pies (refer to Chapter 7).

Though generally considered a rural cuisine, Pennsylvania Dutch fare was well accepted in the early urban centers of the state, such as Pittsburgh, Allentown, Bethlehem, and Reading. Even Philadelphia, which was founded by English Quakers, favored German foods. Scrapple has become so associated with the city that it is often called Philadelphia scrapple, despite its country beginnings. It is eaten for breakfast, often drizzled with catsup, and is used to make deep-fried croquettes or to stuff vegetables like green peppers and cabbage for dinner. Lebanon bologna is a Pennsylvania Dutch smoked beef sausage that has become a state specialty. It is traditionally sliced, battered, or dipped in bread crumbs, fried, and served with sauerkraut and mashed potatoes. Although the origins are lost to history, Philadelphia pepper pot, a soup made with tripe, onions, potatoes, and black peppercorns, is most likely a Pennsylvania Dutch recipe and is sometimes served with dumplings. Cheesesteak (grilled strips of beef topped with American cheese and grilled onions in a toasted Italian roll), the quintessential Philadelphia sandwich, was supposedly invented during the 1930s when Pat Olivieri, a hot dog push-cart vendor, was in the mood for something else to eat and sent his brother to a local butcher shop for meat. Olivieri cooked the chopped beef on his cart's grill, scooping it into an Italian roll with onions, and a new sandwich was born.

The hearty fare of the Dutch and Germans combined with many traditional items also found in New England, such as puddings, savory pies, and seafood soups and stews, to produce Mid-Atlantic cuisine. Later immigrants to the Mid-Atlantic region introduced foods that have become associated with certain cities and states. Notably, southern Italians in New York and New Jersey brought pizza, spaghetti with tomato–meat sauce, calzone, cannoli, gelato, and espresso. Eastern European Jews introduced pastrami, smoked salmon and whitefish, chopped liver, and other deli items. Particularly in New York, other eastern European, Russian, Greek, Chinese, Caribbean Island, and Middle Eastern cuisines became popular, due, in part, to numerous ethnic eateries (refer to chapters on each group for more information). New York is noteworthy for the influence of its restaurant fare. Taverns, boarding houses, oyster houses, and coffeehouses served the needs of those eating out in the late eighteenth and early nineteenth centuries. The first European-style bakery was opened in 1825, and delicatessens serving the Jewish community were established in the 1880s. Full-service continental-style restaurants became popular in the mid-1800s. By the turn of the century, New York City had become the gastronomic center of the nation. And it continued to expand in cuisine offerings: 1920, Nom Wah Tea parlor opened and has since become the oldest continuously run restaurant in Chinatown of Manhattan. Many dishes created for elite diners are now American specialties, such as Waldorf salad (originally a mixture of apples and celery in mayonnaise served at the Waldorf-Astoria), vichyssoise (chilled leek and potato soup from the Ritz-Carlton), Lobster Newburg (lobster tail topped with a Madeira-flavored cream sauce), and the dessert baked Alaska (from Delmonico's).

Food for Thought

Buffalo wings, deep-fried chicken wings drenched in spicy seasoned butter (often using Tabasco® sauce) and served with celery and blue cheese dressing, evolved in Buffalo-area bars during the 1960s. No one has established the exact origins of the appetizer.

The word cookie is derived from the Dutch word for a small cake, koekje.

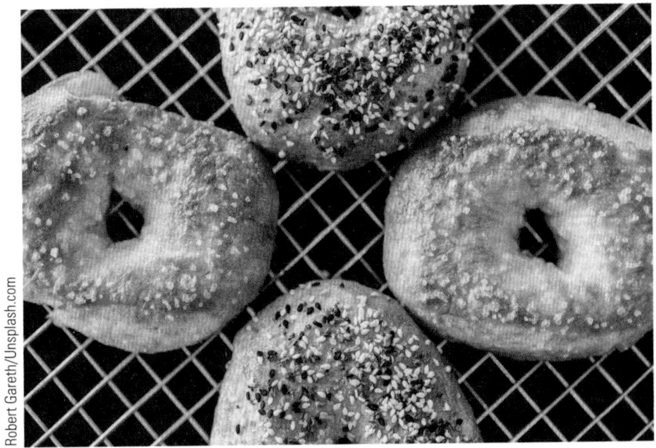

Robert Gareth/Unsplash.com

▲ **Bagels, introduced by Polish immigrants, were paired with an 1872 New York invention, cream cheese; the chewy doughnut- shaped roll was popularized nationwide during the 1990s.**

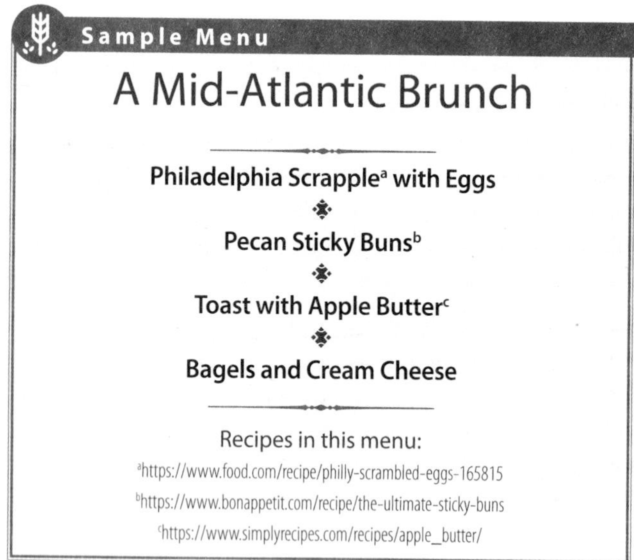
Sample Menu

A Mid-Atlantic Brunch

Philadelphia Scrapple[a] with Eggs

Pecan Sticky Buns[b]

Toast with Apple Butter[c]

Bagels and Cream Cheese

Recipes in this menu:

[a]https://www.food.com/recipe/philly-scrambled-eggs-165815

[b]https://www.bonappetit.com/recipe/the-ultimate-sticky-buns

[c]https://www.simplyrecipes.com/recipes/apple_butter/

New Jersey, often called the garden basket of New York due to its numerous commercial crops, is also known for its contributions to food technology. Scientific work on hybridization has yielded new, improved varieties of peaches, tomatoes, and sweet potatoes. Food-processing techniques developed in New Jersey include condensed, canned soups (the Campbell Soup Company); inspected, bottled milk (the Borden Company); and the first application of pasteurization to milk at a small farm outside Princeton. Black tea, in convenient individually sized bags, was introduced in Hoboken in 1880 (the Thomas J. Lipton Company).

In addition to the Dutch and Pennsylvania Dutch cookies, doughnuts, pies, pancakes, and waffles of the region, other sweets have gained nationwide acceptance, especially those from Pennsylvania. Philadelphia was one of the first cities to enjoy ice cream, perhaps as early as 1782. An ice cream parlor with frozen treats, cakes, syrups, and cordials was opened in 1800, and the following years saw the first wholesale distributor of ice cream and the first ice cream soda. The city gained a reputation for a high-quality product, and ice cream molded into flowers, fruits, animals, or holiday icons is still a specialty. Another confectionery contribution was affordable chocolate. In Pennsylvania, commercial production of chocolate for beverages and bonbons began during the late 1700s, though it was so costly it was considered a luxury item. Milton Hershey of Derry Church was the first manufacturer of chocolate for the mass market beginning in 1905 when he reduced his expenses by making uniform bars instead of fancy novelties. Two years later, he introduced the chocolate candy, Hershey's Kisses.

Food for Thought

Coffee milk, similar to chocolate milk but made with coffee syrup, is the official state beverage of Rhode Island.

Several beverages are associated with the Mid-Atlantic states. American beer, a heavy, top-fermented beverage similar to English ale, was first commercially produced during the late seventeenth century in Pennsylvania. Two hundred years later, a German immigrant to Philadelphia founded the first brewery that made a bottom-fermented beverage. The new, lighter beer known as lager, or pilsner, soon became synonymous with beer in the United States (refer to Chapter 7). New York has been a major wine producer in the Northeast and is third nationally behind California and Washington. Wine varieties such as chardonnay, riesling, and Seyve-Villard, and reds such as cabernet sauvignon and merlot, as well as sparkling wines and some fortified wines, such as sherry and port. New Jersey is the state where hard apple cider was first distilled to produce the apple brandy known as applejack, sometimes called New Jersey lightning.

Health Concerns

Americans continue to experience large disparities by geography, education, race, and ethnicity in the context of health. State-specific data suggest that people living in the New England states are often healthier than the U.S. average, while those in the Mid-Atlantic states are closer to national norms (refer to chapters on each ethnic group for population-specific data). As in all of the regions of the United States, obesity and rates of diabetes have consistently increased in the Northeast and Mid-Atlantic states (refer to Figures 15.3 and 15.4). For the four regions of the United States, five states (Vermont, New Hampshire, Connecticut, Massachusetts, and New Jersey) in the Northeast rank in the top 10 for healthy behaviors. The Northeast region is the healthiest in the United States (refer to Figure 15.5).

The number of cigarette smokers reporting daily smoking is highest among smokers living in the Midwest. The highest death rate due to lung cancer is in the south and the lowest is in the west (refer to Figure 15.6).

Food for Thought

The number of farms in the United States has dropped from 5.7 million in 1900 to 2 million in 2020. During this period, the average size of each remaining farm has more than tripled.

The Midwest

Regional Profile

The Midwest is known as the Great Plains region of the United States. The earliest American settlers and European immigrants in the area found a vast, mostly flat terrain covered by tall prairie grasses. Oak-wooded hills and low mountain ridges ringed the territory. The rich soil irrigated by the extensive Mississippi and Missouri River systems proved ideal for wheat, corn, and numerous fruits. The region is still renowned for its agricultural productivity, which is why it is nicknamed "America's breadbasket."

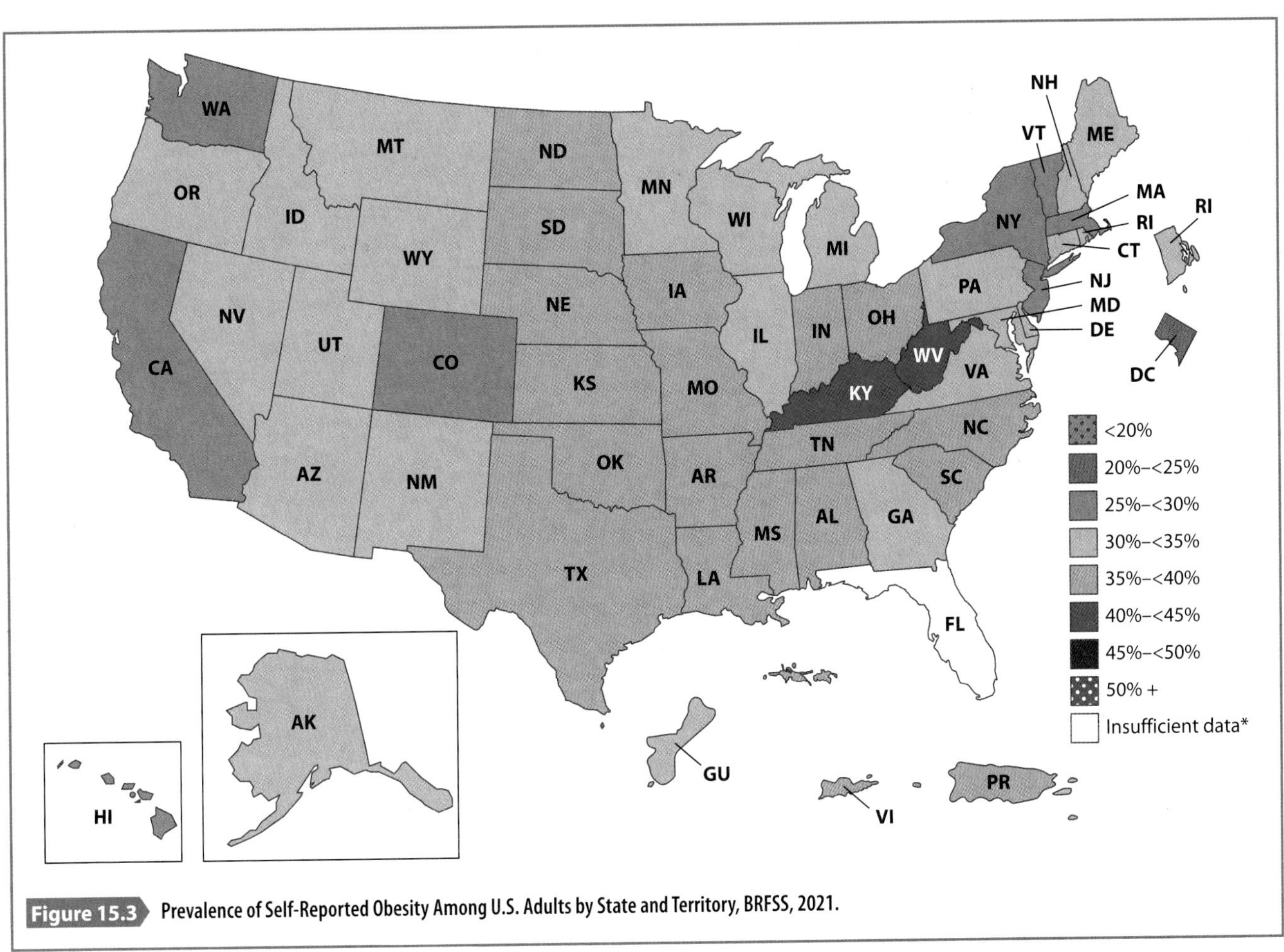

Figure 15.3 Prevalence of Self-Reported Obesity Among U.S. Adults by State and Territory, BRFSS, 2021.

The Midwest encompasses twelve states with 21 percent of the total land area and just over 21 percent of the total U.S. population.[18] It is divided into the east north central region (Illinois, Indiana, Michigan, Ohio, and Wisconsin), and the west north central region (Iowa, Kansas, Minnesota, Missouri, Nebraska, North Dakota, and South Dakota).

The states of the east north central Midwest area are bounded by the Great Lakes, which temper the climate. Although the French were the first Europeans to explore the region, it was Americans from the Northeast states, as well as Virginia and Delaware, who were the first pioneers. Later, immigrants from Germany, Switzerland, Scandinavia, central Europe, and the Cornwall area of England were attracted by the fishing, dairy, mining, lumber, and meat-packing industries. The west north central Midwest states are geographically near the center of North America, exposed to long winters, short summers, and extreme temperatures. Most Americans who settled the territory were homesteaders, interested in the inexpensive land and farming opportunities. They came from New England and the Mid-Atlantic states, followed by new immigrants from Germany, Scandinavia, and central Europe, particularly Poland.

As suggested by the history of immigration to the area, the Midwest has the largest percentage of White communities in the nation. Over half of all U.S. citizens of Czech and Norwegian ancestry live in the Midwest, as well as large numbers of people of Finnish, Croatian, Swedish, German, and Polish heritage. There are below-average numbers of Black Americans (approximately 10 percent of the total population) throughout the Midwest; the exceptions are in Ohio, Michigan, and Illinois, which have slightly above-average Black American populations. Native Americans, Latin Americans, and Asians/residents of Oceania are also underrepresented, although there is a large population of Latinx in Illinois, approaching the national average, and above-average numbers of Native Americans in the Dakotas.

Almost 5 million individuals (7.3 percent) living in the Midwest region were born in another country. One immigrant group that has made the Midwest home are people from Laos, including Hmong, who have arrived since the 1970s (refer to Chapter 12 for immigration history and food habits). About 37 percent of all Hmong counted in 2019 live in Minnesota, Wisconsin, and Michigan.[19] Thirty-four percent are from Latin America. Additional recent immigrant populations

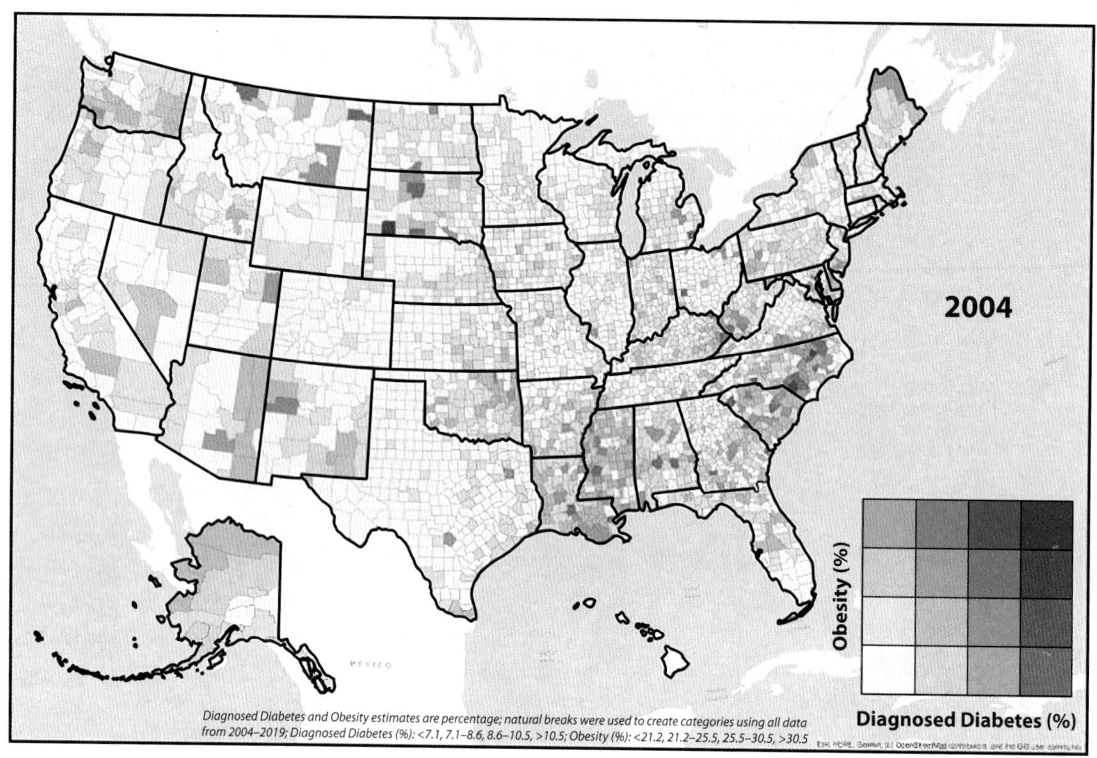

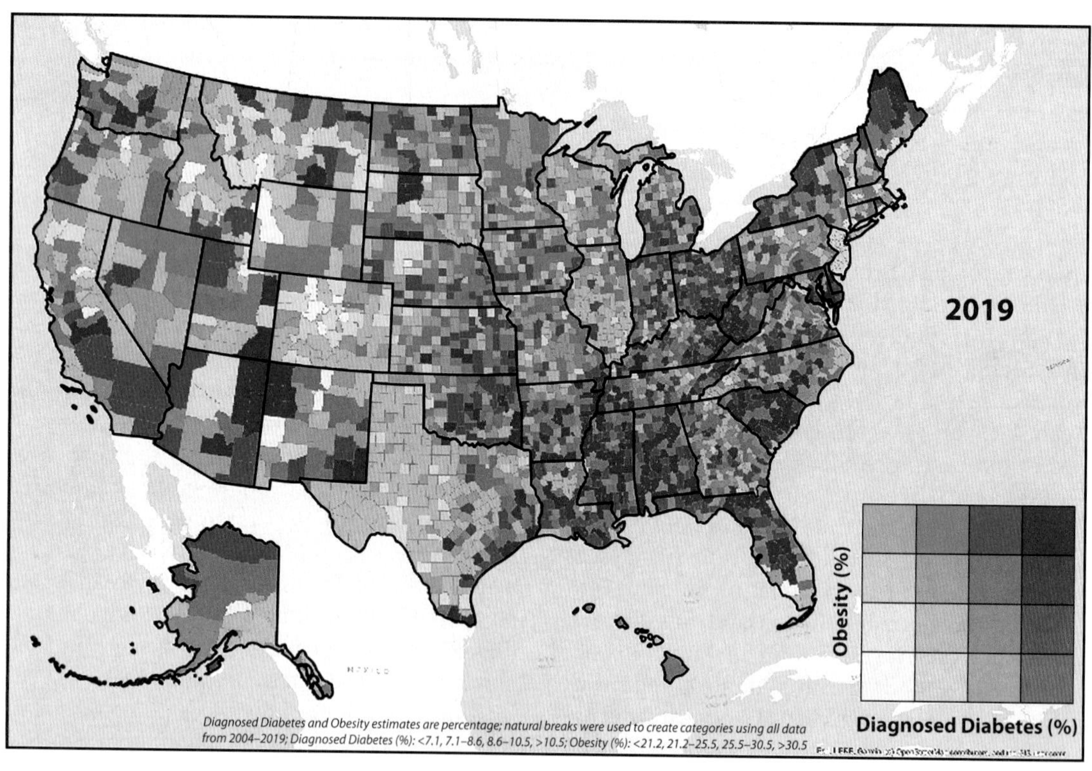

Figure 15.4 Comparison of Obesity and Diabetes from 2004 to 2019.

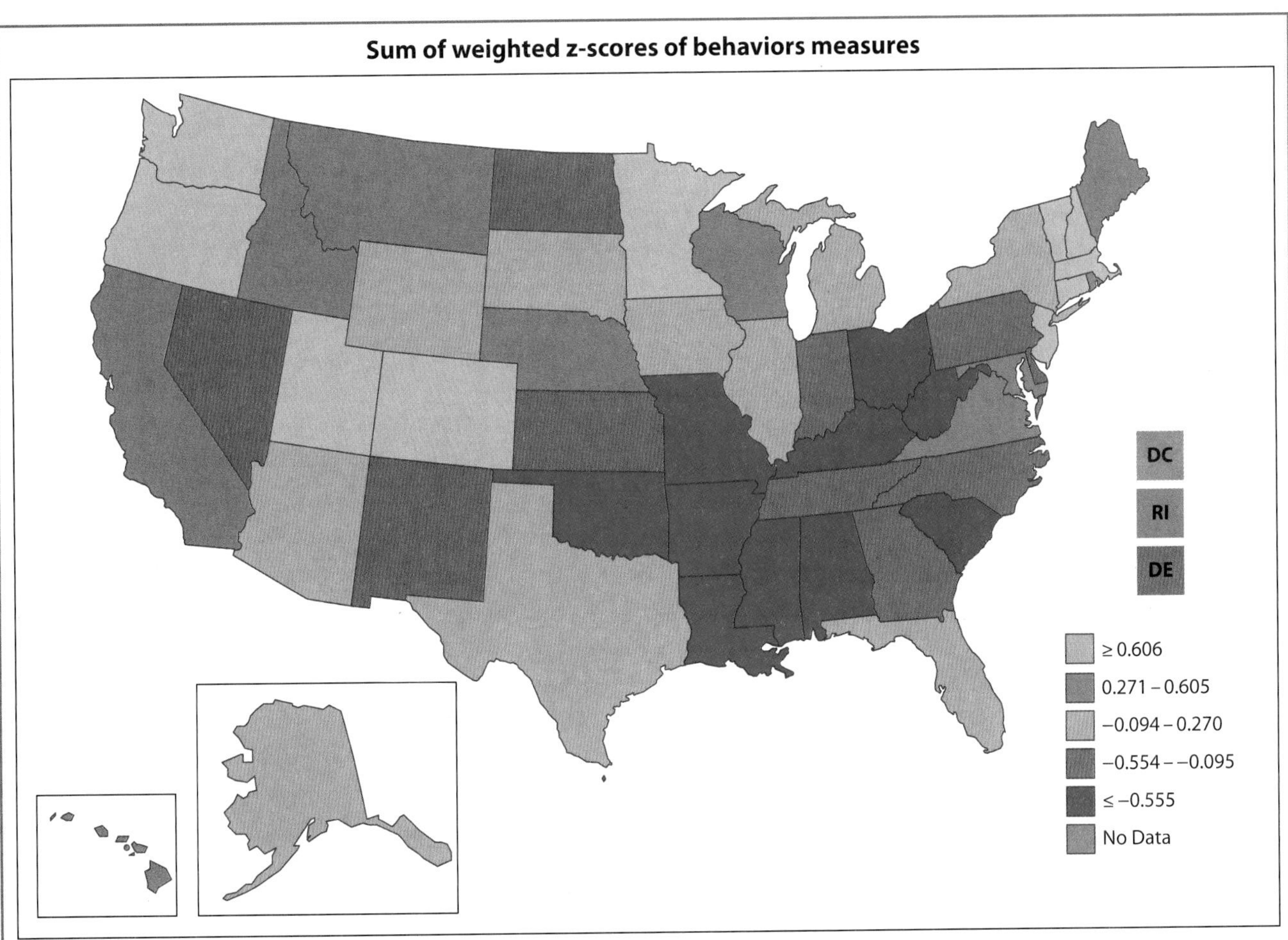

State	Rank	Z-score	State	Rank	Z-score	State	Rank	Z-score
Vermont	1	1.179	Virginia	18	0.334	North Dakota	35	−0.238
Utah	2	1.049	Hawaii	19	0.302	Indiana	36	−0.400
Minnesota	3	0.928	Rhode Island	20	0.271	Georgia	37	−0.435
New Hampshire	4	0.919	New York	21	0.228	North Carolina	38	−0.453
Colorado	5	0.820	Arizona	22	0.189	Nevada	39	−0.532
Connecticut	6	0.733	Texas	23	0.132	Tennessee	40	−0.554
Oregon	7	0.715	Wyoming	24	0.044	Missouri	41	−0.599
Massachusetts	8	0.680	Florida	25	0.008	Ohio	42	−0.615
Washington	9	0.624	Alaska	26	−0.009	South Carolina	43	−0.752
New Jersey	10	0.606	Iowa	27	−0.050	West Virginia	44	−0.889
Maine	11	0.587	South Dakota	28	−0.065	Oklahoma	45	−0.930
Idaho	12	0.501	Illinois	29	−0.068	Arkansas	46	−1.097
Wisconsin	13	0.468	Michigan	30	−0.094	Alabama	47	−1.194
Maryland	14	0.434	Kansas	31	−0.148	Kentucky	48	−1.339
California	15	0.420	Pennsylvania	32	−0.149	Mississippi	49	−1.358
Nebraska	16	0.399	Delaware	33	−0.177	Louisiana	50	−1.374
Montana	17	0.398	New Mexico	34	−0.204			

Northeast Region
Midwest Region
South
West

Figure 15.5 **Ranks of Healthiest Behaviors by State, with 1 being healthiest and 50 being least healthy. Health behaviors are defined by sleep health, physical activity and nutrition, sexual health, and tobacco use.**

Source: America's Health Rankings. 2021. Behaviors by state. United Health Foundation. Retrieved from https://www.americashealthrankings.org/explore/annual/measure/behavior/state/ALL (accessed May 2, 2022).

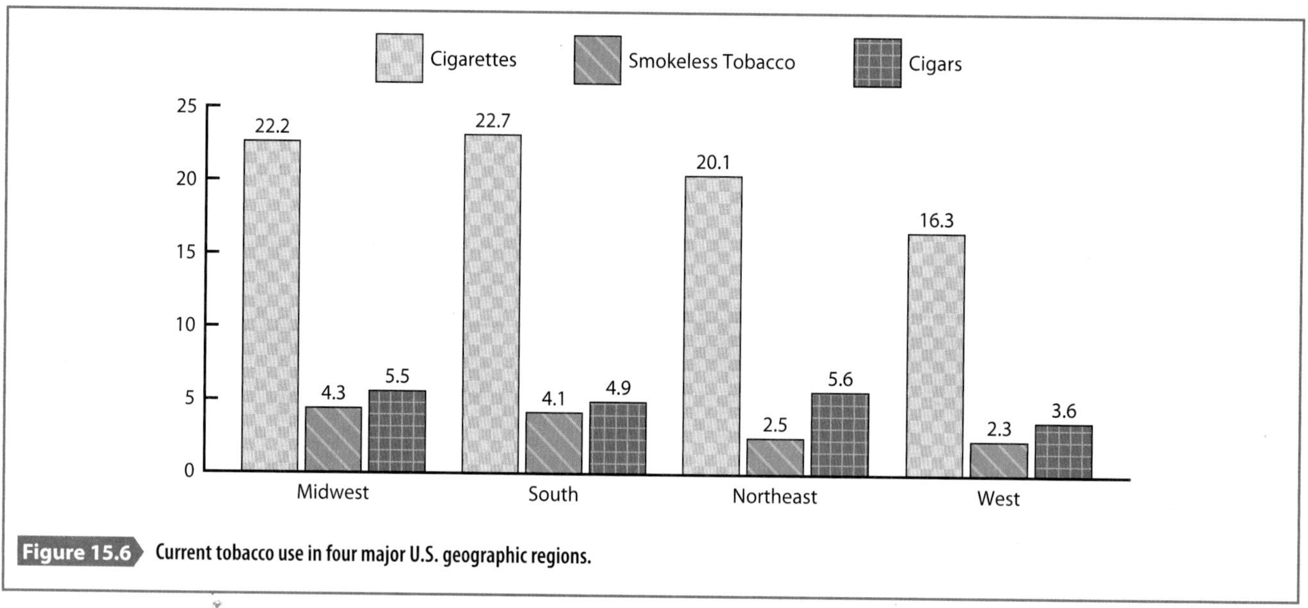

Figure 15.6 Current tobacco use in four major U.S. geographic regions.

include Asian Indians in Illinois and Michigan, Koreans in Illinois, Middle Easterners in Michigan, and Russians in Illinois and Ohio.

The Midwest has the lowest percentage of people living in metropolitan areas in the United States. Median household income is slightly less than the national average, at $62,054 according to 2020 American Community Survey data. Approximately 12.3 percent of individuals living in the Midwest are considered to be living in poverty (refer to Table 15.3).[20]

Traditional Fare

Traditional Midwestern fare is often described as no-frills homestead and farm food, exemplifying what is called typical American cuisine (see Table 15.4). Prime meat or poultry is prepared simply and served with vegetables, potatoes, and fresh bread. In many families, hearty breakfasts start the day, robust soups and stews replenish body and spirit, and homespun desserts round out the meal.

In the Midwest, beef and pork are preferred meats. Canning and freezing to preserve summer's bounty is less common in urban areas today, though traditions persist and are rising again in popularity. Bread is sometimes baked at home, and pies make use of seasonal fruits. Midwestern hospitality, exemplified by festive sorghum harvests, group apple peelings, and canning parties, among other gatherings, is continued through buffets, potluck suppers, ice cream socials, corn roasts, and fish boils popular throughout the region, especially in small towns and rural areas.

East North Central

The earliest American settlement in the east north central region of the Midwest was in Marietta, Ohio, in 1788. The

Table 15.3 Midwest Region Profile 2020

	Midwest Region	United States
Population	68,219,726	326,569,308
Median age	38.6 years	38 years
Median household Income	$62,054	$64,994
Poverty	12.3%	12.8%
Education:		
High School	91%	88.5%
≥ Bachelor's degree	31.4%	32.9%
Place of Birth:		
Europe	17%	11%
Asia	37%	31%
Africa	9%	5%
Oceana	0%	1%
Latin America	34%	50%
North American	2%	2%
Race & Ethnicity:		
White	75%	60%
Black	10%	12%
Native	1%	1%
Asian	3%	6%
Islander	0%	0%
Other	0%	0%
Two Races	3%	3%
Hispanic	8%	18%

U.S. Census Bureau. 2020. *American Community Survey 5-year estimates*. Retrieved from *Census Reporter Profile page for Midwest Region*. https://censusreporter.org/profiles/02000US2-midwest-region/

Table 15.4 Midwestern Specialities

Group	Foods	Preparations
Protein Foods		
Milk/milk products	Milk, buttermilk, butter, cream, cheeses	Cream gravy, fondue, *rømmegrøt*, *skyr*
Meat/poultry/ fish/eggs/ legumes	Native game, including buffalo, venison, beaver, raccoon, opossum, turkey, prairie chickens (grouse), pheasant Pork in all forms, especially salt pork, hams (country ham and Westphalian ham), and sausages (bratwurst, weinerwurst, kielbasa); beef Oysters shipped from the East Coast Freshwater fish, especially smelt, sturgeon, trout, and whitefish Dried beans	Jerky, *booyah, Hasenpfeffer* Ham with gravy, pork chops, barbecued pork, hot dogs, *Bubbat* Beef pot pie, stew, barbecued brisket, bierocks, pasties, Cincinnati chili Fish boils, fried trout or smelt Baked beans with salt pork or bacon
Cereals/Grains	Corn, wheat, rye, oats, wild rice	Cornbreads, porridges; oatmeal; *bannocks*; rye breads, pumpernickel; biscuits, dumplings (including stuffed, such as *pierogi* and *verenikas*) Baked goods, especially fresh fruit pies (apple, cherry, persimmon, rhubarb), iced cakes, strawberry shortcakes, strudel, *kolaches*, butter cookies, pancakes, *aebelskivers*, Danish pastries
Fruits/Vegetables	Apples, berries (blueberries, elderberries, strawberries), cherries, grapes, peaches, persimmons, rhubarb Cabbage, onions, peas, potatoes, rutabagas, turnips, wild mushrooms	Applesauce; apple butter, fritters, bread, salad; fried apples, candied apples; fruit jams and jellies Sauerkraut, sauerkraut balls; coleslaw; potatoes—boiled, fried, baked, as dumplings, salad; onion pie
Additional Foods		
Seasonings	Salt, pepper; parsley, dill; cinnamon, ginger, nutmeg, saffron; molasses	Most foods are preferred mildly spiced
Nuts/seeds	Almonds, black walnuts, hickory nuts, pecans; poppy seeds	Nut pies, almond paste; nut candies; poppy seed cakes and pastries
Beverages	Apple juice, beer, wine, apple brandy	Lager-style (American) beer
Fats/oils	Butter, lard	
Sweeteners	Sugar, honey, molasses, sorghum	

people who came to the area from the original colonies were mostly farmers who survived in their new homes on hogs, corn, beans, squash and pumpkins, cabbage, and potatoes. Corn, a Native American crop, was eaten at every meal as porridge or as baked or fried bread. Sun-dried or smoked meat strips called jerky were also adopted from the Native Americans of the region, used first for game such as venison, then later for beef. Other wild meats, poultry, and fish, such as rabbit, squirrel, woodchuck, opossum, raccoon, skunks, duck, quail, sturgeon, and trout, were widely available. Even bear meat was consumed.[21] Native fruits included persimmons, blueberries, bush cranberries, gooseberries, ground cherries, grapes, and many types of nuts. Later settlers brought wheat and oats, as well as apples, cherries, peaches, and berries. Fishing provided salmon, smelt, trout, and other freshwater fish; dairying, particularly cheese making, offered further food variety.

Today, agricultural products are still significant in the region. In addition to wheat and corn, soybeans are a primary crop in Illinois and Ohio, grown for oil (used in products such as margarine, mayonnaise, salad dressing, and for industrial purposes), meat substitutes, and animal feed. Apples are a major crop in Michigan—local preparations include apple salad, apple meatloaf, and apple bread. The French introduced sour European cooking cherries to Michigan, where nearly all of these nationally consumed fruits are produced. Once unusual, an Illinois specialty is horseradish. German immigrants brought eastern European food to the state, and the pungent, gnarly root thrived. Illinois is the largest producer of horseradish in the United States.

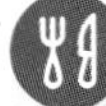

Food for Thought

The origins of meatloaf, the quintessential midwestern beef dish, are unknown. It may have come with German immigrants who sometimes added rye bread as an extender, or sauerkraut for moisture to ground meat dishes, it might have been medieval, or have other tantalizing origins. Regardless, it was first recorded in the 1870s in the United States as a breakfast dish.[22]

Fish boils combining fish, potatoes, onions, and salt were begun by Scandinavians as an efficient way to feed the workers at lumber camps. Today, fish boils at the edge of Lake Michigan are annual tourist events in Wisconsin.

Dairying remains important in some regions as well. For many years, Wisconsin was the leading U.S. producer of milk, sweetened condensed milk, butter, and cheese, although in 2020 and 2021 California topped the country in milk production.[23] Dairying was sparked by the arrival of Swiss farmers to the state in the 1840s. They brought their expertise in breeding livestock and making cheese. Colby, a hard cheese similar to cheddar, is an original Wisconsin cheese that was created in 1885. Another variety developed in Wisconsin is brick, a semisoft cheese with holes and a flavor described as sweet, nutty, and spicy. Italian cheeses, including ricotta, mozzarella, provolone, Romano, and Parmesan, are specialties of northern Wisconsin, while blue cheese is made in the caves near Milwaukee.

Contributions in food processing from the east north central Midwest states have extended beyond regional importance to influence the development of American cuisine. Many of these changes took place in Illinois during the late 1800s and early 1900s. Historical accounts include stories about Philip Armour, who made millions in pork sales when he founded the first large-scale meatpacking plant in Chicago; Gustavus Swift, who made his fortune in hams and sausages; Oscar Mayer, a German immigrant who got his start in the hot dog business as a butcher in Chicago; Louis Rich, a Russian immigrant who became involved in poultry processing and founded a turkey luncheon meat empire; and James Lewis Kraft, a grocery clerk and Canadian immigrant, who came up with the idea that home-delivered, uniform pieces of cheese would be more popular than freshly cut wedges from a large wheel. He later introduced processed and prepackaged cheeses, including Velveeta.

Developments were not limited to Illinois. In Ohio, an Austrian immigrant, Charles Fleischmann, created the first standardized yeast cakes for baking (he later formed a distillery that produced the first American gin). Michigan is probably best known for its role in the creation of the U.S. cereal industry. The city of Battle Creek was home to two health sanitariums during the late nineteenth century. The first was founded by Seventh-Day Adventist leader Ellen Harmon White, who advocated vegetarianism. Her medical director was Dr. John Kellogg, the inventor of cornflakes (refer to Chapter 4). C.W. Post, a former Kellogg patient, started his own health institute in Battle Creek. He created a coffee substitute, Postum (a blend of wheat berries, bran, and molasses), and a cereal based on his own recipe for digestive problems, called Grape-Nuts.[24]

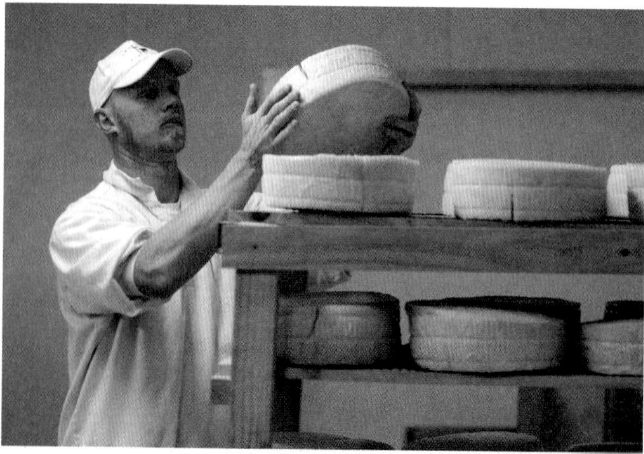

Will Salter/Lonely Planet Images/Getty Images

▲ **Wisconsin is known for its dairy foods, especially cheeses such as Colby and brick.**

Each group of pioneers in the region brought favorite dishes, though some had already been altered by available ingredients such as those Native Americans, Africans, or Latin Americans might use. Baked beans, meat pot pies with biscuit topping, and succotash were preferred by settlers from New England. In Ohio, these settlers stuffed meats with breadcrumbs, a practice still popular in the state. The people from New York and Pennsylvania favored sausages, sauerkraut, pickles, and relishes when they moved westward. In Indiana, where the earliest pioneers came from the South, pork is especially popular, including roasts and chops, and sometimes the whole roasted pig. Sausage patties and ham are common for breakfast, typically served with pancakes or biscuits, cream gravy, and fried apples. The southern influence is also seen in batter-fried chicken served with fried biscuits (made with a yeast dough that puffs up into spheres when dropped into hot oil, then slathered with butter while still warm).

In areas where European immigrants congregated in numbers, regional ethnic fare developed. For example, the Michigan Dutch (actually from the Netherlands, not Germans like the Pennsylvania Dutch) brought ham croquettes, pea soup, saucijzenbroodjes (now known in English as pigs-in-a-blanket), and double-salted licorice. In Ohio, the fare of European immigrants was more broadly integrated into the regional cuisine: Germans popularized sausage, ham, potato, and cabbage dishes, such as the unusual Ohio specialty called sauerkraut balls (deep-fried sauerkraut and ham fritters served with mustard sauce); Polish immigrants introduced pierogis (boiled dumplings traditionally stuffed with potatoes, cabbage, onion, and/or meat, or fruit), kielbasa sausage, and strudel (flaky pastry rolls filled with sweetened fruit, nuts, poppy seeds, or cheese). Fish boils, pickled fish, and meatballs are just a few of the items adopted from Scandinavian immigrants in Wisconsin. Some European foods are so well accepted that their ethnic associations have been forgotten. Eastern Europeans brought to Wisconsin their pork or veal sausages, which are now considered state specialties—Sheboygan is the self-proclaimed "Bratwurst Capital of the World." Missouri also has a strong bratwurst tradition, particularly in areas settled by German immigrants. In other cases, European influence has been more limited, seen mostly in one or two dishes, such as Swiss cheese fondue in Indiana, and in Michigan, a dish with French roots known as booyah (perhaps from the term bouillon), a game stew featuring venison or whatever else was available (including rabbit, woodchuck, squirrel, muskrat, or duck), salt pork, carrots, potatoes, and onions.

Other dishes with ethnic origins have been adapted to midwestern tastes, losing much of their heritage along the way.

For example, Ohio is probably best known nationally for Cincinnati chili. It is an all-beef version created by Slavic-Macedonian immigrants, brothers Athanas (Tom) and Ivan (John) Kiradjieff, in 1922, flavored with a balanced blend of sweet spices (e.g., cinnamon, allspice, cloves, and nutmeg) and hot spices (garlic, cumin, black pepper, and dried chilies). Some researchers note the similarities between the seasoning of Cincinnati chili and dishes such as pastitsio or moussaka (refer to Chapter 13).[25] Chili parlors found throughout Ohio (and parts of nearby Kentucky) serve the mild chili "one-way" (just the meaty stew alone), "two-way" (over spaghetti), "three-way" (spaghetti, chili, grated-cheese topping), "four-way" (spaghetti, chili, cheese, and diced onions), or "five-way" (spaghetti, chili, cheese, onions, and kidney beans).

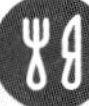

Food for Thought

Wisconsin fare is can favor "white" foods such as whitefish (from the Great Lakes) and white meat (pork, veal, or chicken) combined with white dairy products (such as farmer's cheese, cottage cheese, cream cheese, fresh cream, or sour cream).

Deep-dish Chicago-style pizza is baked in a skillet. It is an American adaptation of the pizza brought to the region by Italian immigrants from Naples.

The origins of some dishes reflect the succession of immigration to an area. Cornish pasties are an example. Miners from Cornwall arrived in Michigan's Upper Peninsula to excavate iron and copper in the 1840s, bringing their traditional lunch specialty called pasties (refer to Chapter 6). This complete meal-in-a-turnover often featured venison in the Michigan versions, with potatoes and turnips as the common vegetable filling at one end. At the other (dessert) end of the pasty, apples were the most popular fruit. When immigrants from Finland came in the following years, they adopted the dish, which was similar to piraat and kalakukko, Finnish pastries filled with meat or fish, rice, and vegetables. The origins of the dish are claimed by many Finns in the region, though those of Cornish descent point out that the Finnish turnovers are not pasties because the filling is mixed instead of layered. Today's pasty shops, often featuring untraditional fillings (e.g., pizza ingredients), are common throughout the Upper Peninsula (UP) and in cities where "UPers" ("Yoopers"), those native to the Upper Peninsula of Michigan, have settled, such as Detroit.

Sweets, especially baked goods, hold a special place in the cooking of the east north central Midwest states. Traditional items such as hickory nut cookies and pies are found in many areas. In Indiana, dessert favorites include steamed or baked persimmon pudding; pork cake, a moist dessert made with sausage or salt pork, molasses, brown sugar, flour, dried fruits, and spices that is a Christmas tradition in some Indiana homes; and sweet cream pie, pastry filled with a

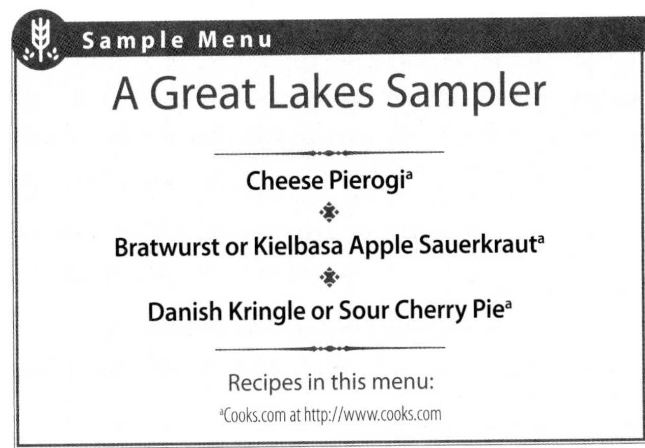

Sample Menu

A Great Lakes Sampler

Cheese Pierogi[a]

Bratwurst or Kielbasa Apple Sauerkraut[a]

Danish Kringle or Sour Cherry Pie[a]

Recipes in this menu:

[a]Cooks.com at http://www.cooks.com

heavily sweetened custard that is popular all year. In Michigan apple fritters, caramel-covered apples, candied apples, and Dutch apple kock (cake) are common. Elderberry-flower fritters dipped in powdered sugar are also a specialty. In Wisconsin, many popular desserts have retained their foreign names, including German kuchen (yeasted coffee cake, often with a fruit and cream filling and crunchy, sugary streusel topping) and schaum torte (meringue topped with ice cream and/or whipped cream and fresh fruit); and Danish kringle (pretzel- or ring-shaped flaky pastry with fruit, nut, cheese, or butterscotch filling).

Beer is especially associated with the Midwest, particularly Wisconsin. The first breweries were located in the southwestern section of the state and produced the ales and stouts favored by English settlers. By the middle of the nineteenth century, however, ten breweries producing German-style lagers and pilsners had been founded in Milwaukee, including plants owned by Frederick Miller, Frederick Pabst, and Joseph Schlitz. At the beginning of the 1900s, there were over 300 breweries statewide, but Prohibition and consolidation in recent years have reduced that number. In 2022, 28 breweries were based in Milwaukee, had a brewery in the city or a Milwaukee taproom.

In St. Louis, too, beer producers influenced the economy in the 1840s and 1850s, when thousands of German immigrants arrived. There, 18-year-old immigrant Adolphus Busch met Eberhard Anheuser, owner of Bavarian Brewery, married his daughter, and went on to create Anheuser Busch Brewing Company. Busch took advantage of the new refrigerated train cars to spread his products beyond the region and used pasteurization in the brewing process. The company introduced Budweiser in 1876.[26,27]

West North Central

Other settlers in the west north central Midwest states in the mid-nineteenth century came to farm the fertile land of Iowa, Kansas, Minnesota, and Missouri. Harsh winters and a scarcity of provisions limited variety in many early pioneer homes. Homemakers of the period describe burying melons in sand, which with luck would stay fresh until Christmas. Other cooks would prepare up to a hundred fresh fruit pies at a time, covering the extras with snow for use throughout the winter months. Parched corn, herbs, bark, or root brews replaced coffee.[28] Prestige foods were often unavailable, so ample, even excessive, amounts of common foods became symbolic of hospitality in the midwestern frontier. The more western areas of the west north central Midwest states, which are drier and less suitable for crops, provided limited opportunities for agriculture. The region attracted trappers, traders, and prospectors. Wild game, such as bear, buffalo, elk, deer, small mammals, as well as turkeys, prairie chickens (grouse), quail, doves, and frogs, was hunted; the meat or oil was often sold in settlement towns. These regional foods were first documented in *Mrs. Seely's Cookbook: A Manual of French and American Cookery* in 1902.[29]

As in the east north central Midwest region, pioneers from New England and the Mid-Atlantic states contributed dishes eaten frequently in their eastern homes: Baked beans and pies of all sorts became as common as sausages and sauerkraut. One northeastern specialty that became surprisingly popular throughout the Midwest was oysters. By the mid-1800s the live shellfish were shipped regularly by express companies to the region packed in barrels filled with wet straw. They were canned as well and sent via the railroads. Scholars write, "An ambitious young congressman, Abraham Lincoln, entertained friends and associates in Illinois with oysters served up in every conceivable fashion"[30] and one 1859 recipe for small birds, such as magpies, suggested stuffing a breaded oyster into each bird before roasting over a fire.[28]

Irrigation improved crop production, and today corn, wheat, soybeans, and sugar beets are widely cultivated throughout the region. Barley, oats, sunflowers, rutabagas, and rye are other crops in some areas. Wild rice, seeds of a native North American aquatic grass found in shallow rivers and lakes, is a Minnesota specialty (refer to Chapter 5). Though Missouri has 15.6 million acres of cropland, nearly 7 million acres are pastureland and over 4 million acres are woodlands, according to the state's agricultural census in 2017. Areas of the state are well-suited for nut trees such as the native eastern black walnut tree. The nuts are strongly flavored with a slightly bitter aftertaste and are the primary ingredient in black walnut pie and flavor other seasonal treats such as black walnut ice cream. Pecans, too, are indigenous to the state. They are popular in pies, candies, cookies, and cakes. Further, beekeepers take advantage of the woodlands in Missouri to provide another specialty of the region—honey.

Iowa is noteworthy for its commercial hog farms and is the number one producer of pork in the nation. Pork is also a favorite in Missouri and the state is well known for its country hams, which are cured with salt, then smoked and hung to age in the cool winter months. The resulting meat is red, salty, and dry in texture. It is traditionally served with biscuits and red-eyed gravy made from ham drippings, coffee, and flour.

While barbeque traditions vary by region, Kansas City barbeque often is seasoned with a dry rub, slow-smoked over a variety of woods, and served with a tomato-based sweet-tangy flavorful sauce. Other traditional styles of barbeque in the United States include Texas style, Carolina style, and Memphis style.[31]

Beef is significant in Kansas, Nebraska, and the Dakotas. Before the introduction of cattle to the region, over 30 million bison roamed the Great Plains, providing sustenance, clothing, shelter, and fuel to the local Native Americans. American settlers and European immigrants also ate bison, what they called hump-backed beef. However, the huge bison herds interfered with expanding settlements, the railroads, and Texas cattlemen, who drove their longhorns through the prairie states to the slaughterhouses of the North and East. In addition to these pressures on the bison herds, their slaughter was also seen by top generals, politicians, and President Ulysses S. Grant as a way Native Americans could be starved into submission.[32] Though completely eradicated as a food at the time, today bison meat has become available again in parts of the Midwest, and the largest buffalo ranches are found in South Dakota. Kansas is famous for its corn-fed beef, and cattle are the most important agricultural commodity in the state. Steaks, beef stews, barbecued beef, and hamburgers are often Kansas favorites. In South Dakota, early settlers introduced longhorn cattle from Texas; they were soon joined by Scottish cattle, including Aberdeen, Angus, and Herefords. Immigrants from Scotland were soon exporting beef to their homeland. Cattle ranching is a major industry in the state, though sheep and hogs are also important commodities. South Dakota is one of the only states in the west north central Midwest that features lamb dish specialties.

Despite a preference for pork or beef, poultry is well represented in west north central Midwest fare. Chicken with dumplings or noodles, pan-fried chicken with cream gravy, and chicken or turkey pot pies (topped with pastry or biscuits) are classic midwestern dishes.

Food for Thought

Dairying is common in several west north central Midwest states. Minnesota is one of the top butter and cheese producers in the nation, and Iowa is known for the development of American blue cheese, introduced in the 1920s by Maytag Dairy Farms.

Pierogi, dough dumplings stuffed with a filling such as meat, potato, or cheese, are known as pelmeni by some Russians, varenyky by Ukrainians, and verenikas by German Russian Mennonites.

Several notable religious communities settled in west north central Midwest states. In Iowa the Amish who established homes around Kalona grew all of their own food and butchered all of their own meat, traditions still practiced today. Cornbread with tomato juice gravy, stews or hashes with potatoes and peas, fried meats and eggs, and fresh fruit pies are common dishes. A group of German Lutherans, known as True Inspirationists, settled in seven Iowa villages in 1859 to form what is known as the Amana Colonies. They lived communally, with everyone eating three generous meals and two coffee breaks each day in a large dining hall. The weekly menu was set and included mehlspeisen (literally "flour desserts," such as simple puddings) on Tuesdays and boiled beef every Wednesday. The Colonies now serve German specialties to visiting tourists in several large restaurants. German Russian Mennonites (who had first migrated from Germany to southern Russia) came to Kansas in the 1870s. They brought German-style foods familiar in Pennsylvania Dutch areas, such as chicken noodle soup, pancakes, sausages, and buttermilk pie. They also introduced verenikas (their term for pierogis) served with cream gravy. Beef rolls stuffed with bacon, onions, and pickles similar to German rouladen, and sausage-filled buns called bubbat are other Kansas dishes brought by the German Russian Mennonites.

Food for Thought

The Danish community of Askov, Minnesota, has an annual festival commemorating the rutabaga. Although the tuber is often called a "Swede" or "Swedish turnip," Danes are believed to have introduced the rutabaga to the region.

European influence was seen in secular settlements as well. German Russian yeast dough turnovers (typically filled with beef, cabbage, and onions) are common throughout the Great Plains. They were derived from the Russian pirozhki. The turnovers are called bierocks in Kansas and the Midwestern regions east and south of that state, and they are known as runsas in Nebraska and the northern Midwest areas.

In Minnesota, German immigrants brought hogs and dairy cattle and introduced their dark rye breads, including pumpernickel, to the region. Specialties such as hasenpfeffer (stewed rabbit), spätzle (tiny dumplings), and maultaschen (a sort of German ravioli filled with ground ham, eggs, onions, and sometimes spinach) were other common German dishes. Preserved fish was a mainstay for the Scandinavians. Pickled fish, smoked fish, and salt-cured fish were popular, particularly the Norwegian dish known as lutefisk (refer to Chapter 7), served with butter and potatoes. Ham, bacon, Swedish meatballs, and Danish frikadeller (fried, breaded ground beef and veal patties) were consumed. Dark breads and the thin Norwegian potato pancake called lefser are still common, as are butter cookies (especially at Christmas) and Danish aebleskivers (pancake balls), traditionally served with chokecherry or blueberry syrup or jam. The Scandinavian concept of the smörgåsbord was introduced to the nation in Minnesota (refer to Chapter 7). Several ethnic communities in Minnesota maintain their culinary heritage at holidays and festivals, including the German Catholic city New Ulm and the Danish town Askov.

In Nebraska, the Swiss introduced plum tarts and a specialty called thuna, breadsticks topped with creamed greens thickened with flour. Czech settlers brought jaternice (pork sausage), jelita (blood sausage), and houska (a sweet, braided bread). Swedish yeasted waffles and Hungarian chicken paprika are other examples of European contributions to the state. In Missouri, the French introduced crêpes and brioche to the region. Germans as well as French and some Italian settlers brought winemaking to the state, as well as hard cider from apples and brandy from peaches. Missouri was the largest grape producer in the United States until Prohibition and the 18th Amendment put an end to the industry.[33] Winemaking has slowly reemerged in the state since the 1970s. In North Dakota, the Norwegians brought spekejøtt (smoked, dried lamb), rullepølse (cold, spicy rolled beef), and søtsuppe (fruit soup) and baked goods, including the large pyramid of almond paste and meringue rings called kransekake. A large population of settlers from Iceland smoked mutton, made skyr (a sweet, cultured milk product similar to yogurt), fried kleinur (doughnuts), and baked vinarterta (a multilayered cardamom-flavored cake with fruit fillings) for dessert. The Scotch Irish introduced colcannon (mashed potatoes, onions, and cabbage), and the French Canadians came with croissants and cassoulet (refer to Chapter 6).

A unique cuisine of the Midwest is found in the Ozark Mountains of Missouri. Contrary to immigration trends in urban areas, the people who came to the Ozarks gradually arrived from other states in small groups and were scattered throughout the region. They subsisted on hunting, fishing, gathering, and cultivating corn, beans, squash, and various tubers.[33] Hogs were let loose to forage until butchering time in December or January. The people of the Ozarks were known for their stews made from opossum, raccoon, or squirrel. Sorghum was used to sweeten foods, ginger root was brewed for beer, and sassafras was steeped for tea. Today, the Ozarks are best known as a vacation and retirement destination.

Popular desserts in the west north central Midwest states include fruit pies and frosted cakes. Czech kolaches are a specialty found throughout the region. These yeasted buns are baked with an indentation on top that is filled with sweetened cheese, poppy seeds, or fruit (apple, apricot, cherry, and prune are traditional) and sprinkled with sugar or streusel before they are baked. The Scandinavian dessert kransekake (an almond ring cake) is also found in many communities.

Health Concerns

Measures of health in the Midwest are high for coronary risk factors and this region has the highest smoking prevalence in the United States (refer to Figure 15.6).[34] For more on the United States' health rankings of Midwest states, refer to Figure 15.5. Significantly higher-than-average rates of heavy drinking are found in Michigan, Minnesota, Wisconsin, North Dakota, Nebraska, Illinois, and Iowa, with the highest rate in Wisconsin.

The South

Regional Profile

Many southerners say the South is more an attitude than a location. This perhaps explains why there are so many definitions of the region, such as those states below the historic

Mason-Dixon Line or those south of the culinary grits line (the divide between where grits are eaten and where they aren't). While few question the U.S. federal government designation that Alabama, Arkansas, Florida, Georgia, Louisiana, Kentucky, Maryland, Mississippi, the Carolinas, Tennessee, Virginia, and West Virginia are part of the South, the borderline states of Delaware, Missouri, Oklahoma, and Texas can be argued for inclusion either way. Using the U.S. government definition, Missouri is considered part of the Midwest, whereas Delaware, Oklahoma, and Texas are part of the South.

The lands of the South are varied. They include the fertile coastal plains along the Atlantic and Gulf Coasts, the rolling hills leading up to the mountains (called the piedmont in most states), the rugged Appalachian and Ozark Mountain territories, the lowlands of the Mississippi Delta, and the high desert plains of the western reaches. The climate also ranges from the warm, moderate Atlantic states and the hot, humid Gulf Coast states to the hot, dry weather in parts of Texas and Oklahoma.

The development of the South was in many ways independent from that of the northern United States. During colonial times, southern states were predominantly agricultural, growing tobacco, wheat, corn, rice, and indigo (a blue dye). The plantation system that emerged in the coastal regions was characterized by commercial farms owned by aristocratic English or French immigrants and worked by Africans, Native Americans, and others. Each plantation was a self-sufficient, independent operation providing cash crops and food products for use by each household. It was a comfortable, leisurely lifestyle for the upper classes, enlivened by occasional visits to the cultural centers of Atlanta, Charleston, or New Orleans.

During the period when the northern areas of the nation became more urbanized and industrialized, the South remained rural and agricultural, adding cotton as a major crop. Differences of opinion regarding the role of the federal government in state issues, particularly slavery, led to the Civil War in the mid-1800s. After losing the war, the South regrouped in the late nineteenth century. The traditions and practices that give the South its character became more important than ever. The South continues to preserve its identity, in part, through its cuisine.

Over one-third (38.3 percent) of Americans make their home in the South, the highest percentage of the U.S. population in any region.[35] It is divided into the South Atlantic states of Delaware, Florida, Georgia, Maryland, North Carolina, South Carolina, Virginia, West Virginia, and the District of Columbia; the East South Central states of Alabama, Kentucky, Mississippi, and Tennessee; and the West South Central states of Arkansas, Louisiana, Oklahoma, and Texas. Overall, the South has below-average numbers of Asians and Pacific Islanders (3 percent), Latinos (18 percent), and Native Americans (<1 percent), but above-average numbers of African Americans (19 percent): 56 percent of all U.S. Black people live in the South, including single-race non-Hispanic Black people, multiracial non-Hispanic Black people, and Black Hispanic people.[36] Over 14 million (12 percent) living in the South region were born in another country. Sixty-one percent of those are from Latin America, 23 percent are Asian, 8 percent are from Europe, and 6 percent are from Africa (refer to Table 15.5).

The population of the South is notable for its high numbers of Protestant Christians and low numbers of people without religious affiliation. Baptist and evangelical faiths are especially popular. Three-quarters of the population in the South live in metropolitan areas. Census data from 2020 shows median household income in the South is about $60,000, approximately $5,000 lower than the national median. Poverty rates for the South are at approximately 14 percent for all individuals, nationally it is 12.8 percent (refer to Table 15.5).[18]

Sample Menu

A Hearty Plains Lunch

Chicken Noodle Soup[a]

Meatloaf[b,c]

Mashed Potatoes

Pickled Cucumbers (Cucumbers in Vinegar)[c]

Apricot or Apple Kolaches[c]

Recipes in this menu:

[a]https://www.tasteofhome.com/?s=chicken+noodle+soup

[b]https://www.tasteofhome.com/collection/midwestern-food-countdown/

[c]https://www.tasteofhome.com/recipes/

Traditional Fare

The foods most associated with the South reflect both the bounty of the plantation and the scarcity of the enslaved; it reflects the techniques of African plantation cooks from various countries using indigenous Native ingredients and those that they brought from Africa. It combines flavors from Europe, Africa, Latin America, and Native heritages to create a flavor profile unique in the world. Corn dishes, pork, sweet potatoes, and greens began are the foundation of southern fare and remain characteristic components today (refer to Chapter 8).

The southern lifestyle has fostered a culture of graciousness and cordiality. The traditional isolation of the plantations meant socialization was limited in frequency but lengthy in duration. Hours of travel to nearby homes typically resulted in overnight visits or extended stays. Parties, balls, picnics, barbecues, and seafood feasts were all occasions for get-togethers. For Black Americans, Sunday meals

Table 15.5 South Region Profile 2020

	South Region	United States
Population	124,605,822	326,569,308
Median age	38 years	38 years
Median household Income	$59,816	$64,994
Poverty	14%	12.8%
Education:		
High School	87.5%	88.5%
> Bachelor's degree	30.8%	32.9%
Place of Birth:		
Europe	8%	11%
Asia	23%	31%
Africa	6%	5%
Oceana	0%	1%
Latin America	61%	50%
North American	2%	2%
Race & Ethnicity:		
White	56%	60%
Black	19%	12%
Native	1%	1%
Asian	3%	6%
Islander	0%	0%
Other	0%	0%
Two Races	2%	3%
Hispanic	18%	18%

U.S. Census Bureau. 2020. American Community Survey 5-year estimates. Retrieved from *Census Reporter Profile page for South Region*, https://censusreporter.org/profiles/02000US3-south-region/

with extended kin were the primary way to maintain family connections. In the hills and mountains of the South, the difficulties of subsistence farming necessitated friendly relationships between neighbors. Less wealthy families often survived through regular sharing of food. As a result of these conditions, the South has become known for hospitality.

The first European explorers in the South Atlantic states were the Spanish, who arrived in Florida in 1513 and founded St. Augustine in 1565. They were soon followed by the English, who started in Virginia and spread north and south along the Atlantic coastline during the seventeenth and eighteenth centuries into Delaware, Maryland, the Carolinas, Georgia, and eventually into Florida. The Native American population at the time numbered in the hundreds of thousands, including the members of the Powhatan, Cherokee, Chickasaw, Choctaw, Creek, and Seminole nations (refer to Chapter 5).

The White settlers discovered a region with plentiful fruits, nuts, game, fish, and seafood. Native strawberries, blackberries, blueberries, huckleberries, ground cherries, persimmons, muscadine grapes, beechnuts, hickory nuts, and pecans covered the land. Bream, catfish, perch, pike, and trout filled the rivers, while oysters, clams, and crabs were abundant along the coast. In Florida pompano, red snapper, shrimp, spiny lobster, and conch were widely available. Diamondback terrapin, sea turtles, and alligators were found in many waterways; and bear, deer, opossum, rabbits, raccoons, squirrels, turkey, grouse, ducks, and quail were prevalent in woodland areas. Native Americans of the region grew corn, beans, pumpkin, squash, sweet potatoes, and sunflowers.

Most of the first White settlers in the region were farmers who established plantations. They brought wheat, hogs, cattle, poultry, cabbage, potatoes, and fruit trees, including apples. Black people introduced southern staples, such as peanuts, okra, watermelon, and sesame seeds, and often taught the farmers of the lowland coastal areas how to successfully grow and harvest rice.[37] It was these traditional foods of the Native Americans, European settlers, and Black Americans that combined to create the foundation of southern fare (see Table 15.6).

South Atlantic

Plantation hospitality was famous in the South Atlantic region. A description of a meal served to guests in Georgia from the early 1800s listed turtle soup, trout, ham with sweet potatoes, turkey with a cornmeal and walnut stuffing, rice, asparagus, and green beans, followed by orange sherbet to cleanse the diners' palates before continuing with cold venison, cheese, corn fritters with syrup, and sweet potato pie.[38] Black Americans were sometimes allowed garden patches to tend for their own use, which supplemented their often meager rations or provided a crop to sell for profit. These gardens were often planted in collard greens, cabbage, turnips, beets, English peas, beans, onions, and garlic.[39] Traditional southern fare, such as Georgia squirrel stew, ham, hoecakes, okra with tomatoes, and biscuits served with preserves, was served at family meals as well.

Hot breads are the cornerstone of every meal in the states of the South Atlantic, primarily cornbread (refer to Table 15.7) or biscuits. In Virginia, spoon bread is a specialty; it is a cornbread enriched with eggs and milk and then cooked until it forms a crust on the top but remains custardy underneath. In Delaware, the biscuits are made with sour milk. Beaten biscuits prepared by hitting the dough repeatedly with a rolling pin to produce pockets of air for leavening are a favorite in many areas.

Country hams, ribs, fatback, cracklings, and chitterlings were traditionally produced from hogs and remain important today. Stuffed ham is found in Maryland, one popular recipe, particularly in the southern sections of the state. It calls for inserting greens (e.g., cabbage, kale, and/or watercress) flavored with onions, mustard seeds, and cayenne into deep slits of the ham. The ham is served cold and is often the centerpiece of the Easter meal. In Virginia, Smithfield ham is a specialty, adapted from the process used by the local Powhatan Native Americans to salt-cure and smoke venison. A Smithfield ham is similar to a country ham (refer to the section "West North Central"), but it is made with the shank end of the leg and with the bone in. It is first rubbed with

Table 15.6 Southern Specialities

Group	Foods	Preparations
Protein Foods		
Milk/milk products	Buttermilk, milk	Cream gravy
Meat/poultry/fish/eggs/legumes	Native game, including buffalo, venison, raccoon, opossum, badger, squirrel, turkey, ducks, alligator, diamond back terrapin Pork in all forms, especially country-cured and Smithfield hams; beef, mutton, kid Chicken Crab (blue, stone), crawfish, conch, oysters, shrimp, spiny lobster; ocean fish, such as mullet, pompano, shad; freshwater fish, particularly catfish Chicken eggs Dried beans; peanuts	Brunswick stew, squirrel stew, possum 'n' taters, turtle soup Ham on beaten biscuits, sliced ham and redeye gravy; barbecued pork; *souse* (head cheese); chitterlings; Texas-style barbecued beef, chili con carne, son-of-a-bitch stew; *cabrito* Fried chicken with cream gravy, chicken and dumplings Crab, shrimp, or crawfish boils; crab cakes; she-crab soup; conch chowder; oyster stew; shrimp pilau; shrimp Creole; jambalaya; gumbo; *étouffée*; fish muddle; fried catfish Scrambled eggs and brains, scrambled eggs and ramps Baked beans, butter bean custard; peanut soup, peanut brittle
Cereals/Grains	Corn, rice, wheat, buckwheat	Hominy, grits, corn pone, hush puppies, cornbread, spoon bread; rice pilaus; beaten biscuits; buttermilk or sour milk biscuits; buckwheat pancakes
Fruits/Vegetables	Apples, huckleberries, key limes, oranges, mayhaw, peaches, watermelon Wild greens (cochan, creases, dandelion, dock, lamb's quarters, poke, sorrel, and ramp), domesticated greens (e.g., mustard, turnip), black-eyed peas, cabbage, okra, ramps, sweet potatoes	Preserves and pickles; fried pies; key lime pie; ambrosia; peach pie Greens simmered with fat back or salt pork, consumed with pot likker; poke salad (sallet); fried ramps; hoppin' John; coleslaw, fried okra, okra stews; sweet potato pie
Additional Foods		
Seasonings	Chili peppers (especially bird's eye); *filé*; celery, garlic, onions, green peppers; bourbon, sherry, whiskey	Pepper sherry, chili powder, hot sauce; High Holy mayonnaise; barbecue sauce
Nuts/seeds	Black walnuts, hickory nuts, pecans; sesame (benne) seeds	Nut cakes, brittles, glazed pecans, pecan pie, pralines; sesame seed candies and cookies
Beverages	Buttermilk; bourbon, corn whiskey, Sherry, Tennessee whiskey	Whiskey and bourbon are added to barbecue sauces, baked goods, candies
Fats/oils	Lard	
Sweeteners	Sorghum syrup	Used over pancakes, grits, cornbread, in coffee

Table 15.7 Southern Corn Breads

Cornbread	Made with white cornmeal, eggs, and water. No sugar is added. Baked in a pan, sliced into squares, served with butter, honey, or sorghum syrup.
Cracklin' bread	Usually yellow cornmeal bread with added pork cracklings for flavor, traditionally cooked in a frying pan on the stove.
Spoon bread	Yellow cornmeal bread made with eggs and milk. Baked slowly in a pan until golden crest forms on top and center remains custard-like.
Corn pone	Yellow cornmeal and water (lard added if available) mixed into a stiff dough, formed into sticks (sometimes called "corn sticks") or patties (sometimes called "hoecakes") and cooked in a skillet.
Hush puppies	Yellow cornmeal and water dough, with added egg and buttermilk if available, formed into balls and deep-fried.

salt, sugar, and pepper for curing then smoked over hickory, and then hung to age. The meat differs from a country ham in that it is saltier, darker in color, and leaner. The flavor is very strong, and it is traditionally eaten in very thin slices on biscuits or fried with red-eye gravy (made with ham drippings and coffee) and served with fried apples. Another Native American game dish adopted by the southern settlers, Brunswick stew, became a mainstay throughout the region.

There are many variations, but most commonly today contain chicken, ham or salt pork, corn, beans, potatoes, onions, tomatoes, and lots of black pepper.

Chicken dredged in cornmeal or flour and fried in lard, traditionally served with cream gravy, is a quintessential dish of the region. Though popular throughout the entire South, poultry is especially associated with Delaware. The first broilers in the nation were marketed in the state during the 1920s when an excess of chicks prompted an enterprising egg producer to sell the birds when they reached about two pounds at 16 weeks of age. This was far younger than most chickens were sold at the time and yielded a tender bird that could be roasted or broiled instead of stewed or fried. It was the beginning of a national industry, and today broiled chicken is the state dish of Delaware. Roasters are also popular in Maryland where other chicken specialties include pot pies and chicken seafood stews.

Seafood is especially important in the South Atlantic coastal areas. Maryland, for example, is famous for its shellfish. The state is indented by the largest estuary in the nation, Chesapeake Bay, which teems with oysters, clams, scallops, and crabs. Oysters were so common that many settlers in the region ate them three times a day: raw, fried, baked, fricasseed, in seafood stews, in chowder, in oyster stuffing for turkeys, and over steaks. Crabs were equally versatile. A regional specialty is blue crabs, a swimming crab so named because the underside of the large claws is blue. They are traditionally steamed over water flavored with vinegar and seasoned with salt, pepper, ground ginger, celery, mustard seeds, and paprika. Because they are small, half a dozen or more are served to each diner, with plenty of beer to wash them down. The meat is used to make one of Maryland's most esteemed dishes, crab cakes. The crab is mixed with a little mayonnaise, cracker crumbs, and a spicy seasoning of cayenne, dry mustard, and hot sauce, and then formed into small patties and fried. They are served with lemon wedges and tartar sauce. Crab soup (with beef stock and bacon) and deviled crabs (baked in the shell and topped with bread crumbs) are other common preparations. Another noteworthy shellfish of the region is soft-shell crab—a blue crab that has shed its hard shell during a molt. The new papery shell is completely edible, but it begins to harden after only a day. Blue crabs are often kept in tanks until they shed their hard shells to time harvesting of the soft-shell crabs. The whole crab is served deep-fried or sautéed.

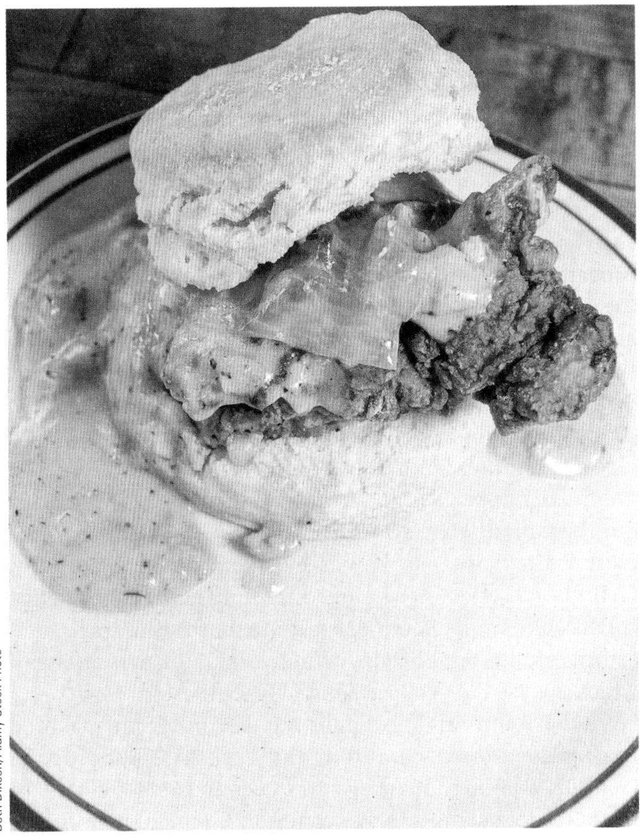

Beth Dixson/Alamy Stock Photo

▲ **Fried chicken is a quintessential dish of the South. It is often served with cream gravy and biscuits.**

The Florida waterways and coastline also offer a profusion of seafood. Red snapper, pompano (a very large, meaty fish), mullet, and tarpon are a few of the fish commonly available; shellfish includes shrimp (several varieties), spiny lobster (similar to those of New England, but without claws), conch (a large mollusk), and stone crabs (only the very large claw is eaten—the claw is removed when the crab is caught, and then the crab is thrown back in the water to grow a new one). Many of Florida's specialties have developed out of this unique ocean larder. Red snapper fillets are baked with orange juice. Pompano is stuffed with shrimp, seasoned with Sherry, and baked, or prepared en papillote (with a nod to the French influence of the Gulf Coast states). Spiny lobster tails are stuffed with fish and grilled, while stone crab claws are traditionally boiled and served with garlic butter or mustard sauce. Rock shrimp, a hard-shelled, white shrimp that tastes like a cross between lobster and shrimp, has become a trendy restaurant item throughout the country. Conch fritters and conch chowder (made with onions and tomatoes, seasoned with Worcestershire sauce, oregano, and bay leaves) are popular.

Elsewhere in the region, oyster roasts (similar to a New England clam bake) are favorites in South Carolina, served with hoppin' John, biscuits, and small sandwiches, such as a crab omelet on slices of bread. Oyster suppers, informal feasts featuring oysters cooked over a fire in the moonlight, then served with melted butter, are popular in Georgia. Shrimp are common in the Carolinas, including shrimp pâté or butter-sautéed shrimp with grits for breakfast, and deep-fried shrimp and rice croquettes. In Delaware, one specialty called muddle (a stew of miscellaneous fish with potatoes and onions) capitalizes on coastal resources. A variation unique to South Carolina is pine bark stew, a muddle flavored with bacon, named for the tiny roots of pine trees that seasoned it traditionally, or because it was cooked over a pine bark fire. Also common in the state are Frogmore stew, a spicy seafood, sausage, and corn combination similar to gumbo, and she-crab soup similar to that of Maryland but garnished with a spoonful of Sherry and a dollop of unsweetened whipped cream.

Long-grain rice is common in many parts of the South Atlantic region. A variety of rice, possibly from a ship wrecked off the coast of Madagascar, was found suitable for the coastal plain climate of South Carolina, and thousands of acres of tidal lands were diked and flooded to support the crop. By 1700, rice was well established, thanks in large part to the farmers from West Africa skilled in rice cultivation. It became known as "Carolina Gold" (due to its amber color when ripe) and became the basis of much of the wealth of the southern U.S. planters who exported it to Europe. There, Carolina Gold competed with rice from India that the colonial British were selling. Cookbooks such as *The Carolina Housewife* by a Lady of Charleston (1847) had 100-plus rice recipes.[40] The rice was traditionally boiled instead of steamed to produce individual fluffy grains that did not stick together. French Huguenots who settled in South Carolina during the seventeenth century may have introduced pilau (also spelled purlow or pullow) which is a rice-based dish that most likely originated in Persia or India and has become a specialty of the region. Gullah Geechee people from West African communities also prepare a similar dish called shrimp perloo. It is characterized by combining a single additional ingredient, such as shrimp or okra, with rice, which is first simmered in an aromatic broth (reserved from cooking the secondary ingredient) until dry, then mixed. African-influenced hoppin' John, made with black-eyed peas and rice, is also a pilau. Molded rice dishes that are baked until they form a golden crust are called rice pies or rice casseroles. Some include layers of meat or fish. One unusual rice dish found in Georgia is Country Captain Chicken, perhaps invented by a sea captain from Savannah who used spices from India to liven up his routine fare aboard ship. It is a chicken with spices and includes tomatoes, green peppers, and dried fruit such as raisins, and is served over rice. In the Carolinas, rice breads, such as philpy (cooked rice added to cornbread), and desserts, such as rice pudding, are also found.

Certain crops historically associated with the South Atlantic states have been in the region so long they are occasionally mistaken as native foods. Some accounts state that Native Americans of the region cultivated melons. Melons are not native to the New World, although it is possible they were brought to Florida by the Spanish explorers of the sixteenth century, in which case the Native Americans may have been growing them for perhaps one hundred years by the time White settlers arrived from the North. Tomatoes are a food that the Spanish may have brought to the region from elsewhere in the Americas. They also introduced peaches to the Carolinas, which at one time were so plentiful they were used as hog feed. Today South Carolina is the second largest producer of peaches in the South, after California, in the nation.

Food for Thought

Hoppin' John is served on New Year's Eve in South Carolina and other parts of the South because eating the rice and black-eyed peas is thought to bring good luck in the upcoming year.

Unlike most states of the South Atlantic, neither corn nor rice grows well in the cool, damp climate of West Virginia. Buckwheat, however, thrives. Buckwheat pancakes served with whole-hog sausage and applesauce are a specialty.

Thomas Jefferson brought many French specialties to his home in Monticello, such as *boeuf à la daube* (jellied beef) and crêpes. He also brought Italian foods, including pasta, to the United States. Although Jefferson or his daughter, Mary Randolph, is credited with introducing macaroni and Parmesan cheese to the United States, it was James Hemings, Jefferson's Black American chef, who likely developed the recipe which evolved into the American dish, mac and cheese.

Oranges, the foundation of the Florida citrus industry, were another early introduction by the Spanish who obtained the tantalizing new fruit from Asia where citrus is native. *Citrus aurantiifolia* was carried across North Africa and introduced to Spain and Portugal, after which European explorers are thought to have brought citrus to the New World in the sixteenth century. Grapefruit were hybridized from pummelos that had been brought from the Caribbean, and other citrus fruits, such as tangerines, tangelos, and Persian (also known as Tahiti) limes, were introduced. Key limes—small, thin-skinned yellowish limes with juicy, green flesh—grew well in the Florida Keys and are often grown in home gardens. They are renowned for their tangy flavor and make a popular pie. Today, 42 percent of the U.S. citrus crop is grown in Florida (nearly all the oranges are processed into juice).[41] Florida is also known for other subtropical crops, such as avocados, guavas, kumquats, mangoes, papaya, and pineapples, as well as early-ripening crops, such as tomatoes and strawberries. Sugarcane is grown in the south of the state, and sabal palmetto palms grow like weeds, providing the delicacy known as hearts of palm. In Georgia, pecans, peanuts, and watermelon are commonly cultivated. Vidalia onions, thought to be exceptionally sweet due to the mild Georgia weather and the low-sulfur soil around Vidalia in Toombs County, Georgia, are a specialty crop sold throughout the nation. Mayhaw jelly, made from the cranberry-like fruit of the native mayhaw tree, is a particular favorite in Georgia and other states along the Gulf Coast. Other native fruits found in the South Atlantic are muscadine grapes and scuppernongs (the bronzy white version of muscadines), which are used to produce jams, jellies, pies, and wine.

In the South Atlantic, English settlers in Virginia favored roasted beef dishes, mutton, and Yorkshire pudding. In Georgia, a French nuance can be seen in the popularity of dishes such as crab soufflé; common German-style dishes include sauerkraut and pepper pot soup; and the Scots brought scones and haggis (hog's stomach stuffed with oatmeal—refer to Chapter 6). In South Carolina, a French influence was seen in many dishes, particularly elaborate desserts like Huguenot torte (a sponge cake with pecans and apples) and charlotte russe (a special cylindrical mold lined with ladyfingers, then filled with Bavarian cream and garnished with strawberries and whipped cream). In Florida, Greek immigrants who came to Tarpon Springs for sponge-fishing jobs at the beginning of the nineteenth century (refer to Chapter 13) introduced traditional dishes such as moussaka (stuffed eggplant), spanakopita (spinach- or cheese-filled phyllo dough pastries), and gyros (pita bread sandwiches). In West Virginia lasagna, fagiole (pasta with beans), minestra (vegetable soup often thinner than minestrone with meat added, if available), and cannoli are popular in the area around Clarksburg where the West Virginia Heritage Festival annually celebrates the history of Italian immigrants in the growth of the state.

One notable ethnic group in North Carolina is the German Moravians, persecuted German Protestants, who had immigrated to Pennsylvania originally but moved south in the early 1700s when they discovered that much of that land was already claimed. The Moravians established an insular German community near the Winston-Salem area, founding a wholesale produce business that sold local fruits and vegetables in markets extending to Philadelphia. They were best known for their baked goods, such as sugar cakes (a yeasted, potato bread dough covered with brown sugar and cinnamon before baking) and citron tarts (tarts with lemon curd filling). Moravians commemorate special occasions, including November 17 (the founding of North Carolina), with Love Feasts featuring wine, creamy coffee, and cakes topped with a nut frosting. At Christmas, paper-thin ginger spice cookies and a sweet bread studded with raisins and candied citron, sprinkled with sliced almonds, are specialties.

In recent years, a more significant culinary influence in Florida has been the contributions of Cuban immigrants to the Miami area (refer to Chapter 9). *Arroz con pollo* is made with chicken and rice, flavored with the Cuban combination of tomatoes, olives, capers, raisins, and chili peppers. Black beans, traditionally prepared with rice and salt pork or ham, are common. Cuban sandwiches, with roast pork, ham, sausage, cheese, and dill pickle filling mounded on Cuban bread, are fast-food favorites. Flan, a baked custard with caramel topping (sometimes flavored with orange), has become a popular dessert.

Cuban cuisine is not the only spicy food found in the South. Many settlers, especially in South Carolina and Georgia, had lived first in Barbados and other Caribbean Islands. They brought a taste for tropical flavors and spicy seasonings. Fruit and vegetable pickles were common, for example, mango chutney from India, which was also made with other local fruits and called "Indian pickle." Today, Jerusalem artichoke, okra, green tomato, squash, and watermelon rind pickles are still popular condiments in the region. In Georgia, very small (one-fourth to one-half inch) scorching-hot bird's eye peppers (also known as tepin chilies) are sometimes crushed and placed at the bottom of a bowl before adding soup or stew. Pepper sherry, made by infusing incendiary Scotch Bonnet chilies in sherry, is a popular condiment added to dishes for zing in South Carolina.

Desserts have always had a place on the South Atlantic table. Tea breads and cakes (such as Sally Lunn cake, best described as a sponge cake–like bread, which is popular throughout the region), fruitcakes, and pies are common. Peach pie is the consummate Georgia dessert, although recipes vary. Some are custard pies topped with sliced peaches, others are two-crust pies, and some are individual deep-fried pies. Pecan pie is popular as well. Key lime pie, a specialty from Florida now found throughout the South, traditionally includes a lime custard filling covered with a meringue topping but can also be made as a chiffon pie (folding the meringue into the custard to lighten it and then topping the pie with whipped cream). Ambrosia, made with sliced oranges and grated coconut, is another Florida dessert common in other states of the region. Puddings and custards were an everyday treat in the early days of settlement, made with leftover cornmeal, rice, or bread; chocolate was a favorite but costly, so it was used only on special occasions. Today, bread puddings are still favorites. Candies, such as divinity with nuts and nut brittles, are specialties.

The cooking of the more rural inland areas of the South Atlantic states differed from the more populated coastal areas. During the early 1800s, Scotch-Irish immigrants searching for religious freedom began making their homes in the Blue Ridge, Cumberland, and Great Smoky mountains of the Appalachians. They also spread west to the Kentucky and Tennessee frontier. English and some Welsh settlers moved from the coastal South Atlantic states inland to the hilly Piedmont areas. Germans from Pennsylvania traveled south along the Shenandoah Valley into Virginia and North Carolina. Hogs 'n' hominy (pork and corn) kept the pioneers going until they established small farms. Frontier meals were robust. For example, the noon meal might consist of ham, bacon or sausage, chicken or grouse, game meat, dumplings or biscuits, cornbread or grits, gravy, sweet potatoes, and boiled greens served with coffee, milk, or corn whiskey.

Traditionally, every bit of the pig was consumed on Appalachian farms, including the snout, or rooter (which was roasted), the tail (which was added to stews), and the brains (which were usually boiled, mashed, and scrambled with eggs). Bacon and cabbage, and ham with cream gravy were typical entrees, while barbecued pork with spicy hot sauce on the side was prepared for special occasions. Most families kept a dairy cow and a breeding cow for a few calves each year. Fresh beef was preferred. When a cow was slaughtered, it would be shared with neighbors, who would later return the favor.

Game supplemented the diet, especially squirrel, rabbit, raccoon, opossum, turtle, and frogs. Badger, considered by some a dish of last resort, was known as bombo in North

Carolina hill country. Brunswick stew is a favorite. Wild greens were well-loved by adults in the Appalachians, but not so popular with children.[42] Poke, creases (similar to watercress), dandelion, lamb's quarters, dock, sorrel, and ramp (a particularly assertive wild onion) were added to soups, stews, potatoes, or eggs, or cooked as a side dish. Poke salad is representative: a cooked salad (from the English tradition) in which the greens are parboiled, then fried in bacon or fatback grease until tender. They are seasoned with salt, pepper, and hot sauce or vinegar. Domesticated greens such as mustard and turnip greens were also common.

Food for Thought

Coca-Cola was invented by an Atlanta pharmacist, John Pemberton, in 1886 as a headache remedy. "Dope" is an older slang term for cola drinks in parts of the South that could stem from the use of cocaine in the original recipe. At the time, cocaine was legal and a common ingredient in small amounts in medicines.

Other than greens, green beans, hominy, sweet potatoes, potatoes, okra, and beets were the most frequently consumed vegetables. Cornbread (sometimes with cracklings added),

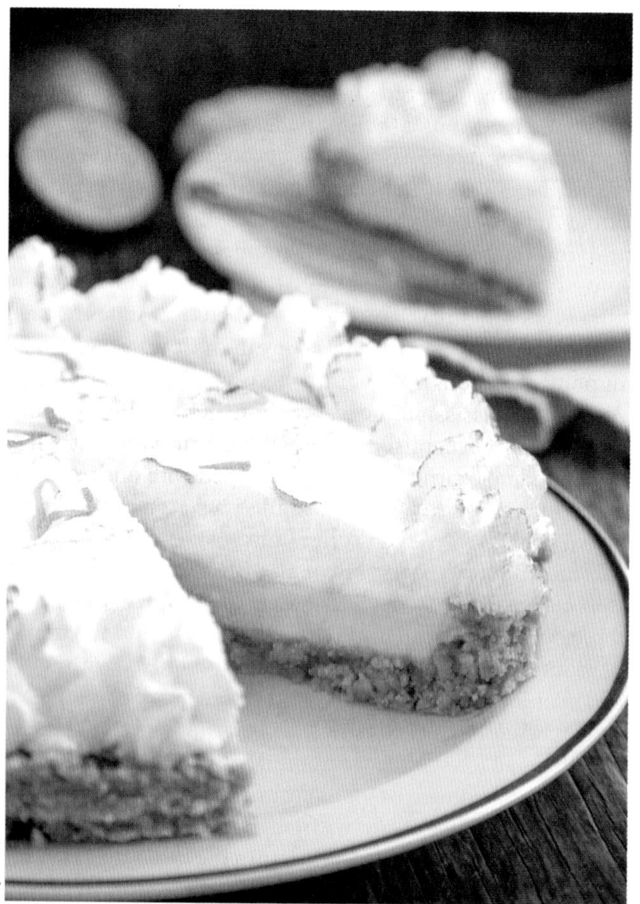

AnjelikaGr/Shutterstock.com

▲ Key lime pie, which has a lime custard filling and is traditionally covered with meringue, can also be made as a chiffon pie (folding the meringue into the custard to lighten it and then topping the pie with whipped cream).

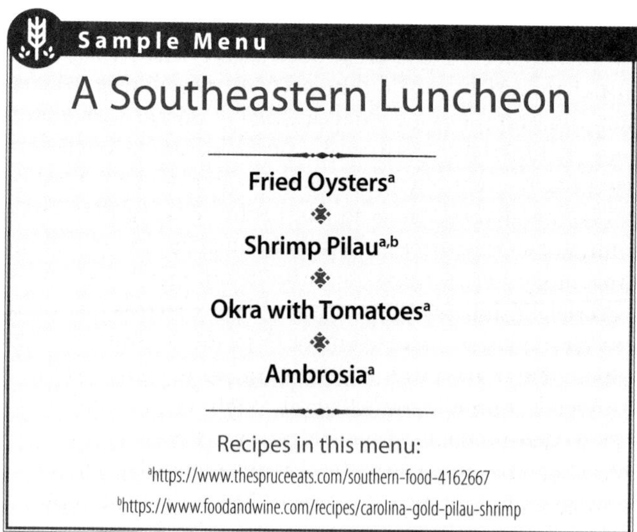

Sample Menu

A Southeastern Luncheon

Fried Oysters[a]

Shrimp Pilau[a,b]

Okra with Tomatoes[a]

Ambrosia[a]

Recipes in this menu:

[a]https://www.thespruceeats.com/southern-food-4162667

[b]https://www.foodandwine.com/recipes/carolina-gold-pilau-shrimp

biscuits, dumplings, and/or grits were served at every meal. Pinto beans, called soup beans, were common, served with cornbread crumbled on top or a dollop of pickled vegetable relish (i.e., cabbage, bell peppers, green tomatoes, onions, chili peppers). Watermelon was a favorite fruit, eaten fresh or preserved as pickles or jam. Applesauce, apple pies, and fried apple slices were popular. Honey was the most common sweetener, even consumed alone as a dessert. Thick, caramel-colored sorghum syrup was also used, poured over cornbread, or used to sweeten coffee.

Many of these foods are still favored in the Appalachians today, though research suggests changes in preparation techniques and the use of convenience food items are increasing as dependence on hunting and farming decreases.[43] A survey of senior adult Appalachians found that they were interested in lower-fat diets and had switched to baking and broiling instead of frying. Shortening has replaced lard in many dishes. Many also use items such as cornbread mixes instead of preparing foods from scratch.[44] However, even those who have relocated to other areas may maintain their heritage by regularly consuming fried chicken with gravy, soup beans, skillet cornbread, biscuits and gravy, fried potatoes, green beans cooked in lard, and other foods typical of Appalachian fare.[42,43,44]

East South Central and West South Central

The early fare of the East South Central and West South Central states was similar to that of the Atlantic states but with more significant French overtones. Immigrants from France settled in the Gulf Coast region during the seventeenth century, and at the end of the eighteenth century, French Acadians from Canada relocated to Louisiana (refer to Chapter 6). They were joined by White American and English settlers arriving from the North. Plantation life in the region was similar to that of the South Atlantic, except that it was more dependent on cotton than on tobacco. The tradition of the big southern breakfast and dinner may have originated in the region and was the norm for plantation owners and their city associates. Coffee and mint juleps were available for early risers. Late-morning repasts included eggs, grits, biscuits, cornbread or muffins, waffles, and several types of meat, such as ham, sausage, or fried chicken. A large dinner with soups, stews, and dishes similar to those at breakfast was consumed in the early afternoon; supper was a lighter version of dinner.

Pork and corn remained key to the cooking of the East South Central and West South Central states. The cornbread in this area is made from white cornmeal without the addition of sugar. The French added their recipes for soups, stews, fricassees, and baked goods to the southern mix, as well as their appreciation for good eating. The resulting cuisine is found in some form throughout the Gulf Coast, from Mobile, Alabama to Beaumont, Texas. The French factor accounts for such adopted and adapted specialties as bouillabaisse (a French fish stew); fish cooked en papillote (in paper packets with a velouté sauce); and *sauce mayonnaise* (homemade mayonnaise), particularly a version similar to aïoli made with fresh garlic and served with shrimp or cucumbers. Creole cuisine, a blending of French, Spanish, African, English, and Native American cooking, is unique to New Orleans. It is a complex fare with many refined dishes; celery, tomatoes, bell peppers, onions, and garlic are the hallmark flavorings.

Cajun fare, created by the French Acadians, is mostly limited to the bayou country of Louisiana, though its gumbos, jambalayas, and étouffées have become popular throughout the region and beyond (refer to Chapter 6). While Oklahoma and Texas are both southern in attitude and enjoy many specialties of the South, such as grits, greens, Gulf Coast seafood, and Brunswick stews, their dishes are also influenced by Native American, central European, and Latinx cooking. Beef is the dominant meat; barbecue is prevalent; and hot, spicy seasoning emboldens their dishes.

The fare of the East South Central states is more homogeneous than that of the West South Central region. Alabama, Kentucky, Mississippi, and Tennessee share many culinary traditions. The French influence is limited to the coastal areas, where dishes feature seafood as the main ingredient. In Alabama, shrimp are especially prevalent, prepared fried, boiled in seasoned water, with rémoulade sauce, and stuffed into mirleton (chayote squash), avocados, and other vegetables. Plump, local oysters, called Bon Secour oysters, are plentiful and popular throughout the Gulf Coast. In Mississippi, rock shrimp and blue crabs are typically boiled and served with an assortment of seasonings, such as vinegar, lemon juice, bird's eye chilies, and cloves. Outdoor oyster bakes and fish muddles served with corn dumplings are other Mississippi coastal favorites.

It is the inland foods of the East South Central states that are most associated with the region, however. Sumptuous breakfasts are still common in some areas. In western Tennessee, for instance, the meal may feature eggs, tomatoes, potatoes, and cornmeal biscuits with sorghum syrup. During the winter, thick slices of Tennessee country ham with grits and red-eye gravy are often served with the meal; in the summer, fried chicken is more common. East South Central dinners and suppers also include many traditional items. Fried chicken is found throughout the region. In Alabama chicken and dumplings, ham balls (fried fritters), and Brunswick stew (made with a whole hog's head) are specialties. In many areas, biscuits and cornbread such as sweet potato biscuits, crackling bread, hoecake bread (cornmeal and water cooked in a frying pan), and beaten biscuits are eaten daily. Tennessee pork sausages are a specialty, as is spiced beef (marinated in vinegar, brown sugar, and seasonings, then simmered and sliced thinly). In the eastern region of the state, barbecued ribs prepared with a tomato-whiskey sauce are a favorite. Hominy, greens, okra, green beans, black-eyed peas, peas, butter beans (similar to lima beans, but slightly smaller), rutabagas, and turnips are typical side dishes of the region. Many of these foods are cooked in lard or flavored with pork. In Kentucky, for example, green beans are simmered with bacon throughout the day to make a smoky, mushy stew.

Game meats are prevalent in some areas. Squirrels and frogs are featured in certain dishes from Alabama. Early settlers in Kentucky depended on game. Bear meat was popular because it could be smoked like pork and was fatty enough to provide bacon. Burgoo, a stew traditionally made with wild birds and game meats such as squirrel, is the signature dish of Kentucky. It is still made this way in some areas, though most current versions use chicken, pork, beef, or lamb; cabbage, potatoes, tomatoes, lima beans, corn, okra, and cayenne—and some variations add filé powder, curry powder, or bourbon. In eastern Tennessee, the diet was historically closer to Appalachian fare than the plantation style of the western half of the state. Deer, raccoon, opossum, squirrel, and wild turkey were primary meats for the settlers of the area and are still consumed occasionally today.

In Mississippi, catfish up to 100 pounds can still be caught in the rivers and lakes of the state, but most are now farmed in ponds. Although the first catfish farms were started in Arkansas, Mississippi harvests about 175 million pounds annually of farm-raised catfish.[45] Traditionally, catfish is deep-fried in a cornmeal crust and served with hush puppies and coleslaw. Newer recipes include fried strips served with barbecue sauce or mustard, and catfish pâté.[42]

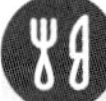

Food for Thought

Moon pies are a Chattanooga, Tennessee, confection that have become an obsession in the South. They are graham cracker sandwiches with a marshmallow filling covered in chocolate, vanilla, banana, or caramel icing. During the Great Depression, a moon pie and an RC Cola were called a "working-class dessert" because both could be had for a dime.

Sweets in the East South Central states are favorites. In Alabama, seasonal pies were popular, especially dewberry (the first ripe fruit of the summer season) and peach. Fried pies, a southern specialty, are thought to have originated in the state. Small circles of pie crust are filled with fruit (typically peaches or peach preserves in Alabama), then folded into a half-moon shape, crimped, deep-fried, and sprinkled with powdered sugar. Rich, chocolaty Mississippi mud pie has become popular nationwide, while butter bean custard pie is a local specialty of the region, made with mashed butter beans cooked as a sweet pudding flavored with cinnamon, cloves, and nutmeg. Banana pudding is another favorite. Pecans are native to Mississippi and added to bread, sugar glazed, orange glazed, and baked in syrupy sweet pecan pie. Many farms in eastern Tennessee had at least one apple tree, providing fruit for apple butter and pies. Funnel cakes, undoubtedly introduced by German immigrants, are topped with sorghum syrup. Fried pies were also popular.[45]

Traditional beverages consumed in the East South Central states include buttermilk and coffee, though iced tea and soda (most often called pop) are more popular now. Sassafras tea is common in eastern Tennessee. Perhaps, the best-known food products of the region are alcoholic beverages. Bourbon was developed in Kentucky. Many of the early Scotch Irish settlers in the state discovered farming corn for corn whiskey was more profitable than farming it for cornmeal. It is thought that the first corn whiskey aged in oak barrels, creating the characteristic flavor of bourbon, was produced in Bourbon County, Kentucky, in the late eighteenth century. In 1860, a further refinement occurred when it was accidentally discovered that charred oak barrels added not only a touch of color but also a favorable smoky taste. A favorite bourbon drink of Kentucky is the mint julep (bourbon sweetened with a touch of sugar or syrup and a hint of fresh mint), traditionally served in a silver cup. Bourbon also flavors stews, hams, pound cakes, fruitcakes, and bourbon balls (a candy made with chocolate, crushed vanilla wafers, pecans, corn syrup, and bourbon). Whiskey is associated with Tennessee. In 1866, Jack Daniel purchased a corn whiskey still and added an extra refinement to the distillation process, using maple wood charcoal to filter the whiskey before aging it in charred oak barrels. This produced a flavor distinct from bourbon, and the liquor became known as Tennessee whiskey.

The foods of the West South Central states (Arkansas, Louisiana, Oklahoma, and Texas) share some similarities due to geographic proximity but also vary due to historical influences. Arkansas exemplifies the region. It is at the crossroads of the South, the Southwest, and the Midwest. The diverse terrain in the state includes the fertile alluvial plains of the Mississippi River in the southeast of the state, the dry pasturelands of the Southwest, the orchards and wheat fields of the Northwest, and the rocky hills and mountains of the Ozarks in the Northeast. Settlers were mostly of English or Scotch Irish heritage, and they brought the foods they prepared in their home states, such as cured hams, sausages, baking-soda biscuits, and molasses pies from the North, and fried chicken, buttermilk biscuits, sweet potatoes, and peach cobblers from the South. Barbecued beef and pinto beans are found in the areas of the state adjacent to Texas,[42] and in the Ozarks, the fare is similar to that found in the Missouri section of the mountains (refer to the previous section on the cooking of the Midwest), with pork, game meats (especially baked opossum and raccoon), corn, beans, and greens the foundation of the diet.

Arkansas specialties include pork chops with cream gravy (sometimes made with bits of sausage in it) and pan-fried chicken that is then baked with a Creole sauce. Arkansas is also the leading producer of rice in the nation. Ducks, which are attracted to the rice paddies, are a specialty in the region, roasted over a fire, baked with bacon and basted with wine or port, and prepared as gumbo. Catfish have long been an Arkansas favorite, dredged in cornmeal and fried, or in catfish stew. Catfish is traditionally served with hush puppies (deep-fried cornmeal biscuits) and coleslaw.

The fare in the other West South Central states overlaps with that of Arkansas. The hilly north areas of Louisiana feature dishes with pork and cornmeal. The southern portions of Oklahoma are called Little Dixie, and a study of foods in the eastern portion of the state found that pork, fried chicken, catfish, biscuits and cream gravy, cornbread, fried okra, and black-eyed peas were frequent items in local eateries. However, grits and buttermilk were rarely offered. In the affluent eastern region of Texas, southern-style dishes frequently feature costly ingredients and tend to be richer (with extra butter, eggs, and cream) than versions from other southern states. Cornbread, biscuits, hominy and grits, black-eyed peas, okra, sweet potato pie, bread pudding, and pralines are a few common items. Rice is an important crop, and southern-style rice dishes are popular.

Other similarities in the West South Central states are found. Cooking in parts of Oklahoma is similar to food in southwestern Arkansas, as seen in the greater use of flour instead of cornmeal. Although the Oklahoma territory was not officially opened up to settlement by Whites until 1889, homesteaders invaded the state early to claim plots in the Land Run (they were called Sooners). The ones that waited for the official starting gun, and had promoted the settlement for years prior, were called Boomers. Black Americans, 3,000 of whom had been enslaved by Native Americans, purchased land in the region after abolition. Slavery in the Indian nations differed from American slavery by most accounts. Black families were not broken apart and usually were allowed to live together even if they had different owners. The Black community gathered in their own religious services. They were permitted to learn to read and write.[46] Most settlers in Oklahoma established small family farms. The plains regions in the state are arid, and droughts occurred regularly. The fare in this region of Oklahoma derived more from scarcity than from the ethnic and regional preferences of the settlers. Rabbit and turnip stew was flavored with flour-thickened gravy, while beef and wheat berries were the primary ingredients of Oklahoma Stew. Baking soda biscuits were common, and black blizzard cake (a pound cake whose name refers to the frequent dust storms in the region) was a specialty.

In the Northeast and panhandle areas of Texas, settlers also scraped out a living on small family farms, surviving on corn, beans, and native game and fish. When wheat proved a successful crop in the region, cornbread was replaced with biscuits. In the western areas of the state, beef has always been popular. It is served traditionally as stews and steaks. Chicken-fried steak was one specialty created to treat tough cuts—the steak is cut thinly, then pounded with a mallet, coated in flour, and fried. It is served with a ladleful of gravy made with coffee. Bread or tortillas and pinto beans often round out the meal. Today, Texas pasturelands are the leading producer of cattle, sheep, and lambs in the nation.

It is the differences in the cuisines of the West South Central states that are most noteworthy. Unlike Arkansas, Louisiana was colonized by the French, who established several fortified settlements along the Gulf Coast, including Nouvelle-Orléans (New Orleans) in the 1700s. African people were brought in to work the plantations, and thousands of French Acadians from Canada and French Creoles from Haiti seeking refuge arrived.

Fish and seafood are more important than pork in the southern regions of Louisiana. The famous stews of the area—bouillabaisse, gumbo (which has African as well as Native origins), and jambalaya—are examples of dishes made from coastal plenty. Shrimp is the primary seafood industry in Louisiana, marketed throughout the nation fresh and frozen. It is commonly served boiled with lemon butter or with sauce piquante (tomatoes, green peppers, onions, bay, vinegar, and hot sauce) over rice, a dish often called shrimp Creole. Shrimp is also added to stews and stuffings for vegetables. Oysters are commonly served raw, on the half shell, and by the dozen in the many oyster bars of New Orleans. They are traditionally slurped with a squeeze of lemon juice and a dash of hot sauce or a sauce mixed to taste by each diner with catsup, vinegar, and horseradish. Oysters, too, are added to soups and stews.

Food for Thought

Chuckwagon fare was a cooking style all its own, dependent on the skills and whims of the cowboy chef often called "Cookie" or "Miss Sally" (who was usually a cantankerous single man). Beans, cornbread, sourdough biscuits, and coffee were the staples, but some specialties were created on the trail, including "son-of-a-bitch stew" (known as "son-of-a-gun stew" in more genteel circles) made with beef organs, including tongue, brain, liver, heart, and kidneys.

The term Creole is often used to describe Europeans born outside Europe. It is applied to the descendants of French, Spanish, and Black immigrants in New Orleans. It is also used to describe a highly seasoned food typically prepared with rice, okra, tomatoes, and peppers.

Crawfish, which look like miniature lobsters, are found in all the fresh waterways of the state. They have become the ethnic emblem of Cajuns and the regional symbol of southern Louisiana. Over 150 million pounds are produced annually. Some are harvested from the wild, but most are cultivated in approximately 1,200 crawfish farms.[47] They are typically served at a crawfish boil, where they are cooked in water seasoned with cayenne, salt, and herbs. Potatoes or corn are often added. The crawfish are placed in a gigantic mound in the center of the table, and each person takes and peels as many as desired. Only the meat in the tail and the claws is edible, along with the fat found in the head, which is extracted with a finger or sucked out appreciatively. Crawfish are also prepared fried, stuffed, as fritters, in soups and stews, in pies, and as étouffée (meaning "smothered") in a spicy tomato sauce.

Other regional specialties include rice dishes, such as fried cakes called calas, red beans and rice, and dirty rice (cooked with gizzards). Rice is also the foundation of dishes like gumbo and jambalaya. Baked goods and sweets are specialties, including French petits fours, crêpes, beignets (deep-fried squares similar to doughnuts), and pralines (pecan candies). Café au lait, a favorite beverage in New Orleans, is a dark-roasted coffee (sometimes flavored with chicory root) prepared with equal amounts of hot milk. Café brûlot is a sweetened dessert coffee flavored with brandy and curaçao (orange liqueur).

Restaurant fare in New Orleans is renowned. Among the nationally recognized dishes created by local chefs are oysters Rockefeller (baked on a bed of salt with a rich spinach sauce), oysters Bienville (baked with a béchamel sauce and green pepper, onions, pimento, and cheese), bananas Foster (sliced bananas cooked in butter, brown sugar, rum, and banana liqueur served over vanilla ice cream—it started as a breakfast specialty), and Ramos gin fizz (a shaken or blended cocktail with cream, gin, lemon juice, orange flower water, and egg whites). Street food is equally tasty in the city. Fried oysters, sliced tomatoes, and onions with tartar sauce on a French bread roll are especially popular. They are called peacemakers, from the nineteenth century, when men would bring one home as a surprise for dinner after a fight with their wives. Po' boy (for "poor boy") is another name for the sandwich, although a po' boy may also refer to a sandwich with deli meats, sausages, and cheeses or shrimp with or without

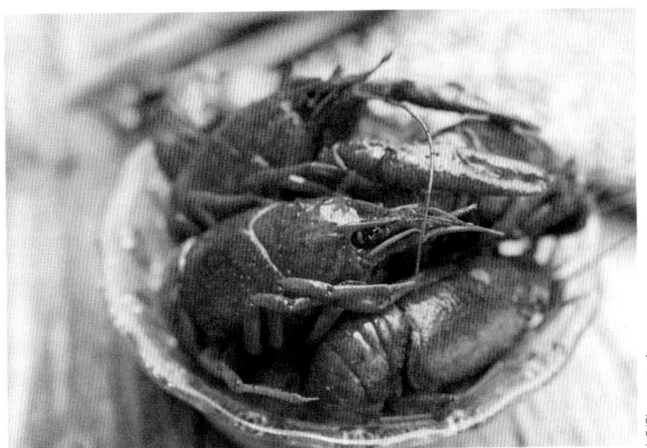

L.F/Shutterstock.com

▲ **Crawfish is a specialty in southern Louisiana that has become popular in other areas of the South.**

gravy or tomatoes. A muffuletta sandwich is yet another version, usually including a chopped olive salad with meats and cheeses on a whole round loaf of seeded Sicilian-style bread.

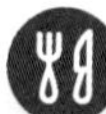

Food for Thought

Sandwiches with deli meats and cheese on a French bread roll are found throughout the country. In addition to being called "po' boys" in New Orleans, they are also known as "bombers" (upstate New York), Cuban sandwiches (made with roast pork in Miami), "grinders" (New England), "heros" (New York City), "hoagies" (Philadelphia), Italian beef sandwiches (Chicago), and submarine sandwiches (from a World War II naval base in Connecticut).

Oklahoma started its U.S. history as Indian Territory, lands set aside in the 1820s for the Native American communities that had been dispossessed of their homes in the Gulf Coast areas. Five major Indian groups lived in the region: Cherokee, Chickasaw, Choctaw, Creek, and Seminole. They were primarily agrarian, growing corn, beans, and squash. They gathered indigenous foods (such as acorns, chestnuts, creases, grapes, Jerusalem artichokes, hickory nuts, persimmons, ramp, and sorghum) and hunted small game (refer to Chapter 5). Today, Native Americans make up approximately 13 percent of the total population in the state, second only to Alaska where Native Americans are 20 percent of the population.[48] Traditional foods, such as a Cherokee soup made with hickory nut cream, called kanuche, and game dishes, are served mostly at ceremonial occasions. Fry bread and adapted dishes, such as scrambled eggs with spring onions, are more common but have not been accepted into the broader Oklahoma cuisine. Europeans, Latinx, and Black people contributed to Oklahoma's food history, with its base resting on staples long domesticated by Native Americans before 1492—beans, squash, and corn in many forms. Ranching and its complex mixture of European and Hispanic customs left an impact on Oklahoma foodways, most obviously in the prominence of beef, according to the Oklahoma Historical Society. Chicken fried steak, a statewide favorite, stands as an example of Oklahoma's dietary heritage—with its southern, originally African, method of cooking, and the beef itself a product of Oklahoma's western heritage.[49,50] Some Italian American foods are consumed, such as spaghetti and meatballs, particularly around the town of Krebs in the southeastern region of the state. Sauerkraut, potato soup, and dark breads are evidence of German Russian influence, and central European traditions are maintained at heritage festivals. A few Tex-Mex items such as chili con carne have become very popular.

Various ethnic cuisines are much more evident in Texas. The state is the size of New England, the Mid-Atlantic states, Ohio, and Indiana combined. It was occupied by Native Americans, claimed by the Spanish and French, ruled by Mexico, and existed as an independent nation before it became part of the United States in 1846. Germans, Czechs, and Poles emigrated from Europe to central Texas, attracted by land grants. Sausages, ham, sauerbraten, sauerkraut, pumpernickel bread, potato salad, potato dumplings, bierocks (meat-filled pocket pastries), and strudel are popular in areas where the Germans and other central Europeans settled.

The most distinctive Texan fare evolved in the south of the state, where Mexican and Spanish influence added their flavors to dishes. Some authentic Mexican foods, such as tortillas, tamales, chalupas, salsas, guacamole, and buñuelos (refer to Chapter 9) were accepted by White settlers in the region. However, most foods in the area are adapted dishes with Mexican overtones, often referred to as "Tex-Mex cuisine." Examples include tamale pie, nachos, and most tacos and enchiladas, which usually feature nontraditional fillings. One regional specialty is chili con carne, known in Texas as "a bowl of red," which began as beans, progressed to beans with beef, and is now typically an all-beef stew flavored primarily with hot chili powder. Barbecue is also favored. Unlike barbecue in other regions of the country (e.g., Kansas City), there are two sauces involved in Texas barbecue. The first, called the *mop*, or sop, is used to marinate the meat before cooking and for basting the meat on the spit or grill. (The term mop for the sauce basted on barbecued meat may have come from the use of a clean mop to slap the sauce on whole carcasses.) The second sauce is served on the side with the cooked meat. Although barbecued beef is most associated with the state, barbecued goat kid (cabrito) is almost as popular in the southern sections. The unifying element in most of these foods is that they are preferred hot and spicy. In addition to chili powder, chili peppers are used in many dishes. Numerous varieties are added, but worth mentioning is the tepín chili, the indigenous precursor to domesticated pequin chilies. They are among the hottest of all chilies (also called bird's eye peppers, described previously). Chilies often flavor foods in Texas not normally associated with the spice, such as cornbread and jelly. In addition to chili peppers, other fresh fruits and vegetables are now prevalent in southern Texas due to irrigation. Cantaloupe, pink grapefruit, peaches, sugarcane, and tomatoes are a few examples of specialty crops.

Health Concerns

Health risk indicators in the South tend to be higher than in the rest of the nation (refer to the chapters on each ethnic group for population-specific data). Florida and West Virginia have average or above-average rates in every health risk and mortality category—Alabama, Arkansas, Kentucky, Mississippi, and Oklahoma show a similar profile, except heavy drinking, which is below average. Southern states have the highest obesity and diabetes rates in the nation. (Refer to Figures 15.3 and 15.4.) Lack of leisure time, inactivity, diabetes, low-birth weight, and mortality rates are of concern in many states. Only the percentage of heavy drinking is substantially lower in some areas. Nine of the southern states are ranked lowest in the nation (41–50) for health indicators (refer to Figure 15.5).[50]

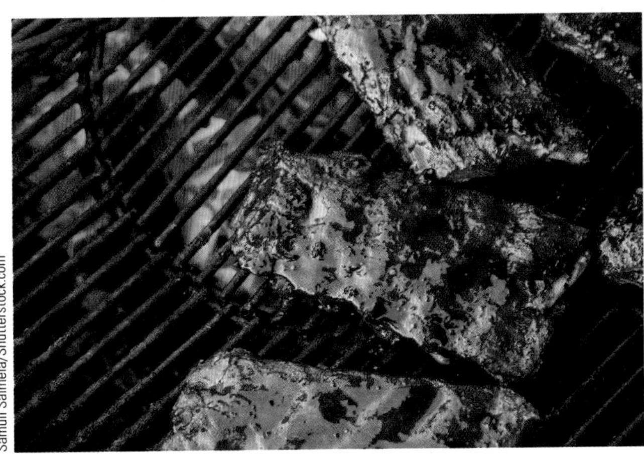
Samuli Salmela/Shutterstock.com

▲ **Barbecue is a traditional Tex-Mex method for preparing food.**

Table 15.8 Western Region Profile 2020

	West Region	United States
Population	77,726,849	326,569,308
Median age	37 years	38 years
Median household Income	$72,464	$64,994
Poverty	12.2%	12.8%
Education:		
High School	87.2%	88.5%
≥ Bachelor's degree	34.2%	32.9%
Place of Birth:		
Europe	8%	11%
Asia	38%	31%
Africa	3%	5%
Oceana	1%	1%
Latin America	48%	50%
North American	2%	2%
Race & Ethnicity:		
White	50%	60%
Black	4%	12%
Native	1%	1%
Asian	10%	6%
Islander	1%	0%
Other	0%	0%
Two Races	4%	3%
Hispanic	30%	18%

U.S. Census Bureau. 2020. *American Community Survey 5-year estimates.* Retrieved from *Census Reporter Profile page for West Region*, https://censusreporter.org/profiles/02000US4-west-region/

The West

Regional Profile

The western United States is the largest region in the nation, encompassing an enormous diversity of lands, from the icy tundra of Alaska and the Rocky Mountain range to the tropical volcanic islands of Hawaii. The tallest mountains in the country, vast fertile valleys and coastal plains, stretches of scenic desert, and temperate rainforest add to the variety. It is the history of the open wilderness that links this region. Indigenous peoples adapted their lifestyles to fit each climate and terrain. Pueblo people made their homes in the cliffs and cultivated corn, beans, chilies, and squash; the Inuit of Alaska lived in ice igloos and hunted sea mammals and fish for food; and the native Hawaiians enjoyed such fresh abundance that they cooked few dishes (refer to Chapters 5 and 12). The first Whites in the West were explorers, trappers, miners, and traders—hardy individuals (mostly men) seeking their fortune. Emigrants came from every direction: the Spanish and Mexicans from Mexico in the South, Russians from the North, Chinese and Japanese from the West, and the numerous pioneers of northern and southern European descent (mostly English, Scottish, Welsh, Danes, Swedes, Slavs, Italians, and Greeks) from the Midwest, looking for new farming, ranching, and fishing opportunities. The West is the most diverse region not only in climate and terrain but also in population (refer to Table 15.8).

The West is divided into the Mountain states of Arizona, Colorado, Idaho, Montana, Nevada, New Mexico, Utah, and Wyoming and the Pacific states of Alaska, California, Hawaii, Oregon, and Washington. Approximately 24 percent of all Americans reside in the Western region and, of these, over half live in California (refer to Table 15.5). Large numbers of many ethnic groups reside in the West. Compared to total U.S. figures, five times as many Pacific Islanders and nearly twice the Asians, Latinx, and Native Americans make up approximately 41 percent of the western population. This includes disproportionate numbers of total Inuit, Japanese, Aleut, Filipinos, Salvadorans, Chinese, Vietnamese, Mexicans, Native Americans, Asian Indians, and Koreans. Blacks and Whites fall below the U.S. average in the region. Among Whites residing in western states, there are large numbers with Danish and Spanish ancestry and Yugoslavian heritage (including those from what are currently Croatia and Serbia) (refer to Table 15.5).

Furthermore, a few individual western states report notable ethnic population figures. Over 15 million individuals

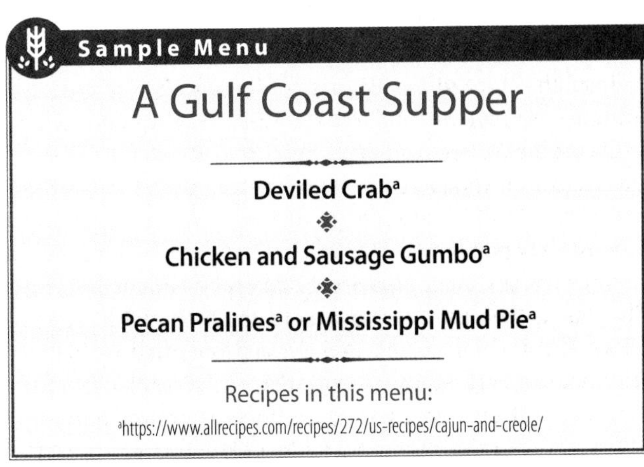
Sample Menu

A Gulf Coast Supper

Deviled Crab[a]

Chicken and Sausage Gumbo[a]

Pecan Pralines[a] **or Mississippi Mud Pie**[a]

Recipes in this menu:

[a]https://www.allrecipes.com/recipes/272/us-recipes/cajun-and-creole/

(19 percent) living in the Western region were born in another country. Forty-eight percent are from Latin America, 38 percent are Asian, and smaller percentages are from Europe and Africa. Asians and residents of Oceania account for over half the population in Hawaii, for example. Latinx are a large percentage of both the New Mexico and California populations. Arizona and New Mexico host large numbers of Native Americans; Alaska Natives, including Inuits and Aleuts, make up a significant percentage of the population in Alaska. Despite the vast open space of the region, over 86 percent of the population lives in metropolitan areas. The average household income according to American Community Survey data is approximately $72,464. People living in poverty are under the national average of 12.2 percent.[13]

History of the Potato

When people think of the state of "Idaho" they think of potatoes. Perhaps, this is because the state license plate says "Famous Potatoes". However, potatoes were not native to Idaho, but to South America. Henry Spalding first introduced potatoes to the state in 1830 to the Nez Perce Tribe as part of his missionary work. He was not a farmer at all. By 1959, potato processing plants in Idaho grew to provide food during World War II and Idaho became the nation's leading producer, which continues to this day. The climate and soil in southern and eastern Idaho are ideal for the crop. Here are a few potato facts:

- The sweet potato belongs to the morning glory family, while the white potato belongs to the same group as tomatoes, chili pepper, eggplant, and the petunia.
- The potato is 80 percent of water, 20 percent of solids, and contains about 100 calories.
- Americans eat around 124 pounds of potatoes each year.
- In 1995, the potato became the first vegetable to be grown in space.[51]

The growth of towns and the success of irrigation increased the food supply. Expensive goods such as wines and chocolates became available, and eastern specialties, including Long Island duck and Smithfield ham, were offered at restaurants. Depending on the region, potatoes, corn, apples, wheat, and hops prospered; cattle, dairy cows, and sheep became plentiful. In Alaska and Hawaii, White settlers faced different challenges. With the arrival of experienced fishermen, more of the Pacific coast seafood was utilized. Salmon, crab, oysters, and clams were especially popular.

Immigrants from other countries came to the West in search of mining and railroad jobs, including the Chinese and Mexicans. Both of these groups enjoyed highly seasoned foods and promoted the use of chili peppers. Other groups, such as the Italians, Japanese, and some Greeks, became involved in fishing and introduced specialties such as seafood cioppino (a seafood stew using local fish and shellfish) and teriyaki. Many immigrants opened restaurants and markets to serve the needs of the booming towns. German sausages, Italian cannoli, and Chinese stir-fried dishes were all available. Still, other immigrants arrived looking for farmland; they planted the fertile Pacific coastal regions and the California Central Valley with temperate fruits and vegetables such as apples, pears, dates, grapes, plums, prunes, cherries, artichokes, avocados, broccoli, brussels sprouts, lemons, grapefruit, and oranges.

Traditional Fare

The West was largely unknown to Whites before the nineteenth century. Adventurous trappers and traders made their way into the territory from the Great Plains, often surviving on dried bison meat. Miners who followed the gold and silver strikes in the California Mother Lode, Pike's Peak in Colorado, Montana's Grasshopper Creek, and the Alaska Klondike prepared their own meals, usually pork, beans, and hardtack (tough, dry, unleavened bread or biscuits) three times a day. Some were dependent on the way stations, hotels, and boarding houses that opened to support the rush. Neighborly hospitality, so common in the Midwest and South, disappeared in the name of profit; miners were charged the maximum for supplies, for example, eggs for $3 each, flour for $13 per bag, and butter for $20 per pound, upwards of $83, $363, and $559, respectively, today, according to historical data from the gold rush. The farmers and ranchers who later made their way westward frequently consumed game with cornbread and potatoes to complete the meal. Sourdough bread and biscuits were common with settlers in the Mountain states, California, and Alaska. A mashed potato or a milk and flour starter was left out to catch wild yeast and begin fermentation. Once going, the starter was kept indefinitely, replenished each time a little was used as leavening (refer to Table 15.9).

The Mountain States

Cuisine in the Mountain states varies considerably between the North and South. Cooking in Idaho, Montana, Utah, and Wyoming was influenced by the American and European settlers and features the foods available in the cooler climates of the northern ranges and plains. Meats are a specialty. The fare in the southwestern states of Arizona and New Mexico is shaped by the limitations of the desert and the significant Native American, Spanish, and Mexican presence in the area. The foods of Colorado and Nevada are mostly patterned by northern states in their cooking, with some southern state influences.

Bighorn sheep, deer, pronghorn antelope, elk, moose, javelina (wild pig), bear, and bison were prevalent in many parts of the North. Recreational hunting is popular in the region, and game meats are favorites. Venison with huckleberry sauce is a specialty in Idaho, and in Montana, it is prepared roasted, or as chili con carne, or into meatballs in a spicy tomato sauce. Both venison and antelope are favorites in Wyoming. Tenderloin, sirloin, and T-bone steaks are cut; the ribs and sirloin tips make roasts (sometimes marinated and braised in wine, vinegar, and spices); the brisket, flank, and plate are used for stews or hamburgers; the hams are smoked; and miscellaneous meat is used to make Polish sausage or

Table 15.9 Western Specialties

Group	Foods	Preparations
Protein Foods		
Milk/milk products	Milk, cheese (Cheddars such as Cougar Gold, Monterey Jack, Tillamook); Basque sheep's milk cheeses	
Meat/poultry/fish/eggs/legumes	Native game, including buffalo, deer, elk, moose, antelope, mountain sheep, mountain goats, bear, javelina (wild pig), beaver, rabbit Beef, mutton and lamb, pork Clams (e.g., geoducks), crab (Dungeness, king, snow), oysters, shrimp, squid Salmon, tuna, halibut, mackerel, sardines, anchovies, mahi mahi, bonito, marlin, snapper; freshwater fish, particularly trout Chicken eggs Dried beans	Game meat steaks, roasts, stews (such as chili con carne), hamburger, sausages; beaver tail Steaks; *beef enchiladas, tamales, chimichangas, pirozhki; teriyaki;* Indian tacos; *Pueblo pozole*; lamb spit-roasted or roasted with chilies; *chorizo*; luau (pit-cooked) pork Clam chowder, Seattle clam hash; *cioppino*, steamed crab, crab cocktails, fried calamari; grilled or poached salmon, *lobimuhenno's* (salmon chowder); *sushi, sashimi, teriyaki*; trout grilled with bacon Hangtown fry Chickpeas with lamb, chickpea pudding; Basque beans; lentil soup with lamb, lentil and sausage casserole, white beans cooked with pimento and cheese; split-pea soup
Cereals/Grains	Wheat, corn	Sourdough breads, biscuits, pancakes; *sopapillas*; fry bread; *panocha*; *capirotada*; whole-wheat Mormon bread; *bara brith*; *malasadas*; Hawaiian bread; tortillas (corn or wheat); *piki*; Asian noodle dishes (e.g., *saimin*) and dough-wrapped foods (egg/spring rolls, *lumpia*, wonton); fortune cookies
Fruits/Vegetables	Apples, apricots, wild and cultivated berries, cactus fruit, cherries, dates, figs, grapes, kiwifruit, lemons, oranges, peaches, pears, pineapple, plums, prunes, sugarcane Artichokes, avocados, asparagus, broccoli, breadfruit, cauliflower, chili peppers, eggplant, *jicama*, *nopales*, olives, onions, specialty lettuces (arugula, radicchio, rocket), tomatoes, *tomatillos*, potatoes, taro root, zucchini	Fresh fruit desserts; fruit added to roasts or poultry stuffings; preserves, jellies, wines; cold fruit soups Fresh vegetable side dishes; mesclun salads; guacamole; Basque potatoes; squash patties; *poi*
Additional Foods		
Seasonings	Chili peppers (especially New Mexico/Anaheim, jalapeño/chipotle, serrano); cinnamon, cilantro, epazote, cumin, garlic, oregano, mint, safflowers (dried petals), *yerba buena*; chocolate; vanilla	Fresh chilies, dried chili powders, smoked chilies, pickled chilies; salsas; red or green chili sauces; mole sauce; fresh, dried, powdered, roasted, pickled garlic
Nuts/seeds	Almonds, hazelnuts, macadamia nuts, pine nuts (piñon seeds), pumpkin seeds	
Beverages	Varietal wines; coffee; tea (chamomile, Brigham Young); hot chocolate	Coffee drinks (lattes, etc.); *picón* punch
Fats/oils	Olive oil	
Sweeteners	Sugar from beets, cane	Sugarcane is eaten fresh in Hawaii

salami. In Nevada and some other states, deer are raised on ranches for consumption. Numerous game birds are found as well, including geese, ducks, pheasants, partridges, grouses, and wild turkeys. Pheasant roasted with apples or in a pie is a favorite in Wyoming. Fish, such as sockeye salmon, bass, and catfish, is available in thousands of freshwater lakes and streams. Mountain trout is a regional specialty.

Cattle and sheep ranching are the dominant agricultural activities of the Mountain states. Colorado is the leading producer in the nation of lamb, known as Rocky Mountain lamb. In addition, bison is raised and processed as a specialty meat in the region. Pork is farmed in Montana, and poultry, especially turkey and eggs, is produced in Utah.

Food for Thought

Colorado is the state with the highest elevation in the nation, averaging nearly 6,800 feet. Pioneer cooks had difficulties making baked goods at high altitudes. Extensive experimentation found that leavening must be reduced and oven temperatures raised to produce satisfactory breads and cakes.

Basques from Nevada may have introduced sourdough bread to San Francisco, where it has become a signature item.

Forage is grown to support meat production in the region, though wheat, oats, barley, sugar beets, hops, lentils, beans, cherries, and apples are cash crops in some areas. Potatoes are synonymous with Idaho. They are grown primarily in the volcanic soils of the Snake River plain, where 10 billion pounds are harvested annually, approximately one-third of national production. Sixty percent are frozen, dehydrated, or milled into flour. Peppermint and spearmint (grown for their oils used in flavorings) are specialty crops in the state. Native berries are a regional favorite, especially in Montana, including huckleberries, which are made into breads and pies, and sour-tasting chokecherries, which are used in pies, cakes, preserves, jellies, and wine.

Settlers of the region often brought their favorite foods. For example, Wyoming attracted a diversity of immigrants, many of whom opened bakeries, confectionery stores, and restaurants. French croissants, Middle Eastern halvah (sesame seed candy), German schnitzel, and Chinese wonton soup were reportedly available in southeastern Wyoming as early as 1900.[52] In Montana, Scandinavians who arrived from Minnesota to work in lumbering brought yellow split-pea soup, cold fruit soups, Swedish meatballs, and ham with cherry sauce. Borscht, cheese-filled pastry shells (vatroushki), and cherry desserts were favored by the Russians. The Scots made oatmeal porridge and Anglo-Indian mulligtawny stew with mutton, and central Europeans brought stuffed cabbage, dumplings filled with fruit or cheese, and pancakes rolled around cherries. In Idaho lohikeitto's (a salmon chowder) was brought by the Finns; and bara brith, a bread studded with currants, was favored by the Welsh. Many dishes in Idaho today feature local ingredients with European nuances, such as split-pea soup, lentil soup with lamb, white beans cooked with pimento and cheese, and ham with apple casserole. Apple jelly is added to mayonnaise to make salad dressing. Prunes are used in preserves and desserts, such as prune-whip pie and prune pudding.[52] In Colorado, chili peppers and other spices came with the Mexicans, and dishes such as chicken or turkey cooked in mole sauce (a rich blend of spices, nuts, and unsweetened chocolate) became popular throughout the state.

One of the most notable ethnic groups in the northern Mountain states is the Basques, who settled in Idaho and Nevada, working first as shepherds and later as land-owning sheep ranchers. Initially, only men came, later bringing their families. Women did most of the cooking, providing meals for the ranchers such as biscuits with sheep's milk cheese and coffee for breakfast, and Basque beans (pinto beans with lamb or pork), lamb stews, or Spanish-style potato omelets for the main meal. They introduced sourdough bread and a pencil-thin version of the spicy Spanish sausage chorizo. Sliced potatoes, onions, and bacon make up a casserole referred to as Basque potatoes, still a favorite in the region. Basques often established hotels, which served as meeting places for Basques doing business in the area and for new immigrants. The hotels became famous for their four- or five-course meals served family-style, and non-Basque visitors often came for the food. Chickpea and meat stews, spit-roasted lamb, and even traditional seafood dishes such as *bacalao al pil-pil* (dried salt cod cooked with garlic, chilies, and olive oil) were offered when the ingredients were available. Red wine, chamomile tea, and picón punch (a beverage no longer common in Spain but still available where Basques live in the United States, made from bitter orange picón liqueur, brandy, grenadine, and soda water) were popular drinks.

In Utah, another group that has maintained many of their food traditions is the Roman Catholic Italians who originally came from Calabria for mining and railroad jobs in the late nineteenth century. They often grow Mediterranean vegetables and seasonings, such as eggplants, tomatoes, endive, fava beans, fennel, zucchini, garlic, parsley, and basil, in home gardens. Everyday fare includes breadsticks, pastas, minestras (refer to Chapter 6), salads, and fresh fruits for dessert. Specialties such as goat meats and goat cheeses, a variety of meats cooked up with eggs in a frittata or a spicy stew, boiled chicken's feet, and deep-fried squash patties made with chopped squash and squash blossoms are traditional favorites. Outdoor baking ovens used by the first settlers are still found in the region.[53,54]

Utah is also home to a large population of Mormons (nearly 80 percent of all residents in the state), who settled there in the early 1800s to escape the persecution suffered in Ohio, Illinois, Missouri, and other areas where the members of the Church of Jesus Christ of Latter-Day Saints had lived. Many were of northern European descent, particularly British and Scandinavians, and they brought a preference for hearty foods. Ham, pot roast, roast beef, stews, and fried chicken remain favorite entrees, often served with homemade whole-wheat bread or buttermilk biscuits. Spicing is usually mild. Hamburger bean goulash, a Utah specialty, is thought to be a denatured version of chili con carne.[52] Milk gravy, made with browned flour, pork drippings, milk, and seasoned with black pepper, was served with so many foods that cowboys riding through the area dubbed it "Mormon dip." Potatoes, red cabbage, green beans, and peas are still common side dishes. There are two types of cooking carried over from frontier days that are still popular in Utah: pit-roasting meat and cooking in Dutch ovens. Dutch oven cobblers featuring the current fruit in season are sold by the serving with vanilla ice cream at many special celebrations.[55] The Mormons are well known for their love of sweets, and desserts are prominent in the diet. Layer cakes, fruit pies, strawberry shortcakes, fruit candies, chocolates, and ice cream are still commonly consumed. Sour cream raisin pie is a popular Utah dessert that recalls the sweetened milk custards and dried fruits of early pioneer days. Another notable favorite is pepparkakor, a Scandinavian ginger cookie often Anglicized as "pepper cookies." Mormons do not drink alcohol or stimulating beverages such as coffee or tea; lemonade and Brigham Young tea (sweetened hot water with milk) are traditional beverages.

In the southwestern regions of the Mountain states, a warm climate conducive to agriculture is combined with insufficient rain to grow most crops without irrigation. Some of the most scenic terrain in the nation, from the majestic

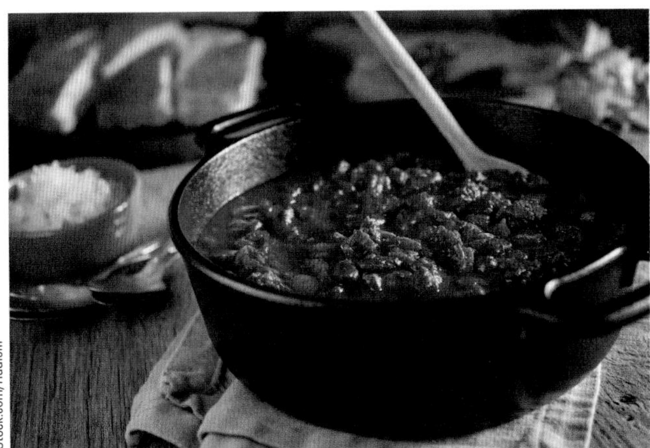
iStock.com/Rudisill

▲ Chili flavored with chili peppers is popular in the West.

Grand Canyon to the broad plains of the Sonoran Desert, is found in Arizona. New Mexico is a mix of high desert plateaus, portions of the Great Plains, and sections of the Rocky Mountains. Southwestern fare reflects the arid conditions and the preferences of the people who settled the region, especially the Native Americans, the Spanish, and the Mexicans.

Native Americans who lived in the region before European contact, particularly Pueblo peoples, cultivated small amounts of corn, beans, chili peppers, squash, and pumpkins. Pine nuts (piñon seeds) were indigenous foods. Juicy fruits (called tunas, or Indian fig) and the young pads (nopales) of the saguaro and prickly pear cactus were other native items. Small game, such as rabbit, provided meat in the diet. They prepared stews flavored with chilies and very thin, blue corn tortillas called piki. Other tribes, such as the Navajo and Apache, were initially hunters who roamed the region in search of big game and wild plants (refer to Chapter 5).

When the Spanish arrived in the sixteenth century, they introduced many of the foods that became elemental in the cooking of the Native people in both the United States and Mexico, including wheat, hogs, sheep, and cattle, as well as chocolate and other items obtained through trade in the Americas. The Spanish explorers were followed by Mexican-born settlers who established small farms called haciendas, ranchos, and estancias beginning in the late 1500s along the banks of the Rio Grande in New Mexico and southern Arizona. Anglo-Americans (those who spoke English) followed, first to New Mexico and then to Arizona, adding to the population of Spanish Americans (mostly of Mexican and Native American ancestry who spoke Spanish) and Native Americans. The ethnic heritage of the region is evident in the many Native American celebrations, adobe villages, and numerous examples of Spanish architecture that still exist.

Nowhere is the blending of Native American, Spanish American, and Anglo-American culture more evident than in southwestern fare. Wheat tortillas became a staple in parts of the American Southwest and in northern Mexico. Hearty beef or lamb stews replaced the mostly vegetarian versions, and fry bread, made with wheat flour and cooked in lard, became common. Popular dishes in Arizona and New Mexico with Native American and Spanish or Mexican roots include menudo (spicy tripe soup flavored with mint), pozole (hominy flavored with pork, chili peppers, and often epazote or oregano), chimichangas (wheat tortillas wrapped around a beef or chicken and vegetable filling, then deep-fried), green chili stew (beef, tomatoes, onions, and a variety of green chili peppers), chickpeas with lamb, and Indian tacos (fry bread folded and filled with meats, cheeses, vegetables, and salsa). Indian roasted lamb with red and green chili peppers, Spanish *arroz con pollo* (updated with chilies), and Mexican chilaquiles, enchiladas, tamales, quesadillas, and flautas are other common dishes in the region. Chili peppers, onions, garlic, oregano, yerba buena, epazote, safflower blossoms (dried and powdered, reminiscent of saffron), and mint sometimes flavor savory dishes. Toasted pumpkin seeds or pine nuts from the native piñon tree were added to spice blends for sauces, providing a nutty flavor to roasted meats and poultry. Today, almonds are used in the same way.

Sweets depend on chocolate, vanilla, cinnamon, and other spices. Popular desserts include anise cookies called biscochitos (a Christmas specialty), the light, deep-fried wheat flour puffs called sopaipillas served with honey or cinnamon syrup, and flan. Puddings are also common, including panocha (similar to Indian pudding from the Northeast, but made with wheat kernels and flavored with cinnamon), and capirotada (bread pudding with pine nuts, raisins, and mild cheese, traditionally served with a caramel sauce).

Agriculture in Arizona has expanded with irrigation. Grapefruit, lemons, melons, and figs flourish in the region. Two vegetables popular in Mexico have found success in the state as well. Tomatillos, a relative of the ground cherry that looks a little like a green tomato in a papery husk, and jicama, a crispy tuber related to the morning glory, have both been transplanted from Mexico to Arizona. Tomatillos are added to salsa verde and other green sauces, and the sweet pea-flavored jicama frequently provides a crunch in local salads. New Mexico is the leading producer of chili peppers in the

Sample Menu

A Southwestern Supper

Posole/Pozole[a,b]

Fresh Flour Tortillas

Jicama Salad[b] or Nopalitos Salad[b]

Biscochitos[a,b] (Butter Cookies) or Flan[b]

Recipes in this menu:

[a]Cocinas de New Mexico at http://www.visitalbuquerque.org/albuquerque/cuisine/recipes/

[b]https://www.simplyrecipes.com/southwestern-recipes-5090768

United States. There is no consensus on the common names for the hundreds of varieties, nor is there a single heat classification system. Mild New Mexican (also called Anaheim) chilies, medium-hot ancho chili (the name for dried, ground poblano chilies), hotter jalapeños (sliced, pickled jalapeños are sprinkled on nachos; smoked jalapeños are called chipotles), and very hot serrano chilies are the most popular in southwestern cuisine.

The Pacific States

No region in the United States is as diverse as the Pacific states. Significant variations in climate, terrain, and settlement history have led to the development of very different cuisines in the three coastal states of California, Oregon, and Washington and that of the two states separated from the continental nation: Alaska and Hawaii.

The climate of the Pacific coast states ranges from cool and moist in the northern areas near the Canadian border to hot and dry in the southern deserts abutting Mexico. Parallel mountain ranges run north–south through the region, dividing the states into different agricultural zones. The food of the Native Americans depended on their location.[48] Those near the Pacific consumed clams, mussels, and fish, with local berries and greens. In inland areas of California, acorns were the foundation of the diet, leached of tannins and processed as a meal or flour. Western Oregon and Washington are endowed with a wealth of native foods, including deer, elk, antelope, rabbits, beaver, muskrats, ducks, geese, greens, wild mushrooms, and a multitude of berries. In the eastern sections of the states, however, high prairie-like plateaus and near-desert conditions exist (refer to Chapter 5). The logging industry was important to the economy of Oregon, Washington, and parts of Idaho and Montana. Logging camps had cooks who were Finnish or Chinese. Hearty meals such as stews made with meat, potatoes, and a vegetable with biscuits were a daily meal. Pie and coffee were also daily staples.[56]

The first Whites to settle in California were the Spanish in the eighteenth century. They built several presidios (forts), pueblos (small farms), and a series of missions (each one day apart in travel time), to protect their claim to the territory. The Spanish cultivated numerous crops, including wheat, olives, grapes, and oranges in the lands surrounding the missions, and planted native foods including corn, beans, and tomatoes as well. Cattle and hogs were raised. Many of the local Native Americans were forced into the missions as laborers. When Mexico took control of the state in the early nineteenth century, much of the mission territory was redistributed as grants to resident families who founded wealthy rancheros producing mostly beef. Despite Spanish claims to the contrary, many other European powers sought access to California's riches. Russia, in particular, established colonies in northern California to support its fur trade along the Pacific coast and in Alaska. Trappers were the first Whites to explore Oregon and Washington. Significant settlement from other states did not occur in the region until the discovery of gold in California during the 1840s and the opening of the Oregon Trail to pioneers from New England, the Midwest, and the South, who came to make their fortunes in the new frontier of the West. Regardless of ancestry, most early settlers adapted their cuisines to the local natural pantry.

Coastal seafood was a mainstay for many settlers. In Oregon, items familiar in Atlantic fare, particularly clams, were favored. Over two dozen varieties (e.g., butter, horse, Japanese littleneck, Manila, and razor) live in the sands of the Pacific Northwest. Clam chowder, adapted with whatever local settlers could rustle up, including rice, tomatoes, and cabbage, was common.[57] Geoduck (pronounced "gooey-duck") clams are large, bivalve native to Oregon and Washington with necks (siphons) that can stretch several feet. A geoduck may weigh up to 15 pounds, although most are in the two- to three-pound range. The body is sliced and pounded into thin steaks (similar to abalone), and the neck is usually minced or ground for soups or stews. Washington also has an abundance of seafood. Beginning in the 1800s, the five species of salmon in the region (king or chinook, sockeye, dog, humpback, and silver) were sent fresh to West Coast markets or pickled and shipped in barrels to Hawaii, South America, the East Coast, and Europe. Iced fish was also sent to Europe, where it was smoked, then returned to the United States. Washington still leads the nation in total salmon catch and products. Oysters are another specialty. The small native Olympia oyster is a favorite, but overharvesting has greatly reduced availability. Pacific oysters, which were imported from Japan in the early 1900s, are the species consumed most often on the West Coast, though European flat oysters are also harvested. Oysters are typically served on the half shell in the region, although bacon-wrapped broiled oysters, oyster fritters, barbecued oysters, oyster loaf, and oyster stew are common cooking preparations. Dungeness crab, named for the town of Dungeness on the Olympic Peninsula, are caught during the winter months. In California, sardines were the leading catch during the early twentieth century. As their numbers diminished due to overfishing, other fish, such as tuna, salmon, halibut, mackerel, and anchovies, became the predominant catch. Dungeness crab, traditionally eaten steamed with melted butter and lemon or in crab cocktails, and squid, served deep-fried or over pasta, are popular. Abalone, a large, flat-shelled mollusk that clings to rocks off the California coast, is a specialty. The tough muscle must be pounded into a thin steak to tenderize it before cooking. It has a delicate, sweet flavor and is typically lightly floured and sautéed in butter.[58,59]

Many early settlers in the Pacific coastal states started small farms, which over the years have grown into a significant industry. California produces more than half the fruits and vegetables consumed nationally and accounts for nearly the entire U.S. production of avocados, artichokes, garlic (some of which are processed as granules and powder), walnuts, almonds, pistachios, apricots, nectarines, olives, dates, figs, pomegranates, prunes, and persimmons. It leads the nation in growing numerous other crops as well, such as lettuce, broccoli, grapes, lemons, strawberries, and

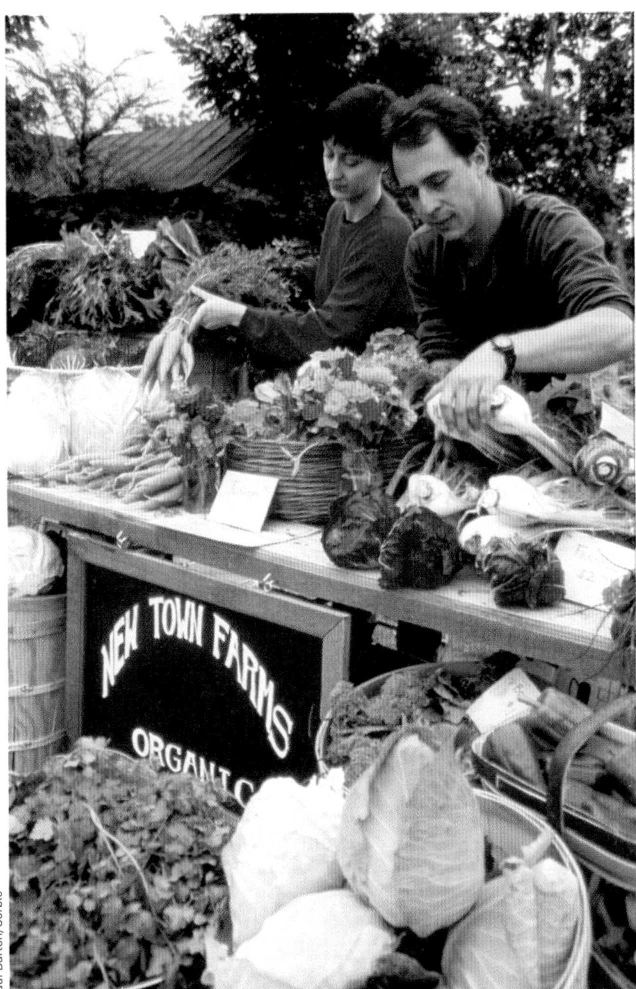

Paul Barton/Corbis

▲ California produces more than half of the fruits and vegetables consumed in the nation and takes pride in a cuisine based on fresh, local ingredients.

melons. One hundred percent of U.S. raisins are produced in California. Specialty fruits, such as kiwifruit and feijoa (a small, green, egg-shaped fruit native to Brazil that tastes a little like pineapple and eucalyptus with mint nuances), are now being grown. In Oregon, fruits such as pears (mostly Bartlett, with some Anjou, Bosc, Comice, Seckel, and Winter), apples, prunes, plums, cherries, and domestic berries, have proved very successful. An Oregon specialty is hazelnuts (also called filberts). The trees were introduced from France in the 1800s, and today nearly all hazelnuts consumed in the United States are grown in the state. Washington leads the nation in the production of both apples and cherries. Apples are especially associated with the state: Grown on the eastern slopes of the Cascade mountains, they require extensive hand labor to thin each cluster of blossoms to a single king blossom and to pick any fruit that appears after the initial crop sets. This process produces exceptionally large, well-formed apples. Nearly the entire crop is devoted to Red Delicious and Golden Delicious varieties, although several other types are grown in small amounts, such as Fuji, Gala, Granny Smith, and Winesap. Hops, Walla Walla onions (a cool weather sweet onion that is a different variety from the sweet onions grown in Georgia and Hawaii), mint, and spearmint are specialty crops.

Dairying is significant in the Pacific states, with California first in milk production nationwide. Best known are the cheeses of the region, including several cheddar styles such as Cougar Gold from Washington, Tillamook from Oregon, and Monterey Jack (a mild, white cheese) from California. More recently, French-style chèvre (goat cheese) and other cheese varieties are being produced.

The abundance of seafood, dairy products, and fruits and vegetables in the region has led to the creation of cuisines that emphasize what is fresh and local. In California, celebrity chefs, such as Wolfgang Puck and Alice Waters, have popularized dishes such as pasta with chanterelles and grilled duck breasts, goat-cheese salad with arugula and radicchio, poached salmon with fresh basil and olive butters, and pears and figs poached in zinfandel with *crème de cassis* (black currant)—all examples of the California approach to cooking. Other trendy items started in California include mesclun salads (made with a mixture of baby lettuces) and roasted garlic, which can be added to salads and stews or spread on bread like butter. Grilled fish, especially salmon and halibut, is a specialty in all three states. In Oregon, abundant use of fruit is seen in both savory and sweet dishes, such as fruit soups, poultry stuffed with prunes or apricots, and salads with fresh berries or dried fruit, as well as various fruit pies, soups, preserves, jams, and jellies.[58,59]

Few distinctively ethnic flavors are found in the cooking of Washington, and limited influence from the settlers of Oregon is seen in German items (schnitzels, sauerbraten, sage sausages, stuffed cabbage, sauerkraut, and strudels) and southern-style fried chicken served with biscuits and hominy. In contrast, thousands of Chinese, Italian, and Japanese immigrants came to California in the early twentieth century, lured by jobs in farming, ranching, fishing, fish processing, meatpacking, and the canning of fruits and vegetables. Agriculture continues to draw immigrants from Mexico and Central America looking for migrant farm work. Other recent immigrants adding to the diversity of the state include Vietnamese, Cambodians, Laotians (particularly Hmong), Koreans, Asian Indians, Ethiopians, Filipinos, and Samoans. Many California specialties are attributable to the ethnic preferences of the population. Mexicans brought corn tortillas, refried beans, guacamole, and popular filled dishes like tacos and enchiladas. Italians introduced northern Italian favorites, such as polenta and pesto, as well as seafood dishes, such as the tomato-based fish stew made with local fish and Dungeness crab called cioppino, as well as fried calamari (squid). The Chinese offered authentic stir-fried dishes, wontons, egg rolls, and adapted dishes such as chop suey and fortune cookies. The Japanese added sukiyaki, teriyaki, tempura, sushi, and other favorites to the mix. Armenians in the Central Valley brought flavorful lamb skewers, dolma (rice- and lamb-stuffed eggplant or grape leaves), and specialty desserts such as baklava. Newer immigrants have popularized hot Thai dishes, Vietnamese pho, Filipino lumpia, and Indian tandoori cooking and flatbreads in the state (refer to the chapter specific to each ethnic group for more details).

California, Oregon, and Washington are famous for their wines. The European settlers of the mid-nineteenth century first introduced the superior varietal grapes used in French and German wine-making to California. Today there are many premier wine regions in the state, including Napa Valley, Sonoma, Santa Cruz, Monterey, San Luis Obispo, and Santa Barbara. The Central Valley accounts for most of the grapes cultivated for the bulk wine market. Successful varietals include Cabernet Sauvignon, Merlot, Syrah, and Zinfandel among red wines and Chardonnay and Sauvignon Blanc among whites. Sparkling wines, which may be made from red or white grapes, and dessert wines are also specialties of the state. Oregon wines have gained a reputation for quality, especially for cool weather varietals such as Pinot Gris (a white wine) and Pinot Noir (a red grape used in French-style burgundies). Washington is best known for its white wines, such as chenin blanc, gewürztraminer, and riesling. In more recent years, fruit wines, such as those made from blackberries, currants, cranberries, or peaches, have become common, especially in Oregon.

The cooking of Alaska has been defined by the climate and terrain, which are by no means uniform throughout the state. Warmer regions are found along the coastal panhandle extending south into Canada, around the Yukon River Delta, and the protected Matanuska Valley in the South-Central region, but there is little land suited for agriculture. The Native Americans, Inuits, and Aleuts of the region lived primarily on seafood and game. Wild berries and roots were harvested in the short summer months (refer to Chapter 5). The first permanent White settlement in Alaska was on Kodiak Island. The Russians arrived in the 1700s to hunt fur seals. They brought kasha, a cooked buckwheat porridge, buckwheat blini, and soups of fish or cabbage. Pirogs, large filled pastries, were made with fish, game, or cabbage. On Easter, they prepared traditional dishes such as the rich fruitcake called kulich (refer to Chapter 7). A rush of prospectors searching for gold arrived in the Klondike area in the 1800s. Supplies were severely limited, and the new settlers lived on little more than flour, bacon, salt pork, lard, and a bit of coffee or tea. Most kept a sourdough culture going to make breads and biscuits. Sourdough specialties included poppy seed potato bread, rye bread with caraway seeds, and whole-wheat bread. Kelp was collected at the coast, and wildflowers were boiled to make syrup. Some miners hunted to supplement their diets, and game, such as deer, caribou, moose, Dall sheep, rabbits, and ptarmigan, was available. Game meats are still popular today, including steaks, roasts, hamburgers made from moose meat, and caribou meat sausages and Swiss steaks.

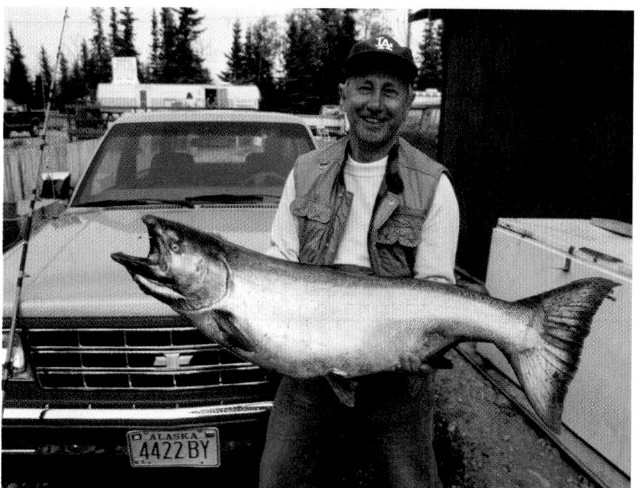

Buddy Mays/Corbis

▲ **Salmon and other seafood are favorites in Alaska and the Pacific Northwest.**

Food for Thought

Coffee drinks such as lattes have become a specialty item associated with Seattle. The city is home to the Starbucks Corporation, which spurred the trend of U.S. coffee bars (modeled after Italian espresso bars) in 1984. There were over 15,149 Starbucks coffee bars nationwide in 2019.

Sheep are now raised on the Aleutian Islands, providing lamb for the mainland. Cattle ranches are found on Kodiak Island and in the Delta and Matanuska. Reindeer herds were imported to Alaska in the late 1800s from Siberia and Scandinavia in the hopes they would become a profitable meat source. Many starved to death when the ranges were overgrazed, and others are thought to have become part of caribou herds. Today, some reindeer in the Seward Peninsula are raised for meat and for supplying antlers to Asia. More important are the dairy operations providing fresh milk, butter, and cream. Potatoes are the most successful crop, but vegetables such as cabbage, cauliflower, and rhubarb also grow in the region. Many of the vegetables attain gigantic proportions in the long daylight hours of summer; for example, cabbages may reach 70 pounds, and rhubarb sometimes grows 4 feet tall.

Seafood is the main commodity in Alaska, ranking first nationally in quantity and value of the yearly catch. Salmon, herring, and halibut are the most prevalent fish. Shrimp and crab, including Dungeness, Snow (also known as Tanner), and limited king crabs, are trapped during the winter months. Most are frozen or canned for export to the rest of the United States and Japan.

In Hawaii, a mild tropical climate and abundant natural food resources greeted the earliest inhabitants. The volcanic islands are believed to have been first settled by Polynesians from the Marquesas Islands and Tahiti in the fifth century. The foundation of their diet was starchy vegetables such as taro root (traditionally made into poi—boiled, pounded into a paste, and slightly fermented), breadfruit, plantains, cassava, and yams. Seafood and possibly pork and chicken were also eaten (refer to Chapter 12). British explorers discovered the islands in the late 1700s; the area became a major American port for whaling ships in the nineteenth century, and Japanese, Chinese, Korean, Filipino, and Asian Indian agricultural workers came to support the developing pineapple and sugarcane industries.

Traditional native dishes and foods introduced to the islands by the many immigrants coalesced into Hawaiian fare. Unlike some areas of the nation, where various foreign contributions have melded into a single cuisine with occasional European, Latinx, or Asian overtones, many dishes in Hawaii maintain their ethnic integrity. Foods from different cultures are commonly served at the same meal, however, representing the state's diverse heritage. Popular Hawaiian foods include those with Japanese origins, such as teriyaki-grilled meats and fish, sashimi (raw, thinly sliced fish), and noodle dishes such as saimin, an island adaptation of ramen noodles, topped with pork and frequently eaten for lunch. The Chinese brought wok cooking, dim sum, long-grain rice, soybeans, bok choy, lotus root, kumquats, litchi, and ginger to the region. Scottish scones and shortbreads are available, and Portuguese sweet bread is so common it is often called Hawaiian bread. Another Portuguese specialty, malassadas (fried doughnuts without a hole), is especially popular, and local variations made with poi or macadamia nuts are novelty items. Filipino fish sauces and lumpia (Filipino-style egg rolls), Korean kimchi (fermented, spicy relish) and spicy beef dishes, and Indian curries are other contributions.

Historically, sugarcane was the most important crop in Hawaii, accounting for 20 percent of the raw sugar produced nationally. But soaring costs and environmental concerns have put most sugarcane plantations out of business. Pineapples have also been a significant commodity, though pressures from Asia are reducing their profitability. Hawaii grows most of the world's supply of macadamia nuts and also exports famous kona coffee, grown on the western slopes of the island of Hawaii. Cattle ranches are found on the islands of Maui, Hawaii, and the privately owned Niihau; most provide beef for local consumption. Seafood, another Hawaiian specialty, is also mostly fished for Hawaiian markets, although some tuna is canned and exported. In addition to tuna, common food fish include mahi-mahi (also called dorado), bonito, mackerel, and snapper.

Health Concerns

In general, people living in the West are healthier than the national average (review chapters on each ethnic group for population-specific data). The western states have the lowest prevalence of cardiovascular diseases and higher rates of healthy lifestyle activities (refer to Figure 15.5). Rates of obesity range from the lowest in Colorado and Hawaii at 20 percent to the highest among the western region in Idaho, Wyoming, California, Arizona, New Mexico, and Alaska (refer to Figures 15.3 and 15.4).

Discussion Starters Reflection

Examination of Ethnicity, Culture, Diet, and Health

For Chapter 1, you described your cultural identity (your race and ethnicity) and the foods that you typically eat (what you like to eat, what foods are eaten in your home). Now, identify the regional area (Northeast, Midwest, South, or West) that your diet most reflects—and any more specific area(s) within that larger region (New England, Mid-Atlantic, East North Central, West North Central, South Atlantic, East South Central, West South Central, Mountain states, or Pacific states). Next, identify any even more specifically localized area and/or culture within that specific area that your diet seems to reflect.

Are the region, area, and culture that your diet seems to reflect the same as the region, area, and culture that apply to you? Do other factors affect your diet, such as ethnicity?

Look at the appropriate table of health concerns for the area that your diet reflects and think about your family members' individual health histories, as well as your racial and ethnic background(s). Next, identify health concerns that you might need to address in the future. For example, if your diet is southern and, in particular, West Virginian, you would identify high blood cholesterol, hypertension, and diabetes as possible future health concerns. On the other hand, if your diet is western and, in particular, Californian, but is also heavily influenced by a Greek heritage, you will want to analyze whether that Greek influence on your diet is strong enough that you should identify overweight and obesity as possible future health concerns, even though studies suggest that Californians generally are similar to the national average in those two categories. In small groups, share your findings. Together, brainstorm about what each person in your group could begin doing now to address possible future health concerns.

Review Questions

1. List and describe three factors influencing regional cuisine. Pick one region and summarize its influences.
2. How did Native American foods/cooking methods influence regional U.S. cuisine?
3. Compare and contrast the preparation of beans, corn, and apples in different regions of the United States.
4. Describe one unique recipe associated with a particular region of the United States that you were not familiar with before reading this chapter. Would you try it? Why or why not?
5. Based on health statistics, which region of the country would you choose to live in to stay healthy? What dietary factors may be influencing these health statistics? If you wanted to eat "unhealthy" one day, which regional cuisine would you try? Why?

6. You have decided to eat locally. What does this mean, and what foods would be available for you to purchase? List some of the arguments for eating local.

Reflection

1. Consider the region where you grew up. What are some foods that you grew up with that are regional specialties?
2. What is the health rank of the state or states that you grew up or reside in currently? In your opinion, what could be done to improve this ranking?

References

1. Ferdman, R.A. 2014. Where the greatest beer, wine, and liquor drinkers live in the U.S. *The Washington Post*. Retrieved from https://www.washingtonpost.com/news/wonk/wp/2014/07/29/where-the-biggest-beer-wine-and-liquor-drinkers-live-in-the-u-s/
2. Bitter, C. 2020. Demographics and wine: The class divide. Vine Economics. Retrieved from https://www.vineconomics.com/blog/demographics-and-wine-the-class-divide
3. Conway, J. April 15, 2021. Number of operating brewpubs in the United States from 2006-2020. Statista. Retrieved from https://www.statista.com/statistics/484651/number-of-operating-brewpubs-in-the-us/ (accessed May 2, 2020).
4. U.S. brewery count by category. n.d. Statistics, Brewers Association. Retrieved from https://www.brewersassociation.org/ (accessed May 1, 2015).
5. USDA. 2021. Food prices and spending. Retrieved from https://www.ers.usda.gov/ (accessed May 3, 2022).
6. French, S.A., Tangney, C.C., Crane, M.M., Wang, Y., & Appelhans, B.M. 2019. Nutrition quality of food purchases varies by household income: The Shopper study. *BMC Public Health*, 19(1), 1–7.
7. Martin, A. 2022. Food prices and spending. USDA Economic Research Service. Retrieved from https://www.ers.usda.gov/data-products/ag-and-food-statistics-charting-the-essentials/food-prices-and-spending/
8. Korsmeyer, C. (Ed.). 2016. *The taste culture reader: Experiencing food and drink*. Bloomsbury Publishing.
9. Stevens, A. 2020. Taste of Place and Provenance. Retrieved from https://cedar.wwu.edu/wwu_honors/349/
10. Carolyn, K. 2017. Nicola Perullo. Taste as experience: the philosophy and aesthetics of food. Reviewed by. *Philosophy in Review*, 37(2).
11. Kobayashi, A. 2019. *International encyclopedia of human geography*. Elsevier.
12. Ashworth, G.J. & Graham, B. 2018. Senses of place, senses of time and heritage. In *A museum studies approach to heritage*. Routledge, pp. 374–380.
13. U.S. Census Bureau. 2020. *American Community Survey 5-year estimates*. Retrieved from *Census Reporter Profile page for Northeast Region*. Retrieved from http://censusreporter.org/profiles/02000US1-northeast-region
14. Klein, C. 2021. Chocolate's sweet history: From elite treat to food for the masses. History. Retrieved from https://www.history.com/news/the-sweet-history-of-chocolate#
15. Oliver, S.L. 1995. *Saltwater foodways*. Mystic, CT: Mystic Seaport Museum.
16. Sonu, S.C. 2003. *The Japanese sea urchin market* (Vol. 40). US Department of Commerce, National Oceanic and Atmospheric Administration, National Marine Fisheries Service, Southwest Region.
17. Division for Heart Disease and Stroke Prevention: Data Trends & Maps, U.S. Department of Health and Human Services, Centers for Disease Control and Prevention (CDC), National Center for Chronic Disease Prevention and Health Promotion. 2013. Retrieved from http://www.cdc.gov/dhdsp/
18. U.S Census. 2020. *American Community Survey*, 2020. Retrieved from https://www.census.gov/data/tables/time-series/demo/popest/2020s-state-total.html
19. Budiman, A. 2021. Hmong in the U.S. fact sheet. Pew Research Center. Retrieved from pewresearch.org/social-trends/fact-sheet/asian-americans-hmong-in-the-u-s/
20. Editors. 2020. Midwest region. Census Reporter. Retrieved from https://censusreporter.org/profiles/02000US2-midwest-region/
21. Wilcox, E.W. 2002. *Buckeye cookery and practical housekeeping*, 1877 (facsimile edition). Bedford, MA: Applewood Books. (Original work published 1887)
22. Bruni, F. & Steinhauer, J. 2017. A history of meatloaf, long may it reign. Bon Appetit. Retrieved from https://www.bonappetit.com/story/history-of-meatloaf
23. Statista. 2022. Top 10 milk producing U.S. states in 2020 and 2021.
24. Deutsch, R.M. 1962. *The nuts among the berries*. New York: Ballantine Books.
25. Woellert, D. 2013. The Authentic History of Cincinnati Chili. Arcadia Publishing.
26. Britannica, T. Editors of Encyclopaedia. 2021. *Anheuser-Busch Companies, Inc., Encyclopedia Britannica*. Retrieved from https://www.britannica.com/topic/Anheuser-Busch-Companies-Inc
27. Ogle, M. 2006. Ambitious brew: The story of American beer. Houghton Mifflin Harcourt.
28. Luchetti, C. 1993. Home on the Range: A Culinary History of the American West. Random House Incorporated.
29. Anderson, J. 1997. *The American century cookbook*. New York: Clarkson Potter.
30. Wills, M. 2021. How oysters became a food fad way out West. JSTOR.
31. Urban Plains Alumni. 2019. American Barbecue styles: a Midwest guide. Urban Plains. Retrieved from https://urban-plains.com/american-barbucue-stules-a-midwest-guide
32. Phippen, J.W. 2016. Kill every buffalo you can! Every buffalo dead is an Indian gone. *The Atlantic*, 13.
33. Matson, M. 1994. *Food in Missouri*. Columbia: University of Missouri Press.
34. Centers for Disease Control and Prevention. n.d. Burden of cigarette use in the U.S. Retrieved from https://www.cdc.gov/tobacco/campaign/tips/resources/data/cigarette-smoking-in-united-states.html?s_cid=OSH_tips_GL0005&utm_source=google&utm_medium=cpc&utm_campaign=TipsRegular+2021%3BS%3BWL%3BBR%3BIMM%3BDTC%3BCO&utm_content=Smoking+-+Facts_P&utm_term=statistics+about+smoking&gclid=Cj0KCQjwyMiTBhDKARIsAAJ-9Vs3PKB6_fpKppFC8bPK0WRIA50ON5NQE55t_lSy_SAOz7sBy1MvWU8aAtKxEALw_wcB&gclsrc=aw.ds
35. U.S. Census. 2021. Retrieved from https://www.census.gov/popclock/data_tables.php?component=growth
36. Tamir, C., Budiman, B., Noe-Bustamante, L., & Mora, L. 2021. Facts about the U.S. Black Population. Pew Research Center. Retrieved from https://www.pewresearch.org/social-trends/fact-sheet/facts-about-the-us-black-population/
37. Carney, J. 2014. The African origins of Carolina rice culture. *Cultural Geographies*, 7(2), 125–149.
38. Lee, H.G. 1992. *Taste of the states: A food history of America*. Charlottesville, VA: Howell.
39. Rose, J. 2016. Food and Slave Communities in the Antebellum South.
40. Rutledge, S. 1847. The Carolina housewife or, House and home: by a lady of Charleston. *Oxford Text Archive Core Collection*.
41. USDA. 2020. Citrus fruits 2020 summary. United States Department of Agriculture. Retrieved from https://www.nass.usda.gov/Publications/Todays_Reports/reports/cfrt0820.pdf

42. Shields, D.S. 2015. Southern Provisions. In *Southern Provisions.* University of Chicago Press.
43. Visocky, S.H. 2016. *Appalachian Foodways from Then to Now: Using Traditional Foods to Enhance Dietetic Practice* (Doctoral dissertation, Appalachian State University).
44. Brock, S. 2019. *The Foxfire Book of Appalachian Cookery.* UNC Press Books.
45. State of Mississippi. 2021. Agriculture fact sheet aquaculture 2021. Mississippi Department of Agriculture and Commerce. Retrieved from https://www.mdac.ms.gov/wp-content/uploads/com_aquaculture.pdf
46. Krauthamer, B. n.d. Slavery. In *The Encyclopedia of Oklahoma History and Culture.* Oklahoma Historical Society. Retrieved from https://www.okhistory.org/publications/enc/entry?entry=SL003
47. Hollister, J. 2022. Crawfish popularity hits new high. Aquaculture North America. Retrieved from https://www.aquaculturenorthamerica.com/crawfish-popularity-hits-new-high/
48. World Population Review. 2022. Native American population 2022. Retrieved from https://worldpopulationreview.com/state-rankings/native-american-population
49. Jackson, J.B. Foodways. *The Encyclopedia of Oklahoma History and Culture.* Retrieved from https://www.okhistory.org/publications/enc/entry?entry=FO014
50. America's health rankings. 2014. United Health Foundation. Retrieved from http://www.unitedhealthfoundation.org
51. Idaho Potato Museum. n.d. Retrieved from https://idahopotatomuseum.com/potato-facts/ (accessed May 8, 2022).
52. Lee, H.G. 1992. *Taste of the states: A food history of America.* Charlottesville, VA: Howell.
53. Notarianni, P.F. 1994. Italians in Utah. In A.K. Powell (Ed.), *Utah history encyclopedia.* Salt Lake City: University of Utah Press.
54. Raspa, R. 1984. Exotic foods among Italian-Americans in Mormon Utah: Food as nostalgic enactment of identity. In *Ethnic and regional foodways in the United States.* Knoxville: University of Tennessee Press.
55. Utah Humanities. 2008 The Beehive Archive. Retrieved from https://www.utahhumanities.org/stories/items/show/76 (accessed May 8, 2022).
56. Mendocino Coast Model Railroad & Historical Society. n.d. Retrieved from https://www.mendorailhistory.org/1_logging/camp-food.htm (accessed May 8, 2022).
57. Jones, E. 1981. *American food: The gastronomic story* (2nd ed.). New York: Vintage.
58. Pillsbury, R. 2018. *No foreign food: the American diet in time and place.* Routledge.
59. Contois, E.J. 2018. Welcome to Flavortown: Guy Fieri's Populist American Food Culture. *American Studies,* 57(3), 143–160.

Glossary of Ingredients

Abalone (paua): Large, flat mollusk with finely textured, sweet flesh in the broad muscular foot that holds it to rocks (must be pounded before use). It is common in the waters off Asia, California, Mexico, and New Zealand. Available fresh, frozen, canned, and dried.

Abiu (caimito): Yellow egg-shaped or round fruit native to the Amazon; popular throughout Brazil and Peru. Translucent white flesh with caramel-like flavor.

Acerola cherries (Barbados cherries): Exceptionally sour Caribbean berries resembling small, bright red cherries with orange flesh.

Achiote: See *Annatto.*

Adzuki bean (aduki, azuki; red bean): Small, dark red bean used primarily in Japanese cooking, often as a sweetened paste.

Ahipa: See *Jicama.*

Ajowan (ajwain; carom; omum or lovage seeds): Similar to celery seeds in appearance and to thyme in flavor. Used in Asian-Indian and Middle Eastern cooking.

Ajwain: See *Ajowan.*

Akee (ackee, ache; seso vegetal; pera roja): Red fruit with three segments containing large inedible seeds and flesh resembling scrambled eggs. Nearly all parts toxic, causing fatal hypoglycemia. Fresh, dried, frozen akee banned in United States; some canned types permitted.

Alligator: Reptile native to rivers and swamps throughout the southern Gulf Coast region, from Florida to Texas. Mild white meat, with texture similar to veal. Tail and other parts eaten.

Almond paste: Arab confection of ground almonds kneaded with sugar or cooked sugar syrup (some brands also contain egg white) used in many European and Middle Eastern desserts. Marzipan is a type of almond paste made with finely ground, blanched almonds.

Amaranth (tampala; yien choy; Chinese spinach): Leafy, dark green vegetable similar to spinach; red and purple leaf varieties, also. The high-protein seeds can be ground into flour and used in baked products, or boiled and eaten as cereal. Popular throughout Asia and Latin America.

Ambarella (hog or Jew plum; kadondong; otaheite or golden apple; vi-apple): Small, oval-shaped fruit with very strong flavor native to Polynesia but also found in Southeast Asia and Caribbean. Used unripe for preserves and ripe in desserts.

Amchoor (amchur; khati powder): Dried, unripe mango slices or powder, with a sour, raisin-like flavor.

Angelica root: Herb with a licorice-flavored root common in European dishes. Usually available candied. Used medicinally in China.

Annatto (achiote, atchuete): Seeds of the annatto tree used to color foods red or golden yellow. Used in Latin America, India, Spain, and the Philippines. In the United States annatto is added to some baked goods, Cheddar-style cheeses, ice creams, margarines, and butter for color. May be cooked whole in oil or lard to produce the right hue or used as a ground spice.

Apio: See *Arracacha.*

Apios: See *Groundnuts.*

Apon seeds (agonbono): Seeds of the wild mango commonly used in West Africa. Basis of the soup known as agonbono.

Areca nuts: See *Betel.*

Arracacha (apio; Peruvian carrot): Starchy white root of the carrot family with flavor similar to chestnuts and parsnips used in South America, especially Colombia, Peru, and Venezuela.

Arrowroot (chee koo): Many varieties of a bland, mealy tuber found in Asia and the Caribbean. When made into a powder, it is used to thicken sauces and stews.

Artichoke (carciofo): Globelike vegetable member of the thistle family, with multiple edible bracts (leaves) crowning the undeveloped edible flower (the heart). The flavor is slightly sweet. Popular in Middle Eastern and southern European dishes.

Arugula (rocket): Small member of the cabbage family native to the Mediterranean; the peppery leaves are popular in salads throughout Europe.

Asafetida (devil's dung): Dried resin with a pungent odor reminiscent of burnt rubber, which nonetheless imparts a delicate onion-like flavor. It is available as a lump or powder and is commonly used in Asian-Indian dishes.

Asian pear (apple pear): Round, yellow fruit from Asia with the crispness of an apple and the flavor of a pear.

Atemoya: Hybrid of the cherimoya and sweetsop. See *Cherimoya; Sweetsop.*

Aubergine: See *Eggplant.*

Avocado (aguacate; alligator pear; coyo): Pear-shaped to round fruit with leathery skin (green to black) and light green, buttery flesh. Native to Central America. Numerous varieties; eaten mostly as a vegetable, though considered a fruit in some cuisines.

Bacalao (bacalhau, baccala): Cod preserved by drying and salting, popular in northern and southern European cooking (especially Portuguese). Must be soaked, drained, and boiled before use.

Bagoong: See *Fish paste.*

Bagoong-alamang: See *Shrimp paste.*

Bambara groundnut (Congo goober; kaffir pea): Legume very similar to peanuts, native to Africa.

Bamboo shoot (juk suhn): Crisp, cream colored, conical shoot of the bamboo plant. Used fresh (stored in water) or available canned in brine (whole or sliced).

Banana flower (plantain flower): Native to Indonesia and Malaysia, bananas are now found in most tropical regions. Male inflorescence of the plant (female inflorescence that develops into fruit not eaten) is sheathed in inedible red-purple petals. Starchy interior must be boiled repeatedly to remove bitterness; used fresh in salads, cooked in curries, soups, or as side dish in palm oil or coconut milk.

Bangus: See *Milkfish.*

Baobab (monkey bread, lalu powder): Slightly sweet seeds from the large fruit of the native African baobab tree. Used roasted or ground. Pulp of the fruit is also consumed.

Basmati rice: See *Rice.*

Bean curd (cheong-po, tempeh, tofu, tobu): Custard-like, slightly rubbery white curd with a bland flavor made from soybean milk. Japanese bean curd (tofu) tends to be softer than Chinese, which is preferred for stir-fried dishes. A chewier version common in Southeast Asia is called tempeh. Cheong-po, a Korean bean curd, is made from mung beans.

Beans: See specific bean type.

Bean sprouts (nga choy): The young sprouts of mung beans or soybeans popular in Asian cooking (sprouts may also be grown from the tiny seeds of alfalfa or peas, also from legumes). The crisp 1- to 2-inch sprouts are eaten fresh or added to stir-fried dishes.

Belgian endive: See *Chicory.*

Berbere: Ethiopian spice mix (typically very hot) used to season many foods, usually including allspice, cardamom, cayenne, cinnamon, cloves, coriander, cumin, fenugreek, ginger, nutmeg, and black pepper.

Bergamot orange: Pear-shaped orange with exceptionally tart flesh. Rind used to flavor dishes in the Mediterranean and North Africa; oil extracted from rind flavors Earl Grey tea.

Betel (areca nuts; catechu): The heart-shaped leaves of the betel vine (related to black pepper) are used to wrap areca nuts (from the Areca palm; the nuts are usually called betel nuts because of their use with betel leaves) and spices for paan in India. Betel nuts and leaves are chewed together in many Southeast Asian countries and in India to promote digestion. May stain teeth red.

Bindi: See *Okra.*

Bird's nest: Swallows' nests from the cliffs of the South China Sea made from predigested seaweed; added to Chinese soups or sweetened for dessert. Must be soaked before use.

Bitter almond: An almond variety with an especially strong almond flavor, often used to make extracts, syrups, and liqueurs. Grown in the Mediterranean region, bitter almonds are used in European dishes. They contain prussic acid and are toxic when raw (they become edible when cooked) and are unavailable in the United States.

Bitter melon (balsam pear; bitter gourd, foo gwa): Bumpy-skinned Asian fruit similar in shape to a cucumber; pale green when ripe. The flesh has melon-like seeds and an acrid taste due to high quinine content (flavor and odor become stronger the longer it ripens).

Bitter orange: See *Seville orange.*

Black bean (frijol negro; turtle bean): Small (less than 1.2 inches) black bean used extensively in Central American, South American, and Caribbean cooking.

Black beans, fermented: Black soybeans salted and fermented to produce a piquant condiment. Used in Chinese cooking as a seasoning or combined with garlic, ginger, rice wine, and other ingredients to make black bean sauce.

Black-eyed peas (cow peas; crowder peas): Small legume (technically neither a pea nor a bean), white with a black spot, native to Africa and southern Asia.

Black mushrooms: See *Mushrooms.*

Blood orange: Old variety of orange with deep maroon-colored flesh, sometimes streaked with white. Intense sweet-tart flavor. Common in Spain and North Africa.

Blowfish (bok; fugu; globefish; puffer): A popular Japanese specialty, blowfish contain a deadly neurotoxin in the liver and sex organs. Must be carefully prepared by expert; flesh has a slight tingle when eaten.

Bok choy (Chinese chard; pak choi; white cabbage): Vegetable of the cabbage family with long, white leaf stalks and smooth, dark green leaves used in Chinese cooking.

Boonchi: See *Long bean.*

Bottle gourd: See *Calabash.*

Boxthorn: See *Matrimony vine.*

Breadfruit: Large, round, tropical fruit with warty green skin and starchy white flesh popular in nearly all tropical regions. It must be cooked. Unripe, green fruits are generally prepared as a vegetable, boiled, fried, or even pickled. In South Pacific may be fermented to make poi-like starchy dish. Ripe, yellow-fleshed fruit usually sweetened and served as dessert. Available canned; frozen.

Breadroot (Indian breadroot; prairie turnips; *timpsila; tipsin*): Hairy perennial plant (*Psoralea esculenta*) with large brown root eaten by Native Americans of the Plains and adopted by European immigrants who knew it as *pomme de prairie.*

Brinjal: See *Eggplant.*

Buckwheat (kasha): Nutty-flavored cereal native to Russia (where it is called kasha), sold as whole seeds (groats) and ground seeds (grits if coarsely ground, flour if finely ground). It is common in Russian and eastern European cooking.

Buffalo berry: Scarlet berry of the *Sheperdia* genus, so called because it was usually eaten with buffalo meat by Native Americans of the plains.

Bulgur (bulghur, burghul): Nutty-flavored cracked grains of whole wheat that have been precooked with steam. Available in coarse, medium, and fine grades.

Burdock root (gobo): Long thin root with thin brown skin and crisp white flesh and an earthy, sweet flavor. Popular in Asian cooking.

Cactus fruit (cactus pears, cholla, Indian figs, pitaya, sabra, strawberry pear, thang long): Succulent fruit of various cacti popular in numerous nations. Red prickly pear cactus fruit—cactus pears, cholla, Indian figs, sabra, tuna—common in Mexico, U.S. Southwest, Central America, Israel and some other Middle Eastern countries, Australia, South Africa, and Italy. Fruit of the organ pipe cactus sold in the United States as strawberry pear or pitaya. Fruit of saguaro cactus, nopales cactus, and apple cactus eaten in desert areas of Mexico and U.S. Southwest. Climbing epiphytic cacti common in South America, Australia, Israel, and Vietnam; one variety called thang long red pitaya or dragon fruit.

Cactus pads (nopales, nopalitos): Paddles of the prickly pear cactus or nopales cactus commonly eaten in Mexico and parts of the U.S. Southwest, fresh, cooked, or pickled. Available canned.

Cactus pears: See *Cactus fruit.*
Caimito: See *Star apple.*
Cajú: See *Cashew apple.*
Calabash (bottle gourd; calabaza; West Indian pumpkin): Gourd-like fruit of a tropical tree native to the New World.
Calabaza: See *Calabash; Cushaw*
Calamansi (calamondin, Chinese or Panama orange, golden or scarlet lime, musk lime): Small sour lime native to China but widely distributed in Indonesia and the Philippines, also available in Southeast Asia, Malaysia, and India. Prized for its sour flavor in Filipino cooking.
Callaloo (cocoyam): Edible leaves of root vegetables, especially amaranth, malanga, and taro. Callaloo is sometimes the name of a dish made from these leaves.
Camass root: Sweet bulb of the camass lily common in the U.S. Pacific Northwest.
Candlenut (kemini; kukui nut): Oily tropical nut sold only in roasted form (toxic when raw). Popular in Malaysia, Polynesia, and Southeast Asia.
Càng cua: See *Peperomia.*
Cannellini: See *Kidney bean.*
Capers: Small gray-green flower buds from a bush native to the Mediterranean; commonly pickled.
Carambola: See *Star fruit.*
Cardoon: Member of the artichoke family resembling a spiny celery plant, popular in Italian cooking.
Cashew apple (*cajú*): The fleshy false fruit attached to the cashew nut. Native to Brazil, it is also eaten in the Caribbean and India.
Casimiroa (white sapote, zapote blanco): Dark green to yellow fruit native to Central America; resembles an Asian pear. Soft, white flesh is eaten fresh or prepared as jellies, ices, milkshakes, and fruit leather.
Cassareep: Caribbean sauce made from the juice of the bitter variety of cassava cooked with raw sugar.
Cassava (cocoyam; fufu; manioc; yuca): Tropical Latin American tuber (now eaten in most tropical areas of the world) with rough brown skin and mild white flesh. Two types exist: bitter (poisonous unless leached and cooked) and sweet. Flour used in Africa (gari), the Caribbean, and Brazil (farinha). Cassava starch (fufu) is used to make the thickening agent tapioca. Leaves also consumed.
Caviar (red caviar, ikura, tarama, tobikko): Fish roe from a variety of fish eaten worldwide, including sturgeon (technically the only roe that is called caviar), salmon (red caviar, ikura in Japan), flying fish (tobikko), carp (tarama, most often made into a paste with lemon juice and other ingredients, in Greece called taramasalata), herring, and mullet. Sturgeon caviar graded according to size and quality.
Celeriac (celery root): Gnarled, bulbous root of one type of celery, with brown skin, tan flesh, and nutty flavor.
Cèpes: See *Mushrooms.*
Chanterelles: See *Mushrooms.*
Chayote (christophine, chocho, huisquil, mirliton, vegetable pear): Thin-skinned, green (light or dark), pear-shaped gourd. Native to Mexico, it is now common in Central America, the Caribbean, the southern United States, and parts of Asia.
Cheong-po: See *Bean curd.*
Cherimoya (anona, custard apple, graviola): Large, dimpled, light green fruit native to South America. White, creamy, flesh has a flavor reminiscent of strawberries, cherries, and pineapple. See also *Custard apple.*
Chicharrónes (pork cracklings): Deep-fried pork skin, fried twice to produce puffy strips.
Chickpeas (Bengal gram dal, chana dal, garbanzo bean): Pale yellow, spherical legume popular in Middle Eastern, Spanish, Portuguese, and Latin American cooking. Can be purchased canned or dried.
Chico: See *Zapote.*
Chicory (Belgian endive, witloof): European chicory plant. Leaves used as salad green; bitter root roasted to prepare a coffee substitute. Often added to dark coffee in Creole cooking.
Chile pepper: Although chile peppers, or chiles, are often called hot peppers, the fruits are not related to Asian pepper (such as black pepper) but are pods of capsicum plants, native to Central and South America. The alkaloid capsaicin, found mostly in the ribs of the pods, is what makes chile peppers hot. In general, the smaller the chile, the hotter it is. More than 100 varieties are available, from less than one-quarter inch in length to over eight inches long. Used fresh or dried. Common types include mild pods (see *Peppers*), slightly hot peppers such as Anaheim (also called *California* or *New Mexico chile*) and Cayenne (used mostly dried and powdered as the spice cayenne); dark green, medium hot Jalapeño (often available canned—when smoked are known as Chipotle); spicy, rich green Poblano (used fresh, or ripened and dried, called Ancho); hot Serrano (small, bright green or red); and very hot Chile de Arbol, Japones, Péquin (tiny berrylike pepper, exceptionally hot, also known as bird or bird's eye peppers), Piri-piri (favored in West Africa for sauces and marinades; also name of dishes that include some form of the pepper) and Tabasco (small, red chiles, often used dried and for sauce of same name). Those with extreme heat include Habanero and Scotch Bonnet; similar varieties native to the Caribbean.
Chile pepper sauce/paste (harissa, kochujang, pili-pili, Tabasco): Fiery condiments based on hot chile peppers. Sauce typically made from fermented chile peppers, vinegar, and salt (Tabasco sauce is the best-known U.S. brand). Pastes often include other ingredients, such as garlic and oil (Chinese-style and North African harissa). Pili-pili used in West Africa made with the piri-piri chile (see *Chile peppers*) and other ingredients such as tomatoes, onions, or horseradish. Korean kochujang includes soybeans and is fermented.
Chili powder: Ground, dried chile peppers, often with added spices such as oregano, cumin, and salt.
Chinese date (dae-chu; jujube): Small Asian fruit (not actually belonging to the date family) usually sold dried. Red dates are the most popular, but black and white are also available.
Chinese parsley: See *Coriander.*
Chitterlings (chitlins): Pork small intestines, prepared by boiling or frying.
Chokecherry: Tart, reddish black cherry (*Prunus virginiana*) native to the Americas.
Cholla: See *Cactus fruit.*
Chrysanthemum greens (chop suey greens, crowndaisy greens, sookgat): Spicy leaves of a variety of chrysanthemum (not the American garden flower), popular in Asian stir-fried dishes, especially in Korea.
Cilantro: See *Coriander.*
Citron: Yellow-green, apple-size citrus fruit. Valued primarily for its fragrant peel that is used raw to flavor Indonesian foods, and candied in European baked goods. Available crystallized and as preserves.

Citronella: See *Lemon grass.*

Clotted cream (Cornish cream, Devonshire cream): Very thick cream made by allowing cream to separate from milk, then heating it and cooling it so that it ferments slightly. Finally, the cream is skimmed from the milk (although Cornish cream is skimmed before heating and cooling). Popular in southwest England, where it is spread on bread or used as a topping for desserts.

Cloud (wood) ears: See *Mushrooms.*

Coconut cream: High-fat cream pressed from fresh grated coconut.

Coconut milk: Liquid extracted with water from fresh grated coconut.

Cocoplum: Bland plum with white flesh native to Central America, found in the Caribbean, Central America, and Florida. Eaten fresh or dried.

Cocoyam: See *Callaloo; Cassava.*

Conch: Large, univalve mollusk found in waters off Florida and Caribbean (where it is sometimes called lambi). Chewy meat valued for its smoky flavor; can be bitter. Used especially in soups and stews.

Copra: Dried coconut kernels used in the extraction of coconut oil.

Coriander (cilantro, Chinese parsley, dhanyaka, yuen sai): Fresh leaves of the coriander plant with a distinctive "soapy" flavor, common in Asian, Middle Eastern, Indian, and Latin American cooking. Seeds used as spice; root used in Thai cooking.

Corn smut (huitlacoche): Fungus (*Ustilaginales*) that grows on corn ears. Prized in Chinese, Mexican, and Native American cooking.

Couscous (cuscus, cuzcuz): Small granules of semolina flour used as a grain in African, Italian, Brazilian, and Middle Eastern dishes.

Cow pea: See *Black-eyed pea.*

Cracked wheat: Cracked raw kernels of whole wheat used in Middle Eastern cooking.

Crawfish (crawdad, crayfish, mudbug): Small freshwater crustacean, 4 to 6 inches long, that looks and tastes something like lobster. Found in Europe and the United States (California, Louisiana, Michigan, and the Pacific Northwest). The names *crawfish* and *crayfish* are also applied to the langostino, a saltwater crustacean that lacks large front claws.

Crème fraîche: Slightly thickened, slightly fermented cream popular in France.

Culantro (bhandhani, ngo gai, recao, siny coriander): Herb (*Eryngium foetidum*) that is close relative of cilantro (see *Coriander*); however, looks more like a dandelion with a pungent flavor reminiscent of crushed beetles. Used interchangeably with cilantro in the Caribbean and Central America, especially associated with Puerto Rican sofrito. Seasons Thai curries, Malaysian rice dishes, Indian chutneys and snacks; larger leaves used as a wrap for foods in Vietnam. Reportedly high in riboflavin, carotene, calcium, and iron.

Curry leaves (kari): Herb with tangerine overtones used throughout India, Sri Lanka, and in parts of Malaysia. Fresh leaves are briefly fried in ghee, then added to dishes before other seasoning. Not usually a component of curry powder.

Curry powder: The western version of the fresh Asian-Indian spice mixture (garam masala) used to flavor curried dishes. Up to twenty spices are ground, then roasted, usually including black pepper, cayenne, cinnamon, coriander, cumin, fenugreek, ginger, cardamom, and turmeric for color.

Cushaw (calabaza, green pumpkin): Round or oblong winter squash with yellow flesh and a flavor similar to pumpkin.

Custard apple (anona roja, bullock's heart, mamon): Green-skinned, irregular (heart-, spherical-, or ovoid-shaped) fruit about 3 to 6 inches in diameter, with granular, custardy flesh. Flavor sweet but considered inferior to related fruits such as cherimoya and sweetsop. See also *Cherimoya.*

Cuttlefish (inkfish): A mollusk similar to squid, but smaller. Available fresh or dried.

Daikon (icicle radish, white radish, mooli): Relatively mild white radish common in Asian cooking. The Japanese variety is the largest, often 12 inches long, and is shaped like an icicle. The Chinese variety tends to be smaller.

Dals: Indian term for hulled and split grains, legumes, or seeds. Many types are available, such as lentils and split peas.

Dashi: Japanese stock made from kelp and dried fish (bonita). *Dashi-no-moto* is the dried, powdered, instant mix.

Dilis (daing): Small fish related to anchovies, dried and salted. Used in Filipino dishes.

Dragon's eyes: See *Longan.*

Drumstick plant (horseradish tree, malunggay, reseda, sili leaves): Small, deciduous tree native to India, now popular in India, Southeast Asia, the Philippines, and West Africa. Fern-like leaves (very spicy flavor), flowers, seeds (resembling bean pods but not a legume), and roots (indistinguishable from horseradish) consumed.

Duhat: See *Jambolan.*

Durian: Football-size spiked fruit with a strong odor reminiscent of gasoline or rotten onions and sweet, creamy flesh prized in Malaysia, Southeast Asia, and parts of China.

Edamame: See *Soybean.*

Eddo: See *Taro.*

Eggplant (ai gwa, aubergine, brinjal, melananza, nasu): Large, pear-shape to round member of the nightshade family with smooth, thin skin (white or deep purple in color) and spongy, off-white flesh. Native to India, where it is called brinjal, it has a mildly bitter flavor. Especially popular in Mediterranean and Asian cuisine. Asian varieties known as Japanese (nasu) and Chinese (ai gwa) eggplant are widely available; the Thai type is small, round, and white with green stripes and is less common.

Egusi: See *Watermelon seeds.*

Elderberries: Small shrubs up to 20 feet. Numerous species found throughout northern hemisphere. In the United States the small, dark purple berries used fresh and in preserves, pies, and wine. Blossoms fried as fritters.

Enoki: See *Mushrooms.*

Epazote (Mexican tea; pigweed, wormseed): Pungent herb related to pigweed or goosefoot (and sometimes called by these names). Found in Mexico and parts of the United States. Often added to bean dishes to reduce gas.

Farinha: See *Cassava.*

Fava bean (broad bean, brown bean, horse bean, Windsor bean): Large, green, meaty bean sold fresh in the pod. Smaller white or tan fava beans are dried or canned and cannot be used interchangeably with the fresh beans. Common in Italian and Middle Eastern cooking.

Feijoa (pineapple guava): Small (up to 3 inches), ovoid fruit with greenish skin and white flesh. Flavor is similar to strawberries and pineapple with minty overtones. Shrub native to central regions of South America, but now also found in California, Australia, and New Zealand.

Fennel (finnochio, sweet anise): Light green plant with slightly bulbous end and stalks with feathery, dark green leaves, a little like celery. Used as a root vegetable, especially in Italy (known as finnochio). Delicate licorice or anise flavor.

Fenugreek (methi): Tan seeds of the fenugreek plant, with a flavor similar to artificial maple flavoring. Essential in the preparation of Asian-Indian spice mixtures. Leaves, called methi, also commonly eaten.

Fiddlehead ferns: Young unfurled fronds a specialty dish of the U.S. Northeast and southeastern Canada. Roots were eaten by Native Americans.

Filé powder: See *Sassafras.*

Fish paste (bagoong, kapi, pa dek, prahoc): Thick fermented paste made from fish, used as a condiment and seasoning in the Philippines and Southeast Asia.

Fish sauce (nam pla, nam prik, nuoc mam, patis, tuk-trey): Thin, salty, brown sauce made from fish fermented for several days. Asian fish sauces vary in taste from mild to very strong, depending on the country and the grade of sauce. Filipino patis is the mildest; Vietnamese nuoc mam is among the most flavorful. Nuoc cham is a sauce made from nuoc mam by the addition of garlic and chile peppers.

Five-spice powder: A pungent Chinese spice mixture of anise, cinnamon, cloves, fennel seeds, and Szechuan pepper.

Fufu: See *Cassava; Yam.*

Fugu: See *Blowfish.*

Fuzzy melon (hairy melon, mo gwa): Asian squash similar to zucchini with peach fuzz-like skin covering. Called fuzzy.

Gai choy: See *Mustard.*

Gai lan (Chinese broccoli, Chinese kale): Thick, broccoli-like stems and large, dark or blue-green leaves, with slightly bitter flavor. Used especially in stir-frying.

Garbanzo bean: See *Chickpea.*

Gari: See *Cassava.*

Geoduck: Large (up to 15 pounds) clam native to U.S. Pacific Northwest, with neck or siphon as long as 3 feet. Neck used in soups, stews; body sliced for steaks.

Ghee: Clarified butter (*usli ghee*) from cow's or buffalo milk used in India. The term *ghee* is also used for shortening made from palm or vegetable oil.

Ginger root: Knobby brown-skinned rhizome with fibrous yellow white pulp and a tangy flavor. Used sliced or grated in Asian dishes. Immature root with milder flavor used in some preparations, particularly pickled ginger popular in Japanese cuisine and candied ginger. Dried, ground ginger provides ginger flavor without the bite of fresh.

Ginkgo nut: Small pit of the fruit of the ginkgo tree (ancient species related to the pine tree), dried or preserved in brine, common in Japan.

Ginseng: Aromatic forked root with bitter, yellowish flesh, used in some Asian dishes and beverages; best known for therapeutic uses.

Glutinous rice: See *Rice.*

Granadilla: See *Passion fruit.*

Grape leaves: Large leaves of grape vines preserved in brine, common in Middle Eastern cooking.

Graviola: See *Cherimoya.*

Gravlax: See *Salmon, cured.*

Greens: Any of numerous cultivated or wild leaves, such as chard, collard greens, creases, cochan (coneflower), dandelion greens, dock, kale, milkweed, mustard greens, pokeweed, purslane, and spinach.

Grits: Coarsely ground grain, especially hominy, which is typically boiled into a thick porridge or fried as a side dish. Served often in the U.S. South.

Ground-cherries (Cape gooseberries, poha, golden berries): Yellow fruit that looks similar to a tiny husked tomato, from a bush native to Peru or Chile. Now popular throughout Central and South America, Central and South Africa, and the South Pacific. Also available in Australia, China, India, Malaysia, and the Philippines.

Groundnuts (apios, Indian potatoes): South American tuber *Apios americana* eaten by Native Americans, adopted by European settlers. Different from Africa groundnuts (referring to either peanuts or Bambara groundnuts).

Guanabana: See *Soursop.*

Guapuru: See *Jaboticaba.*

Guarana (Brazilian cocoa): Shrub, *Paullinia cupana* indigenous to the Amazon. Dried leaves and seeds of the fruit are used to make a stimulating tea (containing caffeine) or mixed with cassava flour to form sun-dried sticks.

Guava (araca de praia, cattley guava, waiwai): Small sweet fruit with an intense floral aroma, native to Brazil. Skin is yellow-green or yellow, and the grainy flesh ranges from white or yellow to pink and red. Many varieties are available, including strawberry guava (also known as cattley guava, araca de praia, and waiwai) and pineapple guava. Guava is popular as jelly, juice, or paste.

Guayo: See *Mamoncilla.*

Guineps: See *Mamoncilla.*

Headcheese: Loaf of seasoned meat made from the hog's head and sometimes also feet and organs.

Heart of palm (palmetto cabbage, palmito): White or light green interior of the palm tree, especially popular in the Philippines. Available canned.

Hickory nuts: Tree indigenous to North America, in same family as pecans. Eaten fresh, roasted, or ground into meal or pressed for a cream-like fluid by Native Americans; used in confections in the U.S. South.

Hog peanut: A high-protein underground fruit that grows on the root of the vine *Falcata comosa* in the central and southern United States. The peanut has a leathery shell that can be removed by boiling or soaking. The nut meat can be eaten raw or cooked.

Hoisin sauce: Popular Chinese paste or sauce, reddish brown in color, with a spicy sweet flavor. It is made from fermented soybeans, rice, sugar, garlic, ginger, and other spices.

Hominy (posole, pozole): Lime-soaked hulled corn kernels (yellow or white) with the bran and germ removed. Traditionally prepared by some Native Americans with culinary ash, which increases potassium, calcium, iron, phosphorus, and other mineral values. Ground, commonly called grits (see *Grits*).

Hot pepper: See *Chile pepper.*

Huisquil: See *Chayote.*

Icicle radish: See *Daikon.*

Ikura: See *Caviar.*

Imli: See *Tamarind.*

Indian breadroot: See *Breadroot.*

Indian fig: See *Cactus fruit.*

Indian potato: See *Groundnuts.*

Irish moss (carrageen): Gelatinous seaweed extract added to milk or rum as a beverage in the Caribbean.

Jaboticaba (guapuru, sabara): Brazilian shrub or small tree with 0.5- to 1.5-inch fruit clustered like grapes. Gelatinous pulp is mild and sweet.

Jackfruit: Large (up to 100 pounds) fruit related to breadfruit and figs, native to India, now cultivated in Asia, Malaysia, and Southeast Asia. Two varieties are widely eaten, one with a crisp texture and bland flavor, the other softer and sweeter. Immature fruit is usually prepared like other starchy vegetables such as breadfruit and plantains, or pickled. Sweeter types are popular as dessert. Available dried or canned.

Jaggery: Unrefined sugar from the palmyra or sugar palm common in India.

Jagua: See *Mamoncilla*.

Jambolan (duhat, Indian blackberry, jaman, Java plum, rose apple, voi rung): Small sour fruit grown in India and Southeast Asia, especially the Philippines. Used primarily in preserves, juices, and sherbets.

Jerusalem artichoke (sunchoke, sunroot): Small nubby-skinned tuber that is the root of a native American sunflower. It is neither from Jerusalem nor related to the artichoke, though the flavor when cooked is similar. It is used raw and cooked.

Jicama (ahipa, sa got, singkamas, yambean): Legume with medium to large tuber with light brown skin and crisp white flesh, indigenous to Brazil. Used raw in Latin American cuisine, it has a sweet, bland flavor, similar to peas or water chestnuts. Also found in Asia, where it is typically stir-fried or added to other cooked dishes.

Jujube: See *Chinese date*.

Juneberries (saskatoons, serviceberries; shadbush): Red to deep purple berries on large bush native to the Great Plains region of the United States and Canada. White blooms in June associated with shad migratory run on East Coast; favorite of Native Americans.

Juniper berry: Distinctively flavored dark blue berry of the juniper evergreen bush, native to Europe. Used to flavor gin.

Kadondong: See *Ambarella*.

Kaffir lime (ichang lime, makrut, wild lime): Aromatic citrus popular in Southeast Asia, especially in Thai cooking. Juice, rind, and leaves used to flavor curries, salad dressings, and sauces.

Kamis: Sour, cucumber-like vegetable native to the Philippines. Used to achieve a sour, cool flavor in Filipino cooking.

Kang kong: See *Water convolvulus*.

Kanpyo (kampyo): Ribbons of dried gourd used mostly for garnishing dishes in Japan.

Kaong: See *Palm nuts*.

Kapi: See *Fish paste*.

Kasha: See *Buckwheat*.

Kava: See *Pepper plant*.

Kemini: See *Candlenut*.

Kewra: See *Pandanus*.

Key lime (dayap, nimbu, West Indian or Mexican lime): Small, tart lime indigenous to the Caribbean, popular in Florida Keys; also used in east and north Africa, India, and Malaysia. Known best as primary ingredient in key lime pie.

Khati powder: See *Amchoor*.

Kidney bean (cannellini, red peas): Medium-size, kidney-shaped bean, light to dark red in color (a white variety is popular in Europe, especially Italy, where they are known as *cannellini*). The flavorful beans are common in Europe, Latin America, and the United States.

Kochujang: See *Chile pepper sauce/paste*.

Kohlrabi (tjin choi tow): Light green or purple bulbous vegetable that grows above the soil and produces stems bearing leaves on the upper part. A member of the cabbage family, it can be eaten raw or cooked.

Kola nut: Bitter nut of the African kola tree (extracts from this nut were used in the original recipe for Coca-Cola).

Kudzu (ge gen, Japanese arrowroot): Japanese vine valued for its tuberous root (up to 450 pounds) that is dried and powdered for a starch used in sauces and soups and to coat foods before frying. Now found in much of Asia and U.S. Southeast where it is best known for its growth rate of up to 1 foot per day. May alleviate hangovers or induce sobriety.

Kukui nut: See *Candlenut*.

Kumquat (kin kan): Small, bright orange, oval fruit with a spicy citrus flavor common in China and Japan. Also available in syrup and candied.

Laverbread: Thick purée of laver (see *Seaweed*) that is baked. Used in sauces and stuffings in Great Britain.

Lemon grass (citronella root): Large, dull green, stiff grass with lemony flavor common in Southeast Asian dishes. Available fresh, dried, or powdered.

Lily buds (golden needles, gum chum): The buds of lily flowers used both fresh and dehydrated in the cooking of China.

Lingonberry (low-bush cranberry): Small wild variety of the cranberry found in Canada and northern Europe. Usually available as preserves.

Litchi (lychee): Small Chinese fruit with translucent white flesh and a thin brown hull and single pit. The flavor is grape-like but less sweet. Available fresh and canned. Dried litchis, also called litchi nuts, have different flavor and texture.

Lobster: Ocean-dwelling crustacean valued for its sweet flesh. Two main species consumed in United States. American lobster (*Homarus americanus*) found from Labrador to North Carolina; meat from large claws and tail, premature eggs called *coral*, and liver eaten. Spiny lobster (*Panulirus argus* and other species) looks similar to American lobster but is a different animal. Found in warm waters from North Carolina to Brazil; small claws, only tail meat eaten.

Longan (dragon's eyes): Fruit of an Asian Indian tree related to litchis. Used fresh, canned, or dried.

Long bean (boonchi, dau gok, sitao, yardlong bean): Roundish Asian bean, 12 to 30 inches long. Similar in taste to string beans, long beans are softer, and chewier, less juicy, and less crunchy than string beans.

Long-grain rice: See *Rice*.

Loquat (nispero): Slightly fuzzy yellow Asian fruit about 2 inches across, easily peeled, with tart peach-flavored flesh. Cultivated worldwide; available fresh, dried, and in syrup.

Lotus root (lian, lin gau hasu, renkon, water lily root): Tubular vegetable (holes, as in Swiss cheese, run the length of the root, producing a flower-like pattern when the root is sliced) with brownish skin and crisp, sweet, white flesh. Becomes starchy when overcooked or canned.

Lox: See *Salmon, smoked*.

Luffa (cee gwa, Chinese okra, loofa, padwal, silk melon): Long, thinskinned Asian vegetable, a member of the cucumber family, with spongy flesh. Immature luffas consumed fresh, stir-fried, and in curries; mature luffa becomes bitter. Also see *Sponge gourd*.

Lulo: See *Naranjillo*.

Lupine seeds (tremecos): Bitter seeds of a legume used primarily for fodder. Must be leached in water before eating.

Macadamia nut: Round, creamy nut native to Australia, now grown in Africa, South America, and Hawaii.

Mahi-mahi (dolphinfish, dorado): A saltwater finfish found in parts of the Pacific and the Gulf Coast (not the mammal also known as dolphin).

Mahleb: Middle Eastern spice made from ground black cherry kernels, which impart a fruity flavor to foods.

Makrut: See *Kaffir lime.*

Malagueta pepper (grains of paradise, guinea pepper): Small West African berries related to cardamom, with a hot, peppery flavor. In Brazil the term refers to a tiny Pequin chile pepper.

Malanga (cocoyam, tannier, yautia): Caribbean tuber with creamcolored, yellow, or pinkish flesh, dark brown skin, and nutty flavor. Name also applied to other tubers (see *Taro*).

Mamey (sapote): Medium-size egg-shaped fruit with brown skin and soft flesh ranging in color from orange to yellowish to reddish. It has a flavor similar to pumpkin. See also *Mammea.*

Mammea (mamey apple): South American fruit with reddish-brown skin and bright yellow flesh that tastes like peaches.

Mamoncilla (guayo, guineps, jaguar, macao, Spanish lime): Small 1- to 2-inch green fruit found in the Caribbean and South America that grow in clusters like grapes but have thicker skin and distinctive sweet, citrusy flesh around a large seed.

Mango (mangoro, mangue): Fruit native to India, now found throughout Africa, Asia, Latin America, and parts of the South Pacific. Yellow to red when ripe, averaging 1 pound in weight. The flesh is pale and sour when the fruit is unripe, bright orange and very sweet when it is ripe. Used unripe for pickles and chutneys, ripe as a fresh fruit.

Manioc: See *Cassava.*

Marzipan: See *Almond paste.*

Masa: Dough used to make tortillas and tamales. Made fresh from dried corn kernels soaked in a lime solution, or from one of two flours available: masa harina (tortilla mix made from dehydrated fresh masa) or masa trigo (wheat flour tortilla mix).

Mastic: Resin from the lentisk bush that has a slightly piney flavor, used to flavor Middle Eastern foods. Available in crystal form.

Matai: See *Waterchestnut.*

Mate: Plant in holly family native to South America. Dried, powdered leaves, called *yerba,* are brewed to make a stimulating tea (containing caffeine) that is popular in Argentina, Brazil, and Paraguay.

Matrimony vine (boxthorn, wolfberry): Asian vine with culinary and medicinal uses; both leaves and fruit are used in China.

Mayhaw: Type of hawthorn tree found in U.S. South. Its fruit looks like cranberries. Tart apple flavor. Used in preserves, syrups, and wines.

Methi: See *Fenugreek.*

Mikan: Japanese citrus related to tangerines and mandarin oranges. Eaten fresh, frozen, and canned in syrup.

Milkfish (awa, bangus): Silvery, bony fish with oily flesh especially popular in Filipino cooking.

Millet: Cereal native to Africa, known for its high-protein, low-gluten content and ability to grow in arid areas. The variety common in Ethiopia is called *teff.*

Mirin: Sweet rice wine used in Japanese dishes.

Miso: Fermented soybean-barley or soybean rice paste common in Japanese cooking. Light or white (shiro miso) is mild flavored; dark or red (aka miso) is strongly flavored. Also available sweetened and as powder.

Mizuna: See *Mustard.*

Morels: See *Mushrooms.*

Mullet (ama ama): Finfish of two families that can be black, gray, or red. The flesh is a mix of dark, oily meat and light, nutty-tasting meat. The texture is firm but tender.

Mung beans (green gram dal, mung dal): Yellow-fleshed bean with olive or tan skin used in cooking of China, India. See also *Bean curd; Bean sprouts.*

Mushrooms: Fresh or dried fungi used to flavor dishes throughout the world. Common Asian types include *enoki* (tiny yellow mushrooms with roundish caps), *oyster mushrooms* (large, delicately flavored gray-beige caps that grow on trees), *shiitake* (dark brown with wide flat caps, available dried as Chinese black mushrooms), *straw mushrooms* (creamy colored with bell-like caps), and *cloud ears* or *wood ears* (a large, flat fungus with ruffled edges, available dried). Popular mushrooms in Europe, available both fresh and dried, include *chanterelles* (a golden mushroom with an inverted cap), *morels* (a delicately flavored mushroom with a dark brown wrinkled cap), and *porcini* or *cèpes* (large brown mushrooms with caps that are spongy underneath; also called *boletus*).

Musk lime: See *Calamansi.*

Mustard (Chinese green mustard, gai choy, kyona, mizuna, potherb): Though best known for the condiment made from its seeds, greens of several varieties are popular in Asia, called gai choy in China (dark green-reddish leaves), mizuna (small yellowish, notched leaves) in Japan. Usually steamed, boiled, or stir-fried. Root also consumed.

Nam pla: See *Fish sauce.*

Nam prik: See *Fish sauce.*

Nance: Small, yellow tropical fruit native to Central America and northern South America. Similar to cherries with a slightly tart flavor. Two varieties are available.

Napa cabbage (celery cabbage, Chinese cabbage, Peking cabbage, wong bok): Bland, crunchy vegetable with broad white or light green stalks with ruffled leaves around the edges. Several types are available, similar in taste.

Naranjilla (lulo): Walnut-size, orange-skinned, green-fleshed fruit indigenous to the Americas, used mostly for its juice. Particularly popular in Central America.

Naseberry: See *Zapote.*

Nigella seed ("black cumin," "black onion," kalonji): Small, black seeds native to Europe, North Africa, and the Middle East. Sometimes used as a substitute for black pepper, the flavor of the seeds (which are related neither to cumin nor onions) is pungent, slightly bitter. Added to spice mixtures in India and the Middle East, sprinkled on savory breads and cakes in both regions, as well as in Eastern Europe.

Nispero: See *Loquat.*

Nku: See *Shea nut.*

Nongus (palmyra): Fruit of the palmyra palm, grown in India, Indonesia, and Malaysia primarily as a source of sugar. See also *Jaggery.*

Nopales, Nopalitos: See *Cactus pads.*

Nuoc cham: See *Fish sauce.*

Nuoc mam: See *Fish sauce.*

Oca: Tuber of Andean plant (*Oxalis tuberosa*). Resembles a pink potato. Tastes lemony when fresh, sweet after storage. Used in South America, prepared like potatoes or eaten fresh.

Okra (bindi, lady's fingers): Small, green, torpedo-shaped pod with angular sides. A tropical African plant valued for its carbohydrates that are sticky and mucilaginous. Used as a vegetable and to thicken soups and stews.

Olive: Fruit of a tree native to the Mediterranean. Green olives are preserved unripe. Large, soft Kalamata olives are a medium size, purplish Greek olive. Dark olives (such as Niçoise) are picked in autumn, often cured in salt, with a tannic flavor. Ripe, black olives are smooth-skinned and mild-flavored or wrinkled with a strong tannic flavor.

Olive oil: Extracted from the olive flesh, it is labeled according to percent acidity, from *extra virgin* to *virgin* (or *pure*). U.S. labeling laws restrict the use of the term virgin to only olive oil made from the first press; virgin olive oils mixed with refined olive oils to reduce acidity are labeled *pure*.

Ostiones: Oyster native to the Caribbean that grows on the roots of mangrove trees.

Otaheite apple: See *Ambarella*.

Oyster mushrooms: See *Mushrooms*.

Oyster sauce: Thick, brown Chinese sauce made with soy sauce, oysters, and cornstarch.

Pacaya bud: The bitter flower stalk of the pacaya palm found in Central America. The edible stalk is about 10 inches long and is encased in a tough green skin, which must be removed before cooking.

Pa dek: See *Fish sauce*.

Palillo: Peruvian herb, used dried and powdered to provide a yellowish- orange color to foods.

Palmetto cabbage: See *Heart of palm*.

Palm nuts (kaong): Seeds from palms; pounded into palm butter in West Africa. Also boiled and added to halo-halo mix in Philippines. Available canned, in syrup.

Palm oil (aceite de palma, dende oil): Oil from the African palm, unique for its red-orange color, used extensively in West African and Brazilian Bahian cuisine. Crude oil contains high levels of carotenoids and tocopherols; refined oil deodorized and decolorized, significantly reducing nutritional value. Oil from the seed of the palm fruit high in saturated fats; should be labeled palm kernel oil, but often mislabeled as palm oil.

Pandanus (flowers—kewra, screw pine; leaves—duan pandan, pandan, rampa, screw pine): Perfume essence of the male screwpine flower *Pandanus fascicularis* used primarily in north Indian cooking. Screw-pine leaves *Pandanus amaryllifolius* reminiscent of mown hay, used to flavor the foods of Southeast Asia, Malaysia, South India, Bali, and New Guinea. Fresh withered leaves used in rice puddings and as wrappers for steaming foods in Thailand. Bright green screw-pine essence also available.

Papaya (kapaya, pawpaw, tree melon): Thin-skinned green (underripe), yellow, or orange fruit with sweet flesh colored gold to light orange to pink; native to Central America, now found throughout the tropics. Mexican (large and round) and Hawaiian (smaller and pear shaped) varieties are commonly available. The shiny round black seeds are edible. Unripe papaya is used in pickles; the ripe fruit is eaten fresh.

Paprika: Powdered red peppers especially popular in Hungarian cooking. Paprika is made from several types of pods related to bell and chile peppers. Paprika is usually designated sweet or hot. Spanish paprika, used in Spanish and Middle Eastern dishes, is more flavorful.

Passion fruit (granadilla, lilikoi): Small oval fruit with very sweet, gelatinous pulp. Its berries are used dried; leaves brewed to make herbal tea.

Patis: See *Fish sauce*.

Pawpaw (Hoosier banana, Poor Man's banana, tree melon): Light orange fruit that tastes like a cross between a banana and a melon. Native to the Americas, it is approximately 6 inches long. See also *Papaya*.

Peanuts (groundnuts, goobers, monkey nuts): Legume native to South America, introduced to Africa by the Portuguese, then brought to the United States in the 17th century by black slaves. Eaten raw, roasted, or pulverized into peanut butter. Popular in Africa and the United States; used in some Chinese, Southeast Asian, and Asian-Indian dishes.

Pejibaye (peach palm): Fruit of a Central American palm, especially popular in Costa Rica.

Peperomia *(càng cua)*: Small plant with heart-shaped leaves *Peperomia pellucida* found throughout Central and South America, Africa, and Southeast Asia. Used as a culinary herb in Vietnam, and as a medicinal herb in the Philippines, Polynesia, and parts of Latin America.

Pepitas (cushaw seeds): Pumpkin or squash seeds, typically from cushaw, common in Latin-American cooking. May be hulled or unhulled, raw or roasted, salted or unsalted.

Pepper plant *(Piper methysticum)*: Leaves of the South Pacific plant used to produce the intoxicating beverage called *kava* or *awa*.

Peppers: Misnamed pods of the capsicum plants native to South and Central America (not actually related to Asian pepper plants, which produce black pepper). Peppers are divided into sweet and hot types (see *Chile pepper*). Sweet peppers include bell peppers (green, red, yellow, and purple), pimentos, and peppers used to make paprika (see *Paprika*).

Perilla (shiso; beefsteak plant; quen-neep): Aromatic herb with distinctive minty flavor; green or red. Available fresh or pickled. Used mostly as a seasoning or garnish in many Japanese and Korean dishes; sometimes served as a side dish or to wrap rice and other items.

Pigeon pea: Small pea in a hairy pod (a member of the legume family, but not a true pea) common in the cooking of Africa, the Caribbean, and India. Yellow or tan when dried.

Pignoli: See *Pine nut*.

Pigweed: See *Amaranth; Epazote*.

Pili nut: Almond-like nut of a tropical tree found in the Philippines eaten raw and toasted. Popular also in Chinese desserts.

Pili-pili: See *Chile pepper sauce/paste*.

Pine nut (pignoli, piñon seed): Delicately flavored kernel from any of several species of pine tree. Pine nuts are found in Portugal (most expensive type), China (less costly, with a stronger taste), and the U.S. Southwest. Common in some Asian, European, Latin American, Middle Eastern, and Native American dishes.

Pink bean (rosada): Small oval meaty bean that is a light tannish pink in color.

Pinto bean: Mottled bean similar to kidney beans, especially popular in U.S. Southwest and Mexico.

Pitanga (Surinam cherry, Brazilian cherry): Small, bright red, ribbed fruit of shrub or small tree *Eugenia uniflora* native to northeastern South America; found also in the Caribbean and Florida. Thin skin with orange flesh that melts in the mouth. Sweet with a slightly bitter bite.

Pitaya, Pitahaya, Pitajaya: See *Cactus fruit*.

Plantain: Starchy type of banana with a thick skin, which can be green, red, yellow, or black. There are many varieties, ranging in size from 3 to 10 inches. The pulp is used as a vegetable and must be cooked. It is similar in taste to squash. Flower also consumed (see *Banana flower*).

Poha: See *Ground-cherries*.

Poi: See *Taro*.

Porcini: See *Mushrooms.*
Posole, Pozole: See *Hominy.*
Prahoc: See *Fish paste.*
Prairie turnips: See *Breadroot.*
Prickly pear: See *Cactus fruit; Cactus pads.*
Pulses: Term used especially in India for edible legume seeds, including peas, beans, lentils, and chickpeas.
Quinoa: Cereal native to the Andes, typically prepared like rice. Also available as flour and flakes (hojuelas).
Radicchio: Magenta-colored, slightly bitter member of the chicory family used throughout southern and northern Europe.
Rambutan: Bristly, juicy, orange or bright red fruit used in Southeast Asian cooking; related to the litchi.
Ramp: Strong-flavored indigenous American onion that tastes somewhat like a leek. Both leaves and bulbs are edible.
Recao: See *Culantro.*
Red bean: Small, dark red bean native to Mexico and the southwestern U.S.
Red caviar: See *Caviar.*
Red pea: See *Kidney bean.*
Rice: Grain native to India. More than 2,500 varieties are available worldwide, including basmati rice (small grain with a flavor similar to popcorn, very popular in India and the Middle East); brown rice (unmilled rice with the bran layer intact; can be short-, medium-, or long-grain); glutinous rice (also called *sweet* or *pearl rice*; very short grain and very sticky when cooked); long-grain rice (white, polished grains that flake when cooked, common in China and Vietnam); and short-grain rice (slightly sticky when cooked, popular in Japan and Korea). Rice flour is used to prepare rice noodle, rice paper, and baked products.
Roseapple (pomarrosa, kopo): Small, thin-skinned pink or red fruit native to Southeast Asia with somewhat spongy flesh that has slightly acidic flavor.
Roselle (Florida cranberry; karkadeh; red sorrel; sorrel): Pods of a hibiscus plant relative, common in Africa, the Caribbean, Southeast Asia, Australia, and Florida. Used to make a tart tea popular in Egypt and Senegal and a rum-laced punch in the Caribbean. Also used for chutneys, preserves, and candies. Young leaves are eaten raw as salad or cooked as greens.
Sabra: See *Cactus fruit.*
Saewujeot: See *Shrimp paste.*
Saffron: Dried stamens of the crocus flower. It has a delicate, slightly bitter flavor and bright red-orange color. Available as threads or powder.
Sa got: See *Jicama.*
Salal: Thick-skinned black berries of a native American plant in the heath family. Used fresh and dried, good for preserves. Leaves used for tea.
Salmon, cured: Salmon fillets cured in a mixture of salt, sugar, and dill weed, common in Sweden (where it is known as gravlax), Finland, and Norway.
Salmon, smoked: Raw, tender salmon slices lightly smoked and cured in salt produced in Norway, Nova Scotia, and Scotland. Smoked salmon soaked in a brine solution is called *lox*, a Jewish specialty.
Salmon roe: See *Caviar.*
Salt pork: White fat from the side of the hog, streaked with pork meat, cured in salt.
Saluyot (jute, okra leaves, rau day): Leaves from Southeast Asian jute bush with slippery texture when cooked (not related to okra). Added to soups and stews in Filipino cooking.
Samphire (beach asparagus, glasswort, sea pickle, pousse-pied): Several species of samphire thought to have originated in Brazil, but now found worldwide, especially in Australia and the South Pacific. Yellow- and purple-skinned varieties are available. Passion fruit is often made into juice.
Sapodilla: See *Zapote.*
Sapote: See *Zapote.*
Saskatoons: See *Juneberries.*
Sassafras (filé powder): Native American herb used to thicken soups and stews.
Screwpine: See *Pandanus.*
Sea cucumber (sea slug): Brown or black saltwater mollusk up to 1 foot in length. They lack a shell, but have a leathery skin and look something like smooth, dark cucumbers. Sold dried, they are rehydrated for Chinese dishes, becoming soft and jellylike, with a mild flavor.
Sea urchin roe (uni): Small, delicate eggs of the spiny sea urchin, popular in Japan.
Seaweed (kim): Many types of dried seaweed are used in Chinese, Korean, and Japanese dishes, including *aonoriko* (powdered green seaweed), *kombu* (kelp sheets), and *nori* (tissue-thin sheets of dark green seaweed, also known as laver). Also popular in the Pacific Islands. See also *Irish moss; Laverbread.*
Serviceberries: See *Juneberries.*
Sesame seeds (benne seeds): Seeds of a plant native to Indonesia. Two types are available: tan colored (white when hulled) and black (slightly bitter). Untoasted sesame paste popular in the Middle East (tahini); toasted sesame paste and powdered seeds common in Asia, especially Korea. Widely grown for their oil. Light sesame oil is pressed from raw seeds, dark oil from toasted seeds; the dark oil has a strong taste and is used as a flavoring.
Seville orange (bitter orange; naranja aria, sour orange): Orange with tough skin and dark flesh native to Mediterranean. Inedible raw; juice used in liqueurs (Grand Marnier, Cointreau, Curaçao) and in cooking of the Mediterranean, Caribbean, Central America, and Korea.
Shadbush: See *Juneberries.*
Shallot: Very small bulb covered with a reddish, papery skin, related to onions but with a milder, sweeter flavor.
Shea nut (bambuk butter, nku): Nut from the African shea tree, grown for its thick oil, called shea nut butter or shea nut oil.
Shiitake mushrooms: See *Mushrooms.*
Shiso: See *Perilla.*
Short-grain rice: See *Rice.*
Shoyu: See *Soy sauce.*
Shrimp paste: Strongly flavored fermented Asian sauce or paste made from small dried shrimp or similar crustaceans. Many types are available (bagoong-alamang is the Filipino variety; saeujeot is the Korean type).
Singkamas: See *Jicama.*
Snail (escargot): Small, edible land snail (a common variety of garden snail, cleansed with a commercial feed), popular in France. Giant, baseball-sized snails popular in parts of Africa and the South Pacific.
Snow pea (Chinese pea pod, ho lan dow, mange-tout, sugar pea): Flat, edible pod with small, immature peas.
Sorghum (guinea corn, kaffir corn): Cereal common to tropical regions of Africa with seeds produced on a stalk. In the Appalachians, Ozarks, and the U.S. South, sorghum is often processed to make sweet syrup.

Sorrel (dock, sour grass, wild rhubarb): Small, sour green popular in Europe and parts of United States. See also *Roselle.*

Sour orange: See *Seville orange.*

Soursop (guanabana): Large (often 12 inches long) rough-skinned fruit with cottony, fluffy flesh that can be white, pink, or light orange. Native to northern South America or the Caribbean, now found in many parts of the Americas, Africa, India, China, Southeast Asia, Malaysia, and South Pacific. Often made into juice or conserves.

Soybean: Small high-protein bean common in Asia. Many varieties of different colors, including black, green, red, and yellow, are available; immature beans in the pod (called edamame) popular in Japan. They are used fresh, dried, and sprouted, most often processed into sauces, condiments, and other products (see *Bean curd; Bean sprout; Hoisin sauce; Miso; Oyster sauce; Soy milk, Soy sauce*).

Soy milk: Soybeans that are boiled, pureed, then strained and boiled again to produce a white milk-like drink.

Soy sauce (shoyu, tamari): Thin, salty, brown sauce made from fermented soybeans. Several types are available. Chinese and Korean soy sauces tend to be lighter in flavor than the stronger, darker Japanese shoyu. Very dark soy sauces, such as Chinese black soy sauce and Japanese tamari may be thickened with caramel or molasses.

Spicebush: Shrub (*Lindera benzoin*) with spicy-smelling bark and leaves; red berries. Used to make Native American teas.

Spiny lobster: See *Lobster.*

Sponge gourd (luffa): Immature vegetable consumed in Asia fresh and in soups; tough fibrous skin used for sponges (loofah), filters, and stuffing.

Star anise: Eight-armed pods from a plant in the magnolia family, with an anise-like flavor. Native to China.

Star apple (caimito): Purple, apple-size fruit with mild, gelatinous, lavender-colored flesh native to the Caribbean. Seeds form a star around the center.

Star fruit (carambola): Small, deeply ribbed, oval fruit with thin skin shaped like a star when sliced. Green and sour when unripe, yellow and slightly sweet (though still tart) when ripe. Unripe fruit is used in Indian and Chinese dishes. Ripe it is eaten fresh.

Strawberry pear: See *Cactus fruit.*

Straw mushrooms: See *Mushrooms.*

Sumac: Sour, red Middle Eastern spice made from the ground berries of a nontoxic variety of the sumac plant.

Sunflowers: Native to the United States (genus *Helianthus*); over 60 varieties. Seeds eaten by Native Americans raw, dried, and powdered (in breads). Unopened flower head can be cooked and eaten like an artichoke. Petals are dried and used like saffron in Southwest.

Sweet peppers: See *Peppers.*

Sweetsop (annona blanca, ata, sugar apple): Sweet, white-fleshed fruit related to the cherimoya, custard apple, and soursop.

Szechwan pepper (fagara): Aromatic berries with a hot flavor popular in some Chinese and Japanese dishes.

Tabasco sauce: See *chile pepper sauce/paste.*

Tahini: See *Sesame seeds.*

Tamarind (imli, tamarindo): Tart pulp from the pod of the tamarind bean. Available in the pod, as a paste, in a brick, or as a liquid concentrate. Unripe pulp used extensively in flavoring numerous foods and beverages, especially Asian Indian and Latino dishes, as well as Worcestershire sauce and prepared salad dressings. Ripe pulp eaten fresh.

Tampala: See *Amaranth.*

Tannier (tannia): See *Taro; Malanga.*

Tapioca: See *Cassava.*

Taramasalata: See *Caviar.*

Taro (cocoyam, eddo, dasheen, tannier, malanga, yautia): Starchy underground vegetable similar to cassava with brown hairy skin and white to grayish flesh, common in the Caribbean and Polynesia. In Hawaii the boiled, pounded taro paste called *poi* is a staple in the traditional diet. The young shoots and large leaves are also eaten (see *Callaloo; Malanga*).

Tarpon: Large silver fish of the herring family found off the coasts of Mexico and Central America.

Teff: See *Millet.*

Tempeh: See *Bean curd.*

Tepary beans: Small, high-protein bean with wrinkled skin. Grows wild in the U.S. Southwest.

Ti: Tropical plant popular in Polynesia (not related to tea). Ti leaves are used to wrap food packets, and the root is eaten and brewed for a beverage.

Tilapia: Small freshwater fish with sweet, firm, white flesh.

Timpsila: See *Breadroot.*

Tipsin: See *Breadroot.*

Tobikko: See *Caviar.*

Tobu, Tofu: See *Bean curd.*

Tomatillo (husk tomatoes, miltomate): Small, light green, tomato-like fruit surrounded by a green or tan papery husk, common in Mexico. The flesh is slightly tart and is eaten cooked, usually in sauces and condiments. Available fresh or canned.

Tremecos: See *Lupine seeds.*

Truffle: Black (French) or white (Italian) fungus found underground. Truffles vary from the size of small marbles to as large as tennis balls and are distinctively flavored, similar to a wild mushroom. Available fresh or canned.

Tuk-trey: See *Fish paste.*

Tuna: See *Cactus fruit.*

Turtle: Popular in Caribbean, Central America, and U.S. South. Diamondback terrapin (*Malaclemys terrapin*) is the primary ingredient in turtle soups of the Atlantic states. Green turtle (*Chelonia mydas*) is a sea turtle, commonly eaten as steaks or stews. Other turtles eaten occasionally (including eggs) are alligator snapping turtle, common snapping turtle, and loggerhead turtle.

Ugli fruit: Citrus fruit that is a cross between a pomelo and a mandarin orange, with a very bumpy yellow-orange skin and a sweet orange-like flavor. Especially popular in Jamaica.

Uni: See *Sea urchin roe.*

Usli ghee: See *Ghee.*

Verjuice: Juice of unripe lemons used in Middle Eastern fare to give a tang to dishes.

Voi rang: See *Jambolan.*

Wasabi: Light green Japanese condiment from root of plant similar to horseradish with a powerful pungency. Available fresh or powdered; green-dyed horseradish often sold as wasabi.

Water chestnut (matai): Aquatic, walnut-size tuber with fibrous brown peel and crunchy, sweet, ivory-colored flesh. Available fresh or canned.

Water convolvulus (kang kong, ong choi, rau muong, water spinach) Plant related to sweet potato valued primarily for its sprouts and young leaves. Natives to China; significant crop in Southeast Asia, Malaysia, and South India.

Watermelon seeds: Seeds often eaten in Africa (called *egusi*, toasted and ground or pounded into meal or paste for thickening soups and stews) and in Asia (toasted as a snack; sometimes flavored or dyed red).
White bean: Three types of white bean are widely used: cannellini (see *Kidney bean*); Great Northern beans, which are large, soft, and mild tasting; and the smaller, firmer navy beans.
White radish: See *Daikon*.
Wild rice: Seeds of a native American grass.
Winged bean: Edible legume called the soybean of the tropics. All parts of the plant are consumed, including the shoots, leaves, flowers, pods and seeds, and tuberous root. The pods are large, from 12 to 24 inches long, and feature wing-like flanges.
Winter melon (dong gwa, petha, wax melon/gourd): Round greenskinned member of the squash family with a waxy white coating and translucent white green or pink flesh. Similar in taste to zucchini, it is used cooked in Chinese dishes. Called fuzzy melon when immature, winter melon when mature. See also *Fuzzy melon*.
Witloof: See *Chicory*.
Wolfberry: See *Matrimony vine*.
Wong bok: See *Napa cabbage*.
Worcestershire sauce: Sauce developed by the British firm of Lea and Perrins including anchovies, garlic, onions, molasses, sugar or corn sweetener, tamarind, and vinegar, among other ingredients.
Yacón (yakon, leafcup): Sweet-tasting root, *Polymnia sonchifolia*, with brown skin and white flesh native to Andes. Eaten throughout South America; in some regions confusingly called *jicama* (See *Jicama*).
Yam (ñame; yampi; cush-cush; mapuey): Tuber with rough brown skin and starchy white flesh (not related to the orange sweet potato called *yam* in the United States). Numerous varieties; may grow quite large, up to 100 pounds. Found in all tropical regions. Yam paste called *fufu* in West Africa.
Yambean: See *Jicama*.
Yard-long bean: See *Long bean*.
Yautia: See *Malanga; Taro*.
Yerba buena: A variety of mint used in some Native American teas.
Yuca: See *Cassava*.
Yucca (Navajo banana): Spiky-leaved desert plant (*Yucca baccata*) with large, pulpy fruit that ripens in summer. Eaten fresh, boiled, baked, or dried into fruit leather.
Zapote (chico, black sapote, naseberry, sapodilla): Drab-colored fruit of the sapodilla tree (which is the source of chicle used in chewing gum). It has granular, mildly sweet flesh, which can be yellow, red, or black. The zapote is a member of the persimmon family. Potato valued primarily for its sprouts and young leaves. Native to China; significant crop in Southeast Asia, Malaysia, and South India.

Index

A

C

G

J

K

L

T

U

V

W